Contemporary Conservative Care for Painful Spinal Disorders

Contemporary Conservative Care for Painful Spinal Disorders

Edited by

Tom G. Mayer, M.D.
Clinical Professor, Department of Orthopaedic Surgery
University of Texas Southwestern Medical Center
and
Medical Director, PRIDE/Dallas
Dallas, Texas

Vert Mooney, M.D.
Professor of Orthopaedic Surgery
University of California San Diego
San Diego, California

Robert J. Gatchel, Ph.D.
Professor of Psychiatry and Rehabilitation Science, Department of Psychiatry
University of Texas Southwestern Medical Center
Dallas, Texas

1991
Lea & Febiger
Philadelphia — London

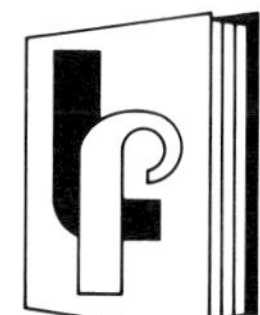

Lea & Febiger
200 Chester Field Parkway
Malvern, Pennsylvania 19355
U.S.A.
(215) 251-2230

Library of Congress Cataloging-in-Publication Data

Contemporary conservative care for painful spinal disorders / edited
 by Tom G. Mayer, Vert Mooney, Robert J. Gatchel.
     p.   cm.
   Includes index
   ISBN 0-8121-1344-6
   1. Spine—Diseases. 2. Backache. I. Mayer, Tom G. II. Mooney,
 Vert. III. Gatchel, Robert J., 1947-   .
   [DNLM: 1. Backache—rehabilitation. 2. Spinal Diseases-
 -diagnosis. 3. Spinal Deseases—rehabilitation.   WE   725 C761]
 RD768.C67   1991
 617.5′64—dc20
 DNLM/DLC
 for Library of Congress   91-9298
                                                        CIP

Reprints of chapters may be purchased from Lea & Febiger in quantities of 100 or more.

PRINTED IN THE UNITED STATES OF AMERICA

Print number: 5 4 3 2 1

This text is dedicated to our wives, Holly Mayer, Ruth Mooney,
and Anita Gatchel, who continue to contribute so much to our
professional and personal lives.

Foreword

This book presents an unusually comprehensive review of the evaluation and care of the painful spine. There is considerable emphasis on basic concepts and also, a parallel emphasis on nonoperative rehabilitation. This, I believe, is a timely expansion of our view of comprehensive care of the spine. We are now at a moment in medical history when there is some disenchantment with spinal surgery. This state of mind probably results from certain excesses in the past. This book will attempt to place in perspective the role of surgery as one element in the care of the deteriorating spine.

This text obviously was organized to carefully review all of the major issues in current spine care. This is truly a comprehensive text in that it is not restricted to the specific interests of just manual medicine, surgery or other subspecialty areas. It is organized into eight parts, which present an algorithm for conceptualizing modern spine care. Thus, each are connected chapters wherein one concept leads to the next. The authors, carefully chosen experts in these various areas, represent respected thinkers in the field. Each author can be said to be on the cutting edge of knowledge in his or her specific area. Moreover, each chapter attempts to focus first on the conceptual framework of the interest area and then progress into practical aspects of assessment and diagnosis. Considerable attention is directed at informing the readers of alternatives for care—not just the author's particular choice. Several areas represent significant departures from traditional thought. For example, the concept of early exercise after back injury is a reversal from previous beliefs that prolonged rest was the way to treat such an injury. The new ideas in anatomy, physiology, and biochemistry are displayed by teachers who are familiar with the subject as well as the audience.

Because this is a comprehensive text, it is appropriate for a wide audience. It intends to be a major resource for primary care physicians as well as medical specialists who are interested in the most updated approach to spinal care. It should be of great value to a variety of therapists such as physical and occupational therapists, as well as psychologists engaged in this expanding field. Students wishing greater depth of knowledge in issues of spine assessment and treatment should find all the basics they need in this volume. Although this text does not go into technical details of spinal surgery, surgical specialists should find many things that are new and valuable for their own comprehensive care of the spine.

It is difficult to supply all of the answers to a problem such as the painful spine. There are so many avenues that need to be explored. So many new answers are emerging. In spite of the complexity and the size of the problem, this text has put together, in a practical and readable manner, the most information available today.

Leon L. Wiltse

Preface

A man "puts his back into it" and "gets his back up." Since time immemorial, the spine symbolizes physical strength, ferocity and stubbornness in much the same way as the heart symbolizes emotion and the head embodies logic. Few other anatomic areas are so frequently represented in literature and artistic expression. The spine is an unusual organ, combining a unique flexible support function and the primary neurological interconnect from our "personal computer's" central processing unit to its peripherals.

Its emergence represents a most fundamental evolutionary step, delivering the vertebrates from the invertebrates. In turn, further evolution provided opportunities for locomotion on land with the emergence of sagittal plane movement rather than the coronal motion common to all fishes. The mammalian re-entry into the water (whales and porpoises) maintains this sagittal motion feature of land-based locomotion. Most recently, efficient bipedal locomotion has been identified as primarily a result of spinal evolution.

Significant changes have occurred in our medical view of the spine over the past decades. Yet, seen in historical perspective, many of our concepts have simply been reinvented, our diagnoses refined and our treatments improved. The recent explosion in medical technology has also contributed to a more refined evaluation of many older concepts. However, because of its complexity and inaccessibility to physical examination, progress in spine treatment has usually lagged behind that of other segments of the musculoskeletal system. This continues to the present, as will become evident when, in the context of painful spinal disorders, we carefully examine the physiology of *pain*, the measurement of *function*, and the sources of *disability*.

This text may be seen as an algorithm for conceptualizing modern spine care, not merely as a series of interconnected chapters. The editors have taken great pains to outline and order the concepts, diagnostic approaches, and treatment options that characterize modern spine care. The authors were carefully selected to represent the most highly respected thinkers in the field in their particular area of expertise. Because they are on the "cutting edge" of each knowledge area, they will be able to provide the most up-to-date summary and interpretation of the clinical and scientific literature, as well as their own personal experiences. Moreover, they were also chosen because of their reputations as apt teachers of contemporary spine care.

This text was organized to carefully review *all* of the major issues in current spine care. Unlike many other texts on this subject, it is not restricted to the specific interests of its editors in surgery, manual medicine, or other subspecialty area of spine care. As such, it cannot cover any of these subspecialty areas in total depth, but must instead rely upon providing a basic understanding and overview. This will lead to the reader's willingness to delve further into the extensive current bibliography in each chapter when interest calls. As much as possible, algorithmic approaches have been used to guide the reader's attention. Each chapter has been arranged to focus first on the conceptual framework for the modalities or procedures that are to be covered. Then, whenever possible, the practical aspects of assessment, diagnosis, and care are covered, with specific attention directed at informing the readers of alternatives for care and the author's particular choice for type, frequency, and duration.

This text was conceptualized and organized to be a major resource for primary care physicians and medical specialists who are interested in the most updated approaches to spinal care. Moreover, it will also be of great value to the variety of therapists (e.g., physical therapists, occupational therapists, and psychologists) engaged in this expanding field. Students wishing greater depth of knowledge on issues in spine assessment and treatment should find all the basics they need in this volume.

Dallas, Texas
Orange, California
Dallas, Texas

TOM G. MAYER
VERT MOONEY
ROBERT J. GATCHEL

Contributors

WAYNE H. AKESON, M.D.
Professor and Head
Division of Orthopaedics and Rehabilitation
University of California San Diego Medical Center
San Diego, California

DAVID AMIEL, DIP. ING.
Division of Orthopaedics and Rehabilitation
University of California San Diego Medical Center
San Diego, California

GUNNAR B.J. ANDERSSON, M.D., PH.D.
Professor
Department of Orthopaedic Surgery
Rush Presbyterian-St. Luke's Medical Center
Chicago, Illinois

JEAN-JACQUES ARBITOL, M.D.
Division of Orthopaedics and Rehabilitation
University of California San Diego Medical Center
San Diego, California

DENNIS BARNES, M.A., PH.D. CANDIDATE
Division of Psychology
University of Texas Southwestern Medical Center
Dallas, Texas

MICHELE C. BATTIÉ, P.T., PH.D.
Assistant Research Professor
Department of Orthopaedics
University of Washington
Seattle, Washington

STANLEY J. BIGOS, M.D.
Associate Professor
Department of Orthopaedics
University of Washington
Seattle, Washington

NIKOLAI BOGDUK, B.Sc., M.B., B.S., PH.D.
Associate Professor
Faculty of Medicine
University of Newcastle
New South Wales, Australia

STEVEN CARTER, M.S., C.R.C.
Private Rehabilitation Consultant
Career Assessment Services
Dallas, Texas

RICHARD A. DEYO, M.D., M.P.H.
Associate Professor
Medicine and Health Services
University of Washington, Seattle
and
Director, Northwest Health Services Research &
  Development Program
Department of Veterans Affairs Medical Center
Seattle, Washington

ALAN L. ENGELBERG, M.D., M.P.H.
Senior Occupational Medicine Physician
Department of Medical and Health Sciences
Monsanto Company
St. Louis, Missouri

DAVID R. EYRE, PH.D.
Professor, Department of Orthopaedics
University of Washington
Seattle, Washington

PAUL L. FLICKER, M.D., A.A.O.S., P.A.C.S.
Assistant Professor
Department of Orthopaedic Surgery
University of Texas Southwestern Medical Center
Dallas, Texas

WILLIAM E. FORDYCE, PH.D.
Professor of Psychology
Department of Psychiatry & Behavioral Science
University of Washington Medical School
Seattle, Washington

JAMES FRICTON, D.D.S., M.S.
Associate Professor
Department of Diagnostic/Surgical Sciences
    and Co-Director, TMJ Clinic
University of Minnesota
Minneapolis, Minnesota

JOHN W. FRYMOYER, M.D.
Professor, Department of Orthpaedics and
    Rehabilitation
                    and
Director, McClure Musculoskeletal Research Center
Department of Orthopaedics and Rehabilitation
University of Vermont
Burlington, Vermont

STEVEN R. GARFIN, M.D.
Associate Professor of Surgery
Division of Orthopaedics and Rehabilitation
University of California San Diego Medical Center
San Diego, California

TIMOTHY A. GARVEY, M.D.
Assistant Professor of Orthopaedic Surgery
University of Minnesota, Twin Cities
Minneapolis, Minnesota

ROBERT J. GATCHEL, PH.D.
Professor of Psychiatry & Rehabilitation Science
Department of Psychiatry
University of Texas Southwestern Medical Center
Dallas, Texas

PHILLIP E. GREENMAN, D.O., F.A.A.O.
Department of Biomechanics
Michigan State University
East Lansing, Michigan

JUDITH GREENWOOD, PH.D., M.P.H.
Director of Research
West Virginia Workers' Compensation Fund
Charleston, West Virginia

SCOTT HALDEMAN, M.D., PH.D., D.C.
Assistant Clinical Professor
Department of Neurology
University of California, Irvine
Orange, California

HAMILTON HALL, M.D., F.R.C.S.(C)
Associate Professor
Department of Surgery
University of Toronto
                    and
Medical Director
Canadian Back Institute
Toronto, Canada

ROWLAND G. HAZARD, M.D.
Assistant Professor
Depts. of Orthopaedics and Rehabilitation, and
    Surgery
University of Vermont
                    and
Director, New England Back Center
Williston, Vermont

HARRY N. HERKOWITZ, M.D.
CoDirector, Section of Spinal Surgery
Department of Orthopaedic Surgery
William Beaumont Hospital
Royal Oak, Michigan

GARY HERRIN, PH.D.
Professor
University of Michigan Center for Ergonomics
Ann Arbor, Michigan

STANLEY A. HERRING, M.D.
Puget Sound Sports Physicians
                    and
Assistant Clinical Professor
Departments of Rehabilitation Medicine and
    Orthopaedics
University of Washington
Seattle, Washington

DONALD W. HINNANT, PH.D.
Program Director
Pain Therapy Center
Charleston, South Carolina

SUSAN J. ISERNHAGEN, R.P.T.
President, Isernhagen & Associates, Inc.
Duluth, Minnesota

CLAUDIA JACKSON, PT, PH.D. CANDIDATE
Director, Physical Therapy Professionals, Inc.
Coral Gables, Florida

PATRICK R. JOHNSON, PH.D.
Acting Assistant Professor
Department of Psychiatry & Behavioral Sciences
University of Washington Medical School
Seattle, Washington

JANICE KEELEY, P.T.
Productive Rehabilitation Institute of Dallas for
    Ergonomics (PRIDE)
Dallas, Texas

WILLIAM KERMOND, M.D.
Medical Director, PRIDE, Braintree
Braintree, Massachusetts

MICHAEL L. KRIEGEL, PH.D
Clinical Director, Pain Therapy Center
Greenville, South Carolina

GERALD S. LAROS, M.D.
Professor of Orthopaedic Surgery
Texas Technical University School of Medicine
Lubbock, Texas

LEONARD N. MATHESON, PH.D.
Director, Employment and Rehabiliation Institute of
    California
Santa Ana, California

TOM G. MAYER, M.D.
Clinical Professor
Department of Orthopaedic Surgery
University of Texas Southwestern Medical Center
                    and
Medical Director, PRIDE, Dallas
Dallas, Texas

ROBIN McKENZIE, P.T.
Consultant in Spinal Therapy
                    and
International Director, The McKenzie Institute
Waikanae, New Zealand

MATTHEW MONSEIN, M.D.
Medical Director
Sister Kinney Chronic Pain Rehabilitation Center
Minneapolis, Minnesota

VERT MOONEY, M.D.
Professor of Orthopaedic Surgery
Department of Surgery
University of California Irvine School of Medicine
Orange, California

PATTY NEWTON, M.ED.
Productive Rehabilitation Institute of Dallas for
    Ergonomics (PRIDE)
Dallas, Texas

PETER B. POLATIN, M.D.
Assistant Clinical Professor
Department of Psychiatry
University of Texas Southwestern Medical Center
                    and
Associate Medical Director, PRIDE
Dallas, Texas

MALCOLM H. POPE, PH.D.
Director of Research
Department of Orthopaedics & Rehabilitation
University of Vermont
Burlington, Vermont

GEORGE PRESTON, J.D.
Hicks, James & Preston
Dallas, Texas

JEFFREY A. SAAL, M.D.
Chief of Physiatry, SpineCare Medical Group
Daly City, California
                    and
Director of Research and Education, San Francisco
    Spine Institute
Daly City, California

JOEL S. SAAL, M.D.
Consultant for Research
San Francisco Spine Institute and SpineCare
    Medical Group
Daly City, California

GEORGE M. SMITH, M.D., M.P.H.
President, G.M. Smith Associates, Inc.
Bethesda, Maryland

E. SHANNON STAUFFER, M.D.
Professor, Department of Surgery
Chairman, Division of Orthopaedic Surgery
Southern Illinois University School of Medicine
Springfield, Illinois

C. DAVID TOLLISON, PH.D.
Program Director
Pain Therapy Center
Greenville, South Carolina

TAPIO VIDEMAN, M.D., DR. MED. SCI.
Senior Researcher
Institute of Occupational Health
TOPELIUKSENKATU
Helsinki, Finland

JAMES N. WEINSTEIN, D.O.
Associate Professor

Department of Orthopaedic Surgery
University of Iowa Hospitals and Clinics
Iowa City, Iowa

ARTHUR H. WHITE, M.D.
Medical Director, San Francisco Spine Institute
Medical Director, SpineCare Medical Group
Daly City, California

SAM W. WIESEL, M.D.
Professor and Chairman, Department of
  Orthopaedic Surgery
Georgetown University Medical Center
Washington, D.C.

SAVIO L-Y. WOO, PH.D.
Division of Orthopaedics and Rehabilitation
University of California San Diego Medical Center
San Diego, California

Contents

**Part III
Psychosocioeconomic Factors Related to
Spinal Disorders**

Part V
Subacute Spinal Disorders

Part VI
The Place for Surgical Treatment

Part VIII
Special Issues in Spinal Care

Introduction and Overview of Degenerative Spine Problems

Tom G. Mayer

Rationale for Modern Spine Care

COST

Why are we interested in painful spinal disorders? The answer is a complex one, associated with factors not usually considered germane in evaluating the importance of medical problems. These disorders defy classification into standard disease categories: no microbe or vascular impediment appears with any regularity as a concomitant of these processes (Table 1–1). Radiographically visualizable degenerative changes have been widely believed to correlate with these disorders, but epidemiological evidence suggests that there is poor correlation between peak incidents of "degenerative" spinal disorders and the appearance of radiographic change. In fact, the high incidence of symptoms in a younger population, without appreciable visualizable structural change, may lead the clinician to doubt the veracity of patients' description of their symptoms, and adds to the adversary process often encountered when caring for these patients.

Moreover, there are few diseases or disorders in which the customary doctor-patient relationship is so compromised. In seeking relief, patients frequently search out evaluations and treatment from multiple physicians while seemingly extraneous, nonmedical factors are often implicated in symptom prolongation. Questions of "Did an injury really occur?" are customarily raised, with consequent involvement of a "disability system" peopled by attorneys, insurance adjusters, employers, and vocational rehabilitation personnel. Physicians are called upon to write reports and make judgments for which they generally feel less than fully prepared. The impact made by these "disability system" professionals, as well as the recognition that they are gatekeepers for the system, often leads to physician frustration. There is even some support for a socioeconomic (as opposed to a medical) frame of reference into which work-related injury might be placed.[1–7] The physician may feel additional resentment as he or she perceives that efforts to return the patient to productivity may conflict in some ways with the goals of other members of the "disability system."[8–13]

Yet, in spite of the lack of clarity concerning this disorder, painful spinal problems produce a devastating social cost in our industrialized society. They create the largest economic cost of any benign condition and represent the primary cause of disability in industrialized countries for patients under age 45. Over this age, spinal disorders represent the third largest cause of disability. As such, the condition robs society of the productive capacity of its most eligible workers, while the worker sustains a series of psychosocioeconomic consequences of work incapacity including financial, social, and personal losses. Cost estimates of this condition have been between 16 and 60 billion dollars.[14–20]

Though accurate statistics are difficult to obtain, in part because the keepers of the statistics (government, industry, insurance) may wish to minimize the impact of these disorders, an estimated 2 to 5% of the adult population has a temporarily disabling low back pain episode annually.[21–24] In the United States, nearly 400,000 American adults attribute their back pain to an occupational injury. Although work-related back injury represents 15 to 30% of all work

Table 1–1
Critical Factors in Modern Spine Care

Cost
Pain
Function
Disability

3

compensation injuries, it represents about 50% of workman's compensation costs. Currently 5.3 million Americans are disabled by low back pain and more than twice that number are impaired; about 1% of the population may have been declared "totally and permanently disabled" through administrative and legal processes.[21,24,25] This disability may lead to various forms of long-term compensation (Social Security Disability Income, Military/Veterans Disability Benefits, long-term disability, workman's compensation benefits) that may be paid for life, or that may be structured into some type of shorter term or lump sum settlement.

Complicating medical care for these patients is the natural history of painful spinal disorders (Fig. 1–1). The vast majority (90 to 95%) of spinal pain incidents resolve spontaneously within 3 to 4 months, with 50 to 60% resolved in 2 weeks. Because these numbers reflect only those patients entering the medical system at some time, the numbers for early or spontaneous recovery are probably higher. After all, the back "twinge" ultimately affects 80% of the population. Most physicians seeing patients in a primary care mode (internal, occupational, and family medicine) are generally confronted only with the acute self-limited condition and treat these patients expectantly. As such, patients who develop more chronic (and costly or disabling) conditions perceive physician neglect. This perception occurs in the face of physician attempts to hold the line against overtreatment and overmedication. The small number of "nonresponders" may further confuse the physician with general lack of objective physical signs, early behavioral changes, and educational gaps that influence the timing of structural diagnostic tests and referrals.

The bill for medical care for all painful spinal disorders appears to be close to 20 billion dollars annually, of which slightly more than one half is expended for surgical treatment.[14] Interestingly, all other musculoskeletal trauma may cost only about 50% of this amount for medical care. The loose definition of injury that identifies 90% of lost time back injuries in the United States (but only 25 to 40% in Scandinavia) has exacerbated the adversarial compensation process. Because much evidence exists that back pain may result more from the normal aging process than from an injury, much resentment arises from employers who bear the brunt of the cost. In fact, however, in the more socialized economies of Northern Europe where a distinction between compensable and noncompensable spinal pain is less abrupt (in terms of availability of medical care and disability payments), the costs are greater.[15] Although the taxpayer in those countries bears a greater share of the burden than in the United States, employers are usually called upon to make a nearly equal contribution to the social welfare benefits.

Thus, low back disorders result in substantial cost to our nations economically and to our most productive young people in the personal consequences of disability. Most alarming, in the latter half of the 1970s, the cost of low back disability grew 1400% faster than the rate of population growth.[26] We next consider the implications of these findings in focusing our attention on the primary issues: *pain, disability,* and *function.*

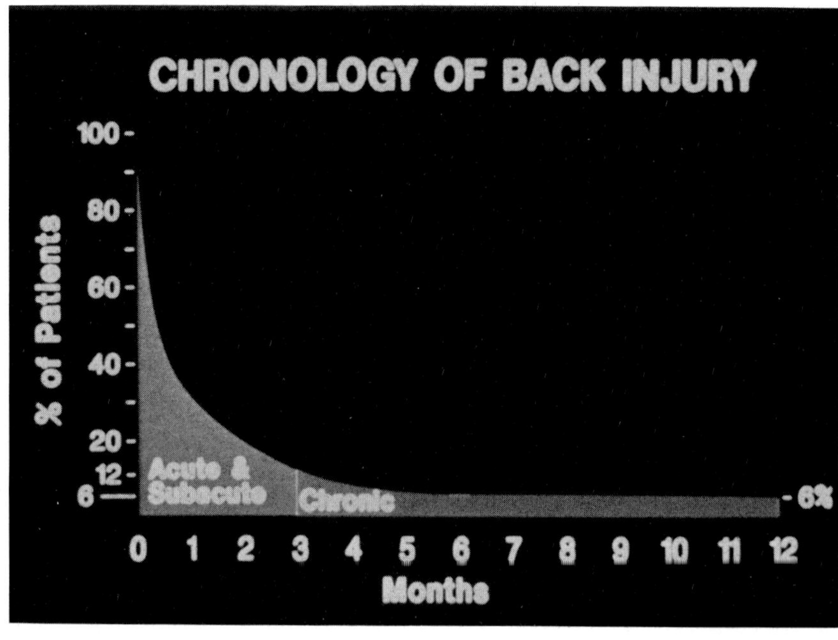

Figure 1–1. Time course of acute low back pain. (From Mayer, T.G., Gatchel, R.J.: Functional Restoration for Spinal Disorders: The Sports Medicine Approach. Philadelphia, Lea & Febiger, 1988.)

PAIN

Causes of back pain are manifold, and can be categorized in many ways. This text attempts to present concepts, diagnosis, and treatment in an orderly sequence. First, we examine the normal anatomy and physiology of the spine, including its biomechanics and biochemistry. The peripheral stimulus to the nervous system has traditionally received the greatest attention because of the opportunities to intervene medically or surgically to correct biomechanical aberrations. Recent evidence suggests that, at least in certain situations, biochemical abnormalities creating a persistently painful disc may contribute to peripheral pain stimuli, opening an exciting new area for investigation. All too often, spinal disorders have been seen as a "law unto themselves." To correct this misperception, several authors point out similarities between pain and function in anatomically distinct areas, the relationship of soft tissue healing and homeostasis principles to spinal pain, and the importance of systemic diagnoses in a small but significant proportion of spine problems initially thought to be caused by injury. Dramatic new technology for assessing structural changes (such as computer tomography, magnetic resonance imaging, magnetic resonance spectroscopy) present ever-increasing opportunities for identifying structural pain sources.

Painful stimuli are transmitted to our central processing unit (i.e., the brain) through an ascending wiring system (the ascending spinal pathways). Physiologic neural modulation occurs as part of this process. Descartes' early concept of pain transmission was modified near the turn of the last century upon recognition of anatomic pathways for transmission of specific kinds of stimulation. A great body of knowledge has accumulated regarding the nociceptive pathways from target receptor to central pain center. Two competing, but ultimately reconcilable theories, termed Specificity (Von Frey) and Pattern (Goldschneider), emerged with partial support for both theories appearing in subsequent publications.[27–30] Neurophysiology of nociception and pain transmission are discussed in depth.

Central phenomena remain the most difficult to analyze, with the widely perceived dichotomy between physiologic and psychologic factors remaining a barrier to understanding. The Gate Control theory[28] first gave credence to the link between these two factors, even at a time when psychological diagnostics and behavior modification were being identified as new modalities for chronic pain intervention.[11,31–33]

Included in neurophysiologic bases for pain are the neurochemical changes occurring in the brain. Endorphins, enkephalins, vasoactive intestinal peptide (VIP), and substance P are among many biochemical neuromodulators. Depression, the symptom aggregate representing multiple neurophysiologic alterations (and a common fellow-traveler of chronic pain), is felt to have serotonin and norepinephrine correlates, a discovery that has led to the use of antidepressant medication in some forms of pain treatment. Conversely, prolonged use of narcotic analgesics leading to habituation, obsessive behavior, and increased pain sensitivity may be related to interaction with the brain's endorphin receptors. Pure psychologic factors, currently not amenable to physiologic description, may substantially impact the experience of pain. Alteration of pain perception by fear, depression, somatization, high anxiety, and different ethnic/cultural factors have all been implicated.[34–37]

Pain is the symptom that brings the majority of patients into the medical system. Yet pain is inherently an unverifiable central phenomenon that cannot be objectively measured. It cannot be experienced either by physician or therapist. In most cases, careful physical examination and structural testing can objectively document the source of pain, leading to a diagnosis and specific treatment. Because of complex neuromusculoskeletal anatomy and physiology in deeply placed structures, such verification may be nearly impossible in painful spinal disorders. Inability to clearly make a structural diagnosis not only affects the physician's ability to intervene specifically, but also prevents adequate reassurance to the patient and confidence in reactivation treatment. Encumbered by these handicaps, the physician's advice may inadvertently become an iatrogenic pain reinforcer.

FUNCTION

Though patients seek medical attention for pain complaints much more frequently than for deficits of physical performance, it is the loss of function that is most closely correlated with the economic cost and human suffering of spinal disorders. This occurs because a small percentage of chronic disabling or chronic episodic spinal disorders produces substantial medical/compensation cost (Fig. 1–2). Patients tend to progressively lose the ability to perform a variety of social functions, with increasing periods of disability as the "deconditioning syndrome" develops.

Function refers to the organism's ability to perform tasks involving homeostasis or in manipulation of the environment. In relation to its external involvement, the organism is provided with a series of tasks including acquiring nutrition, protecting itself from harsh environments, and reproducing itself.

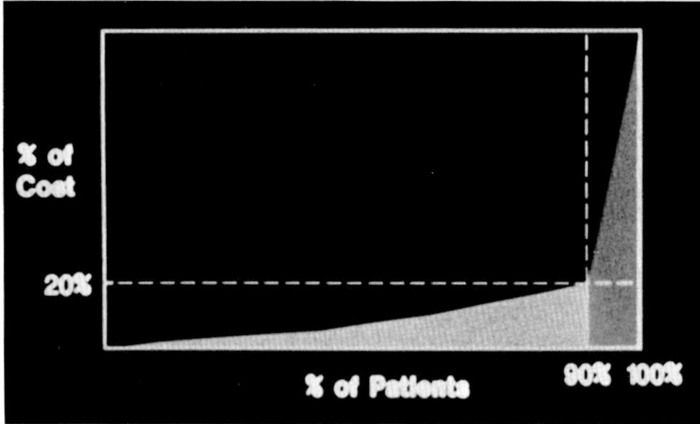

Figure 1–1. Graph of cost increase as length of disability increases.

The musculoskeletal system has an important role to play, as the largest body component in terms of mass, in providing the motors to achieve these goals. Specific tasks may include ambulation, climbing, crawling, and other forms of locomotion, as well as pushing, pulling, lifting, and other forms of manual hauling tasks. The human musculoskeletal system can be defined as an architectural structure composed of a finite set of interconnected functional units that possess the capacity to operate within specific dimensions of performance (e.g., strength, range of motion, speed). Considering all functional units collectively results in the recognition of a finite set of distinct basic elements of performance (BEPs). Human functional units are either a single or a collective set of anatomic structures that work together to realize the respective dimensions of performance.[38,39]

This conceptualization of function leads to recognition of a variety of important functional principles (Table 1–2).[15,39,40] "Conservation of energy" is a critical initial principle. The human will almost invariably seek the most efficient methods for performing a task; i.e., the way that best conserves energy. Even exercise, which appears on the surface to contradict this principle, utilizes the energy conservation principle. Exercise is seen within the context of a cognitive formulation in which social and psychologic factors produce a desire for, or a belief in, periods of increased physical activity to maintain homeostasis in order to increase survival or social benefits ("the healthy lifestyle").

The "safety principle" is the second functional modifier that affects human performance. Normally, neuromusculoskeletal feedback mechanisms permit BEPs to achieve maximum output without harm to the organism. Following injury, the threshold for perception of violation of the "safety principle" may be dramatically lowered, even below the point nec-

essary for maintenance of BEPs homeostasis. At such a point, the deconditioning syndrome becomes progressive.[15] These two basic principles may be modified by the capacity for substitution. One functional unit may substitute for another in performance of specific tasks. An example of this is the normal bending of the spine as the most efficient (and generally self-selected) mechanism for stoop labor. After injury, much bending may be limited by deconditioning, after which the safety principle limits bending further. In this case, squatting with a straight spine may still permit the hands to touch the ground to achieve the same goal of environmental manipulation, albeit with lower efficiency than was apparent prior to injury. Figures 1–3 and 1–4 illustrate the primary principles.

Inactivity and disuse can be modeled in both humans and experimental animals through immobilization. Much work has been done in this area, with a regular finding of negative effects on soft tissue homeostasis.[41–46] Healing tissue that is immobilized tends to produce amorphous, nonfunctional scar with low strength (in its customarily strongest tensile or compressive direction) provided it has been subjected to healing without adequate physiologic stress. This principle might be known as the "generalized Wolff's Law" of collagenous tissue and has been applied to healing of muscle, tendon, and bony tissues.[47,48] Even after healing with permanent loss of function (such as relative instability), increasing the function of one BEP may positively affect performance in others. An example is strengthening muscles to protect both normal and injured joints from further injury.[49]

New technology is also available for measurement in this critical area, just as it is in evaluating structural pathology. Measurement of function, an essential part of obtaining information on spinal deconditioning, is simply not available through self-report or visual means. Because physical capacity measures of BEPs depend inherently on voluntary effort, substantial disagreement remains on use and misuse of assessment tools. Yet, so great is the need for physical evaluation methods of assessing work capacity, guiding rehabilitation, screening pre-employment candidates, and evaluating impairment, that considerable research activity is currently focusing on validating devices and protocols for functional assessment. This text discusses most of these issues in detail.

Table 1–2
Principles of Interaction of Functional Units

1. Conservation of Energy (Efficiency)
2. Safety
3. Substitution

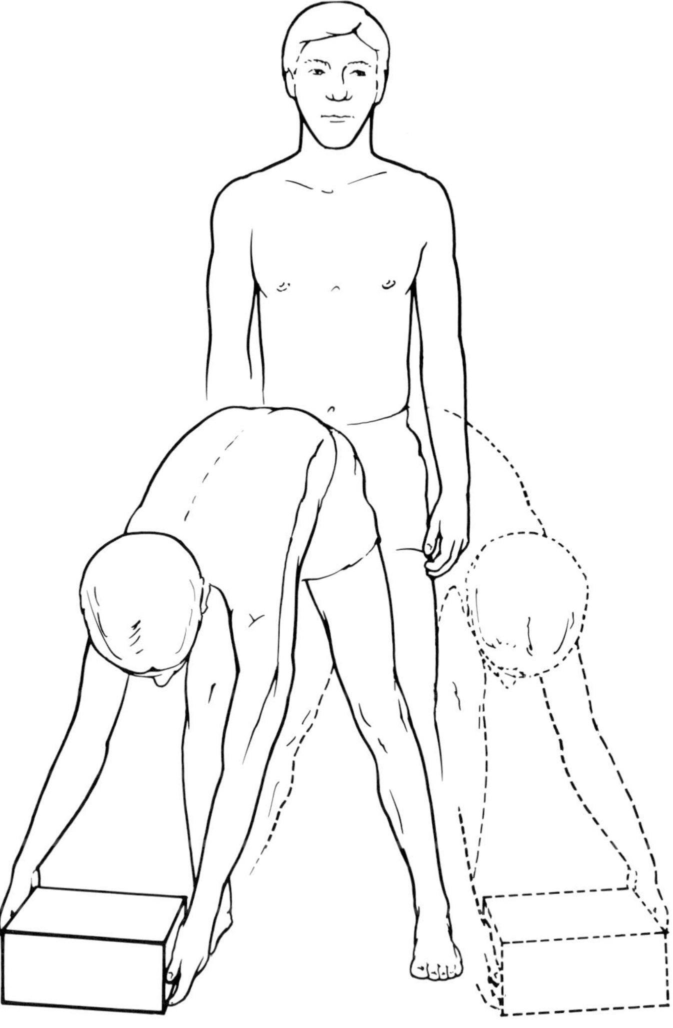

Figure 1–3. The "conservation of energy principle." The subject maintains a stable foot/ground contact and "hands on his ligaments" in maneuvering light to medium loads in an arch. (From Mayer, T.G., Gatchel, R.J.: Functional Restoration for Spinal Disorders: The Sports Medicine Approach. Philadelphia, Lea & Febiger, 1988.)

DISABILITY

Disability is an unfortunate, but nearly inevitable end result of painful spinal disorders. Almost invariably, however, this disability is only partial, associated with a permanent partial impairment. When medical treatment, both passive and active, is concluded in an appropriate timeframe, the ability to perform all physical tasks optimally may be compromised to a variable extent. Such impairment may be compensable if it leads to work incapacity, physical capacity deficits, or chronic pain perception. As such, there is a legitimate paramedical interest among those who represent the professionals of the disability system (attorneys, employers, and insurance and vocational rehabilitation personnel) in issues of retraining, return to work, and compensation. Competing non-medical groups may seek to maximize their sway over their issues of concern.

The medical care system is also the gatekeeper for the disability system. It has been shown that the medical care system may have its greatest impact on disability of patients with painful spinal disorders.[50,51] Though surgical care may play a role in treatment of these patients, it is rarely the sole factor in relieving disability. The role of conservative care as an adjunct to surgical treatment (or vice versa) is discussed extensively in this text.

The medical care system is also the gatekeeper for impairment/disability evaluation.[1,6] Impairment evaluation is a medical specialty that is becoming progressively more codified and refined into standardized protocols, such as the American Medical Association's *Guides to the Evaluation of Permanent Impairment*. Diverse mechanisms exist for evaluating impairment (depending on the principles, rules, and goals of the disability system involved), which may vary greatly on a state or national basis. Multi-

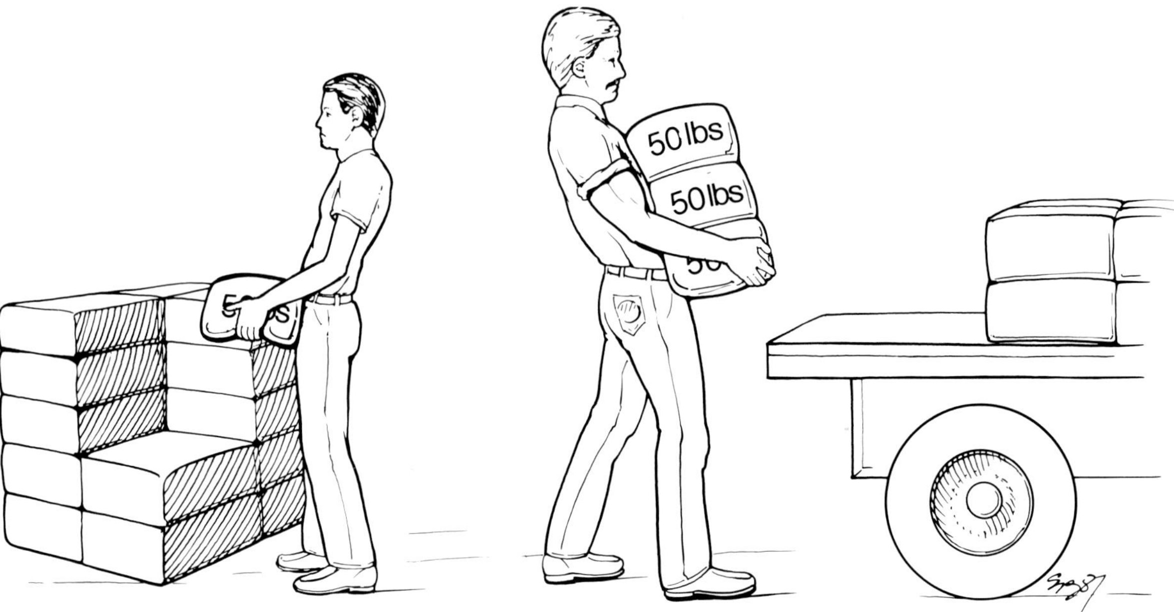

Figure 1–4. "Safety principle" for prevention of overload. Each individual self-selects a "safe limit" based on feedback of physical capacity. The "safe limit" may be considerably greater for one individual than for another, and may be substantially modified by injury or deconditioning. In this example, both individuals utilize their own perception of overload, task substitution opportunities and power output to achieve highest efficiency in conservation of energy. (From Mayer, T.G., Gatchel, R.J.: Functional Restoration for Spinal Disorders: The Sports Medicine Approach. Philadelphia, Lea & Febiger, 1988.)

ple alternative systems exist even within the US Federal System (e.g., SSDI, FELA, FECA, AAFES, Jones Act), all of which may vary substantially in approach, level of indemnity payments, and ultimate cost.[1,7] All of these systems have a fascinating history of their own. This text comprehensively discusses the important principles of impairment/disability evaluation and their application to specific compensation systems.

SUMMARY

Many classifications are possible for evaluating a medical condition, but the unusual nature of painful spinal disorders requires a special formulation. It carefully considers conditions without a recognized pain source, which incorporate a variety of complicating physiologic and psychosocioeconomic modifiers. Human and financial cost outlay is impressive.

Pain brings the patient to the physician, but its usefulness for diagnosis and treatment may be severely limited by lack of objective verification. Much work is documented on identification of actual or potential pain sources and neurophysiologic mechanisms of nociception. New technology and research concepts are expected to increase diagnostic specificity.

Function may be a somewhat ambiguous concept. In attempting to set the definitions for this text, we have looked at identifying physiologic functional units, specific tasks, basic elements of performance (BEPs), and complementary dimensions of human performance. General principles of energy conservation (efficiency), substitution, and safety have also been established, with their attendant modifiers. Deconditioning from disuse or immobilization accompanies painful spinal disorders in time, and parallels the development of the highest cost cases. This correlation provides a clear physical concomitant to psychologic aspects of chronic spinal pain, with measurement through new technology and protocols becoming essential for documentation of functional progress.

Disability refers to physical incapacity. It may result, in part, from physical impairments consequent to painful spinal disorders. These impairments are rarely more than partial, but may lead to higher level disability if accompanied by a variety of deconditioning and psychosocioeconomic factors. Impairment evaluation systems are becoming more standardized, but still are subject to a century of historical development of laws based on diverse goals and principles. The reader can find a cogent discussion of impairment and disability evaluation principles and alternative systems at their state-of-the-art in Part VII of this text.

REFERENCES

1. Greenwood J.: Intervention in work-related disability: the need for an integrated approach. Soc Sci Med *19*:595–601, 1984.
2. Berkowitz M., Johnson W., Murphy E.: Public Policy Toward Disability. New York, Praeger Press, 1976.
3. Howard I., Brehm H., Nagi S.: Disability: From Social Problem to Federal Programs. New York, Praeger Press, 1980.
4. Martinelli R., Dell Orto A.: The Psychological and Social Impact of Physical Disability. New York, Springer-Verlag, 1977.
5. Brand R., Lehmann T.: Low back impairment rating practices of orthopedic surgerys. Spine *8*:75–82, 1983.
6. Carey T., Fletcher S., Fletcher R.: Social Security disability determinations: knowledge and attitudes of consultative physicians. Med Care *25*:267–275, 1987.
7. Report of the Commission on the Evaluation of Pain. SSA Pub 64–031, US Dept of Health and Human Services, Social Security Admin, Office of Disability, March, 1987.
8. Bigos S., et al.: Back injuries in industry: a retrospective study II. Injury factors. Spine *11*:246–251, 1986.
9. Bigos S., et al.: Back injuries in industry: a retrospective study III. Employee-related factors. Spine *11*:252–256, 1986.
10. Spengler D., et al.: Back injuries in industry: a retrospective study I. Overview and cost analysis. Spine *11*:241–245, 1986.
11. Sternbach R., Wolf S., Murphy R., Akeson W.: Traits of pain patients: the low-back "loser." Psychosomatics *14*:226–229, 1973.
12. Nachemson A.: Prevention of chronic back pain: the orthopedic challenge for the 80s. Bull Hosp Jt Dis Orthop Inst *44*:1–15, 1984.
13. Leavitt S., Johnson T., Byers R.: The process of recovery: patterns in industrial back injury. Indust Med Surg *40*:7–14, 1971.
14. Holbrook T., Grazier K., Kelsey J., Stauffer R.: The frequency of occurrence impact and cost of selected musculoskeletal conditions in the United States. Chicago, American Academy of Orthopedic Surgeons, 1984.
15. Mayer T., Gatchel R.: Functional Restoration for Spinal Disorders: The Sports Medicine Approach. Philadelphia, Lea & Febiger, 1988.
16. Rockey P., Fantel J., Omenn G.: Discriminatory aspects of pre-employment screening: low-back x-ray examinations in the railroad industry. Amer J Law and Med *5*:197–214, 1979.
17. Snook S., Jensen R.: Cost. *In* Occupational Low Back Pain, (Edited by J. Frymoyer). New York, Praeger Press, 1984.
18. Florence D.: The chronic pain syndrome. Postgrad Med *70*:217–228, 1981.
19. Nordby E.: Epidemiology and diagnosis in low back injury. Occup Health Safety *50*:38–42, 1981.
20. Waddell G.: A new clinical model for the treatment of low-back pain. 1987 Volvo Award in Clinical Sciences. Spine *12*:632–644, 1987.
21. Abenhaim L., Suissa S.: Important and economic burden of occupational back pain: a study of 2,500 cases representative of Quebec. J Occup Med *29*:670–674, 1987.
22. Andersson G.: Low back pain in industry: epidemiologic aspects. Scand J Rehabil Med *11*:163–168, 1979.
23. Klein M., Jensen R., Sanderson L.: Assessment of workers compensation claims for back strain/sprain. J Occup Med *26*:443–448, 1984.
24. Frymoyer J., Cats-Baril W.: Predictors of low back pain disability. Clin Orthop *221*:89–98, 1987.
25. Peavy J.: Back injuries. Bureau of Mines Technology Transfer Symposia. Reno, New US Dept of Interior, 1983.
26. Frymoyer J., et al.: Risk factors in low back pain. J Bone Joint Surg *65A*:213–217, 1983.
27. Bonica J.: The Management of Pain, 2nd Ed. Philadelphia, Lea & Febiger, 1990.
28. Melzack R., Wall P.: Pain mechanisms: a new theory. Science *150*:971–979, 1965.
29. Melzack R., Wall P.: The Challenge of Pain. New York, Basic Books, 1982.
30. Gatchel R., Baum A.: Introduction to Health Psychology. New York, Random House, 1983.
31. Fordyce W., Fowler R., Lehmann J., DeLateur B.: Some implications of learning in problems of chronic pain. J Chronic Dis *21*:179–190, 1968.
32. Fordyce W., Steger J.: Chronic pain. *In* Behavior Medicine: Theory and Practice. (Edited by O.F. Pomerlau and J.P. Brady). Baltimore, Williams & Wilkins, 1979.
33. Fordyce W., Roberts A., Sternbach R.: The behavioral management of chronic pain: a response to critics. Pain *22*:113–125, 1985.
34. Beecher H.: Relationship of significance of wound to the pain experienced. JAMA *161*:1609–1613, 1956.
35. Hill H., Kornetsky C., Flanguy H., Wilder A.: Effects of anxiety and morphine on the discrimination of intensities of pain. Clin Invest *31*:473–480, 1952.
36. Tursky B., Sternbach R.: Further physiological correlates of ethnic differences in responses to shock. Psychophysiol *4*:67–74, 1967.
37. Zborowski M.: Cultural components in responses to pain. J Social Issues *8*:16–30, 1952.
38. Kondraske G.: Towards a standard clinical measure of postural stability. *In* Proc Eighth Ann Conf IEEE Eng Med Biol Soc (Edited by G. Kondraske, C. Robinson) *3*:1579–1582, 1986.
39. Kondraske G.: Human performance: measurement, science, concepts and computerized methodology. Neurology (in press).
40. Gracovetsky S., Farfan H.: The optimum spine. Spine *11*:543–573, 1986.
41. Woo S., Buckwalter J.: Injury and Repair of the Musculoskeletal Soft Tissue. Park Ridge, IL, AAOS Symposium, 1988.
42. Videman T.: Connective tissue and immobilization: key factors in musculoskeletal degeneration? Clin Orthop *221*:26–32, 1987.
43. Bortz W.: The disuse syndrome. West J Med *141*:691–694, 1984.
44. Akeson W., Amiel D., Abel M., Garfin S., Woo S.: Effects of immobilization on joints. Clin Orthop *219*:28–57, 1987.
45. Booth F.: Physiologic and biochemical effects of immobilization on muscle. Clin Orthop *219*:15–20, 1987.
46. Rubin C., Lanyon L.: Osteoregulatory nature of mechanical stimuli: function as a determinant for adaptive remodeling in bone. J Orthop Res *5*:300–309, 1987.
47. Gelberman R., et al.: Kappa Delta Award Paper: Flexor tendon repair. J Orthop Res *4*:119–128, 1986.
48. Holm S., Nachemson A.: Nutritional changes in the canine intervertebral disc after spinal fusion. Clin Orthop *169*:234–258, 1982.
49. Radin E.: Role of muscles in protecting athletes from injury. Acta Med Scand (Suppl) *711*:143–147, 1985.
50. Mayer T, et al.: Objective assessment of spine function following industrial injury: a prospective study with comparison group and one-year follow-up. Spine *10*:482–493, 1985.
51. Mayer T, et al.: A prospective two-year study of functional restoration in industrial low back injury: an objective assessment procedure. JAMA *258*:1763–1767, 1987.

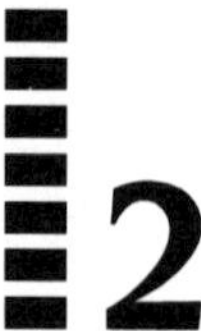

John W. Frymoyer, M.D.

Epidemiology of Spinal Diseases

Spinal diseases have affected mankind well beyond the records of history. Archeologic specimens demonstrate unequivocal evidence of all pathologic processes known to affect modern man, including an equivalent frequency of spinal degeneration. With the exception of tuberculosis, these conditions appear to have had minimal medical or socioeconomic impact until the twentieth century. Today, it is suggested we are in the midst of an "epidemic" of spinal disease based on the prevalence of low back pain and its resultant disabilities and costs.

The purpose of this chapter is to critically analyze lumbar spinal disorders from the epidemiologic perspective, a scientific technique classically applied to the studies of epidemics. This information allows some questions to be answered: How common are spinal disorders? Who is affected? What is the natural history? What is the impact on health care delivery? and What are the costs?

HOW COMMON ARE SPINAL DISORDERS?

Before 1950, there was minimal information regarding the prevalence and incidence of spinal disorders. The earliest studies utilized a cross-sectional experimental design, whereby populations were queried about their current and previous complaints of low back pain. Hult[1] studied different populations derived from subsets of workers. Hult found that 60% of forest workers currently had low back pain or had a history of low back pain. The usual onset of symptoms was in the third decade of life, typically experienced as an aching sensation, a condition which he termed "muscular insufficiency." More significant and disabling symptoms occurred 10 to 20 years later. Although the frequency of these complaints was similar in a less heavy laboring comparison group, the heavy workers were more likely to

have disability as a result of their low back complaint. Similarly, a complaint of low back pain was often accompanied by neck pain.

Kellgren and Lawrence[2] soon thereafter surveyed a more representative cross section of the English population, and included analyzed spinal radiographs. Their data closely paralleled that of Hult, as did a later analysis of a Swedish population surveyed by Horal.[3] Analysis of spinal radiographs revealed age-related degenerative changes in both the cervical and lumbar spine, as measured by disc space narrowing and osteophytes. No conclusions could be drawn about facet arthropathy because of the inter- and intraobserver errors in radiographic analysis.

In the time since these major landmark studies were conducted further cross-sectional surveys have been taken in general populations, as well as in specific age, sex, and occupational subsets in virtually every major industrialized country. The lifetime incidence of low back pain ranges from 51.4 to 70%, when lifetime incidence is determined by the question, "Have you ever had low back pain?"[4] This information, in part, created the impression that low back pain is a very common and potentially serious disorder. However, more critical analysis of these data gives a somewhat different and less ominous perspective. Basically, the information desired is not whether a person has experienced low back pain, but rather its duration, impact on work or activities of daily living, and the resultant disability.

Frymoyer et al.[5] attempted to answer this question by a cross-sectional design study in males age 18 to 55. In an earlier study, 70% of males and females surveyed reported a history of low back pain.[6] In the later study, subjects were asked to quantitate pain using a modified Likert-type scale, which gives five anchor points, ranging from no pain to excruciating pain. Analysis of these data revealed 22% of the subjects had experienced severe or excruciating pain, whereas 48% ranked their symptoms as mild to moderate. This figure is very similar to another cross-sectional survey of males in which 18% ranked their pain as severe.[7] As will be seen later, the patients' self-rating of pain significantly correlated with utilization of health services, loss of function, and disability.

A more representative population sample reported by Deyo[8] has been derived from the NHANES II (National Health and Nutrition Examination Survey). This survey established a sample of participants throughout the United States that was representative of the demographics for the civilian and noninstitutionalized population of this country. Low back pain lasting only more than 2 weeks was identified by 1355 of the 10,404 adults surveyed. An additional subset of 161 subjects reported both low back pain and sciatica of the same duration. Thus, 1516 individuals had low back pain, of which 9% also had sciatica. Only 13.8% of the 10,404 subjects had experienced low back pain of greater than 2 weeks duration during their adult life.

Another method to assess the frequency of spinal problems in our society is to determine how many people have back pain each year (annual incidence), or how many have pain at the time of the survey (point prevalence). Again, there is wide variation according to the population surveyed and how the question is asked. An analysis of both cross-sectional and prospective survey populations determined an average annual incidence is 5%.[9,10] However, the range is great; for example, industrial surveys demonstrate one to 20% of workers report a new episode of low back pain each year.[11] To some degree, this annual incidence varies as a function of the occupational requirements, particularly for heavy lifting. Furthermore, many of these episodes are recurrence of prior complaints, rather than the first episode. Although the data are incomplete, recurrent symptoms affect between 60 and 85% of patients after the initial low back episode.[12,13] Because subsequent episodes are often more severe (as suggested by Hult's original study), it is suggested they represent recurrent injury or progression of a degenerative process.

A third way to examine low back pain is to calculate the resultant disability. It is here that the perception of an epidemic becomes more plausible, although the underlying determinants, as will be seen, probably rest less with structural, and more with psychosocial determinants. The gross population statistics for the United States, in this regard, are staggering. It is estimated that 5.2 million American adults are disabled by low back pain. Of this 5.2 million, one half (2.6 million) are temporarily disabled, and the other one half are permanently dis-

abled.[14] This condition is the most common cause of disability in the working population under the age of 45, and the third most common cause of disability in the working population ages 45 to 65.[15] An even more ominous trend is the disproportionate increase in low back disability as measured against population growth as well as compared to other chronic disease processes. These data are given in Figure 2–1 and demonstrate low back pain disability increased at a rate 14 times population growth from 1957 to 1976.[16] This same situation is occurring in other industrialized societies. Data for Sweden are presented in Table 2–1 to illustrate this point.[17]

All of the information given to this point indicates low back pain as a symptom is very common, affecting 50 to 70% of individuals sometime during their adult life; low back pain, as an impairment, is much less common, affecting approximately 15 to 20% of the population sometime during their adult life; and low back pain, as a disabling health condition, is far less common, but is increasing disproportionally to the population growth. However, the symptom complaint gives only partial information and tells little about disease processes and the prevalence or incidence of the disease. It must be remembered that a high percentage of patients with the complaint of low back pain cannot be given a precise structural causation for their pain. In this analysis one can evaluate other symptoms, which are commonly associated with a specific disease process, or examine conditions for which precise pathologic criteria are available. Examples of the former are sciatica and neurologic claudication, whereas examples of the latter are infections, tumors, and certain arthritic conditions.

Sciatica

The original description of sciatica is ascribed to Cortugno[18] who differentiated leg pain with associated neurologic symptoms of numbness or weakness from less discrete leg pain without associated neurologic symptoms. Since the classic report of

Table 2–1
Subjects on Permanent Disability in Sweden (pop 8.3 millions)

	1952	1982	% Change Working Pop
Rheumatoid Arthritis	9,300	10,300	0
Arthritis	10,100	30,000	170
Low Back Pain	850	37,100	3,800

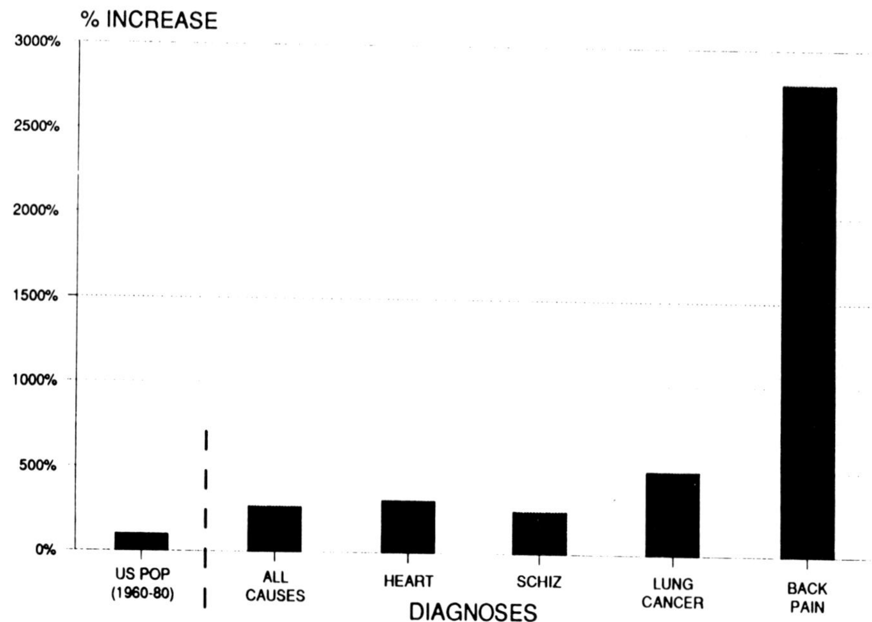

Figure 2–1. Increase in low back pain disability versus other chronic health conditions and population growth.

Mixter and Barr,[19] it has been well recognized that sciatic pain is most commonly associated with lumbar disc herniation, and involves noxious stimulation of the anterior primary rami. The second type of pain has been less well understood, despite the classic experiments of Lewis and Kellgren,[20] replicated by others,[21,22] which demonstrated that this symptom is produced by noxious stimulation of structures innervated by posterior primary rami, such as facet capsules and ligaments. This symptom is often termed sceleratomal pain. This differentiation is important because many epidemiologic surveys have not differentiated the pattern of leg pain or queried about associated neurologic symptoms sufficiently to determine the presence or absence of sciatica. The highest lifetime incidence of sciatica have been reported by Svensson and Andersson,[10] and by Frymoyer et al.[6] Forty percent of their male subjects reported leg symptoms. Table 2–2 demonstrates the relationship between leg pain, numbness, and weakness in the population reported on by Frymoyer.[6,23] This information makes it plausible that the lifetime incidence of leg symptoms were indeed sciatica. However, far lower lifetime incidence rates have been reported. For example, Hirsch et al.[23] reported 13.8% of women had experienced sciatica; in a subset of women ages 45 to 54, the figure increased to 22.4%. These figures are similar to the 11% figure reported by Gyntelberg,[24] who surveyed a Danish population. As previously noted, the NHANES II survey analyzed 10,404 American

adults; 161 had low back pain and sciatica, yielding a lifetime incidence of 1.5%. However, if the subjects reported low back pain of greater than two weeks duration, the lifetime incidence of sciatica was 11%.[8]

Another way to examine the epidemiology of lumbar disk herniation is to examine material derived from imaging studies and autopsy material. Because spinal radiographs are a poor predictor of disc herniation,[25] little information can be derived. However, a weak association has been noted between L4-L5 disc space narrowing and symptoms highly suggestive of sciatica, as shown in Table 2–3.[26] A similar observation has been made by Torgerson.[27] The prevalence of lumbar disk herniations is reported to

Table 2–2

Men Reporting Symptoms in the Lower Limbs Associated with Low-Back Pain

Symptoms in the Lower Limbs*	Men with Low Back Pain (Percent)	
	Moderate (n = 565)	*Severe (n = 288)*
Pain	28.9	54.5†
Numbness	14.0	37.4†
Weakness	17.9	44.0†

*A subject may have reported one or more of these symptoms.
†p < 0.001, chi-square analysis.
(From Frymoyer, J.W., et al.: Risk factors in low back pain. J Bone Joint Surg 65A:213, 1983.

Table 2–3
Association of Severity of Low Back Pain and Number of Symptoms in the Lower Limbs with the Presence of Spinal Osteophytes

	Severity of Low-Back Pain (Percent of Patients)			No. of Symptoms in the Lower Limbs (Percent of Patients)			
	None (N = 96)	*Moderate* (N = 134)	*Severe* (N = 62)	*0* (N = 205)	*1* (N = 35)	*2* (N = 23)	*3* (N = 27)
Claw spurs							
L3-L4	5.2	2.2	8.1	3.9	2.9	4.5	11.1
L4-L5	1.0	5.2	3.2	1.9	2.9	13.6	7.4
L5-S1	10.0	0.3	0.0	0.0	0.0	0.0	0.3
Traction spurs							
L3-L4	1.0	3.0	3.2	1.9	8.6	0.0	0.0
L4-L5	2.1	2.2	11.3	1.9	5.7	4.5	18.5
L5-S1	2.1	0.0	1.6	1.0	1.0	0.0	3.7
Claw or traction spurs							
L3-L4	6.3	5.2	11.3	5.8	11.4	4.5	11.1
L4-L5	3.1	7.5	14.5	3.9	8.6	18.2	25.9
L5-S1	0.7	0.3	0.3	0.7	0.0	0.0	0.7
All levels	11.5	11.9	24.2	10.6	20.0	18.2	33.3

(From Frymoyer, J.W., et al.: Spine radiographs in patient with low back pain. J Bone Joint Surg 66A:1048, 1984.)

be 30 to 40% in myelograms,[28] lumbar CT scans,[29] and magnetic resonance imaging surveys.[30] These figures also closely approximate the 40% prevalence of lumbar disc herniations identified at post-mortem examinations. At first glance these findings seem very closely approximate to the epidemiologic surveys of Frymoyer,[6] and Svensson and Andersson,[10] but herein lies the great paradox. All of these imaging studies have been performed in subjects with NO history of low back pain or sciatica.

Claudication

Neurologic claudication was first recognized as an important part of low back symptoms after the classic clinical studies of Verbiest,[31] which described the spinal stenosis syndrome. Currently, there is little information about the lifetime incidence or prevalence or this symptom. Utilizing the NHANES II survey, we determined that 50% of adults over the age of 50 had leg symptoms suggestive of claudication, but we have interpreted these data cautiously because the questionnaire form was nonspecific.[32]

Others have attempted to define the magnitude of this problem by the analysis of spinal radiographs and ultrasound studies. Valkenburg and Haanen[33] found an age-related increase in the radiographic finding of degenerative spondylolisthesis, which is

the most common structural cause of spinal stenosis. Porter utilized an ultrasonic evaluation of spinal canal diameter, and demonstrated the commonality of spinal stenosis as well as the association between decreased spinal canal diameter and low back symptoms.[34] However, he did not determine the association of these findings to the specific complaint of claudication.

HOW COMMON ARE SPECIFIC PATHOLOGIC ENTITIES AFFECTING THE SPINE?

The previous discussion of sciatica and claudication included some description of the prevalence of lumbar disc herniations, degenerative spondylolisthesis, and spinal stenosis, but it has been emphasized that these anatomic findings are often unassociated with symptoms.

Numerous attempts have been made to test the hypothesis that degenerative diseases are the most common cause of low back symptoms. In this regard, there is certain evidence of age-related degenerative changes affecting the lumbar spine.[3] Attempts to correlate these changes with symptoms, however, have not been fruitful. The most positive assertions were made by Rowe who followed patients in the Eastman-Kodak Company over 10 years. Based on comparisons of radiographs obtained during the decade-long observation period, he concluded that 50% of all symptoms were caused by a degenerative process.[35] Based on little evidence, Moran and King[36] concluded that degenerative segmental instabilities caused 25% of all low back symptoms. Others have analyzed the relationship between radiographs and the probability that a specific abnormality is associated with symptoms. Table 2–4, derived from White and Panjabi,[37] gives one such analysis.

The prevalence of other pathologic conditions is extremely low. The most common nondegenerative condition is spondylolysis, reported to affect between 5 and 20% of the population.[38] The next most common condition is ankylosing spondylitis, variously reported to affect 2 to 40 per 1000 population,[39,40] followed by the much less common pathologic conditions of primary and metastatic tumors of vertebrae (0.12/1000), infections (0.037/1000), and multiple myeloma (0.07/1000).[41] Osteoporosis affecting the spine is also extremely common, and is frequently cited as the reason that females over the age of 60 have low back pain at a greater rate than males.

WHO IS AT RISK FOR LOW BACK DISORDERS?

Numerous studies have attempted to determine the demographic, genetic anthropometric, environmental, occupational, and psychosocial determinants of spinal disorders. Some of the factors identified apply to symptoms such as low back pain or sciatica; others apply to specific pathologic entities, such as lumbar disk herniation; while other factors are specifically associated with resultant disability. In this section, these risk factors are identified. Much of this information has been analyzed in detail elsewhere.[42,43]

Demography

As noted, Hult's[1] early studies identified an age dependency of low back symptoms. Subsequently, this relationship has been carefully analyzed. The prevalence, annual incidence, and point prevalence of low back symptoms increases to the age of 50 and then tapers off in males but not in females. Figure 2–2, data derived from the NHANES survey,[32] demonstrates this relationship. As already noted, osteoporosis is cited as the reason for continued symptoms in females. Females are also affected by a history of childbirth. Multiparous women are three times more likely to have a complaint of low back symptoms. The explanations given include: an in-

Table 2–4
*Radiographic Irregularities of the Spine Likely to be Associated with Spine Pain**

Very Likely
　Spondylolisthesis (moderate or severe)

　Multiple, markedly narrowed intervertebral disk spaces

　Congenital kyphosis

　Scoliosis (severe)

　Osteoporosis

　Ankylosing spondylitis

　Lumbar osteochondrosis (Scheuermann's disease)

Very unlikely
　Spina bifida occulta

　Acute lumbosacral angle

　Single disk narrowing and spondylosis

　Facet arthrosis, subluxation, and trophism

　Disk calcification (except in thoracic spine)

　Extracervical, extralumbar, or extrathoracic vertebrae

　Sacralization of lumbar vertebrae

　Lumbarization of sacral vertebrae

　Hyperlordosis (moderate)

　Intravertebral body disk herniation (Schmorl's nodes)

　Accessory ossicles

Questionable
　Spondylolysis

　Spondylolisthesis (mild)

　Kyphosis (severe)

　Scoliosis (mild to moderate)

　Retrolisthesis of cervical, thoracic, or lumbar vertebrae

　Lumbar scoliosis (>80°)

　Hyperlordosis (severe)

*These data are based on the assumption that there is no other clinically obvious explanation for the spinal pain.
(From White, A.A., Panjabi, M.M.: Clinical Biomechanics of the Spine. Philadelphia, J.B. Lippincott, 1978.)

creased physical demand attendant to lifting young children; loss of abdominal muscular support; and pelvic ligamentous laxity. None of these hypotheses have been examined rigorously.

Sciatica is also influenced by age, but unlike low back pain, its onset is later in life, but then rapidly

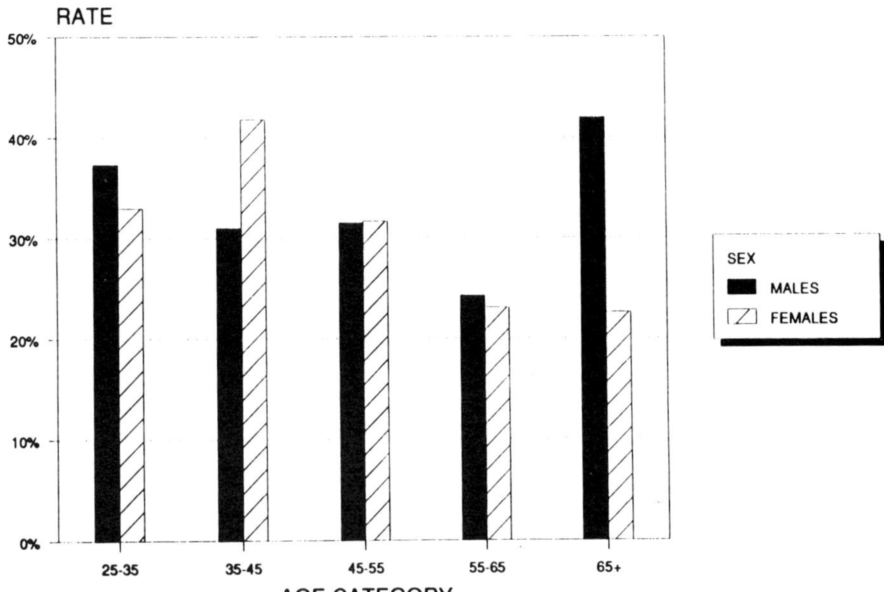

Figure 2–2. The relationship of low back pain to age for males and females. (Courtesy of the Vermont Rehabilitation Engineering Center.)

diminishes in both males and females after the age of 50. This age relationship is paralleled by the peak frequency of surgical interventions for lumbar disk herniation. Spangford[43] analyzed the world's literature, to which he added his own experience. The peak year for lumbar disk excision was 43 in both males and females, as illustrated in Figure 2–3. However, there are distinctive differences between males and females with respect to the risk for surgical intervention, although the prevalence and incidence of disc herniation appears to be similar for men and women. Thus, men are 1.5 to 3 times more likely to be hospitalized[15,44] and 2 times as likely to have a lumbar disc excision than women.[45] The reasons for these differences are uncertain, but perhaps are culturally, rather than medically, determined. For example, it has been proposed the work requirements for men force earlier intervention on the premise that a prolonged period of disability will be less tolerated.

Although the peak incidence for lumbar disc excision is age 43, a smaller subset of patients require in-

Figure 2–3. The peak years for surgical intervention for lumbar disc herniation. (From Spangford, E.V.: The lumbar disc herniation—a computer-aided analysis of 2504 operations. Acta Orthop Scand Suppl 142:17, 1972. Copyright, 1972, Munksgaard International Publishers Ltd., Copenhagen, Denmark.)

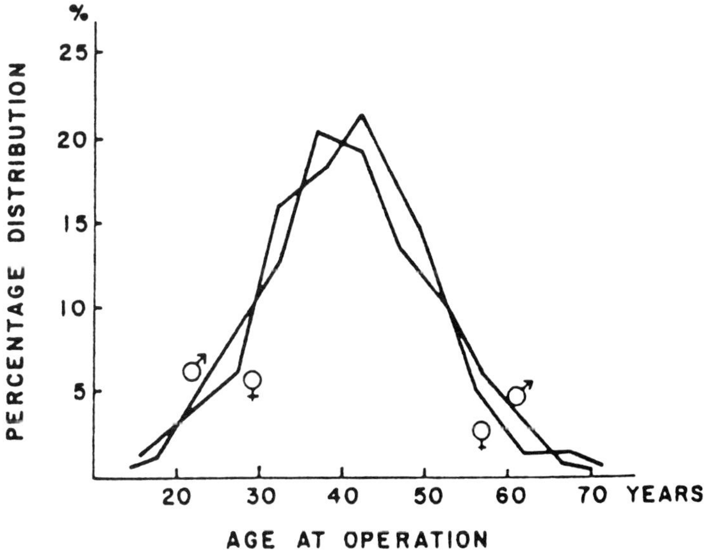

tervention at an older age. In the younger, and largest, group of patients, the vast majority of disc herniations occur at the L4-L5 and L5-S1 levels. With aging, there is an increase in herniations at the L3-L4 level and at higher levels, which continues into the sixth decade.[43] The usual hypothesis states that lumbar degeneration proceeds from the lowest level (L5-S1) and moves cephalad and, therefore, the L3-L4 levels are affected later in life. Against this hypothesis is the observation that disc degeneration is equally prevalent at the L3-L4, L4-L5, and L5-S1 levels.[46]

Although the statistics are incomplete, it seems likely that spinal stenosis and claudication are usually, but not exclusively, a problem in the older age population.[47] Certainly, the radiologic evidence for a predisposition to spinal stenosis is identified in that population over the age of 60, as shown previously in data for degenerative spondylolisthesis. Although the prevalence of that disorder is only modestly different between males and females, the need for surgical intervention in most series is four times greater for females than for males.[48]

Racial differences in spinal disorders have been less well studied, although in certain conditions there are definite major differences between various racial and population groups. Lawrence[49] studied a Jamaican cohort and identified a significantly lower lifetime incidence of low back complaints in that group, when compared to their previously analyzed English population. The reduced complaint of low back pain was paralleled by a significant lessening in radiographic evidence of lumbar spine degeneration. A less well controlled anecdotal survey by Fahrni concluded that these differences resulted from the lessened lumbar lordosis, which he observed in the "primitive" populations he analyzed.[50] As will be seen later, the type of health professionals used by various socioeconomic and racial groups differ significantly.

Specific pathologic conditions of the spine also appear to have significant racial differences. Examples include the fourfold increase in spondylolysis and spondylolisthesis identified in Eskimos and some Asian groups; the increased prevalence of the spondyloarthropathies in some Indian tribes; and the almost exclusive occurrence of idiopathic ligamentous calcification with secondary spinal stenosis in Asians.

Genetic

The preceding information suggests the possibility of a genetic antecedent, which has been proven in family studies of congenital spondylolisthesis. Genetic antecedents also are present in unusual spinal disorders such as achondroplasia and alcaptonuria.

In the broader perspective of degenerative disorders and low back pain, genetic associations have been elusive. Lawrence[49] found a significant increase in suspected disc herniations in the first degree relatives of patients with proven disc herniations, but was unable to demonstrate a mendelian pattern of inheritance. Varlotta and Brown[51] did a similar study, except their patients were adolescents with unequivocal evidence of lumbar disc herniation. Based on their analysis, they concluded a mendelian pattern of inheritance might be operational.

Anthropometry

Physical characteristics such as height, weight, body habitus, leg length, posture, and spinal canal dimensions have been analyzed with varying degrees of observed relationship to complaints of low back pain and sciatica. For example, in their cross-sectional study, Pope et al.[52] showed a modest relationship between low back pain and increased height and weight, but when these were normalized by using the Davenport Index, no differences were identified.[52] Others, such as Heliovaara[53] and Deyo,[54] have noted a more significant association with an increased risk for low back pain and sciatica. For example, Deyo noted an increased risk for patients in the upper fifth quintile of body weight and height, attributed possibly to the increased mechanical stresses placed on the spine. Similar controversy exists regarding the effects of leg length discrepancy.

The role of spinal posture is also controversial. Most surveys indicate scoliosis of less than 60° is not a specific risk factor;[55] if surgical intervention has occurred, the risk of back pain increases as the fusion extends distally into the lumbar spine.[56]

Lumbar lordosis has been more controversial because much of the historic treatment of low back pain, as presupposed, increased lordosis and mechanically disadvantaged the lumbar discs. Many of these conclusions were based on observations of human posture, rather than radiographic measurement. Radiographic analysis, using more precise measurement systems, has demonstrated no relationship between prior or current complaints of low back pain or sciatica and lumbar lordosis.

Finally, the size and shape of the spinal canal is significant to an increased risk of symptomatic radiculopathies and spinal stenosis, although most of the information is derived from clinical observation rather than from controlled epidemiologic surveys. Information derived from ultrasonic studies has already been presented. Heliovaara analyzed radiographs from patients with sciatica and found significant differences in the intra-articular distance at the L5-S1 level, which he interpreted as evidence of spinal stenosis.[57]

Environmental Factors

The external, physical, and chemical environment, particularly as it relates to the occupational setting, appears to have major significance to low back complaints, sciatica, and lumbar and cervical disc herniations.

First, cigarette smoking has been shown to be significantly associated with an increased risk for back pain, sciatica, and disc herniation.[4,5,10,58] Earlier studies of Gyntelberg[24] proposed this association was mediated by coughing, which increased intradiscal pressure. A more direct pharmacologic effect has been observed in experimental animals; the metabolism of the disc is unfavorably altered with reduced incorporation of metabolic precursors for collagen and noncollagenous proteins.[59]

Second, exposure to vibration, particularly vibration caused by motor vehicles, is identified as a significant risk factor for low back pain, sciatica, and disc herniation, increasing the risk for these conditions two- to threefold.[4,5,10,58] Particular populations at risk are commuters driving more than 20 miles per day and truck drivers. The reasons for these differences appear to derive from mechanical, physiologic, and muscular causations. Mechanical studies of the lumbar spine show the resonating frequency is at the 4.5 to 5.5 hertz range.[60,61] Under conditions of resonance, there are increased energy transfers resulting in greater stresses upon tissues and, over time, damage probably caused by fatigue failures. Evidence for this damage is derived from in vitro studies, in which cyclic vibrations of less than 11,000 exposures resulted in disruption of the disc.[63] In laboratory animals, exposure to resonant frequencies results in decreased transfer of nutrients to the disc.[59] Muscular support is also affected, with vibrational exposures causing shifts in the center frequency of paraspinal electromyograms; this finding is consistent with muscular fatigue.[60] Lastly, it has been shown that the concentration substance P (a pain transmitting neuropeptide) is increased in the dorsal root ganglion of experimental rabbits subjected to vibration.[64] Analysis of motor vehicles also shows the 4.5 to 5.5 hertz frequency is common and, thus, the operator is being exposed to a deleterious mechanical and physiologic state.

Third, occupational exposures of other types are clearly implicated. As noted previously, the first epidemiologic study in this regard was that of Hult.[1] Detailed analysis of the workplace environment[65,66,67] demonstrate significant associations between the requirements for lifting, pushing, and pulling and low back pain and sciatica. Of particular importance is the posture adopted during lifting. The most deleterious position is twisting, which in laboratory experiments is a mechanism for the production of radial tears of the annulus fibrosis.[68]

Workers exposed to this posture have a two- to threefold increase in the risk of lumbar disc herniation. Chaffin and associates have further investigated the relationship between the worker and the workplace.[69] He measured, by isometric strength testing, the worker's lifting capacity and compared this strength measurement to job requirements. When the worker's capacity was exceeded, the risk of low back pain increased as much as fourfold. At the other extreme, workers who have sedentary jobs also appear to be at risk, particularly for low back pain.[70,71] In the sitting posture, elevations of lumbar intradiscal pressure increase, which provides a convenient, although unproven, explanation for the increased risk observed. As will be seen, other psychosocial phenomena may be equally operational.

Physical Fitness

A common belief has been that physical fitness, or lack thereof, altered the risk of spinal disorders. The early studies of Cady[72] lent credence to this suggestion. In a prospective study of firefighters, he showed the risk of subsequent back injury was greatest in the least physically fit. Numerous attempts have been made to relate these and other findings to measurements of muscular strength with variable and inconclusive results. The current belief relates physical fitness more to aerobic capacity than to muscular strength. A large body of basic science data has been accumulated in the past decade to support this hypothesis, including the adverse effects of inactivity on disc, diarthrodial joints, ligament, tendon, and muscle. This material has been extensively reviewed in other publications.[73] Similarly, there is growing evidence of a favorable effect of aerobic exercise on these tissues, as well as in the prevention of low back symptoms.

A corollary to the role of physical fitness is the role of athletics. Minimal evidence is available to suggest a major role, although Kelsey demonstrated a significant but marginal effect of golf and tennis on the risk for lumbar disc herniation. A significant association does exist for diving and cervical disc herniations, and for isthmic spondylolysis and spondylolisthesis in football linemen and gymnasts.[40,74]

WHAT IS THE NATURAL HISTORY OF SPINAL DISORDERS?

It should be apparent from the preceding discussion that much of the public and medical concern about an "epidemic" of spinal disease is unfounded. Analysis of the natural history of low back pain confirms this opinion. Figure 2–4 demonstrates the natural history of low back pain derived from studies in

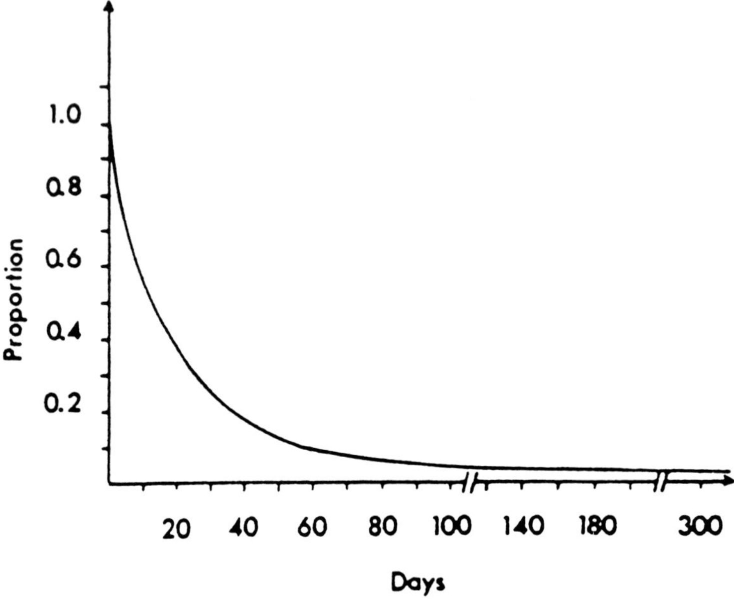

Figure 2–4. The natural history of low back pain, derived from studies in a Swedish population. (From Andersson, G.B.J., Svensson, H.O., and Oden, A.: The intensity of work recovery in low back pain. Spine 8:880, 1983.)

a Swedish population,[75] whereas Figure 2–5 demonstrates the natural history of sciatica.[76] It will be noted that by 3 months, only 5% of the original population has continuing symptoms. This figure closely conforms to NHANES survey data, which showed that 5% of the population had low back complaints of greater than 6 months duration. However, the natural history of this chronically affected subset is distinctly unfavorable, particularly in the historic context. Figure 2–6 demonstrates this natural history.[77] Therefore, the question arises: "What are the determinants of chronic, disabling low back pain?" This question is of the utmost significance because those who suffer from chronic low back pain

constitute 85 to 90% of the total costs attributable to this condition.[78] Here the epidemiologic data strongly implicates psychosocial and occupational factors rather than structural or medical causations. A summary of many publications[65,66,77,78,79] reveals the following information:

1. The disabled subset is characterized by psychologic and psychosocial dysfunction. This dysfunction is measurable by tests such as the Minnesota Multiphasic Personality Inventory (MMPI), which typically reveals elevations in the Hy and Hs scales; by abnormal pain drawings, anatomically nonplausible physical findings (Waddell signs[80]),

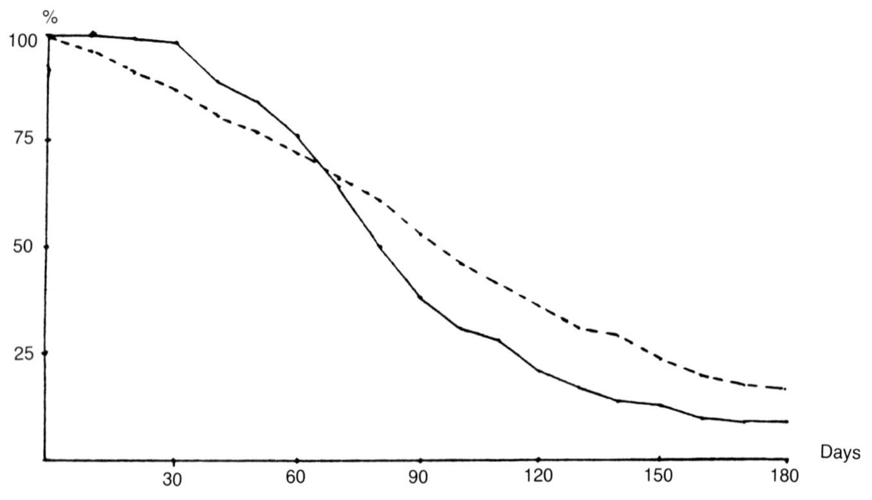

Figure 2–5. The probability of recovery from an acute episode of sciatica caused by lumbar disc herniation. The solid line represents operated patients; the dotted line represents unoperated patients. (From Hakelius, A.: Prognosis in sciatica: a clinical follow-up of surgical and nonsurgical treatment. Acta Orthop Scand Suppl 129:1, 1970.)

PROBABILITY OF RETURNING TO WORK

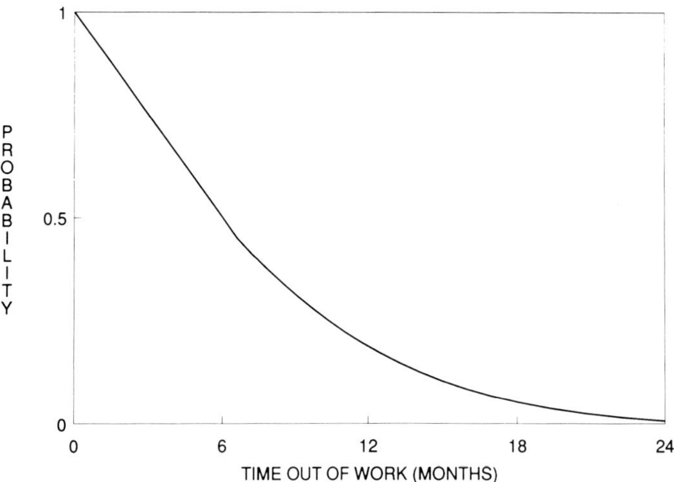

Figure 2–6. The probability of recovery from disabling low back pain.

and other psychological and interview techniques to elicit these behavioral characteristics.

2. The working environment of the disabled individuals is typically described as boring. The work is repetitious, and and the immediate supervisor's opinion of job performance is low.
3. The individual frequently has numerous other health complaints, typically of pain or stress disorders such as ulcers or alcohol or drug abuse.[81]
4. The disabled subset is resistant to conventional treatment, including surgical and non-surgical modalities[82,83] although new, intensive rehabilitation efforts have drastically altered this perspective.[84]

An unanswered question has been, "Are these characteristics antecedent to, or the result of, the disability?" The most informative study in that regard has been the prospective study of Bigos and associates in a large manufacturing plant.[66] Although this study is still in progress, the early analysis showed twenty-six workers who had been disabled for more than three months. The significant predictors were: poor job Apgar (this test measures the relationship of the worker to his job environment); elevations in the Hy and Hs scales of the MMPI; and a poor rating by the immediate supervisor three to six months prior to the onset of symptoms. Strength testing was not predictive; in fact, the disabled subset performed better than their peers in the preliminary testing. However, smoking and decreased aerobic capacity was also identified in this subset.

A different study design yielded similar information.[85] Here, patients with back pain were identified soon after the onset of symptoms, and then followed six months later to determine those who had become disabled. Significant predictors were the perception of fault (i.e., injury), the patient's lack of satisfaction with his/her work environment, and particularly the duration of disability before the patient is examined by a doctor.

Thus, the information strongly supports a predominant psychosocial determinant for disability. However, it must be emphasized that before a patient is relegated to a psychosocial causation, a carefully conceived and controlled diagnostic study must be conducted. In at least one survey, this type of analysis revealed a structurally plausible causation for symptoms in 13% of the patients.[86] Conversely, if the patient's symptoms, signs, and subsequent imaging studies are not unequivocally related and plausible, surgical intervention has a high probability of failure.[82]

WHO TREATS LOW BACK PAIN?

The natural history of low back pain would strongly suggest the need for minimal intervention in the majority of patients. In fact, it can be argued that the majority would be better served by no treatment, particularly if the prescription includes extended bedrest and prolonged work absence.[78] As previously noted, there are significant differences as a function of geographic region, race, and socioeconomic status. This information is given in Table 2–5. The types of treatment also vary as a function of the patient's symptoms and duration of pain. It is worthwhile remembering that many of these treatment modalities have been shown to have little or no effect on the course of the symptom.[87,88]

In the subset of patients who are considered as

Table 2–5
Use of Health Professionals by Race, Region, and Education

	Unweighted (N)	General Practitioner	Orthopaedist	Chiropractor	Osteopath	Internist	Rheumatologist
All subjects	1,516	58.6	36.9	30.8	13.8	7.6	2.5
Race							
White	1,164	59.2	36.4	38.6	17.4	7.9	2.3
Black	96	58.4	45.4	14.1	5.3	5.6	2.5
Other	13	34.7	26.0	22.3	10.5	0.0	12.0
Significance		NS*	NS	<.0001	.006	NS	.001
Region							
Northeast	215	48.6	41.2	29.6	16.6	7.5	1.6
Midwest	349	58.3	34.8	38.1	20.3	7.3	2.4
South	351	63.1	36.6	29.5	14.1	5.8	2.7
West	358	61.0	36.2	44.6	15.0	9.4	3.0
Significance		.004	NS	<.0001	NS	NS	NS
Education							
Elementary or none	351	74.3	28.9	32.8	17.4	5.9	4.7
High school	629	57.5	35.4	37.4	16.4	6.1	1.8
College	283	47.9	45.5	37.2	14.9	12.2	2.3
Significance		<.0001	.0002	NS	NS	.003	NS

*NS = not significant, $P > .05$.
(From Deyo, R.A., Tsui-Wu, Y.J.: Descriptive epidemiology of low back pain and its related medical care in the United States. Spine *12*:264, 1987.)

candidates for surgery, there are also significant regional differences, as well as differences between sexes as previously noted. In the United States, 256,000 operations were performed in 1984, of which three-quarters were for lumbar disc herniation.[89] When these figures are expressed as operations per 100,000, the United States' figure is 69.5/100,000. However, there are significant regional variations, which may be as great as tenfold in the United States. In other countries, the correspondent figures are lower, for example 41/100,000 in Finland, and 10/100,000 in Great Britain.[90] The reasons for these differences is unclear, but it seems unlikely that they are attributable to inherent differences in disease incidence.

WHAT ARE THE COSTS OF SPINAL DISORDERS?

The total costs of low back disorders are estimated to range between $16 and $60 billion dollars or more each year. Such a wide discrepancy strongly suggests the data are incomplete, or that very different analytic approaches have been taken to calculate the costs. Grazier et al.[91] performed the most intensive evaluation of population and economic statistics for the United States. In 1984 they calculated the costs to be $16 billion. The various components of costs can be further divided and include: medical costs, including those attributed to diagnosis and treatment; the direct costs of disability, such as compensation payments and entitlements; and indirect costs due to loss of work time. It is not the intention here to give a detailed analysis of these figures, although a general overview is instructive. For example, the medical costs attributed to plane spinal x rays alone was estimated to be 800 million dollars in 1978.[92] This is a striking figure when some have estimated that only 1/2000 spinal radiographs alter the course of treatment. The costs of disability have been rather extensively analyzed, particularly as they pertain to workmen's compensation. In 1984 this figure was calculated to exceed 5.5 billion dollars,[93] although a much lower figure was calculated in another survey (Table 2–6). The indirect costs are also shown in Table 2–6; however, another survey estimated that the indirect costs in males age 18 to 55 was $11 billion each year. The most instructive information again relates to the disabled subset. As noted previously,

Table 2–6
Some Indirect Costs of Back Pain and Selected Other Medical Problems (Men Only; $ Billion in 1975)

Problem	Earnings Losses for Persons Unable to Work	Productivity Losses Due to Work-Loss Days	Debility Costs	Total Morbidity Costs
Orthopedic impairment: back-spine-neck	1.20	0.15	1.25	2.6
Herniated disk	1.22	0.25	1.03	2.5
Ischemic heart disease	1.70	0.16	0.54	2.4
Respiratory conditions (other than asthma)	0.58	2.77	0.30	3.7

(From Deyo, R.A.: Reducing work absenteeism and diagnostic costs for backache. *In* Clinical Concepts in Regional Musculoskeletal Illness (Edited by N.M. Hadler). Orlando, Grune & Stratton, 1987.)

it is this group that constitutes at least 85% of the total costs of low back pain. In the survey that showed indirect costs of 11 billion dollars, 1.7 percent of the survey population was responsible for 8 billion dollars of the costs.[5] Another instructive analysis was that of Norton.[94] He determined the costs for all workmen's compensation cases who were treated by laminectomy or chymopapain in the state of Oregon. These data are given in Table 2–7. The most striking figure is an analysis of the costs to achieve a successful result, which he showed to be $128,610 for the chymopapain group, and $49,007 for the surgically treated group. These data again enforce the notion that the epidemic of low back disease is dominantly a result of the disabled population, rather than a function of the ubiquitous symptom of low back pain.

SUMMARY

The premise of this chapter is that "spinal disorders have been part of mankind's existence;" yet the epidemic of low back pain is a twentieth century phenomenon. The epidemiology of low back disorders clearly indicates that low back symptoms are extremely common (70%), low back pain of greater than 2 weeks duration is far less common (13 to 22%), serious lumbar spinal pathology and the need for surgery is low, and that disability affects a small, but distinctive subset. The perceived "epidemic" relates to that subset who are increasing at a rate far disproportional to population growth and who contribute the greatest amount of the total socioeconomic burden for society. Although specifics place an individual at risk for current and future low back symptoms and disc herniations, the greatest risk factors relative to the epidemic are psychosocial rather than physical. Because the underlying causations for this subset of patients involve complex social, legal, and industrial factors, it is unlikely that the medical profession alone can create the solution to the problem. However, we can modulate the problem by recognizing the favorable natural history and avoiding overtreatment; we can identify the person at risk for disability and take prompt action for prevention, recognizing low back pain disability does not get better of its own accord; and we can select carefully and according to valid diagnostic criteria, the small number of patients who require surgery recognizing

Table 2–7
Costs of Chemonucleolysis Versus Surgical Discectomy in Workers' Compensation Cases

Category*	I Chemonucleolysis		II Surgical Discectomy	
	Total Costs	*Average/Claim*	*Total Costs*	*Average/Claim*
TTD	$ 979,233	$16,053	$ 456,929	$10,385
PPD	230,153	3,773	223,749	5,085
Total	1,209,386	19,826	680,678	15,470
Medical costs	976,976	16,016	593,511	13,489
Combined compensation and medical costs	2,186,362	35,842	1,274,189	28,959

*TTD = temporary total disability—wage replacement; PPD = partial permanent disability—impairment award.
(From Norton, W.L.: Chemonucleolysis versus surgical discectomy. Comparison of costs and results in workers' compensation claimants. Spine *11*:440, 1986.)

that poorly indicated surgical procedures only add to the magnitude of the disability problem.

REFERENCES

1. Hult, L.: Cervical, dorsal and lumbar spinal syndromes. Acta Orthop Scand 24:174, 1954.
2. Kellgren, J.H., Lawrence, J.S.: Osteoarthrosis and disk degeneration in an urban population. Ann Rheum Dis 17:388, 1958.
3. Horal, J.: The clinical appearance of low back disorders in the City of Gothenburg, Sweden. Acta Orthop Scand 118(suppl):8, 1969.
4. Andersson, G.B.J., Pope, M.H., Frymoyer, J.W.: Epidemiology. In Occupational Low Back Pain (Edited by M.H. Pope, J.W. Frymoyer). New York, Praeger, 1984.
5. Frymoyer, J.W., et al.: Risk factors in low-back pain. An epidemiological study. J Bone Joint Surg 65A:213, 1983.
6. Frymoyer, J.W., Pope, M.H., Rosen, J., Goggin, J.: Epidemiologic studies of low back pain. Spine 5(5):419, 1980.
7. Nagi, S.Z., Riley, L.E., Newby, L.G.: A social epidemiology of back pain in a general population. J Chronic Dis 26:769, 1973.
8. Deyo, R.A., Tsui-Wu, Y.J.: Descriptive epidemiology of low back pain and its related medical care in the United States. Spine 12:264, 1987.
9. Biering-Sorenson, F.: Low back trouble in a general population of 30-, 40-, 50-, and 60-year-old men and women: study design, representativeness and basic results. Dan Med Bull 29:289, 1982.
10. Svensson, H.O., Andersson, G.B.J.: Low back pain in 40- to 47-year-old men: I. Frequency of occurrence and impact on medical services. Scand J Rehabil Med 14:47, 1982.
11. Snook, S.H.: Low back pain in industry. In American Academy of Orthopaedic Surgeons Symposium on Idiopathic Low Back Pain (Edited by A.A. White, III, S.L. Gordon). St. Louis, C.V. Mosby, 1982.
12. Troup, J.D., Martin, J.W., Lloyd, D.C.: Back pain in industry: a prospective survey. Spine 6:61, 1981.
13. Valkenburg, H.A., Haanen, H.C.M.: The epidemiology of low back pain. In American Academy of Orthopaedics Surgeons Symposium on Idiopathic Low Back Pain (Edited by A.A. White, III, S.L. Gordon). St. Louis, C.V. Mosby, 1982.
14. National Center for Health Statistics: Prevalence of Selected Impairments, United States-1977, Series 10, No. 134, DHHS Publication (PHS) 81-1562. Hyattsville, MD, 1981.
15. Kelsey, J.L.: Epidemiology of Musculoskeletal Disorders. Oxford, Oxford University Press, 145, 1982.
16. Fordyce, W.: Back pain, compensation and public policy. In Prevention in Health Psychology (Edited by J. Rosen, L. Solomon). Hanover, VT, University Press of NE, 1985.
17. Nettelbladt, E.: Opuscula Medica (Sweden) 30(2):54, 1985.
18. Cortugno, D.: De Ischiade Nervosa Canmentarius. L. Naples, Simoncos Brothers, 1764.
19. Mixter, W.J., Barr, J.S.: Rupture of the intervertebral disc with involvement of the spinal canal. N Engl J Med 211:210, 1934.
20. Lewis, T., Kellgren, J.H.: Observations relating to referred pain, visceromotor reflexes and other associated phenomena. Clin Sci 4:47, 1939.
21. McCall, I.W., Park, W.M., O'Brien, J.P.: Induced pain referral from posterior lumbar elements in normal subjects. Spine 4:441, 1979.
22. Hirsch, C., Ingelmark, B-E., Miller, M.: The anatomical basis for low back pain: studies on the presence of sensory nerve endings in ligamentous, capsular and intervertebral disc structures in the human lumbar spine. Acta Orthop Scand 33:1, 1963.
23. Hirsch, C., Jonsson, B., Lewin, T.: Low-back symptoms in a Swedish female population. Clin Orthop 63:171, 1969.
24. Gyntelberg, F.: One year incidence of low back pain among male residents of Copenhagen aged 40–59. Dan Med Bull 21:30, 1974.
25. Hakelius, A., Hindmarsh, J.: The comparative reliability of preoperative diagnostic methods in lumbar disc surgery. Acta Orthop Scand 43:234, 1972.
26. Frymoyer, J.W., et al.: Spine radiographs in patients with low-back pain: an epidemiological study in men. J Bone Joint Surg 66A:1048, 1984.
27. Torgerson, W.R., Dotter, W.E.: Comparative roentgenographic study of the asymptomatic and symptomatic lumbar spine. J Bone Joint Surg 58A:850, 1976.
28. Hitselberger, W.E., Witten, R.M.: Abnormal myelograms in asymptomatic patients. J Neurosurg 28:204, 1968.
29. Wiesel, S.W., et al.: A study of computer-assisted tomography. I. The incidence of positive CAT scans in an asymptomatic group of patients. Spine 9:549, 1984.
30. Wiesel, S.W.: Personal communication.
31. Verbiest, H.: Radicular syndrome from developmental narrowing of the lumbar vertebral canal. J Bone Joint Surg 36B:230, 1954.
32. Cats-Baril, W.: Personal communication.
33. Valkenburg, H.A., Haanen, H.C.M.: The epidemiology of low back pain. In American Academy of Orthopaedic Surgeons Symposium on Idiopathic Low Back Pain (Edited by A.A. White, III, S.L. Gordon). St. Louis, C.V. Mosby, 1982.
34. Porter, P.W., Hibbert, C.S., Wicks, M.: The spinal canal in symptomatic lumbar disc disease. J Bone Joint Surg 60B:485, 1978.
35. Rowe, M.L.: Low back pain in industry. A position paper. J Occup Med 11:161, 1969.
36. Moran, F.P., King, T.: Primary instability of lumbar vertebrae as a common cause of low back pain. J Bone Joint Surg (Br) 39B:6, 1957.
37. White, A.A., Panjabi, M.M.: Clinical Biomechanics of the Spine. Philadelphia, J.B. Lippincott, 1978.
38. Fredrickson, B.E., et al.: The natural history of spondylolysis and spondylolisthesis. J Bone Joint Surg (Am) 66A:699, 1984.
39. Hawkins, B.R., et al.: Use of the B27 test in the diagnosis of ankylosing spondylitis: a statistical evaluation. Arthritis Rheum 24:743, 1981.
40. Calin, A., et al.: The prevalence and nature of back pain in an industrial complex: a questionnaire and radiographic and HLA analysis. Spine 5:201, 1980.
41. Deyo, R.A.: Reducing work absenteeism and diagnostic costs for backache. In Clinical Concepts in Regional Musculoskeletal Illness (Edited by N.M. Hadler). Orlando, Grune & Stratton, 1987.
42. Frymoyer, J.W.: Helping your patients avoid low back pain. J Musculoskel Med 1:65, 1984.
43. Spangford, E.V.: The lumbar disk herniation: a computer-aided analysis of 2,504 operations. Acta Orthop Scand 142 (suppl):1, 1972.
44. Thomas, M., et al.: Surgical treatment of low backache and sciatica. Lancet 2:1437, 1983.
45. Kelsey, J.L.: Epidemiology of radiculopathies. Adv Neurol 19:385, 1978.
46. Miller, J.A.A., Schmatz, C., Schultz, A.B.: Lumbar disc degeneration: correlation with age, sex, and spine level in 600 autopsy specimens. Spine 13(2):173, 1988.
47. Arnoldi, C.C., et al.: Lumbar spinal stenosis and nerve root entrapment syndromes: definition and classification. Clin Orthop 115:4, 1976.
48. Rosenberg, N.: Degenerative spondylolisthesis: Pre-disposing factors. J Bone Joint Surg 57A:467, 1975.
49. Lawrence, J.: Rheumatism in Populations. London, Heinemann, 1977.
50. Fahrni, W.H., Trueman, G.E.: Comparative radiological

study of the spines of a primitive population with North Americans and northern Europeans. J Bone Joint Surg *47B*:552, 1965.

51. Varlotta, G.P., Brown, M.D.: Familial predisposition for adolescent disc displacement. Presented at the meeting of the International Society for the Study of the Lumbar Spine. Miami, FL, April 13–17, 1988.

52. Pope, M.H., et al.: The relationship between anthropometric, postural, muscular, and mobility characteristics of males ages 18–55. Spine *10*:644, 1985.

53. Heliovaara, M.: Body height, obesity, and risk of herniated lumbar intervertebral disc. *In* Epidemiology of Sciatica and Herniated Lumbar Intervertebral Disc (Edited by M. Heliovaara). Helsinki, Social Insurance Institution, 1988.

54. Deyo, R.A.: Comparative validity of the sickness impact profile and shorter scales for functional assessment in low-back pain. Spine *11*(9):951, 1986.

55. Collis, D.K., Ponseti, I.V.: Long-term follow-up of patients with idiopathic scoliosis not treated surgically. J Bone Joint Surg *51A*:425, 1969.

56. Kostuik, J., Bentivoglio, J.: The incidence of low back pain in adult scoliosis. Presented at the Seventh Annual Meeting of the International Society for the Study of the Lumbar Spine. New Orleans, May 24–28, 1980.

57. Heliovaara, M., et al.: Herniated lumbar disc syndrome and vertebral canals. *In* Epidemiology of Sciatica and Herniated Lumbar Intervertebral Disc (Edited by M. Heliovaara). Helsinki, Social Insurance Institution, 1988.

58. Kelsey, J.L., et al.: Acute prolapsed lumbar intervertebral disc: an epidemiologic study with special reference to driving automobiles and cigarette smoking. Spine *9*:608, 1984.

59. Holm, S., Nachemson, A.: Immediate effects of cigarette smoke on the nutrition of the intervertebral disc of the pig. Orthop Trans *8*:380, 1984.

60. Wilder, D.G., et al.: Vibration and the human spine. Spine *7*:243, 1982.

61. Panjabi, M.M., et al.: In vivo measurements of spinal column vibrations. J Bone Joint Surg *68A*:695, 1986.

62. Adams, M.A., Hutton, W.C.: 1981 Volvo Award in basic science: prolapsed intervertebral disc. A hyperflexion injury. Spine *7*:184, 1982.

63. Wilder, D.G., Pope, M.H., Frymoyer, J.W.: The biomechanics of lumbar disc herniation and the effect of overload and instability. J Spinal Disorders *1*(1):16, 1988.

64. Weinstein, J., Pope, M., Schmidt, R., Seroussi, R.: Neuropharmacologic effects of vibration on the dorsal root ganglion: an animal model. Spine *13*(5):521, 1988.

65. Svensson, H.O., Andersson, G.B.J.: Low-back pain in 40- to 47-year-old men: work history and work environment factors. Spine *8*:272, 1983.

66. Bigos, S.J., Battie, M.C.: Surveillance of back problems in industry. *In* Clinical Concepts in Regional Musculoskeletal Illness (Edited by N.M. Hadler). Orlando, Grune & Stratton, 1987.

67. Damkot, D.K., Pope, M.H., Lord, J., Frymoyer, J.W.: The relationship between work history, work environment and low-back pain in men. Spine *9*:395, 1984.

68. Kelsey, J.L., et al.: An epidemiologic study of lifting and twisting on the job and risk for acute prolapsed lumbar intervertebral disc. J Orthop Res *2*:61, 1984.

69. Chaffin, D.B., Herrin, G.D., Keyserling, W.M.: Preemployment strength testing: an updated position. J Occup Med *20*:403, 1978.

70. Magora, A.: Investigation of the relation between low back pain and occupation: 3. Physical requirements. Sitting, standing and weight lifting. Indian J Med Surg *41*:5, 1972.

71. Eklundh, M.: Prevalence of musculoskeletal problems in office work. Soc Med T *6*:1, 1967.

72. Cady, L.D., Jr., Thomas, P.C., Karwasky, R.J.: Program for increasing health and physical fitness of fire fighters. J Occup Med *27*:110, 1985.

73. Frymoyer, J.W., Gordon, S.L. (eds): New Perspectives on Low Back Pain. Chicago, American Academy of Orthopaedics Surgeons, 1989.

74. Wiltse, L.L., Widell, E.H., Jr., Jackson, D.W.: Fatigue fracture: the basic lesion in isthmic spondylolisthesis. J Bone Joint Surg (Am) *57A*:17, 1975.

75. Andersson, G.B.J., Svensson, H.O., Oden, A.: The intensity of work recovery in low back pain. Spine *8*:880, 1983.

76. Hakelius, A.: Prognosis in sciatica: a clinical follow-up of surgical and non-surgical treatment. Acta Orthop Scand (suppl) *129*:1, 1970.

77. Beals, R.K., Hickman, N.W.: Industrial injuries of the back and extremities: comprehensive evaluation—an aid in prognosis and management. A study of one hundred and eighty patients. J Bone Joint Surg *54A*:1593, 1972.

78. Frymoyer, J.W.: Back pain and sciatica. New Engl J Med *318*:291, 1988.

79. Vallfors, B.: Acute, subacute and chronic low back pain: clinical symptoms, absenteeism and working environment. Scand J Rehabil Med *11* (suppl.):1, 1985.

80. Waddell, G., McCulloch, J.A., Kummel, E., Venner, R.M.: Nonorganic physical signs in low-back pain. Spine *5*(2):117, 1980.

81. Frymoyer, J.W., et al.: Psychologic factors in low back pain disability. Clin Orthop *195*:178, 1985.

82. Spengler, D.M., et al.: Low-back pain following multiple lumbar spine procedures: failure of initial selection? Spine *5*:356, 1980.

83. Wiltse, L.L., Rocchio, P.D.: Preoperative psychological tests as predictors of success of chemonucleolysis in the treatment of the low back syndrome. J Bone Joint Surg *57A*:478, 1975.

84. Mayer, T.G., et al.: Objective assessment of spine function following industrial injury: a prospective study with comparison group and one-year follow-up. Spine *10*:482, 1985.

85. Frymoyer, J.W., Cats-Baril, W.: Predictors of low back pain disability. Clin Orthop *221*:89, 1987.

86. Pyhtinen, J., et al.: Computed tomography after lumbar myelography in lower back and extremity pain syndromes. Diagn Imag *52*:19, 1983.

87. Deyo, R.A.: Conservative therapy for low back pain: distinguishing useful from useless therapy. JAMA *250*:1057, 1983.

88. Report of the Quebec Task Force on Spinal Disorders, Spine *12*(7S), 1987.

89. Rutkow, I.M.: Orthopaedic operations in the United States, 1979 through 1983. J Bone Joint Surg (Am) *68A*:716, 1986.

90. Pokras, R., Graves, E.F., Dennison, C.F.: Surgical Operations in Short-Stay Hospitals: United States, Series 13, No. 61. DHEW Publication (PHS) 82-1722. Hyattsville, MD, 1978.

91. Grazier, K.L., et al. (eds): The Frequency of Occurrence, Impact, and Cost of Musculoskeletal Conditions in the United States. Chicago, American Academy of Orthopaedic Surgeons, 1984.

92. Scavone, J.G., Latshaw, R.F., Rohrer, G.V.: Use of lumbar spine films: statistical evaluation at a university teaching hospital. JAMA *246*:1105, 1981.

93. Snook, S.H., Jensen, R.C.: Cost. *In* Occupational Low Back Pain (Edited by M.H. Pope, J.W. Frymoyer, G. Andersson). New York, Praeger, 1984.

94. Norton, W.L.: Chemonucleolysis versus surgical discectomy: Comparison of costs and results in workers' compensation claimants. Spine *11*:440, 1986.

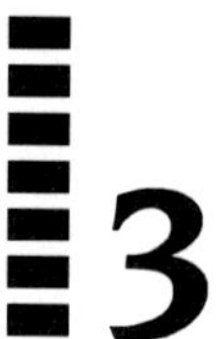

3

E. Shannon Stauffer, M.D.

Relationship Between Cervical and Lumbar Spine Disorders: The Evaluation and Nonoperative Management

INTRODUCTION

Many of the same painful conditions that affect the lumbar spine also affect the cervical spine. The symptoms and the treatment may be similar. However, the symptoms of cervical spine disease tend to be more vague and widespread than the symptoms of lumbar spine disease, which tend to be more localized and discrete. The physical findings of cervical conditions are also more vague and it is more difficult to pinpoint the actual anatomic location of the disorder based on objective physical findings. The symptoms of neck pain, headache, and shoulder pain are more common than objective neurologic physical findings of injury to the distal upper extremity. In contrast, disorders of the lumbar spine frequently have fairly clear cut, specific sensory, motor, and reflex changes in anatomic areas which can be ascribed to specific nerve root, dermatomal, and myotomal areas.

Disorders of the cervical spine involving the neurologic system may cause symptoms from irritation or pressure to destructive lesions of the spinal cord and the nerve roots. In the lumbar spine, there is no spinal cord and neurologic symptoms are more specifically attributed to one or several specific nerve roots. The history, symptoms, and physical examination of a patient with cervical symptoms must include attention to the upper extremities, trunk,

lower extremities, and the genito-urinary system. The examiner should look specifically for evidence of upper motor neuron disorders in the upper extremities, trunk, and lower extremities, and for lower motor neuron disorders in the individual dermatomal areas of the upper extremity. The upper cervical nerve roots supply the sensory distribution to the back of the head (C2) and upper neck (C3, C4), whereas the mid cervical roots (C5, C6) supply the sensory distribution across the upper back and over the shoulders. The mid and lower cervical roots (C5, C6, C7, C8, T1) supply the sensory distribution to the entire upper extremity. Therefore, all these areas must be carefully evaluated for clues to the cause of the symptoms of cervical spine disorders.

The sequence of the diagnostic work-up of cervical spine disorders is similar to that of the lumbar spine, with certain variations that will be discussed in more detail.

THE INITIAL EVALUATION

When confronted with a patient with symptoms relating to the neck, head, shoulders, or upper extremities, the first priority is to localize the anatomic area of the cause of the symptoms. One must consider the nervous system components in the head, i.e., brain, mid-brain, and cerebellum, as well as the

24

cervical spinal cord, nerve roots, trunks, divisions of the brachalplexis, and peripheral nerves, for areas of disease or entrapment. One must also consider the soft tissues adjacent to the joints of the upper extremity for evidence of tendonitis or bursitis, i.e. lateral epicondylitis bursitis, tendonitis, and impingement syndromes of the shoulder, as well as inflammatory nerve irritation or compression at the carpal tunnel and cubital tunnel. One must also consider and examine for boney and articular manifestations on the hand, wrist, forearm, elbow, arm, and shoulder areas.

From the patient's history the examiner should be able to determine the anatomic area from which the symptoms arise and the organs or tissues most likely involved.

The physical examination must be detailed and systematic, including all anatomic areas and organ systems. Begin with an examination of the head, eyes, ears, nose, and throat to rule out intracranial disease. Then proceed with an examination of the range of motion of the cervical spine, specifically documenting the motions that are unique to the occipital-C1 area (head flexion/extension), the C1-C2 area (head lateral rotation), the mid and lower cervical spine area (neck flexion/extension and lateral tilt). Palpation of the neck and upper extremity for tenderness or abnormal masses is performed. Active and passive ranges of motion of the shoulder, elbow, wrist, and hand are recorded. A detailed neurologic examination of each upper extremity is performed to document each nerve root sensory dermatome. Muscle strength is graded on a 5/5 scale. Reflexes of the biceps, triceps, and brachioradialis are compared. The arm and forearm are measured for atrophy. A Jamar grip test is performed to document intrinsic and extrinsic hand muscle strength. Examination is then continued to include the range of motion of the thoracic and lumbar spine, as well as the hips, knees, ankles, and feet in order to rule out systemic or associated conditions. A neurologic evaluation of the lower extremities, particularly looking for hyperactive reflexes or abnormal reflexes, as well as a rectal exam, particularly looking for sensation and sphincter control, are important.

From the history and physical examination, one should be able to rule out conditions arising in the extremities and to localize the cause of the symptoms to the cervical spine. If the symptoms and physical findings point to a disorder of the cervical spine, either the boney articular or neurologic elements, the next priority is to specifically examine for conditions that may be progressive or life threatening, and that require immediate attention. These conditions include neoplasms, infection, myelopathy, and radiculopathy.

The third priority, after localizing the cause of symptoms to the cervical spine and having ruled out a tumor or infection, is to ascertain whether the disorder can be relieved by specific medical treatment or physical measures, or whether it is a condition that requires a surgical intervention. Surgical care is usually required in those cases with evidence of tumor, infection, or neurologic deficit.

Differential Diagnosis

The most common causes of symptoms related to the cervical spine that bring the patient to the physician for medical attention originate from the inflammatory stages of the aging process known as "degenerative disc disease"[1,5] (frequently after it has been aggravated by minor trauma). This diagnosis can be made only after exclusion of all other specific pathologic conditions. The symptoms and signs are often vague, nondescript, and overlap with other conditions. Therefore, one must take a systematic approach to the differential diagnosis in order to rule out specific entities prior to embarking on therapy aimed at alleviating symptoms caused by degenerative disc disease, with or without superimposed trauma. The major categories of conditions to be considered are: congenital and developmental, traumatic (acute and chronic), metabolic, inflammatory (acute infections and chronic noninfectious), degenerative, and tumors (primary and metatastic).

Congenital lesions are rarely diagnosed on clinical examination and are usually discovered by x ray evaluation. The most frequent of these consist of os-odontoidium and failure of vertebral element segmentation. These conditions are rarely symptomatic unless aggravated by trauma or the development of progressive instability of hypermobile segments.

Developmental scoliosis, which results from an idiopathic curve in the thoracic and lumbar spine, does not occur in the cervical spine.

There are certain medical conditions and metabolic disorders which can give rise to symptoms in the cervical spine. Neurologic symptoms can be caused by Guillain-Barre syndrome, which is characterized by a rapid onset of weakness with preserved sensation. Direct progressive cord compression may produce an upper extremity flacid weakness or lower extremity spasticity and weakness, with associated sensory loss, bladder retention, increased lower extremity reflexes, and positive Babinski signs. This may be caused by an extradural lymphoma, leukemic deposits, or an extradural metastasis, which usually is proceeded by pain, then weakness and sensory loss. Acute transverse myelitis produces weakness, neck pain, and loss of bladder function as well as sensory loss. Disc space infection, osteomyelitis of the vertebral bodies, and epidural abscess may not be evident on initial X-rays. Spasmodic torticollis may begin with neck pain and involuntary rotary motion of the spine caused by involuntary spastic contractures.

Tumors can occur in the spinal cord itself, along the nerve roots, in the vertebral bodies, or in the surrounding soft tissue, such as the apex of the lung.

Acute trauma can cause painful cervical disorders by partial tearing of the soft tissue, ligaments, and muscles in the neck or actual disruption of ligaments causing dislocations or fractures of bones. Chronic trauma with repeated rotation, vibration, or prolonged postures in flexed or extended positions may have some role in the production or aggravation of the progressive degenerative disc disease and may cause painful irritative conditions in the cervical spine.

Degenerative disc disease is a condition which causes symptoms to be most pronounced between the ages of 35 and 50. Frequently, these symptoms are initiated or aggravated by a minor trauma, which does not show signs of fracture or dislocation in x rays, but which is associated with narrowing of the disc and pre-existing osteophyte formation around the areas of the attachment of the anulus fibrosis to the body and the joints of Luscha and the neuroforamen (Fig. 3–1).

Hyperextension injuries, which most frequently occur to front seat passengers when their automobile is struck from the rear, frequently cause prolonged pain in the neck, limited range of motion, headaches, and radiation of pain over the shoulders without specific findings of physical confirmation through x rays or other objective means.

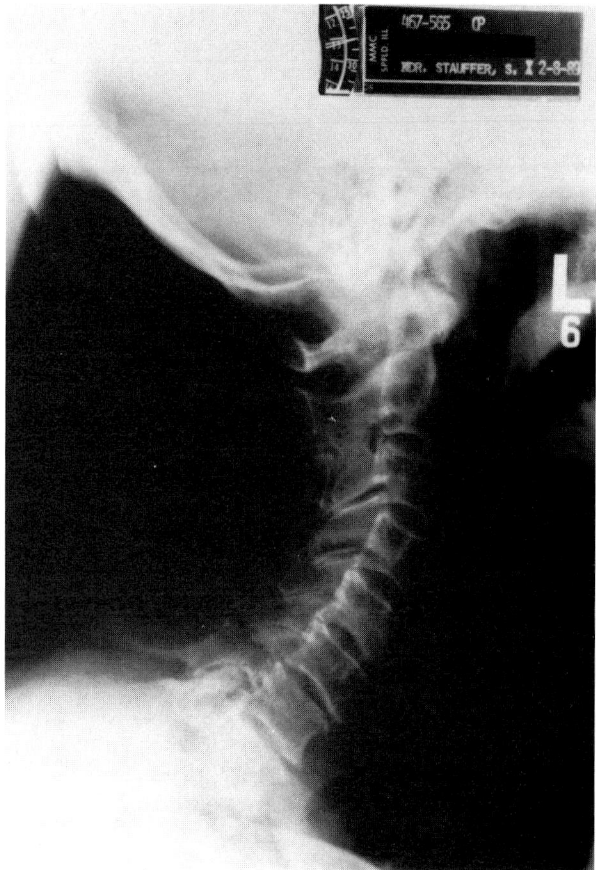

Figure 3–1. Lateral x ray of the cervical spine of a patient with degenerative disc disease.

The Relationship of Peripheral Entrapment Syndromes to Cervical Spine Nerve Root Irritation

Frequently, a person who has symptoms and signs of irritation of the cervical nerve roots also has objective signs of peripheral nerve compression, most commonly at the median nerve in the carpal tunnel. The "double crush" theory implies that a nerve that has a proximal irritation is more vulnerable to producing pain paresthesias and muscle weakness at a peripheral entrapment than a nerve that does not have proximal irritation. Indeed, experience has shown that those patients who were operated on for carpal tunnel release, and who also had cervical spine nerve root irritative disease, experienced poor results from their carpal tunnel release surgery.[4,7,9] It is important, therefore, to include in the physical examination of each patient with neck, shoulder, or arm symptoms, a detailed evaluation of the hand. Evaluate the hand for muscle strength using the Jaymar grip meter and a pinch meter; document the two-point discrimination sensation; and record the response to special tests such as the Phalen wrist flexion test for carpal tunnel compression and the Adson's shoulder abduction test for thoracic outlet syndrome.[1]

Following a thorough evaluation of the patient's history, the examiner should outline a preliminary differential diagnosis list. Following the physical examination the differential diagnosis should be narrowed down to the most likely cause of pain, with several secondary possible causes to be ruled out by further evaluation.

The next evaluation consists of radiographic images. These should include an anterior/posterior x ray of the lower cervical spine to determine whether there is evidence of disc narrowing, body or pedicle destruction, widening of spinous process distance and overall vertebral alignment, as well as evidence of abnormal soft tissue masses. The second x ray evaluation is of the lateral cervical spine in the neu-

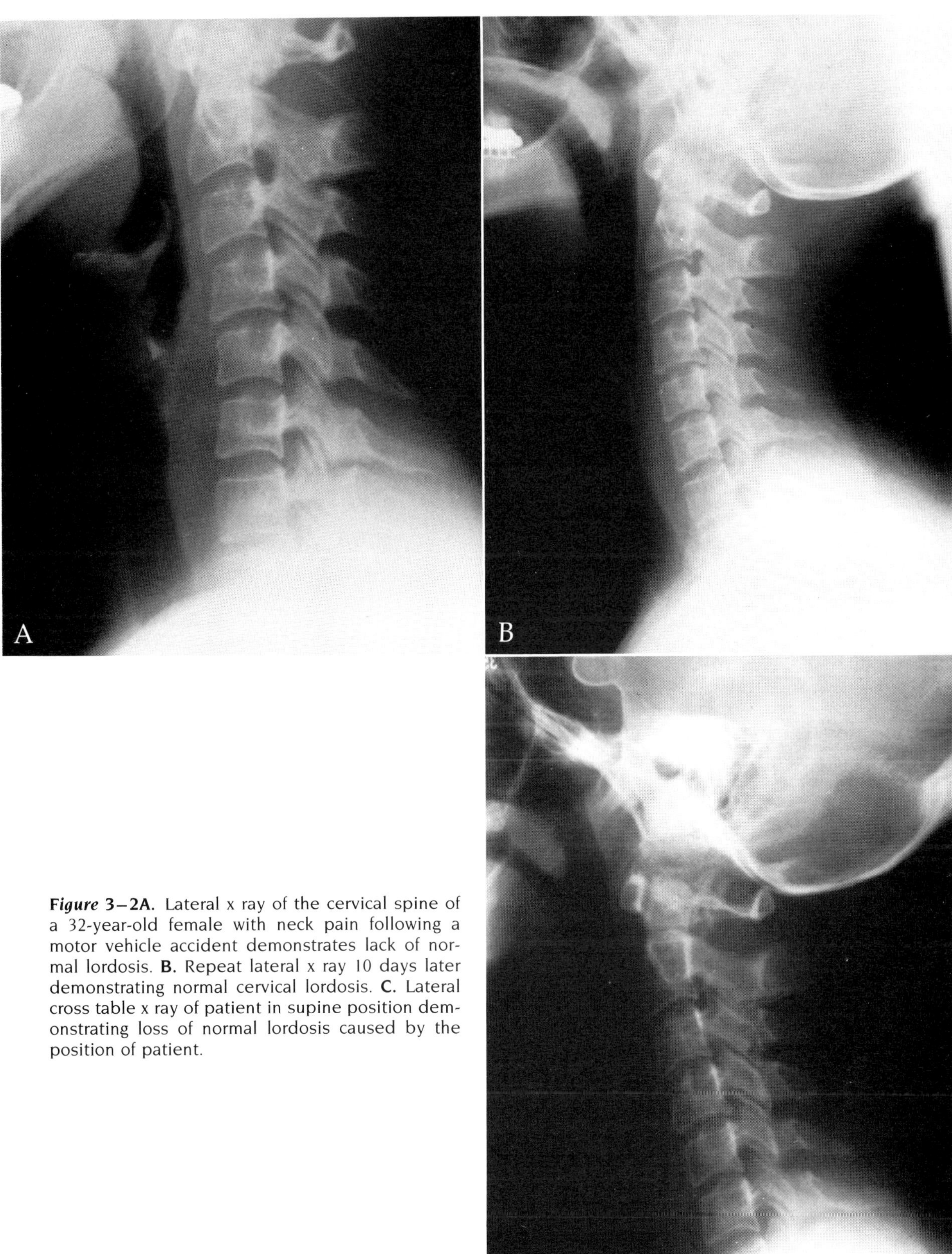

Figure 3–2A. Lateral x ray of the cervical spine of a 32-year-old female with neck pain following a motor vehicle accident demonstrates lack of normal lordosis. **B.** Repeat lateral x ray 10 days later demonstrating normal cervical lordosis. **C.** Lateral cross table x ray of patient in supine position demonstrating loss of normal lordosis caused by the position of patient.

tral position with the patient looking straight forward and the shoulders pulled down. This is the most revealing of the x ray views and should be examined specifically for evidence of loss of the normal lordosis which may be caused by muscle spasm, bone or ligament disruption or destruction, or voluntary positioning by the patient (Fig. 3–2). This position is frequently seen following a sprain injury. It usually reverts to normal in 10 to 14 days. The retropharyngeal soft tissue space should be specifically measured for swelling. A normal space is not more than 3 or 4 mm in the adult—anterior to C3 vertebra. (A crying child may have a large x ray shadow.) Each vertebral body should be carefully checked for alignment and bone detail. Each disc should be checked for height and adjacent osteophyte formation. Ensure that the entire cervical spine of the vertebra is shown and that the dorsal elements can be seen in good detail. A swimmer's view may be necessary to identify C7 and T1 (Fig. 3–3).

The third examination is the open mouth view to identify the integrity of the odontoid and the joint

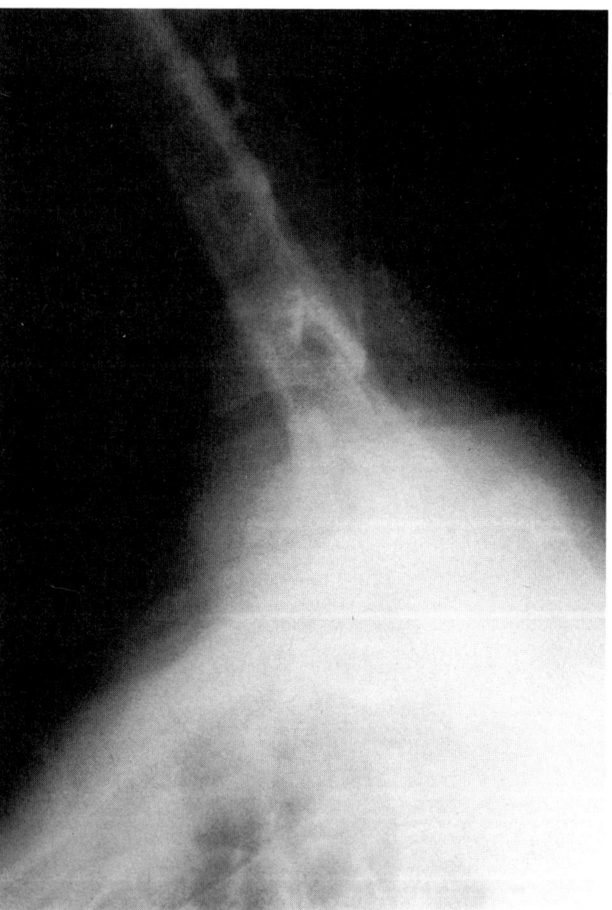

Figure 3–3. Swimmer's view demonstrating normal C7 and T1 vertebrae.

configuration of the occipital C1 and C1-C2 articulations. The fourth and fifth x rays consist of true oblique views to evaluate the neuroforamen, pedicles, and facet joints. These are obtained by turning the entire patient to a 45° oblique angle. Do not rotate only the head.

With the patient's history, physical evaluation, and x-ray evaluation, the diagnosis can be established and treatment initiated.

Occasionally, a laboratory survey of blood values may be advisable to confirm or rule out diagnostic impressions. A hemoglobin, hematocrit, white blood cell count, and sedimentation rate usually suffices to confirm or rule out systemic inflammatory or neoplastic disease.

The Role of Further X Ray Imaging

If the lordodic curve is abnormally aligned, or if a question exists regarding occult instability, a traction x ray may be obtained. The patient should be placed supine on the x ray table and a 20 to 30 pound cervical halter traction applied in order to distract the cervical spine. A lateral x ray is then taken to detect any occult instability. If no instability is shown in this x ray, the examiner can use standing voluntary flexion and extension laterals to appraise the mechanics of the spine and to determine whether each vertebral level is moving as expected. There should be a gradual flexion and extension at each vertebral level.

The CT scan is most valuable in detecting abnormalities at the junction areas of the head and cervical spine. The CT with sagittal and coronal reconstruction will outline the occipit C1 and C2 articulations better than the lateral and open mouth plain films. It also images the cervical thoracic junction at C7-T1 better than the "swimmer's" or oblique views. CT is of less value in the mid-cervical spine and for soft tissue injuries, but it may be used to determine the extent of boney communition and the displacement of fractures.

The Role of MRI

Magnetic resonance imaging has become the method of choice in outlining the soft tissues, particularly the neuro elements, discs, and intravertebral body marrow (Fig. 3–4). The CT and MRI are not indicated in the initial work-up and are only indicated if a question remains regarding the need for surgical intervention after adequate conservative therapy of disc syndromes, or when the possibility of intraspinal cord tumor, syringomyelia, or other soft tissue lesion exists.

A bone scan is frequently valuable if there is no evidence of boney disease on the plain films and if it

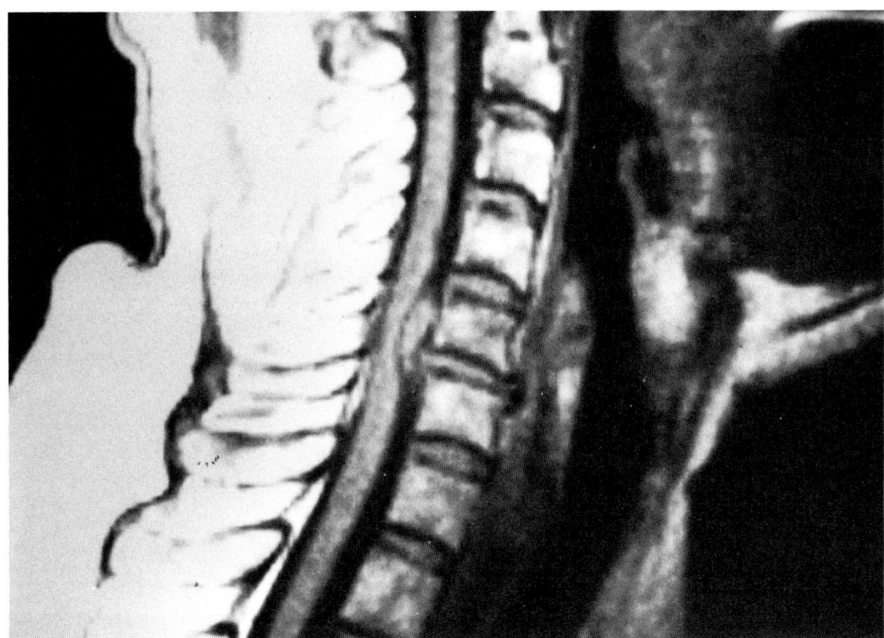

Figure 3–4. Magnetic resonance image demonstrating posterior herniation of C5-C6 disc.

is possible that a metastatic deposit, infectious lesion, or occult fracture is present.

Myelograms of the cervical spine have, in a large portion, been replaced by the noninvasive MRI. Myelograms still have a place in the evaluation of the patient who has a neurologic loss without x ray evidence of boney or ligamentous injury following trauma, or who has persistent neurologic signs, the cause of which cannot be documented by plain films, MRI, or CT scan. A water-soluble myelogram should be performed prior to the CT scan to give better diagnostic images.

The Role of EMG

An EMG of the upper extremities has been found to add little to the clinical investigation, if the motor, sensory, and reflex evaluations are normal. However, if the exact level of positive finding is equivocal, an EMG may localize an irritative phenomenon to one nerve root, which may be helpful prior to consideration for surgical intervention.

Discograms

Discograms are rarely used. The most common indication for a diskogram is a patient who has persistent neck and shoulder pain without localizing physical findings and without objective x ray or MRI evidence of an identifiable nerve root irritation (Fig. 3–5). A disc may have annular tears that are irritating to the dura surrounding the nerve roots, and which can be identified only by placing a needle into the disc area from the anterior approach in the awake patient and then sequentially injecting saline and contrast material into the suspected discs, usually C4-C5, C5-C6, and C6-C7. The two important aspects of the discogram evaluation are pain production and x ray evidence of tears of the anulus. The normal disc will accept only .1 or .2 cc of saline without radicular or radiating pain. A disc that takes .3 or .4 cc of saline without a strong resistance endpoint, is indicative of anular tears and the saline injection should be followed by an injection of .3 or .4 cc of radiographic contrast under image intensification to document escape from the disc. If this injection causes reproduction of the patient's symptoms across the neck, shoulder, or arm, it is indicative of irritation of the nerve root from this specific disc. One must evaluate discograms with caution, however, because the production of the patient's symptoms by internal disc pressure does not necessarily mean that the symptoms of burning, shooting pain across the shoulder and the upper back will be relieved by a surgical discectomy and fusion. If the reproduction of pain is specific to a known dermatome radiating down the arm, this sign is a better prognosis for relief by surgical treatment.

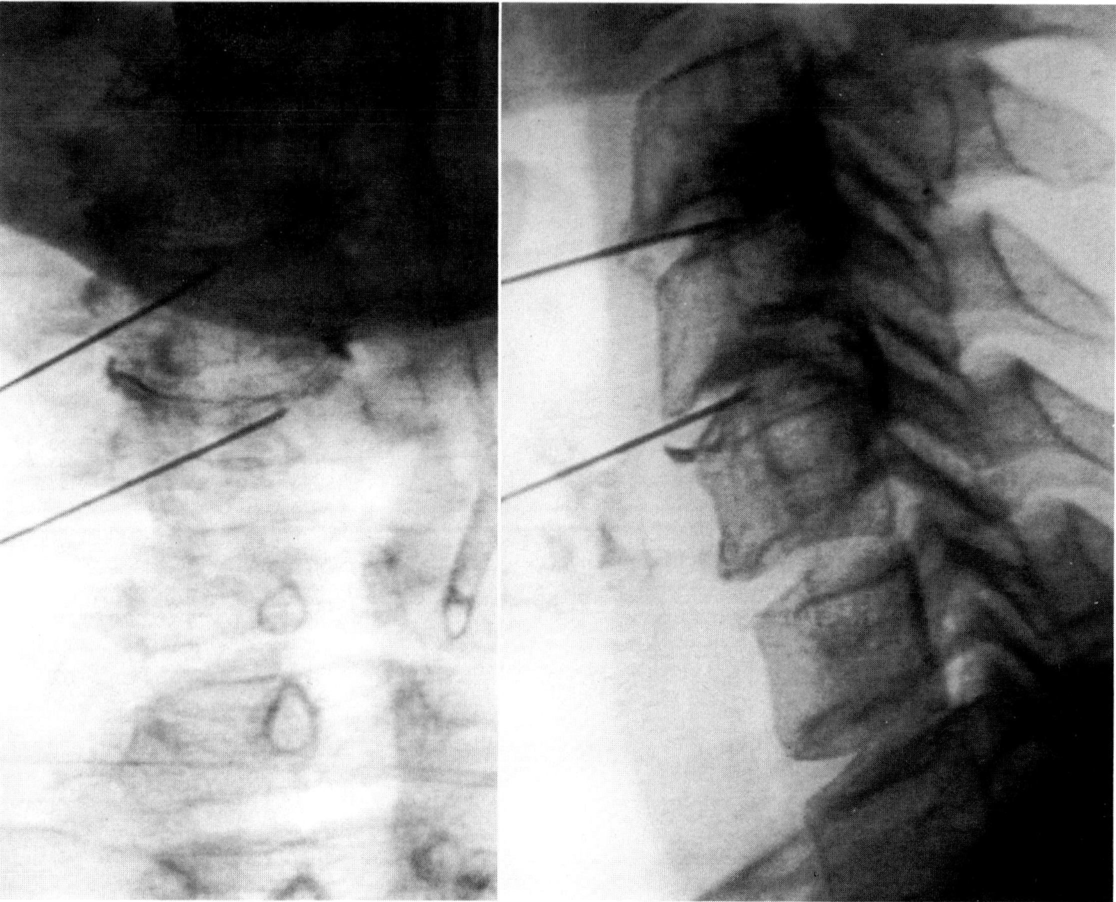

Figure 3–5. Discogram of patient who has persistent neck and shoulder pain without localized physical findings of an identifiable nerve root irritation.

MANAGEMENT OF THE PATIENT WITH SYMPTOMS OF CERVICAL SHOULDER AND ARM PAIN CAUSED BY INFLAMMATORY STAGES OF DEGENERATIVE DISC DISEASE WITH OR WITHOUT SUPERIMPOSED TRAUMA

This patient usually has nonspecific neck, shoulder, and headache pain aggravated by activity and somewhat, but not completely, relieved by rest. Females age 35 to 50 are more affected more often than males. Those with sedentary occupations such as secretaries, computer operators, accountants, and executives are more often affected. The symptoms may be associated with concurrent low back pain symptoms from degenerative lumbar disc disease. X rays are frequently negative for acute changes, and usually, but not necessarily, have one or two narrow disc spaces with mild osteophytosis; this may or may not be significant as their development precedes the onset of symptoms.

The first element of management is education of the patient. The cause of the symptoms is discussed with the patient. The natural history may indicate a persistent condition which may last from 6 weeks to 18 months, but the overall prognosis is that the patient will get over the symptoms with time. Time is the main element, and during this time the patient must remain active to prevent muscle weakness and atrophy. A program consisting of range of motion, stretching, and strengthening exercises should be discussed with the patient along with the explanation that the exercises may, in themselves, be painful and may temporarily increase the symptom of stiffness of the neck. Cervical spine pain aggravated by motion produces a voluntary limitation of range of motion of the cervical spine to prevent aggravation of the pain. This lack of range of motion is increased by wearing a limiting cervical orthosis. Within a short period of time, the facet joints become "stiff" due to lack of motion, and the musculature develops myostatic contractures. Therefore, if flexibility and strength are not maintained while the patient is recovering from his "cervical spine syndrome," a cycle of pain on motion, limitation of motion, and soft tissue contracture occurs. During this period, the patient should be given adequate modalities, including analgesics and surface-applied heat to provide muscle relaxation and allow range of motion and strengthening exercises. Therefore, the rationale for the use of heat and massage must be explained—to relax the muscles and increase the local circulation to allow exercises to be performed with less accompanying pain. During the initial painful, inflammatory period a soft collar may be indicated, particularly after a traumatic episode, to allow the tissues to heal. However, this should not be encouraged for more than 1 to 2 weeks. The patient should then gradually discontinue the use of the collar as exercises are instituted. Traction may be helpful if the patient has constant severe pain.[10] This treatment should consist of longitudinal traction, preferably with the patient at home in bed for periods of 15 to 20 minutes followed by a 10 to 15 minute application of warm bath towels around the neck, followed by gradually increasing isometric exercises.

Trigger point injections of local anesthetic in tender areas, particularly at the medial superior aspect of the vertebral border of scapula, may be beneficial to temporarily relieve the pain cycle and to allow the patient to exercise more freely.[8] It is unclear how trigger point injections relieve the pain, which is a radicular pain caused by irritations of the nerve at the neural foramen area of the spine. Anesthetizing the end organ receptors does not decrease the foramenal irritations of the spinal nerve. Curiously, the injections to the tender areas may be of some benefit for some days to weeks even though the effect of the xylocaine wears off in several hours. Steroids should be used very sparingly, if at all, because of their local effect on soft tissue atrophy and their deleterious effect on tendon and muscle. There is no evidence that an injection of steroids locally into the tender areas has beneficial effect on the efficacy of the xylocaine injection. A TENS unit may be tried for chronic pain that is unrelenting. However, this is not usually as effective in alleviating cervical spine pain as it is in lumbar disorders.

The patient must also be aware that the prognosis varies with the area of the pain. If the pain is mostly arm pain consisting of paresthesias, tingling, numbness, and even some muscle weakness, this has a good prognosis for progressive recovery over a period of time. If the pain does not subside with nonoperative treatment and is caused by persistent irritation of cervical nerve roots by osteophytosis or disc rupture, this area of pain has a good prognosis for relief by surgical intervention. Neck pain itself has a fair prognosis for complete recovery. Headaches have a fair prognosis also. However, if the headaches are caused by cervical spine nerve irritation, the patient may be left with headaches for months or even years.

The interscapular, over the shoulder, burning type of pain with a feeling of muscle "tightness" has the poorest prognosis for recovery. Many times, patients recover from other symptoms but are left with that burning tightness feeling that may last for years. This condition also has the poorest prognosis for relief by surgical discectomy or fusion. After surgery, patients frequently say that their arm tingling and numbness is gone, their arm pain is gone, their neck pain is much better, but they still have this burning pain over the shoulders.

THE ROLE OF MEDICATIONS

A nonsteriodal anti-inflammatory drug such as ibuprofen (Motrin) 800 mg tid, or indomethycin (Indocin) 25 mg tid, or quitoprofen (Oridus) 15 mg twice a day, or piroxicam (Feldene) 20 mg once a day have been found to be effective in controlling symptoms. Muscle relaxants such as meprobamate 400 mg or carisoprodol (Soma) 350 mg may be of value to abate muscle spasm and tightness. Narcotics of the codeine type and stronger type should be avoided because this condition may be prolonged and chronic and the patient will become dependent upon the narcotics for continued pain relief. As the patient becomes addicted to codeine, and the codeine wears off, the patient develops a need for constant administration of codeine to maintain the pain relief level that he expects. Such patients frequently become addicted to codeine and require codeine administration 2 to 3 times a day to maintain a comfortable level. This frequent administration of codeine depresses the circulating level of the patient's endorphins and he will become particularly aware that he has difficulty sleeping and that he wakes up in the middle of the night and has to take another codeine to be able to go back to sleep. If the patient is on chronic codeine medication when first seen, he must be made to understand the necessity of getting off this medication and that it will be difficult for the first several weeks, but that it is in his best interest in the long run.

Sleep is frequently uncomfortable, and it is often helpful to use a special pillow such as the Jackson pillow, which is a very soft, cylindrical pillow about 8 inches in diameter and 18 inches long, filled with soft down or feathers. This pillow keeps the head in a relatively good position whether the patient is lying supine or on his side. The patient should not sleep in the prone position because this places the cervical spine in a rotated position. The patient should avoid constant vibration such as truck driving or riding in an automobile. Work should be performed with the neck in a neutral position, without excessive flexion or extension. Controlled, therapeutic, neck manipulation may provide temporary relief of muscle tightness. However, the risks involved in manipulating the neck and the possibility of causing more damage to the nerve tissue or boney elements outweighs the benefits, and manipulation of the neck, either awake or under anesthesia, is not indicated for this syndrome.

Overall, results indicate that approximately 60% of patients obtain complete relief within 5 years.[3] Forty percent developed late degenerative changes. There was no statistical correlation between those with persistent symptoms and degenerative changes. Symptoms lasted for an average of 21 months in those patients with no degenerative changes and 30 months in those in whom degenerative changes developed. Less than 20% of patients show no improvement, progressing on to the further diagnostic procedures necessary to ascertain if surgical intervention would be beneficial. Frequently, patients will "learn to live with it" if they have no neurologic loss.

There are many unanswered questions in dealing with patients with cervical spine pain syndromes. These questions are fertile areas for future research:

1. What is the effect of genetics on degenerative disc disease?
2. What is the effect of repetitive manual labor?
3. What is the effect of the secondary gain in the patient's recovery?
4. What is the effect of the patient's expectations and the employer's expectations of the patient's ability to go back to work?
5. What is the effect of previous trauma and previous spine fusions on future painful conditions of the neck?

The natural history is that this chronic inflammatory pain syndrome gradually stabilizes. It may take 5 or 10 years. Patients over the age of 60 rarely have significant neck or arm pain regardless of x ray findings of degenerative joint disease. Patients who are retired and who have symptoms of neck pain must be carefully examined for a specific cause such as tumor or infection.

As one discusses the benefits of surgery, one must be aware that successful surgery is that surgery which is performed in a technically expert manner on the right level of the cervical spine for radicular pain, paresthesias, numbness, objective weakness of the arm or hand, and decreased reflexes. These patients have the best results from surgery. Failed surgery is most frequently found in those patients in whom surgery is performed for neck pain only, with no objective signs of radiculopathy. Those patients with scapular shoulder pain frequently have pain postoperatively, not relieved by the surgical procedure. Those patients who are encouraged into surgery because of the inability to modify their work situation or those patients with presurgical litigation for personal injury or workman's compensation claims have a lower percentage of satisfactory results following surgery. The physician and the patient will be disappointed if they are urged into surgery by extenuating circumstances, such as insurance claims or work disability or because of pain rather than bonafide indications for surgery, such as the neurologic finding of sensory loss, muscle weakness, or reflex changes.

REFERENCES

1. Carroll, R.E., Hurst, L.C.: The relationship of thoracic outlet syndrome and carpal tunnel syndrome. Clin Orthop *164*:149–153, 1982.
2. Fisk, J.W.: Myofascial trigger point. *In* Medical Treatment of Neck and Back Pain. Springfield, Charles C Thomas, 1987, pp. 57–70.
3. Hohl, M.: Soft-tissue injuries of the neck in automobile accidents. J Bone Joint Surg *56A*:1675–1682, 1974.
4. Hurst, L.C., Weissberg, D., Carroll, R.E.: The relationship of the double crush to carpal tunnel syndrome. J Hand Surg *10*(2):202–204, 1985.
5. Kraus, H.: Triggerpoints. *In* Clinical Treatment of Back and Neck Pain. St. Louis, McGraw-Hill, *5*:92–111, 1970.
6. Massey, E.W., Riley, T.L., Pleet, A.B.: Coexistent carpal tunnel syndrome and cervical radiculopathy (double crush syndrome). South Med J *74*:957–959, 1981.
7. Melzack, R., Stillwell, D.M., Fox, E.J.: Trigger points and acupuncture points for pain: correlations and implications. Pain *3*:3–23, 1977.
8. Travel, J.S., Simons, D.G.: Myofascial Pain and Dysfunction. Baltimore, Williams & Wilkins, 1983, pp. 27.
9. Upton, A.R.M., McComas, A.J.: The double crush in nerve-entrapment syndromes. Lancet *32*:359–361, 1973.
10. Zylbergold, R.S., Piper, M.C.: Cervical spine disorders, a comparison of three types of traction. Spine *10*:862–871, 1985.

Part II

Anatomy, Physiology, and Biochemistry of Spinal Disorders

Nikolai Bogduk

Structure and Function of the Lumbar Spine

The lumbar spine is that portion of the vertebral column and its adnexae that connects the thorax to the pelvis. It consists of the five lumbar vertebrae and the joints, ligaments, and muscles that bind them together and control their movements. In the upright position, the lumbar spine serves to transmit axial, compressive loads from the thorax and upper limbs to the pelvis and lower limbs (i.e., weight-bearing), and to accommodate certain movements between the thorax and pelvis. Secondarily, the lumbar spine serves to protect the lower end of the spinal cord and cauda equina, which runs through the lumbar vertebrae to gain access to the organs and tissues of the pelvis and lower limbs.

THE LUMBAR VERTEBRAE

With respect to their functions, the various parts of a lumbar vertebra can be grouped in three divisions: (1) the vertebral body, (2) the posterior elements and (3) the pedicles (Fig. 4–1).

The vertebral body is designed to subserve the weight-bearing functions of the vertebra. It consists of a block of bone with flat upper and lower surface areas that are dedicated maximally to sustain axial, compressive loads. Internally, the trabeculae of the vertebral body are arranged as vertical and horizontal struts in a manner designed optimally to maintain compressive strength while minimizing bone density and weight.[1] Each superior and inferior surface of the vertebral body bears a slightly raised circumferential rim, known as the ring apophysis, which serves to anchor the anulus fibrosus of the intervertebral disc (Fig. 4–2).

The posterior elements of a lumbar vertebra consist of the laminae of each side, the transverse processes, the spinous process, and the superior and inferior articular processes (Fig. 4–1). These processes sustain the translatory and rotatory forces applied to

the vertebra through the joints it forms and through the muscles that attach to its processes. In this regard, it is noteworthy that, apart from certain fibers of the psoas major muscle, all the muscles that act on a lumbar vertebra are attached to one or other of the posterior elements of the vertebra. Particular specialized sites of muscle attachment are the mamillary processes on the dorsal edge of each superior articular process, and the accessory processes projecting from the dorsal aspect of the proximal end of each transverse process.

The pedicles project, one on each side, from the posterior surface of the vertebral body and support the laminae and other posterior elements. They receive no muscle attachments, but serve to transmit to the vertebral body the forces applied to the posterior elements, thereby allowing the weight-bearing functions and movements of the vertebral body to be controlled by the joints and muscles acting on the posterior elements.

When viewed from above, the pedicles and laminae are seen to form an arch, known as the neural arch, which together with the posterior surface of the vertebral body, encloses a foramen—the vertebral foramen, which houses the dural sac and its contents.

Each lumbar vertebra forms two sets of joints with the vertebra below: a pair of synovial joints posteriorly and a single joint anteriorly between the consecutive vertebral bodies (Fig. 4–1). The latter is an amphiarthrodial joint formed by an intervertebral disc.

THE INTERVERTEBRAL DISC

Structure

Each lumbar intervertebral disc consists of three parts: a central nucleus pulposus surrounded by an anulus fibrosus, and a pair of cartilaginous plates—

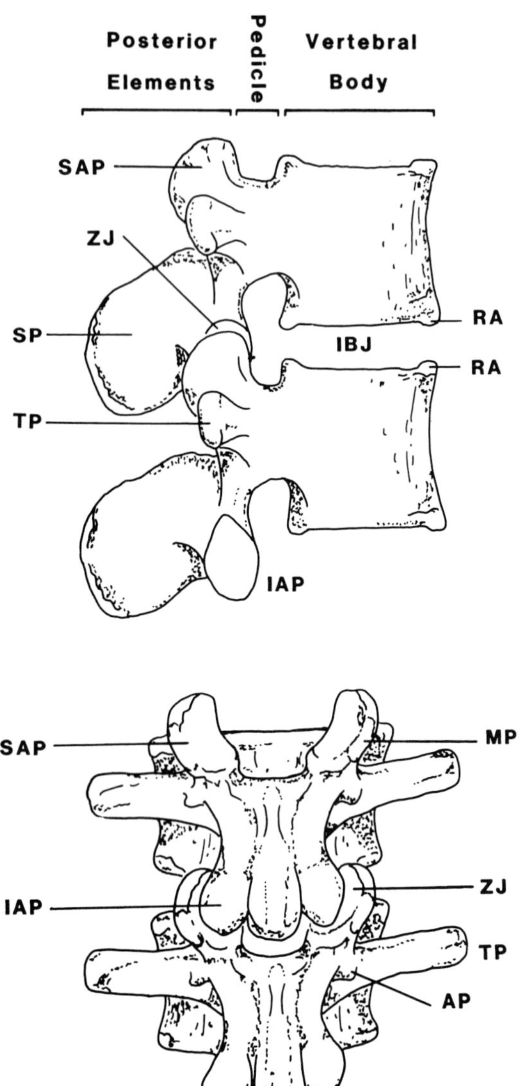

Figure 4–1. The functional divisions and parts of a lumbar vertebra. The vertebral body is the weight-bearing element of the vertebra. It is marked around its upper and lower surfaces by a ring apophysis (RA) and forms an interbody joint (IBJ) with the vertebra below. The pedicles connect the vertebral body to its posterior elements which consist of the transverse processes (TP) and a lamina from which project the spinous process (SP), the superior articular processes (SAP) and the inferior articular processes (IAP). The articular processes form the zygapophysial joints (ZJ). The mamillary processes (MP) and accessory processes (AP) constitute sites of muscle attachments.

the vertebral endplates, which cover the central portion of the upper and lower surfaces of each disc (Fig. 4–2).

The nucleus pulposus consists of a proteoglycan ground substance held together by a modest net-

work of type II collagen fibrils. The proteoglycans bind a large amount of water, which endows the nucleus pulposus with hydrodynamic properties. The water is retained within the nucleus by thermodynamic mechanisms and by electrostatic bonds between the water molecules and ionic radicals on the proteoglycans. The proteoglycans and collagen of the nucleus pulposus are synthesized by cartilage cells, which are located predominantly in the regions of the vertebral endplates.

The anulus fibrosus consists of some 10 to 20 concentric lamellae of collagen fibers (Fig. 4–3). In each lamella the collagen fibers are uniformly orientated at an angle of 65° to the long axis of the vertebral column. However, although the magnitude of this angle remains the same, the direction of inclination alternates in successive lamellae such that where one lamella is orientated 65° to the right, the next deeper lamella is orientated 65° to the left, and so on, with every second lamella having the same orientation.

The vertebral endplates cover the superior and inferior aspects of the nucleus pulposus and the adjacent inner two-thirds or so of the anulus fibrosus. Histologically, each endplate consists of both hyaline cartilage and fibrocartilage. The hyaline cartilage occurs towards the vertebral body, and is best evident in neonatal and young discs. Fibrocartilage occurs towards the nucleus pulposus, and in older discs the endplates are virtually entirely fibrocartilage.

The vertebral endplate constitutes a remnant of the growth plate of the vertebral body.[1] In children, the ends of the vertebral body are completely covered by a thick plate of cartilage, the deepest cells of which calcify and ossify and provide for longitudinal growth of the vertebra. Secondary ossification occurs circumferentially around the growth plate after the age of 7 years to form a ring apophysis by the

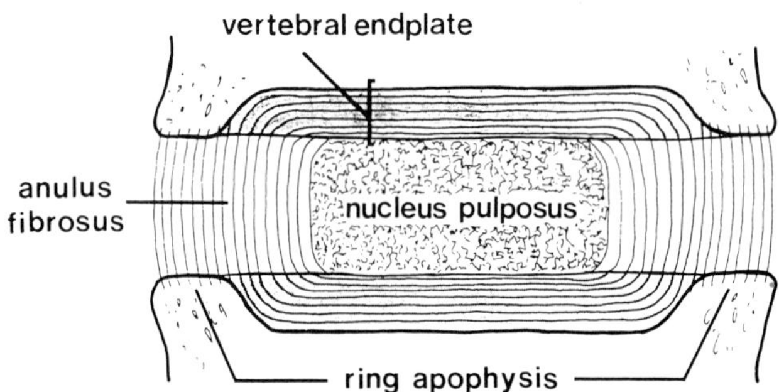

Figure 4–2. A longitudinal section of a lumbar intervertebral disc revealing its internal structure. The inner fibers of the anulus fibrosus encapsulate the nucleus pulposus and form the fibrocartilaginous component of the vertebral endplate; the outer fibers are anchored in the ring apophysis.

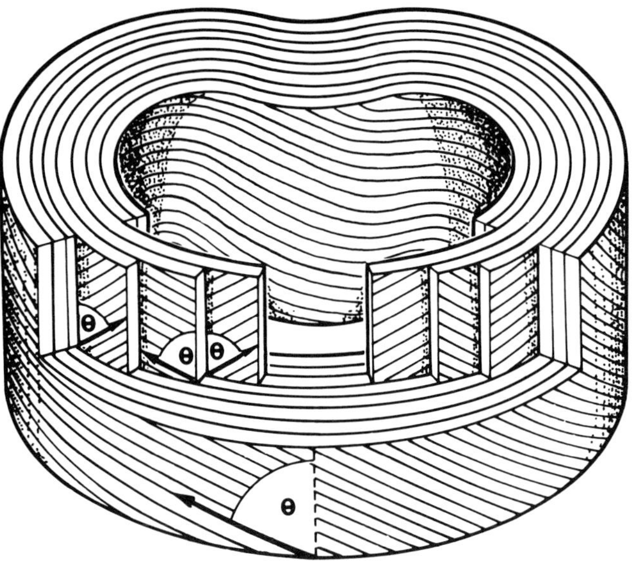

Figure 4–3. The orientation of collagen fibers in a lumbar anulus fibrosus. All fibers in a given lamella are uniformly orientated with respect to the longitudinal axis of the disc ($\theta = 65°$). Fibers in successive lamellae have the same magnitude of orientation but in opposite directions. (From Bogduk, N., Twomey, L.T.: Clinical Anatomy of the Lumbar Spine. Edinburgh, Churchill Livingstone, 1987.)

age of 12, which fuses with the rest of the vertebral body late in adolescence. This leaves only the central portion of the growth plate as the vertebral endplate.

The fibrocartilage of the vertebral endplate is formed by the insertion into the endplate of the collagen fibers of the inner anulus fibrosus. By inserting into the vertebral endplates the collagen fibers of the inner anulus fibrosus effectively form a fibrous capsule that surrounds the nucleus pulposus superiorly, inferiorly, and circumferentially. The collagen fibers of the outer third or so of the anulus fibrosus are not associated with the vertebral endplates, and instead insert into the ring apophysis of the vertebral bodies (Fig. 4–2).

Biochemically, the anulus fibrosus consists principally of type I collagen especially in its outer parts, but with increasing quantities of type II collagen towards the nucleus pulposus. Interspersed among the collagen fibers are proteoglycans and some elastic fibers. The distinction between anulus fibrosus and the nucleus pulposus is not clear, and the intervertebral disc is perhaps best perceived as exhibiting a continuous spectrum of structure consisting of an outer, distinctly fibrous anulus separated from the fluid nucleus pulposus by a transitional zone of fibrocartilage formed by the inner anulus fibrosus.

Function

The foremost function of the intervertebral disc is to separate the vertebral bodies. In the absence of an intervertebral disc the flat surfaces of the vertebral bodies would be directly apposed. This would not preclude a weight-bearing function but would limit the movement of the vertebral bodies to sliding motions and axial rotation. By separating the vertebral bodies the intervertebral disc allows them to tilt with respect to one another, thereby permitting the movements of flexion and extension of the lumbar spine. The intervertebral disc is therefore designed to be sufficiently strong to accommodate the weight-bearing functions of the intervertebral joint while at the same time, sufficiently pliable to accommodate flexion/extension movements.

Efficient weight-bearing by the intervertebral disc relies on a combined function of the nucleus pulposus and anulus fibrosus. When an intervertebral disc is compressed, nuclear pressure rises and the nucleus pulposus attempts to disperse radially, but this dispersion is arrested by the development of tension in the circumferential layers of the anulus fibrosus (Fig. 4–4). A state of equilibrium develops between the radial pressure exerted by the nucleus pulposus and the tension developed in the anulus fibrosus. By restricting nuclear dispersal in this way, the anulus fibrosus allows the nucleus pulposus to transmit the axial force from one vertebra to the next. Moreover, this cooperative action between the nucleus pulposus and anulus fibrosus endows the intervertebral disc with a shock absorbing capacity wherein energy delivered to the intervertebral disc in the form of an axial load can be temporarily stored as tension in the anulus fibrosus, and subsequently released when the axial load is removed.

This description focuses the weight-bearing functions of the intervertebral disc on its nucleus pulposus, but the anulus fibrosus alone is able to sustain the weight-bearing functions of the disc. Indeed, an intervertebral disc from which the nucleus pulposus has been removed initially exhibits essentially the same compression stiffness as an intact disc. However, an isolated anulus fibrosus is susceptible to creep. If loaded under compression for prolonged periods an isolated anulus tends to buckle with consequent narrowing of the intervertebral space; but in an intact intervertebral disc this is prevented by the nucleus pulposus bracing the anulus fibrosus, preventing its fibers from buckling centrally. Thereby, the anulus fibrosus and the nucleus pulposus are able to share the weight-bearing functions of the disc.

A healthy intervertebral disc is more than adequately designed to subserve the weight-bearing functions of the disc, and its strength lies in the abil-

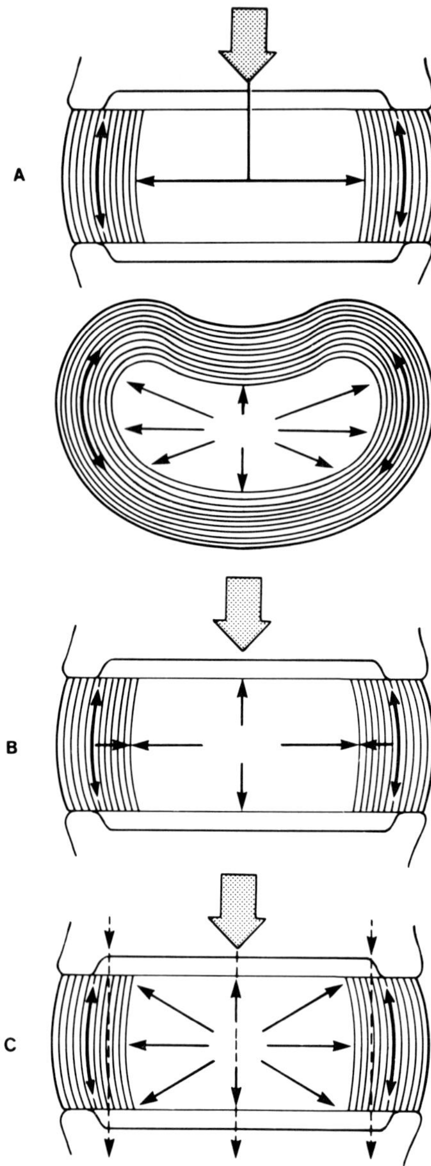

Figure 4–4. Transmission of compressive forces in a lumbar disc. **A.** Axial forces compress the nucleus pulposus which attempts to deform radially, thereby increasing radial tension in the anulus fibrosus. **B.** The tension in the anulus fibrosus resists nuclear expansion. **C.** At equilibrium nuclear pressure is balanced by anular tension, and the axial load is transmitted both by the nucleus and by the braced anulus fibrosus.

ity of the anulus fibrosus to withstand the pressures developed in the nucleus pulposus. Indeed, the strength of the anulus fibrosus is such that under extremes of compression the intervertebral disc fails by fracture of the vertebral endplates and vertebral bodies sooner than by rupture of the anulus fibrosus.[1]

The pliability of the intervertebral disc stems from the fact that the nucleus pulposus is deformable and that the anulus fibrosus can be stretched and compressed. This permits the vertebral bodies to be tilted with respect to one another. During forward flexion, the anterior sectors of the anulus fibrosus are compressed and tend to bulge anteriorly. Meanwhile, the nucleus pulposus is compressed and tends to disperse posteriorly, but its movement is arrested by the posterior fibers of the anulus fibrosus, which are rendered taut by the separation of the posterior margins of the vertebral bodies. A reciprocal series of events occurs during extension of the intervertebral joint. Flexion and extension of the vertebral bodies are limited by the ligamentous action of the posterior and anterior anulus fibrosus respectively. In this regard the anulus fibrosus is one of the largest and strongest ligaments of the body, perhaps ranking second only to the interosseus sacroiliac ligament in cross-sectional area.

During rotation of the intervertebral joint, the nucleus pulposus plays no role. Rotation is resisted solely by the anulus fibrosus, but only half of the collagen fibers in the anulus fibrosus are appropriately orientated to resist rotation in a given direction. Only those collagen fibers orientated towards the direction of rotation develop tension; the remaining 50% of collagen fibers orientated in the opposite direction are slackened by the rotation. Given that collagen fibers can accommodate only about a 4% strain before risking injury, it can be shown that this critical amount of strain occurs if an intervertebral joint is rotated beyond about 3°.[1] The intervertebral disc has no inherent mechanism by which to limit rotation to this range. For protection against excessive rotation, the intervertebral disc relies on the function of the joints formed by the posterior elements of the vertebra.

THE ZYGAPOPHYSIAL JOINTS

Structure

The zygapophysial joints are paired synovial joints formed by the articulation of the inferior articular processes of one vertebra with the superior articular processes of the vertebra below (Fig. 4–1). Each joint exhibits the typical features of a synovial joint including hyaline articular cartilage covering each articular facet, synovial membrane, a fibrous joint capsule, and intra-articular inclusions.[1]

The fibrous capsule of the joint runs transversely from one articular process to the other, but superiorly and inferiorly the capsule is abundant and loose in order to accommodate the upward and downward sliding movements of the articular processes that occur during flexion and extension of the lumbar spine. Ventrally, the joint capsule is formed by the ligamentum flavum.

The intra-articular inclusions of the lumbar zygapophysial joints are of three basic types.[1] The lesser varieties are connective tissue rims found along the dorsal and ventral margins of the joint that simply represent thickenings of the joint capsule that project minimally into the joint near the margins of the articular cartilage; and small fat pads covered by synovium that project into the joint space from its rostro-ventral and caudo-dorsal aspects. The largest type of inclusion is a fibro-adipose meniscoid, typically found at the superior or inferior poles of the joint and, if well developed, may project several millimeters into the joint cavity. The function of these meniscoids appears to be to cover and protect the exposed articular surface during the gliding movements of these joints. Clinically, these meniscoids may be significant if they act as a nidus for the precipitation of intra-articular adhesions in osteoarthritic, immobilized, or hypomobile joints. Additionally, they may be responsible for some forms of "acute locked back" when, after full flexion of the lumbar spine, a meniscoid fails to re-enter the joint cavity and becomes trapped under the joint capsule exerting strain on it, and thereby becoming a source of pain.[1]

When viewed from above, the zygapophysial joints are seen to be either planar or curved,[1] but in either case the articular surface of the superior articular process in each joint tends to face backward and medially, with the inferior articular process facing forward and laterally. In most individuals the joints at lower lumbar levels exhibit a mean orientation of about 45° with respect to the sagittal plane.[1] Joints at upper lumbar levels tend to be oriented closer to the sagittal plane, whereas in some individuals the joints at lower lumbar levels assume a more coronal orientation. The orientation and shape of the zygapophysial joints critically underpins their functions.

Functions

The lumbar zygapophysial joints are designed to resist forward translation and rotation of the vertebra.[1] In obliquely oriented, planar zygapophysial joints the superior articular process of the lower vertebra face backward and medially, thereby presenting a surface which resists forward or lateral movement of the inferior articular process of the vertebra above. The closer such a joint is orientated toward a coronal plane, the greater its resistance to forward translation of the upper vertebra, but the less it is capable of withstanding lateral displacement of the inferior articular processes that occurs during rotation of the upper vertebra. Reciprocally, joints oriented closer to the sagittal plane are suitably positioned to withstand lateral displacement and rotation of the upper vertebra but offer less resistance to forward translation. This relationship is particularly crucial at the lumbosacral level where a predisposition to spondylolisthesis may occur if the lumbosacral zygapophysial joints are oriented in a sagittal plane.

Curved zygapophysial joints subserve a similar function but in a slightly modified way. In curved joints the anterior segment of the superior articular process tends to face directly backward and resists forward displacement of the inferior articular processes of the upper vertebra; the posterior segment of curved superior articular processes tends to face medially and resists rotation of the upper vertebra. The degree to which a curved joint limits forward translation or rotation depends on the size of the anterior or dorsal segment of the joint, respectively, rather than the average orientation of the joint. The wider the anterior segment of the superior articular process the greater the surface area available to withstand forward translation. This has a bearing on the genesis of osteoarthrosis in the zygapophysial joints, because the earliest signs of degenerative joint disease tend to occur in the anterior segments of the joint; and joints with narrow anterior segments are prone to develop degenerative changes sooner because of the relatively greater stresses applied to their smaller surface areas.[1]

THE LUMBAR VERTEBRAL COLUMN

When articulated with one another the lumbar vertebrae form a column of bones that constitutes the skeleton of the lumbar spine (Fig. 4–5). In the upright position, the lumbar vertebral column assumes a curved configuration that is concave posteriorly. This curve adapts the steep anterior slope of the sacrum to the curvature of the thoracic spine, and is known as the lumbar lordosis. The lumbar lordosis can be quantified by measuring the angle formed between planes drawn through the upper surfaces of the L1 vertebra and the sacrum, and this angle can be used as a measure of the posture of the lumbar spine. However, no significant correlations have been established between variations in the size of the lumbar lordosis and the presence or absence of back pain.[1]

THE VERTEBRAL CANAL

In the articulated lumbar vertebral column, the vertebral foramina of the vertebrae are aligned to face one another thereby forming a single continuous channel behind the vertebral bodies known as the vertebral canal (Fig. 4–5). This canal transmits the lower end of the spinal cord and the lumbar, sacral, and coccygeal nerve roots. Between each consecutive vertebra apertures are formed to allow the transmission of nerve roots into and out of the ver-

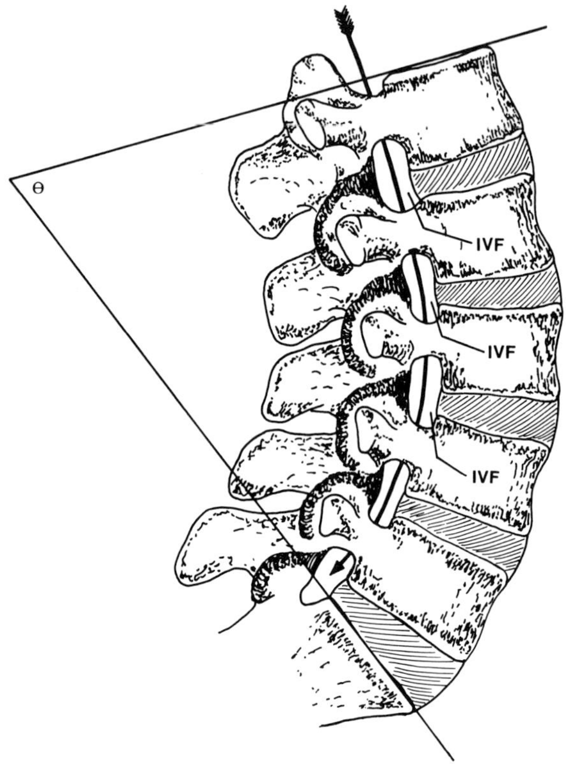

Figure 4–5. The lumbar vertebral column. The lordotic angle (θ) quantifies the curvature of the lumbar spine which encloses the vertebral canal (arrow). Nerve roots and spinal nerves are transmitted through the intervertebral foramina (IVF).

tebral canal. Each such aperture is known as an intervertebral foramen and is bound superiorly and inferiorly by the pedicles of consecutive vertebrae, anteriorly by the intervertebral disc, and posteriorly by the zygapophysial joint and the ligamentum flavum forming its anterior capsule (Fig. 4–5).

LIGAMENTS

Research into the structure and function of the ligaments of the lumbar spine has been particularly intense in recent years; so much so that few ligaments have escaped reappraisal or revision of the classical interpretation of their structure. The named ligaments of the lumbar spine can be grouped into those attached to the posterior elements of the lumbar vertebrae and those related to the vertebral bodies.

Ligamentum Flavum

The ligamentum flavum is a paired segmental ligament that connects the laminae of consecutive ver-

tebrae (Fig. 4–6). On each side, the upper end of the ligament is attached to the lower half of the anterior surface of the lamina and the inferior aspect of the pedicle. Inferiorly, the ligament divides into a medial and lateral portion. The medial portion passes to the posterior surface of the next lower lamina to which it attaches. The lateral portion passes in front of the zygapophysial joint formed by the two vertebrae that the ligament connects where it attaches to the anterior aspects of the inferior and superior articular processes of that joint forming its anterior capsule.[1] Histologically, the ligamentum flavum consists of 80% elastin and 20% collagen. This high elastin content allows the ligament to elongate when the laminae are separated and to contract without buckling when the laminae resume their resting position. Under normal circumstances this lack of buckling protects the underlying neural structures from compression.[1] Pathologic buckling occurs only in extremes of extension or when vertebrae have subluxated vertically as a result of loss of intervertebral disc space.

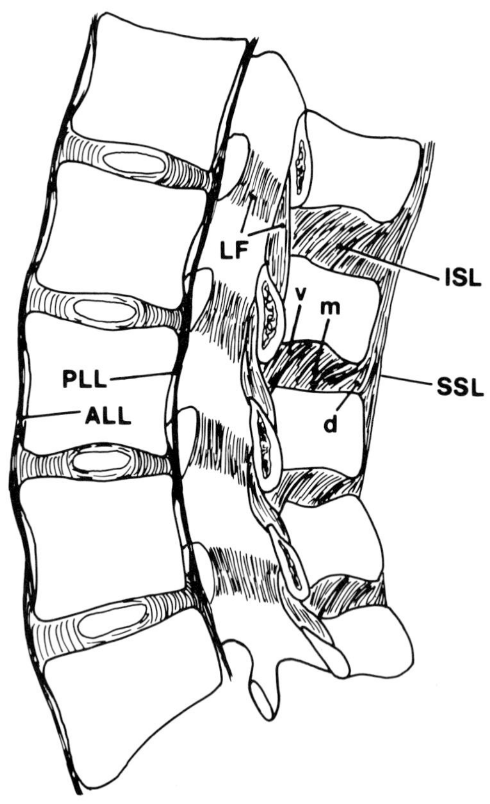

Figure 4–6. The ligaments of the lumbar spine viewed in a midsagittal section. ALL: anterior longitudinal ligament; PLL: posterior longitudinal ligament; LF: ligamentum flavum; SSL: supraspinous ligament; ISL: interspinous ligament and its ventral (v), middle (m), and dorsal (d) parts.

Supraspinous Ligament

Classically, the supraspinous ligament has been interpreted as a ligament connecting the dorsal edges or the spinous processes of the lumbar vertebrae (Fig. 4–6). However, this ligament is regularly present only as low as the L3 spinous process.[2,3] It is variably present between the L3 and L4 spinous processes; infrequently developed at the L4-L5 level; and absent below L5. Even when present, it is questionable whether this structure deserves the title of a "ligament," for microdissection studies reveal that it is virtually exclusively formed by the interlacing of tendinous fibers of the thoracolumbar fascia, the erector spinae aponeurosis, and the multifidus muscle.[2] More strictly its structure is that of a tendinous raphe rather than a true ligament. Similar comments apply to the interspinous ligaments.

Interspinous Ligament

The interspinous ligaments connect adjacent spinous processes, and each consists of three parts (Fig. 4–6).[3] The ventral part consists of fibers passing postero-cranially from the dorsal aspect of the ligamentum flavum to the anterior half of the lower border of the spinous process above. The middle part forms the main component of the ligament and consists of fibers that run from the anterior half of the upper border of one spinous process to the posterior half of the lower border of the spinous process above. The dorsal part consists of fibers from the posterior half of the upper border of the lower spinous process that pass behind the posterior border of the upper spinous process to merge with the supraspinous ligament. Because of this latter association it is evident that the dorsal third of the interspinous ligament is formed by tendinous fibers rather than by ligamentous collagen fibers, the only truly ligamentous portions being the deeper parts passing from one spinous process to the next.

Intertransverse Ligament

The intertransverse ligaments connect the edges of the transverse processes of consecutive vertebrae. Structurally they do not resemble the other ligaments of the lumbar spine and would be more properly referred to as membranes. They are of no mechanical importance, and simply constitute the adult derivative of the embryonic septum that divided the axial musculature into ventral and dorsal compartments.[1]

Iliolumbar Ligament

The classical anatomical literature identifies the iliolumbar ligament as a large ligament that connects the transverse process of the fifth lumbar vertebra to the ilia. This is indeed so in middle aged and elderly individuals, but the iliolumbar ligament is not present in neonates and children.[4] In these individuals it is represented by a band of muscle. This muscle undergoes fibrous metaplasia and is converted into a ligament by the third decade of life. The ventral part of the ligament appears to be derived from the lowest fibers of quadratus lumborum, whereas the dorsal part is a derivative of the fifth lumbar fascicle of iliocostalis lumborum (see below).

Anterior Longitudinal Ligament

The anterior longitudinal ligament is evident as a wide band that connects the anterior surfaces of the lumbar vertebral bodies (Fig. 4–6). Classically, it is said to consist of fibers that span 1 to 4 segments and attach to the margins of the vertebral bodies. However, microdissection of the lumbar spine reveals that many of the fibers of the anterior longitudinal ligament are formed by prolongations of the tendons of the crura of the diaphragm, so that like the supraspinous and interspinous ligaments, the anterior longitudinal ligament is partially tendinous in nature.

Posterior Longitudinal Ligament

The posterior longitudinal ligament covers the posterior aspects of the lumbar vertebral bodies, and presents a denticulate appearance being narrow over the middle portion of each vertebral body but widening over the posterior aspect of each intervertebral disc (Fig. 4–6). The ligament blends with the posterior fibers of the anulus fibrosus and ultimately gains attachment to the margins of the vertebral bodies.

MOVEMENTS OF THE LUMBAR VERTEBRAE

In clinical practice, the standard movements of the trunk are flexion, extension, axial rotation, and lateral flexion. However, these are movements of the trunk, not of the lumbar vertebrae. The fundamental movements of the lumbar vertebrae are sagittal rotation (i.e., X-axis rotation), sagittal translation (Z-axis translation), and axial rotation (Y-axis rotation),[1] and the movements of the trunk are produced by simple and complex combinations of these primary movements of the lumbar vertebrae, either at single or at multiple intervertebral joints.

Flexion of the lumbar spine involves the combination of anterior sagittal rotation and anterior translation, i.e., a forward rocking movement and a forward slide (Fig. 4–7). The lumbar zygapophysial joints are designed to prevent forward translation of the lumbar vertebrae, but when a lumbar vertebra rotates forward its inferior articular processes are lifted out of the zygapophysial joint and a slight gapping of the joint occurs. This allows the vertebra to translate forward for a short distance before its inferior articular processes once again engage the superior articular processes of the vertebra below. During a full range of forward flexion, each lumbar vertebra undergoes 1 to 3 mm of forward translation and 8 to 13° of forward rotation, with a total angular displacement of about 50 to 60°.[5] The range of forward flexion of the lumbar spine is limited by the compression stiffness of the anterior parts of the lumbar intervertebral discs and by tension developed in the posterior anulus fibrosus, the capsules of the lumbar zygapophysial joints, the supraspinous and interspinous ligaments, and in the back muscles and their fascia (see below).

Extension of the lumbar spine involves a reciprocal combination of posterior translation and posterior sagittal rotation. From the upright position each lumbar vertebra undergoes 1 to 5° of posterior sagittal rotation, with the L3 and L4 vertebrae exhibiting the least range of movement, and the entire lumbar spine exhibiting about 16° of angular displacement.[5] Extension of the lumbar spine is limited by the compression stiffness of the posterior portions of the intervertebral discs and by the development of tension in their anterior portions; but at the extremes of motion, movement is arrested by bony impaction. This occurs either between spinous processes or between the tips of inferior articular processes and the underlying laminae; the exact mechanism varies from individual to individual depending on the shape and caudal extent of the tips of the spinous processes or the tips of the inferior articular processes.

Axial rotation of a lumbar intervertebral joint initially occurs about a longitudinal axis passing through the posterior third of the intervertebral disc (Fig. 4–8). As the upper vertebra in a joint rotates, the underlying anulus fibrosus is subjected to torsion, and the posterior elements of the vertebra swing laterally in the direction opposite to the rotation. Axial rotation is arrested by the impaction of the inferior articular process of the upper vertebra against the superior articular process of the vertebra below. This impaction restricts the range of axial rotation at any lumbar intervertebral joint to less than 3°.[1] However, if sufficiently strong rotatory forces are applied to the lumbar spine further rotation can occur about a new axis located in the impacted joint.

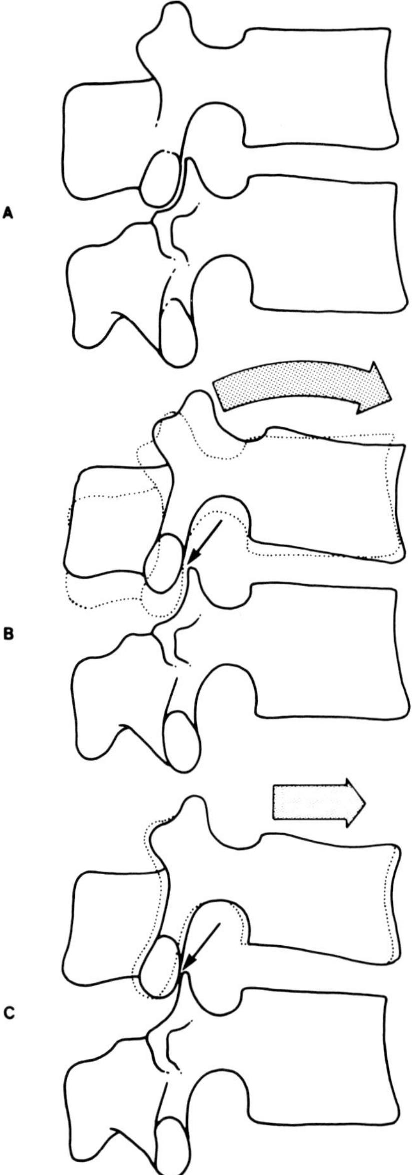

Figure 4–7. Sagittal plane movements of the lumbar vertebrae. **A.** A lumbar vertebra at rest, with the superior articular process of the lower vertebra resected laterally to reveal the contact with the inferior articular process from above. **B.** Flexion involves an intrinsic rotation of the vertebra which lifts the inferior articular out of the zygapophysial joint. A gap develops between the superior and inferior articular processes (arrow) which permits translation to occur. **C.** Translation is arrested as the gap in the zygapophysial joint is closed (arrow). (From Bogduk, N., Twomey, L.T.: Clinical Anatomy of the Lumbar Spine. Edinburgh, Churchill Livingstone, 1987.)

Under these circumstances, movement is accommodated by lateral shearing of the intervertebral disc and posterior subluxation of the unimpacted zygapophysial joint. This extreme form of axial rotation,

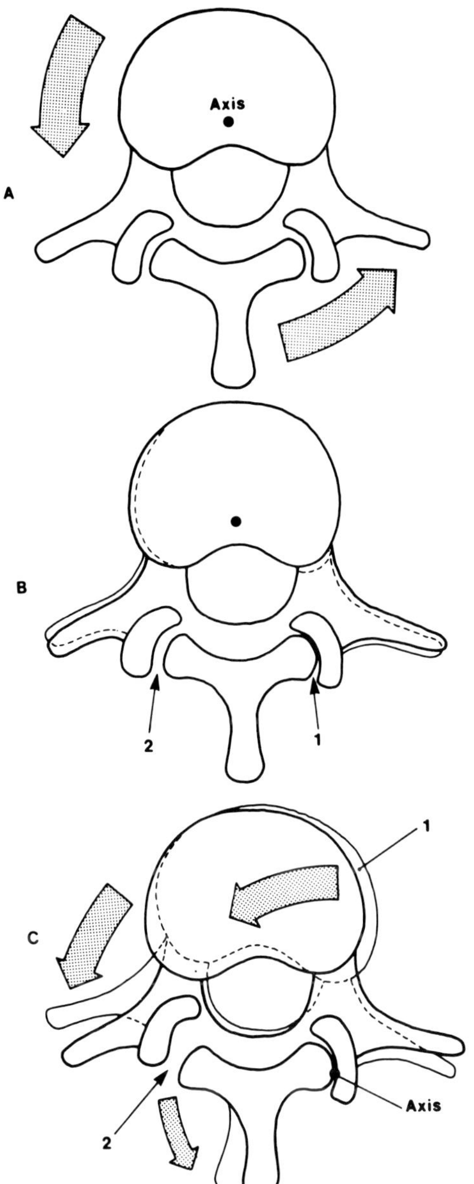

Figure 4-8. Axial rotation of a lumbar motion segment. **A.** Initially the axis of rotation lies in the posterior third of the vertebral body. **B.** Rotation occurs until the contralateral zygapophysial joint is impacted (1). The opposite joint is gapped (2). **C.** Further rotation occurs about an axis through the impacted zygapophysial joint, resulting in lateral shear across the disc (1) and further gapping of the opposite zygapophysial joint (2).

however, is hazardous to the intervertebral joint because it risks injuries to the zygapophysial joints and to the intervertebral disc.

Because of the lumbar lordosis, each lumbar intervertebral joint has a different obliquity with respect to the horizontal plane of the trunk. Consequently, during axial rotation of the trunk, individual lumbar

intervertebral joints do not simply undergo pure axial rotation. Because of the complex way in which twisting forces are distributed through a curved lumbar vertebral column, during trunk rotation each lumbar vertebra undergoes a small amount of flexion or extension and lateral flexion in addition to pure axial rotation. The nature of the combination of these movements is variable and unpredictable; the combination varies from individual to individual in accordance with the size of the lumbar lordosis, the detailed shape of individual vertebrae, and the exact location of the vertebrae within the lordotic curve.

Similar comments apply to lateral flexion of the trunk. The lumbar intervertebral joints are not designed naturally to accommodate pure lateral flexion. Lateral flexion of the trunk involves a complex and irregular combination of axial rotation, flexion, and extension of individual lumbar vertebrae. Although on the average, lateral flexion is usually accompanied by contralateral axial rotation at the L1-L4 segments and ipsilateral rotation at L5, many individuals exhibit contrary or paradoxical combinations at one or more segmental levels.[5]

THE LUMBAR MUSCLES

The muscles of the lumbar spine are the short intersegmental muscles, the psoas major and quadratus lumborum anterior and lateral to the lumbar vertebrae, and the lumbar back muscles posteriorly. Also worthy of consideration are the muscles of the abdominal wall which, although not part of the lumbar spine topographically, nonetheless exert important actions on it.

Intersegmental Muscles

The short intersegmental muscles of the lumbar spine are the interspinales and the intertransversarii. The interspinales are small, quadrangular muscles that connect the opposing edges of consecutive lumbar spinous processes. The intertransversarii connect the transverse accessory and mamillary processes of one vertebra to those of the vertebra below.

What is conspicuous about the short intersegmental muscles of the lumbar spine is that they are too small to contribute appreciably to the forces required to move the lumbar spine, yet they are consistently well developed. However, one feature of these muscles is that they carry high concentrations of muscle spindles, and contemporary thought suggests that their cardinal role is to act as proprioceptors for the lumbar intervertebral joints.[1]

Psoas Major

The psoas major is a seemingly homogeneous muscle located at the anterior surfaces of the lumbar transverse processes at the antero-lateral aspects of the lumbar intervertebral discs (Fig. 4–9). The muscular fibers converge to form a strong tendon that crosses the pelvic brim to insert into the lesser trochanter of the femur. Dissection of the psoas major muscle, however, reveals it to be segmental in nature, with separate bands of fibers arising from the transverse processes, from each of the intervertebral discs from T12 to L5, and from the margins of the vertebral bodies adjacent to these discs.

The lines of action of these various fascicles run close to the axes of sagittal rotation of the lumbar vertebrae; some lie behind and others lie in front of these axes, so that the psoas major exerts a combination of flexion and extension on the lumbar spine. As a whole, the psoas major tends to flex the lower lumbar joints and extend the upper lumbar joints.

Quadratus Lumborum

The quadratus lumborum is a quadrangular muscle that flanks the psoas major and extends from the pelvis to the twelfth rib (Fig. 4–9). It consists of three groups of fascicles. Inferior oblique fibers arise from the iliac crest and iliolumbar ligament to pass upward and medially to insert into the tips of the L1-L4 transverse processes. Superior oblique fibers arise from the five lumbar transverse processes and pass upward and laterally to insert into the twelfth rib. Longitudinal fibers pass directly from the pelvis and iliolumbar ligament to the twelfth rib. The superior oblique fibers and the longitudinal fibers have no direct action on the lumbar spine; essentially they are respiratory muscles designed to fix the twelfth rib. Only the inferior oblique fibers exercise an action on the lumbar spine wherein they exert or control lateral flexion of the lumbar vertebra.

Lumbar Back Muscles

Topographically, the lumbar back muscles are arranged in two groups: the multifidus muscle covering the laminae of the lumbar vertebrae, and the erector spinae covering the transverse processes posteriorly. The erector spinae in the lumbar region has two major components—the longissimus thoracis and the iliocostalis lumborum. A third component is sometimes described—the spinalis thoracis, but this muscle only intrudes into the lumbar region from the thoracic region to gain attachment to the upper two or three lumbar spinous processes, and is of little functional significance for the lumbar spine.

Multifidus

The multifidus muscle is segmental in nature, consisting of short fibers stemming from the laminae of the lumbar vertebrae and five segmental bands arising from each of the lumbar spinous processes.[6] Each band consists of one or more fascicles that are confluent with one another at their origin from the spinous process but which assume discrete and systematic attachments caudally (Fig. 4–10).

Fascicles from the L1 spinous process radiate to the mamillary processes of the L3, L4, L5, and S1 vertebrae, and a slender fascicle gains access to the posterior superior iliac spine. Fascicles from the L2 spinous process radiate similarly to the L4, L5, and S1 mamillary processes and a substantial fascicle reaches the posterior superior iliac spine. From L3, fascicles attach to the L5 and S1 mamillary processes and a large bundle inserts into the upper lateral corner of the sacrum and dorsal sacroiliac ligament. Fascicles from the L4 spinous process reach the S1 mamillary process but largely insert into the dorsal sacroiliac ligament over the intermediate and lateral third of the sacrum. Fibers from the L5 spinous process are inserted into the intermediate third of the sacrum as far caudally as the third sacral segment.

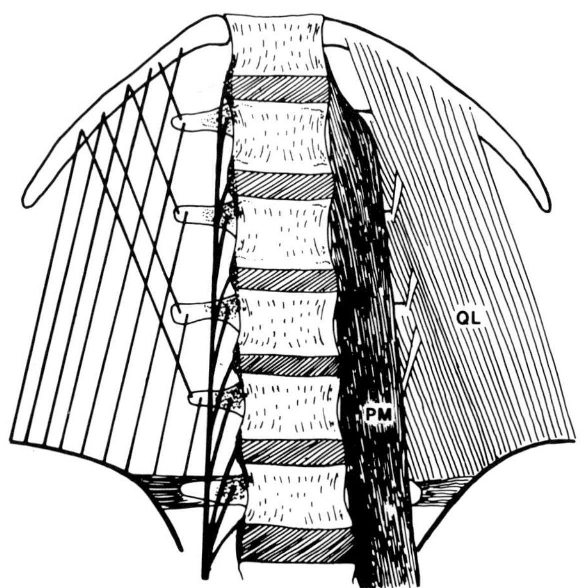

Figure 4–9. Psoas major and quadratus lumborum, viewed from the front. The intact psoas major and quadratus lumborum have been drawn on the right and their fascicular attachments have been drawn on the left. Note how few of the fibers of quadratus lumborum are disposed as lateral flexors of the lumbar spine.

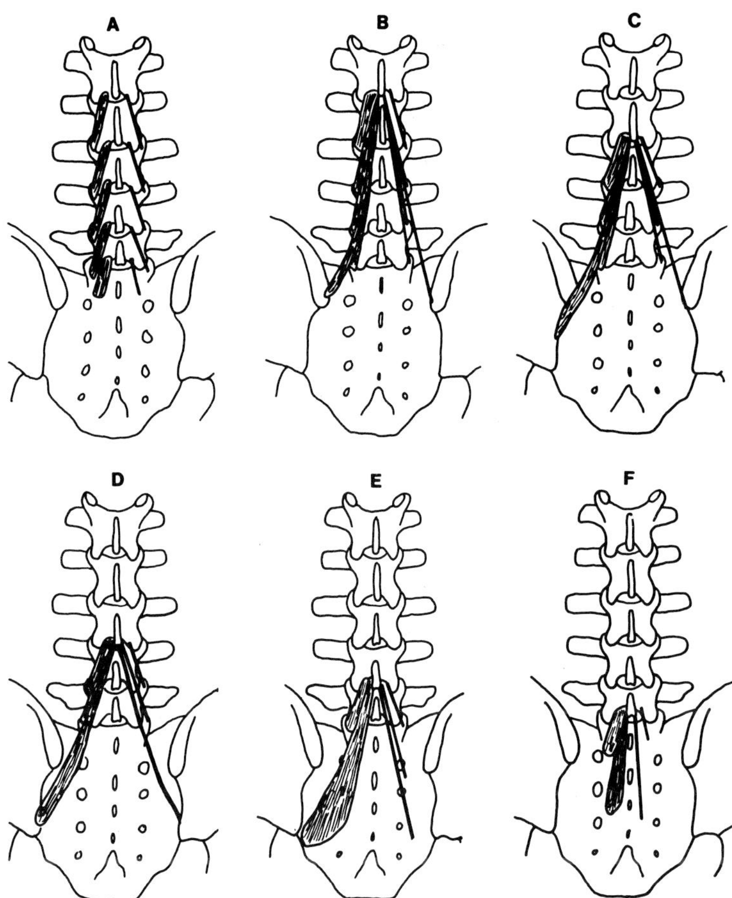

Figure 4–10. The fascicular nature of multifidus. **A.** Segmental fibers arising from the laminae of each of the lumbar vertebrae. **B** to **F.** Segmental bands arising from the spinous processes L1 to L5 each attaching systematically to mammillary processes and the sacrum.

Overall, the fascicular pattern of the multifidus is such that each lumbar segment is independently anchored to caudal attachments of the mamillary processes, posterior superior iliac spine, and sacrum.

Erector Spinae

The lumbar erector spinae is a large muscle lying lateral to the multifidus that not only covers the entire lumbar region, but also extends high into the thoracic region. At thoracic levels its two divisions—longissimus thoracis and iliocostalis lumborum—are clearly separated from one another by the iliocostalis thoracis muscle, but in the lumbar region the two divisions are closely opposed, seemingly forming a single common muscle mass. However, within this muscle mass the two divisions are separated by the lumbar intermuscular aponeurosis, with the longissimus thoracis lying medial to it and the iliocostalis lumborum lateral.[7] Each of the two divisions of the lumbar erector spinae consists of two types of fibers: lumbar fibers which arise from and act directly upon the lumbar vertebrae, and thoracic fibers which arise from thoracic levels and insert into the sacrum and ilium, thereby acting only indirectly on the lumbar spine.

Longissimus thoracis pars lumborum consists of five fascicles that arise from the lumbar transverse processes (Fig. 4–11). Each fascicle arises from an accessory process and the medial half of the posterior surface of the corresponding transverse process. The fascicle from L5 inserts directly into the ilium just above the posterior superior iliac spine, and is covered sequentially by the fascicles from L4-L1. These latter fascicles become tendinous on their lateral surfaces, and the confluence of their tendons forms the lumbar intermuscular aponeurosis which attaches to a narrow area at the rostral end of the posterior superior iliac spine.

The iliocostalis lumborum pars lumborum lies lateral to the lumbar intermuscular aponeurosis, and consists of four fascicles that arise from the tips of the L1-L4 transverse processes and the middle layer of thoracolumbar fascia adjacent to these processes (Fig. 4–12). These fascicles broaden caudally and assume a series of overlapping linear attachments to the iliac crest lateral to the posterior superior iliac

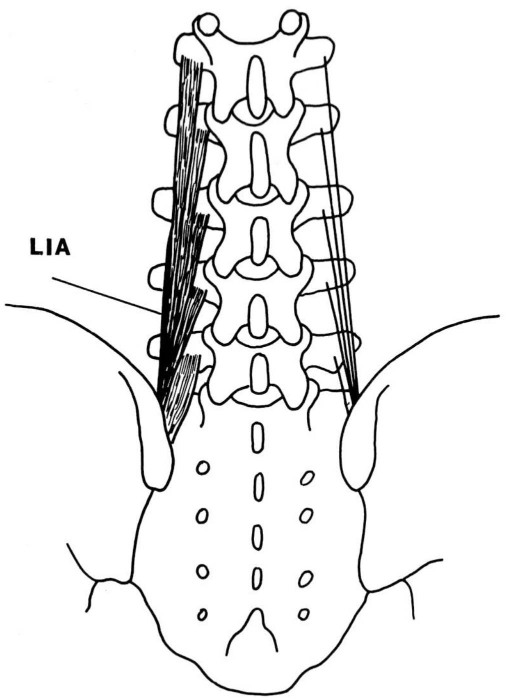

Figure 4–11. Longissimus thoracis pars lumborum. Segmental fascicles arise from the lumbar transverse processes and converge into a common tendon over their lateral surfaces that forms the lumbar intermuscular aponeurosis (LIA).

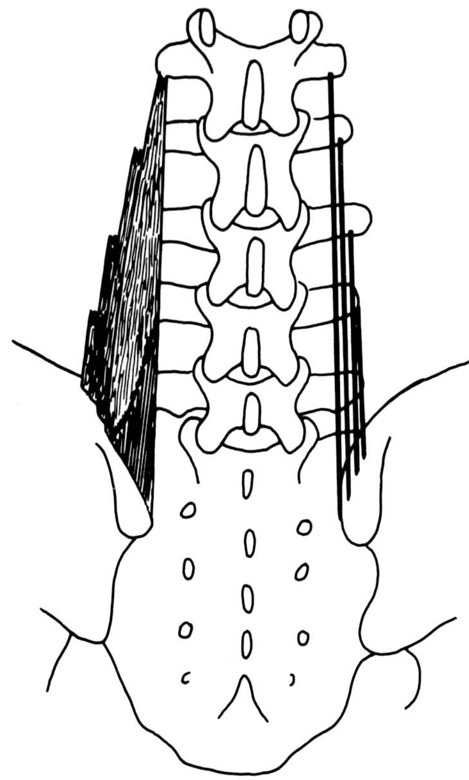

Figure 4–12. Iliocostalis lumborum pars lumborum. Segmental fascicles arise from the tips of the L1 to L4 transverse processes and the adjacent middle layer of thoracolumbar fascia, and are anchored to the ilium.

spine. In adults, the iliocostalis typically lacks a fascicle attached to the L5 transverse process; it is represented in the posterior portion of the iliolumbar ligament.

The longissimus thoracis pars thoracis consists of several, small, individual muscle bellies that arise from the tips of the transverse processes and proximal portions of the respective ribs at levels T1-T12 (Fig. 4–13). Each muscle belly forms a long narrow caudal tendon. The tendons from T1-T12 pass inferiorly to insert sequentially to the lumbar and sacral spinous processes, the dorsal surface of the sacrum below the insertion of multifidus, and to the posterior superior iliac spine. The side-to-side aggregation of these caudal tendons forms the medial half of a wide aponeurotic sheet known as the erector spinae aponeurosis, which covers the lumbar fibers of longissimus thoracis and the lumbar multifidus. In the midline, the tendinous fibers of the erector spinae aponeurosis converge to form the supraspinous ligament.

The iliocostalis lumborum pars thoracis consists of small individual muscle bellies that arise from the tubercles of the lower eight ribs (Fig. 4–13). Each muscle belly forms a narrow flat tendon that passes caudally to insert into a linear area along the iliac crest, with those fibers from higher thoracic levels

attaching medially and those from the twelfh rib attaching laterally. The side-to-side aggregation of these caudal tendons forms the lateral half of the erector spinae aponeurosis which covers the lumbar fibers of iliocostalis lumborum.

Lumbar Muscle Actions

The disposition of the fascicles of the lumbar multifidus is such that they are oriented at right angles to the transverse plane of the vertebra from which they arise. Consequently, they can exert no posterior translatory force on the lumbar vertebrae.[8] Their action is exclusively to produce posterior sagittal rotation or to oppose anterior sagittal rotation.

The lumbar fibers of longissimus thoracis and iliocostalis lumborum are inclined backward and downward from their respective transverse processes and therefore are disposed to produce both posterior and sagittal rotation and posterior translation of their vertebra of origin.[1] This disposition allows these muscles to control not only the anterior sagittal rota-

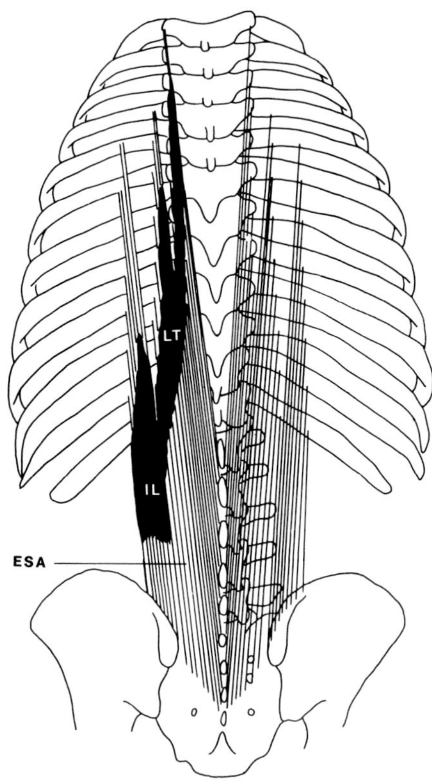

Figure 4–13. The thoracic fibers of longissimus thoracis and iliocostalis lumborum. The fascicles of these muscles have tiny overlapping muscle bellies but long caudal tendons that cover the lumbar region forming the erector spinae aponeurosis (ESA).

tion of the lumbar vertebrae, but also their forward translation.

The primary action of the lumbar multifidus and the lumbar fibers of iliocostalis and longissimus collectively is to produce extension of the lumbar spine or to control the displacement it undergoes during flexion of the trunk. The lumbar multifidus is sometimes said to act as an axial rotator of the lumbar spine, but its fibers are inclined far too vertically for them to be efficient axial rotators. Although the lumbar multifidus is electromyographically active during rotation of the trunk, rather than reflecting any primary action as a rotator, this activity reflects the role of multifidus in preventing unwanted flexion that is produced by the antero-lateral abdominal wall muscles, which are the primary rotators of the trunk.[8]

Acting unilaterally, the iliocostalis lumborum controls lateral flexion of the lumbar spine. Under normal circumstances this movement is not executed by direct muscular action but rather by the influence of gravity on the trunk. Therefore, it is the contra-lateral iliocostalis lumborum that is active to control the movement of the lumbar vertebrae and thorax.[1]

Because the thoracic fibers of the longissimus thoracis and iliocostalis lumborum span the lumbar region posteriorly and are largely inserted into the sacrum and ilium, they have no direct action on the lumbar vertebrae. They act to extend the thorax in relation to the pelvis, and in so doing, exert an indirect extension or antiflexion moment on the lumbar spine.

THORACOLUMBAR FASCIA

The muscles of the lumbar spine are enclosed by the thoracolumbar fascia which consist of three layers: an anterior layer covering the psoas major muscle and quadratus lumborum; a middle layer that springs from the tips of the lumbar transverse processes and intervenes between the quadratus lumborum and erector spinae, where it is continuous with the inter-transverse ligaments; and a posterior layer that covers the erector spinae and erector spinae aponeurosis. The three layers blend laterally to form a thick raphe lateral to the erector spinae (Fig. 4–14).

The posterior layer of thoracolumbar fascia consists of two laminae: a superficial lamina with fibers passing downward and medially, and a deep lamina with fibers passing downward and laterally.[1] The superficial lamina is formed by the aponeurosis of the latissimus dorsi and is well developed throughout the lower half of the thoracic region and the lumbar and lumbosacral regions. It is attached to the tips of the upper three lumbar spinous processes where it contributes to the formation of the supraspinous ligament. At the L4 and L5 levels, where the supraspinous ligament is lacking, the collagen fibers of the superficial lamina cross the midline and interlace with those from the opposite side.

The deep lamina of the posterior layer of thoracolumbar fascia consists of distinct bands of fibers emanating from the L3, L4, and L5 spinous processes, and is formed by fibers of the contralateral latissimus dorsi that have crossed the midline. Those bands from L4 and L5 are attached to the posterior superior iliac spine, and when viewed bilaterally, these bands constitute alar-like ligaments that anchor the L4 and L5 vertebrae to the ilium. The fibers from L3 pass downward and laterally to blend with the lateral raphe just above the iliac crest.

ABDOMINAL MUSCLES

The muscles of the antero-lateral abdominal wall do not attach to the lumbar vertebrae and are clearly separated from the lumbar spine, but nonetheless they are important with respect to the movements of the lumbar spine. Although most of the fibers of the

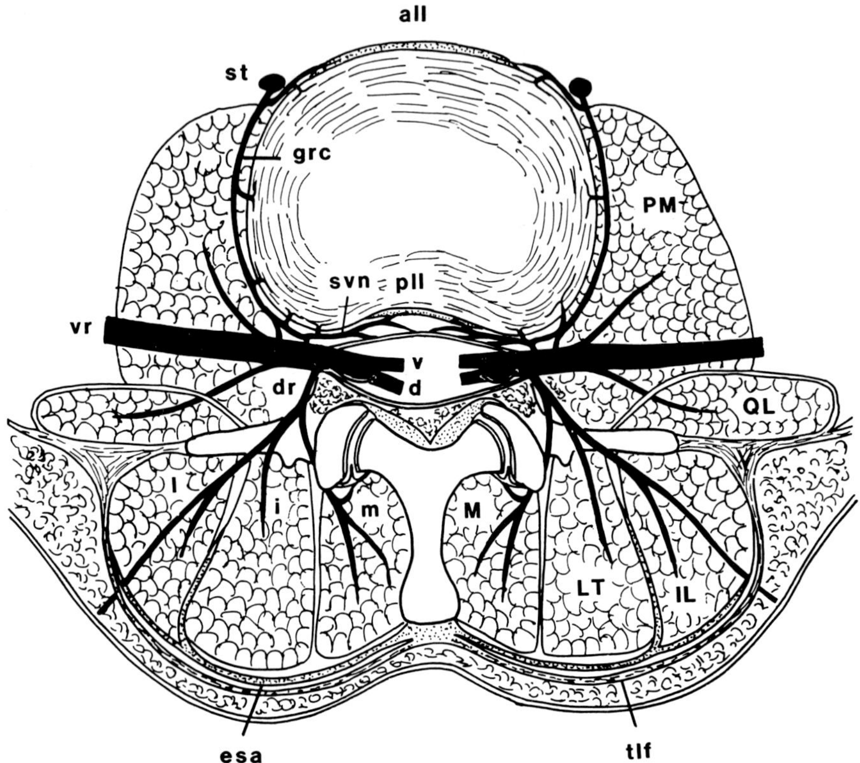

Figure 4–14. Axial view of the muscles and innervation of a lumbar motion segment. Each lumbar spinal nerve is formed by ventral (v) and dorsal (d) roots, and divides into ventral rami (vr) and dorsal (dr) rami. The dorsal rami form medial branches (m), which innervate multifidus (M) and the zygapophysial joints; intermediate branches (i), which innervate longissimus (LT); and lateral branches (l), which innervate iliocostalis (IL) and become cutaneous upon piercing the thoracolumbar fascia (tlf). The ventral ramus innervates the psoas (PM) and quadratus lumborum (QL) before entering the lumbar or lumbosacral plexus. The ventral ramus receives the grey ramus communicans (grc) from the sympathetic trunk (st), and gives rise to the sinuvertebral nerve (svn). The disc is innervated by branches from the ventral ramus, the grey ramus, and the sinuvertebral nerve. The latter also supplies the dural sac anteriorly and the posterior longitudinal ligament (pll). The ligamentum flavum is supplied by the dorsal rami from its external aspect and not by the sinuvertebral nerve. The anterior longitudinal ligament (all) is supplied by the grey ramus communicans. The erector spinae aponeurosis (esa) lies deep to the posterior layer of thoracolumbar fascia (tlf). The latter blends with the middle layer in a raphe lateral to the transverse processes.

external oblique and the internal oblique are involved in the formation of the rectus sheath, and hence in the generation of intra-abdominal pressure, the more posterior fibers of these muscles have bony attachments that enable them to move the thorax in relation to the pelvis, and thereby exert an indirect action on the lumbar spine.

The posterior fibers of the external oblique arise from the outer surface of the lower ribs and insert into the iliac crest. They are oriented downward and forward. The posterior fibers of the internal oblique arise from the posterior end of the iliac crest and pass upward and forward to attach to the lower cos-

tal cartilages. Because of their obliquity the fibers of the internal and external obliques can rotate the thorax, thereby indirectly rotating the lumbar spine. Rotation is executed by the ipsilateral internal oblique and the contralateral external oblique. However, because these oblique muscles also have a downward orientation, whenever they exert axial rotation they must inescapably exert a forward flexion moment on the thorax and lumbar spine. To produce pure axial rotation, this flexion moment must be counterbalanced by a simultaneous extension moment generated by the lumbar multifidus and erector spinae.

The transversus abdominis arises from the inner

surface of the lower six costal cartilages and from the iliac crest, but its middle fibers arise from the lateral raphe of the thoracolumbar fascia. This relationship has given rise to a considerable controversy. In the past, it had been inferred that the transversus abdominis could exert a laterally directed tension on the posterior layer of thoracolumbar fascia, and because of the criss-cross arrangement of fibers in this layer, it seemed possible that the lateral tension could be converted into an extension or antiflexion moment exerted on the lumbar spinous processes.[9] However, revised mathematical calculations in conjunction with a proper appraisal of the detailed anatomy of the thoracolumbar fascia have revealed that although this mechanism does exist, it can contribute little more than 4 Nm of extension force, which amounts to no more than 1 to 2% of the force required for moderate to heavy lifting.[9]

SPINAL NERVES AND NERVE ROOTS

The conus medullaris of the spinal cord occupies the upper reaches of the lumbar vertebral canal. The tip of the conus usually lies opposite the L1-L2 intervertebral disc, but may lie as high as the T12-L1 disc or as low as the L2-L3 disc in the adult. Beyond the conus, the vertebral canal contains the ventral and dorsal roots of the lumbar, sacral, and coccygeal nerves forming the cauda equina. The nerve roots and spinal cord are enclosed by the dural sac and are bathed in cerebrospinal fluid.

At each segmental level, a pair of nerve roots leaves the dural sac and is directed toward the intervertebral foramen on each side, where the roots join to form the short spinal nerve that occupies the intervertebral foramen. Individually, the nerve roots are lined by pia mater as far as the spinal nerve and are enclosed in a common sleeve of dura mater and arachnoid mater which extends from the lateral aspects of the dural sac into the intervertebral foramen where it blends with the epineurium of the spinal nerve. The nerve roots are thus bathed in cerebrospinal fluid as far as the intervertebral foramen. The dorsal root ganglion is located within the dural sleeve just proximal to the spinal nerve and hence occupies the intervertebral foramen. The lumbar spinal nerve roots are nourished by the radicular branches of the spinal arteries (see below) but some 50% of their nutrition is derived from the cerebrospinal fluid that bathes them.[1]

In passing from the dural sac to the intervertebral foramen the lumbar nerve roots assume an oblique course along what is referred to as the radicular canal, which is not truly a canal but rather the lateral extremity of the vertebral canal at each segmental level. Each radicular canal is a curved channel running around the medial aspect of each pedicle of the lumbar spine, and each canal can be divided into three segments.[1] The uppermost segment lies above the pedicle; its anterior wall is formed by the intervertebral disc in this region, and its posterior wall is formed by the uppermost end of a superior articular process. The middle segment lies immediately medial to the pedicle and is related anteriorly to the back of the vertebral body; posteriorly it is covered by the vertebral lamina. This region of the radicular canal is also known as the lateral recess (of the vertebral canal). The third segment of the radicular canal is formed by the upper part of the intervertebral foramen, and is bound by the pedicle above, the back of the lower portion of the vertebral body in front, and the ligamentum flavum behind.

In its course through the radicular canal, each pair of lumbar nerve roots is thus related to an intervertebral disc at the upper end of its canal, and passes just above the intervertebral disc as it enters the intervertebral foramen. At the lateral end of the intervertebral foramen each spinal nerve divides into a small dorsal ramus and a larger ventral ramus (Fig. 4–14). The lumbar ventral rami participate in the formation of the lumbar and lumbosacral plexuses whereas the dorsal rami innervate the posterior structures of the lumbar spine.

INNERVATION OF THE LUMBAR SPINE

Upon leaving the intervertebral foramina the ventral rami of the lumbar spinal nerves enter the psoas major muscle, within which they form plexi (Fig. 4–14). The L1-L4 ventral rami form the lumbar plexus, and major branches of the L4 and L5 ventral rami join to form the lumbosacral trunk, which enters the lumbosacral plexus. Branches of the lumbar ventral rami innervate the psoas major muscle and the quadratus lumborum (Fig. 4–14).

The lumbar sympathetic trunks descend through the lumbar region along the anterolateral borders of the lumbar vertebral column close to the medial edge of the psoas major muscle. In addition to supplying the abdominal and pelvic blood vessels and viscera, the lumbar sympathetic trunks give rise to the rami communicantes of the lumbar ventral rami. White rami communicantes are distributed to the L1 and L2 ventral rami and grey rami communicantes are distributed to every lumbar ventral ramus (Fig. 4–14).

In general, the rami communicantes reach the ventral rami by passing around the concave lateral surface of each lumbar vertebral body deep to the psoas major muscle, but some rami communicantes may also reach the ventral rami by actually penetrating the substance of the psoas major.[1] The rami communicantes typically join the lumbar ventral rami just outside their respective intervertebral foramina (Fig. 4–14). The efferent fibers of the rami communicantes are principally destined to be distributed to the blood vessels and skin in the territory supplied by the lumbar spinal nerves, but in the vicinity of the lumbar spine rami communicantes are involved in the formation of the lumbar sinuvertebral nerves and in the innervation of the lumbar intervertebral discs.

Sinuvertebral Nerves

The sinuvertebral nerves are recurrent branches of the ventral rami that enter the intervertebral foramina to be distributed within the vertebral canal (Fig. 4–14). They are mixed nerves, each formed by a somatic root from a ventral ramus and an autonomic root from a grey ramus communicans. These nerves cross the back of the vertebral body just below the pedicle, and within the vertebral canal each nerve forms an ascending branch which passes upward, parallel to the posterior longitudinal ligament to end in the next higher intervertebral disc. A shorter descending branch ramifies in the anulus fibrosus of the intervertebral disc at the level of entry of the nerve.

In addition to supplying the intervertebral discs and the posterior longitudinal ligament, the lumbar sinuvertebral nerves are distributed to the blood vessels of the vertebral canal and to the ventral aspect of the dura mater. The posterior dura does not receive a nerve supply and is devoid of nerve endings.

Nerves to the Disc

The lumbar intervertebral discs are innervated, not only by the sinuvertebral nerves, which supply their posterior aspects, but also by branches that enter their lateral and postero-lateral aspects. Branches to the lateral aspect of each disc arise from the grey rami communicantes as they cross the vertebral bodies (Fig. 4–14). The postero-lateral corners of the lumbar intervertebral discs receive branches from the terminal portion of the grey ramus communicans and direct branches from the ventral ramus at each segmental level just outside the intervertebral foramen. The intervertebral disc is thus innervated around its entire circumference (Fig. 4–14).

Within each lumbar intervertebral disc nerve fibers and nerve endings are distributed, at least to the outer third of the anulus fibrosus and as far deeply as the outer half of the anulus.[1] The inner portions of the anulus fibrosus and the nucleus pulposus are devoid of nerve endings. The majority of nerve endings found within the anulus fibrosus are simple and complex free terminals, unassociated with blood vessels and presumably nociceptive in nature. On the surface of the anulus fibrosus, various types of encapsulated and complex unencapsulated receptors occur and are presumably proprioceptive in nature.[1]

The Lumbar Dorsal Rami

The lumbar dorsal rami pass backward to enter the posterior compartment of the lumbar spine. The L1-L4 dorsal rami pass through their respective intertransverse spaces where they divide, typically into three branches (Fig. 4–14).

The lateral branch of each lumbar dorsal ramus crosses the transverse process below its level of origin and enters the lumbar fibers of iliocostalis lumborum, which it supplies. The lateral branches of the L1-L3 dorsal rami continue, emerging from the postero-lateral border of the iliocostalis to pierce first the erector spinae aponeurosis, and next the posterior layer of thoracolumbar fascia, to become cutaneous, supplying the skin of the buttock as far caudally as the greater trochanter. The lateral branch of the L4 dorsal ramus has no cutaneous branch.

The intermediate branches of the L1-L4 dorsal rami enter the lumbar fibers of longissimus thoracis and form an intersegmental plexus that supplies this muscle. These branches have no cutaneous distribution.

The medial branches of the L1-L4 dorsal rami cross the junction of the transverse process and superior articular process at each segmental level to enter the multifidus muscle. En route, each medial branch supplies articular branches to the zygapophysial joints above and below its course. Branches also are supplied to the interspinous muscle and interspinous ligament at each segmental level. Within the multifidus the medial branches assume a segmental distribution. Each nerve is distributed exclusively to those fascicles of multifidus that arise from the spinous process with the same segmental number as the nerve. This relationship reinforces the segmental disposition of the muscle, such that those fibers of multifidus that act upon the spinous process of a particular segment are innervated by the nerve of that same segment.

The anatomy of the L5 dorsal ramus differs from that of other lumbar dorsal rami because of its relationship to the sacrum. The L5 dorsal ramus has a prolonged course over the ala of the sacrum and divides into medial and intermediate branches at the base of the lumbosacral zygapophysial joint. A lateral branch is lacking, consistent with the absence of an L5 fascicle of iliocostalis lumborum. Otherwise, like the analagous branches of the other lumbar dorsal rami, the intermediate branch of the L5 dorsal ramus is distributed to the lowest fibers of longissimus thoracis whereas the medial branch innervates the L5 fibers of multifidus and the lumbosacral zygapophysial joint.

BLOOD SUPPLY

The lumbar spine receives an abundant arterial blood supply stemming from the segmental lumbar arteries.[1] These are paired vessels that arise from the aorta at the L1-L4 levels and from the median sacral artery at the L5 level. Each runs around the lateral surface of its respective vertebral body in company with a grey ramus communicans until it reaches the intervertebral foramen. Here, external branches pass in company with the ventral and dorsal rami of the spinal nerves to supply the muscles of the lumbar spine, and a network of small vessels provides an abundant blood supply to each zygapophysial joint.

At the level of each intervertebral foramen each lumbar artery gives rise to posterior and anterior spinal canal branches. The posterior branches supply the laminae of the lumbar vertebrae whereas the anterior branches form an intersegmental arterial arcade along the floor of the vertebral canal. Arising from this arcade are nutrient arteries that enter the substance of each vertebral body through its posterior surface. The other terminal branches of the lumbar arteries are the radicular arteries that accompany the dorsal and ventral roots of each lumbar spinal nerve.

En route to the intervertebral foramen, each lumbar artery supplies many branches that supply the lateral surface of the vertebral body and enter its substance to anastomose internally with the nutrient arteries. However, in contrast to the rich blood supply of the vertebral bodies, the lumbar intervertebral discs receive only a nominal blood supply, with only a few small vessels extending from the lateral surfaces of the adjacent vertebral bodies onto the outer surfaces of the anulus fibrosus. The distribution of these vessels is restricted to the most superficial fibers of the anulus fibrosus and no vessels enter the substance of the anulus fibrosus or the nucleus pulposus. In having no direct blood supply, the intervertebral discs rely critically on diffusion for their nutrition. Half of this nutrition occurs by diffusion from the vessels on the outer aspect of the anulus fibrosus. The remainder occurs by diffusion from a capillary plexus located within each vertebral body immediately deep to each vertebral endplate.[1]

The venous drainage of each vertebral body is largely posteriorly through its nutrient foramen. Veins leaving the nutrient foramina anastomose with one another on the floor of the vertebral canal forming the anterior internal vertebral venous plexus, which drains through each intervertebral foramen into the ascending lumbar vein. A posterior internal vertebral venous plexus lies behind the dural sac and drains the roof of the vertebral canal. The ascending lumbar vein communicates with the inferior vena cava via the lumbar vein that drains the lateral aspects of the lumbar vertebral body.

LIFTING

Lifting is one of the principal activities of daily living that involves the lumbar spine. However, the exact mechanism of lifting still remains controversial despite intensive research over recent years. It is apparent and uncontested that lifting involves extension of the lumbar spine from a flexed position, but the controversy concerns the extent to which various components of the lumbar spine are involved in sustaining the loads imparted on the back during a lift. The act of lifting involves the balancing of the flexion moment, exerted by the weight of the trunk, and the weight to be lifted, by an appropriate extension moment, and arguments still abound concerning the relative roles of the posterior back muscles, the posterior ligaments of the lumbar spine, and intra-abdominal pressure in this regard.

A role for intra-abdominal pressure was conceived when it was noted that the abdominal muscles are active during lifting. It was perceived that raised intra-abdominal pressure could act like a balloon in front of the lumbar vertebral column pushing upward on the diaphragm and thorax to oppose flexion moments, and thereby relieve the load imparted on the back muscles and posterior ligaments. However, recent biomechanical and clinical studies have discredited this notion. Foremost, biomechanical considerations reveal that as the abdominal muscles contract to raise intra-abdominal pressure they simultaneously exert a flexion moment on the thorax, and mathematical calculations reveal that the flexion moment thus produced exceeds the extension moment produced by raised intra-abdominal pressure.[1,9] Furthermore, clinical studies have shown that although patients with back pain have significantly weaker abdominal muscles, strengthening these muscles influences neither back pain nor the magnitude of intra-abdominal pressure generated during lifting.[9]

The back muscles are obvious candidates for the generation of extension moment on the lumbar spine during lifting. However, the maximum force capacity of the back muscles is insufficient to exert an appropriate extension moment other than for small loads of less than about 35 kg. For heavier weights, moments in excess of 400 Nm must be overcome. However, the average maximum strength of the lumbar back muscles is about 200 Nm[10], (this figure is somewhat smaller for older individuals and slightly greater for younger individuals).

The relative weakness of the lumbar back muscles has generated of one school of thought that emphasizes the role of the posterior ligaments of the lumbar spine during lifting.[1] The thesis of this theory is that the gluteal muscle and hamstring are strong enough to overcome the flexion moment exerted by the trunk and any heavy weight to be lifted. The hip extensors exert posterior sagittal rotation of the pelvis, and provided that the lumbar spine remains fully flexed, the trunk can be rotated backward and upward as the pelvis rotates thereby lifting any weight supported by the upper limbs. The lumbar spine must remain fully flexed in order to engage the posterior ligaments of the lumbar spine, which are then responsible for transmitting to the thorax the extension moment exerted on the pelvis. The essence of this theory is that the trunk and lumbar spine are used passively to lift the weight, with the energy being supplied by the hip extensors. The ligaments involved in this process are said to be the supraspinous and interspinous ligaments, the capsules of the zygapophysial joints, and the posterior layer of thoracolumbar fascia. However, on the basis of biomechanical data, appraisal of this mechanism reveals several limitations.

The supraspinous and interspinous ligaments are remarkably weak and can sustain an extension moment of not more than 10 Nm.[11] The capsules of the zygapophysial joints are remarkably strong,[12] but they lie close to the axis of sagittal rotation and can sustain an extension moment of little more than 27 Nm. The ligamentum flavum can sustain a moment of up to 30 Nm. The biomechanics of the thoracolumbar fascia has not been fully studied but data on its tensile strength suggest that it can contribute about 30 Nm of extension moment. Thus, collectively the posterior ligaments of the lumbar spine can sustain only about 100 Nm, which is far less than the 400 Nm required for a moderately heavy lift.

It is evident that no single structure alone can be responsible for the mechanism of lifting. Neither the posterior ligaments nor the back muscles are strong enough to overcome the flexion moment imposed on the lumbar spine during a heavy lift. The actual mechanism of lifting, therefore, remains somewhat of an enigma. However, what has not been considered in detail is the possibility of a concurrent action between the posterior ligaments and passive tension developed in the lumbar back muscles.

When a muscle elongates, the maximum active tension it can generate decreases, but at the same time passive tension develops in the muscle as a result of either stretching of interstitial connective tissues elements in the muscle or as yet unresolved mechanisms within the sarcomeres. Notwithstanding the actual mechanism, the passive tension developed in a muscle is equal to or even exceeds the loss of active tension that occurs when the muscle is elongated. Thus, the combined active and passive tension of an elongated muscle is at least equal to its maximum active tension at resting length.

Transposing this to the context of the lumbar spine, it is evident that the total active and passive tension in the back muscles in the fully flexed position should be approximately equal to their maximum active strength in the upright position, i.e., about 200 Nm. Combining this with the tensile strength of the posterior ligaments yields a total passive extension capacity for the lumbar spine of about 300 Nm, which is close to that required for the execution of a moderately heavy lift.

A further consideration that has not been explored in detail is the possible role of the posterior anulus fibrosus in lifting. Although this structure lies close to the axis of rotation, it is a large and strong ligament. It is therefore conceivable that tension developed in the posterior anulus could supplement the other posterior ligaments of the lumbar spine. However, the actual tensile capacity of the posterior anulus during lifting still remains to be quantified.

MECHANICAL INJURY

The lumbar spine can be affected by a variety of painful disorders such as tumours, infections, and metabolic bone disease, but in Western society these are not particularly common causes of back pain. Troublesome back pain most commonly arises as a result of injuries sustained as a result of repeated or excessive mechanical insults to the lumbar spine, and the nature of the lesions resulting from these injuries can be appreciated by tracing the consequences of excessive normal and abnormal movements of the lumbar spine.

As described above, extension of the lumbar spine is limited by the impaction either of the tips of two consecutive spinous processes or of the tip of an inferior articular process against a lamina. As a result of repetitive or excessive extension, irritation and inflammation of the periosteum can occur at the site of bony contact. When lesions occur between the spinous processes, the condition is known as "kissing spines" or Baastrup's disease. A similar condition can occur on the vertebral lamina but carries no specific name.[1]

Another form of extension injury can occur when inferior articular processes are asymmetrical with respect to their caudal length. Upon extension, the longer inferior articular process contact the underlying lamina first and arrest the movement in the sagittal plane. However, if the extension force continues to be applied, it cannot be absorbed by further extension, and instead is absorbed by rotation of the motion segment. The upper vertebra pivots on the impacted inferior articular process and the contralateral inferior articular process rotates backward, straining or even disrupting the capsule of its zygapophysial joint.[1]

In contrast, the lumbar spine appears to be well protected against injury during flexion, by the posterior ligaments, the intervertebral discs, and the back muscles. Exceptionally, the supraspinous or interspinous ligaments may be strained or ruptured, but interspinous ligament strain has rarely been recorded as a cause of troublesome back pain. Traditionally, it has been held that flexion injuries, particularly the act of heavy lifting in the sagittal plane, can cause acute disc herniation. However, biomechanical studies have shown that this can occur only with severe hyperflexion injuries involving forces and ranges of movement well outside the normal range of activities of daily living. A normal healthy intervertebral disc is well-designed to sustain heavy loads in flexion and is not prone to rupture. In biomechanical experiments, even with severe hyperflexion, only a minority of intervertebral discs fail by herniation.

The lumbar spine is far more vulnerable to injury in axial rotation. Axial rotation is normally limited to less than 3° per segment by impaction of a zygapophysial joint, but injuries can occur to the motion segment if excessive rotatory forces are applied to it.[1] Forced rotation occurs about an axis located in the impacted zygapophysial joint, and results in a posterior displacement of the contralateral inferior articular process and a lateral shear force being applied to the intervertebral disc. In the impacted zygapophysial joint, force rotation can result in fractures of the subchondral bone plates or more extensive fractures through the inferior articular process, the superior articular process or the pars interarticularis of the vertebral lamina; in the contralateral zygapophysial joint sprains or fracture evulsions of the joint capsule can occur. The intervertebral disc is relatively protected by the posterior elements against injury during pure axial rotation.

However, if axial rotation is superimposed on flexion a significant injury can occur to the anulus fibrosus. Flexion pre-stresses the collagen fibers of the anulus fibrosus and renders them less able to accommodate the additional strain imposed on them by the added axial rotation and lateral shear. As a result of flexion and axial rotation, the anulus fibrosus can suffer circumferential tears of its collagen lamellae.

The nucleus pulposus is unaffected by such injuries, because the lesion lies exclusively in the peripheral layers of the anulus fibrosus. The lesion is essentially that of a ligament sprain, and when it lies in the innervated portions of the anulus fibrosus it becomes a potent source of pain just like any ligament injury of the appendicular skeleton.

A single torsional injury to an anulus fibrosus may injure only a few collagen fibers, and therefore does not appreciably compromise the function of the anulus. However, repeated torsional injuries have the propensity to erode the anulus fibrosus by progressively damaging successive lamellae of collagen fibers, thereby producing radial fissures through the thickness of the anulus fibrosus. Because torsional stresses on the anulus fibrosus are concentrated along its points of maximum curvature, radial fissures typically develop across the postero-lateral corners of discs with flat or concave posterior surfaces, and across the posterior midline in discs with convex posterior borders. When present, such radial fissures constitute tracks along which nuclear material may herniate.

Among patients with intractable back pain, such as those presenting to a University clinic, it is emerging that the most common lesion responsible for their pain is internal disc disruption.[13] This condition is characterized by degradation of the nuclear matrix and a centrifugal erosion of the anulus fibrosus, with the perimeter of the anulus fibrosus remaining intact. Although disc bulging or nuclear herniation may be late complications of this disorder, they are not necessarily present at early stages of internal disc disruption when the condition is nonetheless painful. The actual cause of internal disc disruption has not been determined, but the most attractive theory, to date, is that it results from compression injuries to the disc.

When an intervertebral disc is subjected to excessive compressive loads, such as in heavy lifting or in a fall, the disc fails by fracture of one of its vertebral endplates. When nuclear material is exposed to the blood in the vertebral spongiosa it elicits an inflammatory response. At one extreme, this inflammatory response may succeed in sealing the defect or repairing the endplate fracture, but at the other extreme the inflammatory response may continue unabated, and may proceed to erode the nuclear matrix. Initially, this degradative process is confined to the nucleus pulposus, but in time it proceeds to erode the anulus fibrosus in a centrifugal fashion producing fissures that extend first into the inner fibrocartilaginous portion of the anulus and subsequently into the outer fibrous portion. This process becomes painful as a result of two mechanisms.

Although the degradative process is confined to the nucleus and inner anulus, the inflammatory enzymes and exudates have no access to the nerve endings of the intervertebral disc. However, when fissures extend into the middle or outer third of the anulus fibrosus these chemicals gain access to the nerve endings located in those portions. Direct irritation of these nerve endings provides a chemical mechanism by which internal disc disruption can become painful.

As long as the anulus fibrosus remains intact, it can continue to subserve its mechanical functions. However, if the anulus fibrosus is progressively eroded from within, fewer collagen fibers remain intact to sustain the stresses normally imposed upon the anulus fibrosus. Consequently, the relative stress that these remaining, intact fibers bear progressively becomes greater than normal, and in due course the stresses become sufficient to be a cause of pain. This process constitutes a mechanical basis for the pain of internal disc disruption; the pain is not caused by excessive loads being placed on the anulus fibrosus, but is the result of normal loads being placed on fewer and fewer functioning collagen fibers. Moreover, both chemical and mechanical mechanisms may operate concurrently, such that the chemical mechanism is responsible for a constant, dull aching pain unrelated to posture and activity, and also sensitizes the nerve endings in the anulus fibrosus making them more susceptible to mechanical irritation whenever any movement of the intervertebral joint takes place.

Once nuclear degradation has occurred, and if a radial fissure develops through the anulus fibrosus, it is possible for nuclear material to herniate through the fissure as a result of even trivial compressive loads imposed upon the disc by simple activities such as forward bending. However, under these circumstances the forward flexion is not the primary cause of the herniation; it is only a precipitating event. There must have been prior degradation of the nucleus pulposus and erosion of the anulus fibrosus originally triggered by a long forgotten, or unnoticed prior compression injury to the disc.

Therapeutic Implications

Notwithstanding their individual differences, the known mechanical injuries of the lumbar spine have several features in common. All are caused by excessive loads being imposed upon the lumbar spine in one or other of its primary directions of movement. All are potentially potent sources of pain, but most strikingly, all are relatively invisible to conventional radiographic investigations. Small fractures of the articular processes and fractures of the vertebral endplates are not readily apparent on plain radio-

graphs and may even escape notice on CT scans unless multiple, high resolution cuts are taken through the suspected regions. Otherwise, the lesions caused by mechanical injuries of the lumbar spine are located in soft tissues such as the capsules of the zygapophysial joints or the intervertebral disc, which are not demonstrated on plain radiographs or on CT scans. However, the presence of soft tissue lesions in the zygapophysial joints or intervertebral discs can be inferred from the result of provocation and analgesic tests.

Symptomatic zygapophysial joints can be identified by anaesthetizing the responsible joint, whereupon complete relief of all symptoms indicates that the lesion responsible for the patient's pain must lie in that joint. Similarly, provocation discography can be used to stress a putatively symptomatic intervertebral disc, and reproduction of a patient's pain constitutes prima facie evidence that that disc is the source of the patient's symptoms. The diagnosis can be confirmed if local anaesthetic can be injected into the symptomatic disc and succeeds in relieving the patient's symptoms. Furthermore, studies have shown that the pathological features of internal disc disruption can be demonstrated by CT discography.

Axial views of the lumbar spine after discography has been performed demonstrate the internal structure of the intervertebral disc. Discs in which the contrast medium is confined to the nucleus pulposus or to the inner third of the anulus fibrosus are rarely painful, whereas there is a high correlation between reproduction of a patient's symptoms and discs showing extension of contrast medium into the middle and especially into the outer third of the anulus fibrosus.[14] Thus, the presence of internal disc disruption can be confirmed objectively provided that the physician and the patient are prepared to undergo both provocation discography and CT discography.

Another feature that the lesions of mechanical injuries to the lumbar spine have in common is that none are life threatening and none are particularly threatening to the integrity of the lumbar spine. Although any mechanical lesion may be disabling because of the severe pain it produces, in pathological terms it is not prone to extend or disseminate as might a tumor or an infection; and apart from pars articularis fractures, mechanical lesions are not liable to result in instability of the lumbar spine that threatens to compromise the cauda equina. Thus, provided the physician has excluded serious disorders such as infection and tumors, and has properly assessed the mechanical stability of the lumbar spine, the patient can be reassured that they are not suffering a threatening disorder, and that if their injury is not amenable to simple or safe surgical intervention, it should be amenable to healing, or at least functional restoration, despite the apparent severity of the pain that it produces.

REFERENCES

1. Bogduk, N., Twomey, L.T.: Clinical Anatomy of the Lumbar Spine. Churchill Livingstone, Edinburgh, 1987.
2. Rissanen, P.M.: The surgical anatomy and pathology of the supraspinous and interspinous ligaments of the lumbar spine with special reference to ligament ruptures. Acta Orthop Scand Suppl *46*:1–100, 1960.
3. Heylings, D.J.A.: Supraspinous and interspinous ligaments of the human spine. J Anat *125*:127–131, 1978.
4. Luk K.D.K., Ho, H.C., Leong, J.C.Y.: The iliolumbar ligament. J Bone Joint Surg *68B*:197–200, 1986.
5. Pearcy, M.J.: Stereoradiography of lumbar spine motion. Acta Orthop Scand Suppl *212*:1–41, 1985.
6. Macintosh, J.E., Bogduk, N., Valencia, F., Munro, R.R.: The morphology of the human lumbar multifidus. Clin Biomech *1*:196–204, 1986.
7. Macintosh, J.E., Bogduk, N.: The morphology of the lumbar erector spinae. Spine *12*:658–668, 1987.
8. Macintosh, J.E., Bogduk, N.: The biomechanics of the lumbar multifidus. Clin Biomech *1*:205–213, 1986.
9. Macintosh, J.E., Bogduk, N., Gracovetsky, S.: The biomechanics of the thoracolumbar fascia. Clin Biomech *2*:77–83, 1987.
10. McNeill, T., Warwick, D., Andersson, G., Schultz, A.: Trunk strengths in attempted flexion, extension and lateral bending in healthy subjects and patients with low-back disorders. Spine *5*:529–539, 1980.
11. Dumas, G.A., Beaudoin, L., Drouin, G.: In situ mechanical behaviour of posterior ligaments in the lumbar region. J Biomech *20*:301–310, 1987.
12. Cyron, B.M., Hutton, W.C.: The tensile strength of the capsular ligaments of the apophysial joints. J Anat *13*:145–150, 1981.
13. Crock, H.V.: Internal disc disruption: a challenge to disc prolapse 50 years on. Spine *11*:650–653, 1986.
14. Vanharanta, H., et al.: The relationship of pain provocation to lumbar disc deterioration as seen by CT/discography. Spine *12*:295–298, 1987.

5

Malcolm H. Pope

Physiology and Spine Mechanics

Low back pain has been described by White and Gordon[1] as man's most important non-life-threatening disease. The authors went on to say that "once the cause of low back pain is known, more effective means of prevention and treatment are likely to be discussed." Certainly knowledge about the biomechanics and physiology will be helpful in this regard.

PHYSIOLOGY

Disc Structure

The intervertebral disc is composed of the annulus fibrosus and nucleus pulposus (Fig. 5–1). The structure of the annulus is reminiscent of a radial tire with collagen fibers in adjacent sheets crossing each other at approximately 30°.[2] The peripheral portion of the annulus is directly attached to the cortex of the vertebral bodies by Sharpey's fibers and the inner portion is attached to the cartilaginous end plates.[3]

In the young adult the nucleus pulposus has the consistency of toothpaste. The nucleus consists of a relatively random network of collagen and hydrated proteoglycan. Prochop, et al.[4] reported that although the disc contains both type I and II collagen, there is a linear change in the proportion of type I in the outer annulus to type II in the inner. Type II fibers have 25% more water than type I. Grynpas[5] suggested that the type II fibers are better adapted to compressive stress. Coventry, et al.,[6] report that the nucleus and annulus are visually discrete in youth and the annulus becomes more fibrous and progressively less distinct with age. The final result is a fibrotic mass uniting one vertebral body with the next. Degenerative changes increase with age, with most discs being affected by the sixth decade.[7]

In disc disease, the morphologic changes characteristic of aging occur earlier. Disc degeneration has also been noted in a variety of mammals,[8] in diabetic hamsters,[9] in animals with a high salt diet, and in sand rats.[10] The majority of disc herniations occurs in the fourth decade of life and herniations are found in 15 to 30% of autopsy specimens.[11]

Disc Pressure

Water is the most abundant component of the disc and water is retained in the disc, in spite of large compressive loads caused by high osmotic pressure derived from the proteoglycans. An equilibrium state exists between the osmotic pressure, collagen matrix tension, and applied load. The osmotic pressure results from osmotic effects (fixed charge density on the glycosaminoglycans) and is not affected by proteoglycan size.

Virgin[12] first suggested that the nucleus pulposus acts hydrostatically to pressurize the disc. The nucleus pressure is redistributed as tension in the annulus layers. Pressure is present even at rest; some pretension of the spinal ligaments occurs at all times. The normal disc pressure is about 1.5 times the compressive load divided by the cross-sectional area.[13] The pressure is higher in the disc center and decreases toward the exterior.[14] Nachemson[13,15] showed that intradiscal pressure is lowest in the recumbent posture, higher in a standing posture, but highest in unsupported sitting. Using a similar technique Andersson, et al.,[16] showed that disc pressure is significantly reduced when the backrest is inclined to 110°, a 2-cm lumbar support is provided, and armrests are used. Certainly, given such factors as the sedentary nature of occupations in the industrialized nations, the fixed postures induced by key-

56

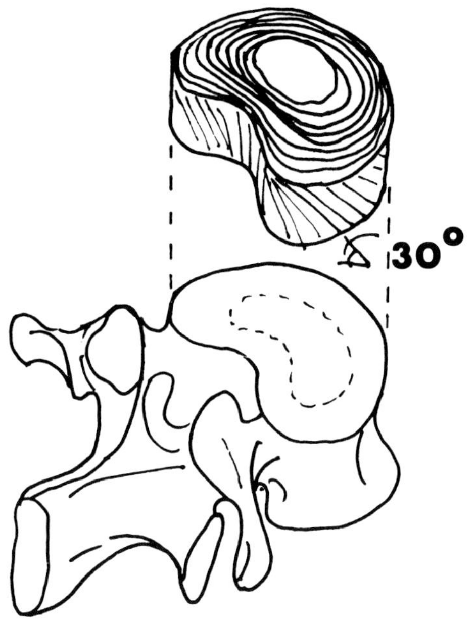

Figure 5–1. The intervertebral disc is composed of the annulus fibrosus and nucleus pulposus. The structure of the annulus is reminiscent of a radial tire with collagen fibers in adjacent sheets crossing each other at approximately 30°.

board use, and the amount of time spent driving, we must consider the occupational stresses induced in the sitting posture. Andersson, et al.,[17] also demonstrated a linear relationship between trunk posture and the measured disc pressure. Twisting and asymmetrical pressures caused greater increases in disc pressure.

A loss of overall height occurs diurnally. Fifty percent of the height loss happens in the first two hours

after waking,[18] but recovery is rapid upon adopting a recumbent posture (Fig. 5–2). In the weightless environment of space height has been seen to dramatically increase by up to 5 cm[19], however it decreases under the influence of lifting loads.[20]

Nutrition

The intervertebral disc is avascular and relies on passive diffusion for both nutrition and the removal of metabolic wastes. Diffusion is via the periphery of the annulus and through the vertebral end plate. The central part of the end plate is most permeable.[21] The blood supply to the annulus stops at approximately 18 years. It is probable that sequelae are the disc herniations usually first seen in the midtwenties. It is likely that this supply is affected by toxic materials such as nicotine[22] and by immobilization.[23] In the latter case, the beneficial effect from the sequence of unloading and loading, which tends to mechanically aid the nutrition, is unrealized. The disc pressure measurements of Nachemson[13] imply an influx of fluid in recumbancy and an outflow when standing or sitting.

Some differences exist in the way that different solutes can diffuse into the disc. Uncharged solutes, such as glucose, can diffuse equally well through either the annulus or the end plate.[24] Negatively charged anions, such as the sulfate anions, can readily diffuse through the annulus but not through the end plate—a result of the many negative anions in the glycosaminoglycan fraction of the annulus. Conversely, the positively charged solutes, such as sodium, are preferentially transported across the end plate.

Figure 5–2. Rapid recovery upon adopting a recumbent posture.

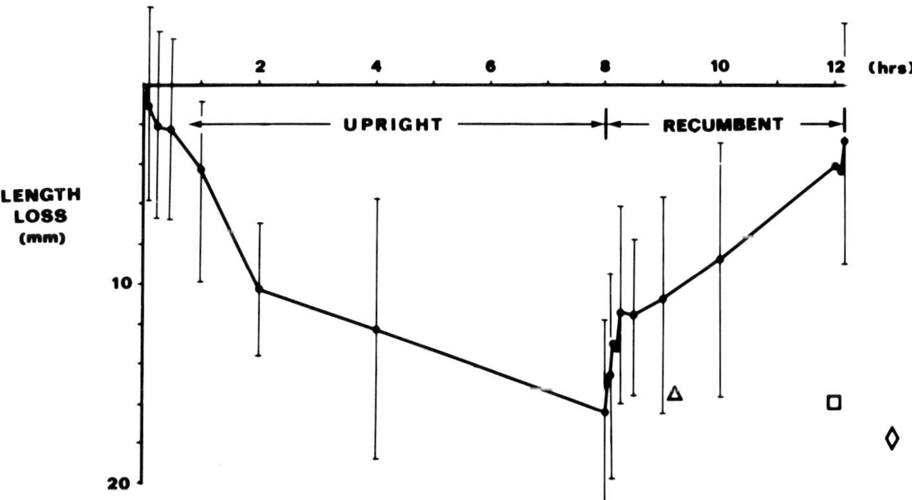

Viscoelastic Behavior

The time-dependent behavior of the disc comes from two sources: the fluid flow of the disc under applied load, and the inherent viscoelastic behavior of the collagen itself and its interaction with the proteoglycan matrix. Time-dependent behavior has been demonstrated both in vivo[25,26] and in vitro.[27,28] The studies of Krag, et al.,[18] indirectly measured the in vivo viscoelastic behavior by measuring the change in overall height of the subjects. Keller, et al.,[25] directly measured the time-dependent characteristics via pins placed into the pedicles of supine pigs subjected to compressive loads. Kaleps and Kazarian[29] fitted the rheological model shown in Figure 5–3 to the time-dependent data. Hirsch and Nachemson[30] reported that higher loads led to greater creep rates. As described earlier, profound changes occur in the structure of the degenerated and aging disc. Kazarian[27] noted that the degenerate disc had a higher rate of deformation and the creep curve stabilized sooner.

BIOMECHANICS

Mechanics of the Motion Segment

Most of the fundamental studies of the lumbar spine are carried out on the motion segment (sometimes referred to as the functional spinal unit or FSU). The FSU is comprised of the superior and inferior vertebral body, the intervertebral disc, and the ligamentous tissues. Several experiments showed that the FSU exhibits nonlinear load deformation behavior, becoming stiffer at higher loads.[31–37] However, some have reported that little difference is evidenced in behavior, as a function of age, gender, and even disc level or amount of de-

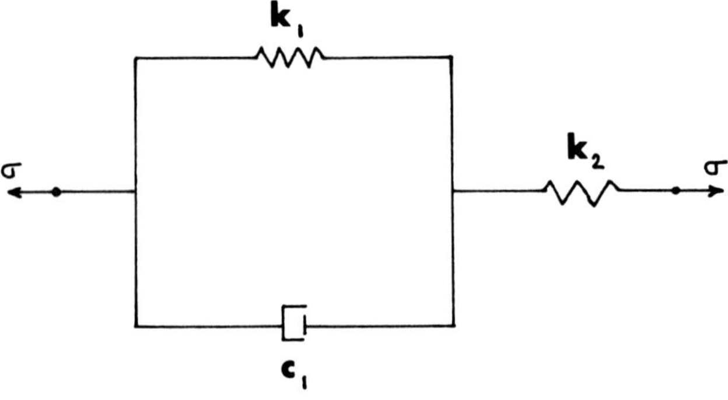

Figure 5–3. The coupled response at the balance point (σ = stress, k_1 = parallel stiffness, k_2 = series stiffness, c_1 = damping).

generation.[31] A curious feature of the FSU mechanical response is the coupled response. The coupled response refers to movement of a load in one direction resulting in motion not only in that direction, but also in other directions.[32] For example, the application of a lateral bending moment might lead to lateral bending, twisting, and shear. The combined stiffnesses under different loading combinations are assembled into a table called a stiffness matrix. Studies show that the lumbar motion segment is viscoelastic, absorbs energy, moves in 6° of freedom (3° of translation and 3° of rotation), and depends upon its bony and ligamentous components for its mechanical response.[33,34,36,37]

The mechanical behavior of the spine is affected by the choice of the point at which the load or torque is applied. Therefore, one can obtain different stiffness matrices at different points of load application and some studies do not contain a description of the location of the loading point. Only Panjabi, et al.,[32] Tencer and Ahmed,[35] and Wilder, et al.,[37] applied loads to the motion segment in locations other than geometrically based reference locations.

The balance point is a mechanically based loading reference, because it is the point at which certain coupled motion is minimized. Tencer and Ahmed[35] described a balance point location based upon minimization of coupled flexion/extension rotation. Wilder, et al.,[37] found the balance point where both coupled flexion/extension and coupled lateral bend rotations were minimized. The coupled response at that balance point is given in Figure 5–3. This was found to be particularly valuable when assessing a response following a mechanical overload leading to instability (Fig. 5–4). Conceivably, it would be possible to find a balance point where all coupled rotations were minimized or all coupled translations were minimized.

In some experiments the FSU is loaded so as to establish motions within the disc itself. When using lateral view, vertebral body corners to define the borders of the disc, Krag, et al.,[18] showed a 20% increase of posterior disc height (Fig. 5–5) as a result of 6° of segment flexion. With radiopaque markers in place it was possible to establish the distortion of the matrix. Stokes[38] found the postero-lateral disc fibers exhibiting a 3.9% tensile strain resulting from a similar flexion rotation. He also noted that it was possible for relatively large height changes to occur between the boney vertebrae while the strain in the disc surface fibers remained relatively small. This discrepancy was attributed to disc bulging.

Other testing has concentrated on the effect of mechanical overloads on the FSU. Perey[39] found the vertebrae can withstand 10 kN of vertical force before failure. Farfan[40] was able to cause annulus inju-

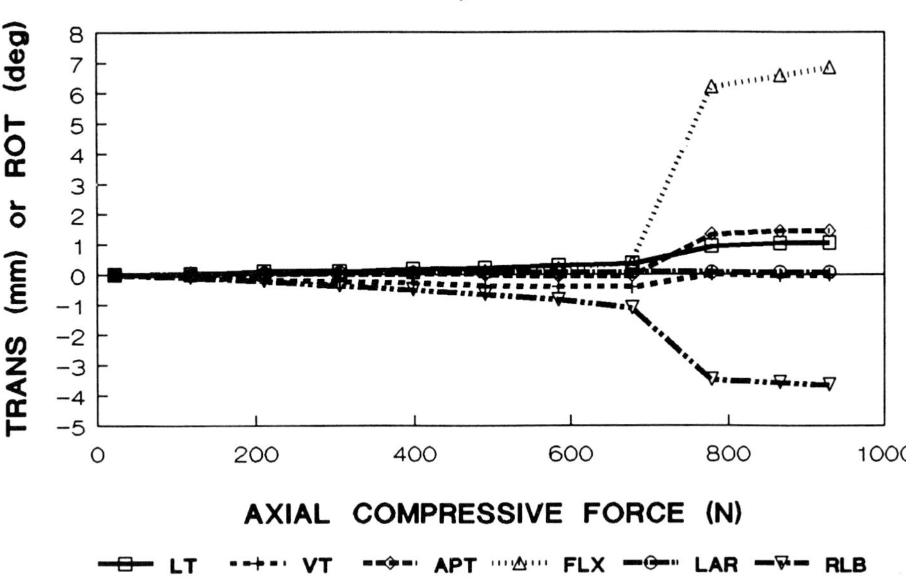

28JNA2M3, 100 seconds

Figure 5–4. Assessing a response following a mechanical overload leading to instability. LT = Lateral translation (+ to the left); VT = Vertical translation (+ upward); APT = Anterior posterior translation (+ anterior); FLX = Flexion rotation (+ flexion); LAR = Axial rotation (+ left axial rotation); RLB = Lateral bend (+ right lateral bend). (From Wilder, D.G., Pope, M.H., Frymoyer, J.W.: The biomechanics of lumbar disc herniation and the effects of overload and instability. J Spinal Disorders 1(1):16, 1988.)

ries with high rate torsion of 20°. A great deal of interest has focused on the role of cyclic loading. Adams and Hutton[41] simulated a day of heavy flexion and torsion loading on the FSU. Many cadaveric lumbar motion segments showed distortions of the lamellae of the annulus fibrosus. It was suggested that the distortion produced was the precursor to a disc herniation tracking tear. Cyclic loading has been reported to cause a tear throughout the annulus.[42] Other workers have reported facet or vertebral body failures, or disc annular or facet capsular ligament tears[43] and disc herniations,[44] caused by cyclic loading.

Relatively less work has been expended on the biomechanics of the facets. The facets can be thought of as an essential part of the three-joint-complex comprised of the two facet joints and the intervertebral disc. The facets have a significant role in load sharing. Farfan[31] has shown that the facets are responsible for half the torsional strengths, with the

Figure 5–5. 20% increase of posterior disc height as a result of 5.6° segment flexion.

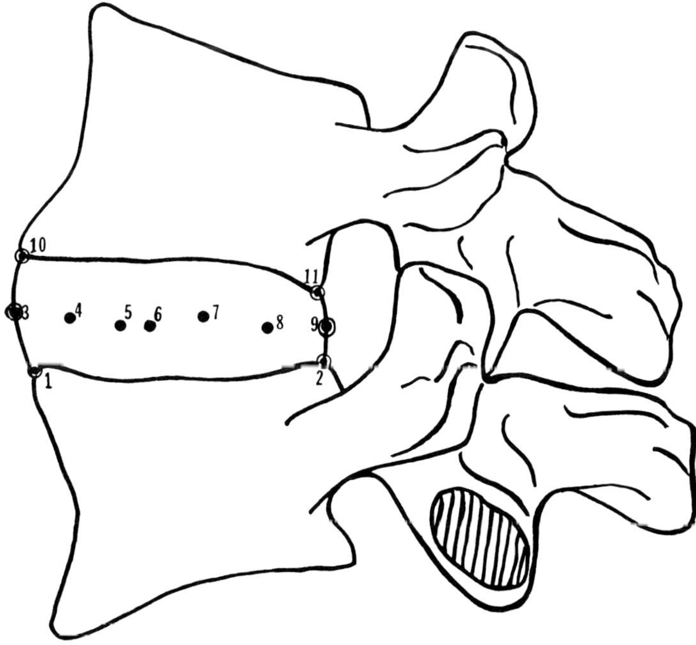

disc and ligamentous tissue responsible for the other half. If the disc is degenerated the facets take up more of the load.

Trunk Mechanics

Both in vivo and in vitro studies have shown that intradiscal pressure (IDP) increases during flexion or when one maintains a seated posture.[16] Flexion postures result in some of the highest intradiscal pressures.[16,21,45] In vitro work by Schultz, et al.,[46] showed that a 10 N-m flexion moment could produce a mean IDP increase of 300 kPa (and a maximum of 700 kPa).

Pelter[47] was the first to report a method for measurement of IDP. Charnley[48] suggested that IDP increases may be related to herniation of the nucleus pulposus. However, it was Nachemson[13] who demonstrated the hydrostatic nature of the disc and who later developed a technique for IDP measurement in vivo. Pressures in young (nondegenerate) discs increase linearly up to compressive loads of 2000 N and is about 30 to 50% higher than the applied load per unit area.

Nachemson, et al.,[31] and Schultz, et al.,[46] subsequently explored in vitro the effects of various loadings on IDP. IDP was not affected significantly by torsion, extension, or shear but was affected considerably by compression, flexion and lateral bending. Such findings will, of course, be affected by the fact that no muscle forces are acting. Schultz, et al.,[46] concluded that IDP reflects the compressive load and can be used to ascertain compressive load in vivo in discs that are not grossly degenerate.

Nachemson, et al.,[15] reported on the IDP in various maneuvers (Table 5–1). Andersson, et al.,[49] found in vivo that IDP increased linearly with an increase of both trunk load and trunk moment. This work confirms the concept that increasing trunk flexion increases the load moment and thus the compressive load. IDP is high in unsupported sitting but can decrease significantly by the use of a backrest inclination greater than 110°, by the use of lumbar supports, and by the use of armrests.[16] Perhaps the most useful attribute of IDP is that it can be used to validate biomechanical models.[50] Such models cannot be directly solved, because of geometric complexity, without the use of optimization schema. In such cases, a validation using IDP is very valuable.

Electromyographic (EMG) Studies

The EMG is based on the electric activity, generated by depolarization of the muscle cell membrane measured either at the surface or deep through the use of needles. In most experiments, the EMG is measured in an attempt to estimate muscle force. Several authors[51,52] report a reasonably linear relationship up to moderate loads. Pope, et al.,[53] report reasonably nonlinear relationships with isometric twisting up to about 75% of maximum voluntary contracture (MVC).

The force/EMG relationship is affected by forward flexion.[51] It has been found that the EMG increases with increasing forward flexion up to a point where the EMG decreases and eventually shuts off completely. At this point, the subject is literally hanging on his ligaments, a finding called the flexion/relaxation phenomenon. A typical curve is given in Figure 5–6. Trunk flexion in the first 50° is flexion of the lumbar spine, whereas further flexion is largely caused by pelvis rotation.[54] As flexion begins, gluteus maximus, gluteus medius, and the hamstrings constrict to lock the hips.[55]

In lateral flexion EMG increases on both sides of the dorsal and abdominal trunk, with the main increase on the contralateral side.[56] The iliocortalis and longissmus are active in lateral flexion whereas the multifidus (probably because of an inefficient lever arm)[56] are largely inactive. Carlsoo[56] reported similar activities of the trunk muscles on either side of the spine in rotation. Pope, et al.,[53] found considerable antagonistic activity in isometric twisting and concluded that the muscular response was postural (i.e., maintenance of stability) as well as torque-generating.

Intra-abdominal Pressure (IAP)

Keith[57] was the first to suggest that intra-abdominal pressure (IAP) is used to support the loads in the trunk by provision of a hyperextension moment. Davis[59] found that IAP increased with forward flexion moment. Davis, et al.,[60] subsequently developed the pressure pill to measure IAP in the workplace

Table 5–1

Computer Loads from Intradiscal Pressure Measurements of a 70 kg Man[15]

Approximate Loads on the L3 Disc in a Person Weighing 70 kg	
Position, Maneuver	*Load (N)*
Supine (awake)	250
Supine (semi-Fowler's)	100
Supine (traction 500 N)	0
Sitting (unsupported)	700
Standing (relaxed)	500
Coughing	600
Straining	600

and used the technique for monitoring spine loads.[61] Andersson, et al.,[62] instructed subjects to voluntarily contract the abdominal muscles to increase IAP. However, this IAP increase did not decrease IDP. Krag, et al.,[63] using IAP measurements and dorsal EMG, found that a voluntarily increase of IAP did not decrease dorsal EMG. Rather, it resulted in a concomitant increase of abdominal EMG activity. Thus, the net load on the spine was increased not decreased. It is probable that IAP increases may help to stabilize the trunk by improving muscle movement and moment but do not help to reduce disc loads substantially.

Occupational Factors

Lifting

Many studies have shown a positive relationship between low back pain and heavy lifting and frequent lifting.[64] Almost one-third of US workers are required to exert near their maximum strength.[64] Thus, manual handling activities, even if performed only infrequently in a job, are still required of a large number of people, placing them at high risk of incurring low back pain. However, some studies[66] have shown that in some industries (i.e., aircraft assembly) no relationship exists between strength and likelihood of injury. The *Work Practices Guide to Manual Lifting*[64] offers specific recommendations on lifting limits. The criteria encompassed include muscle strength and physical work capacities in addition to biomechanical aspects of disc compression. In order to use the guide we must have some knowledge of the object weight, the horizontal and vertical location of the loads, the vertical travel, lifting frequency, and lifting duration. Two limits are defined:

1. *Maximum Permissible Limit* (MPL). This is defined as a lift that produces 7186 N (1430 pounds) of compression on the L5-S1 disc, and average metabolic load of 5.0 kcal per minute. The MPL is only within the strength capabilities of 25% of men and virtually no women.
2. *Action Limit* (AL). This limit is one-third of the MPL. This situation would create 3593 N (770 pounds) of compression on the L5-S1 disc, or require 3.5 kcal per minute and is within the strength capabilities of 75% of women and virtually all men.

In algebraic form the two limits are:

$$AL \text{ (kg)} = 40[(15/H)(1-.004(V-75)] \ (.7+7.5/D) \\ (1-F/Fmax)$$
$$MPL = 90 \ (6/H) \ (1-01 \ [V-30]) \ (.7 \ + \ 3/D) \ (1-F/Fmax)$$
$$AL \ = \ (MPL)/3$$

where:

    H ranges from 15.2 to 81.3 cm
    V ranges from 0 to 177.8 cm
    D ranges from 25.4 to (203.2-V) cm
    F ranges from .2 to Fmax

and

Fmax = 12 for continuous low lifting
                  (P = 8 hr., V < 76.2 cm)
     = 18 for occasional high lifting
                  (P = 1 hr., V < 76.2 cm)
     = 15 otherwise
  P = period of activity

The guide makes assumptions on a number of important variables. It assumes that lifting is two-handed, smooth, and symmetric only in the sagittal plane; that the object has good handles and is not too wide; that posture is unrestricted; that environmental conditions are favorable and that when not engaged in lifting the individual is essentially at rest (i.e., performing no significant carrying, pushing, pulling, or holding).

The weight and dimensions of a load to be lifted are primary risk factors. If a container can be designed to be compact, a worker can minimize the spinal load moment by keeping the object's center of mass close to the body. If the container must be lifted from the floor, and it is too large to pass between the knees, it requires the person to lift the object in front of the knees. This causes a larger spinal load moment than would be the case if the object could be lifted between the knees. Any object larger than about 30 cm cannot easily be lifted between the knees, thus increasing the horizontal distance.

Container design must also include a means by which to grasp the object. This is important not only to lift the container properly, but also to avoid sudden spinal inertial loads that occur when one attempts to regain control of an object slipping from the hands. In general, a forceful grasp of an object is provided by either a "hook grip," whereby the fingers wrap around the object but without thumb opposition, or a "power grip," whereby the thumb assists in retention of the object by overlapping the fingers. If a proper handle is provided, a power grip can be used. This requires less upper muscle action to maintain the coupling because the handle is fully secured between the fingers and the thumb.

Pushing and Pulling

Approximately 20% of overexertion injuries have been associated with pushing and pulling.[64] In these activities, the vertical height of the handle against which one pushes and pulls is important.[65,67-70] The optimal height for a handle to be pushed or pulled has been suggested to be approximately 91 to

114 cm above the floor (i.e., about hip height).[69]

Carts are commonly used to move heavy objects in the workplace. The risk of low back pain induced by the use of such devices arises from two types of hazard. The compressive forces on the L5-S1 disc become quite high, particularly when pulling a heavy load.[68] To avoid this situation, it is important to ensure that the pushing or pulling hand force required is below 200 N[67] and that the hands are at about hip to waist level at the time of maximum exertion, thus minimizing spinal load moments.

The second hazard to the back when pushing or pulling carts comes from the increased risk of slipping during such activities. It is not uncommon for the required coefficient of friction to exceed 1.0 during pushing and pulling activities. Therefore, the floor surface in areas where pushing and pulling activities take place must be kept clean and dry, and workers should be instructed to use, or be provided with, high traction shoes.

Asymmetric Load Handling

Based on biomechanical models, experimental strength studies, and EMG studies, symmetric load handling (i.e., midsagittal plane) is recommended.[53] Asymmetric load handling increases the stress on the spine and most muscle groups and can result in poor postural stability. Unfortunately, asymmetric motions are common in industry. Warwick, et al.,[71] compared symmetric and asymmetric pushing and pulling. In general, the activities in asymmetric postures resulted in decreased strengths (of about 25%). The effects were dependent on the direction of motion and on the specific postures.

Posture

The posture of a worker has been shown to be important in the development of LBP.[16,72–74] Extreme postures can lead to high disc loads caused by the load moments of the body segments, as well as by high loads in other structures such as ligaments, muscles, and facets.

The quantification of potentially harmful postures has been an enigma. Corlett[75] presented a unique approach to recording potentially stressful postures referred to as posture targeting. A worker is observed at random times during the workday and the angular configuration of various body segments is recorded with the aid of the "body diagram." This procedure is useful in evaluating workplace layouts when combined with worker reports of localized musculoskeletal pain obtained at several intervals during a workday.

A computer-based system called ARBAN is a method for ergonomic analysis of work, including work situations with greatly differing body postures and loads.[76] The method consists of recording the workplace on videotape and coding the posture and load situation in a number of closely spaced still frames. The ARBAN system determines the total ergonomic stress for the whole body (as well as for specified body parts) based on rules regarding the relative stress of specific acts. The results are presented as load/time graphs.

Another approach has been the use of measurement devices, worn by the worker, that record postures. Such a device was developed by Nordin, et al.[77] This device measures flexion and divides it into five flexion intervals. The flexion analyzer has been tested and found to be accurate and simple to use.[77] Changes in work techniques and work design can easily be measured and quantified. The advantage of the flexion analyzer is that it is noninvasive, reliable, easily transported, and results are obtained immediately. Most recently, we have developed a three-axis goniometer (flexion, lateral flexion, and axial rotation). The output is preprocessed on a small computer worn by the worker and the day's output is given as a histogram of times spent in a particular posture.

Seated Work

Numerous researchers have reported on the relationship of the seated posture to LBP.[16,60,11] Low back pain is partly caused by high disc loads,[16] but also results from the fixed posture inherent in so many sedentary jobs. Because of the many different opinions that exist and because user requirements vary, the kinds of chairs available vary widely. Regardless of use, however, it is important to be able to adjust any chair to meet basic anthropometric dimensions of the worker.

A proper seat height is desirable and should be adjustable for the individual user. The seat surface should be 3 to 5 cm below the knee fold when the lower limb is vertical. Foot supports can be used with higher than normal chairs. The width of the seat should be sufficient to accommodate the user population. The depth of the seat is also important. It must be possible to use the backrest in order to reduce disc loads. Therefore, the seat pan should not be too deep. Pressure should be avoided on the back of the thigh near the knees. A free area between the back of the lower limb and the seat pan is also useful to facilitate arising and leg movements. About 10 cm is suggested as the minimum clearance.

The work table is also important. The height should be chosen to prevent excessive forward flexion of the neck and of the trunk. An eye focal distance ranging from 20 to 40 cm is appropriate. The height of the table also should be related to the posi-

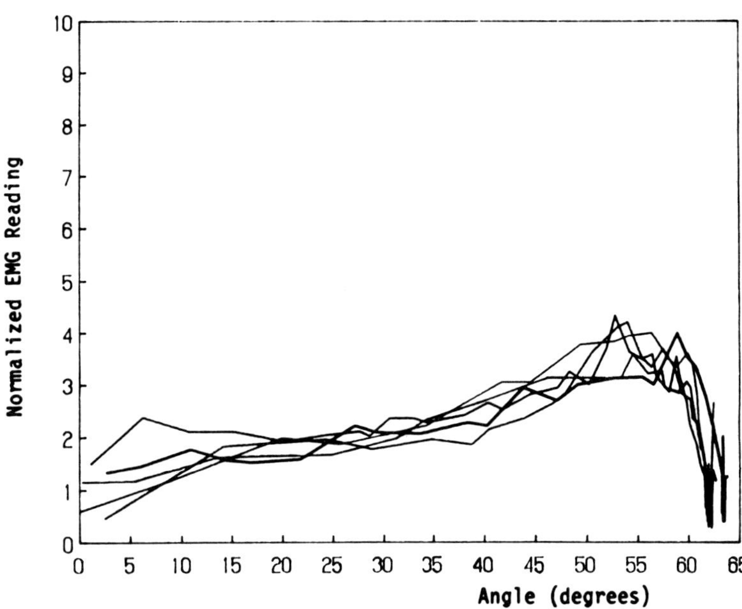

Figure 5–6. Flexion-relaxation phenomenon.

tion of the elbow.[78] It is suggested that workers be provided either an adjustable table or a high table and an adjustable footrest. A table that is too low causes kyphosis of the lumbar spine, increasing the load. On the other hand, a table that is too high causes abduction of the arms and elevation of the shoulder as well as kyphosis of the neck, resulting in fatigue of the shoulder and neck muscles.

Vibration

Workers who drive vehicles are more likely to have LBP[79] and herniated discs.[80] It is probable that vibration is a major factor in the cause, but postural stress, muscular effort, and shock and impact forces are also important. Many vehicles subject the driver to vibrations in the range of resonance of the spine (4 to 6 Hz) and that muscle fatigue also occurs in a vibrational environment. It should be noted that extremely high levels of vibration are found in off-highway vehicles (i.e., military, agricultural, and recreational).

The US standard for vibration measurement is given by SAE J1013 (SAE). Accelerations are measured by a disc made of molded rubber, 250 mm in diameter. The disc has a height of 12 mm and contains a cavity for the accelerometers. The disc is designed to sit comfortably between the ischial tuberosities. The acceleration is usually analyzed in one-third octave band levels.

The natural frequency of a single degree of freedom structure can be determined by two methods: acceleration transmissibility and driving point impedance. Using the acceleration transmissibility method (transmissibility = A_{out}/A_{in}, where A = ac-

celeration), a comparison is made between the output acceleration in the simple structure resulting from the input or driving acceleration. At resonance, the ratio of A_{out}/A_{in} becomes much larger than one. In mechanical driving point impedance studies, when the driving force is compared to the structure's resultant velocity, resonance occurs when both the driving force and resultant velocity are in phase, and the curve in the impedance vs. frequency plot reaches a maximum.

Studies to determine the resonant frequency of the seated human operator subjected to vertical vibration have been reported by many workers.[61,62,63,65,69,81,82] Some of the above-mentioned studies also reported resonant frequencies of standing and supine subjects, and resonant frequencies of seated subjects as affected by side to side or fore-aft vibrations.

One method of reducing whole body vibration is to reduce the vibration input. This can be done by the choice of vehicle and by training operators to choose the terrain over which they drive (if possible) with the objective of reducing vibrations and by changing their driving speed and style. Much of this is within the control of the operator. The principles of good static seating are also important in the dynamic environment.

Andersson, et al.,[83] showed that spinal stress could be minimized in the seated subject. The inclination of backrest was 110° and the seat pan angle was 6°; additional curved support for the lumbar spine was level with the third lumbar vertebra.

Zagorski, et al.,[84] using accelerometers taped to the back of human subjects, found greater acceleration at L3 than at the sacrum in the 2 to 5 Hz frequency range. Wilder, et al.,[70] measured relative motion on the surface of the lumbar region by means of filming seated subjects vibrating at their natural frequency as grid patterns were projected on their backs.

There are other advantages in inclining the backrest at 110°. If the trunk is upright or leaning forward when accelerated vertically, the head and shoulders will bend further forward. This flexor torque adds to the net spinal stress. The psoas muscle activity is reduced, and on vertical acceleration the load is distributed over the backrest as well as the seat.

Wilder, et al.,[85] have shown that the various postural supports can significantly affect the spine's vibrational response. In general, these postural supports shift loads from the lumbar area to other spinal areas. The lumbar, arm, and foot supports were generally helpful, but did affect adjacent structures. The commercially available vibration damping seats that have been tested reduced deleterious vibrations.

To reduce vibrations to less harmful frequencies, soft cushions should be replaced with firm ones. The seat should be suspended to give it a natural frequency of less than 1.5 Hz. Suspension seats made to this specification are readily available commercially, and most of them reduce vibration levels.

SUMMARY

We have found that the disc is a fiber composite structure composed of collagen and hydrated proteoglycan. The structure is well adapted to respond to compressive loads. The disc is viscoelastic, a phenomenon that can be measured in vivo by means of subject height measurements. Disc pressure can be measured in vivo because of the hydrostatic nature of the nucleus. The pressure is indicative of the loads on the spine and these loads can be high in certain postures and certain loadings, as seen in industry. The functional behavior of the motion segment is determined in part by the facets and is described by the compliance matrix. In vivo loads are estimated by intradiscal pressure (IDP), electromyographics, and intra-abdominal pressure. Various occupational hazards such as lifting, awkward postures, sitting, and vibration are discussed.

REFERENCES

1. White, A.A., Gordon, S.L.: Idiopathic Low Back Pain. An A.A.O.S. Symposium. Philadelphia, C.V. Mosby, 1982.
2. White, A.A., Panjabi, M.M.: Clinical Biomechanics of the Spine. Philadelphia, J.B. Lippincott, 1978.
3. Parke, W., Shift, D.: The applied anatomy of the intervertebral disc. Orthop Clin North Am 2:309–324, 1977.
4. Prockop, D.J., Kivirikko, K.I., Tuderman, L., Guzman, N.A.: The biosynthesis of collagen and its disorders: part I. N Engl J Med 301:13, 1979.
5. Grynpas, M.D., Eyre, D.R., Kirscher, D.A.: Collagen of the intervertebral disc: x-ray diffraction evidence for differences in the native molecular packing of types I, II collagens. Trans Orthop Res Soc 5:13, 1980.
6. Coventry, M.B., Ghomley, R.K., Kernohan, J.W.: Part I: the intervertebral disc, its microscopic anatomy and pathology; J Bone Joint Surg 27:233–243, 1945.
7. Farfan, H.F., Heberdeen, R.M., Dubow, H.J.: Lumbar disc degeneration, the influence of geometrical features on the pattern of disc degeneration: a postmortem study. J Bone Joint Surg 54A:492–499, 1972.
8. Sokoloff, L., Setwart, H.: Degenerative changes in Praomys (Mastromys) natalensis. Ann Rheum Dis 26:146, 1967.
9. Silberberg, R., Gerritsen, G.: Aging changes in intervertebral discs and spondylosis in Chinese hamsters. Diabetes 25:477, 1976.
10. Silberberg, R., Gerritsen, G.: Degeneration of the intervertebral disc and spondylosis in aging sand rats. Arch Pathol Lab Med 103:231, 1979.
11. Hult, L.: The Munkfors investigation. Acta Orthop Scand Suppl 16: 1954.
12. Virgin, W.J.: Experimental investigations into the physical properties of the intervertebral disc. J Bone Joint Surg 33B:607–611, 1951.
13. Nachemson, A.: Lumbar interdiscal pressure. Acta Orthop Scand Suppl 43: 1960.
14. Sonnerup, L.: A semi-experimental stress analysis of the human intervertebral disc in compression. Exp Mech 142: 1972.
15. Nachemson, A.: Lumbar intradiscal pressure. In The Lumbar Spine and Back Pain (Edited by M. Jayson). Kent, Pitman Medical Publishing, pp 257–269, 1976.
16. Andersson, G.B.J., Ortengren, R.: Myoelectric back muscle activity during sitting. Scand J Rehabil Med Suppl 3:73, 1974.
17. Andersson, G.B.J., Ortengren, R., Nachemson, A.: Intradiscal pressure, intra-abdominal pressure and myoelectric back muscle activity related to posture and loading. Clin Orthop 129:156–164, 1977.
18. Krag, M.H., Trausch, I.A., Wilder, D.G., Pope, M.H.: Internal strain and nuclear movements of the intervertebral disc. Orthop Trans 7:460–461, 1983.
19. Jayson, M.I.V.: Back pain—the facts. Oxford, Oxford University Press, 1981.
20. Eklund, J.A.E., Corlett, E.N.: Shrinkage as a measure of the effect of load on the spine. Spine 9(2):189–194, 1984.
21. Nachemson, A., Morris, J.: In vivo measurements of intradiscal pressure. J Bone Joint Surg 46A:1077–1092, 1964.
22. Urban, J.P.G., Holm, S., Maroudas A., Nachemson A.: Transport of small solutes into intervertebral discs of moving dogs. Orthop Trans 6(1):47, 1982.
23. Holm, S., Nachemson, A.: Variations in the nutrition of the canine intervertebral disc induced by motion. Orthop Trans 6:48, 1982.
24. Urban, J.P.G., Holm, S., Maroudas A.: Diffusion of small solutes into the intervertebral disc: an in vivo study. Biorheology 15:203, 1978.
25. Keller, T.S., et al.: In vivo creep behavior of the normal and degenerated porcine intervertebral disc. A preliminary report. J Spinal Disorders 1(4):267–278, 1989.
26. Krag, M.H., Cohen, M.C., Pope, M.H.: Load-induced changes in human intervertebral disc height in-vivo: a new and closer look. Orthop Trans 9(3), 516, 1985.
27. Kazarian, L.: Dynamic response characteristics of the human vertebral column: an experimental study of human autopsy specimens. Acta Orthop Scand Suppl 146, 1972.

28. Kazarian, L.: Creep characteristics of the human spinal column. Orthop Clin North Am 6:3, 1975.
29. Kaleps, I., Kazarian, L.E., Burns, M.L.: Analysis of compressive creep behavior of the vertebral unit subjected to a uniform axial loading using exact parametric solution equations of Kelvin-solid models—Part II. Rhesus monkey intervertebral joints. J Biomech 17:131–136, 1984.
30. Hirsch, C., Nachemson, A.: A new observation on the mechanical behavior of lumbar discs. Acta Orthop Scand 23:254, 1954.
31. Nachemson, A., Schultz, A.B., Berkson, M.H.: Mechanical properties of human lumbar spine motion segments. Influences of age, sex, disc level and degeneration. Spine 4:1–8, 1979.
32. Panjabi, M., Krag, M., White, A., Southwick, W.: Effect of preload on load displacement curves of the lumbar spine. Orthop Clin North Am 8:181–193, 1977.
33. Panjabi, M.M., Krag, M.H., White, A.A., III, Southwick, W.O.: Physical properties and functional biomechanics of the spine. In Clinical Biomechanics of the Spine, White A.A., III, and Panjabi M.M. Philadelphia, JB Lippincott, 1978.
34. Schultz, A.B.: Mechanics of the human spine. Appl Mech Rev:1487–1497, 1974.
35. Tencer, A.F., Ahmed, A.M.: The role of secondary variables in the measurement of the mechanical properties of the lumbar intervertebral joint. ASME J Biomech Eng 103:129–137, 1981.
36. Tencer, A.F., Ahmed, A.M., Burke, M.K.: Some static mechanical properties of the lumbar intervertebral joint, intact and injured. ASME J Biomech Eng 104, 193–201, 1982.
37. Wilder, D.G., Pope, M.H., Frymoyer, J.W.: The biomechanics of lumbar disc herniation and the effects of overload and instability. J Spinal Disorders 1(1):16–32, 1988.
38. Stokes, I.A.F., Greenapple D.G.: Surface strain on intervertebral discs. Proc 30th Meet ORS, Feb 7–9:253, 1984.
39. Perey, O.: Fracture of the vertebral endplates in the lumbar spine: an experimental biomechanical investigation. Acta Orthop Scand (Suppl) 25:25–36, 1957.
40. Farfan, H.F.: Mechanical Disorders of the Low Back. Philadelphia, Lea & Febiger, 1973.
41. Adams, M.A., Hutton, W.C.: The effect of fatigue on the lumbar intervertebral disc. Orthop Trans 7(3):461, 1983.
42. Brown, T., Hansen, R.J., Yorra, A.J.: Some mechanical tests on the lumbosacral spine with particular reference to the intervertebral discs: a preliminary report. J Bone Joint Surg 39A:1135–1164, 1957.
43. Liu, Y.K., et al.: Torsional fatigue of the lumbar intervertebral joints. Orthop Trans 7(3):461, 1983.
44. Wilder, D.G., Pope, M.H., Frymoyer, J.W.: Cyclic loadings of the intervertebral motion segment. Proc 10th Northeast Boeing Conf, (Edited by E.W. Hansen), Dartmouth College, Hanover, NH, March 15–16, 1982. New York, Institute of Electrical and Electronic Engineers, 9–11, 1982.
45. Okushima, H.: Study on hydrodynamic pressure of lumbar intervertebral disc. Arch Jpn Chir 39:45–57, 1970.
46. Schultz, A.B., Warwick, D.N., Berkson, M.H., Nachemson, A.L.: Mechanical properties of human lumbar spine motion segments: Part I: responses in flexion, extension, lateral bending and torsion. ASME J Biomech Eng 101:46–52, 1979.
47. Pelter, C.K.: Methods of measuring the pressure of the intervertebral disc. J Bone Joint Surg 15:365, 1933.
48. Charnley, J.: The imbibition of fluid as a cause of herniation of the nucleus pulposus. Lancet 1:124, 1952.
49. Andersson, G.B.J., Ortengren, R., Herberts, P.: Quantitative electromyographic studies of back muscle activity related to posture and loading. Orthop Clin North Am 8:85–96, 1977.
50. Schultz, A.B., Andersson, G.B.J.: Analysis of loads on the lumbar spine. Spine 6:76–82, 1981.
51. Grieve D.W., Pheasant, S.T.: Myoelectric activity, posture and isometric torque in man. Electromyogr Clin Neurophysiol 16:3–21, 1976.
52. Chapman, A.E., Troup, J.D.G.: Prolonged activity of lumbar erectors spinae. Ann Phys Med 6:262–269, 1970.
53. Pope, M.H., Andersson, G.B.J., Broman, H., Svensson, M., Zetterberg, C.: Electromyographic studies of the lumbar trunk musculature during the development of axial torques. J Orthop Res 4(3):288–297, 1986.
54. Davis, P.R., Troup, J.D.G., Burnard, J.H.: Movements of the thorax and lumbar spine when lifting: a chronocyclophotographic study. J Anat 99:13, 1965.
55. Okada, M.: Electromyographic assessment of muscular load in forward bending postures. J Faculty Sci (Univ Tokyo) 8:311, 1970.
56. Carlsöö, S.: The statis muscle load in different work positions: an electromyographic study. Ergonomics 4:193, 1961.
57. Jonsson, B.: The functions of individual muscles in the lumbar part of the erector spinae muscle. Electromyography 10:5, 1970.
58. Keith, A.: Man's posture: its evolution and disorders. The adaptations of the abdomen of its viscera to the orthograde posture. Br Med J 1:587–590, 1923.
59. Davis, P.R.: Variations of the intra-abdominal pressure during weight lifting in various postures. J Anat 90:601, 1956.
60. Davis, P.R., Stubbs, D.A., Ridd, J.E.: Radio pills: their use in monitoring back stress. J Med Eng Technol 1:209–212, 1977.
61. Davis, P.R.: The use of intra-abdominal pressure in evaluating stresses on the lumbar spine. Spine 6:90–92, 1981.
62. Andersson, G.B.J., Herberts, P., Ortengren, R.: Myoelectric back muscle activity in standardized lifting postures. In Biomechanics. 5A (Edited by P.V. Komi). Baltimore, University Park Press, pp 520–529, 1976.
63. Krag, M.H., Gilbertson, L., Pope, M.H.: Intra-abdominal and intrathoracic pressure effects upon load bearing of the spine. Trans Orthop 9(3):358, 1985.
64. National Institute for Occupational Safety and Health (NIOSH): a work practices guide for manual lifting, Tech Report #81-122, U.S. Dept. of Health and Human Services, Cincinnati, OH, 1981.
65. Davis, P.R., Stubbs, D.A.: Safe levels of manual forces for young males. 3. Performance capacity limits. Applied Ergon 9(1):33–37, 1979.
66. Battié, M.: The reliability of physical factors as predictors of the occurrance of back pain reports. Dissertation, Goteborg University, Goteborg, Sweden, 1989.
67. Kroemer, K.H.E., Robinson, D.E.: Horizontal static forces exerted by men standing in common working postures on surfaces of various tractions. AMRL-TR-70-114, Aerospace Medical Research Laboratory, Wright Patterson Air Force Base, OH, 1971.
68. Lee, K.: Biomechanical modelling of cart pushing and pulling. Unpublished doctoral dissertation, University of Michigan, Ann Arbor, MI, 1982.
69. Radke, A.O.: Vehicle vibration, man's environment. Mech Eng July:38–41, 1957.
70. Wilder, D.G., Frymoyer, J.W., Pope, M.H.: The effect of vibration on the spine of the seated individual. Automedica 6:5–35, 1985.
71. Warwick, D., Novack, G., Schultz, A.: Maximum voluntary strengths of male adults in some lifting, pushing and pulling activities. Ergonomics 23(1):49–54, 1980.
72. Andersson, G.B.J., Ortengren, R., Schultz, A.: Analysis and measurement of the loads on the lumbar spine during work at a table. J Biomech 13(6):513–520, 1980.
73. Corlett, E.N., Manenica, I.: The effects and measurement of working postures. Applied Ergon 11(1):7–16, 1980.
74. Karhu, O., Kansi, P., Kuorinka, I.: Correcting working postures in industry: practical method for analysis. Applied Ergon 18:199–201, 1977.

75. Corlett, E.N., Bishop, R.P.: A technique for assessing postural discomfort. Ergonomics 19(2):175–182, 1976.
76. Holzmann, P.: ARBAN—A new method for analysis of ergonomic effort. Applied Ergon 13(2):82–86, 1982.
77. Nordin, M., Ortengren, R., Andersson, G.B.J.: Measurement of trunk movement during work. Spine 9(5):465–469, 1984.
78. Kroemer, K.H.E.: Push forces exerted in 65 common work positions. AMRL-T-143, Aerospace Medical Research Laboratory, Wright Patterson Air Force Base, OH, 1969.
79. Frymoyer, J.W., et al.: Epidemiologic studies of low back pain. Spine 5(5):419–423, 1980.
80. Kelsey, J.L., Hardy, E.J.: Driving of motor vehicles as a risk factor for acute herniated lumbar intervertebral disc. Am J Epidemiol 102:63–73, 1975.
81. Edwards, R.G., Lang, K.O.: A mechanical impedance investigation of human response to vibration. AMRL-TR-64-91, Final Report, AD-609-006, US Air Force, 1964.
82. Pope, M.H., Wilder, D.G., Frymoyer, J.W.: Vibration as an aetiologic factor in low back pain. Proc Inst Mech Eng Conf on Low Back Pain. London, Inst Mech Eng Paper #C120/80, 1980.
83. Andersson, G.B.J., et al.: The sitting posture: an electromyographic and discometric study. Orthop Clin North Am 6:105–120, 1975.
84. Zagorski, J., et al.: Studies on the transmissions of vibrations in human organism exposed to low-frequency whole-body vibration. Acta Physiological Polonica 27:347–354, 1976.
85. Wilder, D.G., Frymoyer, J.W., Pope, M.H.: The effect of vibration on the spine of the seated individual. Automedica 6:5–35, 1985.

James Weinstein

6

Neurophysiology of Pain

PAIN

No matter where it occurs in the body, and no matter what the cause, the unpleasant emotional experience of pain is always an expression of neurological dysfunction. The perception of pain and its modulation occurs through a complex integrated system that receives messages and reacts to them. The reactions are not always of a "fight or flight" nature, but often are an attempt to respond to an unpleasant experience, pain. The intricacies of the central nervous system as related to low back pain are far from understood. Work among different disciplines must continue to put the parts of the puzzle together so that one can remain optimistic about the future of caring for those with back pain.

History

Late nineteenth century psychologists and anatomists recognized that nerve fibers have anatomically distinct endings. A German physician, Max Von Frey, proposed that each anatomically distinct nerve ending responds to a different type of stimulus; touch, temperature, and pain. Pain was considered a specific sensation, transmitted along a unique class of nerve fibers. Well before this, however, a seventeenth century French philosopher Rene Descarte wrote of the existence of specific pathways for transmitting pain information from an injured body part through the spinal cord to a pain center in the brain. This "telephone line" view of how pain messages are transmitted had been accepted for many years. The fact that transecting a nerve path, supposedly carrying pain messages, does not consistently alleviate pain reveals an important message about the generation of pain. Pain is, therefore, a complex perception and depends not only on the intensity of a stimulus but also on the situation in which it is experienced, and more importantly, on the affective component of the individual. Thus, it is a very subjective experience. It is known that in some cultures young men are asked to cross a river with a grappling hook embedded in their stomach to prove their manhood. In pictures of these young men, it is not obvious that they are in pain. However, the expression of pain and the severity of pain differs from one individual to another.

The subjective experience of pain is what makes the study of pain so difficult. Since the days of Descarte, a great deal of information has been accumulated in order to gain further understanding of how messages from injured tissue reach the brain. However, little information is available about the location in the brain where final decisions are made as to whether something is painful or not. In fact, very little is known regarding the cortical mechanisms involved in our perceptions of pain. To date, investigators of pain have been unable to communicate a good understanding of their patients' back pain. To this end, several investigators have themselves submitted to having their nerves crushed, cut, or resutured in order to observe and describe their sensory experiences; but none of these investigators have agreed with each other.

Definition

The taxonomy committee of the International Association for the Study of Pain defined pain as "an unpleasant sensory and emotional experience associated with actual or potential tissue damage, or described in terms of such damage."[1] The committee went on to say that pain is always subjective. Each individual learns the application of the word through experiences related to injury in early life. Pain often occurs in the absence of tissue damage and may in some instances be an emotional experience. If one regards his or her experience as painful and reports it in the same ways as pain caused by tissue damage, then it should be accepted as pain. Thus, pain does not always have to be tied to a damaging stimulus.

67

To understand back pain there must be framework from which to work. The main aim should be an understanding of the mechanisms, the nature of the back pain, and the rationale for treatment. When one understands the mechanisms, one can begin to institute rational treatment with predictable results. Unfortunately, back pain is what the patient feels and how he or she expresses these feelings to us. The limitations of the verbalization of these painful experiences are, as we know, restricting.

The very nature of back pain and its impact on industrialized countries imposes a sense of urgency.[2] Treatment modalities are so varied across health care workers that appropriate analysis of efficacy is difficult, at best. Thus, if one method of treatment fails, another is tried, and it is hard to study the natural history of any one condition or the result of a specific treatment.

It is the intent of this brief chapter to provide some insight into the basic mechanisms of the functional spinal unit.

EFFECTS OF COMPRESSION ON SPINAL NERVE ROOTS

Neurophysiologic studies indicate that nerves of the cauda equina may be more susceptible to compression than are the peripheral nerves. Studies using an animal model have analyzed the effects of graded compression on the cauda equina. The greater the compressive force and duration of compression, the greater the neural impairment and the longer and less predictable the recovery period. Changes in blood flow accompanied by intraneural edema and secondary scar formation may be responsible for changes in axoplasmic transport and nerve atrophy accompanied by Wallerian degeneration and regeneration.[3]

The axons within the dorsal and ventral roots are extensions of the dorsal root ganglion (DRG) and ventral horn neurons, respectively. The survival of these axons, therefore, depends on the integrity of their parent cell bodies, the physiologic connection with the soma and axonal transport mechanisms. Both dorsal and ventral roots contain myelinated and unmyelinated fibers.

The dorsal and ventral roots approximate at the level of the intervertebral foramen wherein the dorsal root merges with the DRG just beneath the pedicle. At each segment, the roots pass just dorsolateral to the intervertebral disc. The subarachnoid space continues out the nerve root sleeve a variable distance to about the level of the DRG. In this region the dorsal and ventral roots are separate structures, each contained within its own dural investment. Continuing peripherally, the distal portion of the DRG fuses with the ventral root to form the "spinal nerve," and the dural sheath becomes continuous with the epineurium.[4]

Dural ligaments have been identified that fix the dura and nerve roots at their exits from the main dural sac to the posterior longitudinal ligament and vertebral body periosteum proximal to the intervertebral disc. Fixation of the root also occurs at the intervertebral foramen where the epineural sheath of the spinal nerve is attached. These findings may explain how disc herniation or anterior compression may produce significant nerve root impingement without compression of the nerve root against the posterior elements.[5]

The dorsal root ganglion (DRG) is critically located at each functional spinal unit just beneath the pedicles and in front of the superior facets. The ganglion may be responsible for the modulation of several known causes of "mechanical low back pain." The ganglion is mechanically sensitive and contains several pain modulators.[6,7] The cells of the DRG terminate mainly in the substantia gelatinosa lamina II of the spinal cord, where the gate described by Melzack and Wall[8] is located. Each functional spinal unit and its adjacent tissues (ligaments, joint capsules, and muscles) receive innervation by a pleurisegmental group of nerves with both sympathetic and dorsal rami components. The sinuvertebral nerve most commonly arises at the distal pole of the DRG (Fig. 6–1). The largest component of the sinuvertebral nerve passes through the antero-superior part of the lumbar foramen cranial to the upper margin of the intervertebral disc and courses superomedially toward the posterior longitudinal ligament. As it approaches the ligament, it divides into superiorly and inferiorly directed rami which, in turn, provide numerous finer branches to the regional tissues.

NOCICEPTOR

A nociceptor is a receptor sensitive to a noxious or potentially noxious stimulus. These nociceptors, once fired, change their properties; some become more sensitive and some less sensitive. Complex unencapsulated endings are thought to be sensitive to tissue or joint position and encapsulated endings respond to pressure. Perivascular endings have vasomotor or vasosensory functions as well as a nociceptor system.[9]

Neural Anatomy (Nerve Endings)

There have been numerous investigations of the type and the distribution of peripheral nerves to and within the spinal tissues around the functional spinal unit or three joint complex (Table 6–1). Three types of myelinated nerve endings have been identi-

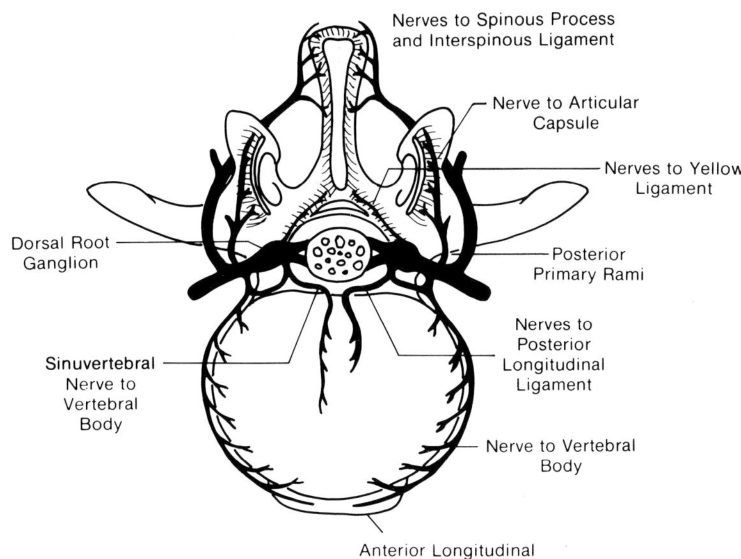

Figure 6–1. The functional spinal unit receives pleuri-segmental innervation by a combination of nerves.

fied:[10,11,12] (1) free nerve endings terminating as single tapered tips, (2) complex unencapsulated endings usually terminating in multiple branches with expanded tips, and (3) encapsulated nerve endings of the Vater-Pacini type. Unmyelinated perivascular nerve networks have also been described. Ma-

Table 6–1
Distribution of Peripheral Nerves to the Three-Joint Complex and Surrounding Soft Tissues

Fiber Type	Function	Location
Myelinated		
Free	Tissue or joint position	Facet joint capsules; anterior and lateral surfaces of annulus fibrosus; anterior/ posterior longitudinal ligaments; supraspinous/ intraspinous ligaments; periosteum
Complex Unencapsulated	Tissue or joint position	Same as listed above
Encapsulated	Pressure	Facet joint capsules; anterior and lateral surfaces of annulus fibrosus; periosteum
Unmyelinated		
Perivascular Simple	Vasomotor Vasosensory	Cartilage endplates; vertebrae; blood vessels
Complex	Nociceptor	
Free	Chemical	Annulus fibrosus; facet joint capsules; ligaments
	Mechanical	
Plexiform	Nociceptor	

linsky[11] identified two types of perivascular nerve endings in the immature annulus fibrosus: (1) simple, free termination of a thin nerve fiber along a capillary wall; and (2) complex branching of a thicker nerve fiber in a blood vessel wall. In addition, plexiform and free unmyelinated nerve fiber terminals, not associated with blood vessels, are present. The structure of these various nerve endings significantly influences the type of sensation perceived as well as its intensity.[4] Plexiform and freely ending unmyelinated nerve fibers respond to chemical or mechanical abnormalities and form the pain or nociceptive receptor system.

Encapsulated endings appear to be located primarily in the facet joint capsules and in the soft tissues along the anterior or lateral surfaces of annulus fibrosus.[10,11] The joint capsules also have free nerve endings and complex unencapsulated endings. The anterior and posterior longitudinal ligaments, the supraspinous ligaments, and the intraspinous ligaments contain free nerve fiber endings and complex unencapsulated endings.[10,13] The posterior longitudinal ligament appears to have the greatest density of nerve endings.[9] The cartilage endplates have perivascular nerves only.[13] The vertebral periosteum is supplied with free nerve endings and complex encapsulated nerve endings,[14] and the vertebrae have perivascular nerves as well as occasional solitary nerves.[15] A number of investigators have reported that the peripheral layers of the annulus fibrosus have free fiber endings, but they did not find nerves in the inner regions of the annulus fibrosus or nucleus pulposus.[10,11,13,16] However, Shinohara reported free fiber endings in the inner regions of the annulus and the nucleus pulposus of degenerated disc.[17] Other authors indicate that although unmyelinated nerves are present in fetal and neonatal disc, these nerves rapidly disappear with growth.[9] Thus, no nerves are present in the substances of the mature human intervertebral disc. Ultrastructural investigations, likewise, have failed to identify nerves in the inner annulus of the disc.

Nerve Fibers

In the peripheral nervous system three types of nerve fibers are found which transmit information from the body to the spinal cord and up to the brain.[18] The largest peripheral nerves, called A beta fibers, are from 5 to 12 micrometers in diameter. These respond to nonnoxious, noninjurious, and nonpainful stimuli. Because of their diameter, they transmit information very rapidly from the peripheral tissues to the spinal cord. A second type of fiber, called A delta fibers, range from 1 to 5 micrometers in diameter and transmit information much slower because of their smaller diameter. The smallest fibers, however, are called the unmyelinated C fibers. They are less than 1 micrometer in diameter and transmit information even slower than the A delta fibers. The A delta and the C fibers are predominantly nociceptors; i.e., they respond to injurious mechanical and thermostimuli as well as to endogenous chemicals released by damaged tissue. When you bump your elbow, the first sharp pain you experience is transmitted by the A delta fibers, whereas the second diffuse throbbing pain, possibly burning pain, is transmitted by the C fibers. One must remember that small diameter C fibers are exclusively activated by painful stimuli. However, large diameter fibers must be present and play a significant role in appreciation of the quality of the stimuli to be perceived. In the absence of large fibers such as A delta, a damaging stimulus might only be perceived as a burning sensation. It is possible, therefore, that in patients who have severe radicular symptoms, burning may be the most common complaint of patients having this peripheral nerve injury. A classic example is "causalgia," which literally means burning.

The low back pain patient often complains of pain when he is up or sitting but may be very comfortable in the supine nonmobile position. If there has been an injury, however, the normal "C" fiber threshold for mechanical, thermal, and chemical stimulation may be altered. Therefore, these fibers may become sensitized, with their threshold for sending a pain signal to the spinal cord and brain being considerably lowered. On the other hand, in the patient who has no history of back pain and no history of injury to the spine or its surrounding structures, ambulating and sitting may never cause pain, whereas those who have had an injury and have an altered thermostatic setting or threshold for pain may experience severe pain with even the slightest motions.

CHEMICAL MEDIATORS

Peripheral

Sensitization of the nerve fibers around the functional spinal unit can be the result of a variety of chemical neurogenic and non-neurogenic mediators from injured and inflamed tissues. Significant work in the area of arachidonic acid released from membranes of damaged cells has been done. Arachidonic acid may be acted upon by two enzymes, cycloxygenase and lipoxygenase, producing prostaglandins and the less well known leukotrienes. Leukotrienes can lower the threshold for activation of peripheral nerves. Most of us are aware of aspirin's effects and the nonsteroidal effects of other drugs that work by blocking cycloxygenase. Leukotrienes are not blocked in this way and, therefore, in an inflammatory state may be the unsuppressed culprit responsible for our sensitization of pain fibers and, therefore, for a lowered pain threshold (Fig. 6–2).

Neurogenic mediators such as substance P communicate with second order neurons in the dorsal horn of the spinal cord, providing information to our brain. Although substance P may be the best known neurotransmitter, it is only one of the neuropeptides used by C fibers to communicate within the central nervous system. It is produced by approximately 20 percent of "C" fibers in the dorsal

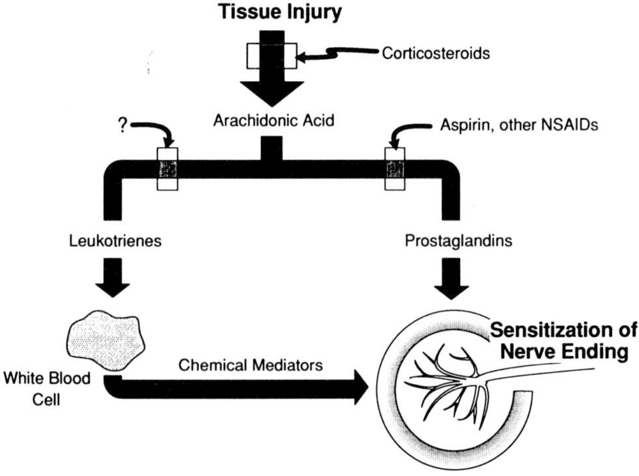

Figure 6–2. In response to tissue injury, non-neurogenic mediators are released from the arachidonic acid of the damaged cell membranes. Two major categories exist: prostaglandins and leukotrienes.

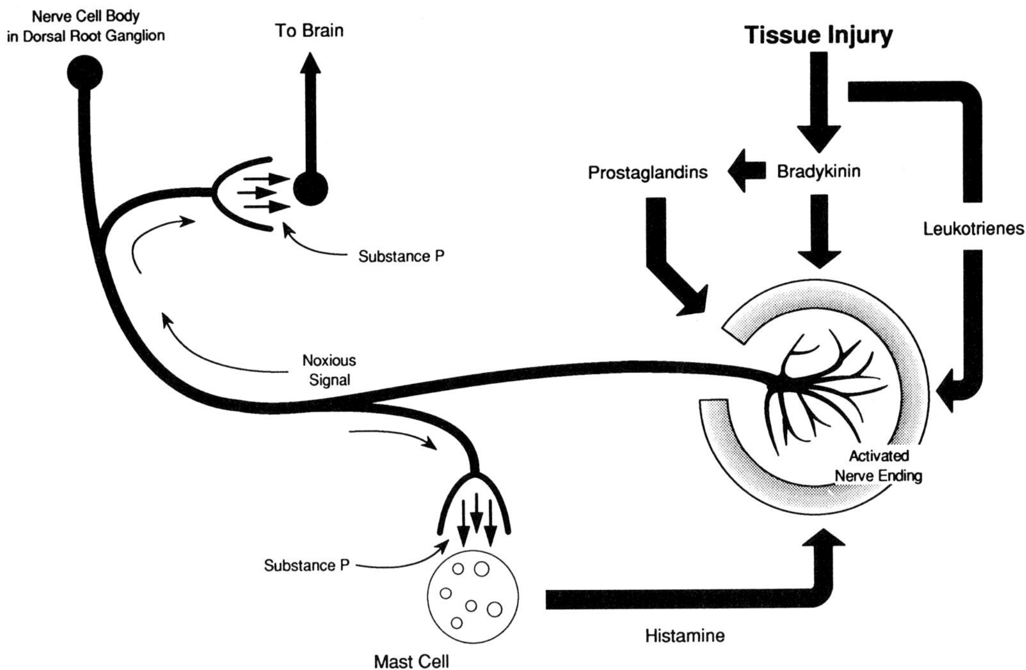

Figure 6–3. Bradykinin can stimulate prostaglandin synthesis as a result of tissue injury. Neurogenic mediators (i.e., substance P) may also be activated by tissue injury and affect both central and peripheral pain and inflammatory mechanisms.

root ganglion and excites spinal cord cells that transmit messages to the brain (Fig. 6–3).

In addition to substance P and the products of arachidonic acid, many other compounds are released from injured tissues. Bradykinin, a non-neurogenic peptide similar in size to substance P but different in structure, is of particular interest because it not only activates "C" fibers to cause pain but simultaneously stimulates the synthesis of prostaglandins, which lowers the threshold of fibers producing enhanced sensitivity to pain (Fig. 6–3).

One can see how inflammation, pain, and the nervous system are intricately related and how the nervous system is a necessary component for the inflammatory response. Tissue injury, therefore, can activate both neurogenic (i.e., substance P) and non-neurogenic (i.e., Bradykinin) systems that in many cases work synergistically to affect local tissue responses, central modulation, and activation of the pain system. These injury and response mechanisms have been well established but not fully understood (Fig. 6–3).

Central

When a nerve (root or peripheral) is injured, dorsal root ganglion cells send an afferent barrage of signals to the central nervous system (CNS).[19] How the CNS handles these messages is critical to our understanding of the relationship of pain to injury. Realizing that these nerve receptors can send false signals when they receive unusual messages from damaged peripheral tissues further confounds the problem. To this end, Melzack and Wall produced the gate control theory[8,18] (Fig. 6–4). Messages concerned with pain are transmitted via central cells in the dorsal horn of the spinal cord. This painful transmission within the spinal cord depends on three factors: (1) the arrival of the nociceptive messages; (2) the convergent effect of other peripheral afferents, which may exaggerate or diminish the effects of the nociceptive message; and (3) the presence of control systems within the CNS, which influence the central cells. Melzack and Wall emphasized that convergent controls decide the fate of the arriving messages as they pass through every level of the CNS and eventually produce reaction, sensation, and movement.[8,18]

From the dorsal horn of the spinal cord, the message ascends to its first level of consciousness, the thalamus. Then, the message ascends to the postcentral gyrus of the brain wherein the nature and location of the pain is interpreted. The frontal lobe provides an affective component, whereas the temporal lobe provides stored memories from previous

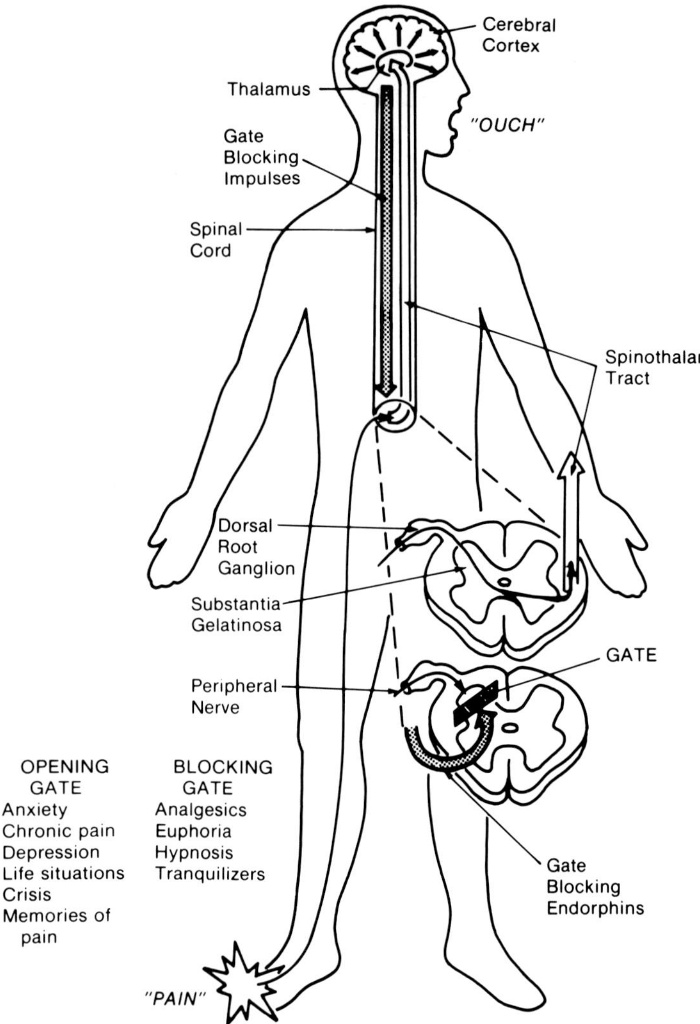

Figure 6-4. A diagrammatic sketch of the gate control theory of pain. Descartes first described such a pathway in 1664. (1) First a toe is injured; this causes a release of various pain modulators, such as substance P. This starts the pain signal on its way as an electrical impulse. (2) The message proceeds to the thalamus, the area of the brain where the painful stimulus first becomes conscious. (4) The message then reaches the cerebral cortex, where the location of pain and its intensity are perceived. (5) Transmission of gate blocking impulses descend from the brain via the spinal cord to provide pain relief. (6) In the dorsal horn, chemicals such as endorphins are released to diminish the pain message from the injured toe.

painful experiences. Some cells within the dorsal horn of the spinal cord (substantia gelatinosa, laminae II) learn to respond not only to a painful stimulus but also to an alerting signal that says a noxious stimulus is about to happen. Thus, the signaling of injury by the central cells in the dorsal horn of the spinal cord depends not only on the arrival of a nociceptive afferent impulse but on other peripheral events and the thermostatic setting of excitability by the various central nervous system mechanisms as well. These controls are contingent on one another and help to explain our variable responses to injury. The presence of such controls means that they themselves may become locked into a pathologic position and exaggerate or create pain.

It is through these control systems that various therapeutic modalities have been used in the treatment of back pain (electrical stimulations, acupuncture, analgesia, manipulation). The challenge is to have a better understanding of this complicated system and its peripheral influences (Fig. 6-4).

CENTRAL PAIN MODULATION

The dorsal horn of the spinal cord, site of the first synapse of the pain pathway, is where neurotransmitters modulate nociceptive processing both pre- and post-synaptically. Both primary afferent neuron input, as well as convergent, peptineurgic input from local circuit neurons and descending bulbospinal neurons of the spinal cord and mid-brain affect responses made at the first synaptic junction.

Much attention has been given to opioidergic neurons in the spinal cord because of their ability to inhibit nociceptive transmission. However, neurotensin, a non-opiod neuropeptide found in the spinal cord, also has inhibitory capacities.[20]

Ascending neurons known to be peptineurgic have been identified in the cerebral cortex and subthalamic, spinohypothalamic-telencephalic pathways. Surprisingly, however, the spinothalamic tract itself may not utilize neuropeptides for neurotransmission.

Families of endogenous, morphine-like, opiods have been described. Most familiar, of course, are the B-endorphins. Other less well known, but not less important, endogenous chemicals are dynorphins. These act at several different types of receptors. Endorphins, typically act at the mu receptors, while the dynorphins have an affinity for k-receptors.[2] In the spinal cord, the principal sources of opiod-like peptides are the intrinsic dorsal horn neurons. Most are local circuit interneurons.

As you can see, "pain" is not a simple perception. Although millions of people suffer because of it and billions of dollars are spent trying to eradicate it, we are only in our infancy of understanding the very complex interactions necessary to perceive or distort our feelings of pain. In the future, we must continue to seek a better understanding of not only our patient's macroscopic expressions of pain, but we also must look microscopically at each cell involved in the whole of the pain process. A time will come when our molecular understanding will provide us with the means to unlock the secrets of pain. Since the time of Descarte, we have come a long way, but we have a great deal more work to do if we are going to provide our patients better remedies in the future.

REFERENCES

1. Merskey, H.: Pain terms: a list with definitions and notes on usage. Recommended by the IASP Subcommittee on Taxonomy. Pain 6:249, 1979.
2. Frymoyer, J.: New Perspectives on Low Back Pain. Chicago, AAOS Publishers, May, 1989.
3. Rydevik, B., McLean, W.G., Sjöstrand, J., et al.: Blockage of axonal transport induced by acute, graded compression of the rabbit vagus nerve. J Neurol Neurosurg Psychiatr 43:690–698, 1980.
4. Sunderland, S.: Nerve and nerve injuries. *In* Peripheral Sensory Mechanism. 2nd Ed. New York, Churchill Livingstone, 1978.
5. Spencer, D.L., Irwin, G.S., Miller J.A.: Anatomy and significance of fixation of the lumbosacral nerve roots in sciatica. Spine *8*:672–679, 1983.
6. Weinstein, J.N.: Mechanisms of spinal pain: the dorsal root ganglion and its role as a mediator of low back pain. Spine *11*:999–1001, 1986.
7. Weinstein, J.N., Pope, M., Schmidt, R., et al.: Neuropharmacological effects of vibration: An animal model. Spine *13*:521–525, 1988.
8. Melzack, R., Wall, P.D.: Pain mechanisms: a new theory. Science *150*:971–979, 1965.
9. Wyke, B.D.: The neurology of low back pain. *In* The Lumbar Spine and Back Pain (Edited by M.I.V. Jayson). 2nd Ed. Kent, Pitman Medical Publishing, 1980.
10. Hirsch, C., Ingelmark, B., Miller, M.: The anatomical basis for low back pain. Acta Orthop Scand 33:2, 1963.
11. Malinksy, J.: The ontogenetic development of nerve terminations in the intervertebral discs of man. Acta Anat 38:96, 1959.
12. Ralston, H.J., Miller, M.R., Kasahara, M.: Nerve endings in human fasciae, tendons, ligaments, periosteum, and joint synovial membrane. Anat Rec 136:137, 1960.
13. Jackson, H.C., Winkelmann, R.K., Bickel, W.H.: Nerve endings in the human lumbar spinal column and related structures. J Bone Joint Surg 48A:1271, 1966.
14. Ikari, C.: A study of the mechanisms of low back pain. The neurohistochemical examination of disease. J Bone Joint Surg 36A:195, 1954.
15. Sherman, M.S.: The nerves of bone. J Bone Joint Surg 45A:522, 1963.
16. Roofe, P.G.: Innervation of the annulus fibrosus and posterior longitudinal ligament. Arch Neurol Psych 44:100, 1940.
17. Shinohara, H.: Lumbar disc lesion with special reference to the histological significance of nerve endings of the lumbar discs. J Jpn Orthop Assoc 44:553–570, 1970.
18. Wall, P.D., Melzack, R.: Textbook of Pain. Churchill Livingstone, New York, pp. 1–15, 1984.
19. Wall, P.D.: Alterations in the central nervous system after deafferentation. *In* Advances in Pain Research 5. Raven, New York, 1983.
20. Ruda, M.A., Coffield, J., Dubner, R.: Demonstration of postsynaptic opioid modulation of thalamic projection neurons by the combined techniques of retrograde horseradish peroxidase and enkephalin immunocytochemistry. J Neurosci 4:2117–2132, 1984.

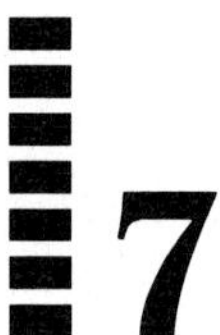

7

David R. Eyre

The Intervertebral Disc and Spinal Disease: Biochemical Concepts

INTRODUCTION

The intervertebral disc is largely an extracellular fabric, based on a complex collagen framework that incorporates at least eight different molecular types of collagen.[1] The strength of the disc rests on the integrity of this collagen architecture. The mechanical properties are also governed heavily by the highly hydrated proteoglycans which inflate and stiffen the collagen.[2] In general, the proteoglycans resemble those of other cartilages but do show distinctive chemical properties. Besides collagen and proteoglycans, the extracellular matrix is rich in various other proteins of poorly understood function.[1] No unique proteins have yet been identified in disc tissue. Such molecules, for example, might be useful as serum markers for monitoring disc degeneration and injury.

Though the disc consists largely of extracellular materials, living cells are essential for maintaining the structure and, hence, normal function of the fabric of the tissue throughout life.[3] Because the tissue is avascular, an adequate supply of nutrients and removal of waste products of cell metabolism by diffusion is also vital for maintaining normal disc mechanical behavior. With aging, signs of progressive degeneration that include decreased hydration, loss of glycosaminoglycans, increasing yellow/brown pigmentation, internal tears, dislocations and prolapses into adjacent vertebral bodies, are typical of adult human spines.[4] These changes, and other biochemical and biomechanical considerations, continue to implicate the disc as a key suspect in the low back syndrome. This chapter summarizes the current understanding of normal disc biochemistry and discusses potential links to back pain. A concept of molecular mechanics is also touched on, namely the fundamental goal of relating the mechanical properties of the disc as a whole to its component structural macromolecules. In this way, changes in biochemical composition that would critically alter material properties and predispose the tissue to mechanical failure might be predicted.

The biochemist's interest in the intervertebral disc has so far tended to focus on understanding the composition and molecular organization of its extracellular matrix. The relevance of matrix biochemistry to the low back syndrome is twofold: (1) the fabric may gradually fail mechanically with increasing age and result in increased stress and damage to other supporting structures of the spine (e.g., the facet joints and assorted ligaments), and thus produce pain; and (2) the matrix may be a source of unique breakdown products that could elicit pain, either directly from nerve endings within the outer annulus or in surrounding ligaments, or indirectly via an inflammatory response.[5] The biochemist is also interested in the metabolism of the cells of the disc in order to understand their role in synthesizing the tissue's unique extracellular fabric and their ability to maintain it during life. Cellular viability could be affected by an impairment in nutrient supply or in waste product removal, thereby shortening the mechanical life of the disc.

NORMAL STRUCTURE AND FUNCTION OF THE DISC

The ultimate strength of the disc, as of most connective tissues, rests on the tensile strength of its extracellular collagen framework. Collagen fibrils are strong in tension because their individual collagen molecules are cross-linked to each other by covalent bonds. The basic form of the collagen fibril has altered little in over 500 million years of evolution, being seen by the electron microscope as a mechanical framework of even the most primitive multicellular animals.[6] It is clear, however, that an extensive variety of molecular modifiers of collagen fibrils have evolved to suit the mechanical needs of different organisms and their specialized tissues. In this context, the collagen fabric of the disc appears to be unusually complex in molecular composition, yet highly organized as a functional mechanical unit.

Collagen content ranges from 10 to 20% of the dry weight of the nucleus to about 70% of the outer annulus.[7] We have known for about 15 years that two main collagen types, types I and II, form the bulk collagen structure, with type I collagen predominant in the ligament-like outer lamellae of the annulus fibrosus and type II predominant in the inner annulus and nucleus pulposus.[8–10] Proteoglycans, and hence water-swelling properties, are most concentrated in the nucleus and inner annulus, where type II is the main collagen, and gradually drop in concentration toward the type I collagen-rich outer lamellae of the annulus.[7] The following summary of current understanding of the biochemical make-up of the disc expands on this basic molecular anatomy.

Cells of the Disc

Cell density in the disc is very low, even for a connective tissue, ranging from about 4000 cells per mm^3 in the nucleus pulposus, 9000 per mm^3 in annulus fibrosus, to 15,000 per mm^3 in the cartilage end plates (the latter density being similar to that of articular cartilage).[1,11] Three cell types have been noted: notochordal cells (seen in the nucleus during development), and fibrocytes and chondrocytes. Notochordal cells disappear from the nucleus in childhood and their synthetic contribution to the extracellular fabric of the nucleus pulposus is determined.[12] The fibrocytes and chondrocytes do not seem to be two distinct cell populations, rather, they are descriptive terms that characterize the changing shape of the disc cells from a more rounded, chondrocytic appearance in the nucleus and inner annulus to a flattened, more fibroblast-like appearance in the outer regions of the annulus.[13]

Whether cohorts of one type of cell (ligamentous fibroblast?) make predominantly one type of matrix (e.g., the type I, collagen-rich, organized fiber bundles of the annular lamellae) and cohorts of another cell type (chondroblast) fabricate inter- and intralamellar collagenous matrix (type II, collagen-rich), is not known. However, neither histologic nor ultrastructural studies have provided convincing signs that such distinct domains are interwoven, each populated by cells of distinct appearance. An alternative concept is of a single, specialized type of disc cell that is modulated in its phenotypic expression (e.g., type I or type II collagen-based matrix) by its environment (e.g., local mechanical stress fields, O_2 tension, cytokine concentrations, influence of matrix molecules through cell surface receptors).[1]

In the mature disc, the cells clearly continue to be active in synthesizing proteoglycans, and presumably other matrix molecules, that are damaged, lost and removed through the effects of normal mechanical wear and tear and enzyme action.[14] The falling levels of sulfated glycosaminoglycans with increasing age, the decrease in hydration, the accumulation of noncollagenous protein and other age-related changes in composition[7] may reflect a failing ability of the disc cells to maintain the fabric in its juvenile state. A failing vascular supply to the end-plates, the main route for nutrition and waste removal for disc tissue, could be a key factor here.[15]

Collagens

Although more than 13 collagen types based on 20 or more genes exist in vertebrate tissues (Table 7–1), little is known about their distinctive functions and why so many types of molecule have evolved.[16] Evidence is growing, however, for an inherent capacity of certain types of collagen molecule to interact and copolymerize, thus forming hybrid fibril structures. This adds a new dimension to understanding how the diversity in material properties of different collagenous tissues might be modulated, and the means by which cells can tailor such variability.

At least eight molecular types of collagen are present in the intervertebral disc (Table 7-2). The nucleus pulposus contains types II, VI, IX and XI, and the annulus fibrosus contains types I, II, III, V, VI, IX, XI and XII collagens. How these collagen types are organized, interrelate, and function in the extracellular matrix is essentially unknown.

Types I and II Collagens

About two-thirds of the dry mass of the disc consists of types I and II collagen fibrils distributed radially in opposing concentration gradients. Type II collagen dominates in the nucleus pulposus and type I collagen in the outermost lamellae of the annulus fibrosus.[7]

Disc type I collagen differs chemically from type I collagen of skin, tendon, and bone in being richer in hydroxylysine and hydroxylysine glycosides and being extensively cross-linked by hydroxypyridinium

Table 7–1
Types of Collagen Molecule

	Molecular Formula	Tissue Distribution
Class 1—300nm Triple Helix (Banded Fibril)		
Type I	$[\alpha1(I)]_2\alpha2(I)$	Skin, Bone, Tendon, etc.
Type II	$[\alpha1(II)]_3$	Hyaline Cartilage, Disc, Vitreous
Type III	$[\alpha1(III)]_3$	Skin, Vascular Tissue, etc.
Type V	$[\alpha1(V)]_2\alpha2(V)$ et al	with Type I
Type XI	$\alpha1(XI)\alpha2(XI)\alpha3(XI)$	with Type II
Class 2—Basement Membranes		
Type IV	$[\alpha1(IV)]_2\alpha2(IV)$ et al	Basal Lamina
Type VII	$[\alpha1(VII)]_3$	Epithelial Basement Membrane
Type VIII	$[\alpha1(VIII)]_3$	Endothelial Basement Membrane
Class 3—Short Helix		
Type VI	$\alpha1(VI)\alpha2(VI)\alpha3(VI)$	Widespread
Type IX	$\alpha1(IX)\alpha2(IX)\alpha3(IX)$	with Type II
Type X	$[\alpha1(X)]_3$	Hypertrophic & Calcified Cartilage
Type XII	$[\alpha1(XII)]_3$	Tendon, Skin, Disc, etc.
Type XIII	Unknown	Endothelial Cells

Table 7–2
Collagen Types in the Intervertebral Disc

			% of Total Collagen
Class I—Fibril Forming			
Type I	$[\alpha1(I)]_2\alpha2(I)$	Annulus	80–0
Type II	$[\alpha1(II)]_3$	Annulus + Nucleus	0–80
Type III	$[\alpha1(III)]_3$	Annulus	<5
Type V	$[\alpha1(V)]_2\alpha2(V)$	Annulus + Nucleus	1–2
Type XI	$[\alpha1(XI)\alpha2(XI)\alpha3(XI)]$	Annulus + Nucleus	1–2
Short-Helix Collagens			
Type VI	$[\alpha1(VI)\alpha2(VI)\alpha3(VI)]$	Annulus + Nucleus	5–20
Type IX	$\alpha1(IX)\alpha2(IX)\alpha3(IX)$	Annulus + Nucleus	1–2
Type XII	$[\alpha1(XII)]_3$	Annulus	<1

residues.[7,10,17] Similarly, disc type II collagen is richer in hydroxylysine, hydroxylysine glycosides, and hydroxypyridinium cross-links than type II collagen of articular cartilage.

It is generally assumed that types I and II collagens are restricted to their own homopolymeric fibril type. However, this may not be so. Indeed, from the complete primary structures of the $\alpha1(I)$ and $\alpha1(II)$ procollagen chains, there is no obvious reason why they cannot substitute for each other in the same molecule let alone in the same fibril. (Their triple-helical domains are of identical length, and their C-propeptides are of closely conserved sequence.)

Types V and XI Collagens

Type XI collagen dominates in the nucleus pulposus and type V collagen in the annulus fibrosus.[1,18–20] The range of molecular formulae that types V and XI collagens represent is still unclear.[21] It has been shown in cornea that types I and V collagens are intimately associated, and so may be copolymerized within the same fibril network.[22] Other evidence for hybrid fibrils that embody types I and V collagens has been reported.[23] One possibility for the disc, therefore, is that type V collagen is copolymerized with type I collagen in the same fibril network, and similarly type XI collagen with type II collagen. Smith, et al.,[24] however, have provided data implying that type XI collagen specifically binds to sulfated glycosaminoglycans and may be more concentrated around the chondrocyte periphery than farther out in the matrix.

An added complexity is the finding that in bone and tendon (and probably other tissues), the $\alpha1(XI)$ chain is present in increasing amounts with developmental age in the isolated type V collagen fraction.[25] The data imply that $\alpha1^{XI}$ can substitute for $\alpha1(V)$ in hybrid type V/XI molecules. Similarly, in articular cartilage, the $\alpha1(V)$ chain appears in increasing amounts with developmental age in the type XI collagen fraction, apparently substituting for $\alpha1(XI)$ chains. The significance of this development-related change in expression of collagen type V/XI gene products and of the suspected hybrid collagen molecules is unknown.

Type VI Collagen

Though a minor protein in the extracellular matrix of many connective tissues, type VI collagen is strikingly abundant in the intervertebral disc.[26] Previous electron microscopic studies of nucleus pulposus had noted an abundance of unusual banded structures with a 110nm periodicity.[27–29] Similar aggregates had been noted in small amounts in other tissues.[27,30] These structures have turned out to consist largely of lateral aggregates of microfilamentous type VI collagen.[30-33] The type VI collagen molecule consists of a short triple helix with a large globular domain at each end. Three gene products [α1(VI), α2(VI), and α3(VI)] have been sequenced as cDNAs, with interesting sequence homologies to domains in von Willebrand factor. They also contain several Arg-Gly-Asp (RGD) sequences that suggest cell binding properties.[34] Though the function of type VI collagen is still not known, it is unlikely that it provides tensile strength akin to that of the 640nm-banded collagen fibrils. No aldehyde-mediated crosslinks were found in purified type VI collagen, and the protein essentially was fully extracted as dimeric and tetrameric molecules by 4M guanidine-HCl.[26] Possible functions include a matrix organizing role through its suspected ability to bind cells and fibrillar collagens, separating and preventing covalent interaction between collagen fibrils, or acting as a cell matrix adhesion protein. Type VI collagen is found in most soft connective tissues, including skin, tendon, aorta and cartilage, is prominent in certain tumors, and is synthesized by fibroblasts in culture.[30,32,33,35] Its abundance in the annulus and nucleus implies that its properties make an important contribution to the distinctive biomechanical properties of the intervertebral disc. No aging changes in type VI collagen content have yet been documented.

Type IX Collagen

Type IX collagen has had several names, being first called type M collagen.[36] It is a form of proteoglycan molecule in the chick (with a chondroitin sulfate chain on the NC3 domain of its α2(IX) chain) and is a heterotrimer of three distinct gene products.[37] It appears in all tissues that contain type II collagen. The concentration of type IX collagen in mature nucleus pulposus (1 to 2% by weight) is similar to that in hyaline cartilages (Wu, J.J. and Eyre, D.R., unpublished observations). The concentration in annulus fibrosus appears to be lower than in nu-

cleus pulposus, and is in proportion to the type II collagen content. In hyaline cartilages, type IX collagen is much more abundant during development than in adult tissue,[38] and this may also be true in the nucleus pulposus.

Monoclonal antibodies have shown that type IX collagen is spread throughout the extracellular matrix of cartilage in close association with type II collagen.[39] The same kind of cross-linking amino acids that polymerize type II collagen molecules were found to be even more abundant in type IX collagen prepared by pepsin digestion.[40] This raised the possibility that type IX collagen may be cross-linked to type II collagen, perhaps as a long suspected interfibrillar "glue" molecule in cartilages.[40] Indeed, immunogold localizations under the electron microscope implied that type IX collagen molecules may be concentrated where type II fibrils intersect.[41] Finally, by amino acid sequence analysis of cross-linked peptides derived from bovine type IX collagen, it was discovered that the molecule did indeed exist in the matrix largely in covalent linkage to telopeptide sequences of type II collagen.[42] Specific helical sites in the COL2 domain of all three chains, α1(IX), α2(IX) and α3(IX), were able to link to α1(II) N-telopeptides,[38,42] and an apparently different helical site in the α3(IX)COL2 domain was linked to α1(II) C-telopeptides.[43] Further sites of intermolecular cross-linking in type IX collagen are evident,[43] and it would seem that type IX collagen functions in covalent linkage as a fibril modifying protein (Fig. 7–1). It remains to be seen whether it mediates links between fibrils or between fibrils and other interfibrillar components of cartilage.

Type XII Collagen

Type XII collagen is another newly discovered short helix collagenous protein. Discovered in embryonic chick tendon as a cDNA sequence with coding homologies to type IX collagen,[44] and as an extractable protein with a prominent band on elec-

Figure 7–1. A type II collagen fibril decorated with covalently linked type IX collagen molecules. Evidence is growing that such heteropolymeric structures between different molecular types of collagen may be a general phenomenon.

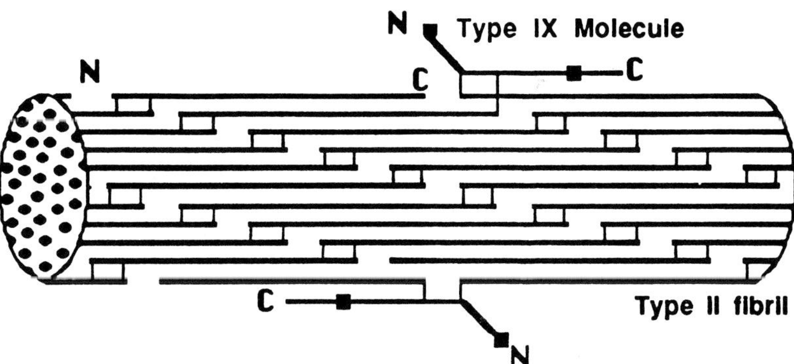

trophoresis at about 200kDa,[45] variant forms of type XII collagen are now indicated in skin and other connective tissues, including the annulus fibrosus.[46] First thought to be the type I collagen fibril's equivalent of type IX collagen, the molecule is now known to share sequence homology with type IX collagen in only one collagenous domain, COL1, with the rest of the molecule having a different appearance.[47] Its concentration in bovine annulus fibrosus is less than 1% of the total collagenous protein (Wu, J.J., personal communication).

Collagen Cross-Linking

Skeletal connective tissue collagens become chemically cross-linked through lysyl oxidase largely by the hydroxylysine aldehyde route.[48] The initial cross-links on this pathway are borohydride-reducible ketoamines. Soon after the fibrils polymerize outside the cell, these crosslinks chemically mature into non-reducible, more complex cross-linking structures. In cartilage and disc tissue, the mature crosslinks appear to be exclusively trivalent hydroxypyridinium residues (pyridinolines).[17,49] Two chemical forms are known, hydroxylysyl pyridinoline (HP) and lysyl pyridinoline (LP) (Fig. 7–2), which are post-translational variants resulting from incomplete hydroxylation of lysine residues at helical domain cross-linking sites (Fig. 7–1). The latter compound, LP, is largely restricted to bone collagen; HP alone is found in significant amounts in the normal disc. In a case of the heritable disorder Ehlers-Danlos Syndrome type VI, LP and HP were equally abundant in disc tissue.[17] One proposed chemical mechanism of formation is an interaction between two ketoamine crosslinks.[50] It is notable that pyridinoline crosslinks are more concentrated in collagens of the disc than in any other vertebrate connective

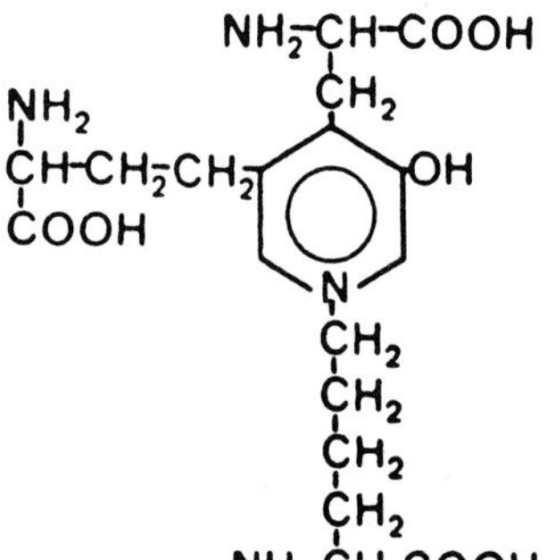

tissue.[17,49] In adult human nucleus pulposus the concentration of HP can reach 3 moles per mole of collagen.[51] Annulus fibrosus and articular cartilage each contain about two HP residues per molecule of collagen.

Proteoglycans

Disc tissue is kept swollen with water in large part because of the physical properties of its sulfated proteoglycans, which are most concentrated in the nucleus pulposus and gradually decrease in concentration from inner to outer annulus as collagen content increases.[27] Disc proteoglycans in general resemble those of hyaline (e.g., articular) cartilage, in that they are the large, aggregating types of molecule (PG-LA), containing chondroitin sulfate and keratan sulfate chains, which form specific, high affinity aggregates with hyaluronic acid that are stabilized by a link protein (Fig. 7–3). There are chemical differences, however, between disc and cartilage proteoglycans, notably in their glycosaminoglycan compositions and in their relative amounts of aggregating and nonaggregating molecules.[2] Thus, disc proteoglycans tend to be richer than most other cartilage proteoglycans in keratan sulfate and to contain a lower proportion of molecules that are capable of forming aggregates with hyaluronic acid. Disc proteoglycans also tend to be smaller and more polydisperse in molecular size than cartilage proteoglycans.[70] In general, proteoglycans from young adult discs more closely resemble proteoglycans of articular cartilage from much older individuals. Small proteoglycan molecules (PG-S1, or biglycan, and PG-S2, or decorin[52]) are also represented in the disc, as they are in many connective tissues. Interesting differences have been seen by electron microscopy using

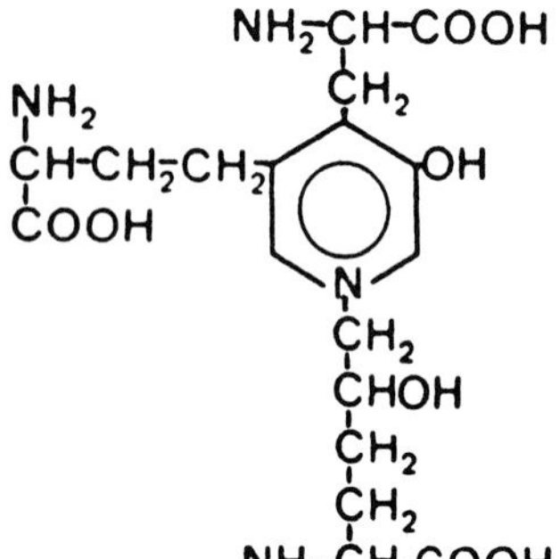

Figure 7–2. Structures of the two known chemical forms of 3-hydroxypyridine cross-link. Mature intervertebral disc collagen is cross-linked almost exclusively by hydroxylysyl pyridinoline (HP) residues (forming the intermolecular bonds indicated in Figure 1). Nucleus pulposus collagen has the highest concentration of any vertebrate connective tissue.

HYDROXYLYSYL PYRIDINOLINE (HP)

LYSYL PYRIDINOLINE (LP)

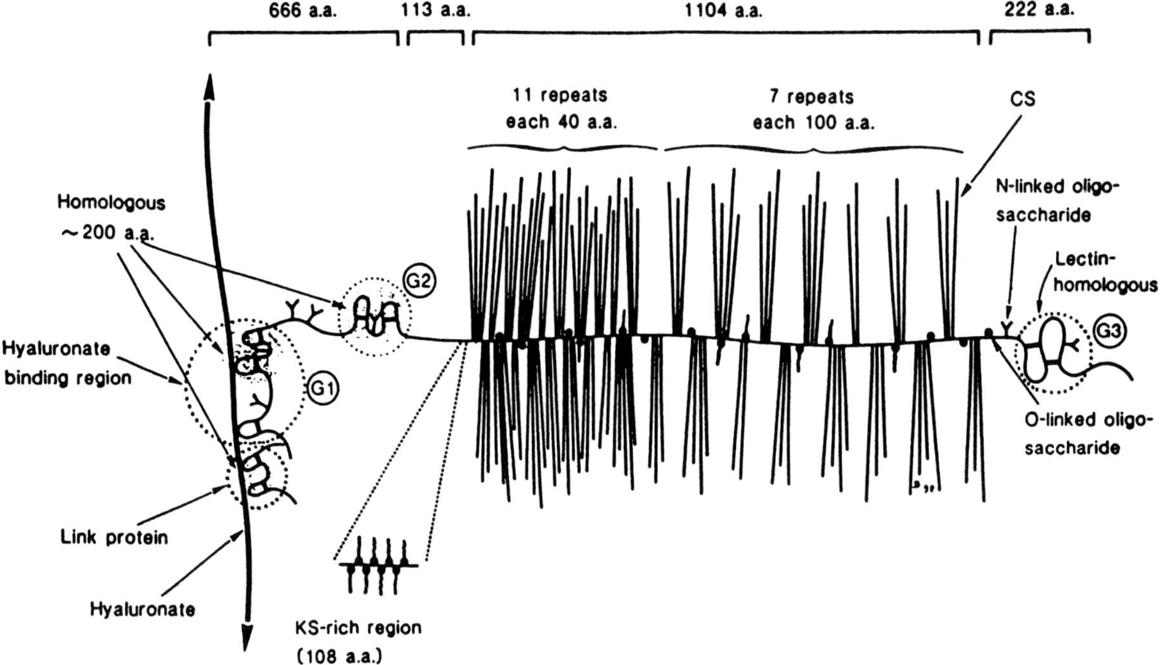

Figure 7–3. Molecular model of a cartilage proteoglycan subunit (PG-LA) aggregated on hyaluronic acid. Disc proteoglycans conform to this model, but the subunits are richer in keratan sulfate (longer chains probably), have a more diverse range of molecular sizes, and include fragments that no longer can aggregate with hyaluronic acid. (From Heinegård, D., Oldberg, A.: Structure and biology of cartilage and bone matrix noncollagenous macromolecules. FASEB J. 3:2042–2051, 1989.)

Cupromeronic blue stain in the orientation of different proteoglycans in association with collagen fibrils in rabbit annulus fibrosus.[80] The full range of genetically distinct types of proteoglycans in disc tissue and their function, however, is not yet well resolved.

Other Matrix Proteins

Though collagens and proteoglycans make up the bulk of disc tissue, various other proteins may be present in the extracellular matrix, including fibronectin,[1] 148 kDa cartilage matrix protein in immature tissue,[53] a 116 kDa subunit polymeric protein,[54] 58 kDa protein, 59 kDa protein (fibromodulin),[55] and a 36 kDa protein.[56] Each of these proteins exhibits preferential binding affinities for collagen, proteoglycans, or chondrocyte attachment, and they may function as specific adhesion proteins in the matrix regulating assembly and interactions of the collagen fibrils and proteoglycans.[57] Sparsely distributed elastic fibers have also been seen in the annulus fibrosus by light and electron microscopy,[58] but apparently only near the sites of attachment to the vertebrae.[59]

No proteins that are unique to disc tissue have yet been identified. Novel molecules that could distinguish the phenotype of annulus or nucleus from other tissues might be very useful as plasma markers for monitoring disc degradation.[1] For example, if low back pain can be the direct result of acute disc injury (not visible by radiography or by other imaging methods), then it would be feasible to seek an increase in plasma levels of disc-specific antigens that correlate with the incidence of the painful episodes. Future biochemical research might achieve such a goal.

Metabolism and Turnover

Collagen in the disc turns over very slowly. Maroudas[61] calculated a turnover time of over one hundred years based on radiolabeled proline uptake into hydroxyproline in adult dogs. However, it would be valuable to know the turnover rate of each collagen type in order to understand the capacity for collagenous matrix remodeling in the adult tissue. It is possible that a minor collagen, e.g., type VI, type IX, or type XII, is turned over more rapidly than the fibrillar collagens as a means of reorganizing the bulk collagen network without replacing it.

Experience with articular cartilage, and to some extent disc tissue, has shown that their cells can rapidly replace proteoglycans, which presumably are being continually lost from the matrix. Intradiscal injection of papain in dogs in vivo led to a significant loss of disc height radiographically.[62] If the papain dosage was adjusted so that the collagen architecture remained substantially undamaged, the disc recovered to normal height, presumably because the cells were able to replace the lost proteoglycans responsible for the decreased osmotic swelling pressure of the collagen architecture.

NUTRITION

The interior of the annulus and the nucleus receive nutrition and have wastes removed purely by diffusion through the end plates of the vertebral bodies, which are supplied with a capillary bed. This is the major route of nutrition and waste removal for the disc.[1,15,63,64] Outer layers of annulus may receive nutrition from a peripheral vascular supply. The end plate route shows evidence of impairment with age.[1,15] The cartilage of the endplates becomes more calcified, perhaps affecting diffusion. The capillary bed architecture also alters, and the commonly seen herniations of disc material into the vertebral bodies (Schmorl's nodes) may further impair nutrition and waste removal with the potential to affect metabolism and result in cell death.

Small solutes (e.g., O_2, CO_2, amino acids, glucose, lactate, sulfate) are transported within the disc largely by diffusion. Pumping or convective transport through mechanical loading are thought unlikely to be significant.[1,65] Lactate gradients produced by the anaerobic metabolism of disc cells have been calculated and indicate that the highest lactate concentration, which occurs at the center of the nucleus, may produce a pH as low as 6.6 in degenerate discs.[1,66] This may be relevant, since acids can trigger nociceptors and cause pain.

AGE-RELATED CHANGES

The disc shows biochemical and material signs of aging faster and earlier than other connective tissues, the accumulation of keratan sulfate rich proteoglycans being an example.[67] A decreased water content of the nucleus and annulus with increasing age is also linked to an overall loss of sulfated glycosaminoglycans from the tissue.[1,7,68] At the same time, noncollagenous protein and hyaluronic acid increase in concentration relative to collagen,[7] which may represent a retention in the tissue of the hyaluronate binding domains of degraded proteoglycans and perhaps of other matrix proteins.[1,7] These changes must alter the material properties of the tissue, especially of the nucleus, reducing compliance and making gross prolapse and internal tears and dislocations of the fabric under load more likely.

In many ways, the degenerative biochemical changes in the disc are comparable to those that occur in articular cartilage with aging and accompanying and perhaps preceding osteoarthrosis. For example, proteoglycan loss is believed to increase the compliance of the collagen network of articular cartilage and may predispose it to mechanical injury with ensuing fibrillation, fissuring and eventual joint failure. There is also a growing awareness of the importance of structural changes at the cartilage/bone interface in both synovial and intervertebral joints in association with degeneration.

Pearce, et al.,[69] have presented evidence from autopsy specimens that the proteoglycan content of all discs in lumbar spines with severely degenerated discs was low compared with age-matched control spines. They proposed that a decreased proteoglycan content preceded degeneration and, moreover, predisposed the disc to failure because of a reduced mechanical competence. Differences between prolapsed and normal disc tissue in collagenolytic and other matrix degrading protease activities have also been noted.[71]

Intervertebral discs, and also other human connective tissues such as articular cartilage, gradually become yellow and eventually brown in old age. Though in the past this was loosely ascribed to deposits of "lipofuscin", or "aging pigment"[72] and also to hemorrhage, this coloration deserves more study as a possible result of the build up of the "browning" reaction products of nonenzymic glycosylation.[73–75] Glucose in body fluids gradually reacts with side chain amines on long-lived proteins such as collagen, a phenomenon that is most pronounced in diabetics because of their elevated glucose levels. The initial glycosylamine adducts that accumulate in native collagen are well documented.[73,76] Work in vitro indicates that these glycation reaction products can go on to form covalent links between polypeptide chains.[77,78] If such reactions progress with age in normal disc tissue (and data say they do[79]), they may affect matrix properties significantly. Morever, if glucose reacts with hydroxylysine residues on the surface of collagen fibrils and blocks potential cross-linking sites, this could alter the ability of the fibrils to add newly made collagen molecules necessary for matrix remodeling and tissue repair. Seeking clinical and pathological evidence of advanced disc degeneration in diabetic patients might test this possibility.

SUMMARY AND FUTURE DIRECTIONS

The disc's unique structure and mechanical properties rely on a remarkably specialized collagen architecture that must be continually inflated by highly hydrated proteoglycans. The matrix combines features of a ligament and hyaline cartilage both molecularly and in gross appearance. Presumably, the complex mix of ingredients is tailored to provide unique mechanical properties. For example, the coarse collagen fibers of adjacent lamellae in the annulus fibrosus, that anchor the vertebral bodies together in the manner of a ligament, may need to be lubricated or elastically tethered to allow limited local slippage between them as they cope with the large bending and torsional deformations that the disc as a whole sustains under load. In cartilage, nucleus pulposus, and annulus fibrosus, the fibrils of type II collagen may have evolved a different requirement for interfibrillar adhesion rather than lubrication. Type IX collagen may fill this role.

Future research should reveal whether the minor types of collagen molecule are a means for such diversity of interactions between collagen fibrils, and between collagen fibrils and the proteoglycan domain. Such details of supramolecular interaction are, of course, crucial for understanding how the distinctive properties of all connective tissues are modulated and maintained. A search for unique molecular markers of disc tissue would also be valuable with the goal of identifying specific serum indicators of disc degradation.

REFERENCES

1. Eyre, D., et al.: Intervertebral Disc-Basic Science Perspectives. *In* New Perspectives on Low Back Pain (Edited by J.W. Frymoyer and S.L. Gordon). Park Ridge, American Academy of Orthopaedic Surgeons, 1989.
2. McDevitt, C.A.: Proteoglycans of the intervertebral disc. *In* The Biology of the Intervertebral Disc, Volume 1 (Edited by P. Ghosh). Boca Raton, CRC Press, 1989.
3. Maroudas, A.: Nutrition and metabolism of the intervertebral disc. *In* The Biology of the Intervertebral Disc, Volume 2 (Edited by P. Ghosh). Boca Raton, CRC Press, 1989.
4. Vernon-Roberts, B.: Disc pathology and disease states. *In* The Biology of the Intervertebral Disc, Volume 2. (Edited by P. Ghosh). Boca Raton, CRC Press, 1989.
5. Parke, W., et al.: Nerve, Basic Science Perspectives. *In* New Perspectives on Low Back Pain (Edited by J.W. Frymoyer and S.L. Gordon). Park Ridge, American Academy of Orthopaedic Surgeons, 1989.
6. Gross, J.: Invertebrate collagens in the scheme of things. *In* Biology of Invertebrate and Lower Vertebrate Collagens (Edited by A. Bairati and R. Garrone). New York, Plenum, 1985.
7. Eyre, D.R.: Biochemistry of the intervertebral disc. Int Rev Conn Tiss Res 8:227–291, 1979.
8. Eyre, D.R., Muir, H.: Collagen polymorphism: two molecular species in pig intervertebral disc. FEBS Lett 42:192–196, 1974.
9. Eyre, D.R., Muir, H.: Types I and II collagens in interverte-bral disc: interchanging radial distributions in annulus fibrosus. Biochem J 157:267–270, 1976.
10. Eyre, D.R., Muir, H.: Quantitative analysis of type I and II collagens in human intervertebral disc at various ages. Biochem Biophys Acta 492:29–42, 1977.
11. Buckwalter, J.A.: The fine structure of human intervertebral disc. *In* Symposium on Idiopathic Low Back Pain (Edited by A.A. White and S.L. Gordon). St. Louis, C.V. Mosby, 1982.
12. Taylor, J.R., Twomey, L.T.: The development of the human intervertebral disc. *In* The Biology of the Intervertebral Disc, Volume 1, (Edited by P. Ghosh). Boca Raton, CRC Press, 1989.
13. Maroudas, A., Stockwell, R.A., Nachemson, A., Urban, J.: Factors involved in the nutrition of the human lumbar intervertebral disc: cellularity and diffusion of glucose in vitro. J Anat, 120:113–130, 1975.
14. Bayliss, M.T., Urban, J.P.G., Johnstone, B., Holm, S.: In vitro method for measuring synthesis rates in the intervertebral disc. J Orthop Res 4:10–17, 1986.
15. Roberts, S., Menage, J., Urban, J.P.G.: Biochemical and structural properties of the cartilage end-plate and its relation to the intervertebral disc. Spine 14:166–174, 1989.
16. Mayne, R., Burgeson R.E., (eds): Structure and Function of Collagen, Volume of Biology of the Extracellular Matrix. Orlando, Academic Press, 1987.
17. Eyre, D.R.: Collagen structure and function: its relevance to spinal disease. *In* AAOS, Symposium on Idiopathic Low Back Pain, (Edited by A.A. White, III and S.L. Gordon). St. Louis, C.V. Mosby, 1982.
18. Ayad, S., Abedin, M.Z., Grundy, S.M., Weiss, J.B.: Isolation and characterization of an unusual collagen from hyaline cartilage and intervertebral disc. FEBS Lett 123:195, 1981.
19. Ayad, S., Abedin, M.Z., Weiss, J.B., Grundy, S.M.: Characterization of another short-chain disulphide-bonded collagen from cartilages, vitreous and intervertebral disc. FEBS Lett 139:300, 1982.
20. Ayad, S., Weiss, J.B.: Biochemistry of the intervertebral disc. *In* The Lumbar Spine and Back Pain, 3rd Ed., (Edited by M.I.V. Jayson). London, Pitman Publishing, 1986.
21. Eyre, D.R., Wu, J.J.: Type XI or 1α2α3α collagen. *In* Structure and Function of Collagen, Volume of Biology of the Extracellular Matrix, (Edited by R. Mayne and R.E. Burgeson). Orlando, Academic Press, 1987.
22. Linsenmayer, T.F., Fitch, J.M., Gross, J., Mayne, R.: Are different collagen fibrils in the developing avian cornea composed of two different collagen types? Ann N Y Acad Sci 460:232, 1985.
23. Adachi, E., Hayashi, T.: Comparison of axial banding patterns in fibrils of type V collagen and type I collagen. Collagen Rel Res 7:27, 1987.
24. Smith, G.N., Jr., Williams, J.M., Brandt, K.D.: Interactions of proteoglycans with the pericellular (1α,2α,3α) collagens of cartilage. J Biol Chem 260:10761, 1985.
25. Niyibizi, C., Eyre, D.R.: Identification of the cartilage α1(XI) chain in type V collagen from bovine bone. FEBS Lett 242:314–318, 1989.
26. Wu, J.J., Eyre, D.R., Slayter, H.S.: Type VI collagen of the intervertebral disc: biochemical and electron microscopic characterization of the native protein. Biochem J 248(2):373–381, 1987.
27. Buckwalter, J.A., Maynard, J.A., Cooper, R.R.: Banded structures in human nucleus pulposus. Clin Orthop 139:259, 1979.
28. Cornah, M.S., Meachim, G., Parry, E.W.: Banded structures in the matrix of human and rabbit nucleus pulposus. J Anat 107:351, 1970.
29. Smith, J.W., Serafini-Fracassini, A.: The distribution of the protein-polysaccharide complex in the nucleus pulposus matrix in young rabbits. J Cell Sci 3:33, 1968.
30. Bruns, R.R.: Beaded filaments and long-spacing fibrils: relation to type VI collagen. J Ultrastruct Res 89:136, 1984.

31. Furthmayr, H., et al.: Electron-microscopical approach to a structural model of intima collagen. Biochem J *211*:303, 1983.
32. Engel, J., et al.: Structure and macromolecular organization of type VI collagen. Ann NY Acad Sci *460*:25, 1985.
33. von der Mark, H., et al.: Immunochemistry, genuine size and tissue localization of collagen VI. Eur J Biochem *142*:493, 1984.
34. Bonaldo, P., et al.: α1 Chain of chick type VI collagen: the complete cDNA sequence reveals a hybrid molecule made of one short collagen and three von Willebrand factor type A-like domains. J Biol Chem *264*:5575–5580, 1989.
35. Bruns, R.R., et al.: Type VI collagen in extracellular, 100nm periodic filaments and fibrils: identification by immunoelectron microscopy. J Cell Biol *103*:393, 1986.
36. Shimokamaki, M., Duance, V.C., Bailey, A.J.: Identification of a new disulphide-bonded collagen from cartilage. FEBS Lett *121*:51, 1980.
37. van der Rest, M., Mayne, R.: Type IX collagen. *In* Structure and Function of Collagen Types, (Edited by R. Mayne and R.E. Burgeson). Orlando, Academic Press, 1987.
38. Wu, J.J., Eyre, D.R.: Covalent interactions of type IX collagen in cartilage. Connect Tissue Res *20*:241–245, 1989.
39. Irwin, M.H., Silvers, S.H., Mayne, R.: Monoclonal antibody against chicken type IX collagen: preparation, characterization and recognition of the intact form of type IX collagen secreted by chondrocytes. J Cell Biol *101*:814, 1985.
40. Wu, J.J., Eyre, D.R.: Cartilage type IX collagen is cross-linked by hydroxypyridinium residues. Biochem Biophys Res Commun *123*:1033–1039, 1984.
41. Muller-Glauser, W., et al.: On the role of type IX collagen in the extracellular matrix of cartilage: type IX collagen is localized to intersections of collagen fibrils. J Cell Biol *102*:1931, 1986.
42. Eyre, D.R., et al.: Collagen type IX: evidence for covalent linkages to type II collagen in cartilage. FEBS Lett *220*:337–341, 1987.
43. Eyre, D.R., Wu, J.J., Niyibizi, C.: The collagens of bone and cartilage: molecular diversity and supramolecular assembly. Proceedings of the 10th International Conference on Calcium Regulating Hormones. Montreal, Elsevier Science Publishers, pp. 188–194, 1990.
44. Gordon, M.K., Genecke, D.R., Olsen, B.R.: Type XII collagen: distinct extracellular matrix component discovered by cDNA cloning. Proc Natl Acad Sci U S A *84*:6040–6044, 1987.
45. Dublet, B., et al.: The structure of avian type XII collagen: α1(XII) chains contain 190kDA non-triple helical amino-terminal domains and form homotrimeric molecules. J Biol Chem *264*:13150–13156, 1989.
46. Surgure, S.P., et al.: Immunoidentification of type XII collagen in embryonic tissues. J Cell Biol *109*:939–945, 1989.
47. Gordon, M.K., et al.: Type XII collagen: a large multidomain molecule with partial homology to type IX collagen. J Biol Chem *264*:19772–19778, 1989.
48. Eyre, D.R., Paz, M.A., Gallop, P.M.: Crosslinking in collagen and elastin. Ann Rev Biochem *53*:717–748, 1984.
49. Eyre, D.R., Koob, T.J., Van Ness, K.P.: Quantitation of hydroxypyridinium crosslinks in collagen by high performance liquid chromatography. Anal Biochem *137*:380–388, 1984.
50. Eyre, D.R.: Collagen: molecular diversity in the body's protein scaffold. Science *207*:1315–1322, 1980.
51. Eyre, D.R.: Collagen crosslinking abnormalities in scoliosis. *In* Pathogenesis of Idiopathic Scoliosis, (Edited by R.R. Jacobs). Chicago, Scoliosis Research Society, 1984.
52. Fisher, L., Termine, J., Young, M.: Deduced protein sequence of bone small proteoglycan I (biglycan) shows homology with proteoglycan II (decorin) and several connective tissue proteins in a variety of species. J Biol Chem *264*:4571–4576, 1989.
53. Paulsson, M., Heinegård, D.: Radio immunoassay of the 148-kilodalton cartilage protein: distribution of the protein among bovine tissues. Biochem J *207*:207–213, 1982.
54. Fife, R.S.: Comparison of a 550,000 dalton cartilage matrix glycoprotein in cartilage from immature and mature dogs. J Rheumatol *16*:656–659, 1989.
55. Heinegård, D., et al.: Two novel matrix proteins isolated from articular cartilage show wide distributions among connective tissues. J Biol Chem *261*:13866–13872, 1986.
56. Sommarin, Y., Larsson, T., and Heinegård, D.: Chondrocyte-matrix interations: attachment to proteins isolated from cartilage. Exp Cell Res *184*:181–192, 1989.
57. Heinegård, D., Oldberg, A.: Structure and biology of cartilage and bone matrix noncollagenous macromolecules. FASEB J *3*:2042–2051, 1989.
58. Buckwalter, J.A., Cooper, R.R., Maynard, J.A.: Elastic fibers in human intervertebral discs. J Bone Joint Surg *58A*:73–76, 1976.
59. Hukins, D.W.L.: Disc structure and formation. *In* New Perspectives in Low Back Pain, (Edited by J.W. Frymoyer and S.L. Gordon). Park Ridge, American Academy of Orthopaedic Surgeons, 1989.
60. Johnson, E.F., et al.: The distribution and arrangement of elastic fibers in the intervertebral disc of the adult human. J Anat *135*:301, 1982.
61. Maroudas, A.: Nutrition and metabolism of the intervertebral disc. *In* Symposium on Idiopathic Low Back Pain, (Edited by A.A. White and S.L. Gordon). St. Louis, Mosby, 1982.
62. Bradford, D.S., Cooper, K.M., Oegema, T.R. Jr.: Chymopapain, chemonucleolysis and nucleus pulposus regeneration. J Bone Joint Surg *65A*:1220–1231, 1983.
63. Brodin, H.: Paths of nutrition in articular cartilage and intervertebral discs. Acta Orthop Scand *24*:177–183, 1955.
64. Crock, H.V., Goldwasser, M., Yoshizawa, H.: Vascular anatomy related to the intervertebral disc. *In* New Perspectives on Low Back Pain, (Edited by J.W. Frymoyer and S.L. Gordon). Park Ridge, American Academy of Orthopaedic Surgeons, 1989.
65. Urban, J.P.G., et al.: Nutrition of the intervertebral disc: effects of fluid flow on solute transport. Clin Orthop *170*:296–302, 1982.
66. Diamant, B., Karlsson, J., Nachemson, A.: Correlation between lactate levels and pH in discs of patients with lumbar rhizopathies. Experientia *24*:1195–1196, 1968.
67. Adams, P., Muir, H.: Qualitative changes with age of proteoglycans of human lumbar discs. Ann Rheum Dis *35*:289–296, 1976.
68. Stevens, R., et al.: Biological changes in the annulus fibrosus in patients with low-back pain. Spine *7*:223, 1982.
69. Pearce, R.H., Grimmer, B.J., Adams, M.E.: Degeneration and the chemical composition of the human lumbar intervertebral disc. J Orthop Res *5*:198–205, 1987.
70. Buckwalter, J.A., et al.: Articular cartilage and intervertebral disc proteoglycans differ in structure: an electron microscopic study. J Orthop Res *7*:146–151, 1989.
71. Ng, S.C.S., Weiss, J., Quennel, R., Jayson, M.I.V.: Abnormal connective tissue degrading enzyme patterns in prolapsed intervertebral discs. Spine *11*:695–701, 1986.
72. Bijslma, F., Copius Peereboom, J.W.: The aging pattern of human intervertebral disc: fluorescent substance and amino acids in the annulus fibrosus. Gerontologia *18*:157–168, 1972.
73. Robins, S.P., Bailey, A.J.: Age-related changes in collagen: the identification of reducible lysine-carbohydrate condensation products. Biochem Biophys Res Commun *48*:76, 1972.
74. Monnier, V.M., et al.: Relation between complications of type I diabetes mellitus and collagen linked fluorescence. N Engl J Med *314*:403–408, 1986.
75. Monnier, V.M., Cerami, A.: Non-enzymatic browning in vivo: possible process of aging of long-lived proteins. Science *211*:491, 1981.
76. Tanzer, M.L., Fairweather, R., Gallop, P.M.: Collagen crosslinks: isolation of reduced N-hexosylhydroxylysine from

borohydride-reduced calf skin insoluble collagen. Arch Biochem Biophys *151*:137, 1972.
77. Eble, A.S., Thorpe, S.R., Baynes, J.W.: Nonenzymatic glucosylation and glucose-dependent cross-linking. J Biol Chem *258*:9406–9412, 1983.
78. Pongor, S., Ulrich, P.C., Bencsath, F.A., Cerami, A.: Aging of proteins: isolation and identification of a fluorescent chromophore from the reaction of polypeptides with glucose. Proc Natl Acad Sci U S A *81*:2684, 1984.
79. Hormel, S.E., Eyre, D.R.: Collagen glycation in the human intervertebral disc: age-related increase in covalently-bound fluorophores and chromophores. Acta Biochem Biophys, in press. Submitted.
80. Scott, J.E., Haigh, M.: Proteoglycan-collagen interactions in intervertebral disc. A chondroitin sulphate proteoglycan associates with collagen fibrils in rabbit annulus fibrosus at the d-e bands. Biosci Rep *6*:879–888, 1986.

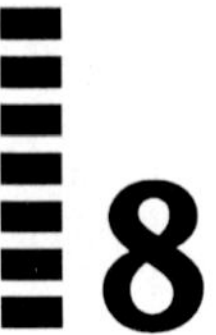

Wayne H. Akeson
David Amiel
Savio L-Y. Woo
Jean-Jacques Abitbol
Steven R. Garfin

8

Concepts of Soft Tissue Homeostasis and Healing

INTRODUCTION

The concepts of soft tissue homeostasis and healing to be described in this chapter have been developed almost exclusively on models of the appendicular skeleton. The experimental models so developed have generally been supported by followup clinical studies in humans. There is little reason to believe that the spine is exempt from the general rules that have been discovered to govern the stress dependence of connective tissue. Clearly, spine fusion models have shown profound effects on the intervertebral disc[1,2] and at least one paper has shown stress dependence of facet joints.[3] This chapter describes soft tissue homeostasis as understood in general terms, and attempts to extend the observations to the rehabilitation of the spine.

Specialized connective tissue cell types clearly respond differently to injury. Fibroblasts respond readily, but cartilage and fibrocartilage respond poorly, if at all. The fact that the annulus fibrosus is fibrocartilaginous in nature may contribute, as in the case of the anterior cruciate ligament (ACL),[4] to its poor healing response.[5] Only a few studies on annulus healing have been reported.[6,7,8] Clinical studies have shown a clear relationship between radial tears of the annulus and disc bulging.[9] Failure of healing of the radial tears may be the central problem in disc protrusion. In this chapter, the ACL healing deficiencies are described as a model, possibly analogous to the annulus. Clearly, more attention should be concentrated on spine ligament and disc healing models to better clarify deficiencies in healing of the human spine.

The concept of the stress dependence of connective tissue is central to this chapter and will be documented in detail as the basis for the discussion on soft tissue healing that follows. For this purpose, effects of both stress deprivation and stress enhancement on joint physiology are outlined and, finally, the existing knowledge of the efficacy of passive motion as a therapeutic modality is summarized.

The understanding of the therapeutic value of motion as an aid to soft tissue healing is a relatively recent development. By contrast, rest has historically been accorded the key role in the management of a variety of disorders of the musculoskeletal system. In this history, the use of an infinite variety of braces, casts, and assorted apparatus to impose the needed immobility on the spine or extremities has a long and colorful tradition. The treatment of fractures and dislocations and the correction of musculoskeletal deformities has provided the most obvious rationale for the use of enforced rest. Additional indications include bone and joint infections, arthritic deformity, and muscle imbalance secondary to neurological dysfunction. However, the basis for treatment decisions utilizing immobility as an essential adjunct has been largely empirical. Giants of early orthopaedic surgery figured prominently in this history.

Both stress deprivation and stress enhancement influence morphological and biomechanical characteristics of connective tissue. Data from experiments on animals and from descriptive clinical studies on humans, which have accumulated over the past two decades, are sufficient to place stress deprivation effects on a secure foundation in qualitative terms.[10,11] Quantitative data on the process remain sketchy, but enough information has been accumulated to suggest a few generalizations that may be used to introduce the subject and provide guidelines for future research priorities. Unfortunately, data on exercise effects on connective tissue other than muscle and bone remain quite meager. The available evidence infers that hypertrophy of tendon and possibly of ligament occurs in exercising animals.[12] Recent studies on exercise effects in humans and animals clearly show that sustained exercise produces bone hypertrophy, an important finding with respect to the osteoporosis of an aging population. Recovery from stress deprivation has been shown to have a much greater time requirement than recovery from the original injury, a matter of frustration to physicians who are required to use casts in the treatment of injuries or deformities, and a matter of even greater frustration to patients forced to undergo prolonged rehabilitation programs to regain prior functional strength, mobility, and agility of the affected extremity.[13] A brief resume of pertinent supporting data for these conclusions follows.

THE STRESS DEPENDENCE OF CONNECTIVE TISSUE

The interrelationship between skeletal form and function has long been accepted. The most explicit expression of the relationship was, of course, Wolff's Law, which states that bone adapts to the applied stresses. In more recent years, the expression has been found to apply equally to the joint composite, including articular cartilage, ligament, tendon, capsule, and synovial membrane, as well as to bone.[13] This broader expansion of Wolff's Law is probably simply recognized with slight editorial license as Wolff's Law of connective tissue. However, others, as is often the rule in science, may have priority in recognizing the broader application of the general interrelationship between form and function as applied to fibrosis connective tissue and the joint composite.[14]

ANATOMIC PATHOLOGY OF STRESS DEPRIVATION OF SYNOVIAL JOINTS

It is instructive to review the protean manifestations of stress deprivation on synovial joints in order to put passive motion therapy into perspective. Sufficient gross and microscopic observations on human anatomic pathology exist to feel confident that reported experimental animal and human changes are closely similar. The changes are conveniently divided into: (1) periarticular and synovial tissue changes, and (2) articular cartilage and subchondral bone changes.

Periarticular and Synovial Tissue Changes

The consistent feature of the gross appearance of the periarticular and synovial tissues of immobilized joints is a fibro-fatty connective tissue proliferation within the joint space.[15,16] In knee immobilization models, this phenomenon is seen prominently in the intercondylar notch, but is also observed in other joint recesses. The proliferative fibro-fatty connective tissue covers exposed intra-articular soft tissue structures such as the cruciate ligaments and the under-surface of the quadriceps tendon. It also blankets the nonarticulating cartilage surfaces. With the passage of time, adhesions develop between the exposed tissue surfaces as the fibro-fatty connective tissue is transformed into more mature scar. The proliferation of this type of tissue is relatively the same in such diverse species as rabbit, rat, dog, and primate. Similar changes also are prominent in human posterior intervertebral joints and in human knee joints.[16]

Articular Cartilage and Subchondral Bone

The changes that occur secondary to immobility affecting articular cartilage can be separated into those in noncontact areas and those in contact areas. The changes in noncontact areas are thought to be secondary to the fibro-fatty connective tissue proliferation described above. The ingrowth of connective tissue that fills the joint space soon covers the joint surfaces. In the rat model studied by Evans, et al.,[15] in which the process was evaluated on a progressive time basis, the articular surfaces were covered within 30 days. The connective tissue became more dense and adherent during the subsequent month and remained relatively constant thereafter. The surface cartilage cells gradually became confluent with the overlying connective tissue. By 60 days, many of the animals had lost the tangential layer of cartilage cells. Evidence was consistent that the thinning of the cartilage began peripherally where the adhesions first occurred. Fibrillation of the cartilage was also seen and variable loss of staining of matrix was observed. Staining changes were also described by Baker, et al.,[17] in human spinal facet joints after anterior spine fusion. These changes included first a zone of loss of staining around the cells peripheral to the cellular lacunae. Ultimately, loss of definition of lacunae occurred, and the cartilage cells became stellate with poorly defined margin. Such change in staining characteristics of cartilage matrix had been described in 1874 by von Reyher.[18] Baker, et al., described similar changes and termed them "Weichselbaum's space."[17,19] Parker and Keefer observed this process in cartilage beneath rheumatoid pannus and proposed that it represented a metaplastic process of cartilage cells transformed into fibroblasts,[20] a view that Baker, et al., endorsed.

In the contact areas, mild to severe changes of articular cartilage are observed depending on the rigidity of immobilization, the position of immobilization, and most important, the degree of compression. Typically, the mild changes consist of loss of intensity of staining of the matrix. In areas of greater compressive forces varying degrees of destruction occur, up to and including full thickness ulceration of cartilage with cellular distortion and necrosis, fibrillation of matrix, and erosion of matrix down to subchondral bone.[21,22]

The major areas of alteration in the subchondral bone occur beneath cartilage lesions in joints immobilized 60 days or longer. Hyperemia in the subadjacent marrow spaces is noted with proliferation of connective tissue. In some areas this tissue penetrated the subchondral plate and entered the calcified layer of articular cartilage. Trabecular atrophy and resorption in the areas subadjacent to cartilage lesions are also seen. Subchondral cysts sometimes develop in this location in animals followed for longer periods. Not surprisingly, such profound alterations in gross and microscopic architecture are associated with significant biomechanical and biochemical changes.

EXPERIMENTAL STUDIES OF THE FIBROUS CONNECTIVE TISSUE RESPONSE TO STRESS ALTERATION

The changes in joint structure and function in immobilized limbs have been the subject of considerable interest with respect to the underlying processes involved, and with respect to the possibility of modifying the responses through the use of hormonal drugs. In an experimental model designed to evaluate the soft tissue response to immobility, the hind limbs of dogs[10] and rabbits[23] were immobilized using internal fixation procedures for up to 12 weeks, and periarticular connective tissues were examined. It should be noted that casts of internal fixation of the flexed knee with a threaded pin placed through the tibia and femur well posterior to the knee joint give similar results. The latter technique has generally been preferred to obviate pressure sores from cast friction.

Biomechanical Changes of the Knee Composite

The knee contracture was assessed immediately after sacrifice utilizing an arthrograph.[24] The arthrograph is designed to measure the joint stiffness in knees in terms of a torque-angular deformation (T-0) diagram. The knees of the experimental and control from each animal were mounted on the arthrograph and cycled at a frequency of 0.2 Hz. Two ranges of motion, five cycles each, were used in sequence: the

first range of knee angles was 50° to 80°, and the second 45° to 95°. Each cycle of flexion and extension was recorded on the X-Y recorder. Recording of the first cycle of the contracture knee was particularly important because subsequent cycles required substantially less energy. In addition, the amount of torque required to extend the knee from 50° to 65° from acute flexion during the first cycle was also significantly higher than that of subsequent cycles. The significant increases in torque and area of hysteresis were used as measures of increase in joint stiffness of severity of joint contracture. A progressive increase in the strength of contracture was observed on serial evaluations between 2 and 12 weeks. Detailed descriptions of the apparatus and technique are given in several earlier papers.[23,24] The arthrograph permits evaluation of the efficacy of therapeutic modalities, such as drug or hormone injections, on the process. Interestingly, hyaluronic acid has been shown to significantly inhibit contracture developed under stress deprivation conditions.[25]

Biomechanical Changes in Ligaments

Following 9 weeks of immobilization, the linear slope, ultimate load, and energy absorbing capabilities of the rabbit medial collateral ligament (MCL)-bone complex during tension decrease to approximately one-third that of the contralateral non-immobilized control. The load-strain characteristics of the MCL substances become inferior. Further immobilization of up to 12 weeks causes additional degradation of the MCL substance.[12] These data are obtained with the aid of the video dimensional analyzer system that can evaluate the mechanical properties of ligament substance and structural properties of the bone-ligament complex simultaneously.[26]

The failure mode is altered and reduced in this model, and modules of elasticity are reduced as well. The bone resorption at the ligament insertion site causes failure by avulsion at the insertion site, a problem noted by several investigators.[27–29]

These mechanical alterations occur after a relatively brief stress deprivation period compared to common clinical treatment programs for fractures and joint injuries. They have important implications to the rationale for selection of treatment options as well as dramatic implications for rehabilitation following recovery from the initial injuries.

Exercise Effects on Specialized Connective Tissue Structure

An animal model has been used to evaluate effects of exercise on bone, tendon, and ligament in normal subjects. In one study, miniature swine were exercised on a track over one year at intervals that created cardiac hypertrophy[30] and increased cardiac output. At the end of one year, cortical bone showed improved structural ' properties of about one-third, indicative of cortical hypertrophy. The material properties were unchanged, indicating that the changes observed were entirely a result of bulk change rather than qualitative improvement. Similar changes were observed for digital extensor tendons. At 12 months after onset of the exercise period, the cross-sectional areas were increased 21% and the load to failure increased 62%.[31] It is important to observe that, at 3 months after onset, differences in bone and extensor tendon were not significant, indicating that a long time and large effort are required to see the improvement in structural properties. Furthermore, site and tissue-specific factors are involved, as indicated by the fact that digital flexor tendons and ligaments were less responsive than bone and extensor tendon to the exercise program.

Recovery from Stress Deprivation

Recovery of the MCL substance following a period of immobilization may be quite rapid. The load-strain curve of the MCL from the experimental knee of animals immobilized for 9 weeks recovered to the same level as that of the control animals after 12 weeks of cage activity. The recovery curve for the 12-week-immobilized knees was slightly inferior to a cage activity recovery period of 12 weeks.[32] The experimental knee ligaments continued to have inferior structural properties as compared to those of the control knees. The P_{max} and the A_{max} for the experimentals were approximately two-thirds that of the controls. The slower recovery of strength of the bone-ligament junction confirmed findings obtained by other investigators.[27,29,33]

The surprising finding, however, is that following remobilization there was a rapid recovery of properties of the MCL substance in the functional range (up to 5% ligament strain), whereas the ultimate load and energy absorbing capability of the MCL-bone complex remained considerably inferior.[32] The tibial insertion sites continued to be the weakest link. These results added to the earlier conclusion made by Noyes, et al.,[33] that up to one year of reconditioning is required (following 8 weeks of immobilization) to regain the strength of MCL-bone complex. In this respect, the results on structural properties are similar. Additionally, our data indicate that the ligament substance recovers rapidly during remobilization and can function normally in the physiologic range.

Therefore, the prevention of stress deprivation effects is paramount to the success of rehabilitation efforts. This conclusion forms an important aspect of the scientific rationale of passive motion in the early phase of rehabilitation.

Biochemical Events Consequent to Stress Deprivation

The biochemical changes of periarticular connective tissue matrix are manifold. Space does not permit a detailed exposition of those changes. However, a summary follows, along with key references to the literature on the subject. An important point, which has evolved from our laboratory, is that notable differences exist between biochemical matrix characteristics of ligaments and tendons and that differences are unfolding between various ligaments. The functional implications of these differences are not yet clear and require further study.

Extracellular Fluid Volume Changes

The water content of fibrous connective tissues is in the range of 65% to 70%. Because the population of cells is relatively sparse in this tissue, the majority of this water is perforce in the extracellular space. On gross inspection, the dissected tissues from the immobilized limb appear less glistening and more "woody" in texture. Chemical analysis shows a 4% to 6% decrease in water content compared to the control side.[34] It seems likely that this amount of water loss is functionally significant. Fluid movement, which plays such an important role in articular cartilage load bearing and lubrication, probably performs the same role in fibrous connective tissue. It has recently been established that hyaluronic acid and its attached or entrapped water is the principal fibrous connective tissue lubricant.[35]

It is presumed that the interstitial fluid in a densely fibrous "connecting" anatomical structure serves as a spacer between individual collagen fibers or fibrils, permitting discrete movement of one fiber or fibril past the adjacent fibers. The importance of interstitial fluid to tissue rheology is obvious; the concept of viscoelasticity of connective tissue rests upon the dual fluid and solid nature of these systems.

Glycosaminoglycan Changes

The largest change found in the composition of the stress deprived periarticular connective tissue is reduction in the concentration of glycosaminoglycans (GAG).[36] The decreases in chondroitin-4 and -6 sulfate (30%) and hyaluronic acid (40%) are statistically significant, whereas the percentage change of dermatan sulfate thought to be associated with fibers is smaller. Decreased concentration of GAG and water would be expected to alter the plasticity and pliability of connective tissue matrices, and to reduce lubrication efficiency. Biochemical analyses of articular cartilage and meniscus from the experimental knees also show a reduction of 24% and 31%, respectively, of GAG content in these tissues.[36]

Water content appeared to parallel the GAG ranges, consistent with the known facts concerning the high water binding capacity of GAG. The preferential loss of GAG is also consistent with known facts about its rapid turnover half life (1.7 to 7 days)[37] as compared with collagen (half life of 300 to 500 days).[38] Turnover studies using tritium-labeled acetate show that the decrement in specific activity of hyaluronic acid with time after preliminary labeling is the same for control and immobilized limbs. The conclusion is, therefore, that degradation does not accelerate, but rather that the synthesis of hyaluronic acid in the immobilized extremities decreases. The fibroblasts of the fibrous connective tissue matrix apparently respond to physical forces by a homeostasis feedback loop to maintain the proper balance of connective tissue constituents.

A gel-like structure created by the interaction between water and glycosaminoglycans is currently well accepted by physiologists working with interstitial fluid flow questions.[39] Clearly, the gel structure is severely compromised in the connective tissue deprived of mechanical stimulation. It is postulated that the GAG and water changes result from qualitative changes in collagen because the fiber-fiber distances must be reduced when water and GAG volumes are reduced.

It is presumed that the lubricating and volume-separating effects provided by hyaluronic acid and water permit the independent gliding of microfibrils past one another, facilitating the tissue adaption to motion permitted by the particular connective tissue weave pattern. Loss of this volume-separating and lubricating property provides for fibril-fibril friction as well as the potential for adhesions or crosslinking between adjacent collagen fibrils. Any newly synthesized collagen is apt to be randomly dispersed and to create interference with the functional gliding between fibers necessary for normal mobility. This is particularly so in the stationary attitude because maturation processes may encourage fibril growth in diameter by including these newly synthesized random fibrils within the fiber structural units. Such mismatch with respect to functional elongation needs and weave without regard to the usual physical force and motion probably is central to the pathomechanics of joint stiffness.

Collagen Changes

The processes seen in the studies described above, which rely on the techniques of anatomic pathology, suggest that connective tissue proliferation or simple granulation tissue production is the basis of joint contractures. However, collagen turnover studies are difficult to reconcile with this concept at first examination. For example, the studies by Brooke and Slack[40] showed that collagen precursor uptake actually was reduced in denervated rat limbs compared to controls. However, collagen synthesis did proceed, but at a reduced level. Peacock[41] used saline solubility of collagen to estimate the amount of new collagen synthesized and found no differences in immobilized and control joints except for the posterior capsular area where collagen solubility increased. However, because he used pin fixation with a placement proximate to the posterior capsule, the significance of finding total collagen mass changes became uncertain. Our laboratory was able to demonstrate reduction in total collagen of only 10% through total joint mass evaluation using the whole periarticular connective tissue unit.[42] Studies of Klein[43] using long-term labeling techniques, which are more sensitive for this purpose, found small increases in collagen mass in denervated limbs.

We feel, however, strategic placement of anomalous crosslinks of newly synthesized collagen fibrils in the contracture process is important. These crosslinks can act as bridges between existing functionally independent fibers with divergent tracking patterns. Using a simplified model, i.e., the Chinese finger trap mechanism, it can be seen that fixed contact at just a few nodal points defeats the functional gliding of the whole apparatus. Demonstration of such changes within the weave of the joint capsule is difficult because of right to left variability in microarchitecture and the small degree of change necessary to effect a mechanical impediment. However, it is easy to be convinced that such a process must play a role in the synovial joint contracture process. Disorganization, which occurs in the cruciate ligament of a rabbit after 9 weeks of immobilization, has been demonstrated in our previous work.[44] The pattern of cellular alignment becomes distorted as well, almost certainly reflecting a more random matrix organization.

COLLAGEN CROSS-LINK ALTERATIONS

The studies of quantitative changes in the crosslinking of collagen from the immobilized rabbit knee periarticular connective tissue show significant increases in the sodium borohydride reducible intermolecular crosslinks.[45] A typical radioactive elution profile from column 1 of a 3N p-toluene sulfonic acid hydrolysate of [3H]NaBh$_4$ reduced periarticular connective tissue from control and immobilized joints and the rechromatography on an extended basic column of the aldolhistidinedihydroxylysinonorleucine peaks show a twofold increase in dihydroxylysinonorleucine (DHLNL) on the immobilized side. It was shown that DHLNL, hydroxylysinonorleucine (HLNL) and histidinohydroxymerodesmosine (HHMD) are the major crosslinks that increase following a period of immobilization. No change in hydroxylysine/lysine ratio between the immobilized and control periarticular connective tissue collagen was detected.

It can be speculated that the increased intra and intermolecular collagen crosslinks are important in the contracture process. How do such crosslinks interact at a molecular level? First, it is unlikely that fiber-to-fiber distance is bridged by a lysine-lysine or a lysine-hydroxylysine reaction. The distances are much too great and the forces too small to create the nodal fiber-to-fiber crosslink that is proposed to hamper joint motion. Rather, it is presumed that the nodal fiber-to-fiber crosslinks result from aggregation of new fibrils with pre-existing fibers of the matrix. The process may proceed in the usual manner of aggregation of fibrils into fibers, then incorporating bridges of newly synthesized collagen fibril elements into pairs of existing fibers. Such structures become mechanically constraining at the time when the joint is freed from constraining devices.

COLLAGEN TYPE CHANGES

Because the formation of reducible crosslinks follows collagen synthesis,[46] and because the presence and relative number of these crosslinks may, in part, depend upon the type of collagen being synthesized,[47] it is important to examine the type or types of periarticular connective tissue collagen synthesized during the period of immobilization. Examination of the densitometric scan of the SDS gel of the CNBr-cleaved peptides from control and immobilized tissue reveals no alteration in the type of collagen being synthesized during the period of immobilization.[42] The peptides $_1$ [III] CV characteristic of Type III collagen are absent in the CNBr-digest of the control and immobilized periarticular connective tissue collagen. Furthermore, these results are confirmed by amino acid analysis and sodium dodecyl sulfate (SDS) gel electrophoresis performed on intact components separated by CM cellulose chromatography. These results provide additional supportive evidence that only type I collagen is found in the dense fibrous structures of normal and contracture knees.

The significance of the changes in collagen type ratios and cross-linking patterns observed secondary to stress deprivation probably reflects the effects of increased collagen turnover. The altered mechanics, in turn, most probably result from the random orientation of newly synthesized fibrous matrix constituents. These new fibrils are disposed without regard to mechanical requirements because of the lack of input from the mechanical signals that normally operate.

THE DEVELOPMENT OF CONCEPTS OF PASSIVE MOTION

The events described above indicate a disturbing and harmful outcome of stress deprivation on synovial joints that threatens the success of rehabilitation after treatment with casts or splints for trauma or other disorders requiring immobilization. It is not unexpected, therefore, that in the past decade and a half, new concepts of treatment emphasizing early motion have developed. The controversy about early motion had, in fact, erupted earlier still. The archetypical protagonists commonly identified as providing leadership for the motion versus rest camps in the century passed were Hugh Owen Thomas, called "Hugh the rester," and Championniere, whose philosophy of treatment was exemplified by his phrase "in motion there is life." The historical advocates of rest versus motion schools relied almost entirely on empirical observation and appeals to authority for the basis of therapeutic decisions. It remained for the clarification of effects of stress on synovial joints to properly prioritize the therapeutic decision on rehabilitation. Equally important in the evolution of modern rehabilitation philosophy were fundamental studies on the influence of stress and motion on repair of bone, tendon, ligament, and cartilage. Furthermore, studies on stress and motion effects on disorders of the synovial joint composite have provided a foundation for musculoskeletal management decisions that are approaching a more logical construct. Technological advances have occurred which, hand in hand with these observations, provided new avenues for treatment that can be coupled with the early motion philosophy of rehabilitation.

In fracture management, for example, it has been possible to achieve improved fracture stability with biomechanically sound internal fixation devices. These devices applied very early in the post-injury period have permitted not only early joint mobility,[48] but mobilization of the total patient. The ability to accomplish patient mobilization after multiple trauma has resulted in a significant improvement in the survival rates in the critically injured patient—a tribute to the modern trauma management system—and a tribute to the philosophy of early mobilization.

The philosophy of early mobilization has adapted passive motion in several forms: (1) occasional, (2) interrupted, and (3) continuous, with various combinations thereof, to the early postinjury or postoperative state when patient compliance with active motion programs cannot reasonably be expected because of postoperative pain or weakness.

For successful application of passive motion to the postinjury state, the integrity of the repair—bone, ligament, or tendon—must be maintained. Details of specific applications await further contributions from basic and clinical science. However, enough is known that it is possible to develop an understanding of some of the general principles of application, which should find universal use in musculoskeletal rehabilitation for the foreseeable future. What follows is a brief outline of the evidence of efficacy of passive motion in a variety of clinical applications and of the scientific basis of those applications.

SYNOVIAL JOINT SPACE CLEARANCE DURING CONTINUOUS PASSIVE MOTION

Studies on clearance rates from synovial joints have demonstrated the value of passive motion in facilitating transport of intrasynovial contents. Cyclical changes in intra-articular pressure during continuous passive motion (CPM) have been documented.[49–51] The clearest example of this application is the paper of O'Driscoll and colleagues[52] on the clearance of blood from the joint space. These data demonstrated convincingly that a hemarthrosis in a model system treated by CPM was more rapidly cleared than in contralateral mobilized joints. The clearance rate of indium-III-oxine-labeled erythrocytes was double that seen in the immobilized joints. After one week there was significantly less blood remaining in the joints treated with CPM. These results were supported by Danzig, et al.[53]

This effect was seen indirectly in a paper by Skyhar, et al., using $^{35}SO_4$ to study nutrition of anterior cruciate knee ligaments under conditions of CPM and rest.[54] It was demonstrated that in CPM knees less $^{35}SO_4$ was taken up than in a cage activity group. The effect of CPM on synovial fluid clearance was so large that the uptake of $^{35}SO_4$ in the CPM treated knees was less than that in the immobilized knees, suggesting, at first, poor diffusion under conditions of CPM, but actually indicating that clearance of isotope occurred before diffusion into the ligament could occur.

These experiments demonstrate the importance of the convection effect of activity to the nutritional support of synovial joint components, especially articular cartilage and ligaments. Furthermore, the clinical application of CPM in the postoperative state is emphasized as a practical step in improved patient care postoperatively or post-trauma. The clearance of blood from the joint space is of undisputed advantage knowing the harmful effects of chronic hemarthrosis in states such as hemophilia.

CONTINUOUS PASSIVE MOTION IN TREATMENT OF SEPTIC ARTHRITIS

The use of motion to favorably influence the outcome of septic arthritis has been demonstrated in papers by Salter, et al.,[55,56] in a model system. The beneficial effect was most prominently seen in articular cartilage, where the damage of the septic process from proteolytic enzymes was reduced by the imposition of a passive motion program. Presumably, clearance of the deleterious lysosomal enzymes that accumulate in joint fluid in septic arthritis was facilitated by motion-induced convection effects. The articular cartilages of joints treated by the activity protocols were presumably spared exposure to high levels of matrix destructive enzymes by the acceleration of clearance of those products from the joint space by CPM. Clinical support for this application has recently been presented by Mooney and colleagues.[48]

PASSIVE MOTION EFFECTS ON REPAIR

Several repair models have been studied for the influence of one of the passive motion modalities. In several applications, the quality of repair appears to be improved under motion conditions as compared to immobility. These applications require stability of the repair line in order for healing to proceed successfully. This is seen most clearly in flexor tendon repair, when failure of the suture line in the early postoperative state can result in tendon disruption. However, if the suture line is maintained, improved outcome has been observed in several respects.[57] In certain circumstances intermittent passive motion has resulted in a successful outcome. In the case of ligament, cage activity has been shown to be superior to the immobilized condition.[58] In other circumstances, especially in cartilage healing, CPM was shown to provide a superior outcome.[59] Generally, the experimental models have indicated improved healing rates of bone, tendon, ligament, and cartilage under motion conditions and also improved quality of repair. Indeed, in the flexor tendon case within the flexor tendon sheath, it has been shown that healing proceeds by different mechanisms under motion conditions (intrinsic healing) as compared to immobilization conditions (extrinsic healing—the one-wound concept).[57] The available data are insufficient to describe optimum clinical protocols of frequency, intensity, or duration of passive motion. We have spoken of the problem as analogous to the drug dosage/response curve. In fact, the optimum values for passive motion may be found to vary in the spectrum of specific applications. Until that data are available, empirical rules apply.

The examples below, however, provide insights into the range of potential applications of passive motion to the problems of specialized connective tissue healing and the broad principles that underly these uses.

Continuous Passive Motion Influence on Cartilage Healing

The interaction between healing of the joint surfaces and motion began with the early concepts of cup arthroplasty. It was recognized that conversion of the new arthroplasty surface to fibrocartilage, after debridement of the degenerative hip and reaming to a concentric sphere of bleeding bone, required motion. Without motion the surface contained only fibrous tissue. In a few instances the opportunity existed to observe surfaces in patients who had not been able to move the hip for unrelated medical reasons. In these patients, conversion of fibrous tissue to fibrocartilage was not observed. Mooney, et al., showed this effect in the rabbit metatarsophalangeal joint, in which immobilized segments did not develop fibrocartilage surfaces as well as mobilized joints.[60] Hohl and Luck were able to demonstrate superior healing in drill hole defects in femoral cartilage of primates if motion occurred as compared to immobilized knees.[61] Convery and Akeson studied drill hole defects of various sizes in horse femoral condyles and observed that relatively small defects (one-eighth in. diameter) healed readily on pasture grazing activity, but larger defects (one-quarter in. to seven-eighths in.) did not heal.[62] The dimensional aspect of cartilage healing is important to recognize because, with or without motion regimens, large defects (one-fourth inch or larger) simply do not heal with hyaline cartilage. Nor do arthroplasty surfaces heal with hyaline cartilage. Rather, large surface defects or craters cover a portion but usually not the entire surface, and the composition of the surface replacement matrix is of fibrocartilage—not hyaline cartilage. This has been demonstrated convincingly by histological and biochemical methods. The biomechanical properties of the replacement tissue are inferior to hyaline cartilage, permitting approximately two times greater deformation on compression as compared to hyaline cartilage. These factors have obvious functional and clinical implications which must temper the interpretation of CPM effects on cartilage healing.

Salter and colleagues have been important contributors to the studies of facilitation of cartilage healing under the influence of CPM. They have shown convincingly that small defects (on the order of magnitude of one-eighth in. diameter) of the femoral articular cartilage in rabbits heal with hyaline cartilage in a significant percentage of knees mobilized by CPM. This is an important observation that relates to several clinical circumstances in which small defects in hyaline cartilage of the joint surface occur. It is important to note that the facilitation of repair of primitive mesenchymal cells to hyaline cartilage occurs in *only* the very small defects, not in large defects or full surface defects.

Continuous Passive Motion Influences on Periosteal and Perichondrial Grafting

Because only small cartilage defects heal with a satisfactory extracellular matrix of hyaline cartilage, several investigators have searched for improved techniques for treatment of such defects. Ohlsen[63] and Engkvist, et al.,[64,65] studied rib perichondrial tissue as a potential source of primitive cells with chondrogenic potential for this purpose. The work was later confirmed by Coutts, et al.,[65] by Salter, et al.,[66-68] and by Mooney, et al.[69] Because experimental studies indicated considerable promise, pilot clinical perichondrial arthroplasty studies for small joints of the hand were soon thereafter performed with some success.[70] Poussa[71] showed similar chondrogenic potential of periosteal grafts. O'Driscoll and Salter confirmed Poussa's work in a rabbit knee joint model.[56] They were able to improve the result from 8% success in immobilized knees to 59% success in knees managed by CPM. Fixation of the periosteal or perichondrial membrane is crucial to the successful outcome of periosteal or perichondrial grafting. O'Driscoll, et al., developed a method of stretching the periosteal membrane over a bone plug sized to fit the defect to be filled. This technique has worked effectively in the experimental application,[66-68] but different methodology will be required for clinical application.

Continuous Passive Motion Influence on Fracture Healing

The development of modern biomechanical devices and modern principles of application of those devices to fracture fixation permits the use of CPM early in the post injury states.[48] CPM is most effectively applied in intra-articular fractures in which fracture lines through subchondral bone and articular cartilage are commonly observed. Following the observations of Salter, et al.,[67] it frequently is the case that the width of the gap between fracture fragments after reduction is less than one-eighth in. If congruence of the joint is established and the cartilage fracture gaps are narrow, CPM should facilitate the cartilage healing process. Additional benefits should be anticipated in terms of facilitation of the rehabilitation program by lessening stress deprivation effects and by providing stress enhancement to guide deposition of matrix components in an orderly and functionally desirable alignment.

Intermittent Passive Motion Effects on Tendon Healing

The application of passive motion to flexor tendon healing in the flexor tendon sheath has been slow to evolve for two reasons: (1) concern about integrity of the suture line and (2) concern about the mechanism of tendon healing requiring ingrowth of connective tissue from the flexor tendon sheath. The paradox of this process, termed the "one-wound concept" by Peacock,[41] was that the very tissue ingrowth that caused healing also caused the tendon to be locked against the flexor sheath and limited the functional tendon excursion. Indeed, the major failures are not with tendon healing, but with tendon adhesions, which significantly reduce the range of motion of the tendon and affected joints. The fundamental studies of Gelberman, et al.,[57] reversed this thinking by demonstrating clearly that tendon healing could occur by an intrinsic mechanism of proliferation of epitenon and endotenon cells when the extrinsic mechanism was blocked by intermittent passive motion. The canine forepaw model was used for these flexor tendon studies. Not only did the tendon heal by the intrinsic route, but the healing occurred more rapidly and with greater mechanical strength while simultaneously preserving mobility of tendon and joints of the affected finger.

It is important to note that the motion required for this effect is not of great duration. The mobilization schedule used was five minutes of careful manual passive motion conducted by a therapist twice a day. The remainder of the time the limb was immobilized in a fiberglass cast. This "mini" passive motion schedule recognized the concerns for the potential rupture of the suture line that occurs with a more aggressive passive motion protocol.

In this instance, motion therapy was able to convert the healing mode from extrinsic to intrinsic, while simultaneously providing improved healing strength and improved mobility—a string of therapeutic bonuses that are seldom so clearly identified after modification of a treatment protocol.

Salter and colleagues have shown, in the patellar tendon laceration model, similar effects of improved healing associated with continuous passive motion. In this case, repair involves both extrinsic and intrinsic mechanisms because of the anatomical differences between patellar and flexor tendons.

Intermittent Active Motion Effects in Ligament Healing

The discussion of ligament healing is confounded by the diversity of structures under the ligament classification with respect to anatomical and physiological idiosyncrasies. For example, the anterior cruciate ligament (ACL) of the knee will not heal for reasons not precisely known, although the "hostile" synovial environment in which the ACL resides is widely presumed to be an important or even decisive factor in that outcome. The ACL receives significant nutrition from synovial fluid and that nutritional source may not be adequate to support fibroblastic proliferation (although it will support a healing response in the case of flexor tendon). Recently, it has been demonstrated in our laboratory that the cells of the ACL have fibro-cartilage characteristics. Failure of fibrocartilage structures to heal is well known. However, it is unknown whether the cellular morphology of the ACL is the explanation for its poor healing. The enigma remains.

Nevertheless, CPM is used by many clinicians in the postoperative period following replacement of the ACL by a grafting technique using a tendon or a synthetic substitute for the ligament. Interestingly, tendon and ligament are not identical biochemically. Distinctive differences between collagen crosslinks and collagen types have been reported.[72] Burks has cautioned that CPM can cause failure of the tendon graft if the graft is not isometric and is not firmly secured.[73] However, if those conditions prevail, the graft is unlikely to survive in a rehabilitation setting whether CPM is used or not. Clinical studies by Noyes support the conclusion that CPM is a safe modality when surgery is properly performed.[74] Tendon grafts actually become weak structurally 3 to 6 weeks after insertion. The tendon cells undergo autolysis in this environment[75] and are replaced by cells from synovial sources. The matrix of the graft is gradually remodeled and assumes the matrix characteristics of ACL.[75]

Unfortunately, none of the animal studies have

shown recovery of mechanical strength of the ACL graft substitute to the level of the original tissue's mechanical and structural properties.

Better experimental and clinical results can be reported for most other ligaments. The medial collateral ligament of the knee, for example, has an abundant surrounding soft tissue blood supply that offers ample nutritional and cellular support of the needed fibroplasia. In this case, the recent work of Inoue has provided strong evidence supporting the concept of early active motion of the knee.[58] When compared to knees that were immobilized the entire postoperative period, or knees that were immobilized the first half of the postoperative period, the early activity group clearly showed superior mechanical and structural strength at the end of 12 weeks. Others have shown a favorable effect of CPM on reorganization of the fibrils of the scar into parallel arrays.[76] It is to be emphasized that in these models the cruciate ligaments are intact, thus providing the stability necessary for early ambulation or CPM.

Continuous Passive Motion After Total Knee Replacement

The total knee replacement procedures now frequently performed for degenerative or rheumatoid arthritis have provided a challenging problem for the application of CPM. Particular needs for improving range of motion postoperatively were felt in the rehabilitation of these patients. Slow recovery of flexion is commonly observed postoperatively, sometimes requiring forceful manipulation under anesthesia.

A multi-institutional study of over 100 total knee replacement cases treated traditionally and compared to similar cases treated with CPM has provided data which clarify the effectiveness of CPM in a clinical rehabilitation setting.[77,78] The patients treated with CPM had a more rapid gain in knee motion and had a shorter hospital stay than patients treated traditionally, a finding supported by other studies.[79-81] Data in Coutts' series showed a lower pain medication requirement than in the traditionally treated series. The theory commonly employed to explain the surprising tolerance of postoperative patients for passive motion is the "gate" theory of Melzack and Wall.[82] This theory postulates that nonpainful afferent input into spinal cord ganglia can overwhelm pain fiber input, thereby blocking a part of the pain perception otherwise experienced. CPM provides considerable afferent input because of the effects of motion on proprioceptive receptors. There is no universal acceptance of this effect in postoperative applications of CPM, but at least it seems clear that CPM does not increase pain medication requirements.

Continuous Passive Motion and Wound Healing

CPM in the postoperative patient does not inhibit wound healing. No wound disruptions have been reported from application of CPM postoperatively, and furthermore, postoperative swelling and joint effusions were reduced.[77] In total, the benefits of a few days of application of CPM postoperatively in this application appear to significantly outweigh questions of cost or risk.

Continuous Passive Motion Prophylaxis Against Thrombophlebitis

The use of CPM in the variety of clinical applications described above has evoked interest in its use in prophylaxis against thrombophlebitis in the postoperative period of high risk.[83] The physiological basis of the wished effect is the pulsation in intramuscular pressure that occurs during passive motion as the muscles of the limb are lengthened and shortened passively.[84] The passive pressure alteration almost certainly has the same functional effect as active muscle contraction in propelling venous blood back to the heart. Because venous stasis is presumed to be an important factor in venous thrombosis, the utilization of CPM, which would significantly reduce venous stasis, would be expected to have a salutary effect on reducing the rate of complications of postoperative thrombophlebitis and pulmonary embolism.

Preliminary results suggesting the validity of this line of reasoning have been presented by Lynch, et al.,[85] and by Vince, et al.,[81] but other studies showed no prophylaxis with respect to incidence of deep venous thrombosis (DVT) as visualized by venogram.[79,80] Several centers have ongoing studies on this problem and considerable information will be forthcoming to document the degree of effectiveness of CPM in this application. As is typical of other studies of DVT postoperatively, the clinical series size must be large in order to be valid.

Other Uses of Continuous Passive Motion

An almost infinite variety of conditions can be treated by CPM. These include use in treatment of elbow contractures post surgical release,[86] treatment of hemophiliac joints post synovectomy,[87] and treatment of knee contractures post arthroscopy.[88] Recent review articles by Salter and by Mooney highlight other related clinical applications.[67,48] The principles of application of CPM are so fundamental as to preclude boundaries with respect to potential future applications, including application to the spine.

CONTINUOUS PASSIVE MOTION AS A POTENTIAL MODALITY TO INFLUENCE CENTRAL NERVOUS SYSTEM ADAPTATION FOLLOWING BRAIN INJURY

Nickel[89] has proposed that CPM may be useful as a rehabilitation modality following stroke. There is an awakening interest in the concept of central nervous system plasticity and in the ability of the central nervous system to recover from injury by development of alternative neural pathways. The clinical question posed is whether passive motion might accelerate this process. The proposed mechanism is increased afferent input from proprioceptive receptors in joints and muscles of the motion segment, which would modulate the central nervous system adaptive response. The local musculoskeletal benefits to be gained are obvious: reduced incidence of joint contracture at a relatively low cost in terms of equipment and therapy personnel. It is expected, for example, that much of the CPM application could be carried out in the home.

It is to be emphasized that this hypothesis is advanced on theoretical grounds and that data from carefully controlled studies are yet to be published.

IMPLICATIONS OF STUDIES ON PERIPHERAL JOINTS TO STRESS DEPENDENCE OF THE SPINE

There are similarities between problems of intervertebral disc healing and healing of other fibrocartilaginous structures, e.g., knee meniscus, glenoid labrum, and the anterior cruciate ligament of the knee. These similarities focus upon problems generated by poor blood supply and by the predominance of fibrocartilage cells in the constituent tissues. Such cells respond poorly to injury, cannot produce scar, and the ability for the chemotaxis mechanism appears limited because of the poor blood supply and limited pool of undifferentiated cellular elements in the vicinity of the injury. One report describes this deficiency of the anulus fibrosus cells[5] in healing. Most of the studies on this problem have focused on meniscus or anterior cruciate ligament. As our experience is with the ACL, that model is described briefly.

The ACL is a fibrocartilaginous structure. Despite the controversy regarding clinical management of the patient with an acute ACL injury,[90–94] most agree that the ACL has a poor capacity for healing. This healing deficiency has been the focus of numerous studies involving various ACL healing models.[93,95–97] Numerous factors are present that may in some way detract from the ACLs ability to repair itself after the proper surgical intervention. Wound healing in general is affected by factors associated with the patient's condition including age, activity level, nutrition, and disease states. Factors that solely affect the healing capacity of the cruciate ligaments include the complex anatomy of these structures, biomechanical forces resulting from motion and muscle action, the nutritional delivery system, the unique biological environment in which these ligaments reside, and the proposed limited intrinsic capacity of the ACL cells to support the healing process.

ACL NUTRITION

The blood supply to various subsections of the cruciate ligament is poor or limited.[95,98] Alm and Stromberg[98] performed early vascularization studies on the anterior and posterior cruciate ligaments in dogs by means of microangiography and histology. A paraligamentous network of vessels was noted coursing through the synovial membrane. These vessels entered the ligaments transversely and anastomosed freely with endoligamentous vessels. The core of the midportion of the cruciate ligaments was less well vascularized than the proximal and distal cores. Arnoczky[95] reported similar findings for normal vascular anatomy of the cruciate ligaments, including less abundant vasculature in the central part of the midportion of both cruciate ligaments. The posterior cruciate ligament, however, was consistently surrounded by a greater density of vessels than the ACL.

Synovial fluid, formed from an ultrafiltrate of blood,[99] has been shown to be a physiologically important though not exclusive nutrient delivery pathway for the ACL.[100] Studies of the nutrient pathway to flexor tendons suggest that diffusion is an important route of nutrient delivery to other fibrous structures immersed in synovial fluid.[101–103]

Our laboratory studied the role of synovial fluid in providing nutrition to rabbit knee ligaments and menisci by intra-articular injection of tritiated proline (a collagen precursor).[100] Incorporated substrate, tritiated hydroxyproline (^{3}H hyp), was measured in the collateral ligaments, cruciate ligaments, and menisci. Autoradiography demonstrated concentration of the isotope (^{3}H proline) and its metabolite (^{3}H hyp) in and around fibroblasts of all these tissues. Measurements of ^{3}H hyp incorporation showed that all knee structures tested utilized synovial-fluid derived proline. The cruciate ligaments demonstrated the highest uptake of ^{3}H hyp. Control ligaments and menisci from the contralateral limb showed no detectable isotope. These findings indicate that these structures can derive nutrition from a synovial fluid source. They also indicate that a major pathway of nutrient delivery is from synovial arterial capillaries to the synovial cavity, and then by trans-synovial bulk flow and diffusion to the knee ligaments and menisci.

It is apparent, then, that the cruciate ligaments derive their nutrition from two sources: (1) its vascular supply which courses from the middle geniculate artery and popliteal arteries to the synovial membrane, and finally to the cruciate ligament structures, and (2) the synovial fluid that continuously bathes the cruciates and allows for trans-synovial bulk flow and diffusion for nutrient delivery. Although a vascular response is noted after injury, the viability of these tissues post injury and repair has been questioned.

BIOLOGIC ENVIRONMENT

The cruciate ligaments reside in a unique environment. Both ligaments are intracapsular, and both are enveloped by a synovial membrane, effectively making them extrasynovial. The synovial membrane, which is only a few cells thick, separates the anterior and posterior cruciate ligaments from the synovial fluid that bathes the other intracapsular knee joint structures.

Of the many factors important in ligament healing such as mechanical forces, blood supply, and local environment, it is the local environment that has often been used as an explanation for the poor healing capacity of the cruciate ligaments.[93] This local environment has been referred to as the "hostile" environment of the synovial joint space. During ACL injury, the synovial membrane is usually torn, exposing the frayed ligament ends to a host of potentially destructive enzymes released by the breakdown of hemarthrosis fluid of the injured joint.

Synovial fluid has been shown to affect ligament fibroblasts, the cells which have crucial importance in ligament healing. Using tissue culture techniques, Andrich and Holmes[104] demonstrated that ACL fibroblast proliferation was diminished when exposed to synovial fluid. Rapid degeneration of the ACL occurs after acute rupture. This phenomenon was described clinically by Warren,[105] who showed that ruptured ACL substance can completely disappear 6 weeks after injury. Kohn[106] confirmed these results,

noting either complete disappearance or only a remnant of the ACL with 32 patients arthroscoped 8 months to 20 years after injury. O'Donoghue,[93] using a dog model of ACL injury, reported inflammatory changes in the unrepaired, released ligaments with significant shortening within 10 weeks of injury.

Results in our laboratory demonstrated a relatively large increase (82%) in injured ACL collagenase content as compared to control ACLs (3 days postinjury). This was consistent with the average net loss of 34% in total collagen mass from the injured ACLs.

Collagenase release has been documented from other articular structures such as synovium[107,108] and articular cartilage.[109,110] These structures synthesize and release a latent form of collagenase. The data from this experiment and others indicate that the ACL and menisci secrete only active enzymes that may be detrimental to the intra-articular structures.[111]

Detractors from the "hostile environment" theory emphasize that tendons are exposed to a fluid similar to synovial fluid in their sheath, and no evidence exists for poor tendon healing in these areas.[112] Flexor tendon fibroblasts appear to utilize synovial fluid for nutrition, and tendon segments that were replaced within a synovial sheath chamber demonstrated histologically that peripheral fibroblasts survived and proliferated.[113–115] Although the cellular elements in tendon appear to show no adverse effects from synovial fluid, one must remember that we cannot validly compare tendons to ligaments in this manner. Tendons and ligaments have different histological and biochemical characteristics.[72] In addition, flexor tendon naturally exists within the synovial fluid filled sheath, whereas the native environment of the cruciate ligaments is extrasynovial.

Post ACL injury, acute hemarthrosis fluid fills the joint space. The sheath enveloping the ACL is generally torn, leaving the frayed ends of the ACL exposed to hemarthrosis fluid, which appears to have a deleterious affect on knee joint structures.[116,117] Fabry in 1982[118] proposed that degradative enzymes were responsible for the degenerative changes seen in hemophilic arthropathy. Pforringer[119] has demonstrated decreases in the mechanical properties of the femur-ACL-tibia complex, as well as histological changes in the ACL after acute hemarthrosis.[120] The slight reduction in mechanical properties with hemarthrosis increased with injury to the synovial sheath.

Studies from our laboratory using a rabbit model of acute hemarthrosis have shown that the menisci, which lack a synovial covering, demonstrated an increase in degradative activity assessed by levels of collagenase activity.[121] Subsequent work found no significant effects of acute hemarthrosis on collagenase activity from ACLs (with intact synovium) and control ACLs.[122]

In contrast to the menisci, the ACL may be a privileged intra-articular structure, as it possesses a synovial covering which allows it to be protected from the intra-articular environment. With acute rupture of the ACL and resultant synovial injury, this protective barrier may be lost. Subsequent exposure of ligament substance to the intra-articular environment may produce changes in the ligament and, in part, explain the poor results reported with attempts to primarily repair the ACL.

A STUDY OF THE INTRINSIC HEALING MECHANISM

Animal Model

To allow us to understand the ACL's intrinsic healing mechanism, a surgical model was developed[123] after numerous surgical repair methods were studied.[123] To limit stump retraction and ensure accurate approximation of the lacerated portions of the ACL, a Z-plasty repair was attempted. Six weeks later no evidence of healing was observed. Failure of this technique was related to the retraction of lacerated ACL stumps, followed by resorption of the exposed ligament ends.

Partial transection of the ACL has been attempted previously in animal models. O'Donoghue[93] described their poor results, and Arnoczsky[95] noted a vascular proliferation in the area of injury, but no evidence of bridging of the gap. Arnoczsky concluded that the inability to heal may be related to the fact that they had lacerated the "anteromedial band" of the ACL, a portion of the ACL that is taut throughout the normal range of motion.

To obviate this problem, the postero-lateral portion of the ACL was transected. An immediate retraction of the incised portion of the ligament was noted. No evidence of gap reduction was shown in any of the animals. A modified Marshall procedure was then attempted to hold the edges of the partially transected ACL together. Six weeks after this operation none of the animals revealed evidence of ACL wound healing. It became obvious that a stent of uncut tissue on one side of the laceration was insufficient to control retraction of the cut ends of the ligament. To circumvent this problem a model was developed in which only the midportion of the ligament was transected. This model minimally disturbs the biomechanical stability of the ligament by retaining lateral and medial ligament continuity. Thus, the lacerated ends stay in close proximity to each other during the post laceration recovery period.

The surface area of the ligament exposed to joint fluid is limited to the site of penetration into the ligament by a 2-mm-wide, razor thin, square-edged Beaver blade. Access to the area of injury by enzymes contained in the synovial space is restricted. The model thereby largely, although not totally, eliminates two mechanisms proposed to be responsible for failure of ACL healing; namely destabilizing biomechanical forces at the injury site, and enzymatic degradation of ligament substance along with inhibition of fibroblast activity by synovial fluid. Using the surgical ACL laceration herein described, we have observed a partial healing response in a small percentage (5%) of ACLs tested.

Healing Response

The intrinsic healing capacity of the cruciates may be the limiting factor in their response to injury. Ultrastructural, histological, biochemical, and biomechanical differences have been described between the ACL and MCL, tissues with strikingly different capacities for healing.[72,124] Light microscopy of the MCL reveals spindle-shaped cells aligned with the long axis of the ligament and interspersed throughout the collagen fiber bundles.[72] The ACL cells are oval shaped and aligned in columns between fiber bundles. Ultrastructurally, MCL collagen fibers are uniformly of large diameter.[124] The fibroblasts have long cellular processes in close apposition to surrounding collagen fibrils. The ACL has a more heterogeneous population of fibril diameters. Oval-shaped cells are surrounded by an amorphous ground substance and have small microprocesses that are not in close apposition to collagen fibrils.

It appears that a spectrum of fibroblast phenotypes exists between the spindle-shaped connective tissue fibroblast of dermis, tendon and fascia on the one hand, and the rounded, nested fibroblast of fibrocartilage on the other. The ACL fibroblast seems to exist near the fibrocartilaginous end of the spectrum in terms of morphologic features. Possibly, the morphological features of these fibroblasts are interrelated with cellular function, and play a determinate role in their response to injury. The form/function suitable for survival in a synovial environment may not be sufficient for mounting and sustaining an effective healing response. The concept that the shape of a cell and its orientation with respect to the surrounding matrix are important factors in modulating its proliferative response to mitogens was mentioned by Wessels[125] in studies on skin. These observations were expanded by Gospodarowicz in a paper entitled "Cellular Shape is Determined by the Extracellular Matrix and is Responsible for the Control of Cellular Growth and Function."[126]

Fibronectin

Fibronectins (Fns) are a class of high molecular weight glycoproteins proposed as a key element in the structural interrelationship of cells to matrix and to other cells.[127,128] They are associated with an array of cellular functions, including cellular adhesion (both cell-to-cell and cell-to-substratum), intra and extracellular matrix morphology, cell migration, and reticuloendothelial system function (i.e., phagocytosis and chemotaxis). By having adhesive domains specific to fibrin, actin, hyaluronic acid, collagen, heparin, and cell surface factors, they function to attract and couple key elements in normal, healing, and growing organized tissue. In fact, Fn has been shown to facilitate wound healing[129] and to be required for normal collagen organization and deposition by fibroblasts in vitro.[130]

The ACL, MCL, and meniscus have stained positive for Fn. The Fn is heavily concentrated in the amorphous ground substance surrounding the ACL cells and meniscal cells, whereas in the MCL the distribution of Fn is spread evenly over the cell membrane, even out along the long cellular processes.

The amount of Fn in rabbit periarticular soft tissues has also been quantitated.[131] The amounts of total extractable Fn found to be present in ACL, PCL, MCL, and patellar tendon (PT), respectively, were 2.0, 1.9, 0.8 and 0.7 μg/mg of dry tissue. While the Fn quantities in ACL and PCL were found to be similar, they were over twice as high as the amounts found in MCL and PT.

While Fn levels have been observed to increase in healing tissue,[132–134] it is not known whether differences in the baseline levels of Fn affect the healing potential of a tissue such as cruciate ligament. Baseline levels in the cruciates are high compared to other periarticular tissues that have a better healing response. While the importance of Fn in various connective tissues is increasingly becoming more evident, further studies are required to clarify its role in normal ligament structure and in the ligament healing response.

ADHESIVE PROTEIN RECEPTORS

Recently, a superfamily of adhesion-mediating cell surface glycoproteins (the integrins) has been identified and partially characterized.[135] A major subfamily called the "very late antigens" (VLA) appears to play a primary role in the adhesion of cells to components of the extracellular matrix including Fn, collagen, and laminin.

The VLA's are transmembrane glycoproteins expressed on a wide variety of cells including fibroblasts, epithelial cells, and hematopoietic cells. A number of functional roles have been assigned to these adhesive protein receptors, including cell migration cell-matrix adhesions, wound contraction, and ligament "tensioning."[136]

The adhesive protein receptors of ligament tissue have received little attention to date. Generalizing from other fibroblast-containing structures, it is reasonable to expect that these receptors exist on cells of the cruciate ligaments and other periarticular tissues. Recently, TGF_β has been found to regulate the cell-surface display of VLA's on a variety of cell types, and modulate the interaction of cells with the extracellular matrix.[137,138] These studies lead us to believe that cell surface receptor distribution and expression may have profound effects on ligament healing capacity. Fundamental studies on these receptors are in progress in several laboratories with respect to distribution in various connective tissue cells and with respect to alteration of expansion during the healing process.

CONCLUSIONS

This review summarizes the existing knowledge on the importance of stress and motion to synovial joint homeostasis. The deleterious effects of stress deprivation occur rapidly and are profound, influencing joint mechanics, biochemistry, and physiology in fundamental ways. The recovery from this process is not symmetrical, requiring many months rather than weeks to re-establish near normal values. In fact, mechanical strength of composite ligament structures have not regained normal strength even after 12 months of resumption of activity.

Exercise at a level producing cardiac hypertrophy and increased cardiac output causes hypertrophy of specialized fibrous connective tissues such as tendons and ligaments. However, that effect occurs slowly at great effort: it requires one year to produce hypertrophy which is at nominal levels of significance.

The use of continuous passive movement (CPM) to bypass some of the deleterious effects of stress deprivation and its application to repair of cartilage, tendon, ligament, and fractures are described. Clinical use in the postoperative management of total joint replacement seems solidly in place and is widely applied to facilitate rehabilitation of the joint affected, to reduce swelling and joint effusion, possibly to reduce incidence of thrombophlebitis and to shorten the hospital stay.

Passive motion places in effect such fundamental cellular and tissue processes that we are probably observing only the infancy of its development. The next decade should see a dramatic increase in its application to problems in the field of synovial joint rehabilitation.

The manner in which cells interpret physical signals is a lively field for fundamental science in conjunction with, and in support of, the clinical efforts. Although few of these experimental or clinical studies have used spine models, there is little reason to believe that soft tissue supporting tissue of the spine would be exempt from such fundamental physiological principles.

CLINICAL APPLICATIONS

Although more and better clinical studies in this field are imperative, the clinical utility of exercise as a therapeutic adjunct for rehabilitation of supporting connective tissues of the spine is on the threshold of a rapid expansion resulting from successes in the several applications described. Facilitation of repair processes by early motion seems an almost universal observation for tendon, ligament, cartilage, and bone. Passive motion appears to be a useful adjunct until active motion can be instituted. In recent years, devices have been developed for application to the hand, large joints of the upper and lower extremities, and the spine. The utility of the passive motion concept to treatment of such widely divergent problems as septic arthritis, hemarthrosis, total joint replacement, and tendon repair indicates the breadth of applications currently employed clinically. The key appears to be the importance of mechanical stimuli as signals to cell receptors that control synthesis of matrix components and other factors that guide extracellular organization of those components. Clearly, additional efforts are required to provide more complete documentation of the importance and relevance of these principles to the spine. The primacy of early application of sound rehabilitation principles in treatment of spinal injury is so far unchallenged.

REFERENCES

1. Cole, T.C., Burkhardt, D., Ghosh, P., Ryan, M., Taylor, T.: Effects of spinal fusion on the proteoglycans of the canine intervertebral disc. J Orthop Res 3:277–291, 1985.
2. Cole, T.C., Ghosh, P., Hannan, N.J., Taylor, T.K.F., Bellenger, C.R.: The response of the canine intervertebral disc to immobilization produced by spinal arthrodesis is dependent on constitutional factors. J Orthop Res 5:337–347, 1987.
3. Akeson, W.H., Amiel, D., Woo, S.L.-Y.: Immobility effects on synovial joints—the pathomechanics of joint contracture. Biorheology 17:95–100, 1980.
4. Lyon, R.M., et al.: The ACL: a fibrocartilagenous structure. Trans ORS 14:189, 1989.
5. Hampton, D., Laros, G., McCarron, R., Franks, D.: Healing potential of the anulus fibrosus. Spine 14(4):398–401, 1989.
6. Key, J.A., Ford, L.T.: Experimental intervertebral disc lesion. J Bone Joint Surg 30A:621–630, 1948.
7. Lipson, S.J., Muir, H.: Proteoglycans in experimental intervertebral disk degeneration. Spine 6:194–210, 1981.
8. Smith, J.W.: Experimental incision of the intervertebral disc. J Bone Joint Surg 33B:612–625, 1951.
9. Yu, S., Haughton, V.M., Sether, L.A., Wagner, M.: Anulus fibrosus in bulging intervertebral disks. Radiology 169:761–763, 1988.
10. Akeson, W.H.: An experimental study of joint stiffness. J Bone Joint Surg 43A:1022, 1961.
11. Akeson, W.H., Amiel, D., Woo, S.L.-Y.: Immobility effects on synovial joints: the pathomechanics of joint contracture. Biorheology 17:95, 1980.
12. Woo, S.L.-Y., et al.: Effect of immobilization and exercise on strength characteristics of bone-medial collateral ligament-bone complex. Am Soc Mech Eng Symp 32:62, 1979.
13. Akeson, W.H., Woo, S.L.-Y., Amiel, D., Frank, C.B.: The biology of ligaments. In Rehabilitation of the Injured Knee. (Edited by L. Hunter and F. Funk). St. Louis, C.V. Mosby, 1984.
14. Frank, C., Akeson, W.H., Woo, S.L.-Y., Amiel, D., Coutts, R.D.: Physiology and therapeutic value of passive joint motion. Clin Orthop 185:113, 1984.
15. Evans, E.B., Eggers, G.W.N., Butler, J.K., Blumel, J.: Experimental immobilization and remobilization of rat knee joints. J Bone Joint Surg 42A:737, 1960.
16. Enneking, W.F., Horowitz, M.: The intra-articular effects of immobilization on the human knee. J Bone Joint Surg 54A:973, 1972.
17. Baker, W.C., Thomas, T.G., Kirkaldy-Willis, W.H.: Changes in the cartilage of the posterior intervertebral joints after anterior fusion. J Bone Joint Surg 51B(4):737, 1969.
18. Von Reyher, C.: On the cartilage and synovial membranes of the joints. J Anat Physiol 8:261, 1874.
19. Weichselbaum, A.: Die feineren verandeungen des gelenk knorpels bei fungoser synovitis und caries der gelenkenden. Virchows Archiv 73:461, 1878.
20. Parker, F., Keefer, C.S.: Gross and histologic changes in the knee joint in rheumatoid arthritis. Arch Path 20(4):507, 1935.
21. Salter, R.B., Field, P.: The effects of continuous compression on living articular cartilage. J Bone Joint Surg 42A:31, 1960.
22. Thaxter, T.H., Mann, R.A., Anderson, C.E.: Degeneration of immobilized knee joints in rats. J Bone Joint Surg 47A:567, 1965.
23. Akeson, W.H., Woo, S.L.-Y., Amiel, D., Coutts, R.D., Daniel, D.: The connective tissue response to immobility: biochemical changes in periarticular connective tissue of the immobilized rabbit knee. Clin Orthop 93:356, 1973.
24. Woo, S.L.-Y., Matthews, J.V., Akeson, W.H., Amiel, D., Convery, R.: Connective tissue response to immobility. Correlative study of biomechanical and biochemical measurements of normal and immobilized rabbit knees. Arthritis Rheum 18(3):257, 1975.
25. Amiel, D., Frey, C., Woo, S.L.-Y., Harwood, F., Akeson, W.H.: Value of hyaluronic acid in the prevention of contracture formation. Clin Orthop 196:22, 1985.
26. Woo, S.L.-Y., Gomez, M.A., Seguchi, Y., Endo, C.M., Akeson, W.H.: Measurement of mechanical properties of ligament substance from a bone-ligament-bone preparation. J Orthop Res 1:22, 1983.
27. Laros, G.S., Tipton, C.M., Cooper, R.R.: Influence of physical activity on ligament insertions in the knees of dogs. J Bone Joint Surg 53A:275, 1971.
28. Cooper, R.R., Misel, S.: Tendon and ligament insertion. J Bone Joint Surg 52A:1, 1970.
29. Tipton, C.M., Matthes, R.D., Martin, R.R.: Influence of age and sex on the strength of bone-ligament junctions in knee joints of rats. J Bone Joint Surg 60A:230, 1978.

30. Woo, S.L.-Y., et al.: The response of cortical long bone secondary to exercise training. Trans 26th Annu Meet Orthop Res Soc 5:256, 1980.
31. Woo, S.L.-Y., Ritter, M.A., Gomez, M.A., Kuei, S.C., Akeson, W.H.: The biomechanical and structural properties of swine digital flexor tendons secondary to running exercise. Orthop Trans 4(2):165, 1980.
32. Woo, S.L.-Y., et al.: The biomechanical and biochemical changes of the MCL following immobilization and remobilization. J Bone Joint Surg, in press.
33. Noyes, F.R., Torvik, P.J., Hyde, W.B., DeLucas, J.L.: Biomechanics of ligament failure. II. An analysis of immobilization, exercise and reconditioning effects in primates. J Bone Joint Surg 56A:1406, 1974.
34. Akeson, W.H., Woo, S.L.-Y., Amiel, D., Coutts, R.D., Daniel, D.: The connective tissue response to immobility: biochemical changes in periarticular connective tissue of the immobilized rabbit knee. Clin Orthop 93:356, 1973.
35. Swann, D.A., Radin, E.L., Nazimiec, M.: Role of hyaluronic acid in joint lubrication. Ann Rheum Dis 33:318, 1974.
36. Akeson, W.H., Amiel, D., LaViolette, D.: The connective tissue response to immobility. A study of chondroitin 4 and 6 sulfate and dermatan sulfate changes in periarticular connective tissue of control and immobilized knees of dogs. Clin Orthop 51:183, 1967.
37. Schiller, S., Matthews, M.D., Cifonelli, J., Dorfman, A.: The metabolism of mucopoly saccharides in animals. Further studies on skin utilizing C14 glucose, C14 acetate, and S35 sodium sulfate. J Biol Chem 218:139, 1956.
38. Neuberger, A., Slack, H.G.B.: The metabolism of collagen from liver, bones, skin and tendon in the normal rat. Biochem J 53:47, 1953.
39. Guyton, A.C., Barber, B.J., Moffatt, D.S.: Theory of interstitial pressures. In Tissue Fluid Pressure and Composition (Edited by A. Hargens). Baltimore. W.J. Wilkins, 1980.
40. Brooke, J.S., Slack, H.G.B.: Metabolism of connective tissue in limb atrophy in the rabbit. Ann Rheum 18:129, 1959.
41. Peacock, E.E.: Comparison of collagenous tissue surrounding normal and immobilized joints. Surg Forum 14:440, 1963.
42. Amiel, D., Akeson, W.H., Harwood, F.L., Mechanic, G.L.: Effect on nine week immobilization of the types of collagen synthesized in periarticular connective tissue from rabbit knees. Trans Orthop Res Soc, p. 5, 1980.
43. Klein, L., Dawson, M.H., Heiple, K.G.: Turnover of collagen in the adult rat after denervation. J Bone Joint Surg 59A:1065, 1977.
44. Akeson, W.H., Amiel, D., Woo, S.L.-Y., Harwood, F.L.: Mechanical imperatives for synovial joint homeostasis: the present potential for their therapeutic manipulation. Proc Third Int Congress Biorheology, p. 47, 1978.
45. Akeson, W.H., Amiel, D., Mechanic, G.L., Woo, S.L.-Y., Harwood, F.L.: Collagen cross-linking alterations in joint contractures: changes in the reducible cross-links in periarticular connective tissue collagen after nine weeks of immobilization. Connect Tissue Res 5:15, 1977.
46. Bailey, A.J., Robins, S.P.: Development and maturation of the cross-links in the collagen fibers of skin. Front Matrix Biol 1:130, 1973.
47. Jackson, D.S., Mechanic, G.: Cross-link patterns of collagens synthesized by cultures of 3T6 and 3T3 fibroblasts and by fibroblasts of various granulation tissues. Biochim Biophys Acta, p. 336, 1974.
48. Mooney, V., Stills, M.: Continuous passive motion with joint fractures and infections. Orthop Clinics of North America 18(1):1, 1987.
49. Pedowitz, R.A., et al.: Intraarticular pressure during continuous passive motion of the human knee. J Orthop Res 7:530, 1989.
50. Baxendale, R.H., Ferrell, W.R., Wood, L.: Intra-articular pressures during active and passive movement of normal and distended human knee joints. J Physiol 396:179P, 1985.
51. Caughey, D.E., Bywaters, E.G.L.: Joint fluid pressure in chronic knee effusions. Ann Rheum Dis 22:106, 1963.
52. O'Driscoll, S.W., Kumar, A., Salter, R.B.: The effect of continuous passive motion on the clearance of a hemarthrosis. Clin Orthop 176:336, 1983.
53. Danzig, L.A., et al.: Increased transsynovial transport with continuous passive motion. J Orthop Res 5:409, 1987.
54. Skyhar, M.J., Danzig, L.A., Hargens, A.R., Akeson, W.H.: Nutrition of the anterior cruciate ligament. Effects of continuous passive motion. Am J Sports Med 13(6):415, 1985.
55. Salter, R.B., Bell, R.S., Keeley, F.: The protective effect of continuous passive motion on living articular cartilage in acute septic arthritis: an experimental investigation in the rabbit. Clin Orthop 159:223, 1981.
56. O'Driscoll, S.W., Salter, R.B.: The induction of neochondrogenesis in free intra-articular periosteal autografts under the influence of continuous passive motion. J Bone Joint Surg 66A(8):1248, 1984.
57. Gelberman, R.H., Woo, S.L.-Y., Lothringer, K., Akeson, W.H., Amiel, D.: Effects of early intermittent passive mobilization on healing canine flexor tendons. J Hand Surg 7:170, 1982.
58. Inoue, M., et al.: Medial collateral ligament healing: repair vs nonrepair. Trans Orthop Res Soc, p. 78, 1986.
59. Salter, R.B., Simmonds, D.F., Malcolm, B.W., Rumble, E.J., MacMichael, D.: The biological effects of continuous passive motion on the healing of full-thickness defects in articular cartilage: an experimental investigation in the rabbit. J Bone Joint Surg 62:1232, 1980.
60. Mooney, V., Ferguson, A.B. Jr.: The influence of immobilization and motion on the formation of fibrocartilage in the repair granuloma after joint resection in the rabbit. J Bone Joint Surg 48:1145, 1966.
61. Hohl, M., Luck, J.V.: Fractures of the tibial condyle. J Bone Joint Surg 38A:1001, 1956.
62. Convery, F.R., Akeson, W.H., Keown, G.H.: The repair of large osteochondral defects. An experimental study in horses. Clin Orthop 82:253, 1972.
63. Ohlsen, L.: Cartilage regeneration from perichondrium. Experimental and clinical applications. Plast Reconstr Surg 62:507, 1978.
64. Engkvist, O.: Reconstruction of patellar articular cartilage with free autologous perichondrial grafts. An experimental study in dogs. Scand J Plast Reconstr Surg Hand Surg 13:361, 1979.
65. Coutts, R.D., Amiel, D., Woo, S.L.-Y., Woo, Y.-K., Akeson, W.H.: Establishment of an appropriate model for the growth of perichondrium in a rabbit joint milieu. Trans Orthop Res Soc, p. 196, 1983.
66. Zarnett, R., Salter, R.B.: Periosteal neochondrogenesis for biologically resurfacing joints: its cellular origin. Can J Surg 32(3):171, 1989.
67. Salter, R.B.: The biologic concept of continuous passive motion of synovial joints. Clin Orthop 242:12, 1989.
68. O'Driscoll, S.W., Keeley, F.W., Salter, R.B.: Durability of regenerated articular cartilage produced by free autogenous periosteal grafts in major full-thickness defects in joint surfaces under the influence of continuous passive motion. J Bone Joint Surg 70(4):595, 1988.
69. Shimizu, T., Videman, T., Shimazaki, K., Mooney, V.: Experimental study on the repair of full thickness articular cartilage defects: effects of varying periods of continuous passive motion, cage activity, and immobilization. J Orthop Res 5:187, 1987.
70. Engkvist, O., Johansson, S.H.: Perichondrial arthroplasty. A clinical study in twenty-six patients. Scand J Plast Reconstr Surg Hand Surg 14:71, 1980.

71. Poussa, M., Rubak, J., Ritsila, V.: Differentiation of the osteochondrogenic cells of the periosteum in chondrotrophic environment. Acta Orthop Scand 52:235, 1981.

72. Amiel, D., Frank, C., Harwood, F., Fronek, J., Akeson, W.H.: Tendons and ligaments: a morphological and biochemical comparison. J Orthop Res 1(3):257, 1984.

73. Burks, R., Daniel, D., Losse, G.: The effect of continuous passive motion on anterior cruciate ligament reconstruction stability. Am J Sports Med 12:323, 1984.

74. Noyes, F.R., Mangine, R.E., Barber, S.: Early knee motion after open and arthroscopic anterior cruciate ligament reconstruction. Am J Sports Med 15(2):149, 1987.

75. Amiel, D., Kleiner, J., Akeson, W.H.: The natural history of the anterior cruciate ligament autograft of patellar tendon origin. Am J Sports Med, in press.

76. Fronek, J., et al.: The effect of intermittent passive motion (IPM) on the healing of the medial collateral ligament. Trans Orthop Res Soc, p. 31, 1983.

77. Coutts, R.D., Toth, C., Kaita, J.: The role of continuous passive motion in the rehabilitation of the total knee patient. *In* Total Knee Arthroplasty—A Comprehensive Approach (Edited by D. Hungerford). Baltimore, Williams & Wilkins, 1983.

78. Coutts, R.D., et al.: The role of continuous passive motion in the postoperative rehabilitation of the total knee patient. Orthop Trans 6:277, 1982.

79. Romness, D.W., Rand, J.A.: The role of continuous passive motion following total knee arthroplasty. Clin Orthop 226:34, 1988.

80. Lynch, A.F., Bourne, R.B., Rorabeck, C.H., Rankin, R.N., Donald, A.: Deep-vein thrombosis and continuous passive motion after total knee arthroplasty. J Bone Joint Surg 70(1):11, 1988.

81. Vince, K.G., Kelly, M.A., Beck, J., Insall, J.N.: Continuous passive motion after total knee arthroplasty. J Arthroplasty 2:281, 1987.

82. Melzack, R., Wall, P.D.: Psychophysiology of pain. Evolution of pain theories. Int Anesthesiol Clin 8:3, 1970.

83. Fisher, R.L., Kloter, K., Bzdyra, B., Cooper, J.A.: Continuous passive motion (CPM) following total knee replacement. Conn Med 49(8):498, 1985.

84. Coutts, R.: Personal communication.

85. Lynch, J.A., et al.: Continuous passive motion: a prophylaxis for deep venous thrombosis following total knee replacement. Amer Acad Orthop Surg 1984.

86. Breen, T.F., Gelberman, R.H., Ackerman, G.N.: Elbow flexion contractures: treatment by anterior release and continuous passive motion. J Hand Surg 13(3):286, 1988.

87. Limbird, R.J., Dennis, S.C.: Synovectomy and continuous passive motion (CPM) in hemophiliac patients. Arthroscopy 3(2):74, 1987.

88. Parisien, J.S.: The role of arthroscopy in the treatment of postoperative fibroarthrosis of the knee joint. Clin Orthop 299:185, 1988.

89. Nickel, V.: Personal communication.

90. Cabaud, H.E., Rodkey, W.G., Feagin, J.A.: Experimental studies of acute anterior cruciate ligament injury and repair. Am J Sports Med 7:18–22, 1979.

91. Feagin, J.A., Abbott, H.G., Rokous, J.A.: The isolated tear of the ACL (abstr). J Bone Joint Surg 54A:1340, 1972.

92. Feagin, J.A., Jr., Curl, W.W.: Isolated tear of the ACL: 5-year followup study. Am J Sports Med 4:95–100, 1976.

93. O'Donoghue, D.H., Rockwood, C.A., Jr., Frank, G.R., Jack, S.C., Kenyon, R.: Repair of the ACL in dogs. J Bone Joint Surg 48A:503, 1966.

94. Palmer, I.: On the injuries of the ligament of the knee joint: a clinical study. Acta Chir Scand Suppl 53:1–282, 1938.

95. Arnoczky, S.P., Rubin, R.M., Marshall, J.L.: Microvasculature of the cruciate ligaments and its response to injury. J Bone Joint Surg 61A:1221, 1979.

96. Butler, D.L., Noyes, F.R., Grood, E.S., Olmstead, M.L., Hohn, R.B.: The effects of vascularity on the mechanical properties of primate anterior cruciate ligament replacements. Trans Orthop Res Soc 8:93, 1983.

97. O'Donoghue, D.H., et al.: Repair and reconstruction of the anterior cruciate ligament in dogs. J Bone Joint Surg 53A(4):710–718, 1971.

98. Alm, A., Stromberg, B.: Vascular anatomy of the patellar and cruciate ligaments. A microangiographic and histologic investigation in the dog. Acta Chir Scand Suppl 445:25–35, 1974.

99. Ropes, M.W., Bennett, G.A., Bauer, W.: The origin and nature of normal synovial fluid. J Clin Invest 18:351, 1939.

100. Amiel, D., Abel, M.F., Kleiner, J.B., Lieber, R.L., Akeson, W.H.: Synovial fluid nutrient delivery in the diarthrial joint: an analysis of rabbit knee ligaments. J Orthop Res 4:90–95, 1986.

101. Manske, P.R., Whiteside, L.A., Lesker, P.A.: Nutrient pathways to flexor tendons using hydrogen washout technique. J Hand Surg 3:32–36, 1978.

102. Potenza, A.D.: Critical evaluation of flexor tendon healing and adhesion formation with artificial digital sheaths: an experimental study. J Bone Joint Surg 45A:1217–1233, 1963.

103. Potenza, A.D.: The healing of autogenous tendon grafts within the flexor digital sheaths in dogs. J Bone Joint Surg 46A:1462–1484, 1964.

104. Andrish, J., Holmes, R.: Effects of synovial fluid on fibroblasts in tissue culture. Clin Orthop 138:279–283, 1979.

105. Warren, R.F.: Primary repair of the anterior cruciate ligament. Clin Orthop 172:65–70, 1983.

106. Kohn, D.: Arthroscopy in acute injuries of anterior cruciate-deficient knees: fresh and old intraarticular lesions. Arthroscopy 2:98–102, 1986.

107. Cheung, H.S., Halverson, P.B., McCarty, D.J.: Release of collagenase, neutral protease, and prostaglandins from cultured mammalian synovial cells by hydroxyapatite and calcium pyrophosphate dihydrate crystals. Arthritis Rheum 24:1338–1344, 1981.

108. Werb, Z., Reynolds, J.J.: Stimulation by endocytosis of the secretion of collagenase and neutral proteinase from rabbit synovial fibroblasts. J Exp Med 140:1482–1497, 1974.

109. Ehrlich, M.G., et al.: Collagenase and collagenase inhibitors in osteoarthritic and normal cartilage. J Clin Invest 59(2):226–233, 1977.

110. Ridge, S.C., Oransky, A.L., Kerwar, S.S.: Induction of the synthesis of latent collagenase and latent neutral protease in chondrocytes by a factor synthesized by activated macrophages. Arthritis Rheum 23:448–454, 1980.

111. Lindy, S., et al.: Increased collagenase activity in human rheumatoid meniscus. Scand J Rheumatol 15:237–242, 1986.

112. Gillard, G.C., Reilly, H.C., Bell-Booth, P.G., Flint, M.H.: The influence of mechanical forces on the glycosaminoglycan content of the rabbit flexor digitorum profundus tendon. Connect Tissue Res 7(1):37–46, 1979.

113. Eiken, O., Lundborg, G., Rank, F.: The role of the digital synovial sheath in tendon grafting. Scand J Plast Reconstr Surg Hand Surg 9:182, 1975.

114. Lundborg, G., Myrhage, R., Rydevik, B.: Original communication: the vascularization of human flexor tendons within the digital synovial sheath region, structural and functional aspects. J Hand Surg 2:417, 1977.

115. Matthews, P.: The fate of isolated segments of flexor tendons within the digital sheath—a study in synovial nutrition. Br J Plast Surg 29:216, 1978.

116. Hough, A.J., Barfield, W.O., Sokoloff, L.: Cartilage in hemophilic arthropathy; ultrastructural and microanalytical studies. Arch Pathol Lab Med 100:91, 1976.

117. Rippey, J.J., et al.: Articular cartilage degradation and the pathology of haemophilic arthropathy. South Afr Med J 54:345, 1978.

118. Fabry, G.: Early biochemical and histological findings in ex-

perimental haemarthrosis in dogs. Arch Orthop Trauma Surg *100*:167, 1982.

119. Pforringer, W.: Hamarthros and kreuzbander—biomechanische untersuchangen teil 1. Unfallchirugie *8*:353, 1982.

120. Pforringer, W.: Hamarthros and kreuzbander—morphologische untersuchangen teil 2. Unfallchirugie *8*:368, 1982.

121. Ishizue, K.K., et al.: Hemarthrosis: a biochemical and mechanical evaluation of effects on the ACL and menisci. Trans Orthop Res Soc *13*:55, 1988.

122. Ishizue, K.K., Amiel, D., Lyon, R., Woo, S.L.-Y.: Acute hemarthrosis; a histological, biochemical and biomechanical correlation of effects on the ACL in a rabbit model. Submitted to J Orthop Res, 1989.

123. Kleiner, J.B., Roux, R.D., Amiel, D., Woo, S.L.-Y., Akeson, W.H.: Primary healing of the ACL. Trans Orthop Res Soc *11*:131, 1986.

124. Lyon, R.M., et al.: The ACL: a fibrocartilaginous structure. Trans Orthop Res Soc Meet *14*:189, 1989.

125. Wessels, N.K.: Tissue Interactions and Development. Menlo Park, Benjamin-Cummings, pp. 213–229, 1977.

126. Gospodarowicz, D., Neufeld, G., Schweigerer, L.: Cellular shape is determined by the extracellular matrix and is responsible for the control of cellular growth and function. Mol Cell Endocrinol *46*:187, 1986.

127. Ruoslahti, E., Pierschbacher, M.D.: Arg-Gly-Asp: a versatile cell recognition site. Cell *44*:517–518, 1986.

128. Ruoslahti, E., Pierschbacher, M.D.: New perspectives in cell adhesion: RGD and integrins. Science *238*:491, 1987.

129. Nagelschmidt, M., Becker, D., Bonninghoff, N., Engelhardt, G.H.: Effect of fibronectin therapy and fibronectin deficiency on wound healing: a study in rats. J Trauma *27*(11): 1267–1271, 1987.

130. McDonald, J.A., Kelley, D.G., Broekelmann, T.J.: Role of fibronectin in collagen deposition: Fab' to the gelatin-binding domain of fibronectin inhibits both fibronectin and collagen organization in fibroblast extracellular matrix. J Cell Biol *92*(2):485–492, 1982.

131. Amiel, D., Foulk, R.A., Harwood, F.L., Akeson, W.H.: Quantitative assessment by competitive ELISA of fibronectin (fn) in tendons and ligaments. Submitted, Biochem Biophys Res Commun, 1989.

132. Kurkinen, M., Vaheri, A.V., Roberts, P.J., Stenman, S.: Sequential appearance of fibronectin and collagen in experimental granulation tissue. Lab Invest *43*(1):47–51, 1980.

133. Lehto, M., Duance, V.C., Restall, D.: Collagen and fibronectin in a healing skeletal muscle injury. J Bone Joint Surg (Br) *67*(5):820–828, 1985.

134. Williams, I.F., McCullagh, K.G., Silver, I.A.: The distribution of types I and III collagen and fibronectin in the healing equine tendon. Connect Tissue Res *12*:211–227, 1984.

135. Hemler, M.E., Huang, C., Schwartz, L.: The VLA protein family. J Biol Chem *262*:3300–3309, 1987.

136. Dahners, L.E.: Ligament contraction—a correlation with cellularity and actin staining. Trans Orthop Res Soc *11*:56, 1986.

137. Roberts, C.J., et al.: Transforming growth factor β stimulates the expression of fibronectin and of both subunits of the human fibronectin receptor by cultured human lung fibroblasts. J Biol Chem *263*(10):4586–4592, 1988.

138. Ignotz, R.A., Massague, J.: Cell adhesion protein receptors as targets for transforming growth factor-β action. Cell *51*:189–197, 1987.

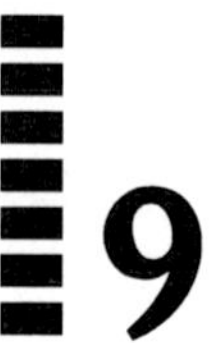

Paul L. Flicker

Potentials of Magnetic Resonance Imaging (MRI) for Spinal Diagnosis

Magnetic resonance is an imaging technique for the visualization of interior body structures that is particularly sensitive to alterations in soft tissue. As such, it is uniquely helpful in the evaluation of central nervous system pathology in general and for spinal diagnosis in particular. As compared to other imaging modalities, the concepts of magnetic resonance are not difficult; however, they are different. In ordinary photography, an image is created by the reflection of light from the surface of an object; in routine x ray imaging, it is the passage of x rays through the body and their subsequent variable attenuation by structures within the body that results in the formation of an x ray picture. For magnetic resonance imaging, the situation is neither the reflection of light energy from the surface nor the passage of x ray energy through the body part, but rather the introduction of low energy radiowaves into, and the reception of small energy signals out of, the part that is imaged in the presence of an external magnetic field.

normal physiologic state of tissues. Whereas plain film x rays and computed tomography are based on attenuation of high energy radiation, and ultrasonography reflects sound waves from surfaces of different densities, MRI depends on basic physical/organic chemistry of internal structures. MR images are ultimately formed from nuclear perturbations in response to introduced low energy radiowaves. It is this basic type of reaction, particularly of the abundant hydrogen proton, which gives MRI its high sensitivity to discriminate pathologic conditions.

In computed tomography, information is collected from the axial plane. To generate reconstructed or reformatted images in the sagittal or coronal planes, the software uses digitally stored data collected from the axial plane. Such sagittal or coronal reformatted images lose some detail and may leave a great deal to be desired. MR imaging can access data directly from either the axial, the sagittal, or the coronal planes, resulting in improved definition of those areas of interest.

GENERAL ADVANTAGES OF MRI

A major advantage of MRI is that this noninvasive technique reflects biochemical changes in addition to providing precise anatomic display of internal body parts. It is this combination of anatomic *and* physiologic imaging that makes MRI unique. Equally important, this result can be accomplished by the manipulation of magnetic fields rather than by the introduction of ionizing radiation; this makes MRI an intrinsically safe procedure with no known harmful effects at the level of clinical usage.

MRI is extremely sensitive to alterations from the

BASIC PRINCIPLES

In order to form magnetic resonance images, it is necessary to establish a strong external magnetic field environment. Within such a magnetic field, certain atomic nuclei within the body become oriented along the lines of magnetic force in much the same manner that a compass needle becomes oriented towards magnetic north pole. The hydrogen atom, which consists of a single proton in its nucleus, is a favored element because of its abundance as well as its high degree of sensitivity for magnetic resonance imaging. In the presence of an external magnetic

102

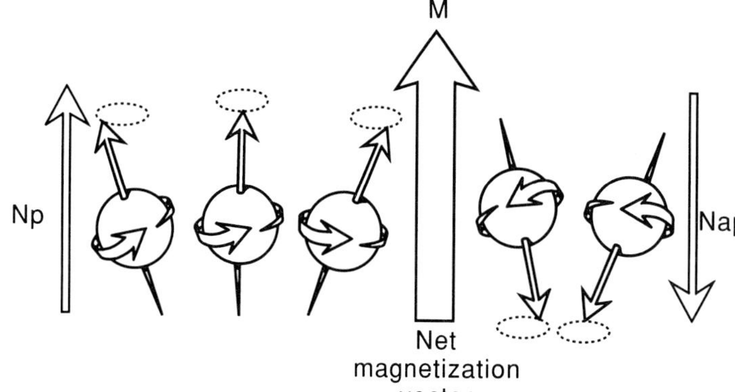

Figure 9–1. At equilibrium, the net magnetization vector (M) points in a parallel direction because more protons point in the parallel direction (N_p) than in the antiparallel direction (N_{ap}).

field environment, hydrogen nuclei (protons) become oriented either parallel or anti-parallel to lines of the magnetic force field; this orientation proceeds in an exponential fashion. At equilibrium, there is a small but important increase in the number of protons that are oriented parallel to the external field. Each proton acts as though it were a small bar magnet. Summation of the magnetic vectors of individual protons results in an overall net magnetization vector (M) that also points in the parallel direction at equilibrium (Fig. 9–1). The term T1 is used to identify time intervals that transpire as this equilibrium situation is approached. Accordingly, T1 characteristics of a tissue describe the behavior of that tissue in a magnetic field environment relative to the time required to achieve an equilibrium condition of protons (Fig. 9–2). It is important to recognize that T1 refers to an exponential *growth* of the net magnetization vector along lines of the external magnetic field. Thus, a particular tissue with a short T1 (on the order of 500 milliseconds) would achieve its equilibrium position faster than another tissue with a long T1 (on the order of 2000 milliseconds) (Fig. 9–3). Orientation of the body within an external magnet

identifies a coordinate system of axes and planes; exponential growth of net magnetization vector (M) occurs along the longitudinal axis (Z) (Fig. 9–4). A magnetic resonance sequence that is established to reflect T1 characteristics of the tissue under study is usually known as a T1 weighted image.

In addition to acting like small bar magnets, individual atomic nuclei also simulate spinning tops or gyroscopes (Fig. 9–5). As in an ordinary spinning gyroscope, the rotation axis of individual nuclei precess or rotate, but at a frequency that is unique to each element. Any external energy which is introduced into such a system will be accepted by the nuclei only if such energy is at the same particular frequency. Energy that is introduced at the correct frequency will cause spinning protons to resonate. This acceptance of energy by spinning protons results in a shift or change in orientation of the overall net magnetization vector (M) relative to the longitudinal axis (Z). When the energy pulse is discontinued, the spinning protons return to their prior orientation under the influence of the external magnetic field. The previously added energy is then released

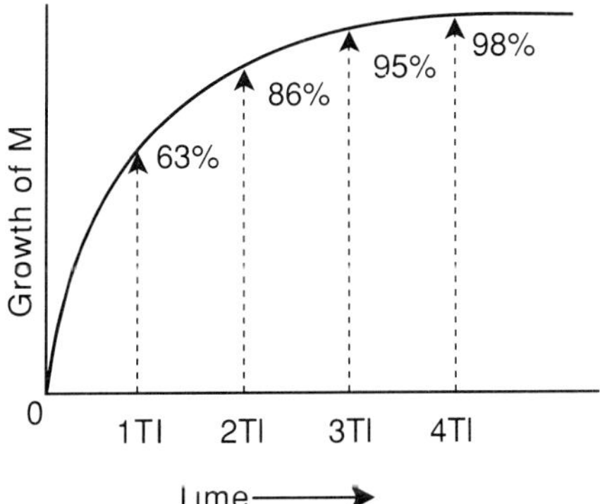

Figure 9–2. One TI represents the time required to achieve 63% growth of the net magnetization vector (M) as described by an exponential curve.

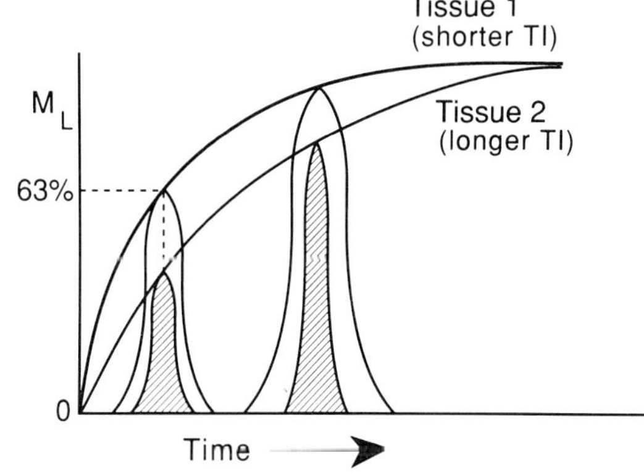

Figure 9–3. Tissues with a shorter TI reach 63% growth of net magnetization (M) along the longitudinal axes (L) at a faster rate than tissues with a longer TI.

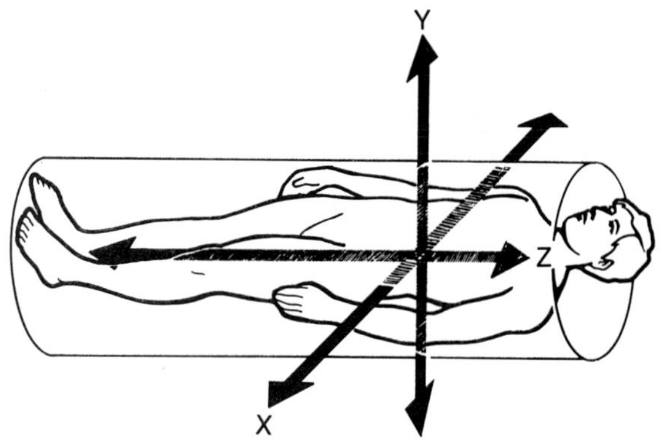

Figure 9–4. The longitudinal axis is represented by the Z coordinate; whereas, the X and Y coordinates describe the transverse plane.

from the system; in fact, it is this latter release of electromagnetic energy that produces the small signals that are collected and processed to form the image in magnetic resonance.

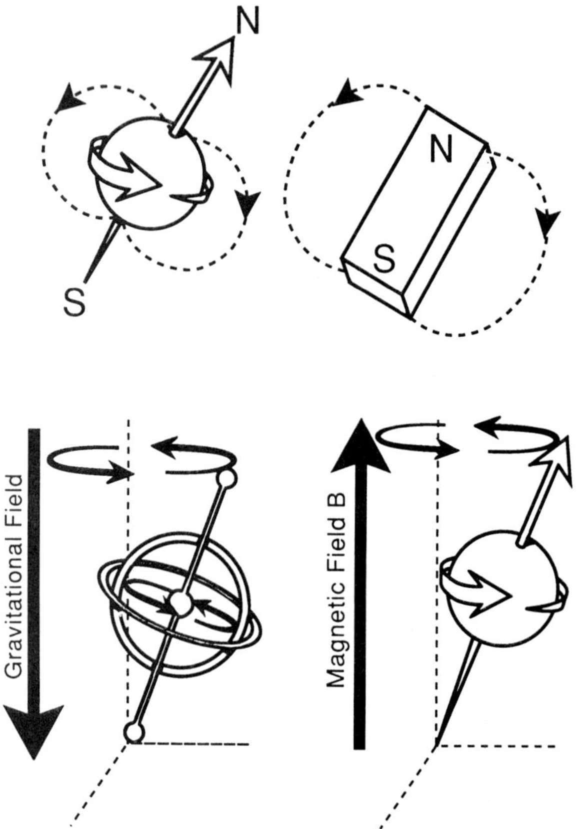

Figure 9–5. In a spinning object, motion of the axis of rotation in an external force field is known as precession.

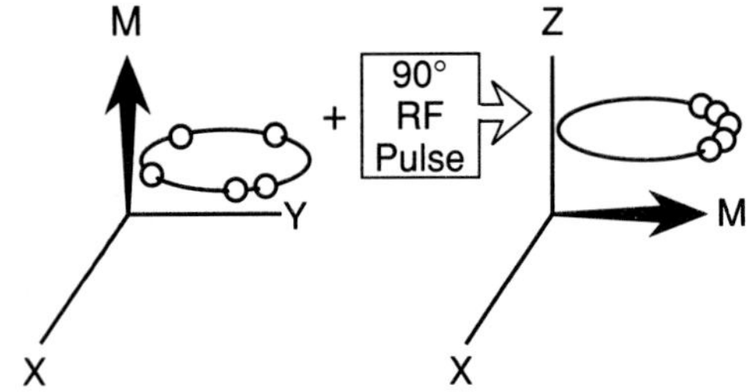

Figure 9–6. After introduction of resonant energy, spinning protons in the transverse plane achieve temporary phase coherence.

Initially, spinning protons have a random phase relationship to each other. However, with the acceptance of resonant energy, phase coherence occurs in the transverse plane (Fig. 9–6). At the cessation of introduced energy, these same protons rapidly lose their phase coherence in the transverse plane. The term T2 is used to identify time intervals that transpire as phase coherence in the transverse plane is lost (Fig. 9–7). Thus, T2 describes an exponential *loss* phenomenon, as distinct from T1 which describes an exponential *growth* phenomenon. Magnetic resonance sequences that emphasize the T2 characteristics of tissues are said to be T2 weighted. Those tissues that have a longer T2 maintain their phase coherence in the transverse plane longer than those tissues with a shorter T2 (Fig. 9–8). The resultant signal intensity on a T2 weighted image reflects differential T2 values such that a tissue with a longer T2 appears brighter (greater signal intensity) than will a tissue with a shorter T2. Water has a long T1 and a long T2. Accordingly, on a T2 weighted image, water, because it maintains phase coherence in the transverse plane for a relatively long time compared to other tissues, appears as a bright signal. However, signal intensity of water on a T1 weighted image (which depends on the rapid growth of net magnetization along the longitudinal axis) is comparatively small and, on such images, water appears dark.

Fat tissue has a short T1 and a long T2. Accordingly, by the same analogy as above, adipose tissue:

- Appears as a bright signal on T1 weighted images because the short T1 of fat favors rapid exponential growth of M along the longitudinal axis.
- Appears as a bright signal on T2 weighted images because the long T2 of fat favors slower loss of phase coherence in the transverse plane.

Muscle tissue has intermediate T1 and T2 as compared to water and fat. As such, muscle generally

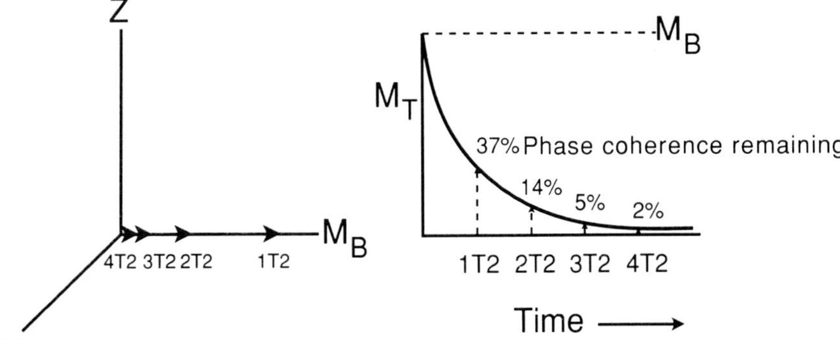

Figure 9–7. M_B is magnetization (M) within the external field (B). One T2 represents the time required for the *loss* of 63% phase coherence in the transverse plane (T) as described by an exponential curve.

appears as a gray signal on both T1 weighted and T2 weighted images (Fig. 9–9).

Energy is introduced into an environment of magnetic equilibrium in the form of low energy radiowaves at the particular frequency of resonance. Radiowaves are nonionizing electromagnetic radiations, and it is this low energy phenomenon that makes MRI an intrinsically safe procedure with no known harmful effects at the levels of clinical use. This introduction of low energy radiowaves into an established equilibrium situation occurs by means of a sequence of pulses which are designed to produce a particular effect on the population of atomic nuclei under study.

One of the commonly used clinical sequences is known as *spin echo* (SE). This protocol initially utilizes an introduction of sufficient energy to displace the net magnetization vector (M) 90° from its equilibrium position along the longitudinal axis. As noted above, this resonant energy also results in transient phase coherence of nuclei in the transverse plane (Fig. 9–10).

Before phase coherence is completely lost, a 180° pulse is introduced that causes phase coherence to

be re-established in the transverse plane. A readable signal results from these rephased protons producing what is known as an echo signal. As phase coherence is again lost, another 180° pulse can be introduced, which results in a second rephasing phenomenon and a second echo signal. Thus, after the initial 90° pulse in a spin echo sequence, subsequent 180° pulses produce echo signals that are collected to form the ultimate image. Time to echo (TE) is the time (in milliseconds) at which the echo occurs; the 180° pulse is introduced at a time of 0.5 TE. Time to repetition (TR) is the time (in milliseconds) at which the entire sequence is repeated by introduction of a new 90° pulse (Fig. 9–11).

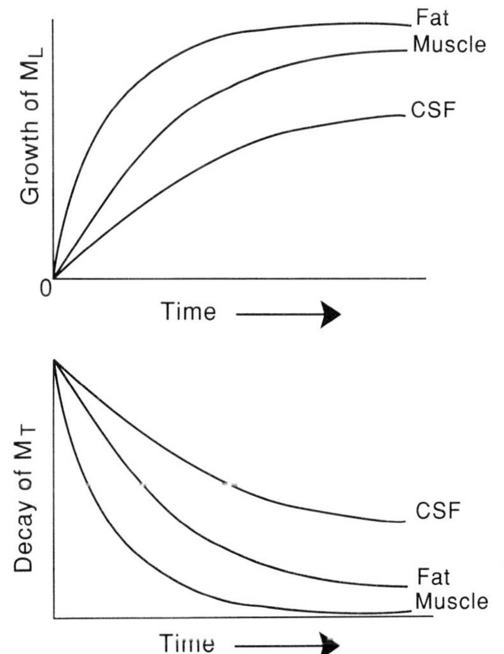

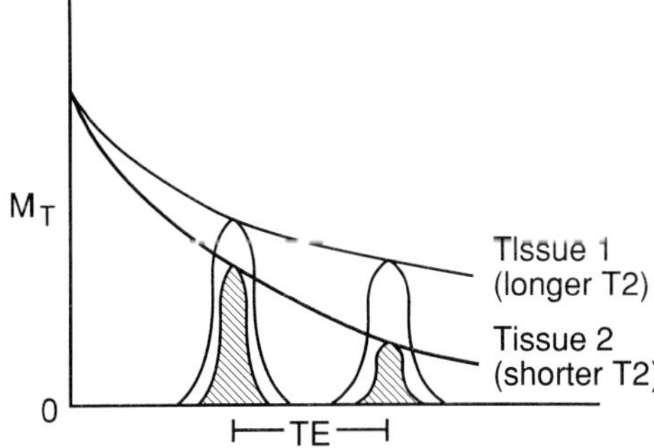

Figure 9–8. Tissues with a longer T2 retain phase coherence in the transverse plane (T) longer than tissues with a shorter T2.

Figure 9–9. CSF has a long T1 and a long T2, whereas fat has a short T1 and a relatively long T2.

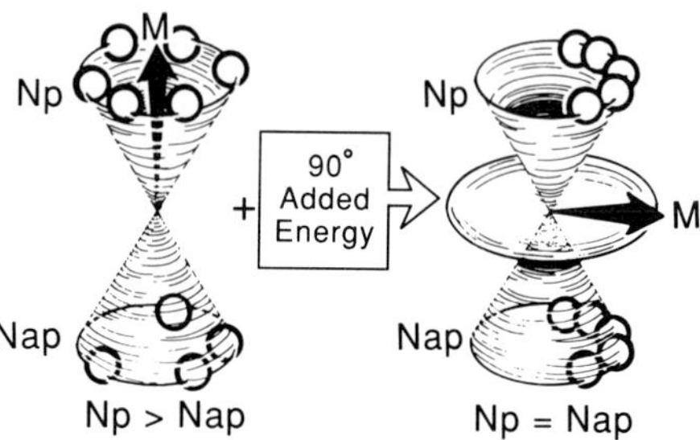

Figure 9–10. A resonant pulse of 90° adds sufficient energy to equalize the number of protons in the parallel (p) and in the antiparallel (ap) directions.

By varying the TR and the TE of an SE protocol, different characteristics of a tissue under study can be emphasized. For example:

1. A T1 weighted SE sequence results when both TR and TE are short, on the order of TR equals approximately 500 milliseconds and TE equals approximately 20 milliseconds. In such an SE sequence, those tissues with a shorter T1 appear bright and those tissues with a longer T1 appear dark.
2. A T2 weighted SE sequence results when both TR and TE are long, on the order of TR equals approximately 1500 to 2000 milliseconds and TE equals approximately 80 to 120 milliseconds. In such an SE sequence, those tissues with a longer T2 appear bright whereas those tissues with a shorter T2 appear dark.
3. A proton density SE sequence (sometimes known as a spin density or partial saturation sequence) results when TR is relatively long, on the order of approximately 1000 milliseconds, and when TE is relatively short, on the order of approximately 40 milliseconds. In this situation, neither T1 nor T2 characteristics of the tissue are favored; the resulting signal is primarily related to the density of protons in the sample.

A second commonly used pulse protocol is known as an *inversion recovery* (IR) sequence. In this situation, resonant energy inserted into an equilibrium environment is sufficient to displace the net magnetization vector (M) 180°. After a time interval (TI), a second pulse of 90° energy is introduced, which results in a readable signal that primarily reflects T1 characteristics of the tissue under study. When the time interval (TI) is short and on the order of 100 milliseconds, the pulse protocol is known as a STIR sequence: *s*hort *t*ime (interval) *i*nversion *r*ecovery (Fig. 9–12). This sequence is particularly useful because the signal from adipose tissue can be selectively suppressed by employing these parameters. Ordinarily, adipose tissue appears as a bright signal intensity both in T1 and T2 weighted images because fat has a short T1 and a long T2. By suppression of the fat signal with a STIR sequence, pathologic tissue changes are often made more apparent.

MAGNETIC RESONANCE SPECTROSCOPY (MRS)

Techniques of magnetic resonance spectroscopy (MRS) have essentially the same conceptual underpinnings as the previous discussion of MRI. In fact, MRS has been utilized in basic chemistry research for many years. It was only after appropriate reconstruction protocols were developed that clinical imaging became a reality.

Atomic nuclei that are spinning behave like small bar magnets and like spinning tops. These nuclei exist in a microenvironment where they are affected by the proximity of other nuclei. In the presence of a strong homogeneous external magnetic field, introduction of low energy radiowaves can reflect positional shift of nuclei such that a spectroscopic analysis can be expressed of one molecule relative to another molecule. For example, the hydrogen nu-

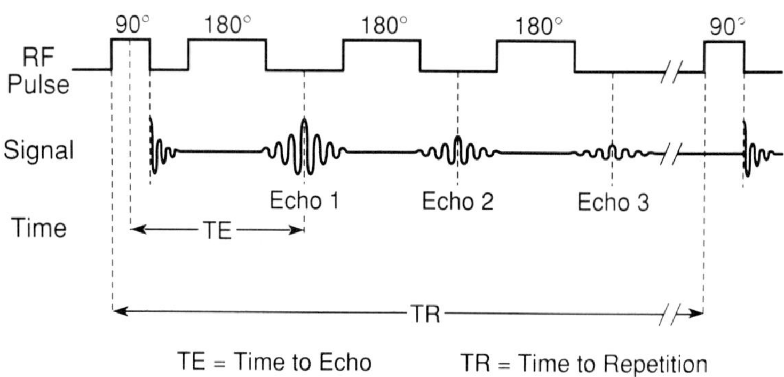

Figure 9–11. Diagram of a spin echo (SE) sequence. Note that progressive echos are of decreased signal intensity.

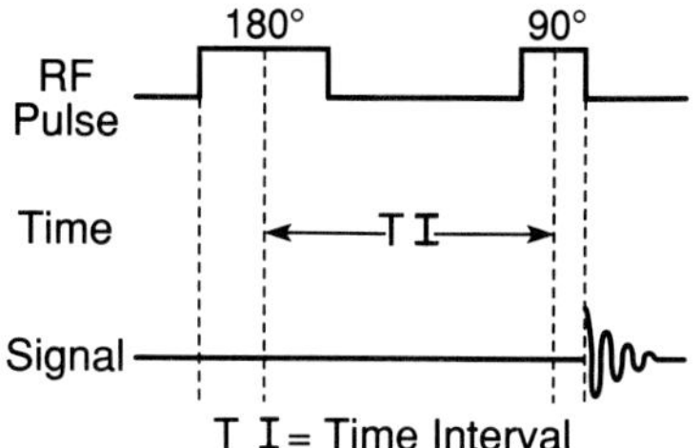

STIR Fat Diagram

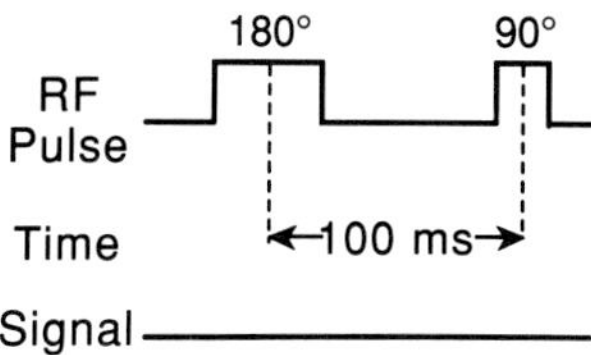

Figure 9–12. The 90° pulse recovers a readable signal after a 180° inversion in an IR sequence. In such a protocol, no signal originates from fat when the time interval is short.

cleus in water does not behave identically to the hydrogen nucleus in fat, and neither behaves in the same manner as the hydrogen nuclei in carbohydrates. In general, the effect of one proton on another proton (or group of protons) depends on the number and the kind of intervening chemical bonds as well as on spatial relationships of the various interacting groups. MRS is a plot of these varying effects producing a fingerprint of the local chemical environment.

High resolution MRS with high intensity magnetic fields has been used extensively to study muscle physiology. Here, phosphorous spectra can be produced that accurately differentiate various molecular compounds in muscle, such as (Fig. 9–13):

   I. Sugar phosphate and phospholipid
  II. Inorganic phosphate
 III. Creatine phosphate
 IV. Gamma-adenosine triphosphate
  V. Alpha-adenosine triphosphate
 VI. Beta-adenosine triphosphate

Flow Phenomenon

Blood moving within vessels provides the opportunity for special imaging techniques using magnetic resonance. The principles outlined previously apply; however, certain variations must be considered. Essentially, flow is a function of the speed with which hydrogen nuclei move through a particular region that is being imaged as well as a function of the percentage of nuclei that are moving. The velocity of blood is a vector quantity with direction and speed that vary both with position within the vessel and with time. Frictional changes produce velocity profiles with slower flow at the periphery than in the middle of a vessel.

When a slice of tissue is selectively excited by introduction of radio frequency energy within a magnetic field environment, ordinarily the return of nuclei towards the equilibrium state produces a signal that ultimately generates an image. However, in the presence of flow, a phenomenon of washout occurs such that the blood in the excited slice of tissue leaves the area of read out before a subsequent excitation or detection occurs. In this situation, flow results in the replacement of previously excited (saturated) protons with less saturated spins, and an alteration in signal intensity occurs. The actual image produced may be of greater or lesser intensity depending on the particular situation. For instance, if the replacing spins are more fully magnetized, then an increase in overall signal intensity occurs; whereas, if the replacing spins are less magnetized than those being washed out of the slice, then signal intensity is decreased. Possibilities are numerous, depending on particular sequences utilized and techniques of data accumulation. Investigation of flow phenomenon will become increasingly important in the evaluation of local obstructions as well as tissue perfusion.

Review of Basic Principles

When biologic tissue is exposed to an external magnetic field, hydrogen nuclei in the sample be-

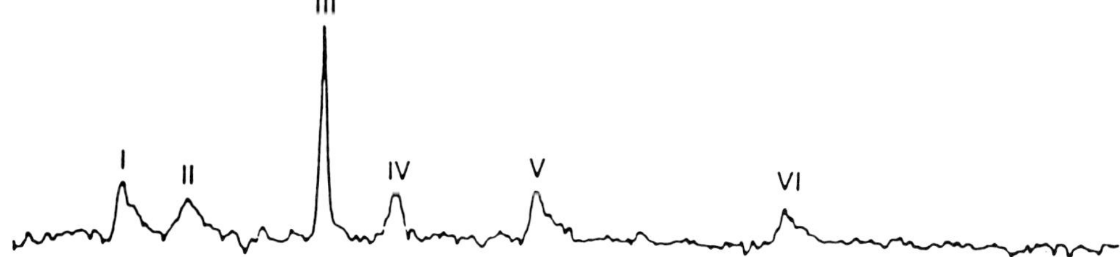

Figure 9–13. Spectrum of phosphorous molecules in normal muscle.

have like spinning tops and precess around the longitudinal axis of the field with a frequency that depends on the strength of the field. Excess nuclei become oriented parallel to the longitudinal force lines such that an overall net magnetization vector points in the direction of the external field lines of force. Radio frequency electromagnetic pulses introduced into these tissues at the proper frequency produce resonance in the precessing nuclei. This acceptance of energy results in a shift of the nuclear population to a higher, excited state of orientation, which is anti-parallel to the direction of the external field lines of force. As a result, the net magnetization vector (M) shifts away from its longitudinal axis orientation. When the radio frequency pulses cease, protons in the tissues relax back toward equilibrium under the influence of the external magnetic field environment. This relaxation occurs in a unique manner which reflects T1, T2, proton density, or flow characteristics. In addition, the local molecular environment of hydrogen nuclei within tissues can result in chemical shift effects. The relaxation of protons after excitation produce electromagnetic signals in a receiving coil. Computer manipulations of this data generate information which contains both spatial localization and signal quantification. From these computations, image displays can be developed. The electrical signals received correspond to a black-gray-white scale such that signals of greater intensity are displayed as brighter images and signals of lesser intensity are displayed as darker images. Overall, any signal must be of significant magnitude to be discriminated from background electrical noise. Also, signal/contrast implications are important for accurate anatomic differentiation.

Spin echo sequences are versatile in that combinations of TR and TE can favor T1, T2, or proton density tissue discrimination according to the general scheme shown in Table 9–1. Thus, a spin echo (SE) sequence of TR/TE: 500/30 represents a T1 weighted sequence in which fat has a bright signal, liquids have a dark signal, and muscle has an intermediate signal. An SE of TR/TE: 2000/80 represents a T2 weighted sequence in which fat has a bright signal, liquids have a bright signal, and the muscle signal is intermediate. An SE of TR/TE: 1500/40 represents a proton density (spin density) sequence in which neither T1 nor T2 characteristics dominate.

The inversion recovery (IR) sequence is particularly helpful for T1 discrimination. It involves an inverting 180° pulse followed by a 90° pulse after a time interval (TI). The 90° pulse produces a component of magnetization that induces a signal in the receiving coil. Inversion recovery also can be used to suppress certain tissue signals by varying the time interval (TI). For instance, the STIR sequence is a short TI (100 millisecond) IR in which adipose tissue signals are suppressed to the point that fat has a dark, rather than a bright, image display.

Instrumentation

The components of a magnetic resonance imaging (MRI) unit consist of (Fig. 9–14):

- The subject under study within a large magnet, so that the system (generally mobile hydrogen nuclei) can be equilibrated.
- Radio frequency transmitter and receiver coils that introduce and pick up pulse signals in the form of electromagnetic energy.
- Gradient coils that permit spatial localization of the signal so generated.
- A computer that controls the pulse sequences and organizes the information received to produce a readable format.
- A video terminal that permits visual display of the computed information and from which hard copies are developed.

The image received is a gray-scale representation of changes within biologic tissue that reflects transfers of electromagnetic energy into and out of the area imaged.

CLINICAL USES OF MAGNETIC RESONANCE

Intervertebral Disc and Adjacent Vertebrae

The intervertebral disc consists primarily of two structures: (1) the annulus fibrosus made up of an overlapping lamellar arrangement of type I collagen fibers which surrounds (2) the nucleus pulposus, which consists of proteoglycans enmeshed in a loose areolar network of type II collagen fibers.

Table 9–1
General Scheme of Tissue Discrimination in Spin Echo Sequences

	Short TR	Long TR
Short TE	T1 weighted: contains T1, T2 and proton density	Proton density weighted
Long TE	No individual discrimination: contains T1, T2, and proton density	T2 weighted: contains T1, T2 and proton density

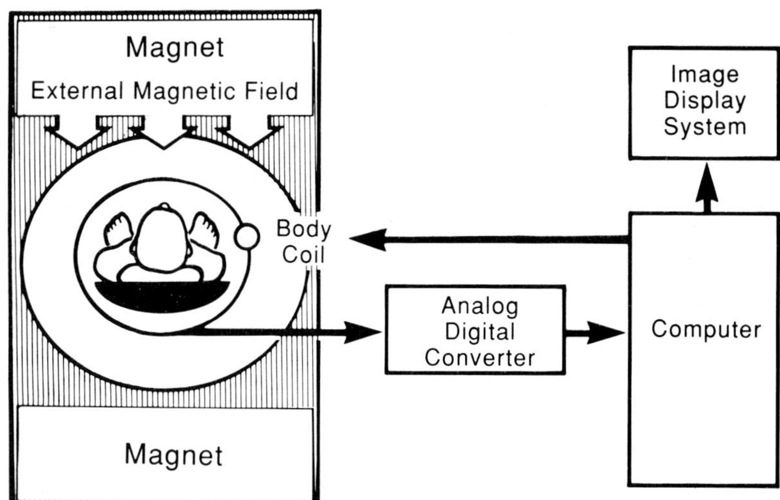

Figure 9–14. Specialized body coils are used to enhance imaging of various areas, e.g., head coils, surface coils, and saddle coils.

The annulus is contiguous with the anterior and posterior longitudinal ligaments and has peripheral fibrous attachments to the vertebral end plates. The lamellar structure of the annulus provides excellent resistance to tensile forces. The chemical structure of the nucleus binds water molecules firmly, and, as such, provides excellent resistance to compressive forces. In health, the combination of intact annular fibers and a relatively central location of the hydrophilic nucleus results in a unique structure that is integral in the functioning motion segment.

Diffusion into and out of the disc occurs primarily by way of the vertebral end plates resulting in metabolic pathways between the disc and the adjacent vertebral marrow.

Magnetic resonance imaging primarily reflects the water content of the nucleus, the overall configuration of the intervertebral disc, and the adjacent bony anatomy. In the healthy back, the disc appears as a bright structure on T2 weighted images because the T2 of water is long. As disc degeneration and desiccation occurs, this bright signal intensity diminishes consistent with a decrease in the water binding capacity of the nuclear proteoglycans. Generally MR images of the lumbar spine consist of sagittal and axial views frequently utilizing spin echo protocols with both T1 and T2 weighted images. The unique ability of MR to perform direct sequential sagittal viewing allows for visualization of the intervertebral foramena as well as midline structures. Similarly, axial sections permit cephalad to caudad visualization from vertebral body through disc substance. In axial sections, good visualization of epidural fat is common because the short T1 and the long T2 of adipose tissue produce bright signal intensity both in T1 and T2 weighted images. Also, position of the thecal sac with its content of cerebrospinal fluid (CSF) is well seen as a result of the long T1 and the long T2 of water. Accordingly, on T1 weighted images, the water content of the thecal sac appears dark, whereas, on T2 weighted images, the water content of the thecal sac appears bright. It is the latter phenomenon that permits a myelographic effect to be obtained without the introduction of radiographic dye material (Fig. 9–15).

Disc protrusions, herniations, and extrusions can be visualized with MR as mass lesions on both sagittal and axial sections. Abnormal disc material ordinarily has diminished signal intensity consistent with decreased water content. Local discrimination of nuclear material can be accurate, and far lateral disc herniations can often be discriminated on high quality imaging sequences. Disc material that contacts the thecal sac or the exiting nerve roots may also be well visualized together with obliteration of the usual epidural fat surrounding nerve roots (Fig. 9–16).

The adjacent vertebral marrow frequently reflects discogenic degeneration. Ordinarily, two types of changes are recognized on T1 weighted sagittal images: Type I alterations are defined as areas of *decreased* signal intensity as a result of an increased fibrovascular infiltration into the vertebral marrow spaces. Type II alterations are defined as areas of *increased* signal intensity as a result of an increased fatty marrow concentration in the adjacent vertebrae (Fig. 9–17).

A purulent process can often be best defined by a short time interval inversion recovery sequence (STIR) wherein the normal fat signal is suppressed. Adipose tissue has a short T1 and a long T2 such that fat appears as a bright signal on both T1 weighted images (short TR/short TE) *and* on T2 weighted images (long TR/long TE). The computer

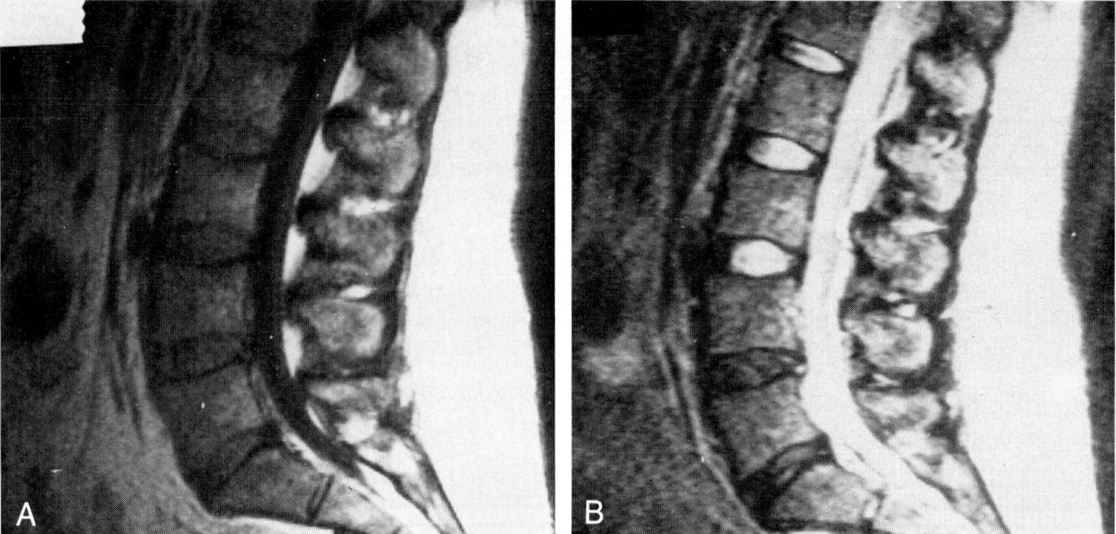

Figure 9–15. A. T1 weighted sagittal of the lumbar spine (TR/TE: 500/30). The CSF is dark and disc water content is not well discriminated. **B.** T2 weighted sagittal of the lumbar spine (TR/TE: 2000/90). The CSF is bright and disc water content is well visualized. Disc dessication is seen at L4-L5 and at L5-S1.

ultimately displays the spectrum of representative signal intensities in a collected data set as a relative black-gray-white scale; thus, the presence of bright signal from fat on both T1 and T2 weighted images has the tendency to skew the relative display scale. If the fat signal is suppressed so that no appreciable information originates from adipose tissue, then, other signals (normal or pathologic) may be better appreciated. Thus, STIR sequences are particularly helpful for the discrimination of proteinaceous fluid collections such as the purulent material of infection, which appears particularly bright when the fat signal has been suppressed.

Muscle

The intermediate T1 and T2 nature of muscle results in a generally gray appearance of the erector spinae in MR images; fibrous planes have decreased signal and fatty infiltrations produce increased signal on routine SE sequences. The high level of sensitivity in MRI generally reveals pathologic conditions quite well, and often as regions of increased signal intensity. However, as discussed below, MR does not (as yet) have a level of specificity that matches its sensitivity.

A unique phenomenon of muscle imaging is the

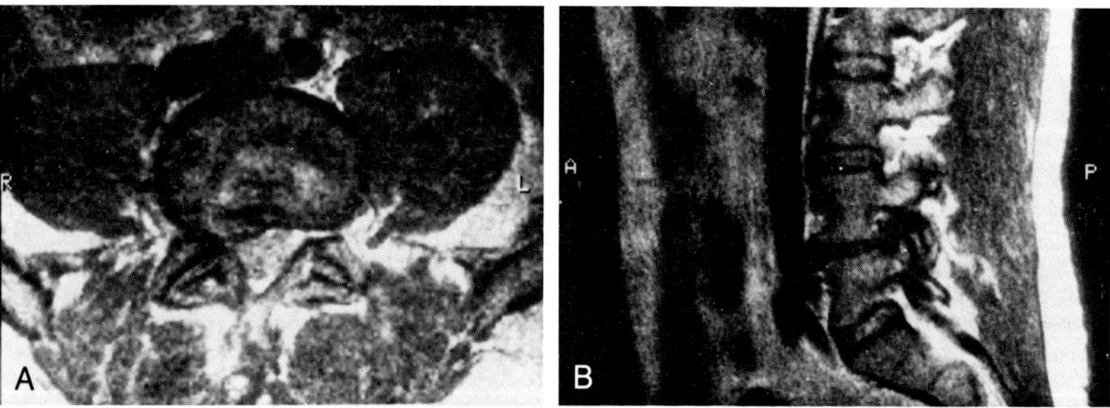

Figure 9–16. A. Axial TR/TE: 2000/40 demonstrating lateral herniation at L4-L5 with obliteration of epidural fat signal on the right. **B.** Parasagittal TR/TE: 1500/40 shows low signal intensity disc material in the L4-L5 foramen obliterating normal high signal of fat.

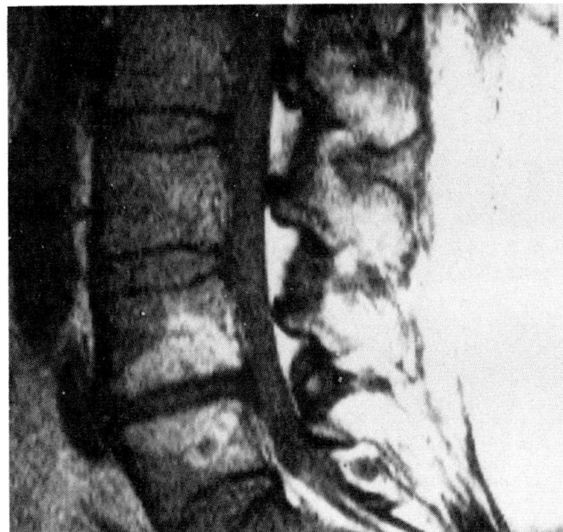

Figure 9–17. Sagittal T1 weighted image (TR/TE: 500/40) demonstrating high signal intensity in adjacent vertebral marrow associated with discogenic degenerative change at L4-L5.

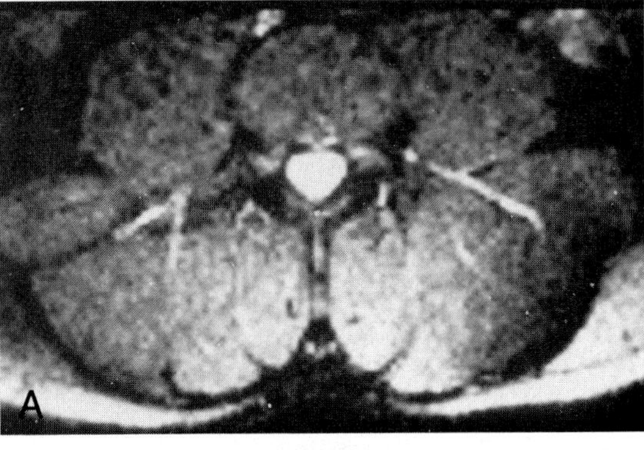

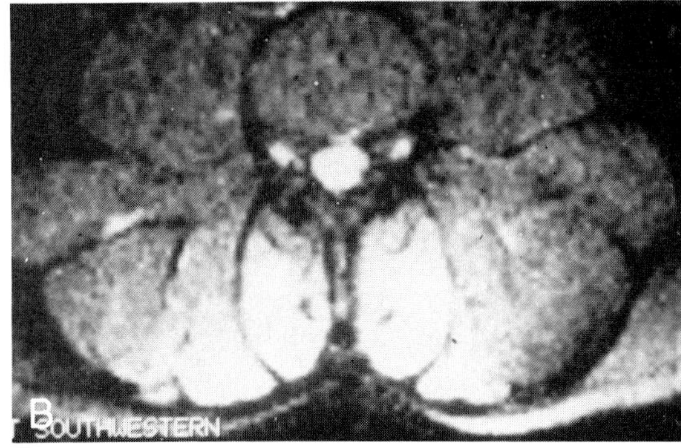

Figures 9–18. Pre **(A)** and post **(B)** extension exercise muscle enhancement demonstrated as high signal intensity in the erector spinae.

response to exercise, which may be visualized by magnetic resonance. Following strenuous muscular activity, there is a defined increase in signal intensity in the exercised muscle mass, which can be demonstrated and corroborated by actual measurements of muscle T1 and T2 (Fig. 9–18).

Nerve

Ordinarily, nerve roots can be routinely defined as areas of dark signal on both lumbar axial and parasagittal views. Within intervertebral foramena the dark exiting nerve is usually seen encased by high signal intensity fat. Also, within the spinal canal area, nerve roots are surrounded by epidural fat, which may be obliterated by protruded nuclear material. Moreover, peripheral nerve abnormalities may be differentiated on selected MR images (Fig. 9–19).

THE FUTURE IS NOW

Clinical MR technology has expanded and continues to expand at a rapid pace. This discussion has set down basic principles of magnetic resonance and has touched on some fundamental applications to low back anatomy and pathology. Important developments continue that will expand the usefulness of this intrinsically safe modality.

Ordinarily, a routine spin echo sequence of the lumbar spine requires approximately 45 minutes of equipment time to acquire the necessary data. Fast and ultra fast techniques have become available such that real time magnetic imaging has become a reality under appropriate conditions. Nevertheless, the more standard protocols continue to dominate the diagnostic scene because of their improved definition of subtle anatomic and pathologic processes.

Controversy exists regarding the merits of higher or lower field strength units. Such a discussion relates to the external magnet itself that establishes an overall environment within which radiowave manipulations occur. The strength of a magnetic field is given in terms of either gauss or tesla. As a point of reference, the magnetic field of the earth is on the order of 0.5 gauss, and one tesla equals 10,000 gauss. Midrange MR units operate at approximately 1.0 tesla whereas lower field magnets operate at 0.15 to 0.5 tesla; higher field units operate at 1.5 tesla and above. In all of these machines there is a problem with patient claustrophobia as well as direct access to very young patients or to critically ill individuals requiring life support systems. Extremely low field operating systems on the order of 600 gauss have been developed with large open areas between horizontally placed magnets. These may offer a sat-

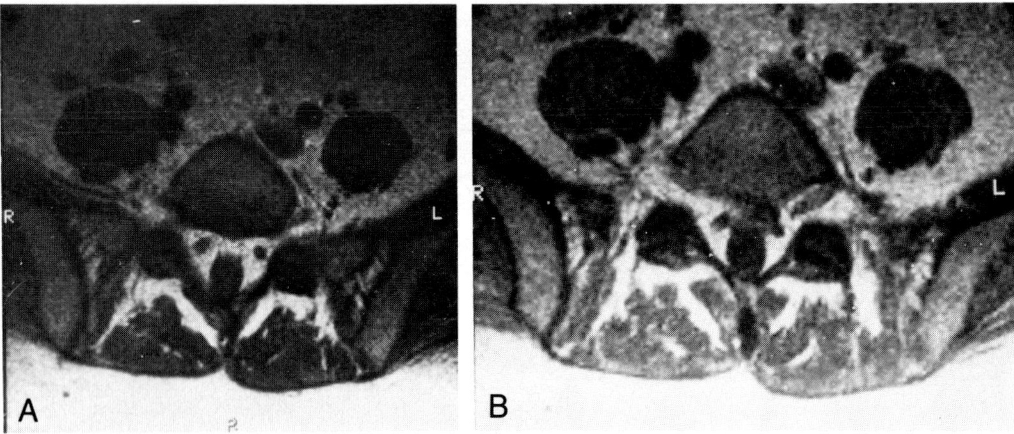

Figures 9–19. Partial saturation axial images (TR/TE: 1000/40) demonstrating normal epidural fat surrounding the nerve roots **(A)** and herniated disc material obliterating epidural fat on the left **(B)**.

isfactory solution to the space constraints of higher field strength units.

On the other hand, it is at higher field strength that the potential of combined imaging and spectroscopy exists. Magnetic resonance spectroscopy requires an external magnetic field of great homogeneity, and this is possible only with higher field strength systems. At the present time MR images are extremely sensitive to pathologic aberrations; however, the level of specificity for diagnosis does not approach the level of sensitivity. The combination of local spectroscopic analysis superimposed on a specific area of anatomic visualization should significantly enhance diagnostic specificity in magnetic resonance. For instance, with regard to the diagnosis of lumbar disc disease, it is recognized that biochemical changes within the disc may produce symptoms of both low back and lower extremity pain. The addition of a reliable in vivo, noninvasive chemical analysis of the disc together with precise anatomic display should enhance diagnostic capabilities in disc disease.

Utilization of paramagnetic contrast agents is a particularly exciting extension of pharmaceuticals for clinical benefit. At the present time, the most widely used such agent is gadolinium (Gd). In general, such agents decrease both T1 and T2 and result in enhanced discrimination of structures. As a chelated compound, Gd-DTPA can be particularly helpful in the evaluation of postoperative changes. The intravenous administration of Gd-DTPA can assist in the differentiation of epidural fibrosis versus recurrent disc herniations. Other intravenous contrast media are under clinical investigation as well.

SUMMARY

This presentation has provided an insight into the fundamental phenomena and imaging techniques of magnetic resonance imaging and spectroscopy to permit the acquisition of a sufficient information base. The reader should be able to discuss pertinent issues with their clinical peers. This chapter makes no claim to being comprehensive; but rather aimed to be an introduction for clinicians and other interested health care providers.

MRI is a beautiful example of science, technology, and design functioning together for the ultimate benefit of people.

REFERENCES

1. Stark, D.D., Bradley, W.G.: Magnetic Resonance Imaging. St. Louis, C.V. Mosby, 1988.
2. Partain, C.I., et al. (eds): Magnetic Resonance Imaging (2nd Ed.). Philadelphia, W.B. Saunders, 1988.
3. Young, S.W.: Magnetic Resonance Imaging. New York, Raven Press, 1988.
4. Bushong, S.C.: Magnetic Resonance Imaging. St. Louis, C.V. Mosby, 1988.
5. Goodwin, P.N., Dandamudi, V.R.: The Physics of Nuclear Medicine. Springfield, Charles C Thomas, 1977.
6. Mulligen, J.F.: Introductory College Physics. New York, McGraw-Hill, 1985.
7. Wood, R.: Understanding Magnetism. Blue Ridge Summit, PA, Tab Books, 1988.
8. Modic, M.T., Masaryk, T.J., Ross, J.S.: Magnetic Imaging of the Spine. Chicago, Yearbook Medical Publishers, 1989.
9. Frymoyer, J.W., Gordon, S.L. (eds.): New Perspectives on Low Back Pain. Park Ridge, American Academy of Orthopaedic Surgeons, 1988.

Tapio Videman
Michele Battié

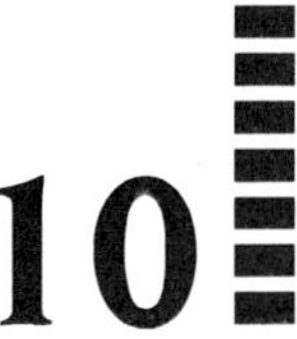

Current Research on Spinal Disorders

INTRODUCTION

The study of ill defined conditions, such as back pain, is difficult. Although the number of scientists studying spinal disorders is small in relation to the significance of the problem, more publications are produced than anyone can keep abreast of. Unfortunately, papers meeting scientific standards are an exception. One of the most systematic, comprehensive evaluations of the state of knowledge about back pain was reported by the Quebec Task Force on Spinal Disorders in 1987. Their initial literature search, encompassing the prior 10 year period, identified more than 7000 articles related to spinal disorders. Yet, less than 3% of the articles were deemed to be of high scientific quality, as judged by an evaluation of the methodology.[1]

Despite the difficulties encountered in conducting proper scientific studies, the potential rewards of increasing our understanding and ability to resolve the problem of painful spinal disorders are great. Thus, quality research needs to be encouraged in all related disciplines.

Personal biases and opinions play an important role in developing hypotheses and motivating research, but they also can lead to varied interpretations of study results and affect conclusions. These inherent personal biases must be kept in mind when reviewing conclusions drawn from study results. Well designed studies reduce the chances for misinterpreting research findings.[2]

The intent of this chapter is to heighten awareness of some important considerations and principles of medical research that allow studies on spinal disorders to be conducted properly. Such an awareness also is essential for evaluating and interpreting studies reported in the literature. Following a discussion of general considerations in the study of spinal disorders, some principles that apply more specifically to epidemiological, clinical, and basic science research are discussed.

GENERAL CONSIDERATIONS

Strategies for Studying "Poorly Understood Conditions"

In Tibet, Buddhists pray while spinning a prayer wheel. One common way of conducting research, what we refer to as the "Tibetan praying wheel strategy," entails putting all possible data into a computer, and allowing it to spin and churn the data with the hope that some statistically significant correlations will result. This can be an expensive and inefficient approach to science. Also, analyzing numerous variables increases the odds of identifying chance associations and drawing incorrect inferences. This strategy, however, is not without value. It can assist in gaining orientation to a problem and in screening for possible interactions between factors, but final conclusions about causality cannot be made.

A well directed, rational approach is needed to gain an understanding of the pathogenesis of spinal disorders. In theory, the classic course of a research project begins with an idea based on clinical or biological experience, followed by forming the hypothesis. The experiment, or investigation, then can be designed and conducted in such a way as to most effectively answer the question posed by the hypothesis. The study design should include identifying the potential causal, modifying, and confounding determinants to be included in the data collection and statistical analysis. The process is completed with the reporting of the study results. All of these steps require careful consideration and skill.

Studying a Long, Complicated Causal Chain

An important principle in studying a complicated chain of events is that all parameters of a step in the chain must be measurable before that step can be fully analyzed. To understand the effects of one parameter on a disorder, the effects of other associated factors must be controlled. The interaction between pathology, activity, and pain in musculoskeletal disease provides an example; we cannot make definite statements about the relationship between pathology and pain if the effects of activity are not controlled (Fig. 10–1). Neglecting to account for the effect of musculoskeletal loading on pain may result in misleading interpretations about the relationship between pathology and pain. For example, in many clinical studies of treatment effectiveness among working populations, the effect of changes in loading, such as work absence, are poorly controlled. In such cases, some observed improvement in symptoms could be explained by decreased obligatory loading and natural healing. Similarly, if incapacity for work is used as an outcome measure, the potentially confounding factor of variations in workloads between jobs held by subjects in treatment and comparison groups must be controlled.

There are other examples of the importance of controlling for the effects of other relevant factors in order to measure the effects of any one factor. Numerous studies have revealed associations between pain and age, but many do not include any reference to the degree of deterioration or loading, which have been related to both age and pain. Although pain may be related to underlying pathology, it may be modified by physical loading and a host of psychosocial factors. Because many older adults, particularly over 60 years of age, no longer work, their activity level typically decreases and their obligatory load demands diminish. Also, an ongoing selection process exists among workers because of individual disease and symptoms on one side and a combination of environmental loading and psychosocial factors on the other. This process may lead to a situation in which individuals with pathological changes and acceptable workloads continue to work, and those with the same pathological changes and heavier workloads retire early. This selection process and differences in loading make the true relationship between age groups and pain difficult to determine.

Also, when studying a complicated chain of events, we must exercise caution in drawing inferences when the outcome parameter is several steps removed from the intervention. If, for example, the definitive diagnosis for study subjects is an entrapped lumbar nerve root, treatment effectiveness optimally would be judged by the percentage of patients in whom the entrapment was released and conductivity restored, as well as relief of pain. The aspect of most back problems that makes this ideal scenario so difficult is that a specific pathoanatomic diagnosis is not available. Thus, we cannot study how a treatment approach directly affects the specific pathologic condition responsible for the back pain complaint because it is unknown. Because of such limitations it may be necessary to adopt a wide range of outcome variables to study the value of treatment. Most studies cannot measure the primary factors of the disease in question.

Back pain is seldom a life threatening condition, but rather a myriad of regional symptoms that can hinder the quality of life. The most severe consequence of this problem appears to be the development of long-term disability with its inevitable impact on the affected individuals, their families, and society as a whole. Thus, considering that we cannot specifically identify the pathologic condition, or directly measure the effect of treatment on an unidentified disease, return to "normal" function and work activities may be a *practical* goal and outcome measure. However, in the absence of objective pathophysiologic tests, we cannot conclude that return to work equates to positive changes in the underlying disease or to relief of back pain. Absence from work has been found to correlate weakly with disease.[3–8]

If studies demonstrate that treatment is less important to outcome than, for example, workers' compensation,[9] the treatment is of questionable value to the outcome measure selected. If the goal is to return people to work, the motivations behind resumption of work should be explored and improved.

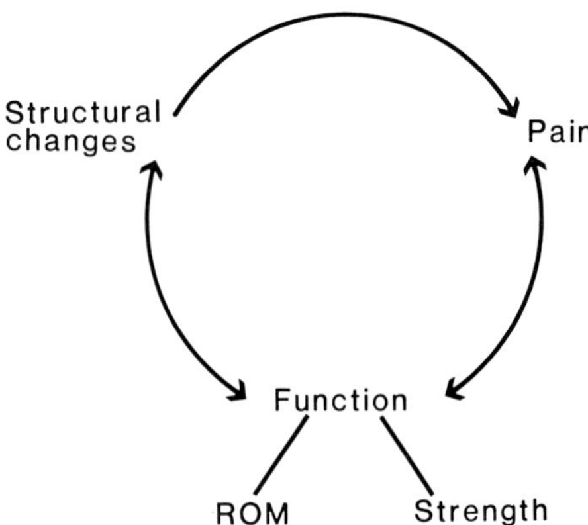

Figure 10–1. Principal parameters of musculoskeletal diseases.

The Value of Exact Diagnoses

We can adequately study the causes, prevention, and treatment only of those disorders that we can recognize and define.[10] Ideally, the diagnosis for a back disorder would provide insights into the pathogenesis, natural history, and appropriate treatment of the disorder, as in other areas of medicine. An exact diagnosis or specific disease would then indicate proper outcome measures for assessing interventions. Unfortunately, providing exact diagnoses for most back problems would not appear to be possible with present evaluation methods. Perhaps in the future, with such technologies as magnetic resonance imaging, we will eventually be able to differentiate normal variations and aging changes from pathologic conditions responsible for certain back pain conditions.

One strategy for future studies is to try to identify different subcategories and perhaps eventually define specific disorders within the general grouping of "back pain." Research could then be applied to the various newly defined subcategories or disorders. We may find, for example, that certain treatments have beneficial effects on some subcategories and detrimental effects on others. However, considering that we lack a clear understanding of the pathophysiology behind most back problems, and significant disagreement exists regarding the diagnostic terms presently used, such categorizations will not be easy.

The nonuniformity in diagnostic terminology, and the inability to define pathological entities, led the Quebec Task Force on Spinal Disorders to propose a classification system for back problems based on clinical symptoms.[1] The system is based on subjective complaints, and thus has limitations. Nevertheless, until more specific disorders can be identified, it does provide for a uniform classification of symptoms that could be used in research to help determine the effects of various treatment approaches on some patient subgroups.

An Analogy: The Study of Abdominal Pain

Although current knowledge allows for few definitive diagnoses of back problems, analogies from other areas of medicine may provide insight and hope. Let us imagine studying abdominal pain 50 years ago. Only a few known diseases such as ulcers, gall stones, and tumors were identifiable. The remaining abdominal symptoms were termed "diag noses" such as "abdominal pain," "abdominal syndrome," or "stress stomach." We did not know that behind this common complaint are a variety of distinct problems, such as: lactose intolerance, irritable

bowel syndrome, gastritis, duodenal ulcer, Crohn's disease, colon cancer, celiac disease (although unusual in its classic form, there seem to be a variety of more common, milder forms), and chronic gastroenteritis.

Today, all of these diagnostic groups are defined and most have a specific cause and treatment. We also know that many of the surgical and conservative treatments used 50 years ago were inappropriate, and in hindsight it is difficult to understand why some came into practice.

If the effect of treatment X on lactose intolerance versus the all encompassing disorder "abdominal pain" were studied, the results might vary greatly. Treatments involving diminishing stress and coffee consumption and increasing fiber in the diet and moderate exercise could be found to affect the occurrence of "abdominal pain." However, for the subgroup of patients with lactose intolerance, for example, a more rational therapy exists: avoiding lactose or substituting the missing enzyme. The diagnosis and treatment of back pain appears to be in a similar stage of evolution as the above example, and thus faces some of the same difficulties.

CLINICAL RESEARCH

Clinical research on low back pain is particularly diffuse because of our limited understanding of the problem at its most basic levels. This has led to a situation in which the dominant theory of back pain pathology, the leading treatment approach, and the most important outcome measure are loosely connected at best. For example, a common belief is that changes in the intervertebral disc are responsible for the pain,[11] a frequent treatment recommendation involves trunk exercise,[12] and the outcome parameter deemed of greatest importance is the length of sick leave.[1]

Determining a Treatment's Successful Completion Rate

The first step in studying treatment effectiveness is to observe how often the treatment technique or regimen is successfully conducted and completed. For example, how often does a surgical procedure such as fusion actually result in bony fusion, or how often is an exercise program completed or achieve its goals of specific gains in strength or range of motion? This success rate is a fundamental issue in studies of exercise and surgical treatments, as well as in drug trials. It is impossible to make final conclusions about the value of a treatment method in terms of outcome measures, such as pain relief, return to work, or recurrence rate without this information.

In order to advance and develop more successful treatments we must look beyond general outcome rates and attempt to understand what is behind treatment results. Let us compare the theoretical treatments A and B for a disease with a natural recovery resulting in excellent outcomes in 10% of cases irrespective of therapeutic approach.

Treatment A is technically difficult and is successful from a procedural standpoint in only 40% of cases, but in those patients for whom the procedure is carried out successfully the outcome is excellent in 90%. Therefore, in 100 patients receiving treatment A, we would expect 36 excellent results because of the treatment (90% excellent results in 40% of the patients = 36) and 6 more because of the natural recovery (10% excellent results in remaining 60 patients = 6). Overall, 42 out of the 100 patients would be expected to have excellent outcomes using this approach.

Conversely, treatment B is less difficult than treatment A and the procedure is conducted successfully in 80% of the cases. However, this method yields excellent outcomes in only 50% of those cases in which the procedure is carried out successfully. Similar to treatment A, the expected excellent outcome for treatment B would be 42 out of 100 cases (80 × 50% = 40 and 20 × 10% = 2).

Treatments A and B have the same success rates in terms of excellent outcomes. Yet theoretically, with improved technique using treatment A, it would be possible to achieve excellent outcomes in 90% of the cases treated whereas only 50% of the cases treated with treatment B would achieve excellent outcomes. A logical conclusion would be to improve the technique of treatment A so that an excellent outcome could be reached in more cases. Examining treatments more closely and recognizing such differences, which may not be apparent on the surface, have obvious ramifications for helping to direct resources and guide future treatment development.

However, if a procedure does not significantly influence the outcomes that have been selected as meaningful, the procedure and its rationale may be of questionable value to the condition. Followup studies of operatively treated spondylolisthesis in adolescence have, for example, shown that the successful fusion rate has little to do with subjective longterm outcome.[13]

Controlled Therapeutic Trials

The limited resources of a society should be used in the most cost effective manner. This principle also applies to the care of back pain. Today, dozens of diverse treatment approaches for spinal disorders exist, particularly for those disorders that lack a specific, verifiable diagnosis. The health care provider, as well as the individual suffering from back problems, is often faced with unclear choices regarding the treatment course to select. Conducting clinical trials comparing approaches can provide useful information as to which treatment offers the best chance for achieving the desired outcome.

Adequate study designs have been developed for comparing treatment effectiveness that center around the concept of randomized clinical trials. This concept also can be successfully used in the study of spine disorders. There have been a number of randomized clinical trials successfully completed with the inclusion of a control group, examining such treatments as discectomy, exercise, bed rest, and medication.[14–18] Clinical studies that include pure placebo groups have the added advantage of revealing how the treatment approach affects the disorder's natural course. While the inclusion of such a group is optimal from a scientific standpoint, in some situations it may not be possible to deny treatment for practical or ethical reasons.

There are a number of issues that can cloud the results of comparison trials. As discussed earlier, the frequent absence of an exact diagnosis or definition of the spine disorder for which the treatments are being applied poses difficulties. Studying poorly defined disorders limits our ability to determine the benefits of a treatment for possible subgroups that may exist within the more generally defined disorder. The selection of appropriate outcome measures also is less clear than if a specific disease were known.

The "Extrac" study comparing traction, McKenzie exercises, and a back school for the treatment of nonspecific back pain revealed no significant differences in pain or functional outcome between the groups. However, patient satisfaction with treatment was clearly highest with the McKenzie approach.[19] Although such studies do not provide information on possible changes in the disorder underlying back pain complaints, the results are important in evaluating practical aspects of patient care. Ideally, changes in the pathologic condition behind the back pain would have been the outcome measure used in comparing treatments, but this was not possible. Until such a goal can be reached, measures of function will probably remain the most meaningful outcome parameters to guide standards of care.

Another issue in designing and evaluating comparison studies relates to minimizing potential differences in the placebo effects of the treatments being compared. For example, contact time with a therapist and the enthusiasm and confidence with which he or she provides treatment may be powerful modifiers of the treatment response. Every effort should be made to make such factors uniform among treatments, otherwise inferences would be invalidated.

In summary, although therapeutic trials related to spinal disorders are presented with a number of difficulties, such as the frequent inability to use a double-blind design, the lack of exact diagnoses, invalidity of outcome parameters, accounting for fluctuations in symptoms and spontaneous recovery, it is important that we make every effort to evaluate the most commonly used treatment modalities. Patients suffering from spinal disorders, and society as a whole, will best be served by scientifically conducted clinical trials of treatments before they are accepted as standards of care. It is difficult to understand how so much money has been dedicated to treatment with so little evidence of effectiveness.[1] The high prevalence of spinal disorders and the limited resources available for health care require a rational approach to medical management.

When treating symptoms for which a specific pathologic condition cannot be identified, one of the cornerstones of medicine, *primum non nocere*, "first do no harm," is particularly relevant. The potential benefits of a treatment or intervention must always be weighed against the risks.

Intervention Studies

The high costs of back pain within the workplace have caused many industries to become interested and active in "prevention" programs. Theoretically, the goal of prevention is to modify risk factors in order to keep "healthy" individuals from acquiring a disease or disorder. Yet, the true effects of most interventions used within industry, and the validity of their rationales, remain undetermined.

To scientifically test the merit of an intervention among healthy individuals, as with therapeutic trials, a control group is needed. A sufficiently long followup period also is necessary to assure that any changes observed are not a brief manifestation of the "Hawthorne effect," a positive response that commonly occurs when any change or intervention is introduced. This effect explains many of the good results observed with interventions.

The term "Hawthorne effect" was coined from an intervention study reported by Roethlisberger and Dickson in 1939.[20] The primary interest of the study involved the relationship between physical conditions and the incidence of monotony and fatigue among the workers. They first studied the relationship between illumination and productivity. The idea to be tested was that an increase in illumination would increase the output of the employees. The results showed no clear relationship between productivity and the degree of illumination. Instead, appreciable gains in production were observed both in the group working under improved illumination and in the control group with constant illumination. In additional experiments the researchers convinced themselves that the basic reason for the positive results was "psychological" and only to a minor extent caused by illumination. Thus, an intervention can demonstrate significant money savings and can be cost effective, but the rationale behind the intervention may still be incorrect. Of course, intervention studies must face a number of other issues if they are to withstand scientific scrutiny, as noted in Table 10–1.

There are a number of other methodology issues that must be considered when planning interventions. As with therapeutic trials, the feasibility of successfully completing the specific intervention

Table 10–1
Other Issues that Intervention Studies Must Face

1. Contamination. It is often difficult to keep the control group from being "contaminated," or exposed to some degree to the intervention. If the control group is so far removed from the study group receiving the intervention as to keep the control group free of contamination, often other dissimilarities between the groups and their conditions exist. Such dissimilarities limit attributing differences in the outcomes purely to the effects of the intervention.
2. Unforeseen Changes in the Environment. A variety of unexpected changes in the environment or conditions surrounding the intervention and control groups frequently occur during a long followup. For example, interventions in industry may encounter substantial subject attrition because of an unstable workforce, or other programs may be introduced during the followup period that potentially affect outcome. Such changes can interfere with the intervention, destroy the validity of the control group, and confound study results.
3. Unintended Changes in Human Behavior Because of the Intervention. The rationale behind an intervention may be sound, but an unexpected change in habits can eliminate the positive effect of an intervention. For example, let us consider an ergonomic intervention for a group of employees with a high incidence of back pain reports, with slips and falls frequently cited as the cause. Observation of the worksite revealed that employees spend much of the day handling large, awkward boxes of supplies that obstruct vision. The rationale behind the ergonomic intervention was that improving the field of vision and decreasing the loads on the spine would result in fewer accidents and subsequent back pain reports. Thus, new packaging of supplies was designed to be more compact, allowing better visualization when carrying the boxes, as well as placing less load on the spine. However, an unexpected outcome of the new packaging was that employees frequently attempted carrying two boxes at a time. This resulted in greater obstruction of vision and greater loads on the spine than had been present previous to the intervention.

must be determined. Appropriate outcome parameters also must be selected based on the main objective of the intervention. For example, is the goal to prevent the occurrence of back symptoms, the filing of industrial back injury claims, the loss of substantial work, or the development of chronic disability?

Practical considerations, including significant time and financial requirements, and potential changes in the workplace or society, make well designed intervention studies difficult to conduct. Despite the need to surmount such challenges, a few intervention studies have been successfully completed.[21,22] Such investigations can provide insights into factors affecting poorly understood problems such as back pain complaints within industry, and can identify practical strategies to assist in managing them.

EPIDEMIOLOGIC INVESTIGATION OF BACK PAIN

In medical science, epidemiology generally refers to the study of occurrence rates of diseases. The scientific value of epidemiologic studies of reports of current or prior pain is limited if the reports deal solely with a complaint rather than with a clearly definable disease.[23] Some of the basic problems facing epidemiologic studies of back pain complaints relate to qualifying and quantifying the pain experience, and controlling for psychological, personal, and cultural effects on pain perception. For example, when a doctor asked the Japanese Emperor Hirohito if he was in pain, Hirohito replied, "What do you mean by pain?"

When first studying a common, poorly defined phenomenon, such as back pain, an epidemiologic approach, such as taking a survey, may be helpful in identifying associations that offer some insight. The results of such approaches are mainly valuable for developing hypotheses and planning further research.

The need for caution in drawing conclusions regarding causation from epidemiologic studies of complaints, rather than specific disorders, can be demonstrated if we again compare low back pain with abdominal pain. Based on answers to the question, "Have you ever had abdominal pain?", we might find that such pain is experienced: "often" by 30%, "sometimes" by 50%, and "never" by 20%. The conclusion would be that 80% of people have "suffered" from abdominal pain. Cross-sectional surveys would demonstrate some clear risk indicators, such as psychological factors (stress, burnout), socioeconomic status, infections, smoking, free time inactivity, and alcohol, coffee, milk, apple, animal fat, and

egg consumption. Depending upon the cultural traditions and attitudes in the society, abdominal pain could be a common reason for disability and an expensive disorder. But back pain is complicated by the fact that it is frequently considered an industrial injury when symptoms occur during the course of work activities, and compensation and issues of fault appear to affect the response to the problem.[9]

We can go one step further with the analogy of abdominal pain and imagine that prevention and rehabilitation programs would be developed, such as: "psychological coping training," or "abdominal school," that teaches the anatomy of the abdomen, how to live with abdominal pain, relaxation, and how and what to eat. This approach may have some value for patients, but clearly would not be the most effective course for managing most disorders causing the pain.

Epidemiology of pain complaints is not the same as that of well defined diseases. The epidemiology of low back pain should follow the principles of studying the occurrence rates of a complaint, rather than a disease.

The Multifactorial Concept

The concept of a multifactorial etiology for back pain is generally accepted. It also is accepted that many of the contributory factors tend to interact with one another.[24–27]

The concept of a multifactorial cause presents major difficulties in drawing conclusions about causation from epidemiologic studies. In order to understand the importance of any identified associations, the factors must be classified in the study design according to whether they are causal, modifying, or confounding. Then, provided that the factors are measurable, one step in the model can be analyzed (Fig. 10–2).

The importance of recognizing associations between variables, and analyzing the data appropriately to assist in determining the nature of the associations, can be demonstrated in the following example. The preliminary cross-tabling of the results of a discographic study revealed statistically significant correlations of pain reproduction with symmetric disc degeneration, annular ruptures, and aging. However, annular ruptures, symmetric disc degeneration, and age are not independent of one another. The connection of one of these factors to pain cannot be analyzed adequately with univariate statistical methods, without controlling for the other two. Subsequent analyses controlling the associations between the factors revealed that the pain re-

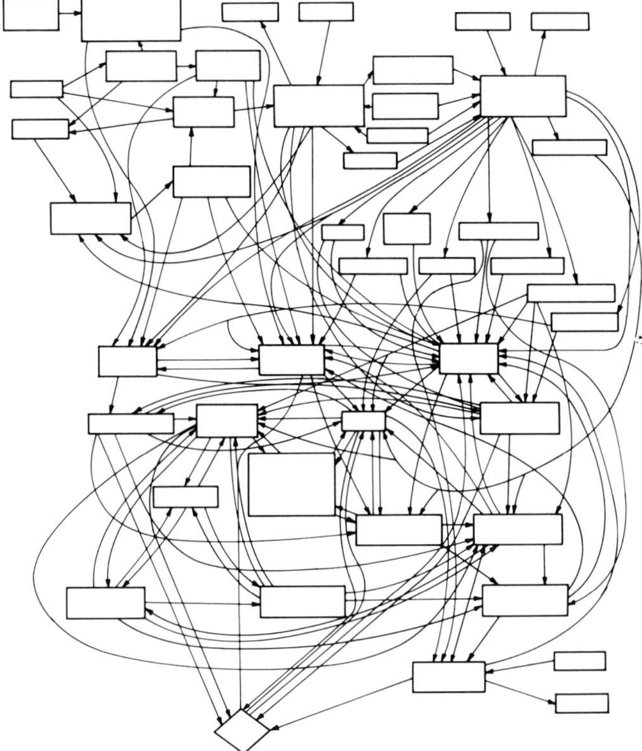

Figure 10–2. This figure displays an imaginary, but plausible, flow chart of the pathogenesis of sickness absence caused by degeneration. Annular degeneration is represented by one box in the middle, and is surrounded by etiological, modifying, and confounding factors, with sickness absence represented by the box at the bottom.

production on discogram is only dependent upon commonly found annular ruptures.[28]

While causal scientific research is possible for some back disorders, such as sciatica, it is more questionable for less clearly defined complaints. The morbidities experienced today may reflect the life events of the prior 15 to 30 years. One hypothesis is that the accumulation of repeated minor tissue injuries over time is the main cause for musculoskeletal degeneration, but this remains unproven.

Physical loading is a very confusing factor, because it has been implicated as both a causal and preventive factor for spinal degeneration. If physical exercise is handled as an aggregate, without assessing any details of the activities, an association with back problems hypothetically could reflect the occasional consequences of excessive loading or injuries, rather than physical activity and exercise itself.

The problems of longterm followup and measurements of lifetime exposures in epidemiologic studies of causal factors for cancer are well recognized.

These difficulties appear small when compared to those encountered in epidemiology of spinal disorders.

BASIC SCIENCE RESEARCH

Basic science offers hope of someday uncovering the pathophysiology behind back symptoms for which no verifiable diagnosis is presently available. Basic science research on back problems is being conducted in a number of areas, including anatomy, biochemistry, and biomechanics. Each of these areas has its own considerations, problems, and opportunities.

Anatomy

Spinal clinicians might benefit from visiting the autopsy theater more often. Some recent anatomy investigations have demonstrated that our knowledge about spinal structures is far from complete.[29] Wolfgang Rauschning, from Sweden, has introduced much new information about basic spinal structures. If we are to use fully and appropriately the new imaging technology, and conduct more precise studies in biomechanics, we need a clear understanding of the anatomy, including changes that are a normal part of the aging process. In the history of medicine, more has been learned from good case reports than through the "Tibetan praying wheel approach."

Biochemistry

Many improvements in modern medicine have occurred through research related to biochemistry. Yet perhaps because of our poor understanding of the cause of back symptoms, research in biochemistry has yielded little affecting the evaluation and treatment of back problems.

There are numerous areas of interest related to biochemistry. For example, if we could measure the degradation of different types of connective tissues, it might be possible to identify different types of connective tissue injuries in a manner similar to the way we diagnose infections today. We then would have possible opportunities for directly evaluating the impact of treatments and prevention programs. Although developments within biochemistry can be rapid, it is difficult to predict when such practical information and applications might be available in the area of spinal disorders.

Biomechanics

This area of research related to back disorders has provided much basic data about factors loading the spine. On the other hand, biomechanics has not produced significant progress for prevention of back pain.[30] The main problem lies in the dual postulated effect of physical loading: causing the disorder and preventing or treating it.[31–38] It is possible to measure the degree of loading for some situations, but the main question is, "What is the relevant question that biomechanics should answer?"

Accident Research

Accident and safety research is an example of applied research based on different basic sciences. One area of this discipline has been directed toward back disorders, but mainly to specific back injuries or accidental traumatic events. This area of study has developed significantly in the past through following the general principles of research. Systems approaches to accident and safety research have brought a new understanding of the problem,[39,40] and the development of accident theories provides a framework for intervention studies. However, most back problems would appear to be multifaceted, with the onset of symptoms being neither of sudden onset nor related to specific traumatic events.[22]

CONCLUSIONS

From a historical perspective, there has been limited development in the treatment of back pain patients during the past 2000 years. Of course, we now recognize a few well defined back disorders and can treat them adequately, but the majority of complaints collected under the label of low back pain are poorly understood. Future progress probably will entail separating the complaint of back pain into more specific, better defined subsets.

Considering that it is likely that there are a number of disorders behind nonverifiable low back pain conditions, answers to the many questions surrounding back pain will probably come from numerous areas. Thus, research relating to painful spinal disorders should be encouraged within all disciplines. Back research must, however, be well designed and properly conducted if meaningful contributions are to be made.

While we attempt to move toward a better understanding of back problems, it may be helpful to remember that the truth is often independent of our beliefs—hence the importance of well conducted research. An expert panel can resolve some issues, but a consensus among experts only means that the group agrees about something. The consensus may be the "truth," but then again it may not. We should not forget that the world was once "known to be flat" by a consensus of experts.

REFERENCES

1. Spitzer, W.O., et al.: Scientific approach to the assessment and management of activity-related spinal disorders. A monograph for clinicians. Report of the Quebec Task Force on Spinal Disorders. Spine 12(7S), 1987.
2. Troidl, H., Spitzer, W.O., McPeck, B., Mulder, D.S., McKneally, M.E.: Principles and Practice of Research. Strategies for Surgical Investigators. New York, Springer-Verlag, 1986.
3. Backenheimer, M.S.: Demographic and job characteristics as variables in absences for illness. Public Health Rep 88:1029–1032, 1968.
4. Bews, D.C.: Monitoring disability absence in an employee group. J Occup Med 14:911–917, 1972.
5. Edstrom, R., Korse, K.G.: Statsanstalldas arbetsforhållanden, trivsel, karriar, sjukfrånvaro, halsa. Lakartidningen 68:939–940, 1979.
6. Hinkle, L.E., Plumer, N.: Life stress and industrial absenteeism. The concentration of illness and absenteeism in one segment of a working population. J Med Industr 21:373–375, 1952.
7. Swann, P.G.: Absence from work attributed to sickness. A review of a recent U.K. conference. Med Bull Stand Oil Co 31:1–22, 1971.
8. Taylor, P.J.: International comparisons of sickness absence. Proc R Soc Lond 65:577–580, 1972.
9. Greenough, C.G., Fraser, R.D.: The effects of compensation on recovery from low-back injury. Spine 14:947–955, 1989.
10. Miettinen, O.S.: Theoretical epidemiology. Principles of occurrence research in medicine. New York, John Wiley & Sons, pp. 11–12, 1985.
11. Frymoyer, J.W., Gordon, S.L. (eds.): New Perspectives on Low Back Pain. Park Ridge, IL, American Academy of Orthopaedic Surgeons, p. 134, 1989.
12. Mayer, T.G., Gatchel, R.J.: Functional Restoration for Spinal Disorders: The Sports Medicine Approach. Philadelphia, Lea & Febiger, 1988.
13. Osterman, K., Seitsalo, S.: Comparison of operative and conservative treatment of spondylolisthesis in adolescents. Paper presented at the annual meeting of the International Society for the Study of the Lumbar Spine. Kyoto, Japan, May, 1989.
14. Weber, H.: Lumbar disc herniation: a controlled, prospective study with ten years of observation. Spine 8:131–140, 1983.
15. Kendall, P.H., Jenkins, J.M.: Exercises for backache: a double-blind controlled trial. Physiotherapy 53:154–157, 1968.
16. Deyo, R.A., Diehl, A.K., Rosenthal, M.: How many days of bed rest for acute low back pain? A randomized clinical trial. N Engl J Med 315:1064–1070, 1986.
17. Videman, T., Heikkila, J., Partanen, T.: Double-blind parallel study of meptazinal versus diflunisal in the treatment of lumbago. Curr Med Res Opin 9:246–252, 1984.
18. Amlie, E., Weber, H., Holme, I.: Treatment of acute low-back pain with piroxicam: results of a double-blind placebo-controlled trial. Spine 12:473–476, 1987.
19. Vanharanta, H., Videman, T., Mooney, V.: McKenzie exercise, backtrac and back school in lumbar syndrome. Paper presented at the annual meeting of the International Society for the Study of the Lumbar Spine. Dallas, TX, May, 1986.
20. Roethlisberger, F.J., Dickson, W.J.: Management and the worker. Cambridge, Harvard University Press, 1939.

21. Wood, D.J.: Design and evaluation of a back injury prevention program within a geriatric hospital. Spine *12*:77–82, 1987.
22. Videman, T., Rauhala, H., Asp, S.: Patient-handling skill, back injuries, and back pain. An intervention study in nursing. Spine *14*:148–156, 1989.
23. Miettinen, O.S., Caro, J.J.: Medical research on a complaint: orientation and priorities. Ann Med *21*:399–401, 1989.
24. Lloyd, D.C.E.F., Troup, J.D.G.: Recurrent back pain and its prediction. J Soc Occup Med *33*:66–74, 1983.
25. Troup, J.D.G.: Causes, prediction, and prevention of back pain at work. Scand J Work Environ Health *10*:419–428, 1984.
26. Troup, J.D.G.: The perception of musculoskeletal pain and incapacity for work: Prevention and early treatment. Physiotherapy *74*:435–439, 1988.
27. Videman, T.: Experimental models of osteoarthritis: The role of immobilization. Clin Biomech 2:223–229, 1987.
28. Moneta, G.B., et al.: Pain during discography in relation to annular ruptures: a re-analysis of 833 discograms. Presented at the annual meeting of the International Society for the Study of the Lumbar Spine. Boston, June, 1990.
29. Macintosh, J.E., Bogduk, N.: The morphology of the lumbar erector spine. Spine *12*:658–668, 1987.
30. Nachemson, A.L.: Chronic low back pain can largely be prevented. Results from a prospective randomized trial in industry. Paper presented at the annual general meeting of the Society for Back Pain Research. London, November, 1989.
31. Rowe, M.L.: Low back pain in industry. A position paper. J Occup Med *11*:161–169, 1969.
32. Frymoyer, J.W., et al.: Epidemiologic studies of low-back pain. Spine *5*:419–423, 1980.
33. Frymoyer, J.W., et al.: Risk factors in low-back pain. An epidemiological survey. J Bone Joint Surg *65*-A:213–218, 1983.
34. Kelsey, J.L., White, A.A.: Epidemiology and impact of low-back pain. Spine *5*:133–142, 1980.
35. Leigh, J.P., Sheetz, R.M.: Prevalence of back pain among full-time United States workers. Br J Ind Med *46*:651–657, 1989.
36. Porter, R.W., Kemp, J.: The relationship between heavy physical work in early life, and the relative incidence of back pain syndromes. Paper presented at the annual meeting of the International Society for the Study of the Lumbar Spine. Rome, Italy, 1987.
37. Mayer, T., et al.: Objective assessment of spine function following industrial injury: a prospective study with comparison group and one-year follow-up. Spine *10*:765–772, 1985.
38. Mayer, T., et al.: A prospective randomized two year study of functional restoration in industrial low back injury utilizing objective assessment. JAMA *258*:1763–1767, 1987.
39. Troup, J.D.G., Videman, T.: Inactivity and aetiopathogenesis of musculoskeletal disorders. Clin Biomech *4*:173–178, 1989.
40. Hale, A., Glendoen, I.: Individual behaviour in the control of danger. Elsevier, Amsterdam, 1988.

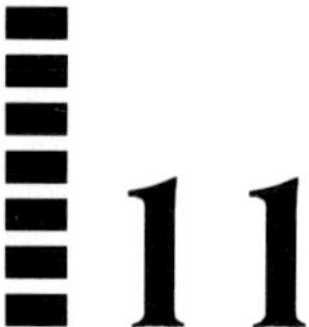 *Gerald S. Laros*

Differential Diagnosis of Low Back Pain

The rational diagnosis and treatment of low back pain syndromes are handicapped by a lack of objective tests that reliably identify the source of pain.[1,2] People who are asymptomatic may have objective tests showing spondylolysis, spondylolisthesis, spinal stenosis, bulging discs, degenerated discs, herniated discs, or spinal osteoarthritis.[3] Symptomatic patients may show these abnormalities on testing and yet their pain may arise from another undemonstrated source. A further diagnostic and therapeutic handicap lies in the frequency of multiple pain sources in the same patient. Mechanisms that result in injury to one tissue in the back often are capable of injurying other tissues as well. If the objective tests (or the over-interpretation of these tests) are accepted uncritically as a guide to treatment, therapeutic failures are certain to occur.

The patient's physical examination and history are increasingly important in reaching a diagnosis upon which treatment can be based because they are the best defense against over-interpretating the superior anatomic imaging available to us through advances in technology. The cause of disability in low back problems is pain. Therefore, pain rather than disturbed anatomy should be the focus of our diagnostic and treatment efforts. The systematic collection of data on the characteristics of the pain, and the mechanical stressing of various anatomic structures to reproduce the pain, can generate a picture of one or more sources that can then be confirmed with appropriate tests for disturbed anatomy.[4,5]

Mechanical injury to low back structures, either from acute trauma or from chronic repetitive trauma, is by far the most common cause of low back pain syndromes. Most mechanical pain can be classified as variants of discogenic or myogenic pain.[6]

DISCOGENIC PAIN: LIGAMENTOUS INSTABILITY

When the innervated ligamentous layer of the outer anulus fibrosus is stretched because of segmental instability, pain results.[7,8] The pain can be acute, often associated with muscle spasm to secondarily splint and stabilize the segment, or chronic with little in the way of physical findings. The acute ligament "sprain" probably represents partial tearing of anular tissue. If the anular tissue becomes weakened to the point of allowing the nucleus to protrude beyond the normal confines of the anulus, it may actually be a prelude to subsequent episodes of frank disc herniation. Or, if the rent in the anulus becomes complete to the point of allowing nuclear liquid to escape, it may lead to a frank anular tear.

Instability or chronic ligament stretch produces discomfort ranging from mild and intermittent to persistent and disabling. Mild discomfort impels us all to reduce lumbar lordosis in order to ease the discomfort. The more persistent variety can be recognized by strengthening spine flexors and correcting lordotic postures.

Pain from chronic ligament stretch is midline and worse with lordotic postures. Like most other mechanical back pain it is worse with bending and lifting. On physical examination, these patients also lack features identifying other pain syndromes. Any diagnostic features to be found are in a positive instability sign or a positive weight relief flexion test.

The instability test is performed with the patient prone with arms at the sides (Fig. 11–1). The examiner's thumb finds an interspinous space and exerts sharp downward pressure seeking a reproduction of pain. Several interspaces are tested to find levels that are not painful for comparison. If no painful in-

122

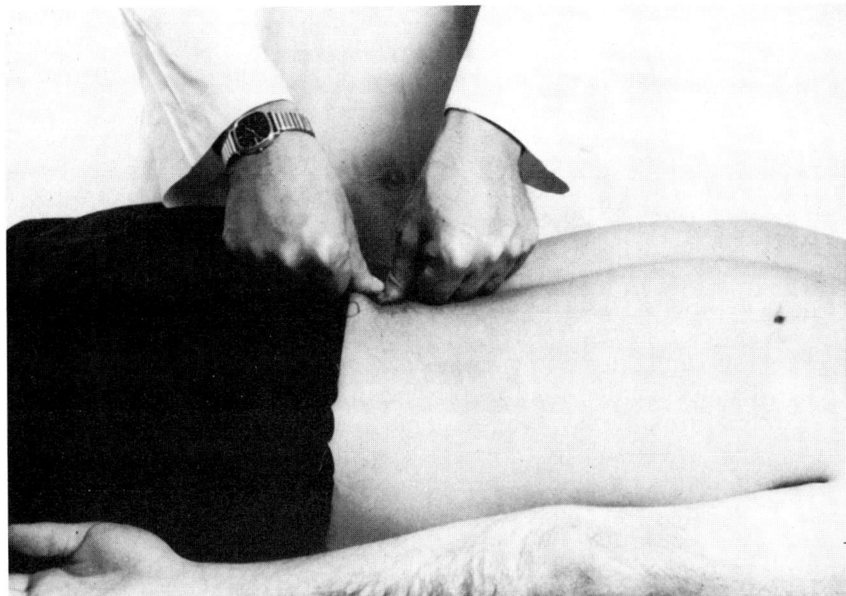

Figure 11–1. Instability test. With the patient prone, the examiner's thumbs seek a painful midline interspinous area. Sharp downward pressure is applied by the thumbs with the patient relaxed and the maneuver is repeated while the patient lifts his head, shoulders and arms up from the table (See Figure 11–6).

terspace is found or if all are painful, the test cannot be performed. If one or two levels are painful, the patient is asked to lift his head, shoulders, and arms and the downward pressure is repeated. If the pain is greater when the patient is prone and relaxed than when extended with paravertebral muscles tight, the test is positive. The test stresses the painful anulus in the relaxed position, but the contracted muscles stabilize the segment, reducing the stress and the pain from pressure. If the pain is greater with the muscles contracted or the pain is equal with both maneuvers, the test is negative.

Weight relief flexion is performed with the patient supine, hips and knees flexed. The examiner places one arm under the patient's knees and lifts the patient's buttocks up from the examination table. If the pain is decreased with this maneuver, the test is positive.

X rays may show a narrowed disc space or a spondylolysis or spondylolisthesis corresponding with the painful interspace; or the x rays may be normal.

The diagnosis of instability depends upon:

1. Midline pain.
2. Positive instability test or weight relief flexion test.
3. Positive response to flexion exercises.

HERNIATED DISC

The herniated disc and its variations of protruded and extruded nuclear material have a well defined clinical picture. The diagnosis of this entity as a cause of pain cannot be made on imaging tests alone in the absence of the clinical picture, and surgical treatment based on imaging tests alone is likely to lead to therapeutic failure. The clinical picture is based on nerve root pressure producing neurologic deficit and nerve root irritability producing nerve tension signs and symptoms.

A critical element in the patient's history is the predominance of leg pain (nerve pain) over back pain (usually anular pain), and that the leg pain is made worse by activities or positions that increase intradiscal pressure. Intradiscal pressure is higher when sitting than when standing. It is elevated by bending forward, bending to the side, lifting, coughing, sneezing, and straining.[9]

The physical findings specific for a herniated disc are nerve tension signs and appropriate neurologic deficit. Straight leg raising, by itself, can produce pain from a variety of sources, including myogenic pain, ischial bursitis, anular tear, and hamstring tightness, as well as herniated disc. The critical distinction is made by the sciatic stretch test. This test is performed after a straight leg raising test by lowering the affected leg a few degrees below the point that produces leg pain and then dorsiflexing the ankle. For the test to be positive for the diagnosis of herniated disc, leg pain must be greater than back pain.

The neurologic examination should demonstrate reflex changes, weakness, or segmental sensory loss. A diminished or absent ankle jerk compared to the opposite side identifies an S-1 lesion. Reinforcement and distraction techniques may be necessary along with repeated testing to confirm this finding.

Weakness of great toe extension identifies an L-5 lesion. Weakness of ankle dorsiflexion may be present with either L-5 or S-1 compression. Strength testing may also require repeated testing and distraction techniques. Some patients will voluntarily relax during testing, simulating weakness. Voluntary relaxation can be recognized if the great toe remains down when the examiner releases the pressure. This may be an effort by the patient to exaggerate findings, but it often results because the test causes pain through nerve tension or because a general muscle tightening increases intradiscal pressure. Weakness can be confirmed by having the patient walk on his heels. With genuine weakness of dorsiflexion of the ankle, the patient is unable to lift the ball of the foot on the weaker side as high as on the normal side. Weakness of the great toe extensor will be apparent if the great toe drops on the weaker side.

Sensation is diminished on the medial side of the foot and lateral calf for L-5 lesions and on the lateral foot and posterior calf for S-1 lesions. A stocking hypesthesia, even involving the entire leg, is not necessarily a sign of hysteria or malingering. It can occur in herniated discs and will disappear after successful treatment of the disc herniation.

Imaging techniques (myelogram, CT, MRI) should demonstrate actual nerve impingement at the level appropriate for the physical findings. A "bulging" disc is often noted in these imaging tests, but unless it is eccentric and actually displacing the nerve root, it does not confirm the diagnosis of herniated disc.

A diagnosis of a symptomatic herniated disc, then, requires:

1. Leg pain worse than back pain.
2. Sciatic stretch test reproduces leg pain greater than back pain.
3. Neurologic deficit consistent with nerve root impingement.
4. Imaging tests confirm nerve displacement at the appropriate level.

ANULAR TEAR

The lesion labeled anular tear or internal disc disruption is based on the concept of a leaking disc, one which permits the irritating liquid material normally restricted to the center of the disc to come into contact with innervated tissue.[10,11,12] The anular tear that permits egress of this liquid has a poor capacity for healing. At most, a thin layer of scar tissue at the periphery of the tear may seal the leak but leave the disc highly susceptible to retearing.[13] The irritating liquid is constantly replenished from living cells in the nucleus pulposus, so it continues to leak indefinitely. Whereas the herniated disc has a significant capacity to be resolved with time, the anular tear continues to produce symptoms indefinitely.

The clinical picture is based on pain related to increased intradiscal pressure and irritability of neural structures. An anular tear is usually produced by an injury that increases intradiscal pressure significantly. Typical injuries are a fall on the buttocks or a sudden straining or lifting injury. However, in some patients, the history suggests that lesser degrees of increased intradiscal pressure may complete a tear in a previously injured disc. The principal element in the history is the predominance of back pain— either alone or in excess of leg pain. Leg pain may be unilateral, as is true of a herniated disc, or bilateral in contrast to the typical herniated disc. Increases in intradiscal pressure exacerbate the pain. The pain is often worse when sitting than when standing. Coughing and sneezing worsen the pain as do forward bending and lifting.

On physical examination, no nerve compression is evident. Motor power and reflexes are intact. Sensory changes may be detected, but usually they are nonanatomic. This feature may lead to the incorrect interpretation that the problem is hysterical. The key physical finding is a positive sciatic stretch test that produces back pain or back pain greater than leg pain. A positive test is presumably produced by tension on irritated dural tissue or possibly by increasing intradiscal pressure. Secondary confirmation of this test may be obtained through a positive "flip" test. For this test the patient is seated on the examining table with the calves against the edge of the table and with hands on the edge of the table. The flexed knee is then lifted to a fully extended position. The test is positive if this maneuver produces more back than leg pain.

Myelogram, CT and MRI imaging will show no compression of neural structures. At most, there may be a central bulging of a disc. Unfortunately, this bulge is too often interpreted as a "herniated disc." The MRI may or may not show evidence of "disc degeneration."

The key diagnostic test is discography with CT discography. A positive examination will show dye extending into the epidural space or extending to the periphery of the disc where it can contact the innervated portion of the anulus fibrosus. A positive test also requires a reproduction of pain accompanying the injection of dye.

In summary, the diagnostic features for anular tear are:

1. Back pain alone or back pain greater than leg pain.
2. Increased back pain with increased intradiscal pressure.

3. Reproduction of back pain to a greater degree than leg pain by sciatic stretch test.
4. No neurologic deficit.
5. Reproduction of pain by discography and discographic dye extending to or beyond the periphery of the anulus fibrosus.

MYOGENIC PAIN

Pain originating in the support muscles of the spine parades under a variety of names. It is called myositis, fibrositis, fibromyositis, myofascial syndrome, and myogenic syndrome. The common denominator is pain related to muscle use or overuse in a muscle that has been rendered susceptible by injury or chronic overuse. Traumatic episodes that injure the disc may at the same time injure the lumbar paravertebral muscles or gluteus maximus muscles, so myogenic pain often accompanies discogenic pain to serve as a complicating diagnostic and therapeutic factor.[6]

Once a muscle becomes susceptible to developing myogenic pain, it apparently remains so permanently. The pain is not necessarily permanent, but the susceptibility is, so that when the muscle is used beyond its threshold point, pain occurs. The irritable and painful area of muscle behaves as though it accumulates fluid during rest because, after inactivity, resumed movement also produces stiffness and pain. This produces the anomalous symptom complex of pain after sustained muscle use as well as pain after rest.

Myogenic pain is intensified by a strong contraction of the involved muscle. Thus, lifting a heavy object causes myogenic pain by stressing the muscle, but it also intensifies discogenic pain by increasing intradiscal pressure. Repetitive bending also stresses the muscle and produces pain. Perhaps the most common muscle use factor causing pain is a sustained contraction of back muscles as seen in patients who work in a partially flexed position or even sit for prolonged periods without back support. Symptoms are also worse with fatigue. Patients working two jobs are likely to exhibit fatigue pain. Weather change or chilling of the muscle which causes pain and "tension" or psychological stress, leading to involuntary muscle contraction, worsens pain.

Pain that is worse when the patient first arises, or gets up from a chair, or gets out of a car, or when the weather changes, is typical of both myogenic pain and arthritis. When combined with x ray evidence of spinal degenerative changes, these symptoms are frequently incorrectly attributed to spinal arthritis. It is worth making the distinction between myogenic pain and pain from osteoarthritis because myogenic pain may be improved with an exercise program and the treatment for osteoarthritis pain (if it exists as a specific pain-causing entity) is symptomatic.

Another source of confusion in diagnosing myogenic pain is myogenic pain radiating into the posterior buttocks and thigh and simulating sciatica. Such radiation is particularly common in gluteus maximus pain that radiates to or occasionally just below the knee. Pain radiating from the buttocks into the calf or foot is not myogenic pain and is most likely to be neurogenic in origin. On physical examination, the key is the reproduction of pain in the involved muscle. The three diagnostic features of myogenic pain are:

1. Local tenderness in a portion of the involved muscle (usually lumbar paravertebral or gluteal muscles).
2. Reproduction of pain in the muscle by passive stretching.
3. Reproduction of pain in the muscle by actively contracting it against resistance.

Eliciting tenderness in the muscle requires finding an area elsewhere in the muscle that is not tender or is substantially less tender because some patients are tender "all over."

The most common site of tenderness in the lumbar paravertebral muscles is near the lumbosacral junction just medial and superior to the posterior superior iliac spine (Fig. 11–2). The tender area is usually lateral to the midline, but may be midline where the muscle fibers decussate across the midline in the low lumbar area. In the more lateral location, the tenderness in the muscle may be difficult to distinguish from facet tenderness.

The most common site of tenderness in the gluteus maximus is medially and superiorly, just lateral and inferior to the posterior superior iliac spine (Fig. 11–3). In this area, the muscle tenderness is often misinterpretted as sacroiliac tenderness. Confirmation of muscle tenderness is sought through reproduction of pain by active and passive stress of the muscle.

Passive stress of the lumbar paravertebral muscles is performed in the supine position (Fig. 11–4). The patient brings both knees to his chest, holding the knees with both hands. The examiner then passively flexes the patient's head and neck to maximally flex the entire spine and maximally stretch the entire paravertebral muscle mass. If this maneuver reproduces pain in the muscle at the site of tenderness, the test is positive.

Passive stress of the gluteus maximus muscle is also performed in the supine position (Fig. 11–5). Each knee and hip are passively flexed indepen-

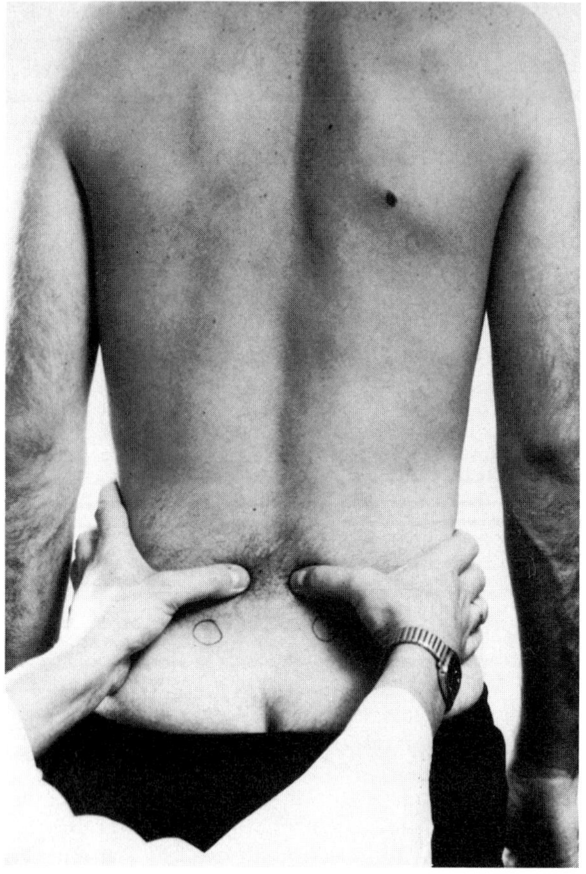

***Figure* 11–2.** The posterior superior iliac spines are marked by circles. The thumbs identify the common areas of tenderness for lumbar paravertebral myogenic pain.

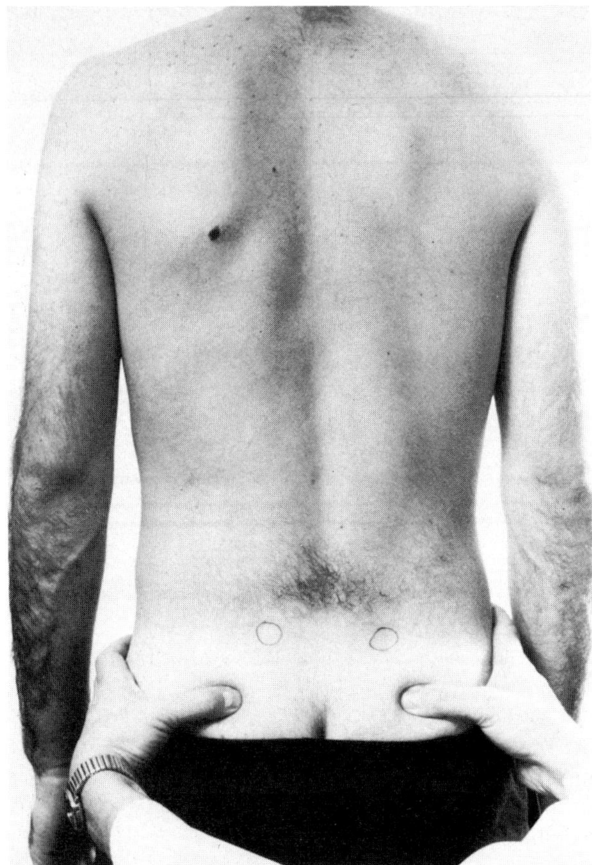

***Figure* 11–3.** The posterior superior iliac spines are marked by circles. The thumbs identify the common areas of tenderness for gluteus maximus myogenic pain.

dently, bringing the ipsilateral knee toward the contralateral shoulder to maximally stretch the muscle. If this maneuver reproduces buttock pain at the site of tenderness, the test is positive. Active stress tests are performed in the prone position with the patient's arms at his sides.

Active lumbar paravertebral stress is performed by asking the patient to lift his head, shoulders, and arms while the examiner provides counter pressure downward against the upper thoracic spine for 5 seconds (Fig. 11–6). Reproduction of pain in the muscle at the tender site constitutes a positive test.

Active gluteus maximus stress is performed by asking the patient to flex one knee and then to lift that knee up from the examining table while the examiner grasps the ankle and presses down (Fig. 11–7). A positive test reproduces pain in the gluteus maximus at the site of tenderness. This test may also cause pain in the lumbar paravertebral muscles be-

cause patients often contract these muscles in the test, but this pain reproduction does not constitute a positive gluteus maximus text.

An additional confirmatory test for muscle pain may be performed with the patient upright. The patient is asked to bend laterally, which causes the muscles on the side opposite the bend to contract (Fig. 11–8). This will reproduce myogenic pain in the contracted muscle. Ipsilateral pain is more likely to be from a facet.

Currently, no laboratory or imaging tests exist to confirm myogenic pain. Diagnosis of myogenic pain is clinical only and depends upon:

1. Increased pain upon resuming activity or with weather change.
2. Identifying tender areas in specific muscles (lumbar parvertebral or gluteus maximus).
3. Reproduction of pain *in these muscles* by active and passive stress tests of the muscles.

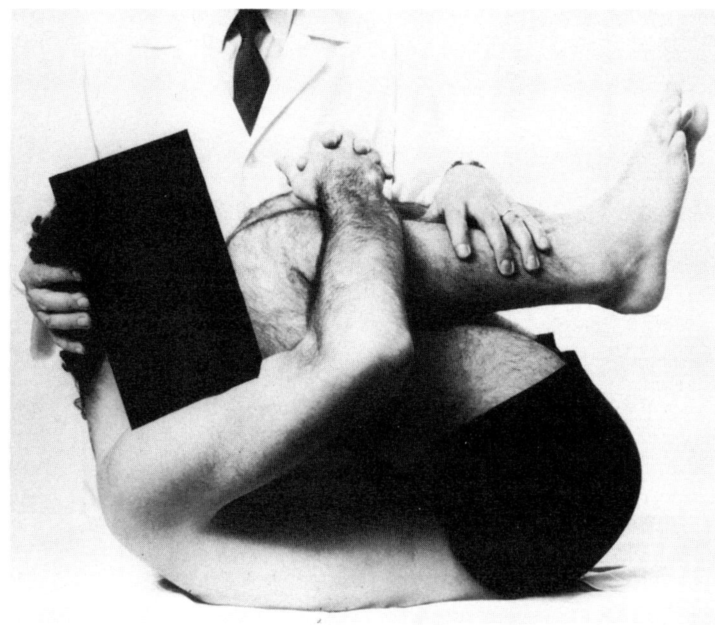

Figure 11–4. Passive lumbar paravertebral muscle stress test. Both hips and knees are flexed. The patient pulls the knees to the chest with his hands. The examiner flexes the neck, bringing the nose toward the knees.

FACET SYNDROME

Pain from an irritable facet joint may be detected by local tenderness directly over a facet, with confirmation by maneuvers to "pinch" or compress the facet joint.[14] The pain tends to be unilateral, with or without radiating leg pain. It may, like myogenic pain, be worse on resuming activity after sitting or lying down or worse with weather change. There is no clearly identifiable diagnostic symptom.

On physical examination, tenderness can usually be identified unilaterally over one or two facet joints. The area of tenderness is relatively circumscribed. Diffuse tenderness over a broader area is more likely to be myogenic pain. In the upright position, the patient is asked to bend backward. This

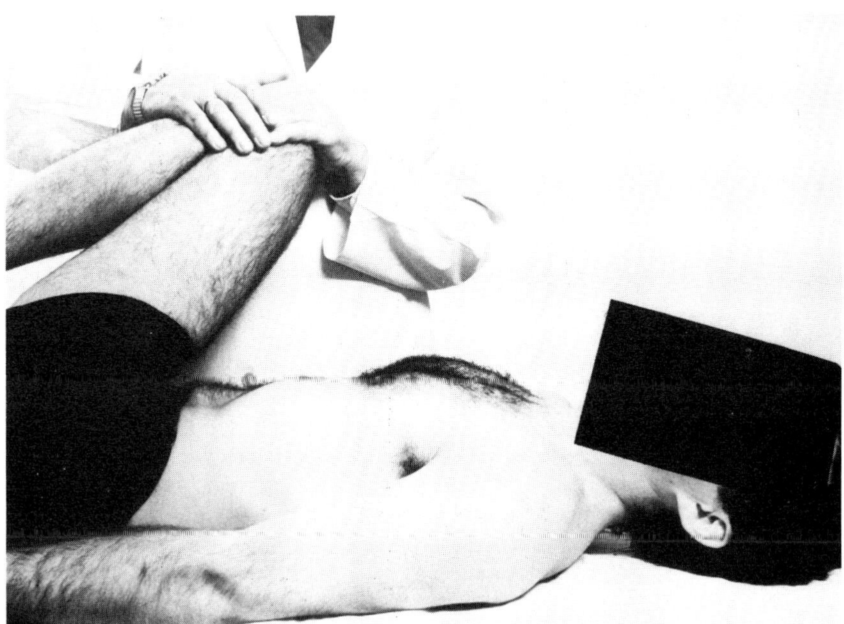

Figure 11–5. Passive gluteus maximus muscle stress test. The hip and knee are flexed and adducted.

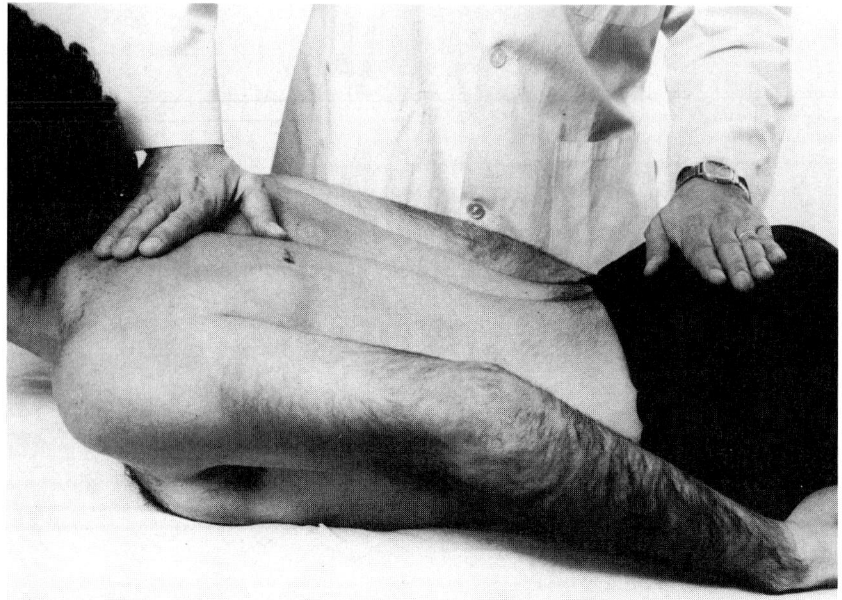

Figure 11–6. Active lumbar paravertebral muscle stress test. From the prone position, the patient lifts his head, shoulders, and arms up from the table while the examiner provides downward pressure against the upper thoracic spine.

maneuver compresses the facet joint and can reproduce facet pain. Pain from an anular tear also may be worsened by this test. Because the lumbar paravertebral muscles are usually relaxed by this movement, myogenic pain may be unchanged or actually improved. On lateral bending, toward the side of pain, the facet is again compressed, reproducing facet pain. Pain on the opposite side is likely to be myogenic. Other elements of the examination may be variable. There may be a positive sciatic stretch test, flip test, or even neurologic deficits. Moreover, oblique spinal x-rays may or may not demonstrate facet arthropathy. Many patients with degenerative changes in their facet joints are symptom free and many with symptomic facet joints show normal x rays.

Relief of pain by facet injection is regarded as the distinguishing diagnostic test, but it may not be definitive in ruling out other diagnoses. Because the clinical picture may simulate a herniated disc, imaging studies are necessary to rule out this diagnosis even if facet injection relieves pain. Some patients with pain relief by facet injection subsequently prove to have anular tears. If the injection is not intracapsular the spread of local anesthetic into surrounding tissues may relieve pain from other sources, such as myogenic pain.

Facet joint pain may be diagnosed by:

1. Local tenderness over a facet joint.
2. Reproduction of pain by extension or ipsilateral side-bending.
3. Relief of pain by facet joint injection.

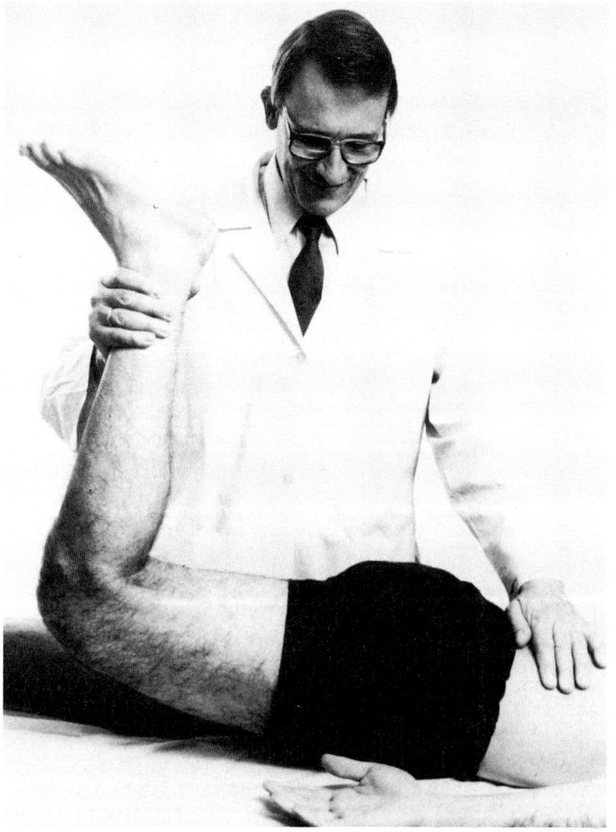

Figure 11–7. Active gluteus maximus muscle stress test. With the patient prone, the knee is flexed and the patient lifts the knee up off the table while the examiner provides downward pressure against the ankle.

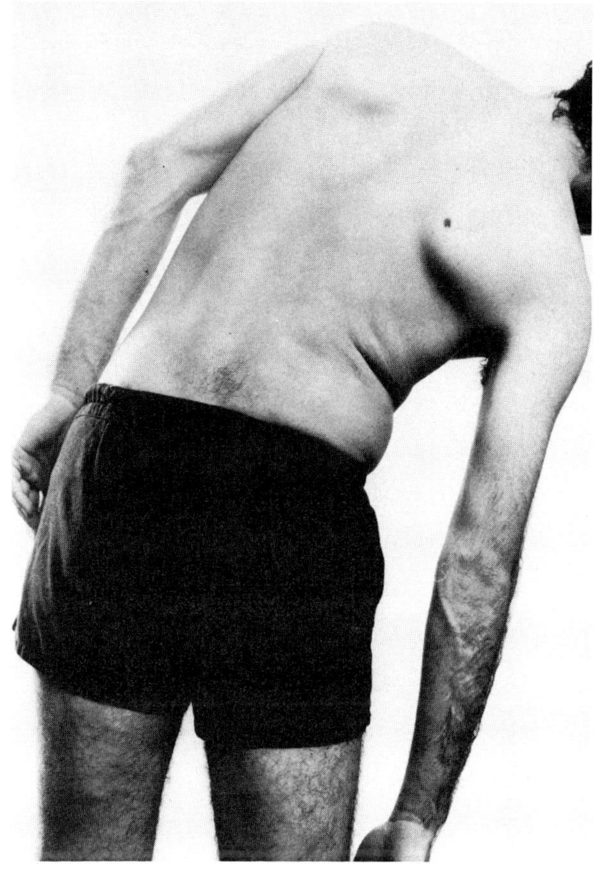

Figure 11–8. With the patient erect and bending to the right side, the left lumbar paravertebral muscle mass is contracted. This is usually uncomfortable if these muscles have myogenic pain.

SPINAL STENOSIS

Spinal stenosis is a diagnosis describing a narrowing of the space available for neural structures in the spinal canal or neural foramina.[7] It most commonly produces symptoms by compressing neural structures rather than irritating them. A herniated disc may be considered a form of spinal stenosis but this lesion produces both compression and irritation of neural structures. In typical spinal stenosis, compression of the neural structures also compresses the vascular supply of the nerves so that the symptoms are predominantly those of neural ischemia. Because both the neural canal and the neural foramen are narrowed with the spine in extension and opened in flexion, neural compression is most often temporary. Pain induces patients to change position and relieve nerve pressure before permanent neurologic damage is done.

The symptoms of spinal stenosis are usually uni-lateral or bilateral leg pain, with or without back pain. Patients are usually sixty years of age or older. The pain develops when the patient is in an upright position and particularly when the patient is walking. The typical symptom is pseudoclaudication characterized by leg pain, numbness, and weakness developing after the patient walks a predictable distance. The patient seeks relief by sitting, leaning forward "to relieve pressure", putting his foot on a raised rest, or lying down. The common denominator is changing the position of the spine from extension to flexion.[15]

Physical examination is most often nonspecific except for the "spinal Phalen" test. Patients usually have a fairly good range of motion of the spine, compatible with age and degenerative changes. Sciatic stretch test results and flip test results are usually negative. Neurologic examination is most often negative but may show changes representing residuals of prior surgery or prior injury.

The spinal Phalen test attempts to reproduce symptoms of leg pain, weakness, or numbness by causing neural ischemia in a manner similar to the Phalen test for median nerve compression. With the patient upright, he is asked to bend backward and sustain this extended position for a full minute or longer (Fig. 11–8). This maneuver accentuates the spinal stenosis. A positive test will produce a crescendo of leg symptoms followed by rapid relief of these symptoms when the patient flexes forward, places his hands on the examination table, and places one foot on a stool.

Routine x ray films often show degenerative changes and may show degenerative spondylolisthesis, but do not offer the degree of diagnostic confirmation needed for surgical treatment. A CT scan may be useful in ruling out other lesions but does not always show the multiple areas of stenosis that must be identified for surgical treatment. A sagital MRI may be more helpful in this regard, but a myelogram with the patient in extension probably offers the best information on the location of stenotic areas.

The diagnosis of spinal stenosis may be made by:

1. Eliciting a history of pseudoclaudication.
2. A positive spinal Phalen test.
3. Imaging confirmation of stenosis.

SPONDYLOLYSIS AND SPONDYLOLISTHESIS

Isthmic spondylolysis and spondylolisthesis are x-ray diagnoses and do not, by themselves, identify clinical causes of symptoms. As such, these x ray findings do not provide a definitive guide to treatment. Patients with back or leg pain and x rays showing these abnormalities usually have symptoms originating from one or more of the six diagnostic categories described here. The standard surgical treatment of fusion is predicated upon a diagnosis of ligamentous instability. Posterior decompression of the neural arch or the isthemic defect is directed toward a variant of spinal stenosis. Neither of these treatments relieves symptoms originating from concomitant diagnoses of myogenic pain, anular tear, or herniated disc at another level. Unless these diagnostic categories are identified or ruled out, surgical failure may occur.

A final diagnostic caveat: Back pain is not necessarily a static diagnostic phenomenon. It can evolve. The character of the pain and its location may change and with it the physical findings and imaging findings. An initial diagnosis of myositis or facet syndrome may subsequently evolve into a diagnosis of anular tear. An initial diagnosis of acute ligamentous injury may evolve into a diagnoses of herniated disc. In patients with chronic back symptoms, periodic re-evaluation is often necessary to reach an appropriate final diagnosis.

REFERENCES

1. Bernard, T.N., Jr, Kirkaldy-Willis, W.H.: Recognizing specific characteristics of non specific low back pain. Clin Orthop 217:266–280, 1987.

2. Nachemson, A.L.: The natural course of low back pain. Proceedings of The American Academy of Orthopaedic Surgeons, Symposium on Idiopathic Low Back Pain, Miami, FL, December, 1980. St. Louis, C.V. Mosby, pp 46–51, 1982.

3. Frymoyer, J.W., et al.: Spine radiographs in patients with low-back pain: an epidemiological study in men. J Bone Joint Surg [Am] 66A:1048–1055, 1984.

4. Hirsch, C., Ingelmark, B.E., Miller, M.: The anatomical basis for low back pain. Acta Orthop Scand 33:1–17, 1963.

5. Kellgren, J.H.: The anatomical source of back pain. Rheum Rehabil 16:3–12, 1977.

6. Laros, G.S., Ozanne, S., McCarron, R.F.: Six categories of low back pain: a prospective study. Submitted to Spine.

7. Kirkaldy-Willis, W.H.: Managing Low Back Pain. 2nd Ed., New York, Churchill Livingstone, 1988.

8. Morgan, F.P., King, T.: Primary instability of lumbar vertebrae as a common cause of low back pain. J Bone Joint Surg [BR] 39B:6–22, 1957.

9. Nachemson, A.L., Elfstrom, G.: Intravital dynamic pressure measurements in lumbar discs: a study of common movements, maneuvers and exercises. Scand J Rehabil Med 1(1):1, 1970.

10. Crock, H.V.: Internal disc disruption: a challenge to disc prolapse fifty years on. Spine 11:650–653, 1986.

11. McCarron, R.F., Wimpee, M.W., Hudkins, P.G., Laros, G.S.: The inflammatory effect of nucleus polposus: a possible element in the pathogenesis of low back pain. Spine 12:760–764, 1987.

12. Mooney, V.: The syndromes of low back disease. Orthop Clin North Am 14:505–515, 1983.

13. Hampton, D., Laros, G.S., McCarron, R.F., Franks, D.: The healing potential of the annulus fibrosus. Presented at the annual meeting of the North American Spine Society, Colorado Springs, CO, July 25, 1988. Spine 14:389–401, 1989.

14. Mooney, V., Robertson, J.: The facet syndrome. Clin Orthop 115:149–156, 1976.

15. Dyck, P.: The stoop-test in lumbar entrapment radiculopathy. Spine 4:89–92, 1979.

Psychosocioeconomic Factors Related to Spinal Disorders

C. David Tollison
Donald W. Hinnant
Michael L. Kriegel

Psychological Concepts of Pain

Over the past 25 years much has been written in support of recognizing pain as a phenomenon in excess of the extent of tissue damage alone. Current thinking positions pain, including pain of spinal disorders, as a complex, perceptual phenomenon comprised of a multitude of psychosocial factors as well as sensory stimulation.[1] However, this present definition has not always held such a favorable position among scientists and practitioners. In fact, although the influence of psychological factors was acknowledged, the historical view of pain has primarily been that of pure sensory stimulation. This currently defunct consideration of pain, thought to have evolved from the advent of sensory psychophysics and sensory physiology during the late nineteenth century, has generated important treatment implications. For example, such thinking spurred efforts to: (1) directly measure pain as a physiological phenomenon uncontaminated by psychological factors, (2) develop sophisticated surgical procedures to ablate the pain pathways from the periphery to the central nervous system, and (3) synthesize more potent analgesic medications.[1]

The relatively recent shift in consideration from pain as a purely sensory phenomenon to pain as a perceptual event was generated in large part by the work of Melzack and his colleagues,[2,3] and Fordyce and his coworkers.[4] Melzack and others, in development of the gate control model, presented a multidimensional model of pain that addressed the inconsistencies of sensory pain theories. He postulated that the experience of pain was the result of the integration of motivational/affective, cognitive/evaluative, and sensory/discriminative contributions. Thus, Melzack proposed that pain was the result of the integration and interpretation of sensory and psychological processes and, therefore, qualified as a perceptual process.[1]

From a different perspective, Fordyce and his colleagues proposed a model of pain that emphasized the subjectivity of the pain experience and the objectivity of behavioral measurement. As shall be discussed in the following section of this chapter, Fordyce avoided attending to pain per se by extending classical learning theory, specifically operant conditioning, to the puzzle of pain. From this perspective, the subjective experience of pain is irrelevant because it cannot be directly observed and measured.

Both the gate control and behavioral or operant models of pain served as catalysts for the current consideration of pain as a multidimensional phenomenon influenced by both sensory and psychological factors. Although a number of models are purported to explain the role of psychological factors in pain, we will restrict our discussion to three perspectives: the behavioral, or operant, model; the cognitive model; and the cognitive-behavioral model. Our objective is to present to readers a brief overview of each model, with a discussion of basic concepts and the application of the models in the treatment of painful spinal disorders.

THE BEHAVIORAL (OPERANT) MODEL

In 1968, Fordyce, et al.,[4,5] published two reports describing the use of behavioral management techniques for treating chronic pain that established both an alternative conceptualization and treatment approach that remains highly visible and utilized more than 20 years later. Instead of automatically presuming an underlying medical or psychological cause for chronic pain, consistent with the traditional medical disease model, the novel behavioral or operant model concentrated directly upon the actions or behaviors of patients with complaints of pain and their families. Established behavior modification principles were then applied to modify selected behaviors emitted by patients and family members in an effort to facilitate patient functioning, rather than to treat pain directly. Following publication of these two articles, the behavioral conceptualization in the treatment of chronic pain increased rapidly and today a more broadly defined behavioral approach is utilized in virtually every recognized pain treatment program in the United States.[6]

Basic Concepts

Prior to discussing the behavioral conceptualization and treatment of clinical back pain, it is important to establish a conceptual and empirical basis for such an application. In this section we offer brief definitions and principles for four basic paradigms critical to the behavioral model (Table 12–1).

Positive Reinforcement

The foundation of positive reinforcement is relatively simple: When a behavior is closely followed in time by a positive consequence or reinforcer (e.g., praise, attention, money, food, etc.), the behavior generating the positive reinforcement will strengthen and increase in rate of future occurrence.[7] For example, a mother follows her child's behavior of removing dirty dinner plates from the dining room to the kitchen with verbal praise. Soon, she sees an increase in the desired behavior as a result of her making positive reinforcement contingent upon the child's demonstration of targeted behavior. This concept has been used extensively to effect desired changes in both child and adult behaviors, and common positive reinforcers may include physical touch, access to pleasurable activities, food, social attention, praise, and a host of other materials and experiences that individuals find enjoyable or pleasurable.[5] Positive reinforcers are routinely identified by observing an individual or asking the patient and family. Although there are common positive reinforcers that most people acknowledge (e.g., money and praise), important individual differences are frequent, particularly with regard to the positive reinforcement of pain and disability behaviors. Identifi-

Table 12–1
Four Basic Paradigms Critical to the Behavioral Model of Pain

Positive Reinforcement

Negative Reinforcement

Punishment

Extinction

cation of cogent and specific positive reinforcers on an individual patient basis is critical to behavioral treatment outcome.

Negative Reinforcement

A second paradigm of the behavioral model is termed negative reinforcement. When a behavior is closely followed in time by a negative consequence, that behavior is likely to occur less frequently in the future and behavior designed to remove the negative consequence or avoid it is likely to increase.[4] This is also known as escape/avoidance conditioning because it is assumed that the behavior is emitted to escape or avoid an aversive situation. For example, the child who whines when asked to take out the garbage and successfully avoids the aversive task may be expected to increase whining behavior whenever the threat of removing the garbage is present. Likewise, an adult may drive within the speed limit in order to avoid the negative consequences of a traffic citation.[8] It is well established that behavior that is maintained or increased because of negative reinforcement can be highly resistant to change and may be maintained even when the aversive experience is not present. For example, an individual may drive within the designated speed limit even when a patrolman is not present. As will be discussed later, negative reinforcement is often important in the behavioral conceptualization of chronic pain.

Punishment

Another important paradigm in behavioral conceptualization is that of punishment. Punishment may be defined as the application of an aversive consequence or removal of a positive consequence in an attempt to reduce the occurrence of a specific targeted behavior. For example, a child who bites his brother may receive a spanking (aversive consequence) or may be sent to his room (removal from a positive social situation). As with positive and negative reinforcers, punishers may be identified by observation or by asking the patient and family. Common punishers include the experience of pain, job and school stress, loss of resources or valuables, social ridicule, interpersonal discord, and loss of social attention or recognition.[8] However, removal of a punisher may result in an increase in the behavior which previously generated the punishing consequence.

Extinction

When a behavior is followed by neither positive nor negative consequences, the behavior will be eliminated or reduced in frequency, a process termed extinction.[7] An exception to the paradigm of extinction is behavior either maintained or increased as the result of negative reinforcement.[8] As previously mentioned, learned escape/avoidance behavior is often resistant to change, particularly if the behavior actually avoids the occurrence of an unpleasant experience. For example, if an individual perceives that driving within the speed limit has successfully avoided a speeding ticket, the driving behavior may be maintained and the actual occurrence of the aversive experience (receiving a traffic citation) is not required because avoidance behavior has been established.

A Behavioral Conceptualization of Clinical Back Pain

Before the behavioral model is applied in the management of chronic back pain, it is important to briefly summarize the behavioral conceptualization of clinical pain based on the existence of learning and conditioning effects upon behavior. In light of a growing body of empirical knowledge over the past 20 years, it has become obvious to most authorities that a significant portion of the "pain experience" involves overt behavior.[8]

Based on the traditional "medical disease model," pain is a neurophysiologic event or sensory system that functions to inform the victim that a noxious stimulus is present. A variety of factors (e.g., pain threshold, stimulus intensity, nervous system integrity, and previous experience) determine whether and to what extent pain is experienced. In essence, there exists a stimulus (pathologic condition) and a response (pain) and the former controls the latter.[6] With few exceptions, when the stimulus is present, pain is experienced, and when the stimulus is removed, pain is eliminated.

The difference between pain as a sensory system (acute pain) and as a chronic condition is critically important.[5] In chronic pain, the response (pain) occurs over a protracted duration of time, thereby affording an opportunity for learned behavior. A patient demonstrates to others that he is in pain by exhibiting behaviors termed operants.[9] For example, a patient grimaces, describes his pain, walks with an antalgic gait, requests medications, and retires to bed. The importance of operants is that they can be modified by the consequences which immediately follow them.[6] The modification of operants is accomplished through the systematic application of positive reinforcement, negative reinforcement, punishment, and extinction.

Practically all pain behaviors are operants.[2] However, it is recognized that antecedent stimuli, as well as consequences, can elicit operants. When a patient complains of sharp, radiating pain down the lower extremity and moves in slow and guarded motions, he may have a herniation or other disorder of a spinal disc. Yet, each of these pain behaviors, as operants, can be modified by the consequences.[9] Presumably, all chronic pain originates with a pathologic stimulus that produces pain responses or pain behaviors. The behavioral or operant model suggests that some victims function in an environment that systematically and positively reinforces pain behaviors and perhaps punishes or fails to positively reinforce well behaviors. Consequently, pain behaviors may persist and increase in intensity over time, as the original pathologic stimulus lessens or even disappears. In either case, the degree of pain behavior has little or no direct relationship to the pathologic factors.[9]

Finally, it is important to emphasize that it is not necessary for the patient to suffer hysteria, hypochondriasis, conversion reaction, personality disorder, or other maladaptive psychological condition in order to learn a pain habit. Learning is known to occur automatically if conditions present are favorable.[9]

Behavioral Treatment of Painful Spinal Disorders

In the behavioral treatment of pain, including chronic spinal pain, it is important to recognize that attention is targeted on the relationship between the demonstration of pain behaviors and the occurrence of reinforcing consequences (sometimes called contingencies). Attention is not directed to the antecedent events subsumed by the term nociception.[6] Consequently, the behavioral model is not intended to treat pain in the traditional sense and does not have as its principle objective the modification of nociception or the direct modification of the experience of pain. Rather, behavioral methods are intended to treat excess disability and the expressions of suffering with the goal of rendering chronic pain victims functional again.

The success of the behavioral model in the treatment of chronic pain is predicated on the clinician first conducting a detailed behavioral analysis. The goals of such an analysis are listed in Table 12–2. In most patients who suffer intractable back pain, the

Table 12–2
The Goals of a Detailed Behavioral Analysis of Chronic Pain

1. Identify the behavior to be generated, increased, maintained, decreased, or eliminated.
2. Determine the types of reinforcers that are likely to be effective with an individual patient.
3. Develop sufficient influence or control over the environment to regulate the consequences of the behavior to be influenced.

specific behaviors to be decreased include the consumption of analgesic medications, excessive medical care utilization, and the response to pain signals by unproductive behaviors. Behaviors to be generated or increased include physical activity and exercise, return to productivity and employment, and other behaviors incompatible with nonproductive behavior.

With the described basics of the behavioral model in mind, let us proceed with a brief discussion of the application of operant techniques in the treatment of chronic pain. For sake of example, we will assume that the patient is an adult male with complaints of chronic lower back pain of 6 months duration and whose pain behaviors are in excess of the degree of diagnosed pathophysiology. We shall further assume that the treatment goals for this patient include: (1) decreasing verbal and overt pain behaviors, (2) increasing physical activity levels, (3) eliminating the consumption of analgesic medications, and (4) effecting long-term environmental change.

The first treatment goal is to decrease verbal and overt pain behaviors. This is primarily accomplished by withdrawing social reinforcers (attention) as a consequence of the target behavior. For example, a nurse walking down the hallway passes our pain patient's room and notes the patient sitting on the edge of his bed with one hand held to the back, as if massaging a painful area. The nurse simply continues past the door without stopping. On another occasion she passes by the room and notes the patient standing at the mirror shaving (and therefore not exhibiting pain behavior). She stops—if only for a brief moment—to make some comment, for example, about a recent political election or even the weather. Another example is the physician making morning rounds who asks our patient, "How's that bad back today?" In the behavioral model, the physician might instead ask, "How long did you walk the treadmill yesterday?"

In the behavioral treatment of chronic pain, all staff must consistently respond to visible and audible demonstrations of pain behavior as if they had not occurred. Furthermore, while social reinforcement is being withdrawn from pain behavior, it is important to diligently reinforce demonstrations of well behavior.

A second goal of behavioral management in our example is increasing physical activity levels. Unfortunately, most health providers encourage chronic pain patients to increase physical activity levels in a work-to-tolerance format. That is, continue walking and exercising until increased pain prohibits continuation and then stop and rest. In this format, rest becomes contingent upon pain and thus constitutes a positive reinforcer for pain behavior. Consequently, we can expect that time spent resting would actually increase, rather than decrease, because of reinforcement.

A behavioral alternative to the work-to-tolerance format is termed working-to-quota and reverses the above scenario. First, the patient demonstrates tolerance limits across a series of trials. Once the level of activity that initiates increased pain has been determined, quotas for physical activity are set that are less than baseline tolerance limits. Next, the patient is presented specific limits for physical activity known not to increase pain, and rest serves as a reinforcer of successful activity completion, rather than for pain behavior. Stated another way, working-to-quota positions rest and attention as activity contingent, rather than being pain contingent as in the working-to-tolerance regimen.

A third behavioral treatment goal is decreasing or eliminating the consumption of analgesic medications. Pain medications are usually dispensed on a prn basis, which has the effect of making medication contingent upon demonstration of pain behavior. If our back pain patient does not grimace, complain of pain, and request "something for pain" the nurses have no reason to dispense the "as needed" relief. Consequently, analgesic medications may serve as a reinforcer of pain behavior because of chemotherapeutic relief and attention following occurrence of pain behaviors.

An operant approach to pain medication management is to shift medications from pain contingent to time contingent, thereby extinquishing the need for medication requests and other associated pain behaviors. During the initial stages of treatment, medications are given prn while accurate records of patient controlled consumption are documented. After several days of baseline recording, all medications are incorporated into a single, orally administered liquid vehicle which is intended to mask taste and color. This process has come to be termed the pain cocktail. The cocktail is then administered at fixed time intervals independent of how the patient feels and intervals are scheduled less than baseline. Across time, the active ingredients of the cocktail are gradually decreased, eventually to zero. When the active ingredients reach a zero level, the patient is informed.

A final treatment goal in our example is effecting long-term environmental change and a number of procedures have been demonstrated as successful in rearranging consequences at home and at work to maintain treatment gains. First, it is necessary that the treatment team work with the patient to insure that employment and leisure time activities yield positive reinforcement. If our back pain patient finds his job at the factory aversive, efforts must be extended to locate alternative employment that is rewarding. The underlying principle is to facilitate patient access to reinforcing conditions in the natural environment which will serve to reinforce maintenance of well behaviors.

An additional requirement of the behavioral model is the active participation of the patient's spouse in regularly scheduled training sessions. These sessions are designed to educate the spouse in the basics of reinforcement and the operant approach and to rehearse alternative responses to future demonstrations of pain behavior on the part of the patient.

Conclusions

The behavioral or operant model has proven to be an effective approach in carefully selected patients suffering chronic pain. However, the approach has been criticized by those who cite the frequent need for extensive control of the patient's environment for a prolonged duration,[10] the clinical intensity required and subsequent cost,[10] and the failure of the model to consider the contribution of cognitive appraisals of pain victims as they affect patients' perceptions and responses to their physical symptoms.[1] Consequently, it is the observation of the authors that the stringent operant approach to pain management has been largely augmented of late with an expansion of behavioral techniques (e.g., biofeedback, relaxation training) and, as we shall determine in the following sections of this chapter, a philosophical shift in the psychological conceptualization of pain.

THE COGNITIVE MODEL

Cognitive theorists in psychology often enjoy quoting the stoic philosopher, Epictetus, who once said, "Men are disturbed not by things, but by the views which they take of them." Early learning theorists[11] emphasized the role of thought and language as cue-producing responses that affect emotional arousal. A significant volume of research has focused in recent years on cognitively mediated affective and physiological responses. Affectively loaded implicit statements have been found to elicit increases in respiration rate and depth,[12] heart rate, subjective anxiety, galvanic skin response,[13] and generalized autonomic arousal.

With the formulation of the gate control theory of pain by Melzack and Wall,[3] pain clinicians and researchers have been able to offer a better explanation of the specialization of fibers and receptors, spacial and temporal patterning, and psychological processes in pain perception and response. Schwartz and Shapiro[13] described two components in the perception and reaction to pain. First is the sensory or information aspect, which is similar to any sense or perception experience. Second is a reactive or motivational or emotional component. The reactive component has been described as the anguish or suffering element in pain. These two components are considered to have separate nerve pathways in the spinal cord and higher cortical regions, with different central projections. The sensory system projects through the neospinalthalamic fibers to the thalamus and somatosensory cortex. The motivational conduction system is by way of an ascending pathway through the reticular formation, thalamus, and limbic system.[3] In other words, the gate control theory holds that the perception of pain and the pain response is a very complex interaction of sensory, motivational, and cognitive components. Somatic input may be modulated by the influence of cognitive, behavioral, and emotional factors prior to pain perception. Thus, the cortex may be involved in the qualitative interpretation of the pain stimulus.[3]

Beecher's well known work with war injuries elaborated on the personal meaning of pain, with particular emphasis on the role of the appraisal process.[14] He found that the pain response of injured soldiers was less than one would consider appropriate for the degree of the injury, and the demand for analgesics was also less than expected. His evaluations indicated that the injured soldiers' view of the wound was interpreted as a means of escaping the danger of war to the safety of home. Studies with placebo effects in pain response suggest that approximately 35% of patients with pathophysiological pain benefit from placebo expectancies of pain relief.[14] Placebo responses have been attributed to possible cognitive processes such as the labeling/appraisal process and, more recently, researchers have suggested that the action of a placebo may be accounted for by the endorphin-mediated system.[15]

A Cognitive Conceptualization of Clinical Back Pain

Cognitive approaches applied to pain control have been greatly influenced by the use of cognitive techniques in the treatment of psychological problems in general. Beck[16] and Ellis[17] have fathered widely accepted utilization of cognitive treatment for psychological problems, and their techniques are commonly used in psychotherapy. Hypnosis has been used for centuries in one form or another and the mechanisms involved are complex and fraught with disagreement by researchers. Hypnosis has been considered to be a form of cognitive distraction and imagery that affects the patient's verbal/cognitive report of pain more than the actual physiological response. Consequently, hypnotic analgesia may be the result of cognitive or motivational factors in the pain experience.[18] Biofeedback researchers using electromyographic training for pain control with back pain patients have determined that patients' pain complaints continued to decrease following treatment for asymmetrical muscle tension and myofascial pain related to spasm. Although pain complaints continued to decrease and ultimately to stabilize post-treatment, patients' EMG readings were elevated upon followup to the level of pretreatment baseline. The researchers suggested that a cognitive feeling of self control, rather than actual physiologic control, is probably crucial for pain reduction with chronic pain patients. Apparently, individuals can develop a feeling of self-regulation for their pain and this confidence in an ability to reduce painful symptoms is a significant component of a positive adjustment to effective pain management.[19]

Cognitive approaches to pain control have focused primarily on some form of guided coping strategy or imagery techniques. Experimental studies that have reported success in reducing pain have included stress innoculation training,[20] distraction with a focus on pleasant scenery,[21] pain acknowledgement while using imagery to change the context of the sensations,[22] along with many variations of pain-reducing imagery.

Cognitive pain-coping strategies have been divided into two major groups, according to Turk, Meichenbaum, and Genest.[23] The authors identified one major group of strategies that attempt to alter the appraisal of the pain stimulation, with a second strategy that attempts to divert attention from the pain. The authors also noted that a person may emphasize the negative aspects and catastrophize the pain experience. Scott and Barber[24] developed a description of cognitive pain coping strategies that included the following: (1) imaging of pleasant events, (2) focusing on other things, (3) disassociating from the pain, (4) imagining pain as numbness, and (5) concentrating on other bodily sensations. In a similar description, Turk,[23] et al., identified major categories of coping strategies, which are listed in Table 12–3.

An overall evaluation of the effectiveness of cognitive strategies for relieving clinical pain has produced promising but inconclusive results. Contrary to the opinion of some, it now appears that chronic pain patients do not automatically have deficits in their cognitive coping skills. In fact, several researchers have suggested that most individuals have basic adaptive skills for coping with pain but that such skills are neutralized by negative cognitive appraisals. If a patient's ineffective coping response results from the interference of negative thoughts and feelings or low feelings of self-efficacy, psychological treatment should focus on amelioration of these in-

Table 12–3
Major Categories of Coping Strategies Identified by Turk,[23] et al.

- Imaginative inattention
- Imaginative transformation of pain
- Imaginative transformation of the context of pain
- Attention focused on the physical surroundings of the pain setting
- Mental distraction (such as counting)
- Somatization or focusing on the body part with a removed, objective view as opposed to an emotional, subjective view of the pain

terferences and on activation of existing skills, rather than on new skills training.[23]

The application of cognitive pain coping strategies to clinical populations is rapidly generating increased support and acceptance. The efficacy of a cognitive strategy in reducing pain is primarily thought to be based on an ability to generate attention-diversion effects, and on its relationship to the experience generated by new interpretation, labeling, and appraisal processes.[24] Many researchers have suggested that the tendency for patients to catastrophize was frequently related to poor emotional adjustment and, in many studies, poor treatment outcome.[25]

Intractable back pain is seldom a purely sensory experience. Chronic back pain is often accompanied by equally persistent emotional and behavioral symptoms that may be addressed by the use of cognitive therapy techniques. Symptoms often include procrastination, hesitation in following through with activity, depression, marital dysfunction, work avoidance, anxiety, anger, and frequent substance abuse. Many of these symptoms may be attributable to self-defeating coping behaviors, which are related to the pain and disability of the pain experience. Proponents of cognitive therapy as a treatment for chronic pain suggest that an evaluation with a focus on cognitive errors or self-defeating thoughts can often lead to psychotherapeutic effectiveness that may offer adjunctive relief of the patient's overall symptoms.[25] Unfortunately, clinical studies utilizing cognitive coping strategies with hospitalized pain patients are few. Several studies with clinical pain populations have, however, demonstrated promising results.[12] The implication of these studies is that effective pain reduction and control may be related to cognitive strategies that allow the patient to acknowledge the nociceptive stimulation but reinterpret the significance of the pain signal. It has also been demonstrated that relevant cognitive strategies that address the sensory, affective, and evaluative interpretations of pain were more effective than irrelevant cognitive strategies. Therefore, patients who display irrational or otherwise dysfunctional beliefs corresponding to their symptoms may benefit from a structured therapeutic program that addresses these issues and offers alternative cognitive processes, which will hopefully engender more adaptive wellness-related behaviors.[26]

Conclusions

Cognitive therapy for the treatment of clinical back pain is a commonly accepted psychotherapeutic practice in many pain treatment centers. The primary objective of this approach is to teach the patient to self-regulate self-defeating cognitions and possible psychophysiological reactions that may contribute to the pain syndrome. However, as will be discussed in the following section, most applications of cognitive theory for pain management occur within the context of a cognitive-behavioral model of psychological intervention.

THE COGNITIVE-BEHAVIORAL MODEL

The cognitive-behavioral approach to pain attempts to weld the behavioral and cognitive therapeutic models into a more efficient assessment and treatment concept with facilitated clinical effectiveness. The model is based, in part, on the idea that combining the powerful behavior change techniques of the behavioral or operant conditioning model, with the cognitive model emphasis on reconceptualization and reappraisal, produces a clinical intervention approach with added comprehensiveness and effectiveness.

The cognitive-behavioral model addresses the two most widely acknowledged psychological components of chronic low back pain—anxiety and depression[27,28,29]—with proven treatment techniques. Behavioral techniques, such as systematic desensitization, have proven effective in the treatment of a variety of anxiety disorders.[30,31] Meanwhile, the cognitive treatment approach has proven equally effective in the treatment of reactive depression.[32] Consequently, the combination of behavioral and cognitive assessment and treatment strategies appears to be a logical and pragmatic step toward the more effective treatment of the psychological disorders associated with a range of painful disorders, including low back pain.

Turk and Rudy[1] propose five basic assumptions that serve as a foundation for understanding the cognitive-behavioral perspective in the treatment of pain. The first is that individuals actively process information in an attempt to evaluate stimuli that impinge upon them from the external environment. The second assumption states that cognitions can be initiated or influenced by behavior, physiology, and

affect—just as affect and behavior can be elicited or modulated by cognitions. The third assumption proposes that an individual's behavior is a result of the reciprocal relationship between the individual and his environment. The fourth assumption states that a person can acquire new ways of thinking, feeling, and behaving that are more effective than previous habits and practices. The last assumption contends that an individual who has learned maladaptive thoughts, feelings, and behaviors should be expected to be involved as an active participant in the transformation to more adaptive patterns.

From the above assumptions, a cognitive-behavioral rationale of pain has developed that characterizes pain problems as multifaceted, with affective, sensory, evaluative, and behavioral dimensions. Treatment is based on the premise that manipulations of these variables can significantly alter the pain experience.[33] The perception of pain is viewed as a dynamic interpretive process that interacts reciprocally between the individual and his environment.[1]

Assessment and treatment utilizing cognitive-behavioral principles focus on the general goal of assisting the patient in modification of pain perception, the ability to control pain, and the extent to which the pain can be controlled or reduced.[35] Specific objectives include educating the patient about the pain problem in order to correct any misinformation or information deficits. Second, the patient is taught specific cognitive and behavioral skills to directly reduce pain, anxiety, and depression. Third, the patient is provided the opportunity to practice these skills in an environment that allows accurate feedback and contingent reinforcement. Finally, the objective is to assist the patient in generalizing specific improvements to the home and work environments. Obviously, it is this last objective that is the truest measure of the clinical effectiveness of the cognitive-behavioral approach.

Clinical back pain, in all of its ramifications, is conceptualized from the cognitive-behavioral perspective as multifaceted in both its cause and treatment.[34] The factors involved include the patient's injury or pain onset, treatment rendered to date (e.g., physical therapy modalities or surgery), the patient's post-injury functional ability, the patient's affect, the extent of interference with his life (e.g., marital, vocational, social, recreational), and the response of significant others to the victim since his injury. Cognitive-behavioral treatment of the patient with clinical back pain would address the patient's level of discomfort by simultaneously educating the patient about back pain and by providing the patient with specific skills to reduce his discomfort, such as relaxation, distraction, improved stress management, cognitive restructuring, and imagery. Once these skills have been acquired, and interference from existing maladaptive habits is neutralized, supervised rehearsal of the patient's new skills is necessary to provide the patient with feedback and to reinforce his effort, as well as to shape directed improvements. Finally, treatment should focus heavily on instilling in the patient an active problem-solving attitude toward back pain, rather than a passive, helpless perspective. Furthermore, efforts should be extended toward preventing future recurrences of back pain by assisting the patient in anticipating potential problems and preparing for them in advance.

Cognitive-Behavioral Treatment of Painful Spinal Disorders

The treatment of painful spinal disorders using the cognitive-behavioral approach may be understood best by presenting an overview of how a treatment program might function. Germane to the cognitive-behavioral approach is a thorough assessment of the following areas: (1) physical examination, to determine the extent of the damage or disease and to determine the extent to which it has affected the patient's functional ability, (2) prior treatment to date and the patient's response to prior efforts, with a focus on how actively the patient has participated in his treatment, (3) the role that compensation may play in the patient's complaints of discomfort and continued dysfunction, (4) a thorough assessment of the patient's pain behaviors; frequently, a patient has an extraordinary focus of attention on his somatic complaints with resulting irrational conclusions based on his symptoms, and (5) an evaluation of the patient's psychopathology. As previously mentioned, anxiety and depression are prevalent in back pain patients. It is expected that an evaluation may indicate relatively high levels of these symptoms. However, more serious psychopathology, such as schizophrenia, is best addressed in a more appropriate psychiatric or psychological setting.

Upon completion of a thorough evaluation, a treatment program may be formulated with guidance provided by several philosophical criteria. The first criteria is an interdisciplinary team that is composed of representatives from medical psychology, medicine, physical therapy, and nursing. An interdisciplinary approach is considered necessary because of the demonstrated propensity for back pain patients to develop chronic pain. For example, one chronic pain program reports that 86% of their patients have a diagnosis of back pain.[10] Obviously, the intensity of an interdisciplinary approach is not necessary during the acute stage of spinal pain, but when normal healing time has elapsed and the patient has not responded, a team approach is considered the treatment of choice.[10]

The second suggested criteria is a general atmosphere of positive appraisal of both the patient's potential for improvement and of the staff's ability to assist the patient in reducing spinal pain and returning the individual to a more appropriate functional level. The level of a patient's motivation is often quite low as a result of depression so frequently encountered in patients with back injuries and pain. The success of the entire treatment program rests, in large part, on the ability of the treatment team to reduce the patient's depression while increasing motivation to a level that will "push" the patient to fully participate in the treatment program. An upbeat, energetic, positive, milieu often helps the patient reconceptualize his feelings of helplessness, and work toward acquisition of pain management skills.

The third criteria is related to the responsibility for treatment outcome. This is a crucial issue that is important both during and after treatment. The cognitive-behavioral model is based on the premise that the patient must alter his self-perception from that of a passive, helpless person, to someone who can be an active and capable participant in the treatment process. In addition, this cognitive restructuring also requires a basic change in the patient's perception of the medical community. The goal is to change the cognition from "Why does my back still hurt?" and "What will my doctor do?," to "My back still hurts. What can I do now to reduce the pain?" This new perception charges the patient with the responsibility of searching for solutions to identified problems.

Our descriptive psychological treatment regimen for the individual suffering back pain emphasizes the previously mentioned foundational components of the cognitive-behavioral model. The treatment program can be offered in either inpatient or outpatient settings and on an individual or group basis. However, it has been our experience that implementation of cognitive-behavioral techniques blends well into the hospital milieu and helps to create a positive group atmosphere.

As the patient demonstrates behavioral skills to reduce pain intensity (e.g., relaxation training or ice massage) and begins to enjoy a general state of decreased pain complaints, cognitive-behavioral skills training is introduced. An introductory technique that we have found easily understood by large numbers of patients is the rather simplistic statement: "Although you can't always control what happens to you, you can control how you respond."

Once cognitive restructuring skills are outlined, opportunities for guided rehearsal become important. The goals of this component in the therapeutic process include providing contingent reinforcement for appropriate behaviors and continued enhancement of the patient's skill and confidence. Cognitive rehearsal provides an excellent treatment for depression, primarily because of the cognitive dissonance it generates. For example, a depressed patients' cognitions often focus on helplessness and an inability to "do anything" about back pain. When the patient is able to significantly reduce his pain through an acquired skill, he is then confronted with a fact that contradicts his helpless feeling. Repeated experiences should rapidly build confidence and self esteem with subsequent reductions in depression and anxiety. In addition, the rehearsal components allow an assessment of the patient's knowledge and skill level, thus providing an opportunity for continuous reformulation of both goals and treatment response.

The final factor in the model is the generalization of the patient's cognitive and behavioral improvements outside the structured therapeutic milieu. This occurs in two phases. The first phase occurs in group therapy sessions while the patient remains actively in treatment.[34] In this phase the therapists assist the patients in anticipating future exacerbations of pain and rehearsing problem-solving strategies required for long-term treatment maintenance. A key ingredient is the rehearsal of the patient's problem-solving strategies and expansion of the targeted response repertoire. The therapist's prediction of future periodic difficulties and a detailed explanation that such exacerbations of pain represent an expected part of continued recovery helps diffuse these partial regressions and reduces the patient's anxiety upon occurrence. The second phase occurs during a structured outpatient followup program that requires the patient to return on a gradual, less frequent basis over several months, perhaps up to a year. During followup appointments, the patient attends both group therapy and physical reconditioning. The focus of followup is to continue the problem-solving strategies during group therapy and the reinforcement of the structured exercise program. In addition, individual reassessment and treatment is provided.

Conclusions

The cognitive-behavioral model for the treatment of back pain incorporates components of both the behavioral and cognitive models of pain management. As such, it addresses two of the more complicating psychological problems associated with back pain—anxiety and depression—with two of the more effective treatment approaches in combination. The cognitive-behavioral model proposes that thoughts, emotions, and behaviors are reciprocally and constantly affected by behavior and environment. Successful treatment largely depends on the skill of the therapist to teach, coach, and motivate individuals to acquire new behaviors and to take responsibility for the treatment of their back pain problem.

REFERENCES

1. Turk, D.C., Rudy, T.E.: A cognitive-behavioral perspective on chronic pain beyond the scapel and syringe. *In* Handbook of Chronic Pain Management (Edited by C.D. Tollison). Baltimore, Williams & Wilkins, 1989.
2. Melzack, R., Casey, K.L.: Sensory, motivational, and central control determinants of pain: A new conceptual model. *In* The Skin Sense (Edited by D. Kenshalo). Springfield, Charles C. Thomas, 1968.
3. Melzack, R., Wall, P.D.: Pain mechanisms: a new theory. Science *50*:971–979, 1965.
4. Fordyce, W.E., Fowler, R.S., DeLateur, B.: An application of behavior modification techniques to a problem of chronic pain. Behav Res Ther *6*:105–107, 1968.
5. Fordyce, W.E., Rowler, R.S., Lehmann, J.F., DeLateur, B.J.: Some implications of learning in problems of chronic pain. J Chron Dis *22*:179–190, 1968.
6. Fordyce, W.E., Roberts, A.H., Sternbach, R.A.: The behavioral management of chronic pain: a response to critics. Pain *22*:113–125, 1988.
7. Fordyce, W.E., et al.: Operant conditioning in the treatment of chronic pain. Arch Phys Med Rehabil *54*:399–408, 1973.
8. Sanders, S.H.: Contingency management in the reduction of overt pain behavior. *In* Handbook of Chronic Pain Management (Edited by C.D. Tollison). Baltimore, Williams & Wilkins, 1989.
9. Fordyce, W.E.: An operant conditioning method for managing chronic pain. Postgrad Med *53*:123–128, 1973.
10. Linton, S.J.: A critical review of behavioral treatment for chronic pain other than headache. Br J Clin Psychol *21*:321–337, 1982.
11. Dollard, J., Miller, N.E.: Personality and Psychotherapy. New York, McGraw Hill, 1950.
12. Novaco, R.W.: Anger and coping with stress: cognitive-behavioral interventions. *In* Cognitive Behavior Therapy: Research and Application (Edited by J.P. Foregt and D.P. Rathjen). New York, Plenum, 1978.
13. Schwartz, G.E., Shapiro, D.: Consciousness and Self-Regulation. New York, Plenum, 1976.
14. Beecher, H.K.: Pain and some factors that modify it. Anesthesiology *12*:633–641, 1951.
15. Fields, H.L., Lewis, J.D.: Pain mechanisms and management. West J Med *141*(3):347–357, 1984.
16. Beck, A.T.: Cognitive Therapy and the Emotional Disorders. New York, International University Press, 1976.
17. Ellis, A.: Reason and Emotion in Psychotherapy. New York, Lyle-Stewart, 1962.
18. Greene, R., Rayber, J.: Pain tolerance in hypnotic analgesic and imagination states. J Abnorm Psychol *79*:29–38, 1972.
19. Nouwen, A., Solinger, J.: The effectiveness of EMG biofeedback training in low back pain. Biofeedback Self Regul *4*:103–111, 1979.
20. Horan, J., Hackett, G., Buchanan, J.D., Stone, C., Demchik-Stone, D.: Coping with pain: a component analysis of stress inoculations. Cognitive Ther Res *1*:211–221, 1978.
21. Bobey, M., Davidson, P.: Psychological factors affecting pain tolerance. J Psychosom Res *14*:371–376, 1920.
22. Blitz, B., Dinnerstein, A.: Role of attentional factors in pain perception: manipulation of response to noxious stimulation by instructions. J Abnorm Psychol *77*:82–85, 1971.
23. Turk, D.C., Meichenbaum, D., Genest, M.: Pain and Behavioral Medicine: A Cognitive-Behavioral Perspective. New York, The Guilford Press, 1983.
24. Scott, D.S., Barber, T.X.: Cognitive control of pain: effects of multiple cognitive strategies. The Psychological Record *2*:373–383, 1977.
25. Hinnant, D.: Cognitive coping strategies with chronic back pain patients. Unpublished Doctoral Dissertation, North Texas State University, Denton, TX, 1985.

26. Keefe, F.J., Rosenstiel, A.K.: Development of a Questionnaire to Assess Cognitive Coping Strategies in Chronic Pain Patients. Presented at the 14th annual convention of the Association for the Advancement of Behavior Therapy, New York, 1980.

27. Wiltse, L.L., Rochico, P.D.: Preoperative psychological tests as predictors of success of chemonucleolysis in the treatment of low-back syndrome. J Bone Joint Surg 57:478–483, 1975.

28. Cashion, E.L., Lynch, W.J.: Personality factors and results of lumbar disc surgery. Neurosurgery 4:141–145, 1979.

29. France, R.D., Houpt, J.L., Skott, A., Krishman, K.R., Varia, I.M.: Depression as a psychopathological disorder in chronic low back pain patients. J Psychosom Res 30:127–133, 1986.

30. Rimm, D.C., Masters, J.C.: Behavior Therapy. New York, Academic Press, 1979.

31. Craighead, W.E., Kazdin, A.E., Mahoney, M.J.: Behavior Modification Principles, Issues, and Applications. Boston, Houghton-Mifflin, 1976.

32. Beck, A.T., Rush, A.J., Shaw, B.E., Emery, G.: Cognitive Therapy of Depression. New York, The Guilford Press, 1979.

33. Turner, J.A.: Comparison of group progressive-relaxation training and cognitive-behavioral group therapy for chronic low back pain. J Consult Clin Psychol 50:757–765, 1982.

34. Holzman, A.D., Turk, D.C., Kerns, R.D.: The cognitive-behavioral approach to the management of chronic pain. *In* Pain Management: A Handbook of Psychological Treatment Approaches (Edited by A.D. Holzman and D.C. Turk). New York, Pergamon Press, 1986.

Dennis Barnes

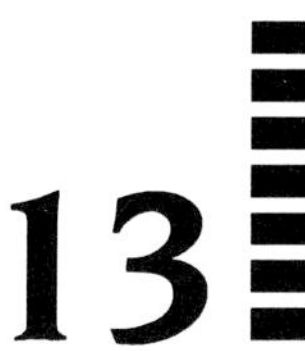

Social Factors Affecting Back Pain

CONCEPTS

Low back pain is a phenomenom that most individuals experience at some point in their lives. Various reports estimate that as many as 85% of all people experience back pain at some point during their adult years.[1] Although the majority of low back pain episodes either spontaneously resolve or resolve with minimal treatment, low back pain still is the most expensive benign condition in industrialized countries.[2] Medical costs for the treatment of low back pain are estimated at $16 billion annually.[3] When legal expenses, costs for compensation and retraining of injured workers, and diminished industrial productivity are added to this medical expense, the result is a staggering exponential economic impact.

In order to fully understand how a benign condition can have such a pervasive economic impact, one must look beyond mere incidence figures and focus on critical qualitative factors of low back pain. Central to this understanding is the distinction between *acute* and *chronic* low back pain. Sternbach[4] noted that acute and chronic pain are distinctively different experiences, which have distinguishable associated affective states. Acute pain is commonly experienced with injury or acute illness; anxiety represents the predominant affective state that corresponds with this experience. However, chronic pain presents a substantially different clinical picture. Chronic pain is typically defined as pain of 6 months duration or longer, which often, although certainly not exclusively, persists with no identifiable organic cause. Many have advanced the simplistic position that acute pain is best conceptualized as a symptom of another wound or injury, i.e., a fracture or a burn, whereas chronic pain is best understood as a complex disease itself rather than as a symptom of something else.[5,6]

It is this chronic phase of low back pain that must be understood and addressed as a complex disease or syndrome in and of itself. Although only 5 to 10% of all low back pain cases ever reach this category, these cases represent a particularly expensive minority, accounting for as much as 75% of all medical costs, lost work days, and indemnity payments attributable to back pain.[7] The disproportionate costs reflect both the refractory nature of the chronic low back pain syndrome and the lack of preparedness of conventional medical systems to deal with this complex situation. Because treatment efforts based upon an acute disease model continue to be used repetitively for the chronic patient, a negative spiral of escalating medical costs and treatment failures ensues. Mayer has referred to this process as the iatrogenic paradox of the chronic low back pain syndrome.[8]

This type of paradox with respect to the chronic low back pain syndrome has led to a much broader conceptualization of the problem. Recently, chronic low back pain has begun to be recognized as a psychosocioeconomic issue as well as a medical problem. This emphasis is consistent with recent trends in medicine in general. More resources are being allocated to identify environmental and social factors that contribute to disease and injury.[9] Identification of such factors not only has an obvious prophylactic significance, but also assists in the design and development of alternative treatment models for particularly refractory conditions such as chronic low back pain.

Why is it important to focus on social factors that affect back pain? The answer to this question is twofold: (1) Back pain, especially chronic low back pain, is a complex syndrome that can only be completely understood when a variety of nonmedical dimensions (e.g., social, psychological, economic) are addressed, and (2) As the chronic low back pain syndrome is more completely understood, more effective treatment models will be developed that should help ease the staggering economic drain of this condition as well as reverse the tremendous waste of human potential, which is the inevitable sequelae of chronic low back pain related disability.

The remainder of this chapter focuses on specific social factors that have been identified as contributory to low back pain and on how a knowledge and understanding of such factors should influence treatment efforts.

DIAGNOSIS

Specific social factors affecting back pain can be divided into three distinct categories. *Primary* factors are those that identify a percentage of an uninjured population likely to develop a low back pain episode. *Secondary* factors identify those individuals with an acute low back pain incident who are likely to develop chronic difficulties (5 to 10% of the injured population), and *tertiary* factors identify those patients, who, once chronic symptoms have developed, are likely to resolve their difficulties and return to productive lifestyles.[10] In general, primary factors are predictive of *who* might suffer a low back injury or episode, whereas secondary and tertiary factors are predictive of *how* individuals will respond once a low back injury is present. We shall examine social factors that have been related to low back pain in each of these general categories separately.

Primary Social Factors

Because low back injuries are a particularly troublesome industrial problem, the work environment has generated more interest and study than all other social factors. A comprehensive retrospective review of 900 back injury cases from Boeing Company employees during a 15 month period of time yielded significant and interesting results.[11–13] Bigos, et al., reported that back injury claims were related to specific types of jobs, particularly those that involve lifting.[12] This is consistent with previous findings that have linked jobs involving lifting, twisting, and bending to back injuries.[14] Bigos, et al., further reported that among this group, previous industrial back injuries were found to be primary predictors of subsequent back claims.[12]

However, other less obvious occupational factors also have been identified as possible primary predictors. Length of time on the job was a significant factor in the Boeing group, with those with less time on the job having a higher incidence of back injuries. Furthermore, previous supervisors' ratings were found to be important as well. A disproportionate number of injured Boeing employees had the lowest

appraisal rating from their supervisor in the 6 month period prior to their injuries.

Epidemiologic studies in Sweden and Denmark have also identified certain occupational factors as possible primary low back pain predictors. Biering-Sorensen and Thomsen[15] reported that longer travel distances from home to work were found to be risk indicators for first time incidence of back injury in a Danish population. Eastrand[16] reported low education (less than 6 years) and lower occupational status as indicative of a higher incidence of low back pain among a group of Swedish males.

Table 13–1 summarizes the direct and indirect occupational factors that have been identified as primary predictors of low back pain. The direct factors involve types of jobs and specific job activities (e.g., lifting) that place individuals at direct biomechanical risk for back injury. However, indirect factors have been identified that suggest that back injury is a more complex phenomenon than once thought. These occupational primary predictors focus on job satisfaction and performance as possible keys to unlocking the mystery of who is susceptible to back injury. The direct associative mechanism of such factors with back injury remains speculative. However, it is clear that these factors must be considered in any attempt to identify individuals at risk for industrial back injury.

A variety of other social factors have been identified as possibly playing a role in the cause of low back pain. Cigarette smoking is one such variable that has been thoroughly examined, and the link between smoking and increased incidence of low back pain is well documented.[17,18] Poor general physical fitness, gender differences, and overall social satisfaction are other factors that have been linked with low back pain.[19,20] However, social factors related to occupation and work environments will likely continue as the primary area of focus for some time.

Secondary Factors

Because of the disproportionate costs associated with a small percentage of the total number of back injuries, much research has been directed at identifi-

Table 13–1
Occupational Factors as Primary Predictors of Low Back Disability

Direct Occupational Factors
1. Physical job demands (lifting, twisting, bending, vibration, etc.)
2. Work environment (noisy vs. quiet, quality of lighting, presence or absence of safety features)

Indirect Occupational Factors
1. Job satisfaction
2. Supervisor ratings of job performance
3. Employee relationships with co-workers

cation of factors that may predict those low back pain episodes which are likely to become problematic. The primary emphasis of such efforts is the early identification of predictive factors of extended and costly disability. These efforts are supported by the hope that such early identification may lead to alternative treatment efforts, which may resolve low back symptoms and substantially reduce the number of cases that ultimately result in chronic disability.

Simply stated, the study of secondary predictive factors relative to back pain is the study of determining those acute episodes which are likely to become chronic. Indeed, such analysis may offer more social benefit than the study of primary predictors. It can be argued that a certain percentage of any industrialized population is going to suffer back injuries each year; identification of primary predictive factors may be successful in determining which groups are most susceptible, but knowledge of such factors, particularly those of social origin, is not likely to yield a significant preventative impact. Conversely, the early awareness of secondary factors may lead to specifically tailored treatment interventions that produce tangible societal benefits. Many such secondary factors are social in nature, and early recognition of these issues is a critical necessity if the difficulties associated with chronicity are to be avoided.

The most systematic research focusing upon secondary predictive factors has been conducted at the Vermont Rehabilitation Engineering Center. Frymoyer and Cats-Baril[21] developed a model designed to assess whether low back disability can be predicted. This model was created deductively by assembling experts in the fields of disability and low back pain and asking them to identify a variety of factors associated with low back disability. These factors were then evaluated, refined, and weighted according to statistical analyses and incorporated into a model designed to predict those patients with low back pain episodes who were most likely to develop extended disability.

A variety of social factors were among those identified by the Vermont group as being predictive of low back disability. In fact, occupational and psychosocial factors were the two categories weighted highest, accounting for 40% of the total weight within the model. Specific factors identified included numerous job-related variables (e.g., job satisfaction, physical demands, stability of work history), injury-related variables (e.g., perception of fault, compensability, attorney involvement) and other social variables (e.g., level of education, previous history of disability, major life events). Early results of this predictive model have been encouraging and demonstrate that such an empirically weighted model can improve considerably upon the performance of experts in predicting disability.[21]

While little research exists to match the systematic efforts of the Vermont group to develop a comprehensive secondary predictive model, many other studies have focused on the identification of social factors that affect the course of a pain episode or low back injury. The role of the family of the low back pain patient is probably the most important social factor to be considered in this regard. Physicians treating low back pain patients have been slow to recognize the importance of family variables on the course and duration of the pain experience. However, documentation of increased stress in families of low back pain patients is plentiful.[22,23]

Research on family involvement in the response to low back pain has focused in many directions, including family of origin studies and the cause of chronic pain, socioeconomic status of families, and chronic pain as an indicator of depression and emotional deprivation within families. Each of these studies represents a significant area of focus in examining family involvement in low back pain episodes. However, of primary importance is the role families play in maintaining the pain experience. Many have conceptualized the low back pain experience from an operant conditioning model with the family as the primary reinforcing agent.[24,25] This point of view characterizes pain, specifically chronic pain, as a group of learned behaviors reinforced by family members. In order for the pain behaviors to be extinguished, they must be exposed to a new set of reinforcement contingencies, i.e., the family must be educated to reinforce "well" and ignore "pain" behaviors.

The experience of prolonged low back pain in a family member almost always necessitates re-evaluation and definition of family roles. In some instances this may be perceived, although not always consciously, as a positive effect (e.g., a working father has a low back injury preventing him from working and enabling him to spend more time at home with the family). In other cases, this impact is decidedly negative, as in the case when a spouse must assume all the household duties of the injured spouse while attending to his or her normal duties as well. In either case, successful resolution of the low back pain episode is not likely unless these family concerns are addressed and appropriately negotiated.

Along with family variables, many occupational factors that were identified as primary predictors also influence response to a low back pain episode. Not only was a low supervisor's rating during the previous 6 month period predictive of a low back pain episode, it also predicted those episodes likely to become most expensive (chronic).[13] Job dissatisfaction, perception of job-related tasks as repetitive and boring, and noisy unpleasant work environments also have been identified as secondary predic-

Table 13–2
Social Factors as Secondary Predictors

1. Occupational:
   a. Job satisfaction
   b. Job type and physical demands
   c. Work history
2. Family response to injury/pain behaviors
3. Attorney involvement in disability case
4. Education level

tors.[21] Table 13–2 summarizes social factors that have been documented as secondary predictors.

Tertiary Factors

Comparatively little effort has focused on the discovery of tertiary predictors, that is, the identification of social factors which predict successful resolution once a chronic low back pain syndrome is present. This undoubtedly results because once a chronic syndrome is manifest, successful resolution becomes less and less likely. A significant number of patients who underwent multiple spinal operations report less than satisfactory relief.[26] Economic pressures and poor surgical results have led to a proliferation of nonsurgical treatment methods (e.g., pain clinics), but results of these efforts have been less than outstanding for the truly chronic patients.[8]

The evidence that does exist relative to tertiary predictive factors is more anecdotal in nature but qualitatively not dissimilar from identified primary and secondary factors. Occupational variables (e.g., job satisfaction) continue to have merit as tertiary predictors. Because by definition a chronic low back pain episode indicates longer periods of disability, the availability of a job to return to and attitudes of employers taking back injured workers become significant tertiary predictors.[2] The perception of the injured worker as "damaged goods" and susceptible to recurrence or reinjury further retards the successful resolution of low back pain disability. Further complicating factors include habituation to narcotic pain relievers (a frequent iatrogenic sequela of treatment for the acute low back pain episode) and social isolation resulting from decreased social contact subsequent to an industrial injury.

Certainly one major factor that is a significant tertiary predictor is the status of the injured worker's compensation. Financial compensation to injured workers during periods of work injury-related disability can become a disincentive to return to employment as disability extends well into a chronic phase. Anecdotes of spontaneous remission of symptoms following financial settlements paid to injured workers abound; however, empirical evidence of the effects of compensation and litigation upon resolution of low back pain disability remains equivocal.[27] One study identified higher compensation payments as a *positive* tertiary predictor, noting higher compensation payments among a group of chronic low back pain patients who successfully completed rehabilitation and returned to work as compared with two groups of similar patients whose rehabilitative efforts were unsuccessful.[10] It was reasoned that the higher compensation payments were reflective of better, higher paying jobs which themselves were the primary incentive for resolution of disability. More specific information regarding the effect of various compensation systems upon low back disability is provided in Chapter 15 of this edition.

Finally, in a recent study by Polatin, Gatchel, and colleagues, a psychosociomedical model was developed to predict success or failure in response to a comprehensive functional restoration program by workers who were chronically disabled with low back pain. (This study is reviewed further in Chapter 26 of this text.)[28] Among the variables found to be significant in this prediction model were availability for a job after treatment, past employment history, and past surgical history. Such results again highlight the important role that job-related and other psychosocial factors can play in the development and progression of chronic spinal disorders.

To summarize, many of the same social factors are important in determining not only who may be at risk for low back injury, but also in predicting how individuals may respond to treatment efforts once injured. Those factors critically important include a variety of occupational features, including job type, job performance and satisfaction, and the role of the family in responding to the injured member. No accurate diagnosis of the total low back pain syndrome can ignore these critically important characteristics.

TREATMENT

We have examined why back pain is indeed a social problem and looked at specific social factors that influence its course. Now we must focus our attention on what can be done to positively affect this complex social and medical problem. We shall first examine strategies for proper assessment of social factors affecting back pain and then turn our attention to efforts aimed at direct intervention.

The foundation of all solid medical treatment efforts is solid assessment and diagnosis. Most benign medical conditions can be successfully treated once they are properly identified. Likewise, the first key to successfully incorporating resolution of social factors into a comprehensive treatment strategy for back pain is to facilitate their accurate diagnosis.

With respect to social factors as primary predictors, this assessment will likely take the form of continued studies in industrial environments. More comprehensive efforts such as the Boeing study cited earlier are necessary to further identify social and occupational factors that are robust enough to predict low back injury in a variety of settings. Consideration must be given to the development of simple and convenient assessment devices that focus upon the factors, such as job satisfaction and performance, currently identified as possible primary predictors of low back injury. Although efforts such as the development of the Work Apgar scale,[18] a brief instrument designed to assess how employees interact in the work environment, represent positive developments, these efforts are preliminary and need revision and refinement. Additional assessment strategies include more frequent formal interviews of employees by their employers, focusing upon discussion of the types of factors previously identified as relevant to potential low back disability.

"Treatment" of the low back disability problem at the primary phase likely will take three forms. The first is to alter the work environment in accordance with identified factors related to low back injury. Just as the physical characteristics of the workplace have been modified to increase safety, so might the social characteristics as well. Admittedly, this may often be difficult and impractical, but more periodic worker evaluations to determine performance and satisfaction might represent an initial step. This might minimize the risk of a disenchanted worker remaining on a particular job for an extended period of time, and thus make the workplace "safer" from a social perspective. Second, criteria used for worker selection can be improved. Pre-employment screening of prospective employees on a variety of physical dimensions is a developing methodology to help ensure that job demands suit employee capability. Such screening efforts could be expanded to include assessment of relevant social dimensions (e.g., previous dissatisfaction in a similar job). With the proper care to ensure that such information is not used haphazardly or in a grossly discriminatory fashion, such efforts could help match employees to jobs in a manner that enhances potential job satisfaction and thus indirectly may have a positive effect on low back pain incidence rates. Finally, general education of the relationship between social occupational factors and back pain must be improved. This education should be presented in as many environments as possible, but certainly should come from medical service providers to their patients and industrial employers to their employees.

Assessment of this problem at the secondary and tertiary phases is equally important. Treating physicians, both primary care physicians and specialists, should be aware of and prepared to recognize the factors that may be early warning signs of chronicity. Involvement of back pain patients' families in the early assessment process may assist treating clinicians in educating patients and their families about what to expect and how to avoid chronic disability. Assessment at this stage, whether families are directly involved or not, must be comprehensive in nature. Attending only to physical findings and the patient's subjective reports of discomfort are insufficient because these reports are influenced by the many social and occupational factors previously discussed. A reminder about base rates is important here. A treating physician who ignores comprehensive assessment and attends only to physical findings and patient self-report of discomfort will likely be totally successful with 90% of low back pain patients. This is because approximately 90% of low back pain episodes either spontaneously resolve or do so with minimal treatment after 3 months. Although this 90% success rate is seductive, it is in many ways artificial. What is critical is early identification of the remaining 10% of cases that go on to become problematic and waste tremendous financial and human resources.

Treatment of the acute low back pain episode is well defined.[2] A small percentage of episodes require surgical intervention, and the majority of the remainder of cases are routinely successfully treated with a regimen of conservative care. It is critical that low back pain care providers are sensitive to indications that treatment does not progress along a customary course. It is at this time that the comprehensive picture of low back disability must be considered and careful decisions must be made regarding the type of continued treatment that is most likely to result in successful resolution. This often results in a shift away from passive treatment modalities to active rehabilitation. If this transition is timed appropriately and the patient is given proper education about what to expect, most cases successfully resolve prior to the development of intractable disability.

How to treat the 5 to 10% of low back pain patients that "slip through the cracks" and develop chronic disability is a more difficult problem. Many pain clinics purport to successfully treat this population, although most such clinics fail to directly address the social contingencies outlined earlier as critically important. A relatively new approach to the treatment of these most difficult cases is the "functional restoration" model.[2,29] This treatment model is multidisciplinary in nature and combines aggressive physical reconditioning and reactivation with direct intervention aimed at the psychosocial sequelae of chronic low back disability. Not only are the physical and psychological aspects of low back injury addressed, but direct social intervention (reg-

Table 13–3
Treatment Considerations by Phase of Low Back Disability

1. *PRIMARY PHASE:*
    a. Workplace alteration to improve safety features
    b. Improved worker selection criteria and pre-employment screening
    c. Improved education regarding the relationship between social factors and incidence of injury
2. *SECONDARY PHASE:*
    a. Surgical treatment when appropriate
    b. Appropriate conservative care
    c. Early identification of problematic treatment course
    d. Appropriate rehabilitation
3. *TERTIARY PHASE:*
    a. Elimination of passive treatment modalities
    b. Aggressive rehabilitation and functional restoration
    c. Disability management and case resolution

ular contact with employer(s), attorneys, insurance representatives, family members) rounds out an effective system of disability management that successfully alters the social reinforcement contingencies and facilitates a direct return to productivity.

Table 13–3 reviews specific treatment considerations for low back disability in the primary, secondary, and tertiary stages.

SUMMARY & CONCLUSIONS

Low back pain and its subsequent disability are critical medical problems facing industrialized societies. A thorough understanding of this complex problem necessitates careful examination of a variety of critical social factors. These include occupational and family variables that influence which individuals are most likely to experience a low back pain episode and how certain individuals are likely to respond to such an episode. Comprehensive assessment and treatment efforts, which include consideration of these social factors, are the keys to reversing the staggering drain of economic and human resources resulting from low back pain related disability.

REFERENCES

1. Beals, R.K., Hickman, N.W.: Industrial injuries of the back and extremities. J Bone Joint Surg *54A*:1593–1611, 1972.
2. Mayer, T.G., Gatchel, R.J.: Functional Restoration for Spinal Disorders: The Sports Medicine Approach. Philadelphia, Lea & Febiger, 1988.
3. Holbrook, T., Grazier, K., Kelsey, J., Stauffer, R.: The Frequency of Occurrence Impact and Cost of Selected Musculoskeletal Conditions in the United States. Chicago, American Academy of Orthopedic Surgeons, 1984.
4. Sternbach, R.A.: Pain Patients: Traits and Treatments. New York, Academic Press, 1974.
5. Hendler, N.H., Fenton, J.A.: Coping with Chronic Pain. Boston, Clarkson N. Potter, 1979.
6. Holden, C.: Pain, dying and the health care system. Science *203*:984–985, 1979.
7. Abenhaim, L., Suissa, S.: Importance and economic burden of occupational back pain: a study of 2500 cases representative of Quebec. J Occup Med *29*:670–674, 1987.
8. Mayer, T.G.: Orthopedic conservative care: the functional restoration approach. Spine: State of the Art Reviews *1*:139–147, 1986.
9. Niemcryk, S.J., Jenkins, C.D., Rose, R.M., Hurst, M.W.: The prospective impact of psychosocial variables on rates of illness and injury in professional employees. J Occup Med *29*:645–652, 1987.
10. Barnes, D., Smith, D., Gatchel, R., Mayer, T.: Psychosocioeconomic predictors of treatment success/failure in chronic low-back pain patients. Spine *14*:427–430, 1989.
11. Spengler, D., et al.: Back injuries in industry: a retrospective study: I. Overview and cost analysis. Spine *11*:241–245, 1986.
12. Bigos, S., et al.: Back injuries in industry: a retrospective study: II. Injury factors. Spine *11*:246–251, 1986.
13. Bigos, S., et al.: Back injuries in industry: a retrospective study: III. Employee-related factors. Spine *11*:252–256, 1986.
14. Nachemson, A.: The lumbar spine: an orthopaedic challenge. Spine *1*:59–71, 1976.
15. Biering-Sorensen, F., Thomsen, C.: Medical, social and occupational history as risk indicators for low-back trouble in a general population. Spine *11*:720–725, 1986.
16. Eastrand, N.: Medical, psychological, and social factors associated with back abnormalities and self reported back pain: a cross sectional study of male employees in a Swedish pulp and paper industry. Br J Ind Med *44*:327–336, 1987.
17. Kelsey, J.L., et al.: Acute prolapsed lumbar invertebral disc: an epidemiological study with special reference to driving automobiles and cigarette smoking. Spine *9*:608–613, 1984.
18. Frymoyer, J.: Helping your patients avoid low back pain. J Musculoskeletal Med pp. 83–101, May, 1989.
19. Boden, S.D., Lestini, W.F., Wiesel, S.W.: Compensation low back pain. Semin Spine Surg *1*:68–75, 1989.
20. Magora, A.: Investigation of the relation between low back pain and occupation: V. Psychological aspects. Scand J Rehab Med *5*:191–196, 1973.
21. Frymoyer, J., Cats-Baril, W.: Predictors of low back pain disability. Clin Orthop *221*:89–98, 1987.
22. Feurstein, M., Sult, S., Houle, M.: Environmental stressors and chronic low back pain: life events, family and work environment. Pain *22*:295–307, 1985.
23. Payne, B., Norfleet, M.A.: Chronic pain and the family: a review. Pain *26*:1–22, 1986.
24. Fordyce, W.E.: Behavioral Methods in Chronic Pain and Illness. St. Louis, C.V. Mosby, 1976.
25. Turk, D., Flor, H., Rudy, T.: Pain and families. I. Etiology, maintenance and psychosocial impact. Pain *30*:3–27, 1987.
26. Zucherman, J., Schofferman, J.: Pathology of failed back surgery syndrome. I. Background and diagnostic alternatives. Spine, State of the Art Reviews *1*:1–7, 1986.
27. Dworkin, R.H., et al.: Unraveling the effects of compensation, litigation, and employment on treatment response in chronic pain. Pain *23*:49–59, 1985.
28. Polatin, P.B., et al.: A psychosociomedical prediction model of response to treatment by chronically disabled workers with low back pain. Spine *14*:956–961, 1989.
29. Mayer, H., Mayer, T.: Functional restoration: new concepts in spinal rehabilitation. *In* Managing Low Back Pain. (Edited by W.H. Kirkaldy-Willis) 2nd Ed. New York, Churchill Livingstone, 1988.

Peter B. Polatin

14

Affective Disorders in Back Pain

INTRODUCTION

Any clinician working with chronic low back pain patients has been impressed with the high incidence of depression in this group. Clinical studies confirm this linkage; the incidence of depression in chronic pain disorders ranges from 10 to 100%. This variability is reflective of differences in the definition and diagnosis of depression[1] and patient selection bias,[2] but nevertheless points to a close association between the two disorders.

Depression may be conceptualized as a symptom, a mood, or a syndrome, and the lack of specificity of the psychiatric diagnosis is a methodologic shortcoming in many of the studies linking it to chronic pain. Is a patient labeled as "depressed" based upon a clinical "guesstimate" with or without the administration of self-report measures such as the Beck Depressive Inventory, the Hamilton Rating Scale for Depression, or the Zung Test for depression? Is he undergoing a comprehensive mental health evaluation by a qualified professional (usually a psychologist or a psychiatrist), after which a specific psychiatric diagnosis is made? If so, which diagnostic criteria are being used (RDC, DSM-III, DSM-III-R, ICDM)? Are all patients with depression lumped together, or are the diagnoses of different depressive syndromes analyzed separately?

Psychiatric Nosology

The most recent American Psychiatric Association classification system, the DSM-III-R illustrates clinically relevant distinctions between psychiatric disorders. A patient with a *major depressive disorder* has core symptoms for a 2-week period, representing a change from previous functioning. Either depressed mood or anhedonia must be present, as well as four of the following: significant weight change, sleep disturbance, psychomotor agitation or retardation, fatigue, guilty ruminations, difficulty thinking or concentrating, and recurrent thoughts of suicide or death. There must be no associated medical illness, recent bereavement, or accompanying psychotic symptoms.

There are, however, several other psychiatric syndromes which present with depression. A patient with a history of previous manic episodes, even with a current presentation suggestive of major depression, is classified as a *bipolar affective disorder* (manic depressive). Someone with a history of depressed mood for the past 2 years or more, with some but not all associated core symptoms and no evidence of any other psychiatric disorder, would be diagnosed as having *dysthymia*. An individual with significant depressed mood occurring within 3 months of an identifiable psychosocial stressor, but not present for more than 6 months, with associated functional impairment, would be classified as an *adjustment reaction with depressed mood*. These are separate and distinct clinical syndromes, with different prognoses and treatment approaches.

Chronic Pain in Depression

There is also a high incidence of chronic pain in depressed patients. An early study of 35 chronic pain patients[3] differentiated one group in which pain preceded the depression, but a larger group in which pain and depression developed simultaneously. In the first group only the depression responded to treatment, whereas in the second both symptoms were relieved by therapy for depression. In a larger, more recent study, 87% of 300 chronic pain patients were found to have clinical depression by comprehensive psychiatric assessment, and 59% of depressed patients were found to have chronic pain.[4] The implication is that patient groups may be

149

differentiated by the sequence of symptoms of pain and depression from the outset, with different responses to treatment.

Relationship of Pain Site to Psychopathology

Studies of the interrelationship of pain and depression have frequently taken a heterogeneous sample of chronic pain patients, i.e., headache, temporomandibular joint dysfunction, diabetic neuropathy, arthritis, chronic low back pain. However, some researchers have suggested that certain pain sites are more commonly associated with depression than others.[4,5] Backache, abdominal pain, and thoracic pain are found to occur in 10 to 15% of depressed patients, whereas pain in genitalia and upper or lower extremities is relatively rarely associated with depression.[4]

Relationship of Sample Site to Psychopathology

A study of chronic pain patients in an outpatient setting may find a different incidence of associated psychiatric illness than a similar study performed on inpatients. This is particularly true of a psychiatric inpatient service, where a higher incidence of more severely depressed individuals will be found.[2]

Organic vs. Functional Pain and Psychopathology

Does the presence or absence of organic disease differentiate chronic pain patients in terms of psychologic characteristics? One study on outpatients with varied pain sites, using a psychiatric diagnostic interview utilizing ICD-VIII criteria, found an incidence of psychiatric disorders of 97% in a group with no organic lesion as compared to 39% in the group with demonstrated disease.[6] Most of the psychopathology was believed to be depression (44% in the nonorganic group and 21% in the disease group). However, two other studies have failed to demonstrate psychologic variation between groups of chronic pain patients differentiated by the presence or absence of demonstrated disease.[7,8]

STUDIES ON THE INCIDENCE OF DEPRESSION IN CHRONIC PAIN

Having identified some of the methodological pitfalls in this area of investigation, we will now review some of the research. One study of 100 outpatients attending a pain clinic that used self-report instruments but no mental health diagnostic assessment, found an incidence of "depression" in only 10%.[9] This was a heterogenous group of pain patients with regard to the site of pain. Conversely, 71 consecutive chronic *low back pain* patients admitted to an inpatient pain program were studied using self-report assessments as well as structured psychiatric interviews.[10] Thirty-one patients were found to have major depression (43%), eight had minor depression, and 18 were diagnosed with intermittent depressive disorder (dysthymia) as defined by Research Diagnostic Criteria (RDC). Therefore, the overall incidence for depression was 80% in this patient group. In another similarly well structured study of 37 chronic pain patients admitted to an inpatient pain program, 32.4% had a current diagnosis of major depressive disorder, 43.2% had a history of major depression, and well over 50% had a family history consistent with depressive spectrum disease (depression, alcoholism, and sociopathy).[11] Magni has reviewed other relevant studies linking chronic pain and depression.[12]

Therefore, although many of the studies on the occurrence of depression in chronic pain are flawed by reason of a heterogeneous pain population or nonstandardized diagnosis of depression, the incidence of depression in chronic back pain is significantly higher than one would expect if these disorders were not in some way related. This has implications for assessment and treatment. The absence of an organic lesion may or may not have psychologic significance.

COMMON FEATURES OF CHRONIC PAIN AND DEPRESSION

Why might these two disorders be related? To understand this better, we will first examine some of the things that chronic pain and depression have in common, and then explore the hypotheses that attempt to explain this close association.

Biological Markers

DST

The dexamethasone suppression test (DST) is one of the most widely used neuroendocrine markers for depression, and is thought to be particularly relevant for melancholia. An initial study of 20 patients with chronic pain found frequent abnormal DST results, suggestive of a close association between the two disorders.[13] However, further research carefully comparing DST results in chronic pain patients with and without psychiatrically diagnosed major depression, found that the abnormal DST results occurred primarily in the psychiatrically diagnosed depressed group.[4,14,15,16]

TRH

The thyrotropin-releasing hormone (TRH) stimulation test, unlike the DST, has been reported to be both a trait and state marker for depression. TRH induced thyrotropin-stimulating hormone (TSH) response is blunted in patients with depression in many studies.[1] Twenty-four patients with chronic pain were tested for TRH response. Fourteen had major depression; six had blunted TSH responses, 4 in the depressed group and 2 in the nondepressed group. One of the nondepressed patients who tested positive had a past history of major depression. Although these results were obtained from a sample that was too small to be statistically significant, they do suggest that the TRH stimulation test may be a biologic correlate between pain and depression.[1]

REM

Abnormally shortened rapid eye movement (REM) latency (less than 60 minutes) on sleep EEG, indicative of abnormal "sleep efficiency" is found frequently in depressed patients. Twenty patients with chronic indeterminate pain were studied with sleep EEGs, and 40% were found to have an altered REM latency. However, these patients were not differentiated into depressed and nondepressed groups.[13] Further research is indicated.

Catecholeamines

Most depressed patients show evidence of low brain turnover of either serotonin or norepinephrine, as manifested by either lower than normal levels of 3-methoxy-4-hydroxyphenylethyline glycol (MHPG) in a 24-hour urine specimen, or abnormal levels of 5-hydroxyindole-acetic acid (5-HIAA) in cerebrospinal fluid. MHPG is a metabolite of norepinephrine and 5-HIAA is a metabolite of serotonin. Research suggests that an inverse relationship exists between these two markers in depressed patients, i.e., when one is below normal, the other is normal or above normal. It is hypothesized that depressed patients with high norepinephrine and low serotonin metabolism are more frequently irritable, anxious, and aggressive, and also have a lower pain threshold. Patients with high serotonin and low norepinephrine metabolism may have less agitation and anxiety, and also have a higher pain threshold.[17] Although this is speculative at present, it has been demonstrated that drugs which increase central nervous system (CNS) serotonin, such as serotonin precursors in high doses (L-tryptophan) and tricyclic antidepressants, also increase pain threshold, whereas substances that increase CNS norepinephrine lower pain threshold. This suggests another common biologic substrate between pain and depression involving biogenic amines.

Others

Other biologic markers that may link pain and depression include decreased platelet density for tritiated imipramine binding sites and reduced platelet monoamine oxidase activity (MAO), although their exact significance is unclear.[12]

Response to Pharmacological Agents

There is a large body of scientific literature documenting the therapeutic effects of antidepressant drugs in the treatment of chronic pain.[10,18] (See Chapter 38.) Several studies have focused specifically on chronic low back pain patients. Positive response has been seen with the heterocyclic antidepressants such as doxepin, desipramine, amitriptyline, clomipramine, and imipramine, as well as with the MAO inhibitors such as phenelzine. Chronic pain appears to improve within days, whereas depression responds within 2 to 4 weeks, and at higher doses. The mechanism of action may be the same or different, and is thought to be related to alterations in serotonin concentrations at specific sites in the central nervous system. Chronic low back pain patients with depression demonstrated transient pain relief following challenge with fenfluaramine, a pure releaser of serotonin. This was predictive of pain mitigation in subsequent treatment with either doxepin or desipramine. Although pain relief was most frequently associated with depression relief, several patients had improvement in only pain or depression. These results were felt to be supportive of a low serotonin hypothesis in chronic pain and depression.[19]

Family Studies

Family studies of depressed patients have revealed high incidence of depression and depressive spectrum disease. Similar investigations of family psychopathology in chronic pain patients has demonstrated depression and depressive spectrum disease in 11 to 69% of first degree relatives.[8,11,20–22] Failure to distinguish the groups of chronic pain patients with and without current or previous depression is a methodologic flaw in some of these studies.

One study does, however, separate out depressed from nondepressed chronic low back pain patients.[8] First degree relatives of the depressed group have a significantly higher incidence of depression than the nondepressed group, but both groups have the same family incidence of alcoholism, which is higher than one would expect to see in a normative population. These findings are inconclusive; nevertheless they do suggest that the occurrence of major depression in chronic pain patients may relate to genetic vulnerability to depression.

Cognitive Distortion

Beck's cognitive theory of depression called attention to the cognitive distortions, such as catastrophizing, overgeneralization, personalization, and selective abstraction, which lead to and perpetuate depression. Chronic low back pain patients also demonstrate a greater number of cognitive distortions.[23] This appears to be associated with general distress, but not somatization in this group.[24] Increased cognitive distortions are most prominent, however, in depressed chronic low back pain patients,[25,26] who have greater distortion when questioned about low back pain[1] than nonpainful depressed patients. Cognitive distortion may be an important mediator between chronic low back pain and depression, and may somehow determine why some, but not all, of these patients become depressed.[26] However, the exact relationship has yet to be clarified.

Anxiety

Symptoms of anxiety are common in patients with major depression. However, there has been only one research study on the presence of anxiety in chronic pain.[27] Seventy-one chronic low back pain patients demonstrated frequent symptoms of anxiety as manifested by anxious mood, tension, fearfulness, difficulty with concentration and memory, muscle aches and pains, and symptoms of sensory, gastrointestinal, genitourinary, and autonomic dysfunction. Patients with major depression were particularly affected. This raises additional questions about the role of anxiety in altering the perception of pain. Patients with anxiety neurosis tend to have a lower pain threshold, whereas depressed patients' thresholds may vary. Melancholics have been found to have an elevated pain threshold, i.e., less reactivity to pain, whereas other depressives have increased reactivity. Is anxiety another modulating link between depression and chronic pain? Further investigation is indicated.

HYPOTHESES ABOUT THE RELATIONSHIP BETWEEN CHRONIC PAIN AND DEPRESSION

Chronic pain and depression are closely associated and linkages have been identified in the clinical research, leading to hypotheses which attempt to explain this interrelationship.

Depression as "Normal Illness Behavior"

Hendler reviews the stages of chronic pain in patients who have had premorbidly normal psychological profiles and evidence of an organic lesion.[28] As noted in Table 14–1, he suggests that there is a normal response over a period of months and years in which clinical depression clearly evolves and then gradually resolves as the patient accepts the permanence of his pain and then attempts to cope. Depression is maximal between 6 months and 3 years after the onset of pain.

Pain as "Masked Depression" or "Depressive Equivalent"

The incidence of depression in pain is high, but the incidence of pain in depression is also high, and some investigators suggest that the two entities are a part of the same spectrum of symptoms, i.e., the "depression-pain syndrome."[4] In some patients, particularly those with poor premorbid psychiatric adjustment, chronic pain may represent "masked depression" or "depressive equivalence."[29] One might expect these patients to have a higher incidence of "functional pain," i.e., with no demonstrated pain generator,[7,28] although studies do not confirm consistent psychiatric differences between the organic and functional pain groups.[7]

Table 14–1
Proposed Stages of Pain

Acute Stage (0 to 2 months): The patient expects to get well and is not clinically depressed. MMPI is normal.

Subacute Stage (2 to 6 months): Hypochondriac concerns begin to emerge. The MMPI shows elevations on scales 1 (hypochondriasis) and 3 (hysteria).

Chronic Stage (6 months to 8 years): The patient realizes that the pain may be permanent and becomes depressed. The MMPI demonstrates elevations on scales 1, 2 (depression) and 3, with scale 2 particularly elevated.

Subchronic Stage (3 to 12 years): The patient accepts that the pain may persist and begins to adjust. Depression lessens. The MMPI shows low scale 2 (depression), but persistent elevations on scales 1 and 3.

In some of these patients, greater conviction of disease, somatic preoccupation, and unwillingness to acknowledge psychologic distress suggest a pattern of abnormal illness behavior[9] in which depression is denied and may be replaced by somatization. It is of particular interest, then, to delineate which came first in this group, the pain or the depression.[3]

The Dysthymic Pain Disorder

Based upon some of the previous observations, Blumer has defined a clinical syndrome, the dysthymic pain disorder.[13] These patients more frequently come from the lower middle class, with a history of excessive work performance (workaholism). There is a high family incidence of troubled marriages, with alcoholism, depression, or chronic pain in family members. The individuals have had to assume precociously adult roles, sacrificing their own needs for the well being of the family. They are intolerant of success, and often develop chronic pain just when they are close to achieving some measure of financial or emotional independence. In their clinical presentation, they tend to be somatically focused, wanting their pain to be taken away by any means.

They present as anergic, anhedonic, and insomniac, and may even admit to despair, but attribute all symptoms to pain and frequently deny depression. It has been theorized that the experience and focus on pain mitigates the depressive symptoms, and that if this defense was not present, these patients might experience even more severe depression and suicidality.

Depression and Chronic Pain as Separate Processes with Overlapping Symptoms

Certainly chronic pain and depression appear to have a number of features in common, but does this necessarily mean that they are on a continuum or that they represent the same process? They both respond to the same pharmacologic agents, and it is thought that common biogenic amines (particularly serotonin) may be involved in both. Cognitive distortion is found in both processes, but particularly in chronic pain with associated depression. Common biological markers have been found primarily when these two processes occur together. Family histories tend to be similar, but not identical, with "depressive spectrum disease" and particularly alcoholism, found in the families of chronic pain patients without depression, in contrast to the higher incidence of major depression in families of individuals with both depression and pain. Not all patients with chronic pain are depressed, and not all depressed patients have chronic pain. The similarities are intriguing

and have generated much creative scientific thought, but perhaps the individuals with chronic pain *without* clinical depression need to be examined more closely, to determine whether they are a subgroup or an exception that proves or disproves the rule.[30]

SUMMARY

A high percentage of chronic low back pain patients are clinically depressed. Although the details of the depression are sometimes not clearly delineated in the research, the association is beyond dispute. Whether chronic pain and depression are clinically, biochemically, genetically, or psychodynamically related has not been unequivocally established. Studies suggest some direct relationships, however, with regard to biologic markers, response to pharmacologic agents, family studies, and other associated clinical features such as anxiety and cognitive distortion. These common features have clear implications for treatment, particularly with regard to the use of antidepressant medications and cognitive therapy techniques. Additionally, some research suggests that better prognostic assessment might result from separating chronic pain patients into groups based upon psychologic characteristics. In one study, variables predicting treatment response differed as a function of depression even though depressed and nondepressed patients did not differ in their response to treatment.[30]

Further investigation is required on depressive subtypes and chronic low back pain, and how these may affect outcome measures. Additional study of biologic markers will be helpful to clarify ambiguities that currently exist. Future research on cognitive distortion may lead to some exciting new ideas about treatment and prognosis, and will contribute to our understanding of the evolution of the disease process of chronic low back pain, with its associated disability and depression.

REFERENCES

1. Krishnan, K., France, R., Davidson, J.: Depression as a psychopathological disorder in chronic pain. *In* Chronic Pain, (Edited by R. France and K. Krishnan). Washington, D.C., American Psychiatric Press, 1988.
2. Merskey, H., et al.: Screening for psychiatric morbidity. The pattern of psychological illness and premorbid characteristics in four chronic pain populations. Pain 30:141–157, 1987.
3. Bradley, J.: Severe localized pain associated with a depressive syndrome. Br J Psychiatry 109:741–745, 1963.
4. Lindsay, P., Wyckoff, M.: The depression-pain syndrome and its response to antidepressants. Psychsomatics 22(7):571–577, 1981.

5. France, R., Krishnan, K.: Pain in psychiatric disorders. *In* Chronic Pain, (Edited by R. France and K. Krishnan). Washington, D.C., American Psychiatric Press, 1988.

6. Magni, G., Merskey, H.: A simple examination of the relationships between pain, organic lesions, and psychiatric illness. Pain *29*:295–300, 1987.

7. Trief, P., et al.: Function vs. organic pain: a meaningful distinction. J Clin Psychol *43*(2):219–226, 1967.

8. France, R., Krishnan, K., Trainor, M.: Chronic pain and depression III: family history, study of depression and alcoholism in chronic back pain patients. Pain *24*:185–190, 1986.

9. Pilowsky, I., Chapman, C., Bonica, J.: Pain, depression, and illness behavior in a pain clinic population. Pain *4*:183–192, 1977.

10. Krishnan, K., et al.: Chronic pain and depression I: classification of depression in chronic low back pain patients. Pain *22*:279–287, 1985.

11. Katon, W., Egan, K., Miller, D.: Chronic pain: lifetime psychiatric diagnoses and family history. Am J Psychiatry *142*(10):1156–1160, 1985.

12. Magni, G.: On the relationship between chronic pain and depression when there is no organic lesion. Pain *31*:1–21, 1987.

13. Blumer, D., et al.: Biological markers for depression in chronic pain. J Nerv Ment Dis *170*:425–428, 1981.

14. Atkinson, J., et al.: Neuroendocrine markers of affective disorders in chronic pain. Pain Suppl *1*:1–474, 1984.

15. France, R., Krishnan, K.: The dexamethasone suppression test as a biological marker of depression in chronic pain. Pain *21*:49–55, 1985.

16. France, R., Krishnan, K., Trainor, M., Pelton, S.: Chronic pain and depression IV: DST as a discriminator between chronic pain and depression. Pain *28*:39–44, 1987.

17. Ward, N., et al.: Psychobiological markers in co-existing pain and depression: toward a unified theory. J Clin Psychiatry *43*(8):32–41, 1982.

18. Tollison, C., Kriegel, M.: Selected tricyclic antidepressants in the management of chronic benign pain. South Med J *81*(5):562–564, 1988.

19. Ward, N.: Tricyclic antidepressants for chronic low back pain: mechanisms of action and predictors of response. Spine *11*(7):661–665, 1986.

20. Blumer, D., Heilbron, M.: Dysthymic pain disorder: the treatment of chronic pain as a variant of depression. *In* Handbook of Chronic Pain Management, (Edited by C. Tollison). Baltimore, Williams & Wilkins, 1989.

21. Chaturvedi, S.: Family morbidity in chronic pain patients. Pain *30*:159–168, 1987.

22. Krishnan, K., France, R., Houpt, J.: Chronic low back pain and depression. Psychosomatics *26*(4), April, 1985.

23. Smith, T., et al.: Cognitive distortion and disability in chronic low back pain. Cog Ther Res *10*(2):201–210, 1986.

24. Smith, T., et al.: Cognitive distortion and psychological distress in chronic low back pain. J Consult Clin Psychol *54*(4):573–575, 1986.

25. Lefebvre, M.: Cognitive distortion and cognitive errors in depressed psychiatric and low back pain patients. J Consult Clin Psychol *49*(4):517–525, 1981.

26. Maxwell, T., Gatchel, R., Mayer, T.: Cognitive Distortion: An Important Mediator in the Relationship Between Chronic Low Back Pain and Depression. Presented at ISSLS, Kyoto, Japan, May, 1989.

27. Krishnan, K., et al.: Chronic pain and depression II: symptoms of anxiety in chronic low back pain patients and their relationship to subtypes of depression. Pain *22*:289–294, 1985.

28. Hendler, N.: Depression caused by chronic pain. J Clin Psychiatry *45*(3):30–36, 1984.

29. Forrest, A., Wolkind, S.: Masked depression in men with low back pain. Rheum Rehabil *13*:148–153, 1974.

30. Dworkin, R., et al.: Predicting treatment response in depressed and non-depressed chronic pain patients. Pain *24*:343–353, 1986.

Judith Greenwood

15

Socioeconomic Factors in Back Pain and Compensation Systems

To begin to understand the interplay between socioeconomic factors and any recognized physical or functional impairment, it is necessary to look at the origins of government sponsored programs to compensate disability. An outstanding work that documents government's role is Deborah Stone's *The Disabled State*.[1] In the first section of this chapter, the major tenets that she sets forth in her book are briefly reiterated. Readers of this book are recommended to pursue her work in full.

Following the overview of the government's role in compensating work disability, the issues in compensating back pain from the perspectives of the two major US governmental programs, workers' compensation and Social Security Disability Insurance, are discussed. Next, the relationship between extended work disability and monetary compensation are examined. Lastly, the argument is made that legal constructs of disability and social interpretations of these constructs have created an expanding system wherein disability is clearly a socioeconomic, not a medical, issue.

COMPENSATING DISABILITY AS A GOVERNMENTAL FUNCTION

Essentially in all societies, resources are distributed according to work, or level of economic participation, and according to need. Among modern European societies, England was the first to provide genuinely disabled people with public assistance through the English Poor Law of 1601, which codified earlier laws in an effort to control the problem of vagrancy and begging. Within the law, five categories were used to define those in need: children,

the sick, the insane, "defectives," and the aged and infirm. Of these, all but the first are part of today's concept of disability, and even the first category, as in the seventeenth century, contains handicapped children.

The English Poor Law had a variable history, but essentially the basic premise of the distribution of economic resources according to work remained the cornerstone of policy for over two centuries. During that time more elaborate systems were developed for classifying those unable to work and those who would turn vagrant or beg if government (then local government) did not provide relief. Because the concept of need was the counterpart of the concept of work, the most common institution of help developed under the Poor Law was the workhouse for paupers where people would live and perform what work they could for the parish.

At its strictest, the Poor Law prohibited alms or "outdoor relief," except for the acutely sick, in the parish at large. Thus, the Poor Law not only attempted to provide for the needs of the poor, but also served to inhibit the migration of able-bodied laborers in search of higher wages who might be temporarily dependent on "outdoor relief." The common denominator binding the categories of people offered relief under the English Poor Law from its inception to the end of the nineteenth century was the inability to work and to maintain employment in a competitive labor market. The least able-bodied persons, persons least desirable to employers, could receive public relief

In Germany, in the late nineteenth century, disability became a category in its own right, and the German model then became implicitly or explicitly the model for all subsequent social insurance plans.

155

From the beginning the German pension policy for invalidity and industrial accidents anchored the concept of disability in a competitive labor market to the inability to earn a certain amount rather than the total incapacity to earn because of any given condition. Thus, the German model used disability to define the nature and degree of labor mobility within the German occupational and social structure.

The difference between the English and the German policies can be understood only in the political context in which Germany became a unified empire with a national government headed by Otto Von Bismarck, a conservative. Bismarck had three explicit political rationales for a national social insurance program: it tied the future of the worker to the future of the state thereby quelling political activism and rebellion; it reinforced the monopoly of the state; and it relieved the burdens of poor relief from local governments. National social insurance was a major means through which Bismarck established a strong central government; material benefit begat political loyalty, a positive *quid pro quo.*

The use of disability to maintain social order and hierarchy and at the same time to let people out of a work-based reward system is clearly seen in the original German Invalidity and Pension Law of 1889. A person would be considered disabled when he or she, because of a mental or physical condition, ". . .could no longer earn at least one third as much as a mentally and physically healthy person with similar work education and experience in the same region, in any suitable job corresponding to his strengths, and capabilities, and taking into reasonable consideration his education and former education." This premise led to separating the insurance program for white collar workers from that for blue collar workers in 1922 and considering alternate job options much more narrowly for white collar workers.

The German model was in contrast to the English Poor Law, which restricted welfare benefits as a financial drain on government and attempted to enforce employment and reduce the non-working population during industrialization. German policy used benefits as a political tool and defined disability in such a way as to enforce a social and occupational structure. The basic policy difference between the British laissez-faire government and German nationalism showed up in Great Britain's Workmen's Compensation Act of 1897 which placed responsibility exclusively with the employer who could carry insurance with a private company, leaving no role for national government.

The United States was a laggard in establishing social insurance for disability. The first programs were established by state workers' compensation laws, which were passed in all but six states between 1911 and 1920. Most resembled the British Act in so far as relying on employers obtaining coverage through private insurance. In the beginning, state statutes required only notably hazardous industries to provide coverage; nevertheless, the rapid growth of the system of state workers' compensation programs has been called the most dramatic event of the twentieth century history of United States civil justice.[2] The last state to enact a workers' compensation law was Mississippi in 1949. During the mid-century, states began to adopt compulsory coverage for all occupations in contrast to earlier elective coverage for hazardous occupations and to include occupational diseases, but progress was gradual and variable; and variability among states was great.

In 1969, the federal government stepped in with the Coal Mine Health and Safety Act which established the first national program for nonfederal employees: the Black Lung Benefits Program to award disability and death benefits to coal miners and their dependents. In the next year, the Occupational Safety and Health Act was passed and with it the National Commission on Workmen's Compensation Laws was created to evaluate the state programs.

In 1972, the Commission's Report was issued containing 19 recommendations considered by the Commission to be essential for an effective and equitable system. These recommendations became the basis of reform efforts for over a decade. Uniformity among state programs began to emerge, particularly with compulsory coverage for all major employers, with maximum disability benefits standardized in most states to be at least two-thirds of the state average weekly wage, and with full coverage of medical and rehabilitation services. However, considerable variability still exists among states in program administration. Six states with exclusive state funds do not permit private insurance carriers to cover workers' compensation, and thus are similar to the German nationalistic model. Seventeen states permit state insurance funds to compete with private insurance. The remainder of the states rely on employers carrying coverage with private insurance. All but three states, two of them exclusive state fund states, permit employers to self-insure if they can meet certain bonding requirements.

Dispute resolution, litigation rates, and appeals procedures differ widely among states. Even nomenclature is inconsistent. However, enough equity exists now among the state programs with regard to benefits to make it unlikely that the threat of federalization that existed in the 1970s will materialize. Also, the controversies that have centered around the administration of the federal Black Lung Program have detracted from nationalizing workers' compensation.

The federal administration of Social Security Disability Insurance was born out of controversy. Not until the mid 1950s was disability added to the Social Security Administration's programs and only then after two decades of debate over the definition of disability and the mode of disability determination in individual cases. The debate was fueled by testimony from private insurance carriers that had commonly covered disability through life insurance policies from the decade of 1910. The favored definition of disability was a conservative one that stated a person was entitled to disability benefits if he or she was permanently prevented from performing any work for compensation or profit. The courts, however, tended to interpret disability leniently or broadly by reasoning that strict interpretation would deny adequate protection to some policy holders. One court offered a vivid hypothetical example: "If a person should suffer the loss of his arms and legs, his eyesight and his hearing, he might have his trunk conveyed to a busy street corner and make a little money by selling small objects such as post cards, candy, and cigars."[3]

Private insurance testimony before Congress during the late 1930s and the 1940s warned against expansion of a social disability program once enacted. However, proponents of the program had faith that there could and would be "strict tests" and "strict eligibility requirements" to eliminate awards on a purely subjective basis. The crux of the plan was to use "objective medical determination" according to the 1948 Advisory Council to the Social Security Board. Many physicians who had experience in certifying people for other disability programs—private insurance, workers' compensation, veterans administration—testified that clinical determination of disability was problematic. Nevertheless, Social Security program advocates insisted that disability

occurred at some medically determinable point and Social Security Disability Income was established.

COMPENSATION FOR BACK PAIN: THE ISSUES

The Social Security Disability Insurance (SSDI) program is responsive to individual need if a medical condition exists that is deemed to prevent "substantial gainful activity . . . for a continuous period of not less than 12 months." Figure 15–1 illustrates how the program can function for workers who are under 65 and have paid into Social Security long enough to have earned disability protection, usually for at least 5 years of the 10 proceeding the onset of disability. The medical evaluation that verifies any disability, including that related to back pain, must follow the Social Security Administration's "listing of impairments."

The listing for disorders of the spine is restricted to the following:

1.05 Disorders of the Spine:
A. Arthritis manifested by ankylosis or fixation of the cervical or dorsolumbar spine at 30° or more of flexion measured from the neutral position, with X ray evidence of:
  1. Calcification of the anterior and lateral ligaments; or
  2. Bilateral ankylosis of the sacroiliac joints with abnormal apophyseal articulations; or
B. Osteoporosis, generalized (established by X ray) manifested by pain and limitation of back motion and paravertebral muscle spasm with X ray evidence of either:
  1. Compression fracture of a vertebral body with loss of at least 50 percent of the estimated height of the vertebral body prior to the compression fracture, with no intervening direct traumatic episode; or
  2. Multiple fractures of vertebrae with no intervening direct traumatic episode; or
C. Other vertebrogenic disorders (e.g., herniated nucleus pulposus, spinal stenosis) with the following persisting for at least 3 months despite prescribed therapy and expected to last 12 months. With both 1 and 2:
  1. Pain, muscle spasm, and significant limitation of motion in the spine; and
  2. Appropriate radicular distribution of significant motor loss with muscle weakness and sensory and reflex loss.[4]

With regard to §1.05C, other vertebrogenic disorders, the listing includes four paragraphs of specific

Table 15–1
Significant Laws Related to Compensating Disability

1601-	English Poor Law
1889-	German Invalidity and Pension Law
1911 to 1920-	US Workers' Compensation Laws (all but 6 states)
1949-	Mississippi Workers' Compensation Law (last state to enact)
1954 to 1960-	Social Security Amendments for coverage of disability
1969-	Coal Mine Health and Safety Act
1970-	Occupational Health and Safety Act (Report of the National Workmen's Compensation Commission, 1972)

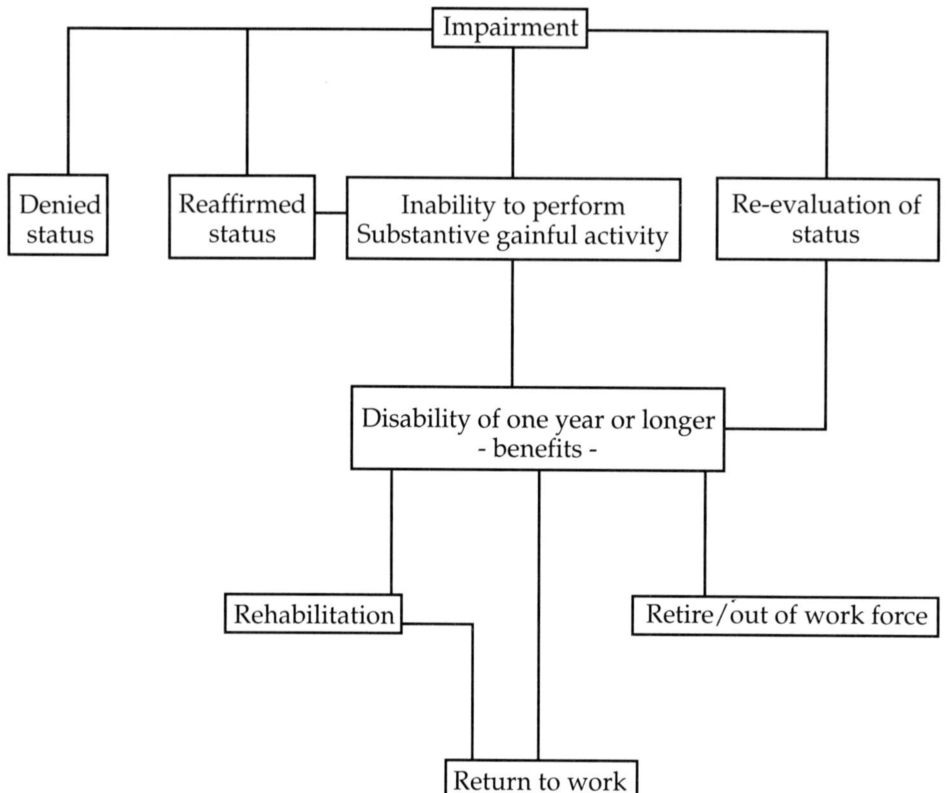

***Figure* 15–1.** Social Security disability.

instructions for making the evaluation and documenting the history and the clinical findings. Subjective low back pain is not even mentioned as a consideration in the medical evaluation. However, in ruling on disability claims, the courts have in general held the view that subjective pain can be objectively determinable. In practical application of the findings of Social Security Disability Insurance disability evaluations, disability remains a flexible construct that does include subjective pain to some extent.

The workers' compensation determination of disability begins with a medical assessment following an alleged work-related injury. The first thing to determine is if, in fact, the history that the injured worker gives comports with the demands and requirements of the job. State laws have wording to the effect of "arising out of and during the course of employment" in order to bar injuries that are not work-related. After causality is determined, often a controverted matter with back injuries, the question to be answered by medical assessment is how long is the person incapable of working at the job held at time of injury. Once that determination is initially made, medical coverage and temporary total disability benefits can begin, as shown in Figure 15–2. Medical coverage begins with the first treatment of injury and continues for the duration of the effects of the injury. Most state laws, however, require that lost time disability, or temporary total disability, begin only after a worker is off work for 3 to 7 days because of an injury.

The next critical juncture in medical assessment of a work-related injury is when maximum medical improvement is gained. At this point, temporary total disability benefits cease and permanent disability benefits may then be awarded. The alternative bases for awarding permanent disability benefits are shown in Figure 15–2 and are more extensively described elsewhere by Burton.[5]

Most state statutes include a schedule for physical loss or loss of the use of body parts that designates the benefit amounts to be paid for each loss. Divergences among states are numerous. For instance, in terms of number of weeks for which permanent disability benefits can be awarded, the loss of an arm equals 225 weeks in Ohio and 500 weeks in Wisconsin. Many disabling injuries and diseases today, however, are not covered in the schedules. In a few states (e.g., Florida and New York), if an impairment is coupled with actual post-injury wage loss, benefits are awarded based on the extent of the wage loss. If no wages are lost however, no benefits are awarded. In other states, if the impairment is permanent, benefits are awarded based on the extent of lost future earning capacity, even if no

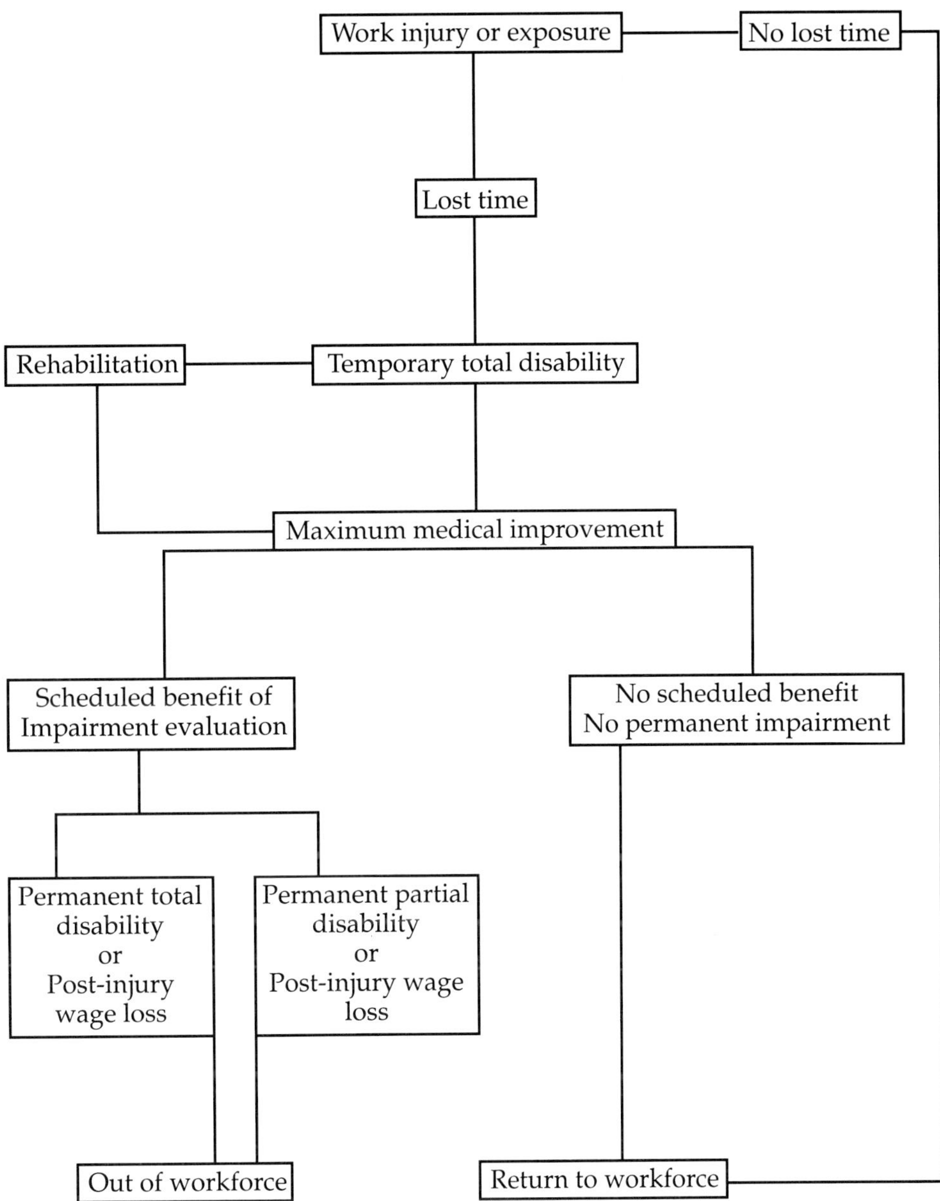

Figure 15−2. Workers' compensation.

present wages are lost. And in other states, if the impairment is permanent, then permanent partial disability benefits are awarded based on a physician's rating of the percentage of "whole man" that is impaired even if no wages are lost. In these ways, workers' compensation differs significantly from Social Security disability benefits. One does not have to be totally and permanently disabled from substantial employment to receive workers' compensation benefits.

Whatever the basis for awarding permanent disability benefits, back injuries produce the most controversy. In making impairment evaluations of the back, physicians commonly rely on a variety of factors, both subjective and objective.[6,7] Although at least 14 states (in 1987) report required use of the AMA *Guidelines for Evaluation of Permanent Impairment*, neither the requirement nor the evaluation criteria are impervious to a physician's modifying the criteria or introducing additional findings in rating the percentage of impairment. In some states, "dueling" physicians representing the claimant and the employer can cause the disability rating to be split between two impairment ratings.[8,9] The workers' compensation permanent disability benefit is without a doubt controversial, and the nature of back disability and the difficulty of measuring back impairment intensifies controversy.

EXAMINING COMPENSATION NEUROSIS

The term "compensation neurosis" evolved from writings by European physicians in the late 1880s who observed that accident laws were "the soil upon which traumatic neuroses have grown" and that "many malingerers had been cured by successful suits of law. Many claimants were suspected of malingering or of exaggerating symptoms in order to obtain benefits."[10] Compensation neurosis is not, however, a valid diagnosis in the DSM-III-R but "traumatic neurosis" is.[11] Generally, compensation neurosis would include somataform disorder, conversion type hysterical neurosis, psychogenic pain disorder, hypocondriasis, and psychological factors affecting physical condition. The objective of this section of the chapter is to review studies showing a relationship between disability and compensation and to discuss the multifactorial nature of disability. Because the studies available focus primarily on workers' compensation, the discussion is limited to that area.

In 1958, Krusen and Ford studied 509 low back pain patients, 54% of whom received workers' compensation and 46% of whom received no workers' compensation for their injuries.[12] All patients were treated in the physical medicine department of Baylor University and all patients studied had at least five physical therapy treatments. Hospitalization rates were about identical between the two groups as a rough indicator of severity. Results of treatment were measured by the patient's report of improvement and by attained level of function. Only 55.8% of patients receiving workers' compensation were considered improved at time of discharge, whereas 88.5% of the patients not receiving workers' compensation were considered improved. In part, these results related to the fact that over two-thirds of the noncompensation patients were treated during the first month of their symptoms, whereas only one-half of the workers' compensation patients had been seen at this point. However, workers' compensation patients seen within one week of injury did only slightly better than those noncompensation patients seen three months or more after injury. Also, all workers' compensation patients received significantly more treatments than the noncompensation patients. The authors concluded that workers' compensation patients seemed to be suffering from a compensation neurosis.

In 1966, in contrast to the above conclusion, White reported on the results of treatment at the Compensation Board Rehabilitation Centre of Toronto and results obtained by medical treatment at home. Satisfactory improvement was achieved in 15 of the 95 patients treated at home, but in 42 of the 99 treated in the Centre, a two-and-a-half times greater success rate. Satisfactory improvement was based on work records during the first 90 days after discharge from the study. White concludes, "The possibility that compensation payment per se has an unfavorable effect on the result of treatment is often suspected . . . It is reasonable to assume that this difference [between the Centre and the home care groups] would not have been so marked if payment for being disabled delayed recovery to a significant degree."[13] Subsequent studies, however, have not supported this assumption.

In 1984, Sander and Meyers studied 126 cases of back injuries among railroad workers of the Southern Pacific Transportation Company in which injuries were classed as either "injury on duty" or "injury off duty" and either as "lumbosacral strain/sprain" or "operated back." They found a statistically significant increase in work absence after injury on duty compared to the off duty for both types of injuries.[14]

In discussing the New Zealand no fault system of compensating all types of accident whether they happen at home, on the road, at the workplace, or during recreation, Bury and Gilkison point out that payment of compensation, especially in a lump sum for claim settlement, can be regarded as positively therapeutic in that "many [claimants] will learn to accept and live with their disability only at that point."[15]

Beals has looked broadly at compensation and recovery from back injury and notes that studies of the frequency of back injury as a cause of sciatica show widely discrepant findings with reported frequency rates of 92% in the United States, 59% in Great Britain, and 22% in Sweden.[16] Beals concludes, "The obvious explanation for this discrepancy lies in our compensation laws, which require an injury before compensation. When injuries are not required for coverage, they 'occur' less often."

The largest national workers' compensation data base is the Detailed Claim Information (DCI) data base of the National Commission on Compensation Insurance (NCCI). The DCI 1981 data base of 71,486 claims shows 95% of all work disability is the result of injuries. One quarter of all claims are low back injuries; 95% of these are strain/sprain injuries. All low back claims account for over one-quarter of all benefits paid, and average benefits for claimants with low back injuries are 40% higher than the average benefits for claimants with an injury to any other body part.[17]

Webster and Snook estimated that the total workers' compensation cost for back pain in the United States, including medical and disability benefits, was nearly 11.1 billion dollars in 1986.[18] The average cost per case was 6807 dollars whereas the median cost was 391 dollars, indicating that back pain claim costs are skewed to high costs.[18] Compared to reported 1981 data, costs escalated 241% in the six year period compared to a 184% increase in total workers' compensation costs during the same time period.[19,20] Snook and Webster and others in separate data sets show that 25% of the cases account for between 87% and 93% of the costs.[19,21–23]

Using a complex economic estimation procedure, Worrell and Appel show that level of benefits affect low back claims in a statistically significant way. For example, according to one estimation procedure, a 10% increase in benefits would be expected to lead to a 3.03% increase in disability claim duration. Applied to an average claim duration of 23 weeks, that increase would translate into 0.70 of a week or about five days greater duration.[24] In an earlier study, Butler and Worrell estimated that a 10% increase in benefits would lead to a 4% increase in disability claims.[25] Thus, if there are 1.4 million disability claims filed annually of which 25% are for low back injuries and if average low back claim duration is 23 weeks and if the average weekly disability benefit is 250 dollars, a 10% benefit increase would result in 14,000 new low back claims filed and a one week extension in duration of disability for all claims. Increased costs alone for these new claims and for the 350,000 old claims would be 171.5 million dollars. Total costs are in the billions of dollars.

Beyond this theoretical look into the relationship between an increased benefit level, certainly an economic factor, and increased frequency and duration of claims, Volinn, et al., analyzed disability claim rate for back sprain in the state of Washington in order to determine the effect of three socioeconomic factors: the unemployment rate, percentage of population receiving food stamps, and per capita income. For two of the three years studied, these socioeconomic factors account for about one-third of the variance in the claim rate. And even though claimants are employed when they are injured, the unemployment rate was significantly related to the claim rate in the three years studied. The authors conclude that ". . .disability is another symptom of distress. Where there is a rise in job insecurity and an attendant rise in economic insecurity, there is greater likelihood that back pain will become disabling . . . . regional economic factors to a considerable extent exert pressure on small social units and individuals."[26]

In a demonstration project focusing on early intervention to limit extended disability and facilitate return to work, Greenwood, et al, found that the case management intervention among underground coal miners reporting back injuries in southern West Virginia was not cost-effective and, in fact, medical costs increased significantly.[27] Although the intervention begun within two weeks after injury may have been too early, the authors speculate that "the general milieu in which the project took place provided few or no incentives to support an advocacy and case management intervention approach. . ." In an economically depressed region where unemployment is high, food stamps are common, and per capita income is low, compensated disability is not viewed as negatively as it may be in strong or expanding regional economies.

Finally, Deyo and Tsui-Wu using national survey data examined correlates of disability caused by low back pain in 1516 persons. Among men, greater educational level correlated significantly with fewer disability days of activity limitation, absence from work, or confinement to bed.[28] Education was a stronger correlate than self-rated pain severity, age, or income. This finding may relate to the fact that men with less education have more physically demanding jobs and sustain more injuries and suffer back pain. Educational level may also affect motivational level, intrinsic abilities, health habits, and compliance. The authors suggest that knowledge of a patient's educational level may be clinically useful in estimating prognosis for patients with back pain.

Considering the above studies and the information presented in the other chapters in this section of the book, we can correctly conclude that compensated spinal disability is not merely a musculoskeletal problem, but a multifactorial problem of which musculoskeletal dysfunction or abnormality is only one component and frequently is not sufficient in itself to cause the disability. The schematic in Figure 15–3 graphically shows the multifactorial nature of spinal disability as involving social and psychological factors, general health, education, age, medical care, legal, and economic factors. Not only are these factors related to disability, but in given cases certain factors or combinations of factors are indeed causative of disability. One can speculate that even without a particular musculoskeletal dysfunction or abnormality, persons would receive disability compensation for other disorders.

Hadler has written extensively about the disservice Mixter and Barr did to clinical practice, compensation administration, and conventional wisdom in 1934 by introducing the concept of "rupture" to explain pathogenesis of backache by "ruptured disc."[29–31] Rupture is a term that clearly invites the concept of trauma or single incident occurrence rather than a disease process exposed. Since Mixter and Barr's report, then, backache has become back injury and subject to the laws of workers' compensation. And compensation administrations have willingly, if reluctantly, accepted the economic consequences.

Many physicians and allied health providers practice common competing treatment modalities, including overtreatment, and receive legally assured payment through medical benefits for their efforts, even though state of the art evaluation of all available treatment modalities shows a minority of these

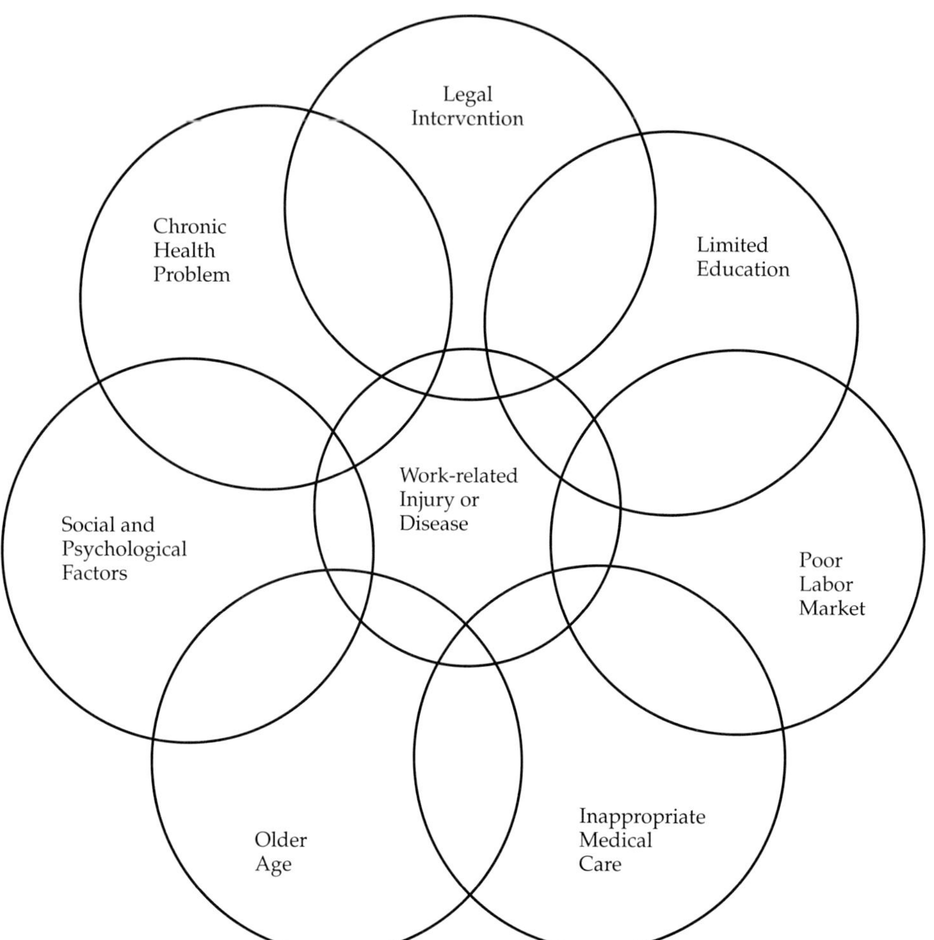

***Figure* 15–3.** The trap. Work-related disability—a multi-modal problem.

modalities to be of demonstrated usefulness.[32] However, even if Hadler could reverse the course of more than 50 years of medical and legal history concerning back injury and ruptured discs and return us to a simpler approach of accepting and dealing with backache through analgesics and modified activity, it is highly unlikely that such a reversal would reverse or significantly lessen the expansion of the compensation system. Even without Mixter and Barr, the back was an anatomical region vulnerable to increased inclusion in an expanding disability system. The following is taken from the report of the Chief Medical Examiner in the *First Annual Report: Public Service Commission, West Virginia, Workmen's Compensation Department, 1914.*

SPRAINED BACKS

There were reported during the nine months of the first fiscal year, one hundred eighty-one cases of so-called sprained backs; of this number eleven were rejected by the Commission, and one hundred seventy allowed. Some of the latter class lost less than one week, and were not a charge against the Fund.

The causes of this class of injuries as stated upon the reports, are varied. They include lifting lumps of coal, retracking mine cars, foot slipping in pushing mine cars, carrying a too heavy load, taking certain positions quickly, etc.

I am of the opinion that in fully 90 per cent of these cases the disability is due to muscular rheumatism and cannot be charged to any injury received in course of employment or otherwise, and that they are not entitled to benefits from the Workmen's Compensation Fund.

I think that before compensation is paid in this class of cases, the claimant should be required to prove that an injury was received as evidenced by objective symptoms or the happening of some untoward condition over which he had no control.[33]

There were a total of 10,544 temporary disability injuries reported that year. Back sprains were thus less than 2% of the total case load in 1914, whereas today they are between 25 and 30% of the total case load. Certainly Mixter and Barr's publication on ruptured discs eased the conceptual categorization of back disorders as arising from definable injuries, but they did not invent back injury. Because the structure and movement of the back is not readily observable and because relating signs and symptoms to structure and movement of the back are readily arguable, back pain was sure to discover accident and injury once a compensation system existed.

THE DISABILITY SYSTEM

The Social Security Administration amendments of the mid-twentieth century, which introduced cash benefits for totally disabled persons of preretirement age, and the state workers' compensation statutes enacted during the decade of 1910, which provided cash benefits for wage replacement and medical care for workers injured on the job, are neutral statements of societal responsibility and obligation. Out of these neutral statements, however, has evolved a highly dynamic disability system comprised of individuals, workers, physicians, health care providers, state and federal administrators, public and private insurers, lawyers, adjudicators, labor representatives, employer and business representatives, vocational rehabilitation specialists, physical testing equipment vendors, and, most recently, medical utilization review organizations. The dynamism of the system results because the popular conception of disability is much broader than the official statements or definitions of disability.[34] Thus, the legal construct of disability is socially manipulated and becomes a de facto socially created economic construct with an inherent characteristic for expansion. Judicial interpretation of the statutory definitions of disability in both workers' compensation and Social Security Administration has, for the most part, been liberal, coinciding with the popular conception (see Berkowitz, Johnson, and Murphy).[35]

The characteristic of the disability construct to expand has been, in part, because of the disability program's tendency to respond to economic conditions, e.g., downturns in regional and state economies, which appear to cause both claim filings and awards to increase (see Howards, Brehm, and Nagi),[36] and, in part, because of increasing medical precision in diagnoses of impairments with an attendant medicolegal attribution of disability, or the inability to work or to work at full capacity. The Mixter and Barr "discovery" of the ruptured disc has been followed by greater specification in cardiologic disorders, psychiatric disorders, and cancers. Consequently the tracking of work-related disabilities has increased, and workers' compensation administrations handle increasing caseloads. Total disability awards under the Social Security Administration are made with

more diagnostic categories relating to work incapacity.

A third and relatively new reason for expansion of the disability construct in workers' compensation is epidemiologic research that places workers "at risk" because of occupational functions, e.g., video display terminals and toxic exposures, most dramatically exposure to asbestos, although in the wake of asbestos many other chemical compounds are considered suspect. As Stone notes: "It is not hard to imagine the process by which epidemiological research makes possible the identification of *potentially disabled* people who are then disadvantaged in the labor market."[37]

Returning the discussion to back disability in particular, it is easy to see how an inherently expanding disability construct has involved back pain from the outset of socially mandated economic compensation for work incapacity. Although clinical research has shown that back degeneration is part of the life cycle and occurs during the prime work years, the degeneration is not necessarily or always symptomatic. When it becomes symptomatic, a cause is sought, and for anyone employed in manually intensive occupations, an occupational incident may trigger the symptoms of degenerative disc disease. With every worker between the ages of 20 and 64 at risk for symptomatic degenerative disc disease,[38] the disability system, in most instances following the rule of liberality and popular conception, will respond to symptoms if the symptoms can be related to a work-related incident or if they can be diagnosed as so severe that work capacity is totally impeded.

Some current workers' compensation reform proposals would eliminate the work relatedness test for compensation of back disorders and other diseases of uncertain cause. Hadler[39] invites consideration of 24-hour coverage for occupational, sports, automobile, and home accidents as exists in New Zealand. Regarding back pain, the current operating definition for the New Zealand Accident Compensation Commission is that a precipitant must have occurred within three months of filing a claim, which virtually assures that any individual with back pain can qualify for benefits.

Burton, as well as Hadler, supports a 24-hour concept, and as consultant to the Senate/House Joint Select Committee on Workers' Compensation, encouraged the adoption of a 24-hour health care provision by the Florida legislature in 1990.[40] The provision is optional for employers in lieu of traditional workers' compensation insurance covering both medical and disability benefits. The optional 24-hour plan would cover all employee injuries and illnesses, including work-related back injuries. Unlike traditional workers' compensation medical coverage, the 24-hour health insurance policy could use co-insurance and deductibles. A separate insurance policy would be needed to cover disability benefits.

Burton[40] also proposes that a few states that have temporary disability insurance programs experiment with Workers' Disease Protection Acts, which would provide benefits for selected diseases such as cancer, back disorders, and heart attacks after the temporary disability insurance has expired, usually after six months. Under Burton's scheme both permanent partial and permanent total disability benefits would be tied to actual wage loss because of disability. Initially there would be no work-related test for receiving benefits, and after maximum medical improvement, benefits would cease unless wage loss at the time could be verified.

Reforms, however, even though resolving certain thorny issues such as eliminating causality or the work-relatedness test and eliminating the extent of permanent partial disability as a proxy for wage loss, would almost certainly bring new problems to the fore. As experience in Florida has shown, the wage loss basis for awarding permanent disability benefits "involves complex legal issues that are neither immediately obvious or easily solved."[42] And as Ha-

dler notes, although the contest for receiving benefits for back pain in New Zealand has been defused from the perspectives of workers and administrators, physicians remain dissatisfied because they are still required to certify that back pain is the result of an accident, albeit work or nonwork related, and they must quantify permanent work disability.[44]

The fundamental tension inherent in the disability system was stated at the beginning of this chapter: the distribution of resources according to work and according to need. In the United States, the legal constructs behind social disability programs that define need attempt to reserve and preserve economic benefits, whereas the popular disposition surrounding the programs is to gain and use economic benefits. Thus, the boundary between work and need blurs, shifts, and bends. It is not fixed by the objective requirements of either individuals or economic circumstances. For example, entire categories of people (e.g., the blind) can be brought into the system as disabled, or a disease or circumstances of a disease (e.g., complicated pneumoconiosis among coal miners) can be presumed totally disabling. Ratings of permanent partial impairment are a presumption

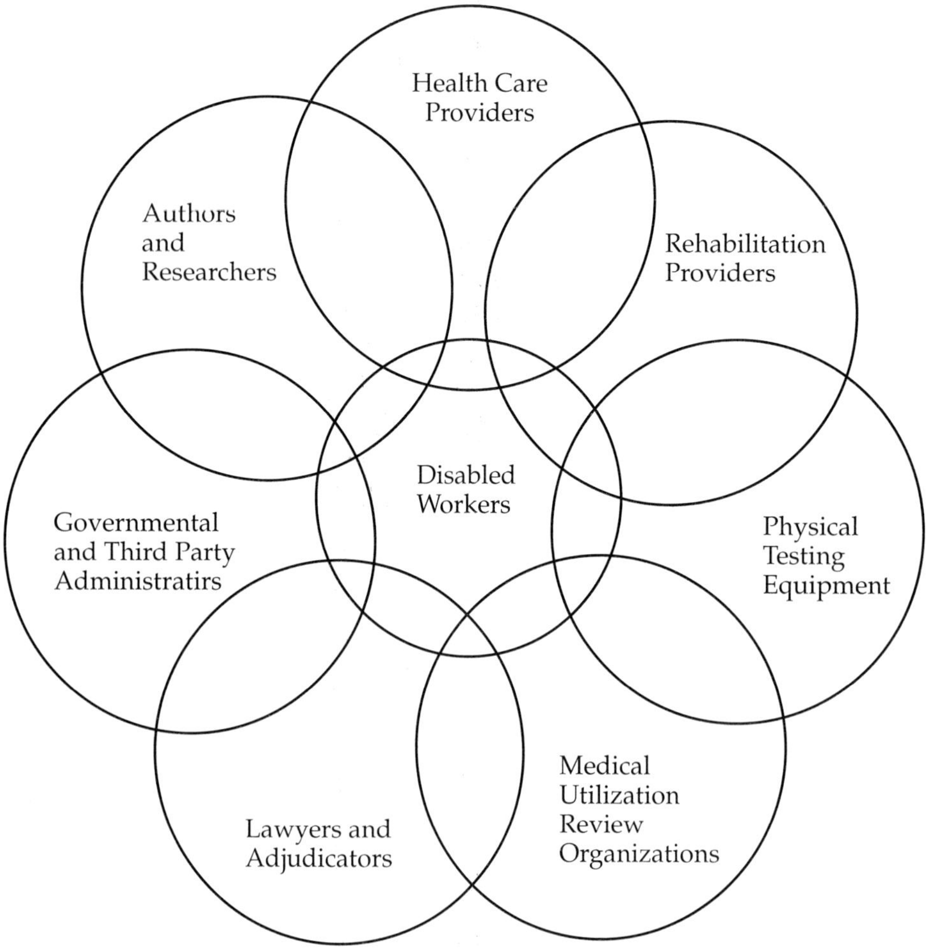

Figure 15–4. Disability system income: Who is dependent?

or proxy of wage loss because of impairment, even if there is no actual wage loss. Once presumptions are in place, they are hard to remove.

Social disability programs in the United States have become full fledged industries, which are now understood to be in the national interest and provide a livelihood for a variety of professional people, not just disabled workers as shown in Figure 15–4. Like the defense industry, the flow of dollars through the system increases its strength. If one takes this perspective, then back disease is a mainstay of the system, not only for disability benefits, but for medical practice fees, attorneys' fees, rehabilitation vendors' fees, profit from durable medical goods, including physical testing equipment, profits for medical utilization review programs, livelihoods of government and private insurance administrators, academic and private sector research grants, and even profits on book sales such as this book. The difference regarding income from the disability system is that the benefits to injured workers and to Social Security beneficiaries are awarded according to a generally restrictive, even if liberally interpreted, "need" based concept, whereas the remuneration and profits to all others involved in the system occur as a reward for socially sanctioned work. The categorical economic difference, therefore, is that all others are required to pay taxes on their earnings, whereas Social Security beneficiaries and injured workers do not have to pay taxes on their benefits, which are derived from taxes: i.e., premium taxes on employers' payrolls for workers' compensation, unless a company is a self-insurer and directly pays benefits itself, and general revenue taxes for the Social Security Administration.

In conclusion, we can clearly postulate that we are all in the disability system together. In wanting a predictable system, we are part of the problem by creating and enforcing regulations and requirements including presumptions; in wanting a flexible system, we are part of the solution by changing and reforming regulations and requirements. And finally we must recognize and understand that income within the disability system includes far, far more than cash benefits to disabled beneficiaries; livelihoods and profits to many abound. One workers' compensation expert has stated: "The sheer flow of dollars through the system will likely be its greatest strength to any challenge to its survival in the future."[44]

REFERENCES

1. Stone, D.: The Disabled State. Philadelphia, Temple University Press, 1984.
2. Darling-Hammond, L., Kniesner, T.J.: The Law and Economics of Workers' Compensation. Santa Monica, CA, The Institute for Civil Justice, 1980.
3. Marshall, V.: Metropolitan Life Insurance Company Statistics. Washington, DC, Social Security Administration, 1935.
4. Disability Evaluation under Social Security. Washington, DC, Social Security Administration, 1986.
5. Burton, J.: A primer on permanent disability benefits. Workers' Comp Mon 1:2, 1988.
6. Brand, R.A., Lehman, T.: Low back impairment rating practices of orthopedic surgeons. Spine 8(11):75, 1983.
7. Greenwood, J.G.: Impairment rating practices of orthopedic surgeons and neurosurgeons. Spine 10(8):773, 1985.
8. Workers' Compensation Research Institute. Use of medical evidence: low back permanent partial disability claims management in Maryland. WCRI Research Brief 2:9, 1986.
9. Workers' Compensation Research Institute. Performance indicators for permanent disability: low-back injuries in New Jersey. WCRI Research Brief 4:3, 1988.
10. Beals, R.: Compensation and recovery from injury. West J Med 140(2):233, 1984.
11. Diagnostic and Statistical Manual of Mental Disorders, 3rd Ed. Washington, DC, American Psychiatric Association, 1987.
12. Krusen, E.M., Ford, D.E.: Compensation factor in low-back injuries. JAMA 166(10):1128, 1958.
13. White, A.W.M.: Low back pain in men receiving workmen's compensation. Can Med Assoc J 95:50, 1966.
14. Sander, R.A., Meyers, J.E.: The relationship of disability to compensation status in railroad workers. Spine 11(2):141, 1986.
15. Bury, H.C., Gilkison, M.S.: The conceptualization of low back pain as compensable accident. In Clinical Concepts in Regional Musculoskeletal Illness (Edited by N.M. Hadler). New York, Grune & Stratton, p. 317, 1986.
16. Beals, R.: Compensation and recovery from injury. West J Med 140(2):233, 1984.
17. Borba, P.S., Nagel, M.J.: The high cost of low back injuries. NCCI Digest 1(3):1, 1986.
18. Webster, B.S., Snook, S.H.: The cost of compensable low back pain. J Occup Med 32(1):13, 1990.
19. Snook, S.H.: The costs of back pain in industry. Spine: State of the Art Reviews 2(1):1, 1987.
20. Social Security Bulletin, Annual Statistical Supplement. Washington, DC, Social Security Administration, p. 305, 1988.
21. Leavitt, S.S., Johnson, T.L., Beyer, R.D.: The process of recovery: patterns in industrial back injury. Part 4. Mapping Health Care Process. Ind Med Surg 41(2):5, 1972.
22. Snook, S.H.: Unpublished data. Hopkinton, MA, Liberty Mutual Insurance Company, 1980.
23. Snook, S.H., Webster, B.S.: Unpublished data. Hopkinton, MA, Liberty Mutual Insurance Company, 1987.
24. Worrall, J.D., Appel, D.: The impact of workers' compensation benefits on low back claims. In Clinical Concepts in Regional Musculoskeletal Illness (Edited by N.M. Hadler). New York, Grune & Stratton, p. 281, 1987.
25. Butler, R.J.: Wage and industry rate responses to shifting levels of workers' compensation. In Safety and the Workforce: Incentives and Disincentives in Workers' Compensation (Edited by J.D. Worral). Ithaca, ILR Press, p. 61, 1983.
26. Volinn, J., et al.: When back pain becomes disabling: regional analysis. Pain, 33:33, 1988.
27. Greenwood, J.G., et al.: Very Early Intervention Project, Management Report II. Charleston, WV, West Virginia Workers' Compensation Department, June, 1988.
28. Deyo, R.A., Tsui-Wu, Y.J.: Functional disability due to back pain: a population based study indicating the importance of socioeconomic factors. Arthritis Rheum 30(11):1247, 1987.
29. Mixter, W.J., Barr, J.S.: Rupture of the intervertebral disc with involvement of the spinal canal. N Eng J Med 211:210, 1934.
30. Hadler, N.M.: Regional musculoskeletal diseases of the low back: cumulative trauma versus single incident. Clin Orthop 221:33, 1987.

31. Hadler, N.M.: To be a patient or a claimant with a musculoskeletal illness. *In* Clinical Concepts in Regional Musculoskeletal Illness (Edited by N.M. Hadler). New York, Grune & Stratton, p. 7, 1987.

32. Quebec Task Force on Spinal Disorders: Scientific approach to the assessment and management of activity-related spinal disorders. Spine *12*(7S), 1987.

33. West Virginia Public Service Commission: First Annual Report. Charleston, WV, Workmen's Compensation Department, p. 194, 1914.

34. Stone, D.: The Disabled State. Philadelphia, Temple University Press, pp. 140–148, 1984.

35. Berkowitz, M., Johnson, W.B., Murphy, E.H.: Public Policy Toward Disability. New York, Praeger Publishers, pp. 53–57, 1976.

36. Howards, I., Brehn, H.P., Nagi, S.Z.: Disability: From Social Problem to Federal Program. New York, Praeger Publishers, pp. 110–132, 1980.

37. Stone, D.: The Disabled State. Philadelphia, Temple University Press, p. 179, 1984.

38. Kelsy, J.L., Shite, A.A.: Epidemiology and impact of low back pain. Spine *5*(2):133, 1980.

39. Hadler, N.M.: Industrial rheumatology: the Australian and New Zealand experiences with arm pain and backache in the workplace. Med J Aust New Zealand *144*:191, 1986.

40. Burton, J.: Health care cost sharing: is there a role in workers' compensation. Workers' Comp Mon *3*(4):18, 1990.

41. Burton, J.: Compensation for back disorders. Workers' Comp Mon *1*(4):8, 1988.

42. Burton, J.: The wage-loss approach: lessons from Florida. Workers' Comp Mon *1*:5, 1988.

43. Barth, P.S.: Can Workers' Compensation Survive the 21st Century. Paper presented at the Eastern Association of Workers' Compensation Boards and Commissions. San Juan, Puerto Rico, January, 1989.

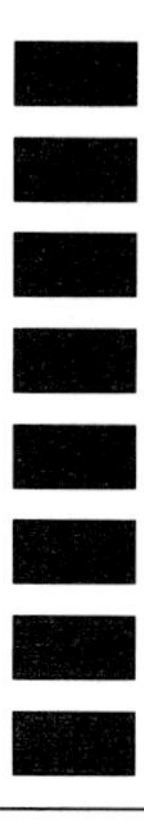

Part IV

Acute Spinal Care Options: Evaluation and Treatment

Richard A. Deyo

Historic Perspective on Conservative Treatments for Acute Back Problems

16

This chapter attempts to trace the recent medical literature on common treatments for acute back problems, but does not delve deeply into the historical roots of these treatments, which are sometimes found in antiquity. Instead, the emphasis is on the evolution of our understanding of these treatments through modern scientific investigations, with a focus especially on the most rigorous available studies of these treatments.

WHY ARE WE INTERESTED IN THE EFFICACY OF CONSERVATIVE THERAPY?

Because most conservative treatments for low back pain are relatively inexpensive and safe, it may seem unnecessary to scrutinize the evidence for their efficacy. Important reasons for doing so exist, however. First, acute low back pain is not primarily a surgical problem. Many authorities believe that most episodes of acute low back pain will never receive a definitive diagnosis.[1] Furthermore, even among patients with herniated discs, nearly all patients require a trial of conservative therapy before the use of invasive interventions (except those with cauda equina syndrome). Although it is difficult to estimate national rates of back surgery among all persons with low back pain, this rate appears to be around 1 or 2% in many European countries.[2] Most patients seek medical care for this problem from primary care physicians such as family doctors.[3] In fact, among family physicians and internists, back problems are the second leading reason for all office visits.[4] Second, many of these treatments entail substantial costs because they are labor intensive (physical therapy), require hospitalization (traction),

or involve work absenteeism and income loss (bed rest). Third, most have potential side effects, such as drug-induced ulcers, aggravation of pain by exercise, and complications of spinal manipulation.

Finally, a large number of conservative treatments are advocated, suggesting that none is clearly supe-

Table 16–1
Non-Surgical Treatments Advocated for Low Back Pain

Oral Drugs	*Counterstimulation*
"Muscle relaxants"	Cold massage
Analgesics	*Percutaneous radiofrequency
Non-steroidal	facet denervation
anti-inflammatory	*TENS
drugs	*Acupuncture
Corticosteroids	
Colchicine	
*Antidepressants	
Physical Measures	*Others (Usually For Chronic Pain)*
Bed rest	*Biofeedback
Corsets, braces	*Back school
Manipulation	*Behavioral therapy
Local heat	*Hypnosis
Massage	
Traction	
Exercise: Flexion,	
Extension, Stretching,	
Aerobic	
Weight loss	
Ultrasound	
Diathermy	
Injected Drugs	
Epidural steroids	
Epidural anesthetics	
Chymopapain	
Facet joint injection	
Trigger point injections	
Sclerosants	

*Usually reserved for chronic pain syndromes.

rior. Conflicting and competing claims for the efficacy of these treatments are common. Table 16–1 is a partial list of the nonsurgical treatments that have been advocated for low back pain. This list does not include the large number of unorthodox treatments (e.g., accupressure, reflexology), which are widely offered but unexamined in scientific literature. Even orthodox practitioners are sometimes guilty of uncritically promoting unproven therapies (e.g., laser stimulation of trigger points). The long history of disproven remedies that were once advocated by well meaning physicians should dissuade us from accepting new practices without rigorous evidence of efficacy.

An important trend, which this chapter documents, is a move away from passive treatments such as bed rest and traction.[5] Growing evidence supports the value of early mobilization, several exercise regimens, and treatment prescriptions that occur on a fixed schedule, regardless of some pain symptoms.

HOW DO WE DECIDE WHAT WORKS?

Treatments are not necessarily effective in clinical practice even though they appear efficacious in research studies. The effectiveness of a treatment in actual practice is a complex function of whether or not the physician has made an accurate diagnosis, the efficacy of the treatment in ideal circumstances, the physician's skill in applying the treatment, and the patient's compliance with the regimen. The failure of any of these factors is likely to result in a poor therapeutic response. However, the conventional clinical trial tests only the efficacy of the treatment under ideal circumstances, and does not consider the other three factors in this equation. Unfortunately, there is little way to predict how these factors will behave in most situations, and data in many cases are nonexistent. Thus, from the medical literature, we can generally only learn about the efficacy of a treatment under ideal circumstances, and this is the focus of this chapter. The other factors are discussed only briefly.

How are we to sort among the conflicting claims that are made for various treatments? The natural history of acute low back pain is that it improves rapidly, and this can mislead casual observers into believing something they have done is efficacious. Indeed, Wadell points out that it is difficult to demonstrate that most treatments are better than the effects of a placebo plus the natural history of the condition.[5] In this circumstance, it is especially important to conduct randomized clinical trials to assess the treatment efficacy. Recent medical history is replete with treatments that enjoyed a brief vogue but were subsequently abandoned when rigorous,

controlled trials were completed. Examples include gastric freezing for peptic ulcer disease, internal mammary artery ligation for angina, and bed rest for hepatitis. Unfortunately, many patients were subjected to the complications and costs of these procedures before they were shown to be useless.

Could historical or nonrandomized control groups suffice to demonstrate efficacy? Unfortunately, nonrandomized control groups are usually demonstrably biased in favor of new treatments, even though this is unintentional on the part of the investigators.[6] Demonstrable biases occur even when randomization is used but is performed in a manner that allows the investigator to identify upcoming patient assignments.[6] When a physician knows the next group assignment, he is likely to be unconsciously biased in acting on the entry criteria and in seeking informed consent. A common objection to randomized trials is that they do not account for the individual patient who may have an unusually favorable response. Nonetheless, randomized trials are well suited to subgroup analysis, and cogent clinical subgroups can often be isolated to examine the effects of treatment in particular circumstances. Thus, randomized trials are necessary, but not sufficient to assure valid results.

Several other methodologic criteria are important to reduce biases and assure the most valid assessment. Although a detailed list of such criteria would be lengthy, Table 16–2 presents a brief list of the more important factors, and a brief explanation of each, adapted from recommendations of several methodologists.[6–8]

There are a variety of barriers to rigorous research of low back pain, some of which are unique to this particular problem. For example, it is relatively easy to blind a drug trial with placebo medication, but more difficult to blind studies of physical therapy. Nonetheless, efforts should be made to assure that the outcome assessors are blinded to the treatment the patient received, to ensure that all patients receive equal contact and attention from the research staff, and to make the control treatments as similar in nature as possible to the active treatments. Another problem is that compliance with physical treatments is hard to measure, and is typically worse than medication compliance.[9] Nonetheless, efforts to quantify compliance may be useful if they employ nonthreatening questions to elicit the level of compliance, the use of patient diaries, family validation of compliance, and reports of appointment keeping compliance. The measurement of outcomes in this area is problematical because patients typically neither die nor are completely cured by medical intervention. A good deal of attention has been given to ways of measuring pain, but greater attention is needed to quantifying patient functional status and

Table 16–2
*Criteria for Assessing the Validity and Applicability of Clinical Research on Conservative Treatments for Low Back Pain**

Validity
1. Random allocation: the best way to achieve equal distribution of prognostic factors (even when they are unknown) between active treatment and control groups.
2. Minimal patient attrition: Those who do unusually well or unusually poor are most likely to drop out, biasing the remaining study sample.
3. Blind outcome assessment: The best way to reduce investigator bias in measuring outcomes. Even if patients cannot be blinded, the examiner usually can.
4. Equal cointerventions: A wide variety of treatments for back pain are readily available and may be obtained by subjects in a clinical trial.
5. Compliance measured: Therapy cannot work if it is not received. Compliance with physical measures and lifestyle changes is often particularly poor.
6. Minimal contamination: Unintended "crossovers" may occur if patients can obtain a study treatment elsewhere.
7. Both statistical and clinical significance considered: a statistically significant result may be clinically trivial. On the other hand, a substantial clinical effect may fail to be statistically significant if the sample size is too small.

Applicability
1. Good demographic description: At least age, sex, and source of patients.
2. Good clinical description: Duration of pain, neurologic deficits, sciatica, prior surgery, work disability, other entry criteria.
3. Treatment adequately described: Dose, duration, frequency, technique, etc.
4. Reporting all relevant outcomes: Physiology, function, symptoms, satisfaction, and costs may all be important.

**Adapted from Deyo, R.A.: Conservative therapy for low back pain: distinguishing useful from useless therapy. JAMA 250:1057–1062, 1983.*

medical care utilization. Finally, investigators are faced with the problem of diagnostic ambiguity about the causes of low back pain. Rather than attempting to determine a specific diagnosis (which may be impossible), it is important to report the clinical characteristics of patients in some detail, and it may be useful to stratify results according to clinical subgroups (for example, age, symptom duration, presence of sciatica, or neurologic deficits).

A REVIEW OF THE EVIDENCE FOR VARIOUS TREATMENTS

Bed Rest

As shown in Table 16–3, rest is the most commonly prescribed therapy for low back pain in the United States. This prescription may directly affect the time patients lose from work or their other activities, but the optimal duration of bed rest has been unclear. The traditional rationale for recommending bed rest was to provide symptomatic relief and to

minimize intradiscal pressure.[10] However, nearly 50% of patients with low back pain report little relief with bed rest,[5] and many episodes of back pain may be unrelated to prolapsed discs. In this circumstance, it is uncertain what the pathogenetic role (if any) of intradiscal pressure may be. Furthermore, many patients who are prescribed bed rest undoubtedly sit up reading or watching television in bed. This raises intradiscal pressure above even the standing position,[10] and probably subverts even the physiologic rationale for this treatment.

Only recently have actual clinical trials been conducted to test the efficacy of bed rest. The first of three randomized trials suggested that bed rest was superior to continued ambulation, but this study was conducted in an unusual setting (military recruits in basic training) and the assessment of outcomes was apparently not blinded.[11] In our study of 203 persons with back pain in a walk-in clinic, subjects were randomized to a recommendation of 2 days or 7 days of bed rest. Those given the two day recommendation missed 45% fewer days of work than those given a seven day recommendation, but there were no other significant or substantial differences in functional, physiologic, or perceived outcomes at 3 weeks or 3 months. Patients reported an average of 11 days of pain following the index visit in both groups, but most had returned to their usual activities well before this time.[12] Gilbert and his colleagues went even further in reducing the bed rest recommendation. In a study of 270 patients in a family practice clinic, subjects were randomized to receive a recommendation of four days bed rest or none at all. There were no detectable differences in the speed or extent of pain resolution, but the bed rest group required 42% longer to return to their normal activities.[13] These studies suggest that for patients without neurologic deficits, brief (if any)

Table 16–3
Common Treatments for Low Back Pain: Frequency of Use Among 1516 Persons with Back Pain in the Second National Health and Nutrition Examination Survey[3]

Treatment	Percent Who Ever Used	Percent of Users Who Thought it Helped
Rest	81%	86%
Heat	74%	80%
Aspirin	58%	77%
Exercise or Physical Therapy	41%	71%
Brace	27%	71%
Traction	21%	63%

bed rest is generally sufficient, and that bed rest does not affect the natural history of the illness.

The common recommendation of staying at rest until pain is resolved may even have adverse psychological and physical consequences. Fordyce and colleagues found that such pain-contingent recommendations resulted in more sick role behavior and claims of impairment than recommendations given with a fixed schedule independent of symptoms.[14] Lengthy bed rest may suggest to patients that they are severely ill, since even a week is longer than currently recommended for patients recovering from acute myocardial infarction or childbirth. In our study, the physician's bed rest recommendation was more important in determining the length of work absenteeism than characteristics of the medical history, examination, or therapy.[12] Finally, bed rest fosters bone demineralization, muscle weakness, and cardiovascular deconditioning.[15–17]

Thus, there is growing evidence that for patients without neurologic deficits, bed rest should be brief (approximately 2 days) and early mobilization should be encouraged. As always, clinical judgement is required and recommendations must be individualized.

Exercise

Controversy persists about the most appropriate exercise regimens for patients with various back pain syndromes. Advocates of flexion exercises, extension exercises, stretching regimens, and aerobic conditioning all compete for professional favor. Whatever the specific regimen, there is a consensus that exercise plays an important role in the treatment of mechanical low back pain, and many centers actually prescribe a combination of regimens. Indeed, the recommended treatment of low back pain is undergoing a shift from passive to more active therapy.[5] Bed rest recommendations are shortening, while early return to activity is encouraged, and increasing exercise is often part of the therapeutic prescription.

Aerobic exercise is often prescribed for patients with back pain, with the primary goal of improving muscular endurance. This reduces fatigue when performing repetitive tasks and results in some strengthening of lower extremity and abdominal muscles. Regular aerobic exercise probably improves neuromotor control, coordination, and mechanical efficiency, all reducing the likelihood of back injury or recurrence of back pain. Reduction of obesity, elevation of plasma endorphins, and psychological benefits may be additional effects of aerobic exercise.[18] Intravital measurements suggest that disc pressure is lower in the standing position than in the sitting

position, so that exercise such as walking would be safe even early in an acute episode of back pain.

Stretching exercises are prescribed with the rationale of improving spine mobility and limbering muscles and ligaments that had been restricted in motion in response to pain. A typical regimen is that developed by Kraus and widely popularized by the Young Men's Christian Association (YMCA).[19] Perhaps the most widely recognized exercises for back pain are the isometric flexion exercises popularized by Williams. His work in the 1930s proposed several rationales for this treatment: to widen the intervertebral foramen and facet joints, to stretch hip flexors and back extensors, and to strengthen the abdominal and gluteus muscles. Measurements of intradiscal pressure have raised some concerns that flexion maneuvers could occasionally be harmful, as they are associated with substantially increased pressure.[10]

Extension principles have been most widely advocated by McKenzie,[20] and his program is outlined in more detail in a separate Chapter 20. Extension exercises are intended to increase spinal mobility, restore lumbar lordosis, strengthen paraspinal and hip extensors, and shift the location of the gelatinous nucleus pulposus within the intervertebral disc. In some cases, spinal extension can reduce or eliminate sciatic pain, leaving only lumbar discomfort. This has been referred to as "centralizing" the pain, and suggests that for such an individual, extension exercises will be beneficial. If sciatica worsens with extension, this program would be contraindicated.

Because there are conflicting opinions about various regimens and a reasonable physiologic rationale for each, it is essential to examine the clinical evidence for treatment efficacy. In doing so, we should remember that encouragement, clinician enthusiasm, placebo effects, and the excellent natural history of acute low back pain all favor improvement regardless of treatment efficacy. Unfortunately, there is a paucity of controlled exercise trials, and most published studies have important methodologic limitations.

To date, no randomized trials of aerobic exercise for back pain have been published. The enthusiasm for this regimen is largely based on the cohort study of Cady, et al., among Los Angeles firefighters. Although the duration of followup was uncertain, it was observed that the incidence of back pain was least among the most fit firefighters, based on bicycle ergometry, isometric strength testing of selected muscles, and spine flexibility. In a small group of uncertain size with previous back problems, no recurrences were observed among the most fit, whereas one-third of the least fit had recurrences.[21]

The major evidence for the value of stretching exercises comes from the program of the YMCA.[22,23] In a followup of nearly 12,000 persons who participated in this 6-week program, 80.7% reported improvement in pain.[22] Unfortunately, no control group was used. We have reported on a randomized trial of a program adapted from that of the YMCA. Subjects with chronic back pain (n = 125) were randomized to receive a stretching exercise regimen or no exercise, although all received instruction in back care, local heat, and frequent followup. The exercise group reported significantly greater improvement in pain severity, pain frequency, and self-assessed activity level. Unfortunately, most subjects did not continue exercising after the 4-week intervention, and group differences were lost 2 months later.[24]

At least three randomized trials of isometric flexion exercises have been reported. Unfortunately, these provide conflicting results. In the late 1960s Kendall and Jenkins studied patients with chronic low back pain and reported that after 3 months of therapy, improvement in symptoms was significantly greater among subjects receiving flexion exercises than among those receiving mobilizing or extension exercises.[25] A decade later, Davies and colleagues sought to replicate several aspects of this study. In their trial, subjects were randomized to receive isometric flexion exercises, extension exercises, or no exercise. The subjects were young adults with subacute back pain, most of whom were actively employed. Although no significant differences were observed among the groups in outcome, both exercise regimens resulted in a larger percentage of improved subjects than the nonexercise regimen.[26] Low statistical power may have prevented the results from achieving significance. A very slight advantage for extension exercises over flexion exercises was observed, and three patients were said to be initially worse with the flexion regimen (none with the extension regimen). The most recent trial was conducted in a family practice setting, in middle-aged adults with acute low back pain. Subjects were randomized to receive isometric flexion exercises or no exercises. Those in the exercise group reported a slower recovery of activities of daily living, and there was a nonsignificant trend against the exercise regimen for range of motion and pain severity.[13] Together, these trials suggest a possible benefit for flexion exercises among persons with chronic or subacute pain, but no benefit in primary care patients with acute back pain.

McKenzie has reported a large case series of experience with extension exercises, but no controlled trials.[20] The studies reported above gave ambiguous results with regard to extension regimens. A recent study compared an updated McKenzie regimen (which includes some flexion exercises) with a certain form of traction and with a "back school" intervention. Patients with pain up to 12 months were included, so that presumably a mixture of both acute

and chronic syndromes were included. The trial was reportedly randomized, but the unequal group assignments cast uncertainty as to whether the method of allocation successfully resulted in true randomization (62 assigned to exercise, 40 to traction, 34 to back schools). Because group assignment was based on birth date, there may have been opportunity for unconscious bias in entering subjects. Though not completely reported in the peer-reviewed literature, this trial reported an advantage of the McKenzie exercise regimen over alternative treatments.[27] The most recent study of extension principles, conducted in Denmark, tested a very intensive regimen for 105 subjects with chronic low back pain. Although the median pain duration in these subjects was 15 years, 78% were still employed. They were randomized to receive either: (1) a moderate 1-month combined regimen of extension and flexion exercises, (2) a very intensive extension regimen given in 30 sessions over 3 months, or (3) a milder version of the extension regimen with one-fifth the repetitions. The intensive exercise regimen proved superior to the other regimens with regard to pain relief, activity limitations, and physiologic measures. The authors emphasized that improvement was only apparent after about 2 months of treatment, and many patients noted increased discomfort from muscle fatigue and tenderness in the first month.[27] The value of this regimen for acute back pain remains to be demonstrated.

In summary, at least some evidence exists for the efficacy of several different exercise programs, although several trials included only patients with chronic back pain. All of the regimens described here require a substantial degree of patient motivation and compliance, and the subjects included in these clinical trials were apparently not typical of those found in most chronic pain treatment centers. Thus, although these programs may be efficacious, the challenge for clinicians is to elicit compliance with referral and ongoing supervision of these exercise treatments.

Other Lifestyle Modifications

Smoking and obesity have been identified as risk factors for low back pain in several epidemiologic studies.[29–32] Though randomized trials of smoking cessation and weight reduction as treatments for back pain have not been conducted, there is physiologic and epidemiologic evidence to suggest potential benefit.

The biologic link between smoking and back pain remains uncertain, but could be related to (1) increased coughing, with elevated disc pressure and risk of herniation; (2) vasoconstriction by nicotine, jeopardizing discal metabolism; (3) an association with psychologic traits (depression, anxiety), which amplify and prolong pain symptoms.[32] There is at least suggestive evidence that smoking cessation may reduce the risk of back pain.[29,31]

In studies that examined true indices of obesity such as body mass index or skinfold thickness, an association has been observed with back pain in general and disc herniation in particular.[29,30] Truncal obesity probably increases mechanical strain on the lumbar spine, and its reduction may help to treat or prevent low back pain, though this hypothesis has not been carefully tested.

Drug Therapy

A variety of oral drugs are used in the treatment of low back pain, most commonly including pure analgesics, nonsteroidal anti-inflammatory drugs (NSAIDs), antidepressants, and "muscle relaxants." Although scientifically adequate trials of analgesic drugs such as codeine and other narcotic analgesics have not been conducted specifically for low back pain, their general properties and clinical experience suggest that they are efficacious in relieving acute back pain and sciatica. Most clinicians would agree, however, that narcotic analgesics should be used only in cases of severe acute pain, and not for chronic pain syndromes.

A variety of NSAIDs have been tested for low back pain, and several acceptable trials have been published (see Table 16–4).[33–36] The apparent success of several NSAIDs in these well designed trials suggests that probably most drugs in this category are efficacious. Unfortunately, many of these trials did not provide an adequate description of patients

enrolled, limiting our ability to generalize about the types of patients who benefit most. Though NSAIDs are generally safe and efficacious, recent action and new product labeling required by the Food and Drug Administration highlight the substantial risk of serious gastrointestinal bleeding with these drugs, especially in older patients.[37]

Muscle relaxant drugs are often prescribed with the intent of reducing muscle spasm, although in conventional oral doses muscle relaxation is probably minimal. Furthermore, there is substantial controversy about the importance of skeletal muscle spasm in producing back pain,[38] and evidence that clinicians cannot agree on the presence of spasm in individual patients.[39] Unfortunately, many trials of muscle relaxant drugs have included patients with both low back pain and cervical or extremity pain. When lumbar pain comprises only a small proportion of the total subjects, it is hazardous to assume that the overall results necessarily apply to patients with low back pain.[7]

Among the studies that focused on back pain, two suggested that carisoprodol was superior to alternative treatments, including butabarbital, diazepam, or placebo.[40,41] In one other study of diazepam for back pain alone, it was not superior to placebo, but statistical power and functional outcomes were not reported.[42] In a trial that included both cervical and lumbar pain, diazepam was superior to placebo overall, but the results for lumbar pain were not separated. In the same trial, cyclobenzaprine was superior to placebo but had more side effects than diazepam.[43] Adequate trials of oral methocarbamol that focused only on low back pain were not identified. A study of baclofen for acute low back pain was plagued by a high dropout rate, a 68% rate of side effects, and failure to report results for all the subjects randomized.[44] Two recent trials examined the

Table 16–4
Well-Designed Trials of Nonsteroidal Anti-Inflammatory Drugs in the Treatment of Low Back Pain

Drug	Randomized	Patient Attrition, %	Blind Outcome Assessment	Adequate Patient Description	Results
Diflunisal	Yes	6%	Yes	No	Diflunisal superior to placebo
Diflunisal	Yes	11%	Yes	No	Diflunisal superior to placebo on only one measure
Naproxen Sodium	Yes	11%	Yes	No	Naproxen superior to Diflunisal or placebo
Piroxicam	Yes	6%	Yes	Yes	Piroxicam superior to placebo
Piroxicam and Indomethacin	Yes	3%	Yes	No	Piroxicam and Indomethacin similar

new drug tizanidine. The first trial was well designed and demonstrated that patients receiving tizanidine could reduce their aspirin use more than subjects receiving placebo, although with the rescue medication, pain relief was similar.[45] Among those receiving tizanidine, 22% experienced drowsiness. A second study compared tizanidine plus ibuprofen with ibuprofen alone. In some subgroups, the combination resulted in better pain relief than ibuprofen alone, but with significantly more subjects on tizanidine "upset by their treatment."[46] With a few exceptions, these studies of muscle relaxants did not provide adequate patient descriptions; therefore it remains unclear to whom the results are most applicable.

Tricyclic antidepressants are generally reserved for patients with chronic pain, and are not considered here. Colchicine has generated some interest as a treatment for acute back pain, but a recent randomized trial of the oral drug demonstrated no advantage over placebo.[47] Poor compliance, a high dropout rate, and a small sample prevent firm conclusions from this trial.

None of the medications discussed here have been demonstrated to be superior to aspirin alone. Although aspirin's efficacy has not been definitively demonstrated, there is at least one suggestive small trial.[11] It is clear that enteric coated forms avoid many of the gastrointestinal side effects of plain aspirin,[48] and this inexpensive drug should probably remain in the first line of treatment for patients with low back problems.

Spinal Manipulation

This form of treatment remains highly controversial, in part because it is strongly associated with the chiropractic profession. The philosophy of chiropractic care remains unattractive to physicians because it rests on unproven pathophysiologic assumptions and often includes claims of therapeutic efficacy for conditions outside the musculoskeletal system. Nonetheless, a number of randomized trials of manipulation for back pain have been conducted, with the manipulation usually provided by physicians or physical therapists. The rationale for manipulation remains unclear, with suggested mechanisms including reduction of a bulging disc by tightening of the posterior longitudinal ligament, freeing of adhesions around a prolapsed disc, mechanical stimulation of certain nerve fibers that inhibit nociceptive transmission, and modification of facet joint alignment. Unfortunately, manipulative techniques vary widely, and the treatments delivered even in clinical trials are probably very heterogeneous. In some cases, the manipulation has not been described adequately.

Five reasonably well designed trials of manipulation suggest that this treatment may have some short-term benefit for selected patients, but that after 2 to 3 weeks, results are comparable to those of alternative treatments. Even a brief benefit may be important, however, if patients experience earlier relief of pain and return to normal activities. Farrell and Twomey demonstrated faster pain resolution among manipulated patients than among those given diathermy, flexion exercise, and patient education.[49] Similarly, the study of Hoehler, et al., suggested greater immediate improvement in patients receiving manipulation than among those receiving massage.[50] Hadler's group demonstrated an advantage of manipulation over "mobilization" for a very specific subgroup of persons with low back pain: those with pain of 2 to 4 weeks duration.[51] Among those with pain for less than 2 weeks there was no advantage for manipulation, perhaps because of the overall highly favorable prognosis in this group. The study of Godfrey, et al., reported no significant differences between manipulation and alternative treatments (massage or electrostimulation), but a short term trend substantially favored manipulation, and the statistical methods may have been inappropriate.[52] The trial of Mathews, et al., compared manipulation with local heat for a total of 291 patients with pain of less than 3 months duration. Manipulation resulted in better outcomes, most significantly among subjects with limited straight leg raising or a positive femoral nerve stretch test.[53]

Several negative trials of manipulation have also been reported, although these suffered variably from heterogeneous interventions, unequal cointerventions, high attrition, and often the inclusion of patients with chronic pain.[54–59]

In the case of chronic back pain, there is no evidence for the efficacy of manipulation. A well designed trial comparing short wave diathermy with manipulation in this setting found no difference in treatment effect.[59] The two trials by Jayson's group unfortunately combined manipulation with traction, which was not provided to the control group. Nonetheless, the experimental treatment was found to be efficacious among primary care outpatients with acute back problems, but not among referred patients with problems of longer duration.[55]

Complications of lumbar spine manipulation appear to be extremely rare, but can be disastrous when they occur. Thus, isolated reports exist of cauda equina syndrome, vertebral fractures, and new disc herniations.[60–62] The occurrence of pathologic fractures in patients with undiagnosed malignancy (but normal x rays) emphasizes the need for careful diagnostic evaluation prior to manipulation.[63]

Traction

Although traction has been used to treat low back pain since the time of Hippocrates, surprisingly little evidence exists to support its value in this setting. Indeed, the weight of the evidence suggests that spinal traction for lumbar pain is not efficacious, although its use for other syndromes (e.g., cervical spine disease) may be more appropriate. The principle of traction is to stretch the back so that vertebrae are pulled away from each other, and it is possible to demonstrate radiographically that the disc space is increased with adequate spinal traction. Physiologic studies suggest that an applied weight of 25% of body weight is necessary to overcome the inertia and resistance of the supine body, and to achieve distraction of lumbar vertebrae.[64]

Table 16–5 lists several randomized clinical trials of traction for lumbar spine disease, including patients with sciatica, back pain plus sciatica, and radiographically proven disc herniations.[53,54,65–70] These trials suffered from a variety of methodologic flaws, with some having high patient attrition or no description of patient attrition, some being unblinded, and some employing unequal cointerventions for the treatment groups. None of these trials reported on statistical power. Nonetheless, the degree of concordance in results is striking. Among all the trials of conventional traction (using weights or motorized traction) the results are uniformly negative. The only positive randomized trial we identified was a trial of "autotraction," in which the tractive force was applied by the patient himself by pulling with the arms. In this trial, autotraction appeared to be superior to a corset with regard to pain and straight leg raising, but functional outcomes were not reported.[70] The use of a corset as the control group is also problematical because patient blinding was obviously impossible, and because the use of sham traction as in other studies would have been preferable. The study of Weber included an autotraction arm in which the results were negative.[69]

A variety of devices utilizing gravity to apply the tractive force (e.g., tilt tables and gravity boots) are currently marketed, but no controlled trials of these devices could be identified. Furthermore, it is clear that gravity inversion has a number of adverse ocular and cardiovascular consequences that could be important for individual patients.[71,72] Other devices, such as the "90-90" traction method,[73] also appear not to have been evaluated in truly randomized trials. Overall, a consensus panel of the Quebec Task Force on Spinal Disorders concluded that there was no scientific evidence to support the use of spinal traction.[74]

Spinal Orthoses

Lumbosacral supports have been used since 2000 years BC, primarily for enhancing the female form. Medical use to support the lumbar spine dates at least from 1530, when an iron corset was fabricated for Catherine of Medici.[75] Rigid lumbar supports (including corsets and braces) are now widely used for pain relief. These devices are prescribed with a variety of rationales, including restriction of lumbosacral motion, abdominal support, and postural correction.

Table 16–5
Randomized Trials of Traction for Lumbar Spine Disease

First Author	n	Traction Method	Patient Description	Blind Assessment	Results
Coxhead	292	motorized*	sciatica	No	Negative
Lidstrom	62	motorized*	LBP + sciatica	Yes	Negative
Weber	86	motorized*	herniated disc	No	Negative
Mathews	27	weight	sciatica	Yes	Negative
Pal	41	weight	LBP + sciatica	Yes	Negative
Weber	72	motorized*	herniated disc	Yes	Negative
	44	"Spina-Trac"	"	"	Negative
	49	Autotraction	"	"	Negative
	50	Manual traction	"	"	Negative
Larsson	82	Autotraction	LBP + sciatica	Yes	Autotraction better than corset
Mathews	143	weight	LBP + sciatica	Yes	Negative (except for women < 45 years)

*Tru-Trac Device

These pathophysiologic concepts have been challenged, and some authors have raised a concern about exacerbating disuse atrophy of important muscle groups.[64] Radiographic studies demonstrate that various supports can reduce angular movement of the lumbar vertebrae, with the most effective devices essentially being body casts, which are applied to the trunk and sometimes to one leg as well.[75]

Randomized trials of these immobilizing devices are sparse. One randomized trial suggested that the use of a corset with a rigid supportive insert was more successful in reducing pain than a similar corset without the insert.[76] Unfortunately, the study included only 19 patients, did not assess patient compliance, and did not blind the outcome assessments. A second trial suggested that use of corsets was less effective than "autotraction."[70] A third trial showed no benefit of a fabric corset, but also suffered from unblinded assessment and no measure of compliance.[54] The Quebec Task Force concluded that there was no scientific evidence to support the efficacy of corsets for lumbar spine disorders, and definitive clinical trials have not been forthcoming.[74]

RECOMMENDATIONS FOR CONSERVATIVE CARE

The tentative nature of these treatment recommendations should be emphasized. In most cases, definitive trials are unavailable, and these recommendations are based on fragmentary evidence. A number of important studies are currently in progress, and their results may certainly modify the recommendations provided here. Nonetheless, the treatment strategies described here are based on the best available clinical data.

General Considerations

Patients with acute low back pain should be reassured of the good prognosis of back pain and informed that the vast majority of back problems are not disabling. They should be advised of the excellent prognosis for return to normal activities and usual work. Second, patients should be reassured that mild or moderate pain as they resume increasing activities will not cause permanent harm. A return to strict activity limitation is in most cases inadvisable. When patients are advised to "let pain be your guide" the outcomes appear to be worse than when specific activity goals are prescribed regardless of discomfort.[14] Furthermore, lengthy activity limitation in the form of bed rest appears not to reduce the duration of pain in most acute episodes.[12,13] Third, the clinician should remember that compli-

ance with many regimens (especially exercise or lifestyle changes) is difficult. It is often true that sedentary persons may benefit most from lifestyle changes, but be least likely to comply with them. Compliance-enhancing strategies that appear to be successful include the provision of both verbal and written instructions and closer patient supervision with more frequent followup. Other general compliance improving strategies are detailed elsewhere.[77]

Bed Rest

Bed rest recommendations for persons without neurologic deficits should generally be brief; 2 to 3 days are sufficient for most. Some ambulation can probably be permitted during this time, to limit muscular and cardiovascular deconditioning. A more detailed set of recommendations concerning bed rest is provided in Table 16–6.

Exercise

Physiologic data demonstrate that standing results in smaller loads on the intervertebral disc than sitting, so that patients can be encouraged to begin walking regularly almost as soon as bed rest is complete. After the most acute pain has subsided (usually within 2 weeks), aerobic conditioning can be recommended for most patients. The intent is to improve muscle endurance and reduce the likelihood of subsequent strain and recurrence. Aerobics may also help to reduce obesity and improve the patient's sense of well being.

The clinician must consider a patient's current level of fitness and other illnesses (e.g., vascular disease or extremity arthritis), when initiating an aerobic fitness program. Readily obtainable goals for the exercise program should be clear at the beginning and directed at achieving the functional ability necessary for work or recreational pursuits. A specific type of exercise is probably unnecessary, with swimming, jogging, walking, and bicycling all generally

Table 16–6
Recommendations Concerning Bed Rest

1. Prolonged bed rest (even 1 to 2 weeks) is inadvisable for most patients without neurologic deficits.
2. Brief rest (1 to 3 days) offers symptom relief for some, but probably does not improve the course of recovery.
3. Reassure the patient that moderate activity is not harmful, even if there is some pain.
4. Patients in physically demanding jobs may require more than 1 to 3 days off work, even if not at bed rest beyond this time.
5. For patients with neuromotor deficits, longer and stricter bed rest is probably appropriate.

appropriate, according to patient preference.[18] Exercise programs that could result in major twisting or bending forces on the spine, such as rowing or certain types of aerobic dance, should be avoided. Exercise sessions should include warmup and cooldown periods, and these may usefully include muscle stretching exercises such as those recommended by the YMCA.[19,22,23] For patients with subacute back pain (6 to 12 weeks) aerobic conditioning and stretching exercises are probably still appropriate, but closer supervision may be necessary. For those with pain that "centralizes" on extension, an extension regimen, such as that outlined by McKenzie, should probably be added. Such a regimen would be avoided if the pain were aggravated by extension or if the patient clearly had spinal stenosis, spondylolisthesis, or moderate scoliosis.

Lifestyle Modification

Although there is no clinical trial evidence to support the efficacy of weight loss and smoking cessation, there is both epidemiologic and physiologic evidence to suggest that these interventions may be useful in preventing recurrences of back pain. Both obesity and smoking are risk factors for back pain, and there is fragmentary observational evidence that smoking cessation may reduce the likelihood of recurrent back problems.

Medication

Good evidence exists to support the efficacy of most nonsteroidal anti-inflammatory drugs (probably including aspirin) for patients with acute low back pain. Some patients with acute severe sciatica may benefit from narcotic analgesics such as codeine, but these drugs should be used very selectively because of their side effects and potential for habituation. Some patients with severe back pain may benefit from muscle relaxant therapy, and carisoprodol may be particularly effective in this regard. Again, side effects, sedation, and the potential for habituation should make the use of these drugs highly selective.

For elderly patients, use NSAIDs cautiously and carefully monitor the patient. The risk of major gastrointestinal bleeding and adverse renal effects appears to be highest in this subpopulation.

Spinal Manipulation

Physicians should keep an open mind about the potential value of spinal manipulation. There is accumulating evidence that some types of spinal manipulation may have short-term, but not long-term benefits. Nonetheless, if patients are able to return to work or their usual activities sooner than would otherwise be possible, manipulation may be an important treatment modality. It is incumbent on the physician, however, to conduct an adequate diagnostic evaluation prior to referral for manipulation, to ensure that patients with systemic diseases (e.g., malignancy) or neurologic deficits are detected. On the basis of existing evidence, it appears unlikely that patients with chronic back pain or those with very acute back pain (those with the very best prognosis) will benefit from spinal manipulation. Current trials may shed further light on this ongoing controversy.

Traction, Orthoses, Heat, Massage, and Ultrasound

Almost no scientifically acceptable evidence exists to support the efficacy of these treatment modalities. Clinicians should be circumspect in their use, recognizing that many apparent responses may well be due to placebo effects plus the favorable natural history of the condition. Despite their long traditions of use, these treatments cannot be considered to have demonstrated efficacy.

REFERENCES

1. White, A.A., Gordon, S.L.: Synopsis: workshop on idiopathic low-back pain. Spine 7:141–149, 1982.
2. Currey, H.L.F., et al.: A prospective study of low back pain. Rheumatol Rehabil 19:94, 1979.
3. Deyo, R.A., Tsui-Wu, Y.-J.: Descriptive epidemiology of low-back pain and its related medical care in the United States. Spine 12:264, 1987.
4. Cypress, B.K.: Characteristics of physician visits for back symptoms: a national perspective. Am J Public Health 73:389–395, 1983.
5. Waddell, G.: A new clinical model for the treatment of low back pain. Spine 12:632–644, 1987.
6. Chalmers, T.C., Celano, P., Sacks, H.S., Smith, H.: Bias in treatment assignment in controlled clinical trials. N Engl J Med 22:1358–1361, 1983.
7. Deyo, R.A.: Conservative therapy for low back pain: distinguishing useful from useless therapy. JAMA 250:1057–1062, 1983.
8. Department of Clinical Epidemiology and Biostatistics, McMaster University Health Sciences Centre: How to read clinical journals: V. To distinguish useful from useless or even harmful therapy. Can Med Assoc J 124:1156–1162, 1981.
9. Deyo, R.A.: Compliance with therapeutic regimens in arthritis: issues, current status, and a future agenda. Semin Arthritis Rheum 12:233–244, 1982.
10. Nachemson, A.: The lumbar spine: an orthopaedic challenge. Spine 1:59–71, 1976.
11. Wiesel, S.W., et al.: Acute low back pain: An objective analysis of conservative therapy. Spine 5:324–330, 1980.

12. Deyo, R.A., Diehl, A.K., Rosenthal, M.: How many days of bed rest for acute low back pain? A randomized clinical trial. N Engl J Med 315:1064–1070, 1986.

13. Gilbert, J.R., Taylor, D.W., Hildebrand, A., Evans, C.: Clinical trial of common treatments for low back pain in family practice. Br Med J 291:791–794, 1985.

14. Fordyce, W.E., Brockway, J.A., Bergman, J.A., Spengler, D.: Acute back pain: a control-group comparison of behavioral vs. traditional management methods. J Behav Med 9:127–140, 1986.

15. Krolner, B., Toft, B.: Vertebral bone loss: an unheeded side effect of therapeutic bed rest. Clinical Science 64:537–540, 1983.

16. Muller, E.A.: Influence of training and of activity on muscle strength. Arch Phys Med Rehabil 51:449–462, 1970.

17. Convertino, V., Hung, J., Goldwater, D., DeBusk, R.F.: Cardiovascular responses to exercise in middle-aged men after 10 days of bedrest. Circulation 65:134–140, 1982.

18. Nutter, P.: Aerobic exercise in the treatment and prevention of low back pain. Spine: State-of-the-Art Reviews 2(1):137–145, 1987.

19. Kraus, H.: Backache, stress, and tension: cause, prevention, and treatment. New York. Simon and Schuster, 1965.

20. McKenzie, R.A.: Prophylaxis in recurrent low back pain. N Z Med J 89:22–23, 1979.

21. Cady, I., Bischoff, D.P., O'Connell, E.R., Thomas, R.C., Allan, J.H.: Strength and fitness and subsequent back injuries in firefighters. J Occup Med 21:269–272, 1979.

22. Kraus, H., Nagler, W., Melleby, A.: Evaluation of an exercise program for back pain. Am Fam Physician 28:153–158, 1983.

23. Kraus, H., Melleby, H., Gaston, S.R.: Back pain correction and prevention. National voluntary organizational approach. NY State J Med 77:1335–1338, 1977.

24. Deyo, R.A., Walsh, N., Martin, D., Schoenfeld, L., Ramamurthy, S.: A controlled trial of transcutaneous electrical nerve stimulation (TENS) and exercise for chronic low back pain. N Engl J Med 322:1627–1634, 1990.

25. Kendall, P.H., Jenkins, J.M.: Exercises for backache: a double-blind controlled trial. Physiotherapy 54:154–157, 1968.

26. Davies, J.E., Gibson, T., Tester, L.: The value of exercises in the treatment of low back pain. Rheumatol Rehabil 18:243–247, 1979.

27. DiMaggio, A., Mooney, V.: The McKenzie program: exercise effective against back pain. J Musculoskel Med December:63–74, 1987.

28. Manniche, C., Hesselsoe, G., Bentzen, L., Christensen, I., Lundberg, E.: Clinical trial of intensive muscle training for chronic low back pain. Lancet 11:473–476, 1988.

29. Deyo, R.A., Bass, J.E.: Lifestyle and low-back pain: the influence of smoking and obesity. Spine 14:501–506, 1989.

30. Heliovaara, M.: Body height, obesity, and risk of herniated lumbar intervertebral disc. Spine 12:469–472, 1987.

31. Kelsey, J.L. et al.: Acute prolapsed lumbar intervertebral disc: an epidemiological study with special reference to driving automobiles and cigarette smoking. Spine 9:608–613, 1984.

32. Frymoyer, J.W., et al.: Risk factors in low-back pain. J Bone Joint Surg 65A:213, 1983.

33. Hickey, R.F.J.: Chronic low back pain: A comparison of diflunisal with paracetamol. N Z Med J 95:312–314, 1982.

34. Amlie, E., Weber, H., Holme, I.: Treatment of acute low-back pain with piroxicam: results of a double-blind placebo-controlled trial. Spine 12:473–476, 1987.

35. Aoki, T., et al.: Multicentre double-blind comparison of piroxicam and indomethacin in the treatment of lumbar diseases. Eur J Rheumatol Inflamm 6:247–252, 1983.

36. Berry, H., et al.: Naproxen sodium, diflunisal, and placebo in the treatment of chronic back pain. Ann Rheum Dis 41:129–132, 1982.

37. Roth, S.H.: Nonsteroidal anti-inflammatory drugs: gastropathy, deaths, and medical practice. Ann Intern Med 109:353–354, 1988.

38. Johnson, E.W.: The myth of skeletal muscle spasm. Am J Phys Med Rehabil 68:1, 1989.

39. Waddell, G., et al.: Normality and reliability in the clinical assessment of backache. Br Med J 284:1519–1523, 1982.

40. Hindle, T.H.: Comparison of carisoprodol, butabarbital, and placebo in treatment of the low back syndrome. Calif Med 117:7–11, 1972.

41. Boyles, W.F., Glassman, J.M., Soyka, J.P.: Management of acute musculoskeletal conditions: thoracolumbar strain or sprain. A double-blind evaluation comparing the efficacy and safety of carisoprodol with diazepam. Today's Therapeutic Trends 1(1):1, 1983.

42. Hingorani, K.: Diazepam in backache: A double-blind controlled trial. Ann Phys Med 8:303–306, 1966.

43. Brown, B.R., Womble, J.: Cyclobenzaprine in intractable pain syndromes with muscle spasm. JAMA 240:1151–1152, 1978.

44. Dapas, F., et al.: Baclofen for the treatment of acute low-back syndrome: A double blind comparison with placebo. Spine 10:345–349, 1985.

45. Berry, H., Hutchison, D.R.: A multicentre placebo-controlled study in general practice to evaluate the efficacy and safety of tizanidine in acute low-back pain. J Int Med Res 16:75–82, 1988.

46. Berry, H., Hutchison, D.R.: Tizanidine and ibuprofen in acute low-back pain: results of a double-blind multicentre study in general practice. J Int Med Res 16:83–91, 1988.

47. Schnebel, B.E., Simmons, J.W.: The use of oral colchicine for low-back pain: a double-blind study. Spine 13:354–357, 1988.

48. Lanza, F.L., et al.: Endoscopic evaluation of the effects of aspirin, buffered aspirin, and enteric-coated aspirin on gastric and duodenal mucosa. N Engl J Med 303:136–138, 1980.

49. Farrell, J.P., Twomey, L.T.: Acute low back pain: Comparison of two conservative treatment approaches. Med J Aust 1:160–164, 1982.

50. Hoehler, F.K., Tobis, J.S., Buerger, A.A.: Spinal manipulation for low back pain. JAMA 245:1835–1838, 1981.

51. Hadler, N.M., Curtis, P., Gillings, D.B., Stinnett, S.: A benefit of spinal manipulation as adjunctive therapy for acute low-back pain: a stratified controlled trial. Spine 12:703–706, 1987.

52. Godfrey, C.M., Morgan, P.P., Schatzker, J.: A randomized trial of manipulation for low-back pain in a medical setting. Spine 9:301–304, 1984.

53. Mathews, J.A., et al.: Back pain and sciatica: controlled trials of manipulation, traction, sclerosant, and epidural injections. Br J Rheumatol 26:416–423, 1987.

54. Coxhead, C.E., et al: Multicentre trial of physiology in the management of sciatic symptoms. Lancet 1:1065–1068, 1981.

55. Jayson, M.I.V., et al: Mobilization and manipulation for low back pain. Spine 6:409–416, 1981.

56. Doran, D.M.L., Newel, D.J.: Manipulation in treatment of low back pain: a multicentre study. Br Med J 2:161–164, 1975.

57. Glover, J.R., Morris, J.G., Khosla, T.: Back pain: a randomized clinical trial of rotational manipulation of the trunk. Br J Ind Med 31:59–64, 1974.

58. Evans, D.P., et al.: Lumbar spinal manipulation on trial: I. Clinical assessment, II. Radiological assessment. Rheumatol Rehabil 17:46–59, 1978.

59. Gibson, T., et al: Controlled comparison of short-wave diathermy treatment with osteopathic treatment in non-specific low back pain. Lancet 1:1258–1261, 1985.

60. Dan, N.G., Saccasan, P.A.: Serious complications of lumbar spinal manipulation. Med J Austr 2:672–673, 1983.

61. Malmivaara, A., Pahjola, R.: Cauda equina syndrome caused by chiropraxis on a patient previously free of lumbar spine symptoms. Lancet 2:986–987, 1982.

62. Gallinaro, P., Cartesegna, M.: Three cases of lumbar disc rup-

ture and one of cauda equina associated with spinal manipulation (chiropraxis). Lancet 1:41, 1983.

63. Austin, R.T.: Pathological vertebral fractures after spinal manipulation. Br Med J 291:1114–1115, 1985.

64. Quinet, R.J., Hadler, N.M.: Diagnosis and treatment of backache. Semin Arthritis Rheum 8:261–287, 1979.

65. Lidstrom, A., Zachrisson, M.: Physical therapy on low back pain and sciatica: An attempt at evaluation. Scand J Rehabil Med 2:37–42, 1970.

66. Weber, H.: Traction therapy in sciatica due to disc prolapse. J Oslo City Hosp 23:167–176, 1973.

67. Mathews, J.A., Hickling, J.: Lumbar traction: A double-blind controlled study for sciatica. Rheumatol Rehabil 14:222, 1975.

68. Pal, B., Mangion, P., Hossain, M.A., Diffey, B.L.: A controlled trial of continuous lumbar traction in the treatment of back pain and sciatica. Br J Rheumatol 25:181–183, 1986.

69. Weber, H., Ljunggren, A.E., Walker, L.: Traction therapy in patients with herniated lumbar intervertebral discs. J Oslo City Hosp 34:61–70, 1984.

70. Larsson, U., et al.: Auto-traction for treatment of lumbago-sciatica: a multicentre controlled investigation. Acta Orthop Scand 51:791–798, 1980.

71. Gianakopoulos, G., et al.: Inversion devices: their role in producing lumbar distraction. Arch Phys Med Rehabil 66: 100–102, 1985.

72. Friberg, T.R., Weinreb, R.N.: Ocular manifestations of gravity inversion. JAMA 253:1755–1757, 1985.

73. Cottrell, G.W.: New, conservative, and exceptionally effective treatment for low back pain. Compr Ther 11(11):59–65, 1985.

74. Quebec Task Force on Spinal Disorders: Scientific approach to the assessment and management of activity-related spinal disorders: a monograph for clinicians. Spine (Suppl) 12(7): S22–S30, 1987.

75. Fidler, M.W., Plasmans, C.M.T.: The effect of four types of support on the segmental mobility of the lumbosacral spine. J Bone Joint Surg 65A:943–947, 1983.

76. Million, R., et al.: Evaluation of low back pain and assessment of lumbar corsets with and without back supports. Ann Rheum Dis 40:449–454, 1981.

77. Sackett, D.L., Haynes, R.B., Tugwell, P.: Compliance. In Clinical Epidemiology, A Basic Science for Clinical Medicine. Boston. Little, Brown, 1985.

Philip E. Greenman

17

The Osteopathic View of Acute Spinal Disorders

Back pain continues to be a major problem to society and to the health care professionals providing for its care. Eighty percent of the population will have at least one disabling episode of low back pain in their lifetime. Low back pain becomes a challenge to the physician because 60 to 80% is idiopathic in nature.[1] I concur with Farfan who said: "I believe that the etiological factor of back pain is mechanical in nature." Farfan further stated that " . . . there are many side effects of excessive mechanical stress in a tissue, which may be involved singly or severally in exciting the central nervous system."[2] Extensive nociceptor receptor systems are located in the skin, subcutaneous tissues, capsules of the apophyseal facet joints and sacroiliac joints, ligaments, periosteum, dura mater, blood vessels, and muscles.[3] The challenge is to identify the site of the nociception and to identify the pathologic process present. One must search for not only the anatomical pathologic condition but also that condition which interferes with function. Anatomic, structural, and functional pathologies can occur either singly or in combination.

CONCEPTS

The osteopathic profession has long clinical experience in identifying and treating functional alterations of the musculoskeletal system. The osteopathic physician uses structural diagnosis and manual medicine procedures within the context of total patient care (Table 17-1).[4] The diagnostic principle is to identify the altered functional capacity and restore it as much as possible. The identifiable altered functional capacity can be in the presence of normal anatomy, or in anatomy that is altered because of developmental variations, trauma, or previous surgical intervention.

The osteopathic physician seeks the manipulable lesion, which is currently termed somatic dysfunction.[5] It is defined as impaired or altered function of related components of the somatic (body framework) system; skeletal, arthrodial, and myofascial structures; and related vascular, lymphatic, and neural elements. The structural diagnostic process seeks to identify areas of somatic dysfunction that may contribute to the patient's back pain complaint.

The goal of therapy is to maximize the structural and functional posture balance to the musculoskeletal system. To achieve that goal one looks to balance the vertebral and bony pelvis mechanics with particular emphasis on developing a balanced base of support. This includes attention to leg length and pelvic obliquity. Attention is given to the achievement of equal length and strength of the muscles of the lower extremity and of the trunk. Any identifiable muscle disorders, such as myofascial trigger points, must be effectively treated to enhance muscle function. The use of postural exercises to enhance the functional capacity of the musculoskeletal system is included in the treatment plan, as is aerobic conditioning. It is useful to institute a program of proprioceptive training to assist in the achievement of the goal (Table 17-2).

Another concept of patient management is appropriate education. The patient must be aware of the natural course of the disease and that 90% of back pain patients find their condition to be self limiting.

Table 17–1
Concepts

1. Diagnose somatic dysfunction.
2. Integrate structural diagnosis into total patient evaluation.
3. Apply appropriate manual medicine procedures to significant areas of somatic dysfunction.
4. Maximize functional capacity of the musculoskeletal system.

Table 17–2
Goals of Osteopathic Treatment

1. Enhance postural balance of the musculoskeletal system.
2. Enhance vertebral, segmental, and sacroiliac mobility.
3. Develop a balanced base of support including attention to anatomic short lower extremity.
4. Achieve balance in length and strength of muscles of trunk and lower extremities.
5. Increase aerobic conditioning.
6. Enhance appropriate body posture in activities of daily living.

The patient must become a partner in the treatment plan. Instruction is provided for appropriate body postures to avoid aggravating the condition, both in the activities of daily living at home, as well as the ergonomics of the work site.[6] It is important that the patient understand the activities that might aggravate the condition and that he performs those activities that will assist in the restoration of maximal functional balance. When using therapeutic exercises in the treatment plan, the patient must be aware of the difference between hurt and harm. Frequently during the restorative phase, some increase in symptoms occurs because of the activity in the dysfunctional areas of the musculoskeletal system. It is important that the patient understand that these activities are not causing additional harm, but in fact are important in the treatment of the condition. Long-term management also requires that the patient is aware of self-help programs that can be used to prevent nondependence upon the health care delivery system.

DIAGNOSIS

The diagnostic process starts with a complete history and physical examination. A rapid triage decision must be made to determine if the condition is life threatening; if it has the potential for severe disability; or if it can be evaluated by a standard examination. Few conditions of the musculoskeletal system are life threatening. However it is not uncommon for a patient to present with back pain caused by a disorder of an internal organ system, such as a dissecting aneurysm, myocardial infarction, or acute pancreatitis. Conditions that might result in severe and permanent disability are those such as acute caudal equina syndrome. These conditions are rare.

History

The patient's history is probably the most important part of the diagnostic process for those presenting with back pain. The history should be comprehensive and include assessment of the family history with particular interest in any genetic tendency toward musculoskeletal problems. A system review is made to rule out disease processes within the organ systems and particularly to identify organic, metabolic, inflammatory, or neoplastic disease that may involve the musculoskeletal system. The past personal history for serious illnesses, operations, and particularly injuries, is necessary. Most patients will have many minor injuries, which seem to them to be of little consequence, but in the overall analysis of their problem can be significant. It is necessary to obtain a work history, particularly if there appears to be an occupational element to the onset and persistence of the back pain complaint. It is useful to get a history of life events, which frequently causes the patient to recall factors that are valuable in determining the origin of the patient's problem.

A detailed history of the back pain is carried out with particular emphasis on the type and time of onset. Did a single injury or a series of microtrauma precede the pain complaint? Was the onset insidious? It is essential to probe the mechanism of injury, whether it is single or multiple. Significant dysfunction can occur with awkward body postures, particularly simultaneous forward bending and twisting, which induces non-neutral coupling mechanics of the lumbar spine. Relatively insignificant trauma, such as a slip and fall, can traumatize the sacroiliac joint resulting in disability far in excess of that anticipated by the minor trauma. Have there been previous episodes that are similar or dissimilar? Where is the pain located? Useful information can be gained from having the patient point directly to the pain. Does the patient point with a single finger or with the whole hand? Where does the pain radiate? Does it proceed into the lower extremities, and if so, what is the distribution? What relieves the pain? Factors such as rest, activity, over-the-counter medication, application of heat or cold, are useful data. Similarly, what makes the pain worse? In making a diagnosis of functional disease, it is most valuable to understand those body postures which help or worsen the pain.

Amount of Disability

As part of the acquisition of the data base, some assessment should be made regarding the amount of disability that the back pain is causing. Instruments such as the Roland Morris scale[7] can be used to quantify the amount of disability caused by the back pain. A baseline pain drawing[8] can be useful in identifying whether the pain pattern is anatomical in nature and in identifying the rare patient presenting with a psychological cause. Some assessment of the patient's perception of pain should be made as part of the data base. Items such as the visual analogue pain scale can provide a baseline from which assessment can be made throughout the treatment plan.

Physical Examination

The physical examination is guided by the history and leads one to focus upon the definition of the areas of somatic dysfunction that would be most amenable to osteopathic manipulative treatment (Table 17-3). The physical examination should be comprehensive and integrate the evaluation of the total patient. One is particularly interested in ruling out any related or nonrelated disease states that may require direct attention, including those that require referral to a specialist. In addition to the general physical examination, particular attention is given to vascular, neurologic, and orthopaedic testing.

The integrity of the vascular system is evaluated by palpation of central and peripheral pulses. Integrity of the vasculature of the upper extremity is made by palpating the brachial, radial, and ulnar arteries with provocative tests like the Adson maneuver. Palpation and auscultation of the carotid arteries bilaterally checks for the vascular integrity to the head and neck. The abdominal aorta is palpated and auscultated for the presence of bruits and enlargement. The femoral, popliteal, dorsalis pedis, and posterior tibial arteries are palpated for the presence of normal peripheral pulsation.

Neurological Tests

The neurological examination tests for the presence of symmetric deep tendon reflexes of both the upper and lower extremities. The presence or absence of pathologic reflexes, such as Hoffman or Babinski sign, is elicited. Vibratory and position sense are tested to identify posterior column disease. The Rhomberg test and tandem walking are useful in evaluating primary spinal tract disease. Strength testing is made of both the upper and lower extremities using the traditional zero to five scale seeking muscle function that is normal or reduced. The sensory examination is viewed by some as the most important part of the neurological examination, and by others as being of little assistance.

The sensory examination is useful in determining specific dermatomal change in sensation, as well as differentiating nerve root from peripheral nerve sensory changes. A great deal can be learned from a well performed pinwheel examination. Root tension signs are then sought. Particularly valuable is the straight leg raising test. Straight leg raising can be used to identify four different conditions. First is straight leg raising to the limit of hamstring tightness. The extended leg is lifted while the opposite anterior superior iliac spine is monitored until the pelvis first begins to rotate in a posterior direction. The procedure is reversed on the opposite side and comparison is made to determine which leg has the greatest amount of excursion before pelvic rotation occurs as a function of shortened hamstring on the ipsilateral side. The same test can be used to elicit pain of a radicular nature extending throughout the lower extremity in a dermatomal pattern. A positive straight leg raising test for radicular pain must be corroborated by at least one other root tension sign. The exacerbation of radicular type pain by dorsiflexion of the foot (Braggard's sign), or the classic Lasegue sign of extension of the lower leg from the position of 90° flexion of the hip and knee, are two of the more useful root tension signs.[9] Straight leg raising that elicits pain at motion of the sacroiliac joint or lumbosacral conjunction can also be useful in differentiating dysfunction at these joint levels. The test can be given by simply monitoring the sacroiliac joint or lumbosacral junction while the straight leg raising maneuver is performed. One of the more pathognomonic signs of discogenic radiculopathy is the elicitation of radicular pain by straight leg raising of the contralateral leg.

Orthopaedic Test

In addition to neurologic testing, some orthopaedic tests exist that can assist in the identification of the pain generator. The Patrick Fabere (figure of four) test identifies disorder within both the hip and the sacroiliac joints. Most of the orthopaedic tests are used to identify anatomic disease; identification of functional disorders requires additional testing (Table 17-4).

The structural diagnostic process seeks to identify functional disorders within the musculoskeletal system. It begins with the evaluation of the gait with particular reference to the function of the lower ex-

Table 17–3
Principles of the Osteopathic Physical Examination

1. Integrate with total general physical examination.
2. Incorporate standard neurologic and orthopaedic tests.
3. Emphasize the evaluation of present somatic dysfunction using the diagnostic triad of:
   a. Asymmetry of form and function of components of MSK system.
   b. Range of motion tests particularly of vertebral and sacroiliac joints seeking hypomobility, normal mobility, and hypermobility.
   c. Tissue texture abnormalities including muscle spasm and hypertonicity; skin and subcutaneous tissue change of temperature, moisture, tension and tenderness.

tremities, pelvis, vertebral axis, upper extremities, and head during walking. In addition to giving attention to the neurologically disordered gait, the physician is interested in identifying alteration in symmetric function within the musculoskeletal system, particularly the symmetry of mobility of the pelvis and hip joints, the alternating sidebending and rotation of the trunk, and the cross-patterning of the upper extremities with the lower extremities. Tandem walking and walking on the heels and toes provide information regarding both the nervous system function and the muscle strength of the lower extremity.

The second step is to analyze the static posture of the patient in all four directions. One is particularly interested in identifying areas of asymmetry from right to left and in the integrity of the lateral posture as identified from the plumb line from the ear to the anterior aspect of the medial malleolus. One looks for the presence or absence of the normal cervical and lumbar lordosis, the thoracic kyphosis, and the position of the posterior sacral convexity against the weightbearing line. Increase or decrease of the lumbar lordosis can be most significant in patients presenting with lower back pain, and a common finding in patients with cervical and upper extremity pain syndromes is forward carriage of the head on the trunk. Palpate the heights against the horizontal plane of the shoulder girdles at the acromion process, at the iliac crests, and at the greater trochanters to identify areas of unleveling. Unleveling of the iliac crests and greater trochanters in the loaded standing weightbearing position alerts one to consider the possibility of the short leg and pelvic tilt syndrome.

The next step is to evaluate performance of the pelvis and vertebral column in forward bending with the feet separated at acetabular distance and with the knees straight. The physician monitors the posterior superior iliac spine and follows mobility during forward bending. This standing flexion test is viewed as negative if the posterior superior iliac spines move symmetrically in a ventral and cephalic direction. If one posterior superior iliac spine moves further in a ventral or cephalic direction, the test is viewed as being positive, and indicates restricted mobility on that side of the pelvis. The usual cause is restricted motion of the ipsilateral sacroiliac joint. False positive standing flexion tests can be present with organic disease of the sacroiliac joints (e.g., sacroiliitis), a tight quadratus lumborum on the ipsilateral side, or a tight hamstring on the contralateral side.

Evaluation is also made of the rhythmic or dysrhythmic behavior of the lumbar and thoracic spines in the forward bending challenge, with particular interest in the development of sidebending or rota-

Table 17–4
Tests for Sacroiliac Mobility

1. Standing and seated flexion tests.
2. Gillet's one legged stork test.
3. Springing tests.
4. Gapping tests.

tional irregularities. The one legged stork test of Gillet[10] is performed by monitoring the posterior superior iliac spine and the sacral crest on each side while the patient lifts the knee past horizontal hip flexion. This is a more specific test for sacroiliac mobility on one side as compared to the other. The patient is then asked to actively sidebend the trunk and an evaluation is made of the range of excursion down the lateral thigh and calf on each side. In addition to the range of motion, the physician observes the behavior of the lumbar spine. Normally there is a smooth sidebending curve to the same side with fullness on the opposite side of sidebending and each sidebending effort demonstrates symmetrical behavior. One evaluates the normal coupling function of the lumbar spine with sidebending and rotation to opposite sides. The patient is then seated with the feet supported on the floor and again the trunk is bent forward while the physician monitors the posterior superior iliac spine on each side (Fig. 17–1). This seated flexion test is interpreted similarly to that while standing and a unilateral increase in ventral or cephalic mobility is interpreted as resulting from restricted mobility of the ipsilateral sacroiliac joint. The behavior of the lumbar and thoracic spine during this forward bending challenge is compared to that which was observed while standing.

In the seated position the straight leg raising of the lower extremity is performed to look for nerve tension signs. The reflexes of the patellar and Achilles tendons are checked for symmetry. In the supine position the relative levels of the anterior superior iliac spines, pubic tubercles, and medial malleoli are evaluated. Muscle testing of the lower extremity is performed for symmetry. One is interested in comparative length as well as strength of the muscles of the lower extremities with particular reference to those of the hips and thighs. Straight leg raising and other root tension signs are performed in the supine position. The patient is then placed prone on the table and comparative levels of the medial malleoli, ischial tuberosities, inferior lateral angle of the sacrum, sacral base, and posterior superior iliac spine and tension of the sacrotuberous ligaments, are determined. The trunk is placed in an extended position to challenge the capacity of the facet joints to close and relative asymmetry of the position of the transverse processes of the lumbar spine and relative tension of the paravertebral musculature, par-

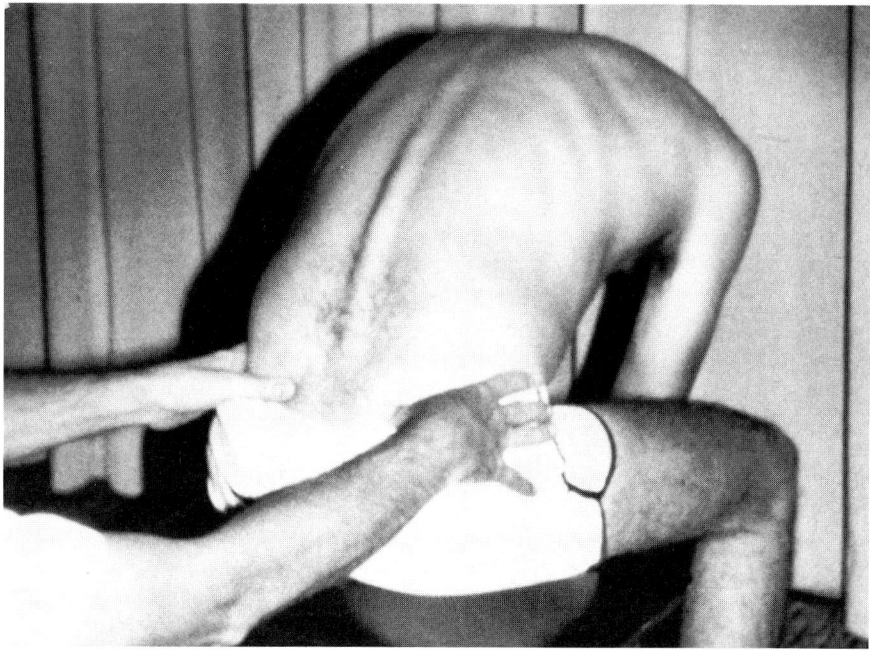

Figure 17–1. Seated flexion test.

ticularly the deep fourth layer muscles, is evaluated.

Based upon data accumulated in this examination, the diagnosis of somatic dysfunction is made from the presence of asymmetry of form and function, altered range of motion (primarily hypomobility), and tissue texture abnormality (particularly muscle hypertonicity). One is particularly interested in identifying the presence of restriction within the normal range of motion within the vertebral segment or region of the body. The restrictive barrier can be caused by altered muscle tone, altered fascial tension, edema, or abnormal joint congruence and mobility. Different restrictive barriers call for different types of manipulative therapy interventions. Areas of somatic dysfunction can appear in combination with anatomical diseases, such as degenerative and herniated lumbar discs, or can occur singly in the absence of many demonstrable anatomic pathologic processes. One must also determine if the defined somatic dysfunction is in fact significant in the patient's complaint; correlation of symptoms, the structural diagnostic findings of the somatic dysfunction, and other diagnostic procedures must be made.

Supplemental Tests

The diagnostic process also includes supplemental studies which should confirm the working diagnosis identified from the history and physical examination. Radiographic studies include the plane films with attention to the anatomy present, whether it is altered by developmental variation, trauma, or gross osseous disorder. Erect films can be used for postural analysis including leg length and level of the sacral base plane together with analysis of the lumbar scoliosis if present. These films can be supplemented by stress films of forward and backward bending and sidebending right and left. These dynamic studies assist in the evaluation of both hypomobility, hypermobility, and the presence or absence of normal coupling movement of the lumbar spine. Additional imaging techniques include bone scan, CT scanning, CT/myelogram, myelography, discography, and magnetic resonance imaging. All of these imaging procedures have their strengths and weaknesses and the appropriate choice is important in identifying the disease present. Electrodiagnosis, including EMG and nerve conduction studies, and additional somatosensory tests can provide evaluation of neurologic function to supplement the evaluation of the anatomy by imaging studies. Laboratory testing should include a CBC, a Westegren SED rate, a SMAC 20 and urinalysis. Based upon those results, additional supplemental laboratory studies may be made to identify inflammatory bone and joint disease.

TREATMENT

The goal of treatment of spinal disorders depends upon the diagnosis made. The basic principles however consist of pain relief, rest from function for a short term with acute situations, and restoration of

Table 17–5
The Manipulative Medicine Methodology

1. Soft tissue procedures (e.g., massage, deep pressure).
2. Articulatory procedures (mobilization without impulse).
3. High velocity, low amplitude thrust procedures (mobilization with impulse).
4. Muscle energy procedures.
5. Functional/indirect procedures.
6. Craniosacral procedures.
7. Release by positioning procedures.

function (the rehabilitative process) as soon as possible.

The use of manual medicine procedures depends upon the number and type of somatic dysfunctions present and their relationship to other disorders, the acuteness or chronicity of the problem, and the age and physical capacity of the patient. A broad variety of manipulative procedures are available and are classified according to the method of their engagement of the restriction present (barrier concept) including the type and location of the barrier, and the activating force used (Table 17-5).

The most common types of manipulative procedures are those classified as *direct action.* In direct action procedures the restrictive barrier is engaged by a process of localization and an activating force is generated, either by the physician or from within the patient in the direction of motion loss. *Exaggeration* techniques are those which move away from the restrictive barrier and engage the barrier in the direction opposite to the motion loss. *Indirect* procedures are those which identify the point of maximum ease in the range of motion between the normal barrier at one side and the restrictive barrier on the other.

The activating forces are classified as *intrinsic,* those generated from within the patient such as muscle contraction, respiration, and inherent body rhythms, and *extrinsic,* such as operator induced effort, gravity, or appliances (e.g., belts or traction).

EXAMPLES OF MANIPULATIVE PROCEDURES

Mobilization with Impulse (High Velocity, Low Amplitude Thrust) (Fig. 17–2).

Diagnostic Procedure: Posterior Rotation of the Right Innominate.

Motion Restriction: Anterior Rotation of the Right Innominate.

1. Patient lies in the left lateral recumbent position.
2. Patient's left shoulder is pulled forward and caudad introducing the neutral mechanics of left sidebending and right rotation of the trunk down to and including the sacrum.
3. Patient's lower extremity is extended to the first motion of the sacrum. Patient's right leg is flexed and placed in front of the lower left leg.
4. Operator's right hand monitors the sacral base with the right forearm controlling the upper trunk.
5. Operator's left hand contacts the posterior superior illiac spine and all slack is taken up.
6. A high velocity, low amplitude thrust is made by the operator's left forearm in an anterior direction

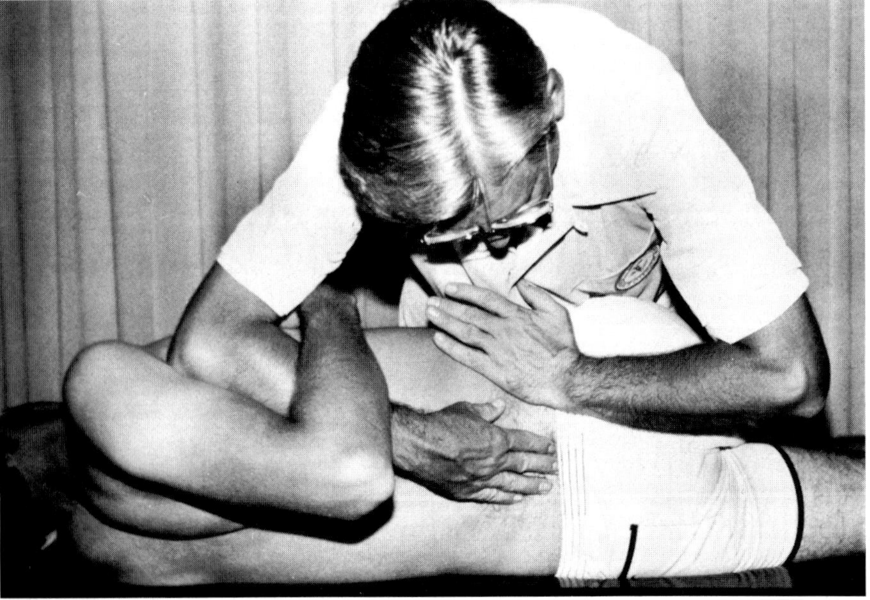

Figure 17–2. Mobilization with impulse (high velocity, low amplitude thrust) technique for right sacroiliac joint dysfunction.

causing the right innominate to rotate anteriorly in relation to the sacrum.

7. Re-examine for efficacy.

Muscle Energy Procedures (Fig. 17–3).

Diagnosis: Right Anterior Innominate.

Motion Restriction: Posterior Rotation, Right Innominate.

1. Patient prone on the table with the right knee and right hip flexed and with the foot held in position between the knees of the operator.
2. Operator monitors the right sacroiliac joint and stabilizes the sacrum with the left hand.
3. Operator's right hand controls the patient's right lower extremity and flexes, internally-externally rotates, and adducts/abducts to point of localization at the right sacroiliac joint.
4. Operator resists hip extension effort by the patient.

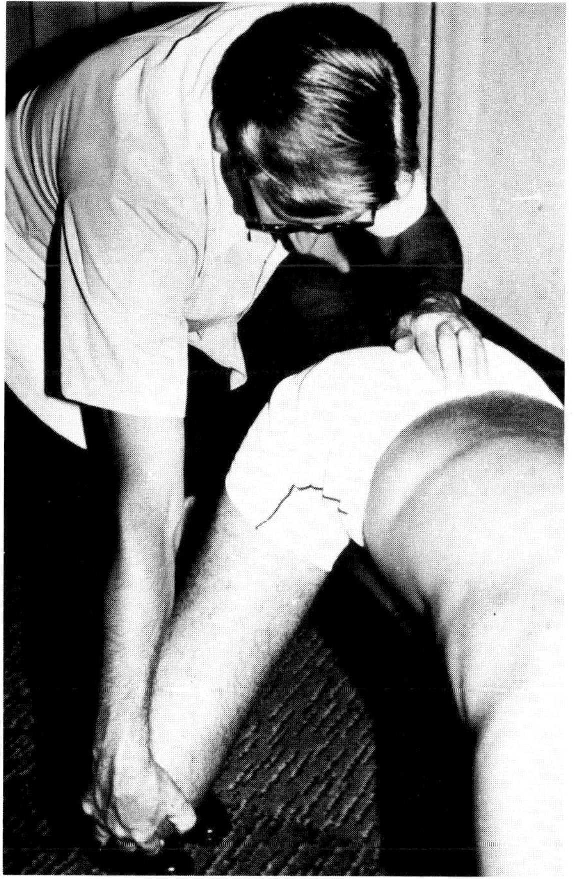

Figure 17–3. Muscle energy technique for right sacroiliac joint dysfunction.

5. The muscle energy effort is repeated three to five times until maximum posterior rotation of the right innominate is achieved.
6. Re-examine for efficacy.

Myofascial Release Technique.

Craniosacral Technique (Fig. 17–4).

Diagnosis: Restricted Posterior Nutation of Sacrum.

(Nutation is defined as the nodding movement of the sacrum between the two innominates. Anterior nutation results in the sacral base moving ventrally and the apex dorsally. Posterior nutation results in the sacral base moving dorsally and the apex ventrally.)

Motion Restriction

1. Patient prone on the table.
2. Operator monitors sacral base with left hand.
3. Operator's right hand overlying sacral apex.
4. Operator monitors inherent sacral nutation and counter nutation.
5. Operator enhances posterior nutational movement of the sacrum during the extension phase of inherent sacral motion.
6. A series of repetitions are followed until maximum posterior nutational movement of the sacrum is accomplished.
7. Re-examine for efficacy.

Mobilization Without Impulse (Articulatory Technique) (Fig. 17–5).

Diagnosis: A Lumbar Facet Dysfunction.

Motion Restriction: Lumbar Sidebending Left and Rotation Right.

1. Patient lies in lateral recumbent position.
2. Patient's left shoulder is directed anteriorly and caudally, introducing trunk left sidebending and right rotation to level of dysfunction.
3. Patient's right leg is flexed at the hip and knee with the right foot in the left popliteal space.
4. Operator's right forearm controls the upper trunk and left forearm controls the pelvis with both hands monitoring at dysfunctional segment.
5. Oscillatory motion is developed by either the operator's right or left forearm, exaggerating the patient's position to enhance mobility at dysfunctional segments.
6. Re-examine for efficacy.

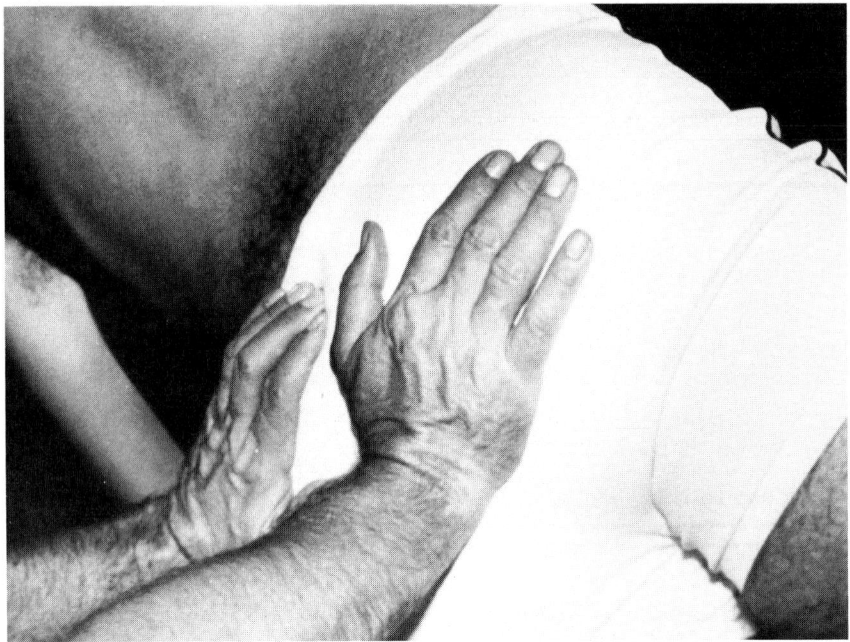

Figure 17–4. Craniosacral technique for bilateral sacroiliac joint dysfunction.

Functional, Indirect Technique (Fig. 17–6).

Diagnosis: Lumbar Facet Dysfunction.

Motion Restriction: Extension, Left Sidebending, Left Rotation.

1. Patient sits astride the table with operator controlling the upper trunk with the right forearm.

2. Operator monitors at the dysfunctional segment by finger or thumb.
3. Motion is directed by the operator in the directions of forward bending, right sidebending, and right rotation until a point of maximum ease is obtained.
4. Patient is instructed to inhale or exhale to point of maximum ease and to hold for 20 to 30 seconds.
5. Operator fine tunes the position of maximum

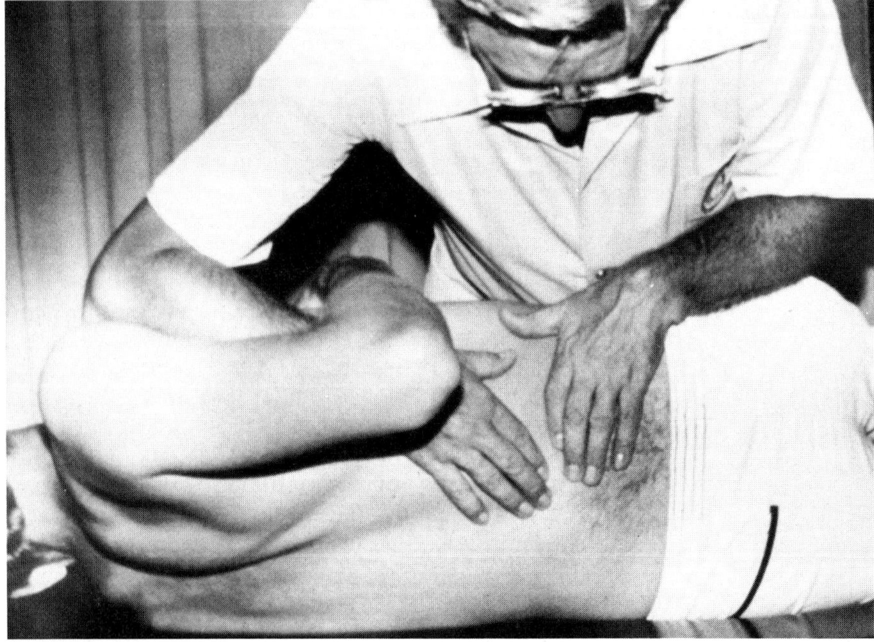

Figure 17–5. Mobilization without impulse (articulatory) technique for lumbar facet dysfunction.

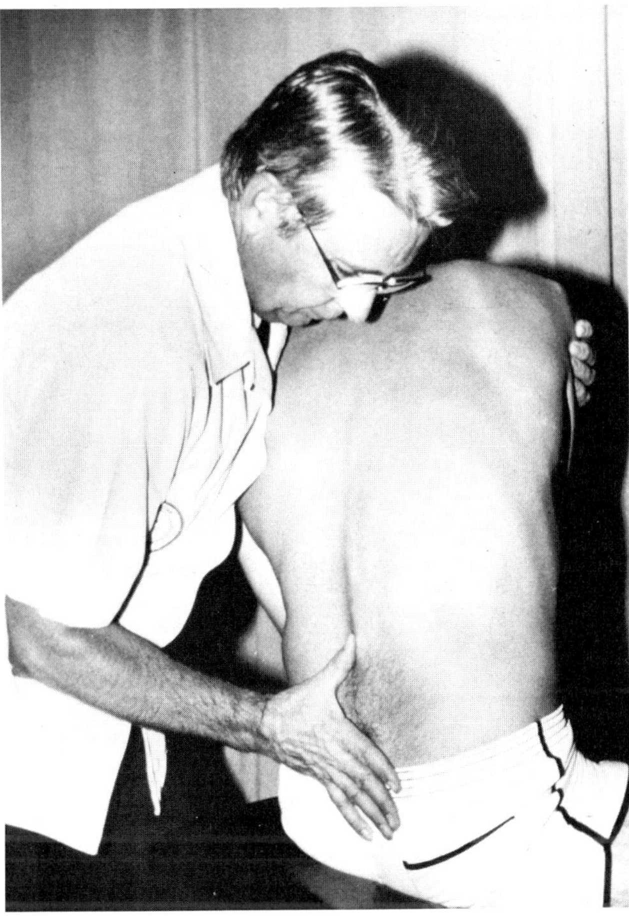

Figure 17–6. Functional/indirect technique for lumbar facet dysfunction.

ease of the dysfunctional segment in the directions of forward bending, right sidebending, right rotation, anterior/posterior translation, right/left translation, cephalic/caudad translation, and again respiratory effort is introduced to a point of maximum ease and held.
6. A series of repetitions are made until maximum release of the tissue surrounding the dysfunctional segment has occurred and the patient is then returned to neutral position.
7. Re-examine for efficacy.

One or more of these treatment modalities may be used at any one therapeutic session as appropriate.

Treatment Prescription

The manual medicine procedure should be prescribed just as any other therapeutic intervention.[11] One determines the type of manipulation, the length of treatment per visit, the frequency of applications, and the duration of the treatment program. The more acute the condition the shorter the treatment time and the shorter the interval between treatments. The more chronic the condition becomes, the more extensive is the treatment time per visit and the longer the time between visits to allow for change to occur. It is frequently noted that following a manipulative intervention there is a short term exacerbation of symptoms because of aggravation of inflamed connective tissues. Each subsequent evaluation should demonstrate improved functional capacity and better postural balance.

Adjunctive therapies include the appropriate use of ice and heat. Ice is particularly useful in acute injuries following a manipulative intervention, to reduce the amount of swelling of the connective tissues. In the later treatment phases appropriate use of intermittent heat can be useful in reducing muscle tension and tissue tightness and to enhance normal blood flow to the part. Overuse of heat can be detrimental in that application can congest the part and contribute to the tissue inflammatory process. Appropriate use of analgesics and nonsteroidal anti-inflammatory agents provides for pain control. Structured dosage schedules are preferred rather than a PRN basis. Occasionally, muscle relaxants are valuable, but caution must be used in those that particularly have central depressive actions. In the chronic phases amitriptyline or similar compounds are useful in both pain control and in restoring a more normal sleep cycle. Infrequently, corsets or supporting belts are used and then for only short periods of time, because the goal is to restore motion and not to restrict it. One favorite is the Hackett Cinch Sacroiliac Belt which provides dynamic tension around the bony pelvis and assists in the treatment of the sacroiliac syndrome. Orthotic and prosthetic devices are occasionally used, the most common being adjustment of heel and sole height in the presence of anatomic shortening of the leg or pelvic obliquity with the goal to level the weightbearing surface of the sacrum.

Most valuable is the use of individualized exercise programs to maximize the effectiveness of the manual medicine procedures to enhance mobility. Many exercise programs are available but the basic principle is threefold. First is to provide exercises to enhance sensory proprioception. These exercises include balance beam, rocker board, and rebounder techniques. With enhancement of proprioception input, the second phase is then initiated; it calls for the stretching of shortened and tightened muscles and muscle groups. When length has been restored then a strengthening program can be initiated. All three phases are directed toward restoration of maximal length and strength in postural balance of all muscle groups within the body. Appropriate aerobic conditioning is an essential component of the treatment plan and can be accomplished with cycling, treadmill, swimming, or other activities. Caution must be used in advocating running and jogging programs because of the observed aggravation of low back conditions in many individuals with degenerative disc and facet joint disease in the lumbar spine. An aerobic pep walk can be almost as effective for aerobic conditioning and is much less stressful to the lower back than jogging or running. Additionally, it provides a good stimulus for symmetrical sacroiliac and lumbar spine mobility. An individualized exercise program should also be prescribed for the workplace and for activities of daily living in the home. Appropriate instruction regarding body posture, movement, and the ergonomics of the workplace can all assist in the treatment of the current condition and the prevention of recurrence.

SUMMARY

From the osteopathic perspective, one is interested in evaluating and treating to achieve maximum functional balance of the musculoskeletal system, in addition to identifying and appropriately treating alterations in the anatomy caused by the disease that is present. Symptoms from dysfunction can occur in the presence or absence of other significant anatomic disorders. The structural diagnostic process is designed to evaluate the presence or absence of somatic dysfunction and its relative significance in the patient's presenting complaint. If somatic dysfunction is found to be significant, then appropriate manual medicine procedures are employed to restore maximum biomechanical function. This therapy is provided in conjunction with other medical, surgical, and physical therapy interventions as deemed appropriate. The key to the osteopathic approach is restoration of maximum functional capacity.

REFERENCES

1. Nachemson, A.: The lumbar spine—an orthopedic challenge. Spine 1:59–71, 1976.
2. Farfan, H.F.: The scientific basis of manipulative procedures. Clinics in Rheumatologic Diseases 6(1):159, 1980.
3. Wyke, B.: The neurology of low back pain. In The Lumbar Spine and Back Pain (Edited by M. Jayson) 2nd Ed. Kent, England, Pittman Medical Publishing, pp. 265–339, 1980.
4. Greenman, P.E.: Differential diagnosis of back pain. In Empirical Approaches to the Validation of Spinal Manipulation (Edited by A.A. Buerger and P.E. Greenman). Springfield, Charles C Thomas, pp. 87–105, 1985.
5. Ward, R.C., Sprafka, S.: Glossary of osteopathic terminology. J Am Osteopath Assoc 80:522–567, 1981.
6. Kirkaldy-Willis, E.S.H.: The back school. In Managing Low Back Pain (Edited by W.H. Kirkaldy-Willis). 2nd Ed. Churchill Livingstone, New York, Edinburgh, London, Melbourne, pp. 265–285, 1988.
7. Roland, M., Morris, R.: A study of the natural history of back pain. I: Development of a reliable and sensitive measure of disability in low back pain. Spine 8:141–144, 1983.
8. Ransford, A.O., Cairns, D., Mooney, V.: The pain drawing as an aid to the psychological evaluation of patients with low back pain. Spine 1:127–134, 1976.
9. Eaton, J.M.: The differential diagnosis of the low back syndrome. New York, Academy of Applied Osteopathy Yearbook 2:122–128, 1965.
10. Gillet, H.: Clinical measurements of sacroiliac mobility. Annals of Swiss Chiropractic Assoc. 6:59–70, 1976.
11. Kimberly, P.E.: Formulating a prescription for osteopathic manipulative treatment. J Am Osteopath Assoc 75:486–499, 1976.

George M. Smith

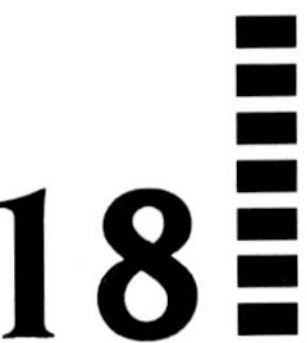

The Role of the Occupational Medicine Physician in the Management of Industrial Injury

INTRODUCTION

This chapter addresses the role of the occupational medicine physician (OMP) in managing injured employees in the industrial setting from a nonclinical perspective. The clinical aspects of managing the acute pain patient are well covered in the other chapters in this section, and, accordingly, here we review the essential nonclinical functions and responsibilities of the OMP and the methodology available to the OMP for carrying out those functions.

In confronting the occupational and employment-related issues surrounding an injured patient, a principle challenge to both the employer and the OMP arises out of the need to assemble sufficient reliable information about *both* the patient's medical condition and the work situation so that the relationship between them becomes clear and understandable. Consequently, although the occupational medicine physician may contribute essential services to an injured worker as a provider of medical care, the OMP is also identified and relied on as an expert source, processor, manager, and communicator of specialized information, and the employer looks to the OMP to assist in managing such nonclinical issues as immediate duty status, long-range employability, and work-relatedness of the medical condition. Because of the critical importance of these types of determinations, we will explore in some depth the nature of the communicating relationship between the OMP and the employer and other non-medical parties, and the unique technical features of the medical decision process that underlies the management of information about employees as acute pain patients in the industrial setting. We begin by looking at the interface between "medicine" and "management," followed by a discussion of the nature of medical information that can be communicated outside the medical domain.

CLINICAL VS. NONCLINICAL—WHAT ARE THE BOUNDARIES OF THE MEDICAL DOMAIN?

It is useful to begin by identifying the boundaries of the medical domain (Table 18–1) so that we may analyze the nature of the interface between the medical and the nonmedical world and the information that must flow across it. A physician possessing the expertise to manage medically technical information does so within a framework of established medical diagnostic criteria and generally accepted medical principles and practice. The capacity of physicians to perform effectively in the practice of medicine depends fundamentally on communications that take place within this professional reference framework. These communications take place in a structured manner that enables all participants to come to agreement about what is and what is not known regarding a patient, and about what additional information is needed to resolve medical uncertainty. In managing their patients, physicians depend upon

191

Table 18–1
The Medical Domain

Established medical diagnostic criteria

Generally accepted medical principles and practice

and cooperate with each other. This is not to say that physicians do not or should not disagree about medical technical issues. However, because of the professional reference framework for communications and decision making, the practice of medicine is not an adversarial process.

Then, why should our expectations of the physician be different in the industrial arena? Why, in the industrial arena, should a physician be asked to function in an adversarial role and to substitute his or her judgement for that of another physician about any matter, clinical or nonclinical? In general, this occurs when a physician is asked to render an opinion about a matter that is not fundamentally medical in nature. However, as long as physicians function within the boundaries of the medical domain, there is no need for them to be adversaries about medical matters, inside or outside the industrial setting.

THE NATURE OF MEDICAL INFORMATION

In addition to communicating medically technical information about patients, principally to each other, physicians also make medical statements, which contain medically nontechnical information, to communicate outside the medical domain (Tables 18–2 and 18–3).

Both medically technical and medically nontechnical information have a well defined place in the industrial environment. Although, in managing patients, a physician works primarily with medically technical information, in the industrial setting particularly, it is essential that the physician is cognizant of the nonmedical consequences of a medical condition. Also, he must be able to communicate accurately, clearly, and completely about those consequences to nonmedical users of information in medically nontechnical terms. Because of the need to incorporate medical information into nonmedical

Table 18–2
Categories of Medical Information

Medically Technical Information—the information used by medical professionals for managing patients.

Medically Nontechnical Information—information communicated by medical professionals to those outside the medical profession.

Table 18–3
Definitions

Medically Technical Information refers to the information used by medical professionals for managing patients. Patient-specific information includes the medical history, review of systems, clinical findings, results of laboratory tests and diagnostic procedures, and diagnoses. General information includes established medical diagnostic criteria, generally accepted medical principles and practice, and the information contained in the medical and scientific literature and textbooks.

Medically Nontechnical Information refers to information communicated by medical professionals to those outside the medical profession. Patient-specific information includes statements about the presence or absence of a medical condition, the consequences of a medical condition with respect to life activities, and whether an individual meets medical standards.

Employable refers to an individual who has the capacity to meet the job demands and conditions of employment defined by the employer. An individual who is employable has the capacity to travel to and from work, be at work, and accept assignment of appropriate tasks and duties.

Impairment means the loss of, loss of use of, or derangement of a body part, system, or function.[5]

Disability refers to the limiting loss or absence of the capacity of an individual to meet personal, social, or occupational demands or to meet statutory or regulatory requirements.[6]

Medical Occupational disability means that an individual's medical condition precludes or warrants restriction from travel to and from work, precludes being at work, or precludes completion of assignments of appropriate tasks and duties.

Medical Documentation refers to copies of existing clinical records. Documentation from a physician's office or clinic includes progress notes, consultation reports, reports of laboratory tests, and diagnostic studies. Documentation from a hospital includes (at a minimum) admission and discharge summaries, consultation and operative reports, and reports of laboratory tests and diagnostic studies.

Certification of a Medical condition (self-certification) refers to an employee's statement that a medical condition precludes the employee working.

(management) decisions, a successful outcome in the management of a patient in the industrial environment depends partly on the occupational medicine physician's integration of both medically technical and medically nontechnical considerations into the management plan and into communications with a patient's employer.

These matters are sufficiently important in the practice of occupational and industrial medicine to warrant examination of the way in which medical information is acquired, processed, and communicated for use by nonmedical users. (Although this chapter focuses on "industrial disability," the concepts developed below are applicable to nonindustrial cases as well, for an individual's capacity to meet job demands and conditions of employment does not depend on the origin of a medical condition.)

THE MANAGEMENT/MEDICAL MODELS

The following three management/medical models were devised to provide a systematic framework within which to develop and implement medical support operations in an industrial setting and have been used in their current form for 8 to 12 years.

Model for the Use of Medical Information in a Nonmedical Setting

Figure 18–1 illustrates the concepts underlying the process by which medical information is communicated from a medical source to a nonmedical user. The model identifies the two categories of medical information referenced above and depicts the interface across which medical information must pass.

Formulation of a medically nontechnical statement must take into account the medically technical concepts and the terms must be precise, for, in effect, the medical source offers a statement of opinion that the nonmedical user receives and uses *as if it were fact*. To be accepted and used, the information contained in the statement must meet the four conditions shown at the bottom of the figure: it must be understandable, supportable, reasonable, and useful. Surprisingly, the information does not have to be *correct*. In general, a nonmedical user will not question the doctor, and, in any particular instance, the weaker condition of supportability is enough. However, correctness is critically important in the long run, for if the information provided by a medical source is incorrect often enough to cause problems for the nonmedical user, the user will either tend to discount its value or ignore it altogether. But, the user's decision problem must, nevertheless, be resolved. Consequently, a primary function of a medical information source in the industrial setting is to provide well structured, nontechnical medical input to management decision processes so that

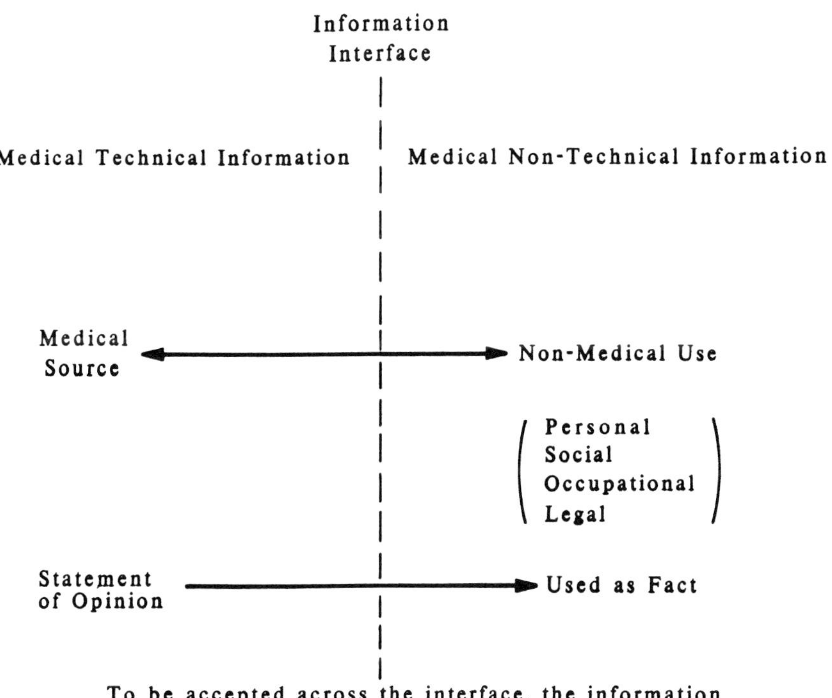

Figure **18–1.** The use of medical information in a non-medical setting. *Copyright, 1983, George M. Smith, M.D.

management is able to make informed decisions about management matters. However, there is an important caveat: the medical information must be formulated in nontechnical terms and must be structured in such a way that management is not bound by what the medical source says.

Model for Medical Determinations Related to Employability

As noted above, in the model for use of medical information in a nonmedical setting, it is necessary to distinguish between medical and nonmedical matters in management decision procedures.

Although every job in an organization is defined by some sort of job description,* a job description alone does not contain sufficient information with which to understand the nature of a job. Beyond the functional description, a job must be analyzed to define tasks, duties, and conditions of employment

---

*Many job descriptions are not formal, written, or complete. As a consequence, major difficulties are encountered in dealing with questions about the relationship between an employee's health and the job because the job itself is not well enough defined.

specifically related to the particular job in its organizational location. However, these specifications do not contain all the information necessary to complete the picture of the job. Ultimately, the job is defined by management's expectations of the incumbent as set forth in performance standards, requirements for reliability, expected duration of useful service life and whatever other factors are deemed to be important. These expectations, which are called "demand criteria" in the model, are comprised of the set of requirements against which the individual's qualification and suitability for employment are initially assessed at the time of hiring and recurrently reviewed during the course of employment. Knowledge of the employer's decision regarding demand criteria is essential input to the OMP's employability determination, for by specifying demand criteria, management makes a clear statement regarding the specific occupational activities for which it is willing to pay wages.

Once established, the demand criteria may be analyzed to determine the kinds of information needed regarding the health of an applicant or employee, and the degree of specificity required to make decisions about the health with respect to those criteria. The results of this analysis serve as the basis for a

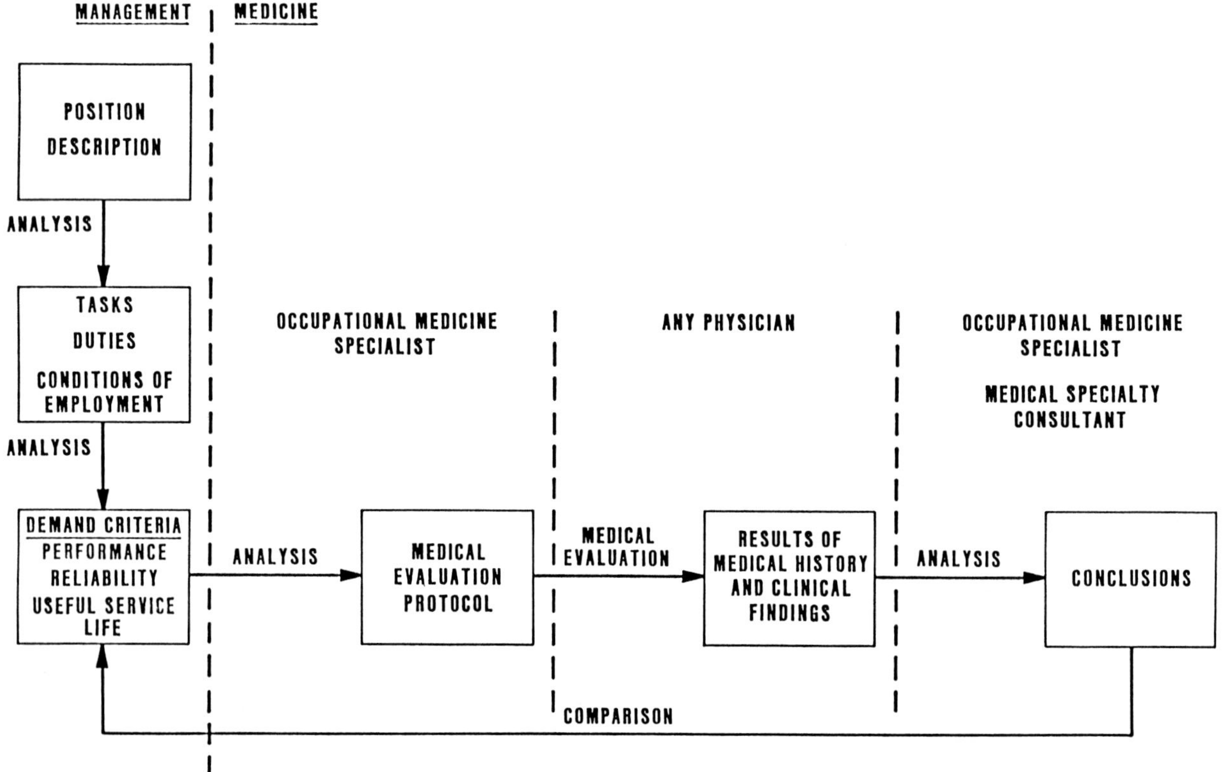

Figure 18–2. Medical determinations related to employability. *Copyright, 1983, George M. Smith, M.D.

medical evaluation protocol, a specific set of instructions to a physician setting forth the specific observations to be made, and, as appropriate, the specific techniques to be used when examining the individual. Because techniques of medical examination are well enough standardized for this purpose, it is reasonable to expect that two physicians examining the same person at the same time using the same protocol would reach the same conclusions. Accordingly, any physician can perform the evaluation and provide clinical information about the individual's health status. The results of the evaluation are then analyzed to reach conclusions about the health of the individual for comparison with the demand criteria, and, because the evaluation protocol was specifically devised to obtain the medical information necessary to make the comparison, it is possible to reach a valid decision about the individual's health with respect to the demand criteria.

It is clear that the processes shown in the upper left portion of Figure 18–2 are administrative, belonging appropriately to management, and that the processes described in the lower right portion of the figure are medical in nature and belong in the medical domain. Accordingly, the boundary between management and medicine in the model is drawn vertically along the left-hand column of boxes.

Closer inspection of the model, however, offers an important clue to the origin of problems commonly encountered in the relationship between a physician and the patient's employer. Consider what happens when the boundary between management and medicine is drawn horizontally above the bottom row of boxes and accountability for the demand criteria (the box in the lower left-hand corner) is placed in the medical domain. When the demand criteria are not defined by management, the physician must guess whether or not management would be willing to pay wages for a particular occupational activity.

In addition, commonly the three medical steps are operationally collapsed into one, and the applicant or employee is sent for a medical examination without a set of instructions to the evaluating physician. In this case, without knowledge of the demand criteria (i.e., without sufficient information about the job and knowledge regarding expectations acceptable to management), the OMP is asked to determine whether or not the individual is "medically" qualified for the job. The physician is asked, in effect, to make management decisions. The value of this model in avoiding these pitfalls lies in its methodology for clearly distinguishing between medical issues and management issues and for well structured communications across the management/medical interface.

Application of these concepts to the management of employees highlights the critical need for management to carry out a current employability determination for the purpose of making decisions regarding day-to-day duty status and retention in employment when an employee is injured or experiences a change in health status for any reason. Having developed information about the change in health and its consequences, it is necessary for the OMP to reassess the correlation between the demand criteria and the employee's present health status. If the results of the OMP's analysis provide a basis upon which management may conclude that the medical condition precludes the employee from meeting the job demands or conditions of employment because of unacceptable risk, it becomes necessary for management to reassess and consider modification of the demand criteria in light of the medical condition. Accommodation, in the form of work or work site modification, temporary assignment of alternative tasks and duties, or the use of assistive devices, also must be considered. Then, the OMP re-evaluates the correlation between the employee's health and the job demand criteria. This iterative process of communication between the OMP and management continues until management determines that the limit has been reached on its capacity to modify the demand criteria. At that point, the last assessment of the relationship between the employee's health and the job demands by the OMP becomes final and serves as the basis for management's action.

Model for Verification of a Medical Condition to Support an Employee's Request for Sick Leave, Accommodation, Special Treatment, or Benefit

Although an employer may ask the OMP for a diagnosis, the diagnosis itself is less important than other information about the employee, for knowledge of a diagnosis alone does not provide a basis upon which to determine whether or not an individual is employable. Rather than knowing a diagnosis, in the industrial setting, an employer has a need to determine whether or not an employee has a medical condition that must be taken into account in making business-related decisions about the employee, and it is the employer who must initiate the process of acquiring the medical information. Although the OMP plays an undeniably critical role in assisting with this decision, the OMP must be astutely responsive to the employer's needs for pertinent and properly structured medical (nontechnical) input to a management decision. Sometimes, this entails answering the question that the employer *should* have asked instead of question that he did ask.

This management/medical model sets forth the essential steps in an information gathering process that enables an employer, with the assistance of the OMP, to capture control over decisions regarding the day-to-day duty status of an employee whose health comes into question, such as in the case of the patient with an acute back injury. The process starts when an employee makes a request, explicitly or implicitly, for a benefit, accommodation, or other special consideration. A request for approval of sick leave or short-term disability is an explicit request. A visit to the occupational medicine clinic to report an injury incurred on the job, or an employee's submission of a first report of injury, represent an implicit request. In either event, the employer must know whether the medical condition precludes travel to and from work, if it precludes being in the workplace, or if it impairs the employee in carrying out his assignment of appropriate tasks and duties.

The model also provides for appropriate use of two fundamental types of medical documentation, self-certification by the employee and full justification based on information contained in the existing medical office and hospital records. The flow chart in Figure 18–3 illustrates the management steps and communications pathways needed for timely and ef-

fective decision making. Implementation of policy and procedures based on this model can assist management in using information about the employee's medical condition in making fully informed, rapid, fair, and defensible decisions regarding the approval of an employee's request for a benefit.

EMPLOYABILITY VS. DISABILITY— THE EMPLOYERS' PERSPECTIVE

In the assessment of an individual's employability, an employer considers both performance capability and risk when determining whether the individual has the capacity to meet both the demands of a job and the conditions of employment. The assessment of performance capability takes into account the individual's knowledge, skills, and abilities, as well as education, training, experience, and other relevant factors, so that the employer may estimate the likelihood of a performance failure. To assess risk factors, the employer estimates the likelihood of incurring some kind of liability or cost in the case of human failure. If the likelihood of incurring liability

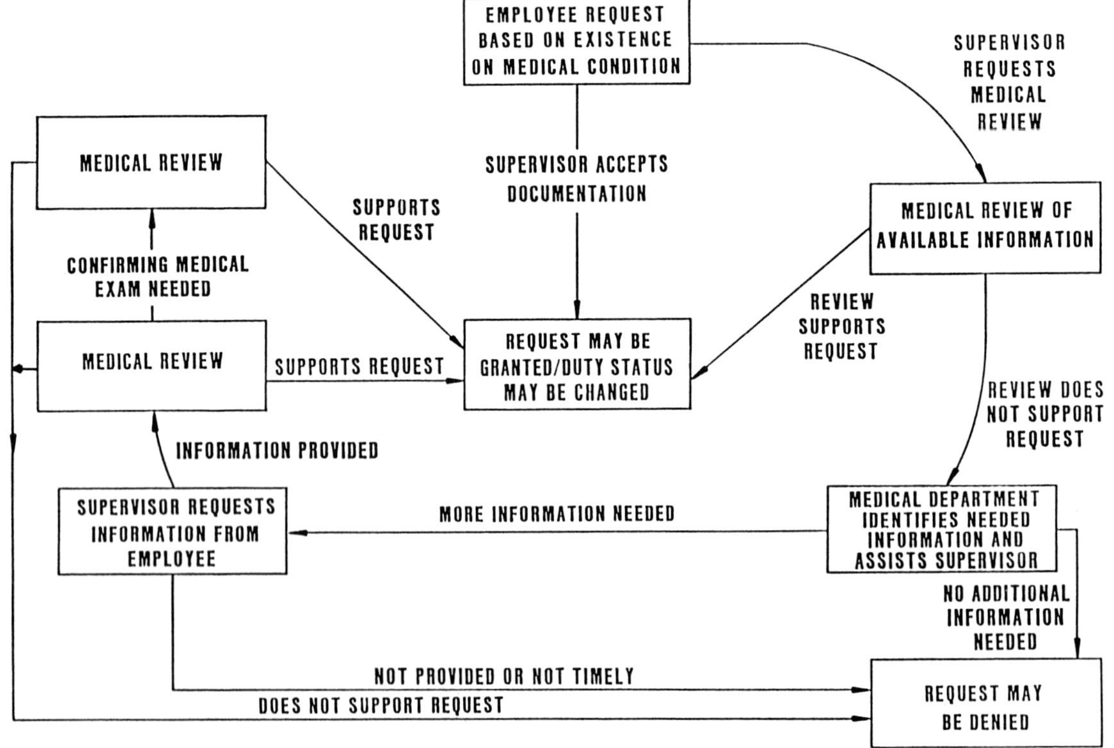

Figure 18–3. Verification of a medical condition to support an employee's request for accomodation, sick leave, special treatment, or benefit. *Copyright, 1983, George M. Smith, M.D.

because of human failure exceeds the employer's limit of acceptability, the employer will conclude that the individual is not employable in that job.

This risk oriented assessment of employability is different from a "desirability" determination; it is an assessment of the degree of correlation between the individual's qualifications and suitability, on the one hand, and the job demands and conditions of employment on the other. The individual is "employable" when the disparity is acceptably small.

During the course of employment, the employer continues (implicitly, as a rule) to weigh performance and risk issues in dealing with questions about the day-to-day duty status of an employee as well as questions about retention in employment. To remain employed, an employee must continue to meet performance standards based on criteria for quantity, quality, and timeliness of production and to meet expectations for reliability. In addition, no matter what the level of the employee's skill and capability, the employee must be sufficiently available for duty to justify retention. Being at work is a matter of prime importance. Accordingly, whether or not an employee is under medical care, if the employee has the capacity to travel to and from work, to be at work, and to accept assignment of tasks and duties (within the boundaries of the job and the medical condition and for which the employer will pay full wages), then the employer can reasonably expect the employee to report for duty. Herein lies the key to an operational understanding of employability and disability.

The presence of a medical condition for which the employee is under the care of a physician, of itself, does not create a presumption of "disability," even if the physician recommends work absence or if the physician asserts, without an explicit medical rationale, that the employee is "disabled" for work. It makes sense, then, to define "employable" to mean an employee who has the capacity to travel to and from work, be at work, and accept assigned tasks and duties for which full wages will be paid. By "accept assignment of tasks and duties" we mean first, no medical reason exists to imply that the employee is at greater risk than an individual without a similar medical condition for injury, harm, or aggravation of the condition by carrying out assigned tasks and duties and, second, that no medical reason exists to question the individual's ability to perform. Therefore, if an employee is employable, there is no basis upon which to consider the employee to be "disabled."

If an employee's medical condition does not preclude travel to and from work and does not preclude the employee from being at work and the employer is willing to pay wages for work the employee is able to do, there is no justification for excusing the absence or paying a benefit. On the other hand, if the OMP's assessment of the available medical information supports a conclusion that the employee's medical condition, for the time being, precludes or warrants restriction from travel to and from work or precludes being at work, there is no question about excusing the absence and paying the benefit for the duration of unemployability. In either instance, OMP's report must specify a date beyond which additional medical documentation is required for further approval of absence. This procedure is effective for both occupational and nonoccupational medical conditions, for *the origin of the medical condition has no bearing on the relationship between the medical condition and the employee's capacity to meet job demands.*

This approach has proven to be valuable because it accounts for the role of the physician in providing input to management's employability determinations. Both the AMA *Guides*[2] and the Federal Civil Service regulations regarding medical determination of employee health conditions[3] recognize that physicians do only two things in their unique capacity as physicians: They ensure that a diagnosis or clinical impression is justified in accordance with established medical diagnostic criteria, and they ensure that conclusions and recommendations are consistent with generally accepted medical principles and practice. For any determinations past those boundaries, a physician is not necessary. It is not that physicians do not go past these boundaries; they do so frequently, either because they volunteer to do so or because they are asked to do so. But, when they go past the boundaries of the medical domain, they are no longer acting in their unique capacity as physicians, and it does not make sense to give greater weight to the opinion of one physician over that of another about a nonmedical matter. Accordingly, it is important to structure the communications between management and medicine to avoid the pitfalls that arise when a physician is asked to answer management questions such as "Can the employee do the job?" Or "Is this employee disabled?" Management should not ask the physician to answer these questions; however, management should ask the physician to answer clearly medical questions, as discussed below.

With respect to performance, there is no way a physician, or anyone else, can determine, on the basis of medical information alone, what an individual can or cannot do. For example, consider the individual with a broken ankle who sees an orthopedic surgeon, who applies a cast. He asks, "Doctor, will I be able to dance when the cast comes off." The doctor replies, "Yes," and the patient says "That's great! I can't dance now and never could." Or, similarly, "Will I be able to sing after you take my tonsils out?" Or, "Will I be able to play tennis after my broken wrist heals." The doctor does not know the answers to these questions.

However, a physician *can* determine whether the medical condition is static or well stabilized. If it is, then there is no medical reason to believe that the individual will gain or lose ability for medical reasons. Therefore, with respect to the performance issues, the medical question becomes, "Is the medical condition static or well stabilized?" If it is, then management can carry out its assessment of performance capability in full confidence knowing that any ability the individual has will not be lost for medical reasons, nor will any ability currently lacking be gained.

It should be evident, then, that the "can" in the question, "Can this individual do the job" should not be taken as a request that the physician make a judgement about ability. It is appropriate, rather, to understand the question as meaning, "Doctor, if we ask the individual to do the job, is anything bad going to happen?" It is, in reality, a risk-related question. However, although a physician may be able to place boundaries on the degree of risk associated with a particular medical condition, only management can decide how much risk is acceptable. Therefore, the physician must be asked only to assess the likelihood that the particular individual will experience an undesirable medical event as a result of the presence of the medical condition compared to an individual who does not have the medical condition,† and to state the likelihood in such a way that management can decide whether or not that degree of risk is acceptable with respect to its willingness to incur a liability or cost.

THE ACUTELY INJURED EMPLOYEE

The Employability Determination and the Employee's Return to Work

Once clinical assessment of the acutely injured employee has been completed and appropriate treatment begun, the OMP will have sufficient clinical information to initiate an assessment of the individual's employability in coordination with the employer. This should be done at the first visit with the intention of avoiding lost time. A determination that the employee is employable would be based on a

conclusion that the medical condition does not preclude travel to and from work or does not preclude being at work, and that the employer is willing to assign tasks and duties for which the employee will receive full wages. If, however, it is determined that the medical condition does preclude travel to and from work, being at work, or assignment of appropriate tasks and duties, the OMP should estimate the expected date of sufficient recovery to warrant reassessment; close monitoring of the clinical status enables the OMP to intervene sooner if appropriate.

The employability determination is based on the same criteria whenever it is carried out, and the decision must be neutral with respect to the employee's motivation to return to work and the employer's willingness to assign tasks and duties. Accordingly, the OMP should consider whether or not there would be a medical basis to recommend against employment if the employee wanted to return to work or had applied for the job in the case of an applicant. The "Employability/Disability Verification Form" is a useful tool to assist the OMP in making this determination and in communicating the outcome to the employer.

When it appears that the medical condition is likely to render the employee unemployable for more than an extended period of time a (more than 7 to 10 days), consideration should be given to obtaining further tests and diagnostic procedures, and the employee is best served by early referral for medical specialty evaluation and treatment.

Duty Limitations

Duty limitations are warranted when a medical basis exists to conclude that the employee would be likely to suffer injury, harm, or aggravation of the condition as a result of engaging in activity beyond a certain level of demand. However, the limitations would have to apply to nonwork-related activities as well. A recommendation for duty limitations by a "treating physician" would be subject to the same standard of documentation and review.

In some instances, duty limitations become a problem, for some managers are unwilling to take an employee back to work unless the employee is "100%." Frequently, in such instances the problem is not "pain in the back" but rather "pain in the butt," and the employer does not want a problem employee in the workplace. The OMP must be sensitive to such issues, and when a case doesn't make sense medically, or when there appears to be unreasonable rejection of the OMP's recommendations, the OMP should verify the employee's work history and performance appraisal record with a manager.

---

*The question is one of relative, not absolute, risk. For example, an individual with epilepsy who has not experienced a seizure within a year is considered no more likely to have another seizure that an individual who has never had one. An individual who has never experienced a seizure has a 1 in 100 chance of having one some time during his or her lifetime, for the incidence of seizure disorders is about 1% in the general population.

Medical Information

Dear Employer:

ANY CLINIC has assessed your employee to determine whether or not a medical reason exists to believe that his or her medical condition precludes travel to and from work, being at work, or assignment of appropriate tasks and duties. However, when an employee has the capacity to travel to work and to be at work, ANY CLINIC anticipates that the employer will expect the employee to report for duty unless an appropriate assignment is not available. To assist you in deciding whether or not to excuse your employee's absence of less than five days, and to help you enable your employee to return to work when he or she is ready, we have provided the following information. This form is provided for information purposes only and is not an official medical record. A copy of the medical record and workers' compensation forms will be provided as appropriate.

TYPE OF MEDICAL CONDITION: ___ Illness ___ Injury ___ Surgery

    ___ Maternity ___ Antepartum ___ Post Partum
    Type of Delivery: ___ Caesarian Section
        ___ Normal

DIAGNOSES: ____

PROBLEM LIST: 1. ____
        2. ____
        3. ____

DATE OF ONSET: *Of Current Condition* _____________

    Of Current Problems 1. _____________
        2. _____________
        3. _____________

WORKERS' COMPENSATION FORMS COMPLETED? _________

IF YOUR PATIENT UNDERWENT SURGERY:

1. Procedure: ____
2. Date _____________ 3. Complications _____________________________
4. Findings at Surgery ____
____

5. Usual recovery period: _________ days/weeks

DATE OF LAST OFFICE VISIT: _________ ___ Improved ___ Not Improved

    If not improved, what is the reason? ___________________________
____

    What is the current treatment? _______________________________
____

DOES ANY PROBLEM PRECLUDE OR WARRANT RESTRICTION FROM:

1. Travel to and from work or similar activities such as travel to and from therapy or shopping? ___ No ___ Yes

    If so: For what medical reason? _______________________________
____

    Date the employee is expected to have recovered sufficiently to travel to and from work: _____________

2. Being at work? ___ No ___ Yes

    If so: For what medical reason? _______________________________
____

    Date the employee is expected to have recovered sufficiently to be at work: _____________

Table 18–4 (continued)

3. **Assignment of any tasks and duties?** ___ Yes ___ No

   If so: For what medical reason? ____

   ____

   Date the employee is expected to have recovered sufficiently to be assigned limited duties: _______________

   Date the employee is expected to have recovered sufficiently to be assigned duties without restriction: _______________

   Signature ____,   Date _____________
   Name ____   Phone _____________
   Address ____
   City, State, Zip ____

Information Management

The physician who first sees an employee after an injury is presented with a singular opportunity to collect information and to make observations of the patient that will never again occur in the course of managing that individual's medical condition or disability claim. Complete and accurate recording of this information has the dual value of protecting both the employee and employer, and along with the clinical responsibilities that are inherent in seeing acutely injured patients, there is a responsibility to ensure that all available information is recorded in anticipation of the variety of medical and nonmedical questions that inevitably arise following an injury at work. The supplemental checklist in Table 18–5 will serve as a guide to items of information that are particularly valuable in industrial disability cases.

Table 18–5
Supplemental Checklist for Management of Information Regarding an Acute Injury

In addition to the information that would ordinarily be obtained by performing a standard history and physical examination, the OMP has an opportunity to record essential information to protect the interests of both the employer and employee. The following checklist may be used to supplement the OMP's own medical evaluation protocol. It is strongly suggested that the OMP use body diagrams to illustrate specific locations of pain, contusions, abrasions, and lacerations.

1. **Verification of the circumstances under which the injury is alleged to have occurred.**
   a. What happened?
   b. What date?
   c. What time?
   d. Where?
   e. What was the specific mechanism of injury?
   f. Were there any witnesses?
   g. How did the employee get to the medical facility?
   h. How was the employee getting along with supervisor and job?
2. **Verification of the Employee's Current Clinical Status.**
   a. Specific location of all complaints of pain, no matter how minor.
   b. Specific location of all contusions, lacerations, and abrasions.
   c. Range of motion of all joints.
   d. Range of motion of spine segments with reference to flattening, straightening, and reversal of lumbar curve on forward bend.
   e. Mental status evaluation with specific attention to factors that may predispose to development of a post traumatic stress disorder.

DISABILITY CASE MANAGEMENT

From the employer's point of view, a case involves employment related issues and is closed when definitive disposition is made of both the employee and the employee's position because, in reality, when absence caused by disability is extended over time, management of the position eventually becomes the most critical concern of the employer.

As noted above, when an employee claims to have a medical condition and requests that his employer gives him something because of it, management wants to know whether or not the employee has a medical condition, and, if so, whether or not the medical condition must be taken into account in making business-related decisions about the employee. If an employee is not present for duty or is not meeting the full range of job demands and conditions for any other reason, management must find ways to restore the lost productivity. Accordingly, from the employer's perspective closing the case can best be understood as a fair, justifiable, and defensible management decision that resolves the employee's employment status and duty status and that results in restoration of the employee's position to full productivity.

From the claims manager's perspective, a case is brought to closure only when the claim for temporary total disability or permanent partial disability is settled or the Workers' Compensation Board or Commission has made an award; apportionment has been decided; all other legal and administrative matters have been addressed; and all appeals have been resolved. The employer, however, has no control over these processes, which may continue for years depending on the issues of the case. Nevertheless, as explained above, it is not necessary or appropriate for the employer to wait for closure of the claim to reach closure on the human resource and position management issues. In fact, management closure with respect to employability and duty status involving a determination that the employee is or is not employable, and if not, a determination that the employee will or will not again be employable, is often critically important to closing the claim.

Temporary total disability comes to an end when the employer has offered the employee suitable employment and is willing to pay full wages to the employee. As noted above, when the employee's medical condition, as defined by the employee's treating physician, does not preclude travel to and from work, being at work, or assignment of tasks and duties for which the employer is willing to pay full wages, an order to report for duty is not a denial of an entitlement. It is not against an employee's interest to be paid a day's wages for a day's work.

When is Injury or Illness Work-related?

In general, under the provisions of a workers' compensation law, an employee is entitled to benefits when he or she incurs an injury or illness that arises out of and in the course of employment. Clearly, only a physician may determine whether or not the employee suffers from an injury or illness. Nevertheless, while medical information is necessary to support claim-related decisions, determinations regarding the "work-relatedness" of the medical condition and justification for payment of benefits are not medical matters.

Verification that an injury or illness has arisen out of and in the course of employment requires sufficient information to support a conclusion that:

1. An event occurred during the course of employment at a particular time and place or that exposure to a particular set of conditions occurred over a defined period of time;
2. The employee suffers from injury or disease;
3. The injury or disease could have been caused by the event or exposure; and, if so,
4. The injury or disease was caused by the event or exposure.

Technically, the burden of proof rests with the individual submitting a claim. However, as a matter of practicality, most often the employer and the occupational medicine physician or treating physician provide the information to support claim.

In carrying out an investigation of the circumstances under which the illness or injury occurred, the employer would appropriately gather information with respect to item 1. above; in practice, however, this does not occur until well after the fact, and, unfortunately, in many cases, it is not done at all. As a consequence, the employee's statements to employer and physician become the primary, and often the only, source of information about the circumstances.

CONCLUSION

The Occupational Medicine Physician acts in an essential transitional role in the industrial setting with responsibility and accountability both within and outside the domain of medicine. Beyond providing clinical services to employers and employees, the OMP serves to ensure that appropriate communications take place in such a way that decisions about injured employees, rather than being presented as opinion, are based on sufficient information to justify the decisions. In managing the injured employee, the OMP has a unique opportunity to protect the interests of both employee and employer by ensuring that medical care is rendered in a timely manner and that information about the employee is complete and accurate.

REFERENCES

1. Guides to the Evaluation of Permanent Impairment, 2nd Ed. Chicago, American Medical Association, 1984.
2. Medical Determinations Related to Employability, 5CFR 339.
3. Guides to the Evaluation of Permanent Impairment, 3rd Ed. Chicago, American Medical Association, pp. 236, 1987.

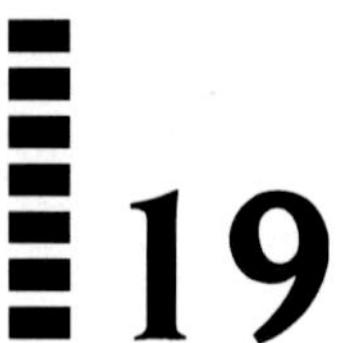

19

Scott Haldeman

The Chiropractic View of Acute Spinal Disorders

Chiropractic is unique among the health professions in that its primary and practically exclusive interest is the spine. Whereas other professions and specialties such as orthopedic surgery, neurology, physical medicine, and physical therapy have a wide scope of practice encompassing the entire musculoskeletal and nervous systems, chiropractors have elected to make the spine and its related structures the focus of their training and clinical practice.

Although modern chiropractors use a wide variety of conservative modalities in the treatment of the spine, they have been most closely associated with the practice of spinal manipulation. It was Daniel David Palmer, on opening the first school of chiropractic in 1895, who emphasized spinal manipulation, or the "spinal adjustment" as he called it, as the primary treatment modality of chiropractors. This emphasis has continued over the past 95 years despite major attacks and the exclusion or relegation of spinal manipulation to a minor part of medical and osteopathic training and practice. Increased research over the past 15 years, however, has led to increased acceptance of manipulation as a treatment option for the management of patients with spinal pain. This has led to the progressive integration of chiropractors into the health care team. Chiropractic training institutions are being incorporated into state public and private colleges and universities while chiropractors increasingly are joining group practices, hospitals, and health maintenance organizations.

CHIROPRACTIC CONCEPTS

Chiropractors see more patients with back pain than either orthopedic surgeons or family physicians.[1] One reason for this, beyond the perceptions that they are spine doctors and the beneficial effects of spinal manipulation, is that chiropractors are better received by patients with back pain than family physicians.[2] This, in turn, may be partly due to the laying on of hands and its soothing effect on patients with back pain. However, according to a survey by Kane, et al.,[3] chiropractors are perceived as having greater ability to make patients feel welcome and are more likely to explain problems and treatment than medical physicians. This intimate interaction of chiropractors with their patients is one of the fundamental concepts of chiropractic practice.

Chiropractors have achieved a close relationship with their patients by emphasizing three distinct yet complementary processes. These processes, having been labeled by many early chiropractic leaders,[4] are philosophy, science, and art. Although the basic concept is not much different than the theory and practice of other professions, it is only within chiropractic that these three topics are emphasized as entities that can exist separately and sometimes seemingly even in conflict with each other. This may be partly because of the different rate at which the three processes have developed.

Chiropractic Philosophy

D.D. Palmer and the early chiropractors took a very old procedure, spinal manipulation, which had been rejected by the medical profession, and incorporated it into a fairly simplistic, naturalistic concept of health and disease. The original concept that disease may be related to disturbances within the nervous system was not primarily a chiropractic concept but had been proposed by a number of eighteenth and nineteenth century physicians.[5] In the early twentieth century B.J. Palmer systematized the philosophy of chiropractic. Gibbons, in his historical analysis of that time,[6] concluded that the inherent ignorance of physicians and the dangers of many medical treatments prior to the universal usage of sterile surgery, antibiotics, and properly researched medication created a strong demand for an alternative health care system.

Chiropractic philosophy, which emphasized the natural ability of the body to heal itself and de-emphasized surgery and drugs, became very popular. This naturalistic philosophy allowed chiropractic to grow despite wide opposition, relatively weak educational standards, and lack of inclusion in health insurance plans, both private and governmental.

Over the past quarter of a century there has been a resurgence of national interest in natural healing methods. Recent medical and biological research has demonstrated the importance of such factors as diet, exercise, and psychological factors in health and disease and has relegated drugs and surgery to increasingly more specific indications. This movement fits well into the philosophy of chiropractic.

Chiropractic philosophy today can be summarized as stating that the body has a strong innate capacity to heal itself of many disorders given a proper internal and external environment. Patients treated by chiropractors are often given information stressing a normal, natural way of life including advice on proper diet, exercise, and stress management. This willingness to talk to patients not only about their complaints but about their general health and well being has helped to generate a feeling that the chiropractor is genuinely concerned about them as a person. This can be considered one of the primary strengths of chiropractic care.[2]

Chiropractic Science

Chiropractors have perhaps been criticized more often on their lack of science than on any other issue. This criticism was at the same time both true and self-fulfilling. Admittedly chiropractors, until recently, had few resources and expertise to spend on research. On the other hand chiropractors were systematically excluded from all scientific institutions, journals, and meetings. As recently as 1980 this author was forced to remove his chiropractic credentials from scientific papers presented at meetings or published in peer-reviewed journals.

Despite, or perhaps because of the constant pressure, chiropractic science has flourished and grown. Today, every chiropractic college is required to have an active research program and at least two chiropractic journals are indexed in the major indexing systems. This has led to a preponderance of research papers presented at chiropractic meetings and a gradual supplanting of philosophical explanations for the effectiveness of specific chiropractic modalities by scientific theory. The naturalistic philosophy of chiropractic is being relegated to its proper position as a true philosophy or guide to chiropractic overall approach to thinking. The theory about why the chiropractic adjustment or spinal manipulation may be successful, on the other hand, is based increasingly on scientific thought processes.

The current chiropractic theory on the mechanism of action of spinal manipulation is multifactorial. It assumes that manipulation has the potential to have a number of different effects. The following theories are currently gaining the greatest attention.

Restricted Motion

This theory suggests that a lack of motion between vertebrae can be a source of disease and symptoms. Evidence from research on peripheral joints suggests that lack of motion can cause deterioration of joint cartilage and perhaps other degenerative changes.[7] Similarly, decreased motion has been shown to have a detrimental effect on the nutrition and metabolism of the intervertebral discs.[8] Mobilization exercises after manipulation are increasingly recommended based on the observation of a correlation between restricted motion and spinal pain. This theory has gained momentum with the observation that, in clinical trials, spinal manipulation can increase range of motion and at the same time reduce pain scores.[9,10]

Muscle Spasm

The determination of paraspinal muscle spasm and the suggestion that this may have some relationship to back pain has a long history in the annals of medicine. Despite the lack of conclusive evidence a great deal of treatment is still directed toward the muscles in patients with back pain. Such modalities as heat, ice, ultrasound, and trigger point therapies are based on this assumption. As expected, therefore, one of the primary effects of manipulation is perceived to be stretching or mobilization of muscles. This, in turn, is thought to cause relaxation and thus relieve pain and improve spinal function. The observation that manipulation can reduce muscle spasm in two small uncontrolled trials has been used to substantiate this theory.[11,12]

Pain Tolerance

A number of controlled clinical trials have demonstrated a reduction in low back pain immediately following spinal manipulation.[13,14] This has led to speculation that there may be an immediate change in pain tolerance rather than a purely biomechanical effect of manipulation. Glover[15] described areas of paraspinal hyperesthesia that he felt could be relieved by manipulation. Terrett and Vernon[16] using more conventional skin pain tolerance measuring techniques and blinded observers found that patients undergoing direct thrust chiropractic adjustments demonstrated progressive elevation of paraspinal skin pain tolerance. This process was noticeable within 2 minutes of the manipulation and lasted for at least 10 minutes. Wyke[17] has proposed that joint afferent input may be a potent modulator of pain. It has been proposed that spinal manipulation activates peripheral receptors presumably in the joint or skin. This results in activation of central inhibitory mechanisms and thereby increases pain tolerance. The report by Vernon, et al.,[18] of a release of beta endorphins following spinal manipulation has lent credence to this theory.

Disc Herniation

Practitioners of spinal manipulation such as Cyriax[19] and Maigne[20] have for years postulated that the primary effect of manipulation is on the disc. This has been picked up by a number of chiropractors who have incorporated it into chiropractic theory. This has led chiropractors to emphasize specific manipulative techniques using traction or distraction to treat patients with disc disorders.[20] Specific manipulative equipment has been developed to combine manipulation and distraction, rationalizing the procedure on reported effects of traction on the disc. Most research, however, has not been able to demonstrate changes in disc positions or herniation following manipulation.

Chiropractic Art

Although specific procedures followed by chiropractors are covered under appropriate headings it must be kept in mind that the art of chiropractic practice cannot be separated completely from the philosophy and science. Many of the diagnostic and treatment methods appear to be directed at specific spinal entities much like specific medication is directed at specific disease processes. To follow the classic medical model of treatment and disease, however, is to miss the essence of chiropractic care and often results in misunderstanding of what chiropractors hope to achieve with their treatment approach.

The art of chiropractic spinal adjustments is to improve spinal function to the best of the chiropractor's ability. The concept of ideal spinal function remains elusive and is constantly undergoing modification as new research becomes available. The

difficulty in determining normal spinal function, however, is not exclusively a chiropractic problem as can be witnessed by the wide variety of opinion by medical or osteopathic authorities on the significant pathologic conditions encompassed in back pain. Despite this difficulty the chiropractor, nonetheless, feels that improvement of spinal function is an essential part of patient care. Thus, spinal adjustments as well as physical modalities and specific exercises are used to mobilize vertebrae, relax muscles, and change neurologic receptor and reflex function.

The chiropractic management of spinal problems, however, does not stop at simply the correction of spinal dysfunction. The naturalistic philosophy compels the chiropractor to advise the patient on general health matters. The spine is perceived as part of the body and not an isolated organ with isolated disorders. Thus, the art of chiropractic includes the close observation and, when possible, attempts to correct environmental factors such as diet, exercise, and psychological stress. The importance of overall posture and movement has long been part of chiropractic history. The sponsorship of good posture contests and events has always included the concept that proper spinal posture and function can only exist in a healthy environment and body.

CHIROPRACTIC DIAGNOSTIC METHODS

There has been some confusion and disagreement between chiropractors regarding the components of an adequate chiropractic diagnosis and the diagnostic limits of a practicing chiropractor. This is partly because of the substantial variability in state laws regarding what chiropractors may or may not do. In certain states chiropractors are limited to the use of the clinical examination and x rays, often only of the spine. In other states chiropractors are permitted to perform or order virtually any diagnostic procedure or test. As a basic principle, however, Gitelman[22] has best described the chiropractic diagnostic thought process as having two components, described below.

The Pathologic Lesion

The first component is the diagnosis of the lesion and its local tissue responses. This process closely mimics the medical model. It is an attempt to identify specific disease such as disc herniation, fracture, tumors, or rheumatoid disease. Chiropractic courses in colleges and at the postgraduate level commonly use standard medical textbooks on this topic. As the chiropractic profession integrates into the general health care system this component is gaining greater importance. Access to institutions, hospitals, and laboratories has helped to increase the general diagnostic skills of chiropractors, which, in the past, were often fairly limited.

There is no point in describing each of the standard tests used by chiropractors to reach a pathologic diagnosis. The history and physical examination, as in the practice of medicine, forms the mainstay of this process. Standard vital signs, cardiovascular, neurological, and orthopedic examination techniques are commonly used by chiropractors on the initial visit of a patient. The basic clinical examination is then supplemented by x rays, basic hematologic, metabolic, and urinalysis screening when necessary. Often chiropractors order CT, MRI, or bone scans to complete a diagnosis.

There is, at this time however, a limit to chiropractic testing. Few, if any, chiropractors would order a myelogram, angiogram, spinal tap, arthrogram, or other invasive test. When such testing is potentially indicated, chiropractors tend to work closely with a medical specialist usually in the fields of neurology, orthopedic surgery, neurosurgery, or physiatry.

The goal of the specific diagnosis is multiple.

a. To determine the presence of an unrelated disease process that may require a direct medical referral. Examples include diabetes mellitus and thyroid disturbances.
b. To diagnose a progressive or traumatic bony lesion requiring immediate specialist referral. Examples include bony tumors, progressive neurological deficits, and unstable fractures.
c. To rule out any contraindications to specific chiropractic treatment.
d. To attempt to localize the pathologic process causing the patient's pain or other symptoms.
e. To assess the patient's overall physical and psychologic health.

The Mechanical Lesion

The second diagnostic step proposed by Gitelman is the assessment of the static and dynamic mechanical status of the locomotor system and specifically the spine. Traditional chiropractors have often referred to this process as a "chiropractic spinal analysis." The end result of this process is the localization of the entity that is to be treated directly by the chiropractor. This entity was labeled a "subluxation" by D.D. Palmer and that term is still widely used within chiropractic practice. It has been defined in a number of ways, usually with both a structural and functional component to the definition. The term "clinically significant manipulable lesion" has been used also.[23]

The primary means for the diagnosis of subluxation are a variety of palpation methods combined with x ray and postural analysis. The detailed analysis of the radiologic relationship between vertebrae, although still used, is no longer the primary mechanism of determining the presence of a symptomatic subluxation. Instead, flat x rays are now used to rule out disease and to document biomechanical relationships between vertebrae. The assumption is made that a manipulation or adjustment that takes into account the angles of the disc spaces and the orientation of facets is likely to require less force than one that doesn't.

The specific components of spinal analysis are:

Structural Alignment

As mentioned above, determining the structural relationships between vertebrae helps the chiropractor to visualize how an adjustment should be performed. Static palpation, postural analysis, and x-rays form the basis for this determination.

Range of Motion

Gross range of motion is determined commonly in front of a plumbline or a mirror. The determination is not simply the limit of range of motion in degrees but the fluidity of motion and the muscular changes during motion. In addition, the shifting of pain in different postural positions provides information regarding the manner in which mechanics influence a source of pain.

Intersegmental Motion

One of the primary determinants of where an adjustment should be directed is the localization of specific intersegmental restricted motion. This is the so-called "fixation." This is performed by the examiner placing his hands on specific aspects of the spine while the spine is moved through its range of motion. The movement of one vertebra on its neighbor is felt (Fig. 19–1).

Joint Play and End Feel

These terms, borrowed from John Mennell,[24] refer to the way a joint feels to the examiner when it is stressed in the neutral position and at the limit of range of motion. So-called hard or soft, painful or painless, solid and springing end feel or joint play are described.

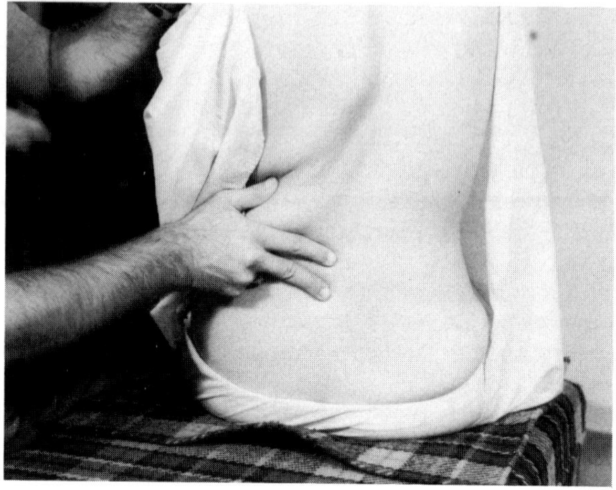

Figure 19–1. Motion palpation of the lumbar spine in the sitting position.

Soft Tissue Palpation

The palpation of muscles and ligaments have been described by early chiropractors as searching for "taut and tender fibers." Muscle spasm or tightness, tenderness over ligaments, muscles, tendons, and trigger points are noted.

It is the combination of these five examination findings together with x rays, other testing procedures, and the patient's symptoms that defines the subluxation or manipulable lesion.

CHIROPRACTIC TREATMENT

The chiropractic approach to the treatment of acute spinal pain follows a number of steps. In this section we assume that both pathologic diagnostic and mechanical diagnostic tests have been performed. All contraindications to chiropractic treatment have been eliminated and the patient is assumed to be an appropriate candidate for chiropractic care. Under these circumstances chiropractic treatment can be placed under a number of subheadings.

Nonmanipulative Acute Pain Relief

Chiropractors are limited in acute pain relief by their inability to prescribe pain relieving drugs. This has forced them to rely on nonmedical, nonsurgical techniques to achieve pain control. This has the advantage of avoiding the side effects of medication and is often appreciated by patients. On the other hand, patients in severe incapacitating pain often have to be managed in conjunction with a medical practitioner.

Methods of achieving acute pain relief commonly used by chiropractors are listed below. It is generally acknowledged that these procedures give only temporary relief. However, because most acute back pain resolves spontaneously, procedures that give temporary relief often are sufficient.

Rest

Chiropractors, as a rule, are not enthusiastic about prolonged bed rest. Philosophically, activity has been perceived as more beneficial than inactivity. This may explain observations that patients under chiropractic care tend to have relatively shorter disability periods. On the other hand, accepting that the innate feedback mechanisms in the body should not be ignored, chiropractors tend not to force patients with acute pain to carry out activities that increase pain. Thus, periods of decreased activity compatible with the patient's physical capacities often are recommended.

Physical Modalities

The pain relieving effect of heat, cold, electrical stimulation, and similar modalities has been recognized since the inception of chiropractic. Initially hot baths, with or without salts, hot towels, and hot water bottles were used. With the growth in the technology of physical therapeutic machines, modalities such as ultrasound, microwave, and galvanic and other electrical currents have been incorporated into many chiropractic practices. Again, from a philosophical point of view, these procedures often are considered preparatory or complementary to the chiropractic adjustment rather than inherently curative or the primary treatment.

Massage

The soothing effect of soft tissue massage in relieving muscle spasm and perhaps increasing local circulation is intrinsic to any manipulative therapy. The simple laying on of hands is, by itself, relaxing. Massage can cause further relaxation, which permits the chiropractor to perform an adjustment with less force and discomfort.

The Chiropractic Adjustment

The "adjustment" has been differentiated by many chiropractors from the more generic term "manipulation." The adjustment is considered a short amplitude, direction- and depth-specific, con-

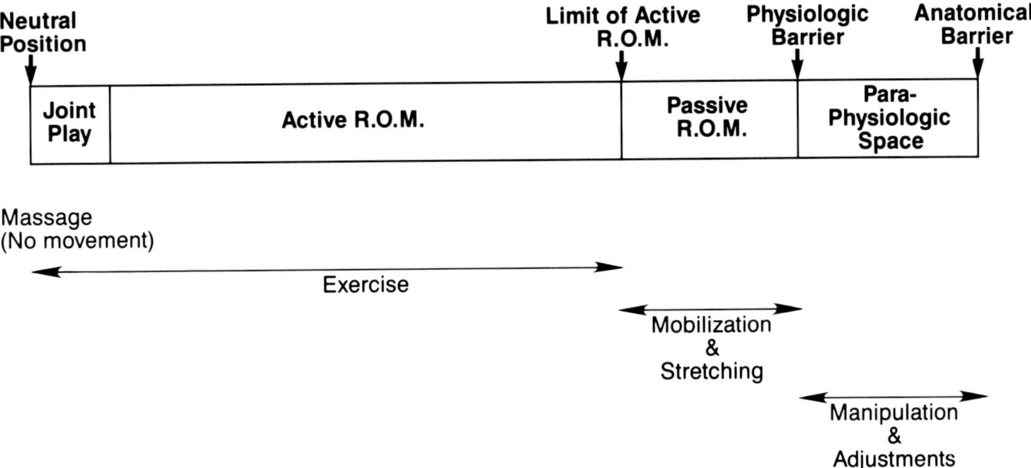

Figure 19–2. Range of motion when exercise, mobilization, and manipulation or adjustment is applied.

trolled manipulative force directed at a vertebra that is found to be dysfunctional or subluxated by the diagnostic tests noted above.

The most common form of adjustment is the high velocity thrust in one of its multiple variations. A number of "nonthrust" or "nonforce" techniques have been developed, although many have been controversial and may actually be specific mobilization techniques. Figure 19–2 is a common diagnostic representation of the effects of exercise, mobilization, and manipulation as it relates to range of motion. There are, however, multiple techniques and methods of spinal adjustment, which have been developed by chiropractic clinicians. These techniques, which are often named after the chiropractor who developed them, utilize different tables or other equipment to reduce force or to allow for specific positioning of the patient.

Following are some of the more common chiropractic adjusting methods for acute low back pain.

The Prone Body Drop

This technique is often referred to as part of the diversified or Meric method and is one of the oldest adjusting methods. The patient is placed prone on a table with or without elevation of the hips or an abdominal piece of the table which falls away. The clinician makes either bilateral or unilateral thenar contact on the appropriate vertebral segment. The adjustive force is achieved by a coordinated drop of the clinician's body past his own shoulders. This allows for a high level of control of both direction and amount of force. Figure 19–3 illustrates a modification of this technique using a knee posture table developed by Gonstead.

The Toggle Recoil

This technique varies from the body drop in that the shoulders and trunk are held stable and a quick approximation of the clinician's elbows is used to deliver the adjustive thrust. This technique requires a great deal of training and experience but when used properly can deliver a rapid thrust in a very specific direction and with a defined depth of approximately one centimeter. Thompson[25] developed a segmental table with a mechanism that allows one segment to drop about one centimeter when a force is applied to it. The combined use of the Thompson table and the toggle recoil can result in much less impact or jarring of the adjustment and requires less strength on the part of the clinician.

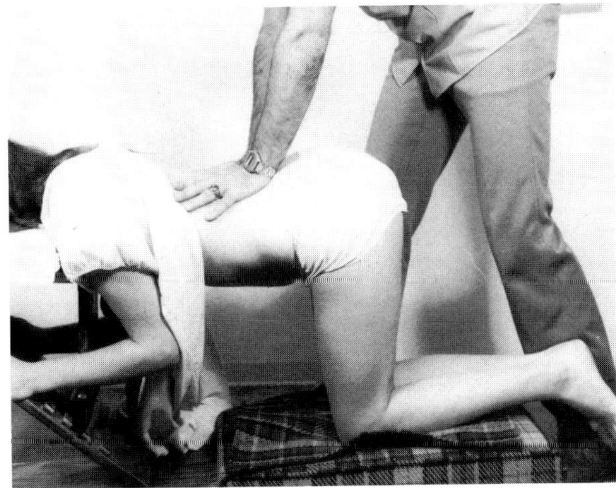

Figure 19–3. Posterior to anterior adjustment of the lumbar spine using a knee posture table.

The Side Posture Adjustment

This is probably the oldest form of manipulation used by early medical, osteopathic, and chiropractic schools. The original technique was a relatively long lever rotational thrust using the shoulder and hip of the patient as levers. If one uses the leg as a lever, a very strong rotational force can be exerted. Because of concern over potential injury, however, a number of chiropractors, notably Gonstead, have modified this technique to make it much more specific and less traumatic. By specific placement, rotation can be reduced to a minimum. A localized thrust can be given using contacts on specific areas of the pelvis, sacrum, or lumbar vertebrae (Fig. 19–4).

Traction-distraction Adjustments

These techniques have been developed over the years with more recent modification by Cox.[21] Specific tables have been developed that allow for strapping of the trunk and legs and the application of traction forces to the lumbar spine. Because these techniques combine directional traction and adjusting thrusts they have been recommended for patients with disc herniation.

Point Pressure Manipulations

Multiple variations of trigger point massage or manipulation techniques have been developed to treat tender areas within muscles. Some of these techniques have been proposed for balancing muscle groups; however, little research has been done to determine exactly what happens when these techniques are applied.

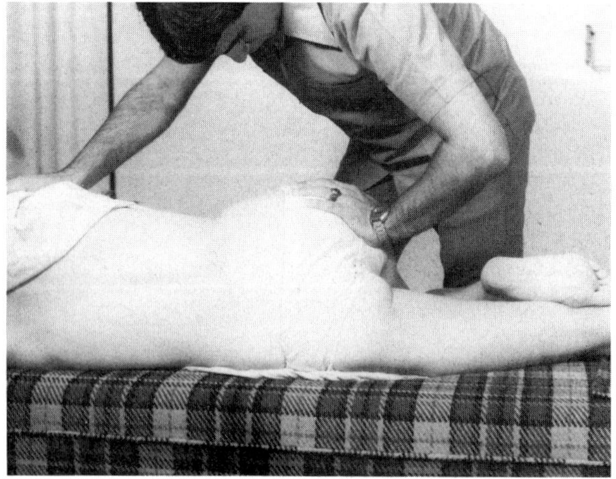

Figure 19–4. Side posture adjustment using specific contact to greatly reduce the amount of applied rotation.

Miscellaneous Techniques

A wide variety of techniques have been developed that fall beyond the scope of this chapter. These techniques use body weight to support spinal segments on blocks, various mechanical plungers to exert a force, and so-called stretch-relaxation and muscle energy techniques.

Post Manipulation Management

Once the manipulation or adjustment has been given chiropractic management tends to focus on improving the internal and external environment of the patient. The assumption is that recurrences of back pain are less likely if the patient is healthy and maintains a healthy lifestyle. This requires a series of steps.

Education

Chiropractors have always spent time educating patients on such subjects as the mechanism of their pain and proper sleeping and lifting habits. More recently chiropractors, along with other health care professions, have tended to formalize this process into back schools.

Exercise

The basic chiropractic premise that proper physical fitness and exercise is beneficial to both the general and spinal health has led to strong recommendations for daily exercise. As with other fields, the nature and type of exercise has changed with recent developments in kinesiology. In recent years it is becoming increasingly common for chiropractors to incorporate exercise and rehabilitation equipment into their practices.

Orthotics

The modification of sitting and standing postures with proper seats, lumbar supports, corsets, and foot orthoses is commonly used to allow patients to perform daily activities with greater ease and less pain.

Diet

Combined with exercise, proper diet is advised to maintain weight and ensure proper nutrition and overall health of the patient.

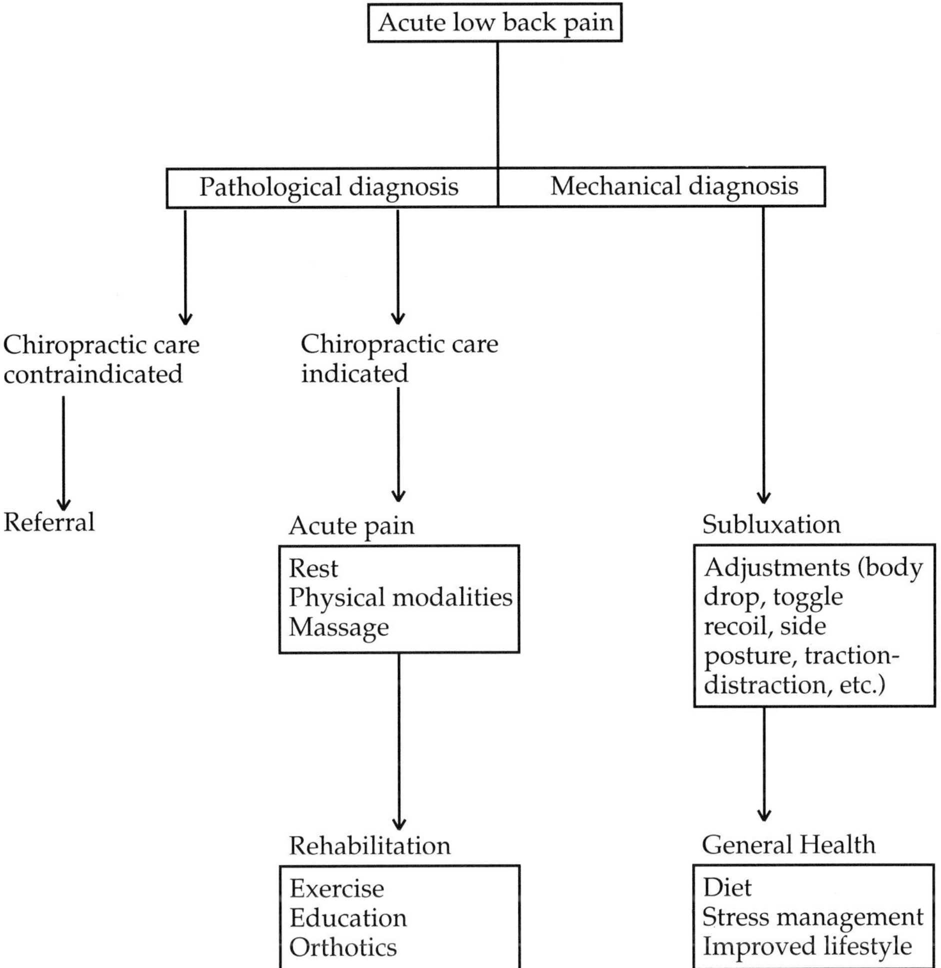

Figure 19–5. The chiropractic approach to acute back pain.

Relaxation

Recognizing a close relationship between excessive psychological stress and ill health, specifically increased incidence of back pain, chiropractors tend to advocate stress management and relaxation.

SUMMARY

The chiropractic approach to acute back pain is a combination of naturalistic philosophy, scientific theory, clinical art, and the skill of spinal manipulation or adjustment. These components cannot be satisfactorily separated as each affects the other. Figure 19–5 summarizes the specifics of chiropractic management of low back pain.

REFERENCES

1. Wood, P.H.N., Bradley, E.: Epidemiology of back pain. *In* The Lumbar Spine and Back Pain (Edited by M.I.V. Jayson). Kent, Pittman Medical Limited, pp. 29–55, 1980.
2. Cherkin, D.C., MacCornuch, F.A.: Patient evaluation of low back pain care from family physicians and chiropractors. West J Med *150*:351–355, 1989.
3. Kane, R.L., et al.: Manipulating the patients. A comparison of the effectiveness of physicians and chiropractic care. Lancet *1*:1333–1336, 1974.
4. Palmer, D.D.: The science, art and philosophy of chiropractic. Portland, Portland Printing House, 1910.
5. McHenry, L.C.: Garrison's History of Neurology. Springfield, Charles C. Thomas, 1969.
6. Gibbons, R.W.: The evolution of chiropractic: medical and social protest in America. Notes on the survival years and after. *In* Modern Developments in the Principles and Practice of Chiropractic (Edited by S. Haldeman). New York, Appleton-Century-Croft, 1980.
7. Akeson, W.H., Aniel, D., Woo, S.: Immobility effects on synovial joints. The pathomechanics of joint contracture. Biorheology *17*:95–110, 1980.

8. Holm, S., Nachemson, A.: Variations in the nutrition of canine intervertebral disc induced by motion. Orthop Trans 6:48, 1982.
9. Evans, D.P., et al.: Lumbar spinal manipulation on trial. I. Clinical assessment. Rheumatol Rehabil 12:46–53, 1978.
10. Nwuga, V.C.B.: Relative therapeutic efficacy of vertebral manipulation and conventional treatment in back pain management. Am J Phys Med 61:273–278, 1982.
11. Diebert, P., England, R.: Electromyographic studies. 1. Consideration in the evaluation of osteopathic therapy. J Am Osteopath Assoc 72:162–169, 1972.
12. Grice, A.A.: Muscle tone changes following manipulation. J Can Chiropractic Assoc 19:29–31, 1974.
13. Glover, J.R., Morris, J.G., Khosla, T.: Back pain: a randomized clinical trial of rotational manipulation of the trunk. Br J Ind Med 31:59–64, 1974.
14. Hoehler, F.K., Tobis, J.S., Buerger, A.A.: Spinal manipulation for low back pain. JAMA 145:1835–1838, 1981.
15. Glover, J.R.: Back pain and hyperesthesia. Lancet 1:1165–1169, 1980.
16. Terrett, A.C.J., Vernon, H.: Manipulation and pain tolerance. A controlled study of the effects of spinal manipulation on paraspinal cutaneous pain tolerance levels. Am J Phys Med 63:217–225, 1984.
17. Wyke, B.D.: Articular neurology: a review. Physiotherapy 58:94–100, 1973.
18. Vernon, H.T., Dhami, M.S.I., Howley, T.P., Annett, R.: Spinal manipulation and beta-endorphin: a controlled study of the effect of a spinal manipulation on plasma beta-endorphin levels in normal males. J Manipulative Physiol Ther 92:115–123, 1986.
19. Cyriax, R.: Textbook of Orthopedic medicine. Vol. 1: Diagnosis of soft tissue lesions. 6th Ed. London, Bailliere Tindall, 1975.
20. Maigne, R.: Orthopedic medicine—a new approach to vertebral manipulation (Translated by W. T. Liberson). Springfield, Charles C. Thomas, 1972.
21. Cox, J.M.: Low back pain. 3rd Ed. Fort Wayne, self-published, 1985.
22. Gitelman, R.: A chiropractic approach to biomechanical disorders of the lumbar spine. In Modern Developments in the Principles and Practice of Chiropractic (Edited by S. Haldeman). New York, Appleton-Century-Croft, 1980.
23. Haldeman, S.: Spinal manipulative therapy in the management of low back pain. In Low Back Pain (Edited by B. E. Finneson), 2nd Ed. Philadelphia, J. B. Lippincott, 1980.
24. Mennell, J. McM.: Back pain—diagnosis and treatment using manipulative therapy. Boston, Little, Brown, 1960.
25. Thompson, J.C.: Thompson technique. Davenport, self-published, 1973.

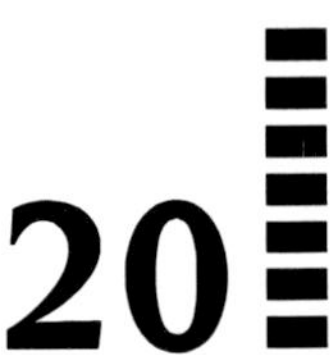

20

Robin McKenzie

A Physical Therapy Perspective on Acute Spinal Disorders

INTRODUCTION

The great majority of patients with activity-related spinal disorders have nonspecific back pain. Over 90% of these problems are mechanical in origin and respond to conservative care. Ninety-two percent are better in 2 months.[1]

Clinical studies into the effectiveness of ultrasound, shortwave diathermy, interferential therapy, and laser therapy have shown that these treatments do not alter the natural history of mechanical back pains. Acupuncture has been shown to be as effective as a placebo, and transcutaneous electrical stimulation modulates pain but has no effect on the disease.[2]

The most frequently used conservative therapies are mechanical treatments delivered by either physiotherapists, chiropractors, or osteopaths. Mobilization or manipulative therapy, often called Spinal Manipulation Therapy (SMT), are probably the most widely dispensed of the mechanical therapies in use today. These treatments provide short-term benefit only;[2] there are no long term benefits. The Quebec Task Force (QTF) reports few treatment strategies that significantly alter the natural history of common mechanical spinal disorders.

In our search for a better method of treatment, we should target one that has the potential to provide the patient with a long term benefit. Such a treatment would ideally be carried out by the patient, and therefore should be simple in design and application. It must be cost effective, and must not create patient dependency. It must have the potential to make the patient independent from therapists whenever possible. It also must be available from the therapist who should be required to teach it.

Once identified, every patient should be entitled to receive such a treatment and every therapist should be obliged to provide it. The question is, "Does such a treatment exist?"

THE QUEBEC REPORT

In 1987, a report entitled "Scientific Approach to the Assessment and Management of Activity Related Spinal Disorders" was published in *Spine*.[2] This Report of the Quebec Task Force (QTF) was commissioned by the Quebec Institute for Workers Safety and Health. One of the main concerns of the Institute was the escalation of costs for the treatment of spinal disorders, especially the cost of physiotherapy. The QTF was required to report on the current status of diagnosis and treatment of activity-related spinal disorders. The QTF report states: "Of the numerous pathologic conditions of the spine, nonspecific ailments of back pain in the lumbar, dorsal, and cervical regions, with or without radiation of pain, comprise the vast majority of problems found among workers (and the incidence in general populations can only be greater)."[2] It is estimated that over 90% of spinal mechanical disorders fall into this category, thus only about 10% of patients can be specifically diagnosed with our present technology and understanding.

To improve our methods of diagnosis the QTF recommends the universal adoption of a system of classification for nonspecific mechanical spinal problems based on simple clinical criteria. The QTF has recommended that pain patterns be used as the basis for this universal classification. The QTF reasoned that such a system could be used by all health professions and would thus speed the process of accurate identification of the problems. This in turn would enable us to improve our current treatment methods. The QTF classification for nonspecific spinal disorders follows.

1. Pain in the lumbar, dorsal, or cervical areas, without radiation below the gluteal fold or beyond the shoulder, respectively, and in the absence of neurologic signs. The Report states "We believe that this category represents most cases. The pain is intermittent or constant, its intensity varying with the patient's tolerance, and is almost always aggravated by mechanical factors.[2]"
2. Pain in the lumbar, dorsal, or cervical areas, with radiation proximally (i.e., to an upper or lower limb but not beyond the knee or the elbow, respectively) and not accompanied by neurologic signs. In this category, the pain that radiates to the proximal part of the limb can be neurogenic, but it originates most often from the deep structures of the rachis, as demonstrated by the studies of Kellgren[3] and McCall, et al.[4]
3. Pain in the lumbar, dorsal, or cervical areas, with radiation distally (i.e., beyond the knee or the elbow, respectively) but without neurologic signs. In this instance, the pain radiates to the whole limb. It may occupy a specific dermatome, thereby suggesting a radicular origin, or it may be more diffuse.
4. Pain in the lumbar, dorsal, or cervical areas, with radiation to a limb and with the presence of neurologic signs (e.g., focal muscular weakness, asymmetry of reflexes, sensory loss in a dermatome, or specific loss of intestinal, bladder, or sexual function). This category includes the radicular syndromes, which are well described in classic textbooks. These radicular syndromes may result from various affections, the most frequent being the discal hernia.

The first classification recommended by the QTF describes uncomplicated problems causing back pain only. Classifications two and three are applied as the picture becomes more complex and the symptoms peripheralize and move progressively below the knee. Classification four applies to those patients with additional neurologic complications.

Having found a useful and highly recommended system for classification of nonspecific spinal disorders, all that is required is a treatment protocol that can be used in conjunction with the QTF categories. A useful system of treatment should aim at changing the patient's classification from a more complex to a less complex status. Thus, if pain *below* the knee can be made to relocate *above* the knee, the patient would move from class three to class two. If the pain could then be made to move from the upper leg to

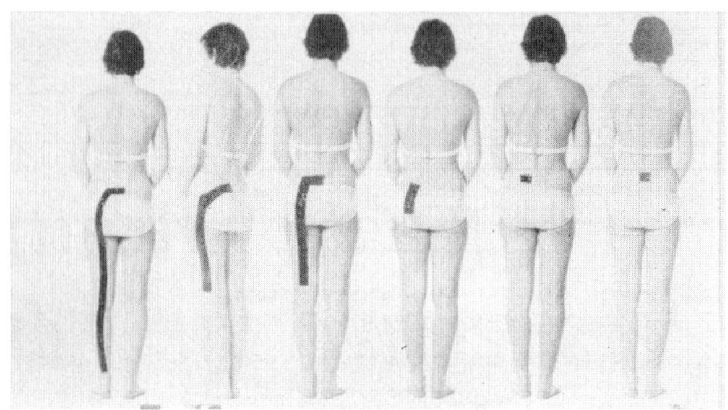

Figure 20–1. The centralization of pain.

the back, the patient would move from class two to class one, again a less complicated classification. The pain in these examples can be seen to be moving progressively from a distal location to a more proximal location as the complications resolve. In other words, the pain "centralizes" as the condition improves (Fig. 20–1).

The system of assessment I described in 1981[5] identifies selected repeated movements that centralize the patient's pain. These movements then form the basis for the treatment program. As the patient's pain centralizes it progressively alters the patient's classification, from a more complex to a less complex category. Repeated movements that cause the pain to increase and move distally are considered inappropriate and are avoided. The treatment method is therefore ideal for use in conjunction with the QTF classification by pain patterns.

By analyzing the effects that repeated movements have on the location of the patient's pain we can identify the direction of therapeutic motion. Several studies now demonstrate the efficacy of the system when used to treat disorders of the lower back.[6–11] Similar studies have yet to be completed in upper spinal regions. Patients whose symptoms peripheralize or centralize in response to repetitive motion demonstrate characteristics of internal derangement described elsewhere.[5,12] I have therefore chosen to classify them as having the "derangement syndrome." Other identifiable subgroups exist within the nonspecific family of spinal disorders.[5,12] Their characteristics are clarified below.

SUBGROUPS IN THE NONSPECIFIC SPECTRUM

The Derangement Syndrome

The Conceptual Model

As long as the annulus fibrosus remains intact and unaffected by the static loading present in everyday life, the patient will experience no more than the normal postural back or neck pains experienced by us all. The annulus fibrosus will restrain the nucleus pulposus from any tendency to displace beyond its normal inner boundaries.[13] However, progressive overstretching, creep, and hysteresis,[14,15] weakens the annulus and impairs its ability to restrain the nucleus. The process of displacement now begins.[13] The embryonic stages of displacement are manifest in complaints of minor back and neck pains only. At this stage displacement is not yet sufficient to cause referred or radicular pain.

Pains felt in the embryonic stages of displacement arise intermittently, and are short-lived, lasting perhaps for 2 or 3 days. The majority of such episodes arise from minor well contained posterior or postero-lateral displacements, which in turn are caused by prolonged or repeated flexion. Displacement causes tension in the annulus, provoking pain that may sometimes appear in the center of the back or to the right or left side, depending on the site of the displacement. When the patient reports that the location of his pain can change from day to day, it is my contention that the location of the displacement has also changed.

With the passage of time and progressive increase in the degree of displacement, *episodes* of recurring pain are experienced. These inflict increasingly severe symptoms, which may be referred or radicular. Such episodes may indicate the breaking of successive layers of the annulus. The available space created by the developing fissure will be occupied by fluid, gel, or sequestrum. Some movements become obstructed by the volume or nature of the displacement within the intact outer annulus. It is at this point that the patient experiences acute pain and locked postures.

In each of these apparently different disorders the patients suffer an obstruction to curve reversal (Figs. 20–2 to 20–4). Indeed, it is the obstruction to curve reversal that is the common factor in all acute disorders, thus providing a clue to the likely mechanism of derangement.

From the application of continuing insult, the annulus will eventually fail completely and either rupture, allowing the extrusion of disc material into the canal, or protrude excessively and irreversibly onto the dura or nerve root. In either situation, the incompetency of the annulus rules out the possibility of reversing the displacement. The application of mechanical therapy is futile and contraindicated at this stage. With time, following repair and fibrosis, the acute symptoms subside. In some patients nerve root adherence may develop and in these cases some sciatic pain may persist for months.

It can be seen that as displacement increases, the symptoms worsen, and the pain moves distally. The derangement model described here is based on the

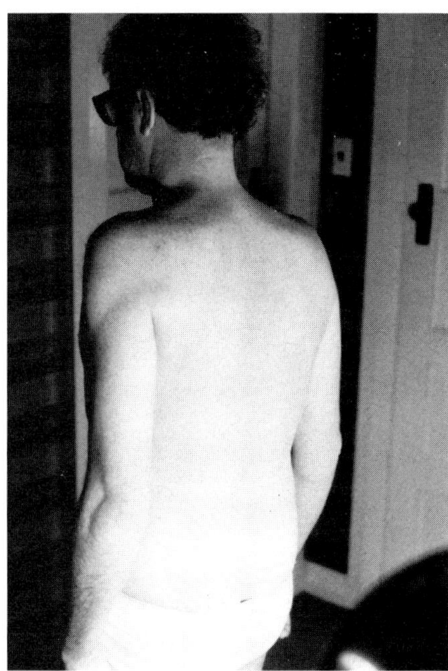

Figure **20–2.** Kyphosis (posterior displacement).

assumption that such displacement is reversible as long as the annulus remains intact. The rationale for the treatment of the derangement syndrome is to apply movements that reverse displacement. The pain will centralize as the displacement is reduced. Centralization of pain occurs only during the reductive process in the derangement syndrome.[5,12]

Acceptance of the conceptual model for the derangement syndrome allows reliable predetermination of the direction of the required therapeutic motion. A better explanation may exist and the present model may eventually be altered, but in the meantime, until that new explanation is forthcoming, this

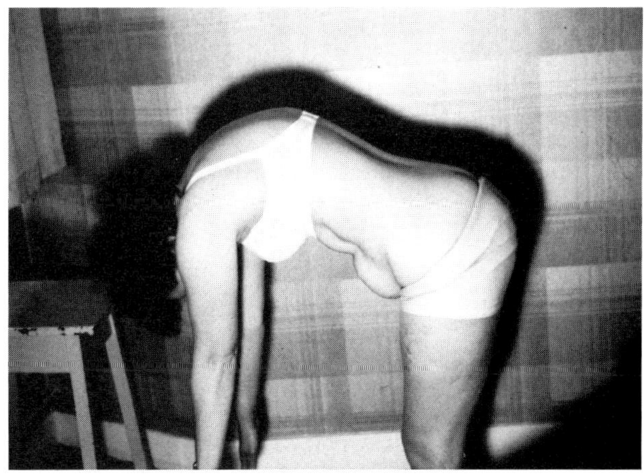

Figure **20–3.** Lordosis (anterior displacement).

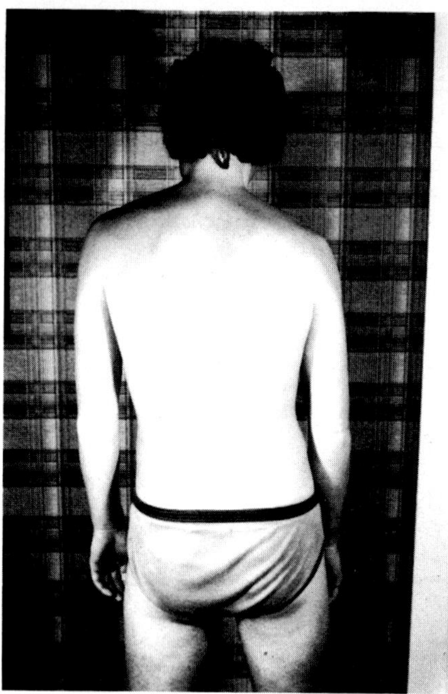

Figure 20–4. List or lateral shift (posterolateral displacement).

is a reasonable and reliable model upon which to base mechanical therapy. Several investigations provide support for the displacement/derangement model described here.[13,16–20]

The Dysfunction Syndrome

The Conceptual Model

Patients within the dysfunction syndrome have contracted, fibrosed, or adherent soft tissues that limit normal motion. The usual cause is cross linkage of collagen formed either adaptively or as a consequence of repair. When symptoms persist long after injury, it is possible that although complete, the repair itself is the cause of the persistent symptoms. These patients do not experience a change in the location of their pain when exercised repetitively.

If poor postural habits persist through the first two or three decades, the annulus and the other overstretched ligamentous and capsular structures begin to fail. The majority of these injuries probably heal quickly and little consequence is felt at the time. However, the cycle of recurring microtrauma and repair eventually leads to loss of elasticity and a reduction of the range of motion. The patient will recall no significant reason for the resulting loss of motion.

A significant injury to the annulus may result in fibrosis within the outer annulus and this too may

result in impaired function. The patient loses full range of motion and experiences discomfort or pain if he or she moves to the now limited end range. We have no way of knowing which structures are affected in such cases. All we can say with confidence is that although repair is complete, soft tissues have contracted, fibrosed, or become adherent in the process. The rationale for the treatment of dysfunction is that an exercise program must be introduced to remodel the tissue by regular stretching of contracted areas.[5,12]

The Postural Syndrome

The Conceptual Model

Some patients complaining of pain of nonspecific origin experience no pain during movement. Their pain occurs only from prolonged static loading. The conceptual model proposes that from the time we commence our early schooling, poor postural and frequent flexion habits cause overstretching of periarticular structures in and near the spine. By the late teens, some individuals have already developed minor back and neck pains. Postural pains arise near the midline of the spine and do not radiate to the extremities. They appear after static loading such as occurs with prolonged sitting, standing, or bending. Such pains are felt only when the stresses are present, and disappear immediately after the structure is released from tension. Providing the patient is active and moving, he experiences no pain. Such patients have pain of postural origin. The rationale for the treatment of the postural syndrome is to educate the patient precisely in the methods required to avoid potentially damaging postures.[5,12]

To identify which of these syndromes may be responsible for the patient's symptoms, it is necessary to apply a dynamic mechanical evaluation.[5,12] This is achieved by having the patient perform repetitive movements in different planes. This will affect the symptoms in different ways depending on the nature of the problem as defined above.

DYNAMIC MECHANICAL EVALUATION

Repeated Movements

When evaluating the effects of repeated movements we are trying to identify changes in the intensity or location of the patient's pain. The manner in which the pain behaves provides us with the clues required to identify the syndrome as well as the direction in which to apply therapeutic motion.[5,12]

Repeated Movements and the Dysfunction Syndrome

Repeated movements, applied in a direction that *stretches* the structures that were shortened, fibrosed, or contracted in dysfunction causes pain to be felt only at the end of the range. Repetition of the movement does not make the patient progressively better or worse. The shortened structure cannot rapidly lengthen so the range of motion will not increase. The pain at end range does not reduce in intensity with repetition; however, when the patient returns to the neutral position the pain ceases. No rapid changes occur. A response such as this indicates the presence of the dysfunction syndrome.[5,12]

Repeated Movements and the Postural Syndrome

Patients with the postural syndrome do not experience pain with any of the test movements or their repetition. These patients must be positioned so that static loading is applied for a sufficient period of time to reproduce pain. Once this has occurred, alteration of the posture stops the pain immediately.

Repeated Movements and the Derangement Syndrome

In derangement, repeated movements applied in the direction that *increases* displacement or flow of fluid, gel, or sequestrum, causes pain to appear, increase, peripheralize, or change location. The pain will be felt during the movement itself. Repetition makes the patient progressively worse. At the same time, a rapid reduction in the range of motion can occur. The patient will feel worse as a result of repeating the movements and, on returning to the neutral position, remains worse as a result.

On the other hand, repeated movements that *reduce* displacement or flow of fluid, gel, or sequestrum, cause pain to disappear, decrease, or centralize. At the same time, a rapid improvement in the range of motion can occur. The patient will feel better as a result of repeating the movements and, on returning to the neutral position, remains better as a result. Rapid changes occur. Thus, repeated movements are diagnostic in derangement disorders (Fig. 20–5).[5,12]

Although most patients with low back pain experience centralization from the performance of extension exercises carried out in the prone unloaded position, others, identified by dynamic mechanical evaluation, must perform extension from a prone laterally flexed position. Another group of patients must repeat flexion movements in order to cause centralization of pain.

TREATMENT

In order to apply mechanical therapy logically, we must treat each syndrome as a separate entity, requiring special procedures that often are unsuitable for the other syndromes. We must correct posture in patients with the postural syndrome; stretch, by remodelling shortened or contracted tissue in the dysfunction syndrome; and apply reductive pressures to displaced tissue in the derangement syndrome.[5,12] It must be emphasized that most patients develop pain and seek assistance as a result of derangement. However, they may also have poor postural habit and after the reduction of derangement and resolution of the symptoms, an underlying loss of function may be exposed. This can often be traced to some previous injury.

To identify the subgroups in the nonspecific spectrum, a good understanding of the centralization of pain phenomena is necessary. In addition, it is necessary to apply the repeated movements accurately and interpret the findings precisely. In the long run and irrespective of the amount of data obtained from the patient's history, clinical examination and paraclinical tests, the final decision with regard to the mechanical approach to be adopted is determined by the patient's response to the mechanical forces applied. The clinician's conception of the appropriate treatment must always be overruled by the emergence of an adverse painful reaction (a frequent occurrence) in response to the initiation of that treatment.

Treatment of the Derangement Syndrome

Sagittal movements performed in the loaded and unloaded positions are likely to affect most pain patterns in nonspecific spinal disorders. Exceptions occur and movements in other planes may be required in some cases.

For disorders affecting the lower back, repetitive flexion, (Figs. 20–6, 20–7) and then repetitive extension (Figs. 20–8, 20–9) are applied. These movements are performed first standing and then lying. Any changes in the intensity or location of pain are recorded. Once the movement that reduces or centralizes the patient's pain is identified, the patient should be instructed to repeat the exercise 8 to 10 times, every 2 hours. Correction of the sitting posture is required in those patients who must extend to reduce the derangement. The maintenance of a

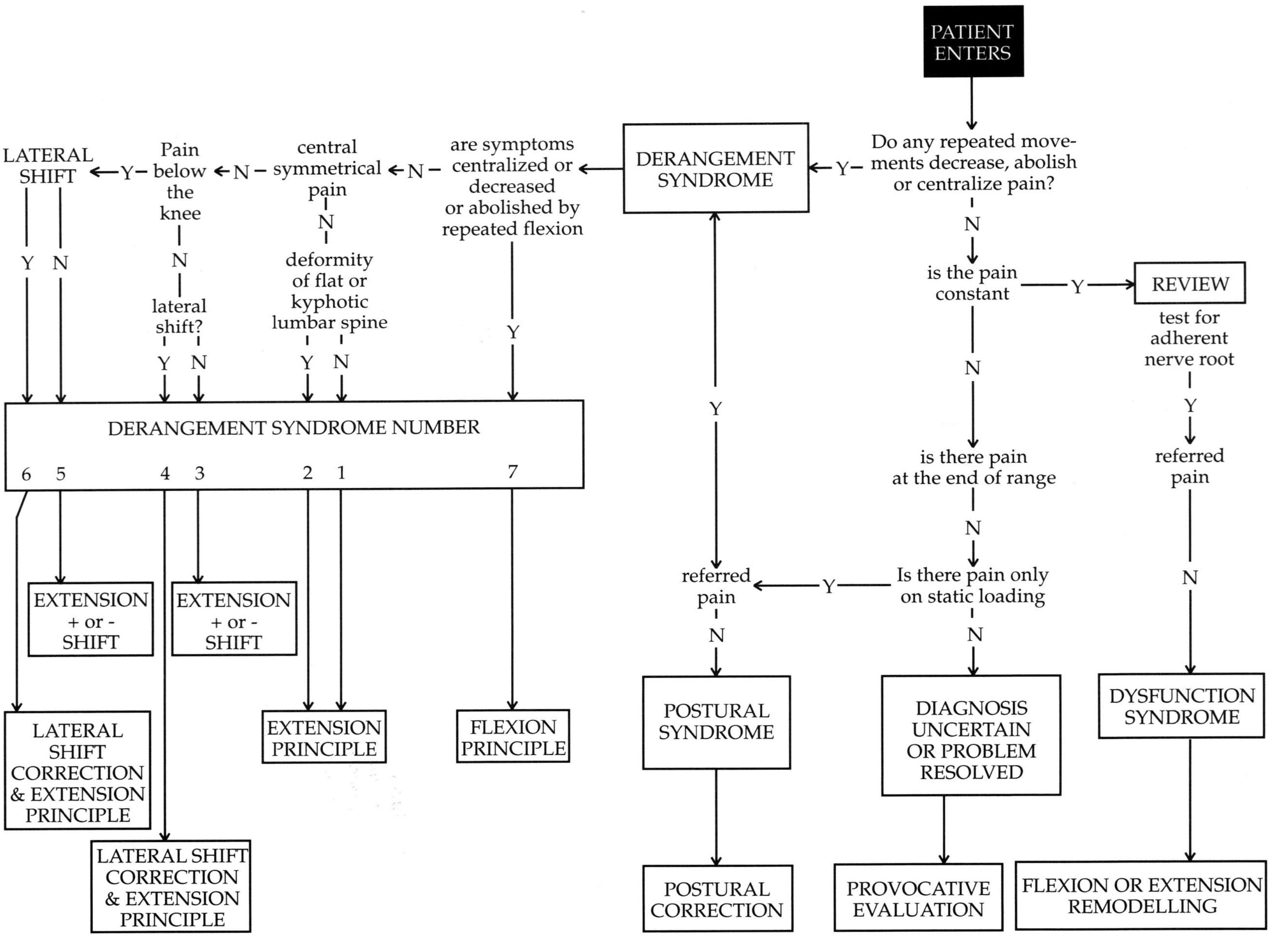

Figure 20–5. The McKenzie Assessment Algorithm.

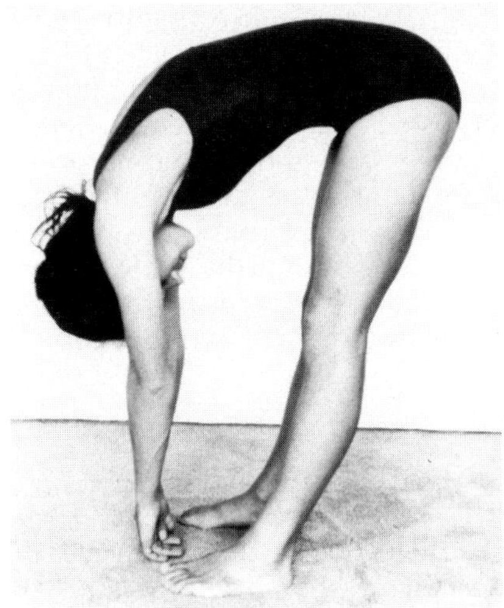

Figure 20–6. Repetitive flexion exercises are applied for the treatment of derangement syndrome.

lordotic sitting posture is essential to the maintenance of reduction of derangement (Fig. 20–10). Any flexion occuring within the first 48 hours after onset immediately results in further displacement.

Treatment of the Dysfunction Syndrome

Once restricted movements are identified, and the integrity of repair has been established, the patient must be given a simple description of the problem. He must be made aware that healing is complete, that pain persists because the repair is inelastic, that to restore the extensibility of the scar he must stretch regularly. He must be made aware that this process will cause some pain with each exercise session, but

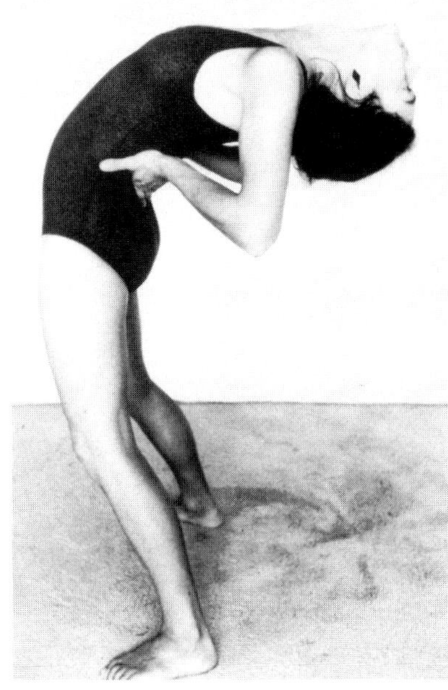

Figure 20–8. Repetitive extension is applied after flexion exercises.

the pain should subside after a few minutes. He also must know that the process of stretching and remodelling will take up to 10 or 12 weeks. Only after the explanations have been provided should the patient commence the exercise program, which has been specifically tailored to his needs.

Treatment of the Postural Syndrome

Postural pains most commonly arise from prolonged sitting, lying, and standing environments. It is necessary to deal with each problem on an indi-

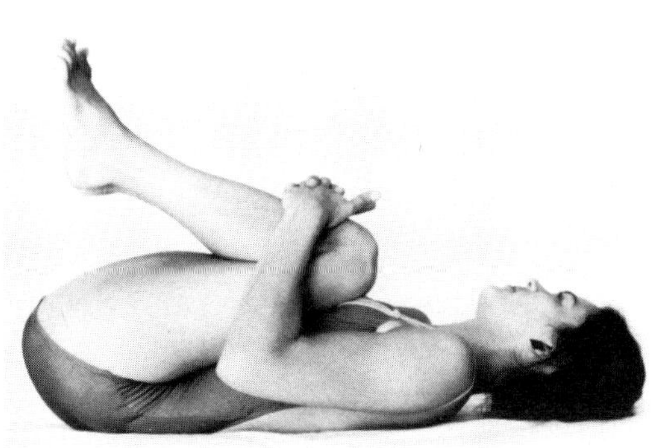

Figure 20–7. A repetitive flexion exercise applied for the treatment of derangement syndrome.

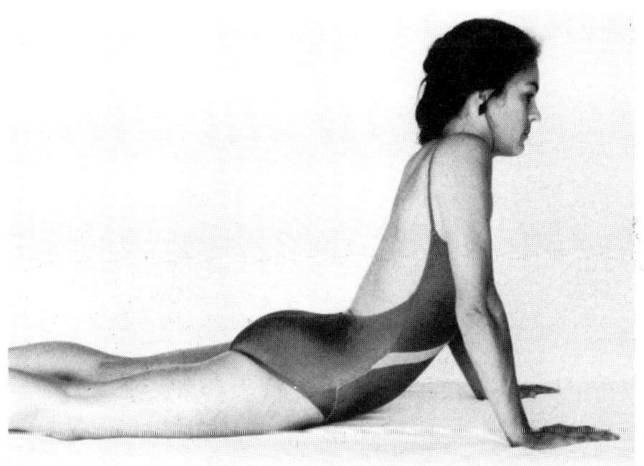

Figure 20–9. A type of repetitive extension exercise applied after flexion.

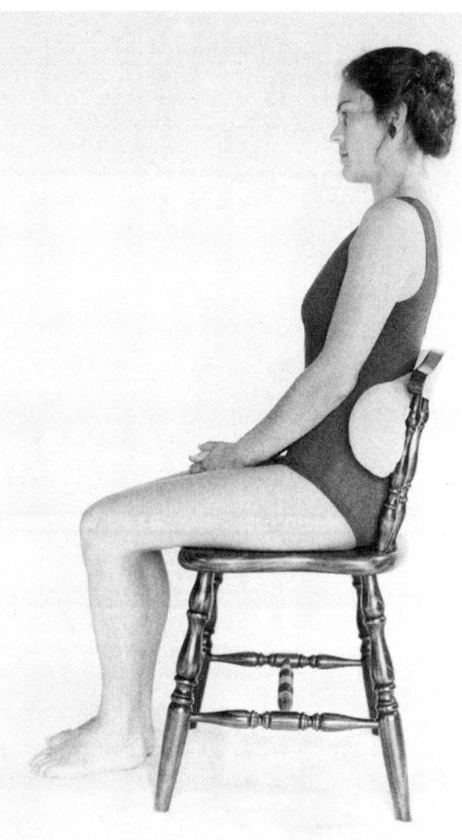

Figure 20–10. Most patients benefit from the use of a portable lumbar roll in all sitting environments.

vidual basis. If the patient has pain that becomes worse with prolonged sitting, the use of a lumbar support to maintain a lordosis is certainly indicated. Most patients benefit from a portable lumbar roll used in all sitting environments.[21] If the patient has pain that becomes worse when lying down, a lumbar roll designed for use in bed frequently solves the

problem (Fig. 20–11). A firm base but soft mattress may also be necessary.[22] If the patient has pain that becomes worse with prolonged standing, it is likely that the lordosis is excessive. If this is the case, instruction in correction of the standing posture is necessary. The patient must be taught to stand erect. This is best achieved by tilting the pelvis to reduce the lumbar lordosis and at the same time raising the chest. A detailed description of the procedures required to treat these three syndromes is published elsewhere.[5,12]

A BRIEF LITERATURE REVIEW

Several studies support these concepts of mechanical diagnosis and therapy. These are briefly reviewed below.

1. Ponte[9] found the McKenzie extension exercises alone to be superior to Williams flexion exercises in the treatment of low back pain.
2. Nwuga[8] found the entire McKenzie protocol superior to the Williams protocol for the treatment of low back pain.
3. Kopp[7] studied a population of 67 patients with the diagnosis of herniated nucleus pulposus. All had loss of extension and an associated neurological deficit. All had previously failed six weeks of conservative care before being placed on the extension exercise program. Conservative care consisted of strict bed rest, followed by protected activity, analgesics, muscle relaxants, deep heat and massage, and attendance at back school.
   Kopp found that 35 of 67 patients responded to the application of repeated extension exercises within 1 and 5 days from the commencement of exercise, with one exception. All 35 achieved normal range of extension and did not require surgery. The remaining 32 patients required surgery.

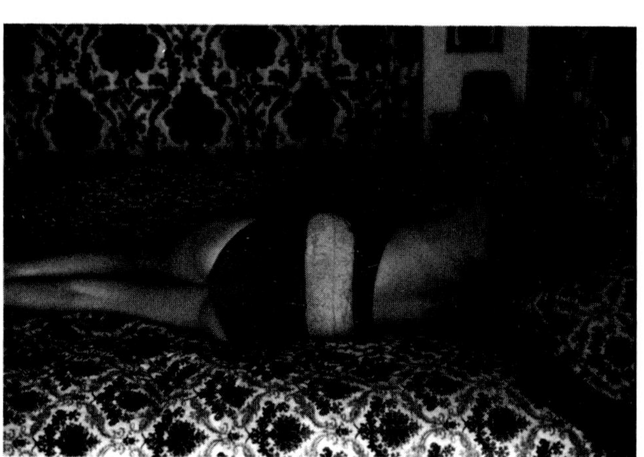

Figure 20–11. A lumbar roll designed for use in bed frequently solves the problem of pain worsenting when lying down.

None of the remaining 32 patients were able to achieve extension prior to surgery. At operation, a high incidence of free disc fragments or nerve root displacement was found.

4. Donelson[6] examined the value of centralization of pain in the assessment and treatment of sciatica. Close correlation was found between the occurence of centralization and a satisfactory outcome, and conversely, between the absence of centralization and an unsatisfactory outcome with mechanical therapy. The centralization of pain was found to be reliable in determining the correct direction of treatment exercise. None of the patients whose pain centralized required surgical intervention; all surgical patients were noncentralizers.

5. Stankovic,[10] in a controlled prospective clinical trial, found that in 100 acute back and referred pain patients, the McKenzie system was superior to mini back school in 5 out of 7 outcome variables. The research group that practiced the McKenzie exercises had significantly fewer recurrences of pain, and fewer patients had to seek help with treatment. The McKenzie group also returned to work sooner at all stages of reporting, and by six weeks 100% had resumed employment. At 11 weeks, 100% of the back school group returned to work. These results are presented in Table 20–1.

In 1986 Vanharanta[11] compared McKenzie exercises with back school and 90/90 traction. One hundred and thirty six patients were randomized to the three groups. Patients crossed to one of the other treatment groups if there was no improvement at the end of one week. It was found that at one week 97% of the McKenzie group improved compared to a success rate of 50% for the 90/90 traction and 38% for the back school group. No patients treated by the McKenzie group were transferred and none were made worse by treatment. Overall, 29 of the patients undergoing 90/90 traction or attending back school were required to transfer to another treatment group

because of treatment failure. All were transferred directly or eventually to the McKenzie program, where all were successfully treated.

McKenzie, Williams, et al.,[21] compared two sitting postures and their effects on back and referred pain. Patients sitting in lumbar lordosis with a support experienced significantly reduced back pain intensity than patients sitting with a flexed posture. The lordotic posture also reduced the intensity of pain felt in the leg and the centralizing of referred pain that occurred in this group was statistically significant.

REFERENCES

1. Fry, J.: Back Pain and Soft Tissue Rheumatism. Proc Advisory Services Colloquium. London, Advisory Services (Clinical & General), 1972.
2. Spitzer, W.O.: Scientific approach to the assessment and management of activity-related spinal disorders. A Monograph for clinicians: Report of the Quebec Task Force on Spinal Disorders. Spine *12*(7S), 1987.
3. Kellgren, J.H.: The anatomical source of back pain. Rheumatol Rehabil *16*:3–12, 1977.
4. McCall, I.W., Park, W.M., O'Brien, J.P.: Induced pain referral from posterior lumbar elements in normal subjects. Spine *4*:441–446, 1979.
5. McKenzie, R.A.: The Lumbar Spine. Mechanical Diagnosis and Therapy. Waikanae, NZ, Spinal Publications, 1981.
6. Donelson, R., Murphy, K., Silva, G.: Centralization Phenomenon: Its Usefulness in Evaluating and Treating Sciatica. Presented at the annual meeting of International Society for the Study of the Lumbar Spine. Dallas, TX, 1986.
7. Kopp, J.R., Alexander, A.H., Turocy, R.H.: The use of lumbar extension in the evaluation and treatment of patients with acute herniated nucleus pulposus. A preliminary report. Clin Orthop *202*:211–218, 1986.
8. Nwuga, G., Nwuga, V.: Relative therapeutic efficacy of the Williams and McKenzie protocols in back pain management. Physiother Pract *1*:99–105, 1985.
9. Ponte, D.J., et al.: A preliminary report on the use of the McKenzie protocol versus Williams protocol in the treatment of low back pain. J Orthop Sports Physical Ther *6*:(2)130–139, 1984.
10. Stankovic, R.: McKenzie method of treatment versus patient education in "mini back school" for acute low back pain, a controlled prospective clinical trial. Proc Int Fed Orthop Manipul Ther Cambridge, UK, September, 1988.
11. Vanharanta, H., Videman, T., Mooney, V.: Comparison of McKenzie Exercises, Back Trac and Back School in Lumbar Syndrome; Preliminary Results. Presented at the annual meeting of International Society for the Study of the Lumbar Spine, Dallas, TX, 1986.
12. McKenzie, R.A.: The Cervical and Thoracic Spine: Mechanical Diagnosis and Therapy. Waikanae, NZ, Spinal Publications, 1989.
13. Kramer, J.: Intervertebral Disk Diseases. Causes, Diagnosis, Treatment and Prophylaxis. Year Book Medical Publishers, 1981.
14. Hickey, J.A., Hukins, K.I.: Relationship between the structure and function of the annulus fibrosus and the function and failure of the intervertebral disc. Spine *5*:2;106, 1980.
15. Twomey, L., Taylor, J.: Flexion creep deformation and hysteresis in the lumbar vertebral column. Spine *7*:2;116–122, 1982.

Table 20–1
Results of McKenzie Versus Back School Comparison Study

Return to Work	McKenzie	Back School
At 1 week	42%	22%
At 2 weeks	84%	46%
At 3 weeks	94%	72%
At 4 weeks	98%	82%
At 6 weeks	100%	90%
At 11 weeks		100%

16. Adams, M.A., Hutton, W.C.: Prolapsed intervertebral disc: a hyper-flexion injury. Spine 7:3;184, 1982.
17. Adams, M.A., Hutton, W.C.: Gradual disc prolapse. Spine 10:6;524–531, 1985.
18. Krag, M.H., Seroussi, R.E., Wilder, D.G., Pope, M.H.: Internal displacement distribution from in vitro loading of human thoracic and lumbar spinal motion segments: experimental results and theoretical predictions. Spine 12:10;1001, 1987.
19. Stahl, C.: Experimentelle Untersuchungen zur Biomechanik der Halswirbelsaule. Dusseldorf, Med. Diss., 1977.
20. Vogel, G.: Experimentelle Untersuchungen zur Mobilitat des Nucleus pulposus in lumbalen Bandscheiben. Dusseldorf, Med. Diss., 1977.
21. McKenzie, R.A., Williams, M.M., Hawley, J.A., et al.: A Comparison of the Effects of Two Sitting Postures on Back and Referred Pain. International Society for the Study of the Lumbar Spine. Miami, FL, April 1988.
22. McKenzie, R.A.: Treat Your Own Back. Waikanae, NZ, Spinal Publications, 1981.

Claudia P. Jackson

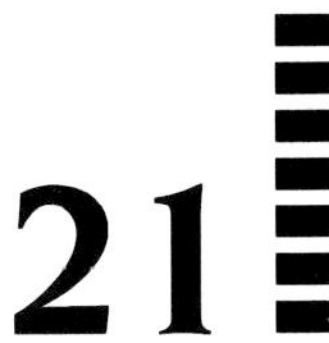

21

Historic Perspectives on Patient Education and Its Place in Acute Spinal Disorders

A back school is an educational program designed to teach patients how to help care for their low back problem. By definition, it does not include diagnosis or treatment, although it may serve as an adjunct to them. Classes may cover basic anatomy, terminology, spinal function, posture, body mechanics, first aid, exercises, ergonomic advice, pain control measures, coping skills, or relaxation techniques. Regardless of the emphasis of any particular program, all back schools share the common goals of reducing patient anxiety, helping patients to share responsibility for their back rehabilitation, and decreasing medical costs.

Back schools have become a critical part of the management of patients suffering from low back pain. Although the idea of educating low back patients has gained wide acceptance, the principles that govern a successful program have often been ignored or forgotten, leading to disappointing results. The goal of this chapter is to acquaint the reader with a back school program for acute patients and to examine the methodologies involved in achieving a successful outcome.

HISTORIC PERSPECTIVE

Patient education is a concept as old as Hippocrates. However, credit for the first "back school" educational program goes to Delpech, who reported on classes for patients with scoliosis and poliomyelitis as early as 1828.[1] The contemporary form of a low back school was introduced by Zacharisson-Forssell in 1970.[2] Known as the Swedish Back School, it was developed to help get the acutely injured worker back to work. The program consists of four 45-minute lessons supervised by a physical therapist (PT). It is built around a slide show, which focuses on factors that cause mechanical stress to the low back. Rest positions and body mechanics for work and activities of daily living (ADLs) are taught based on the principle of minimizing lumbar disc pressure. Maintenance and support of the lumbar lordosis in both sitting and work activities is stressed. A practice session is provided in ADLs and work mechanics. Isometric abdominal exercises and quadriceps strengthening exercises are taught. An optional supervised session of swimming is offered and patients are encouraged to pursue this activity to stay fit. The program is taught at the worksite and its primary goal is to speed the injured worker's return to work.

The Canadian Back Education Unit was introduced by Hall in 1974.[3,4] Hall modified the back school concept for a chronic population, adding elements such as coping skills, drug use and abuse information, and relaxation exercises. Classes range in size from 15 to 25 patients and are taught by a health care team made up of a physical therapist, orthopedist, psychiatrist, and psychologist. The original program consists of four 90-minute classes, with a one hour review class 6 months later. Topics covered include basic anatomy, spinal terminology, common forms of treatment, emotional factors related to pain, and coping mechanisms. Flexion exercises intended to strengthen the abdominal muscles and reduce pain are taught. Body mechanics based on minimizing the lumbar lordosis to reduce stress to the low back are taught. A practical session is held to teach flexion and relaxation exercises. The program is taught in a classroom setting removed from the work environment. A primary goal of this program is to change patients' attitudes about pain.

In 1976, White introduced the California Back School.[5,6] The program is highly individualized, with class size ranging from 1 to 4. The school consists of three 90-minute classes with a one hour followup class one month later. A PT supervises all instruction. Designed for the acute low back patient, this program introduced the concept of an obstacle course to both evaluate functional status and train patients in proper body mechanics. Proper rest positions are taught as a means of reducing pain. Exercises are taught to strengthen the abdominal and quadriceps muscles. Normal posture and spinal function are explained. ADLs are taught with emphasis on a posterior pelvic tilt to minimize pain and stress to the low back.[5] Recreational, work, and sports activities are taught and practiced based on the abdominal corset theory. The program emphasizes psychomotor skills to minimize reinjury. Unlike the Canadian program, which uses a pre- and post-test of cognitive skills, the California School uses the obstacle course to test mastery of motor skills at entry and exit. The program is often run simultaneously with a diagnostic and physical therapy program. A primary goal of this program is to prevent recurrence of the patient's acute back pain.

Back schools were originally designed for patient management. However, in more recent times, they have been used in the industrial setting to prevent injury from occurring. Although it is difficult to single out any one preventive program as being the first or offering an innovative approach, the Back Dynamics Institute offers an industrial program that serves as a appropriate model for this type of program.[7] A research team spends 80 hours in the company to identify injury hazards, inadequate working practices, and training needs. The next phase involves meeting with company management to identify the injury hazards and to provide ergonomic recommendations. The third phase is a 1-hour employee training program in posture, fitness, work practices, and ADLs, which is taught in small groups. A refresher course is offered to all employees 7 months later, adding stress management and nutrition to the original information. This program is carried out at the industrial site and stresses management involvement and co-worker role models to

ensure success. Its goal is to reduce the amount and extent of back injuries by preventing their occurrence.

Although hundreds of back school programs exist today, the three patient-oriented programs mentioned are the historic models upon which most other programs are based. They demonstrate not only differences in teaching methods, content, and goals, but also how programs can and must vary in approaching different populations.

DO BACK SCHOOLS WORK?

Bergquist-Ullman performed the landmark study on the Swedish Back School that stimulated modern interest in this treatment approach. In a controlled, prospective study of acute, industrial patients, the Swedish Back School was found to be superior to PT and placebo in reducing time off from work in the year following injury.[8] Further, back school was as effective as PT in achieving pain reduction. The back school, teaching several patients at a time, also minimized the cost of achieving these results. A more recent controlled prospective study of subacute patients attending a back school with a conditioning component found a decrease in pain intensity, fatigue, anxiety, helplessness, pain behavior, and absenteeism in the back school group.[9] Controlled studies of chronic patients indicate back schools can increase function[10] and decrease the incidence of recurrence.[11] Clearly, the back school has established a beneficial role in the care of acute, chronic, and industrial back injuries, while minimizing the cost of medical care.

Several longitudinal, uncontrolled studies have been performed on the preventive back school used in industry. Followup data on these programs, collected at one-and-a-half to 2 years after back school training, indicates a significant decrease in absenteeism from back related injuries (43–70%) and in cost of disability claims (70%).[5,7,12] Although these initial findings are favorable, further study with control groups is needed to eliminate the influence of economics, maturation, and the Hawthorne effect.

THE ACUTE BACK SCHOOL

The remainder of this chapter focuses on the acute back school, its contents, and methodology. Although some of the principles examined apply to any type of back school, it should be remembered that content areas must be specific to the target population: acute, chronic, or industrial.

Content: The Miami Back School

The Miami Back School was started in 1982 by Jackson.[13] The program is taught by a PT and psychologist and consists of four 2-hour classes and a review class after 6 months. The Miami Back School is divided into acute and chronic programs. The acute program focuses on minimizing anxiety, identifying physical and emotional factors that cause stress to the low back, establishing guidelines for aerobic and endurance exercises, examining simple methods of environmental adaptation to reduce mechanical stressors, and teaching and practicing ADLs based on principles of minimizing disc pressure and muscle fatigue. The program includes a 2-hour practical session on body mechanics and several shorter sessions on relaxation techniques. Table 21–I provides an outline of the acute program.

The primary goals of the Miami program are to minimize recurrence and reduce the risk of chronic disability. Recurrence is thought to be reduced by eliminating or minimizing contributing physical and emotional factors. The risk of chronic disability is reduced by decreasing anxiety and pain, giving patients a sense of control over their condition, educating patients on the true goals and effects of various treatments to help them avoid potentially harmful ones, and reducing the patient's sense of isolation. The Miami Back School uses techniques of education, group support, and anxiety reduction to achieve these goals.

Class 1

This class focuses on the reassuring aspects of low back pain. The natural history of back pain is discussed, with emphasis on full recovery in most cases.[8] Patients are told recovery is partly under their control and it is the goal of the back school to teach them how to take this control. The need for active patient participation in their own care is emphasized.

Removing the mystery surrounding back pain is the next goal, and this is addressed via discussions on anatomy and terminology. Basic elements of spinal anatomy are examined: disc, vertebrae, nerve, muscle, and facet joints. Emphasis is on the functional aspects of anatomy as they apply to back function, pain, and treatment. Normal posture is demonstrated, emphasizing the three physiologic curves. Terminology related to spinal disease is explained. Frightening jargon and misconceptions are eliminated. The emphasis is on de-mystifying medical terms with simple descriptions. It is stressed, for example, that discs do not slip, radiculopathy is not a progressive nerve disease, lumbago simply means the back hurts, and degenerative disc disease does not mean the entire spine is deteriorating. These topics are essential in reducing patient anxiety.[14]

Risk factors are discussed next, with emphasis on how to counteract them. A summary of risk factors presented throughout the program is found in Table 21–2. The dangers of prolonged bed rest are first discussed.[15-19] Patients are told the amount of time spent on bed rest is a better predictor of how many days will be lost from work than the intensity of their pain, the number of prior episodes, their spinal motion, or physical tests such as SLR.[15] A 2-day-limit on bed rest is suggested for any acute attacks of pain.[15] The effects on the low back of smoking,[20-24] sedentary life style[21,25] and obesity[21] are explained. Patients are taught how each of these factors affects the development or persistence of low back pain.

Mechanical stress, emotional stress, and unnecessary treatment are next discussed. Mechanical stress is described in terms of postural habits, body mechanics, and job demands.[20,26-30] The relationship of emotional factors to pain is introduced and is a theme carried through the four classes.[18,31-38] This is discussed in more depth by the psychologist later in the class. The physical and emotional risks of pro-

Table 21–1
Acute Back School Outline

Class 1	Class 3
Anatomy	Common forms of
Terminology	treatment
Risk factors	Exercises for low back
Practice: posture	pain
Benefits of activity	Review and test: ADLs
Emotional aspects	Practice: kneel-standing
Practice: visual imagery	Recreational activities
	Sex
	Practice: visual imagery
Class 2	
Biomechanics: posture	**Class 4**
and body mechanics	Practical session: rest
Environmental	positions, body
adaptations	mechanics, serial
Practice: sitting posture	relaxation
Pain: sources and	
management	Q & A session
Benefits of exercise	
Practice: serial relaxation	

Table 21–2
Risk Factors

Prolonged bed rest	Mechanical stress
Smoking	Emotional stress
Sedentary lifestyle	Unnecessary treatment
Obesity	Drug abuse
Height	Motor fatigue

longed or unnecessary treatment is the last risk factor introduced at this time.

Poor postural habits were identified as a risk factor, so the first practice session focuses on normal posture in standing and sitting. This is the first step in giving patients a sense of control over their condition.[39] Practice is followed by a juice break for rest and socialization.

The benefits of activity, be it housework, walking, a hobby, or office duties, are discussed and suggested as a method to counteract the risk factors of bed rest, inactivity, obesity, and anxiety.[40,41] The theme of activity and exercise to combat back pain is gradually developed through the four classes.

The psychologist is now introduced, and for a half-hour discusses the relationship of emotional factors to pain. Because this is an acute back school, the focus is on the effects of anxiety on pain.[31,32] Prolonged drug use is described as a risk factor to mental and physical health.[42] In place of sleeping pills, L-tryptophan, found in milk and potatoes, is suggested as a method to reduce pain and aid sleep.[43–45] The concept of self-management of pain is introduced. Visual imagery for relaxation and pain control is presented as an example.[46] The class ends with a practical session in visual imagery.

Class 2

This class requires an instructor with a sound working knowledge of spinal biomechanics.[29,47–50] Even more essential, however, is the ability to convey this information in practical terms for patient use.

Normal posture is reviewed, with emphasis on the protective mechanism of the normal physiological curves.[50] Disc pressure changes that result from various postures and activities are then introduced.[29] The final component upon which functional tasks are built is trunk muscle function and fatigue.[51–55]

The basic principles of body mechanics are then presented (Table 21–3). Each principle is followed by practical examples. Slides demonstrating both right and wrong techniques are used for emphasis. A word of caution: handouts, slides, and verbal instruction are insufficient techniques to teach motor skills.[56] A practical session must be provided at some point to ensure understanding and mastery.

An attempt is made to advance functional examples from simple to complex. For example, principle 1 recommends maintaining the normal physiologic curves in most activities.[29,50] The kneel-standing position (Fig. 21–1) is introduced as the preferred method to help maintain a lordosis when working at low areas, such as cleaning an oven, working at a

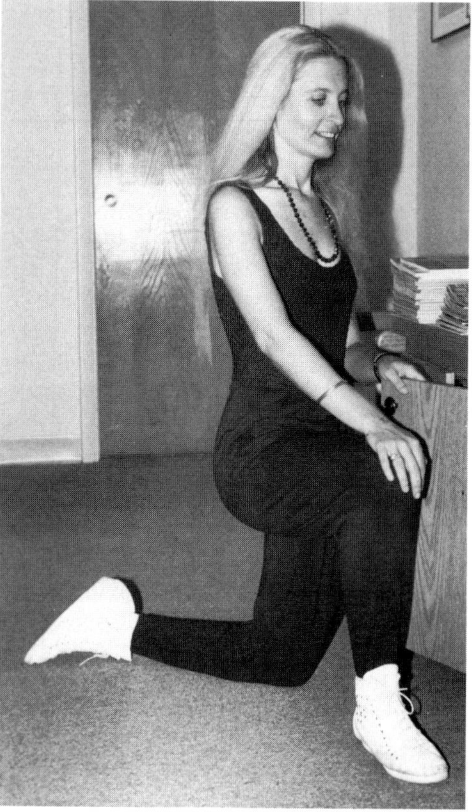

Figure 21–1. The kneel-standing position prevents loss of the lumbar lordosis when working at low heights.

file cabinet, or adjusting the controls on a television or stereo. Patients are firmly instructed *not* to stand against a wall and flatten their backs as a way to maintain good upright posture.

Principles 1, 2, and 6, maintaining the lumbar lordosis and bending the knees to lift,[29,50,57,58] are applied to such situations as picking up the morning paper from the front steps and unloading the dishwasher. Principle 11, the use of adaptive equipment to minimize lumbar loads, has many applications in the home. A long-handled sponge is recommended for washing the car or cleaning the bathtub. A neck-hung mirror prevents bending over the sink during shaving. An extended shoe horn is suggested to avoid lumbar flexion early in the morning,[59,60] a combination of principles 11 and 12. A more complex example is storing and removing bags of groceries from the car. This involves application of principles 1, 3, 5, 6, 7, 9, and 13.[28,29,49,57,58,61–65]

Sitting posture can play a major role in producing or increasing low back pain.[66,67] Proper seating and adaptations to maintain lumbar lordosis are discussed for home, auto, office, and air travel. An arm chair with an inclined back rest of 110 to 120° is the best selection.[66] For the office, a chair with shortened arm rests is recommended to allow adequate access to the desk top while maintaining back support. Alternating sitting with standing is also recommended.[67]

Environmental factors that contribute to back stress are covered next, with emphasis on workplace design.[68,69] Functional reach is defined and suggested as the area of placement for frequently used items (Fig. 21–2). Practical examples of principle 8, avoid repetition,[68,70] are abundant in the work place. We recommend periodic rest breaks from activities such as posting accounts, stapling multiple reports, typing memos, or writing reports. Adaptive devices for the office include a speaker phone, electric stapler, and electric pencil sharpener.

Above average patient height has been identified as a risk factor for low back pain.[3,71,72] This has particular application in the work environment, where everything from chairs, desks, counter height, sinks, and toilets have been selected or designed for the individual of average height. Additional seat cushions, blocks under desk legs and use of a standing or architectural desk are some of the adaptations discussed.

A practical session is then conducted to work on sitting posture. Several different types of office chairs and adaptive lumbar seat supports are made available for patient trials. Patients quickly grasp the progression from the first class, which emphasizes proper sitting posture, to the second class, which emphasizes adapting the seat to achieve proper body posture and support. This session is followed by a juice break.

Pain is an important topic for all back pain patients. We begin by stressing the normalcy of the pain experience in postural and mechanical disorders of the low back. This is essential in reducing anxiety, and therefore pain.[32,73] The judicious use of rest, aspirin or ibuprophen, and ice are suggested for back "first aid."[31] For management of tension, anxiety, and pain, diversion techniques, relaxation exercises, and mechanoreceptor stimulations are recommended.[46,74–80] Our favorite recommendation is the use of a rocking chair, an inexpensive and accessible method of pain control. Rocking can be slow, soothing the sympathetic nervous system,[81] or fast, decreasing pain through mechanoreceptor stimulation.[75] Table 21–4 provides a list of the pain-reducing techniques discussed.

The general benefits of exercising are discussed next. These benefits include improved cardiovascular health,[82–84] improved disc nutrition,[25,85] decreased tension and anxiety,[86–89] reduced absenteeism from work,[90–92] decreased use of health care services,[93,94] and pain reduction.[95] Aerobic exercise is mentioned as a means of reducing both pain intensity and the risk of recurrence.[91,96,97] Patients have been known to resist exercise programs, either from fear of pain or inability to change old habits. We attempt to foster behavioral change[56] by a gradual progression of the concept: class 1, benefits of activity; class 2, benefits of general exercise; and class 3, specific exercises for the low back.

A practical session in serial relaxation ends class 2. Patients are then given a copy of The Body Mechanic, a booklet designed by the author to reinforce course instruction on body mechanics.

Table 21–3
*Principles of Body Mechanics**

1. Normal physiologic curves should be maintained in most activities.[29,50]
2. When bending for any activity, bend knees to reduce stress from hamstrings below and from gravity above.
3. Objects should be brought close to body and near waist height before lifting.[29,61,62]
4. A slow lift produces less intradiscal pressure than a fast one.[61]
5. A wide base of support and staggered foot position aids stability in counterbalancing activities.[57,63]
6. Light to moderately heavy compact objects should be lifted with knees bent and lordosis maintained.[57,58]
7. Avoid twisting the trunk when carrying a load.[28,64]
8. Avoid repetitive or sustained activities.[68,70]
9. Use symmetrical upper body motions to carry or move objects.[68]
10. Pushing an object makes use of the more powerful leg muscles whereas pulling recruits the smaller trunk extensors.[65]
11. Use adaptive devices to extend your reach rather than stooping, reaching, or stretching.
12. Disc is hyperhydrated upon waking and more susceptible to injury. Avoid flexion soon after waking.[59,60]
13. Avoid sudden movements that can overload the muscles.[28,63]
14. Organize work areas so frequently used items are close at hand.
15. When in doubt, ask for help in performing a task.

**Adapted from Jackson, C.P., Klugerman, M.: How to start a back school. J Orthop Sports Phys Ther 10:1, 1988.*

Table 21–4
*Pain Control**

1. Mechanoreceptor stimulation[75]
   massage
   vibration
   rocking chair[75,81]
2. Diversion from pain focus[74,75,78,79]
   counterirritants
   hobby
   hypnosis[79]
3. Relaxation training[46,76,77]
   visual imagery
   serial relaxation
   breathing exercises
   yoga
4. Ice massage or ice packs[80]

**From Jackson, C.P., Klugerman, M.: How to start a back school. J Orthop Sports Phys Ther 10:1, 1988.*

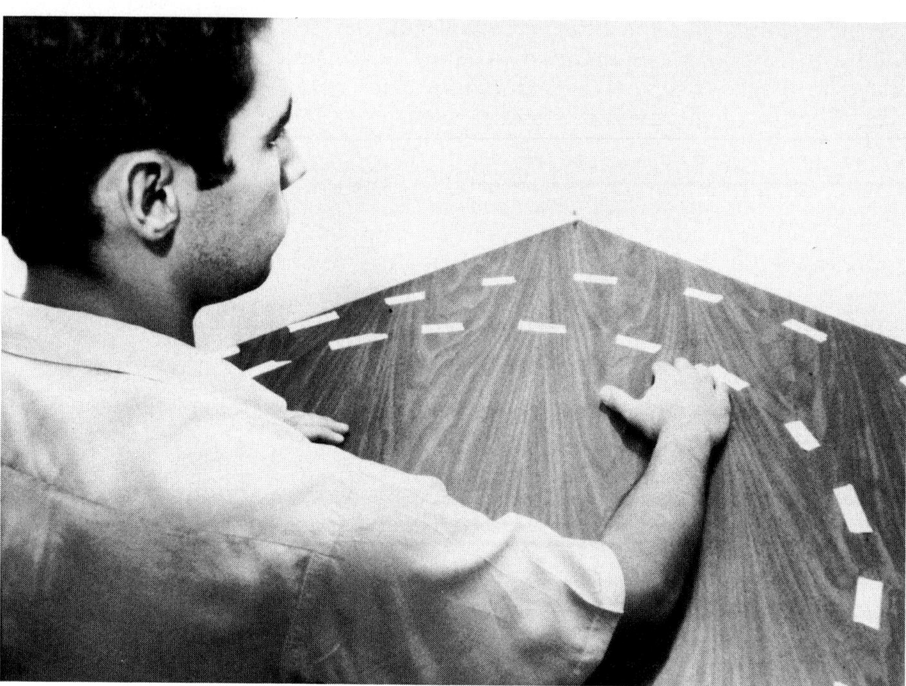

Figure 21–2. Functional reach, indicated by inner broken line, is the arc formed by the hand with the elbow in 20 to 30° of flexion.

Class 3

This class strives to develop the educated health care consumer. Patients are taught about the pros and cons of common forms of treatment for low back pain.[98,99] Because the goal of many forms of treatment is to reduce pain, self-management techniques are again discussed. The psychological and economic benefits of self-management are stressed. Patients are taught the warning signs that indicate medical evaluation is necessary so as not to carry self-management to a detrimental end. The goal of this section is to help patients avoid unnecessary or prolonged treatment.

Specific exercises for low back dysfunction are now introduced.[98] Aerobic exercises are presented as a method to minimize the risk of recurrence and disability.[91,96,97] The specific needs and advantages of various aerobic exercises are discussed.[100] Swimming, bicycling (with proper sitting posture), and walking are recommended as the safest methods of aerobic conditioning for back patients. Target heart rate and training parameters (30 minute sessions performed three to five times a week) are carefully explained.[101] Not every person will be able to start such a program at the same level or progress at the same pace.[102,103] Patients not already on a fitness program are referred to PT to help them safely start and pursue this activity.

The concept of muscle endurance is explained and related to postural habits. The importance of muscle endurance of the trunk extensors is emphasized.[51,52,54,55,104] Patients are taught how motor fa-

tigue leads to altered motor performance.[53] Taking precautions against provoking any signs of increased pain or symptoms, patients are shown two exercises that can aid in trunk extensor endurance: bridging and alternate arm and leg lifts (Figs. 21–3, 21–4). A PT referral is considered for patients who are unable to perform these exercises adequately in the practical session.

The risks of Williams' flexion exercises (delayed recovery and increased intradiscal pressure) are taught.[98] Patients are taught the difference between passive and active exercise and why passive exercise does not improve strength or endurance. The questionable value of a preprinted exercise handout sheet is discussed, and patients are instructed to request an evaluation and individualized program if confronted with such a sheet during the course of future treatment. This is followed by a juice break.

A review session is conducted next, covering ADLs, work activities, and environmental adaptations. Slides showing correct and incorrect techniques are shown out of sequence and patients are asked to score the procedure as right or wrong. The results are tabulated and any misconceptions are reviewed in class 4.

The first practical session for class 3 involves practice of the kneel-standing posture (Fig. 21–1). This position allows patients to get close to their work and maintain a lordosis while avoiding excessive torque forces at the knees that occur in squatting.

Patients are encouraged to return to an active life-

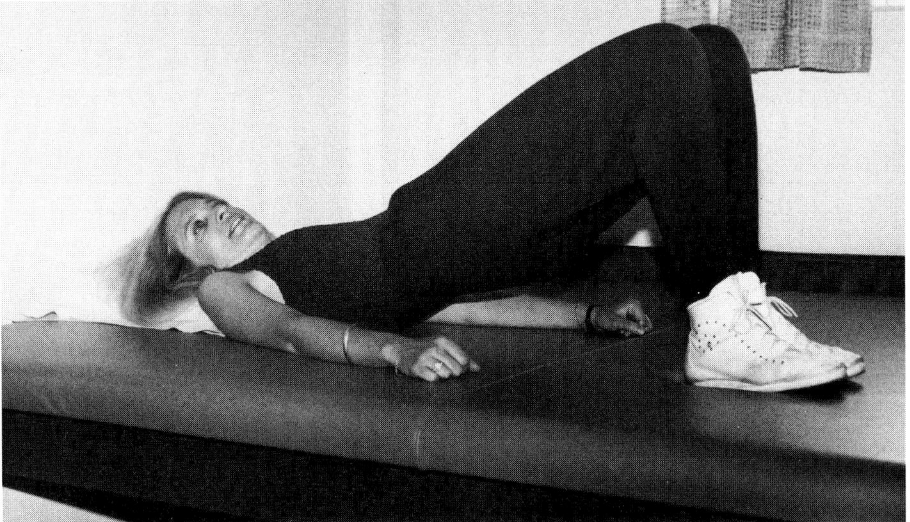

Figure 21–3. The bridging exercise, performed by the gluteus maximus and quadriceps femoris, is used to improve postural endurance.

style that includes sports and recreational activities. Activities such as tennis, golf, dancing, gardening, boating, diving, and canoeing are examined for possible hazards and safe methods of participation. Patients are warned of the risks of activities that require simultaneous trunk flexion and rotation, such as golf (Fig. 21–5). In boating, maintenance of the lumbar lordosis, a wide base of support, and slight knee flexion are suggested for counterbalancing activities (Fig. 21–6). The principles of body mechanics (Table 21–2) are related to all instructions.

Sex is the final topic for class 3. Sexual arousal has been found to reduce pain, and patients are encouraged to resume normal activity in this area.[105] Our "how to" advice extends only to this: be willing to explore. References are given if patients desire more specific information.[106]

The class ends with a practice session in visual imagery. Patients are told to bring questions or problems from the home and work environments for the final class.

Class 4

This class is a practical session covering rest positions, body mechanics, endurance exercises, and relaxation training. Attendance of family and friends at this session is encouraged, at no extra cost.

Tasks practiced or simulated include placing materials into a low cabinet, getting into and out of a car, washing a car, organizing work areas, sitting postures, reaching, and lifting tasks. As both a precaution and teaching technique, patients practice differ-

Figure 21–4. Alternate arm and leg lifts provide endurance training for the paraspinal muscles and trunk extensors.

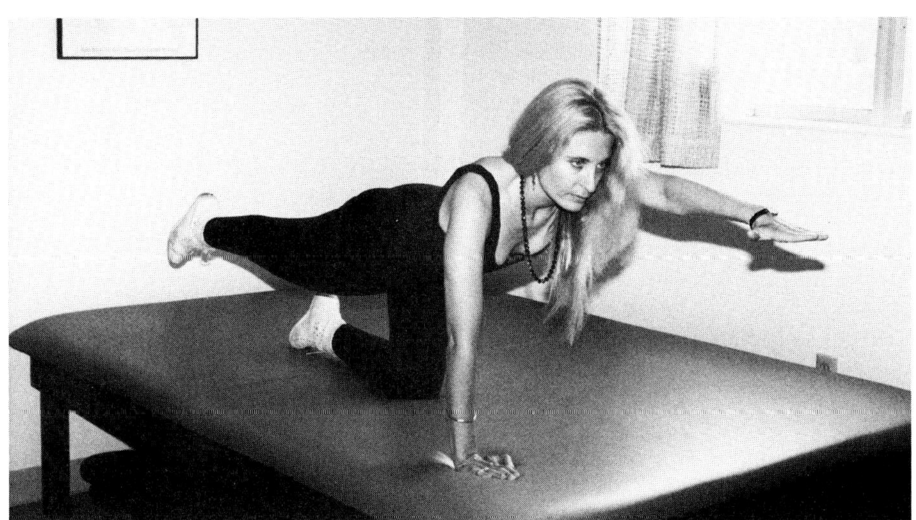

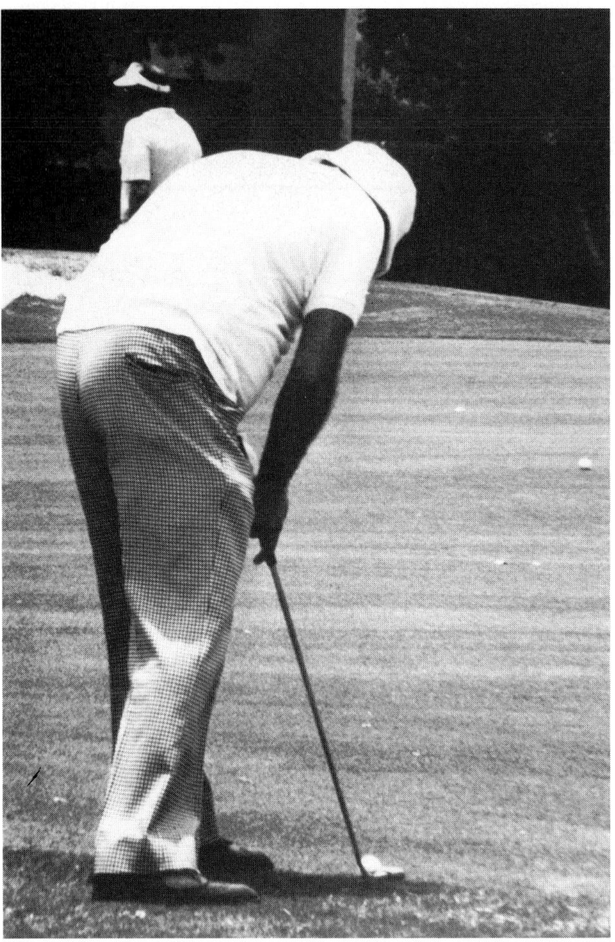

Figure 21–5. Recreational activities are examined for their benefits and risks. Golf is used as an example of the risk of simultaneous trunk flexion and rotation.

ent lifting techniques on a dynamometer prior to real lifting tasks (Fig. 21–7). This allows patients to safely see for themselves the additional stress that occurs in various positions. A 10-point check list is used to evaluate patient performance of various practical skills.

Serial relaxation training is then performed. Relaxation training has been carried out at all four sessions to facilitate patient skill, which is essential if these techniques are to work. Commercial tapes that teach imagery and serial relaxation are suggested to enhance efforts at home.

A question and answer session is conducted to discuss particular home and work situations that patients feel they haven't mastered. The group discusses possible solutions. After all questions are resolved, patients are invited back in 6 months for a free review class, an excellent idea introduced by Hall.[3]

Methodology

A back school does not achieve successful results simply by covering a few relevant topics with flashy media presentations. To ensure success, careful consideration must be given to issues of patient selection, educational principles, goal achievement, and patient compliance. Failure to address these issues can lead to disappointing program results.

Patient Selection

One method of ensuring a successful back school is to select the proper patient for the program. Factors that should influence patient selection include pain behavior, level of education and comprehension, involvement in disability or legal proceedings, depression, and coping style.

Patients who experience intermittent episodes of pain are good candidates for a back school,[3,9] whereas those with unremitting pain appear to benefit less.[3] Severity and duration of pain do not appear to influence outcome. Patients with severe intermittent pain can expect to benefit.[8,3] Duration of pain is not a factor because patients with both acute and chronic pain benefit from back school programs.[3,6,8–11]

High educational level and comprehension skills are strongly correlated to successful outcome. Studies on back school outcomes have found a positive

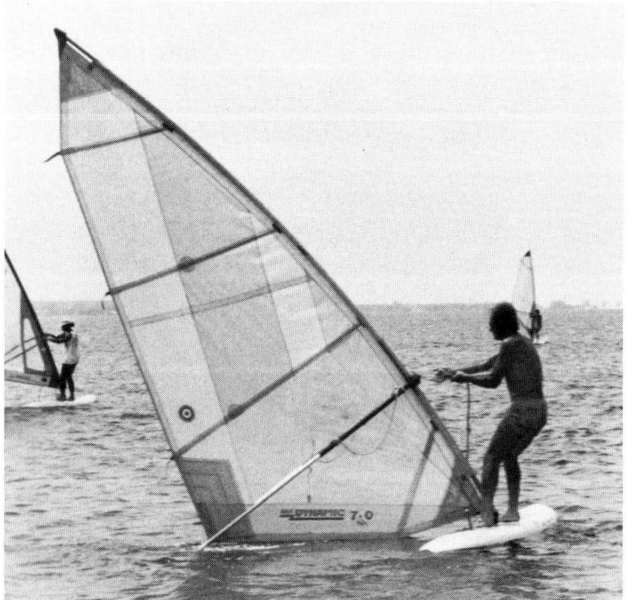

Figure 21–6. Patients are taught to take a wide stance, bend the hips and knees slightly, and keep the back upright during counterbalancing activities, such as wind surfing.

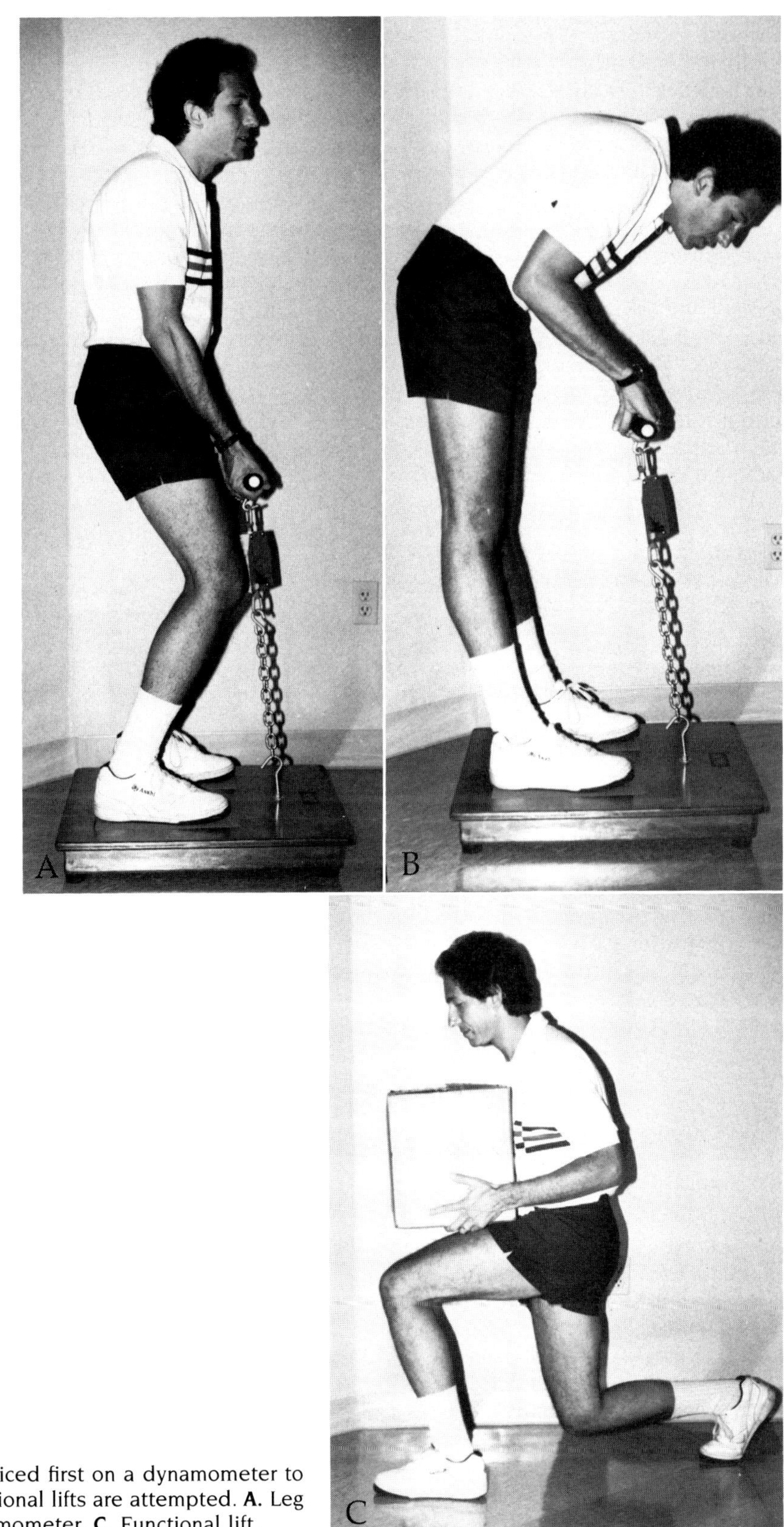

Figure 21–7. Lifting techniques are practiced first on a dynamometer to determine style and capacity before functional lifts are attempted. **A.** Leg lift on dynamometer. **B.** Back lift on dynamometer. **C.** Functional lift.

correlation between mental ability to comprehend and pain relief.[3,107] In global studies of socioeconomic factors and low back outcome, level of education is negatively correlated with the development of disability.[108,109] Thus if the goals of a back school are to relieve pain or avoid chronic disability, they are less likely to be met in the patient with limited comprehension skills.

Involvement in disability compensation or legal proceedings related to back injury reduces the likelihood of symptomatic improvement in low back patients.[110] Although this issue has not been well studied in back school programs, its presence, particularly when coupled with other negative factors, warrants strong consideration before a back school referral is made.

Untreated depression should preclude referral to a back school. Multiple studies indicate depression may be the most important predictor of the degree to which a pain patient's activities are impaired.[33,36–38] Until depression is successfully treated, there is little likelihood of benefit from a back school.

Patients who ask many questions and seek out information are good candidates for a back school. Those who avoid explanations and use denial as a coping skill tend not to benefit from instructional programs.[111]

Educational Principles

Because a back school is an educational process, adherence to certain educational principles is necessary for the program to be effective. Although it is not within the scope of this chapter to teach educational skills, certain salient points warrant mention.

Learning can be cognitive (learning the rules of tennis), psychomotor (practicing a backhand shot), or affective (enjoying winning a set). The more multidimensional the learning process is, the greater the retention of material. A good back school program should therefore address the three learning processes.

Factors that enhance cognitive learning are repetition of key concepts, feedback, teacher access for questioning[112] and time spent in instruction.[112,113] Major themes of the back school should be repeated each session to ensure long term retention. Patients must be given feedback during question and answer and practical sessions. Classes should be taught live (rather than by automated slide or tape show) and by a knowledgeable clinician who can address patient concerns about the material presented. Because time spent in instruction is directly related to amount of recall, a well designed program should consist of 3 or 4 sessions, 1 to 2 hours in duration, depending on the amount of material to be pre-

sented. A program that consists of only one hour-long session is unlikely to achieve long term results.

Psychomotor learning is enhanced by the presence of role models and when tasks are actively carried out under supervision.[56] In a back school, the instructor or successful "graduates" of earlier back schools can serve as role models to show that skills taught can be successfully mastered. When motor skills are taught, such as body mechanics or exercises, adequate practice time is mandatory to insure proper performance and increase feelings of competence,[56] which facilitates learning.

Affective learning is enhanced by the presence of role models,[56] by a positive instructor-patient relationship,[114] and by making material relevant to class participants. Teaching a class of office workers how to lift heavy materials, or a group of luggage handlers how to ergonomically set up an office working area, lessens attention and learning. This aspect of relevance emphasizes the need for adapting back school content for varying patient groups.

Patients with a low prior knowledge of disease perform better with a directed, systematic health education program conducted by a health practitioner, than with a self-directed program.[115] This finding, coupled with the need for teacher access and feedback, highlights the limits of an unsupervised, automated, slide or tape program. Such programs ignore the basic tenants of learning and are unlikely to yield good results.

Even the best learned material will not be maintained forever if it is not periodically reinforced. A decline in retention of material occurs over time, with a substantial loss in only 6 months.[116] A review class, held at least every 6 months, should be a part of any back school program that strives to maintain gains for the long-term.

The last principle of health behavior education is empowerment. Giving the patient a sense of control through the educational process enhances the likelihood of behavioral change.[39] Situations should be provided to give patients an early and real sense of control over their condition. Practice in postural skills, body mechanics, or pain control techniques can meet this need.

Achieving Goals

The goals of a back school program may vary according to the target population (acute, chronic, or industrial), but all programs share three common goals: increase patient participation in and responsibility for his own care, reduce anxiety associated with back pain, and decrease medical costs. Four simple methods can aid in achieving these goals: (1) present concepts in a progression from simple to complex, (2) provide a full (though not highly technical) explanation of important concepts, (3) avoid frightening medical jargon or labels, and (4) provide a nonthreatening atmosphere that facilitates questions and the exchange of ideas.

In attempting to reduce patient dependency and increase participation in their own care, we are asking for a behavioral change. Progressing material from simple concepts (muscle, disc, vertebra) to more complex (function of the spine, disc pressure, and body mechanics) facilitates behavioral changes.[56] The program that stresses complex notions without covering the basics often confuses patients and may increase anxiety and dependence.

Providing a full explanation of important concepts aids in reducing anxiety,[32,117,118] dependency,[119–121] and medical costs.[121–124] This again emphasizes the need for classes of ample duration so that topics can be adequately covered, not simply introduced.

Avoiding medical jargon or labeling conditions can greatly reduce patient anxiety.[14] Care must be taken in designing lectures to avoid terms such as slipped disc, lumbago, and degenerative disease, or to replace them with more simple, accurate, and less frightening concepts.

A nonthreatening environment that facilitates questions and the exchange of ideas is essential in reducing anxiety. This may include sitting at eye level for discussions rather than towering over seated patients, removing the traditional medical white lab coat, including humor in lectures and/or slides, having a juice or coffee break during class when instructors can mingle with participants, adopting a low key but enthusiastic teaching style, and ensuring that the classroom setting is free from outside noises and interruptions. As a practical consideration, the environment should also be comfortable. Because the "students" are suffering from low back pain, appropriate seating is critical to minimizing physical discomfort and distraction.

Compliance

For a back school to be effective, patients must actively pursue the skills they have been taught after they leave the program. Compliance, however, is not automatic. It has been shown that neither intent to change a health behavior nor degree of satisfaction with the health area are consistent with participation in a health promotion program.[125] Even when patient compliance can reduce serious health risks, 50% drop out.[126,127] When the risks are even less, as with back pain, behavioral changes may be neglected shortly after treatment or the initial episode of pain stops.

Methods to improve patient compliance include written referral to the program,[126] easy access to methods of compliance,[126,128] an enthusiastic and

knowledgeable clinician-teacher,[114,126,128,129] periodic feedback on results,[126] reinforcement of course material with written materials,[130] and spouse support.[126–128,131] Once again, the knowledge, enthusiasm, and physical presence of the course instructor is emphasized.

The concept of spouse or family support should be clarified. Studies have shown that a general supportive attitude, rather than encouraging specific behaviors, is the most effective means of gaining patient compliance.[131] Encouraging specific actions can sometimes be interpreted as nagging. Family members should be apprised of how they may best help.

Increased contact with medical personnel also increases compliance.[132,133] This further reinforces the limits of a self-directed or unmanned program as well as the need for a review class. Telephone followup is another method of achieving increased contact.[133] This is particularly important when patients fail to show for the review class.

CONCLUSIONS

We began this chapter with a simple concept of educating back patients. Historically, a task that was performed one-on-one by the doctor or therapist, it has given birth to a whole industry, with little in the way of guidelines for how this educational process should occur.

In 1988, the North American Back School Association formed a committee on back schools to attempt to establish guidelines on such issues as content, teacher credentials, duration of program, and format. Such guidelines are clearly needed to insure that a sound concept is not abused. In the absence of such guidelines, a few suggestions for operating a back school follow.

Selection of the instructor is critical. Ample evidence has been offered in this chapter on the need for a knowledgeable, enthusiastic, and supportive clinician to serve as the instructor for a back school program. The health practitioner who is enthusiastic and believes in the effectiveness of the program will improve outcome.[114,134,135]

Do not confuse education with treatment. A back school is an excellent method to cover common educational needs of low back patients. Yet, even when a common diagnosis exists, each patient presents with different symptoms and functional changes that require their own type of management. Even when common goals exist, such as fitness and trunk endurance, not every patient can begin these endeavors at the same point or achieve the same results. The back school program should emphasize this difference and the need for individual evaluation and treatment outside the program.

Sound educational principles must be followed in designing a back school to ensure that education does, in fact, take place. Factors such as ample time, repetition of key concepts, teacher access for questioning, and practice for psychomotor learning all demonstrate the need for live presentations and multisession programs.

The back school is not a panacea. Even with proper patient selection, some patients still "fail." The instructor must be able to discern the patient who is not learning and refer them to an individual treatment program.

There should be some flexibility in course emphasis to accommodate the population of each class. For example, a class composed primarily of luggage handlers, stock boys, and paramedics should give more instructional and practical time to materials handling than office design. A quick survey of patients' occupations at the beginning of the first class can help direct the instructor in such curriculum choices.

The content of a back school must be sensitive to advances in research. Materials taught must be reviewed periodically to ensure they still reflect current knowledge in back pain and its management, both physical and psychological.

Although it is important to show respect for a patient's pain, this does not mean a back school must maintain an air of solemnity. Humor is an appropriate device to ease tension and aid retention of material. Humorous slides can be effectively used to introduce topics such as stress, aerobics, environmental adaptation, even anatomy. Do not be afraid to be creative and have a little fun.

REFERENCES

1. Peltier, L.: The back school of Delpech in Montpellier. Clin Orthop *179:*4, 1983.
2. Zachrisson-Forssell, M.: The Swedish Back School. Physiotherapy *66:*112, 1980.
3. Hall, H., Iceton, J.A.: Back school. An overview with specific reference to the Canadian Back Education Units. Clin Orthop *179:*10, 1983.
4. Hall, H.: The Canadian Back Education Units. Physiotherapy *66:*115, 1980.
5. White, A.H., White, L.A., Mattmiller, A.W.: Back School and Other Conservative Approaches to Low Back Pain. St. Louis, C.V. Mosby, 1983.
6. White, A.: AAOS Instructional Course Lectures, Back School. St. Louis, C.V. Mosby, 1979.
7. Tomer, G.M., Olson, C.N., Lepore, B.: Back injury prevention training makes dollars and sense. Natl Safety News, *January:*36, 1984.
8. Bergquist-Ullman, M.: Acute low back pain in industry. Acta Orthop Scand Suppl *170:*5–20, 1977.
9. Linton, S.J., et al.: The secondary prevention of low back pain: a controlled study with follow up. Pain *36:*197, 1989.
10. Moffett, J.A.K., et al.: A controlled, prospective study to evaluate the effectiveness of a back school in the relief of chronic low back pain. Spine *11:*120, 1986.
11. Lindequist, S., et al: Information and regime at low back pain. Scand J Rehabil Med *16:*113, 1984.
12. Johnson, C.D.: Safety forum. Ind Safety Prod News, June 21, 1981.
13. Jackson, C.P., Klugerman, M.: How to start a back school. J Orthop Sports Phys Ther *10:*1, 1988.
14. Hadler, N.M.: To be a patient or a claimant with a musculoskeletal illness. *In* Clinical Concepts in Regional Musculoskeletal Illness (Edited by N.M. Hadler). Orlando, Grune & Stratton, 1987.
15. Deyo, R.A., Diehl, A.K., Rosenthal, M.: How many days of bedrest for acute low back pain? A randomized clinical trial. N Engl J Med *315:*1064, 1986.
16. Gilbert, J.R., et al.: Clinical trial of common treatments for low back pain in family practice. Br Med J *219:*791, 1985.
17. Hansson, T.H., et al.: Development of osteopenia in the fourth lumbar vertebra during prolonged bed rest after operation for scoliosis. Acta Orthop Scand *46:*621, 1975.
18. Waddell, G.: A new clinical model for the treatment of low back pain. Spine *12:*632, 1987.
19. Bortz, W.M.: The disuse syndrome. West J Med *141:*691, 1984.
20. Biering-Sorensen, F., Thomsen, C.: Medical, social and occupational history as risk indicators for low back trouble in a general population. Spine *11:*720, 1986.
21. Deyo, R.A., Bass, J.E.: Lifestyle and low back pain: the influence of smoking, exercise and obesity. Clin Res *35:*577A, 1987.
22. Frymoyer, J.W., et al.: Risk factors in low back pain. J Bone Joint Surg *65A:*213, 1983.
23. Kelsey, J.L., et al.: Acute prolapsed lumbar intervertebral disc: an epidemiological study with special reference to driving automobiles and cigarette smoking. Spine *9:*608, 1984.
24. Holm, S., Nachemson, A.: Nutrition of the intervertebral disc: acute effects of cigarette smoking: an experimental animal study. Int J Microcirc Clin Exp *3:*406, 1985.
25. Holm, S., Nachemson, A.: Variations in the nutrition of the canine intervertebral disc induced by motion. Spine *8:*866, 1983.
26. Andersson, J.A.D.: Back pain and occupation. *In* The Lumbar Spine and Back Pain (Edited by M.I.V. Jayson). London, Pittman Medical, 1980.
27. Bigos, S.J., et al.: Back injuries in industry: a retrospective study. II. Injury factors. Spine *11:*246, 1986.
28. Magora, A.: Investigation of the relation between low back pain and occupation. 4. Physical requirements: bending, rotation, reaching and sudden maximal effort. Scand J Rehabil Med *5:*186, 1973.
29. Nachemson, A.L.: The lumbar spine. An orthopaedic challenge. Spine *1:*59, 1976.
30. Schultz, A.: Mechanical factors in the etiology of low back disorders. *In* Symposium on Idiopathic Low Back Pain (Edited by A.A. White and S.L. Gordon). St. Louis, C.V. Mosby, 1982.
31. Phillips, G.D., Cousins, M.J.: Neurological mechanisms of pain and the relationship of pain, anxiety and sleep. *In* Acute Pain Management (Edited by M.J. Cousins and G.D. Phillips). New York, Churchill Livingstone, 1986.
32. Peck, C.L.: Psychological factors in acute pain management. *In* Acute Pain Management (Edited by M.J. Cousins and G.D. Phillips). New York, Churchill Livingstone, 1986.
33. Keefe, F.J., et al.: Depression, pain and pain behavior. J Consult Clin Psychol *54:*665, 1986.
34. Waddell, G., et al.: A concept of illness tested as an improved basis for surgical decisions in low back disorders. Spine *11:*712, 1986.
35. Pope, M.H., et al.: The relation between mechanical and psychological factors in patients with low back pain. Spine *5:*173, 1980.
36. Haley, W.E., Turner, J.A., Romano, J.M.: Depression in

chronic pain patients: relation to pain, activity and sex differences. Pain *23*:337, 1985.

37. Dworkin, R.H., Richlin, D.M., Handlin, D.J., Brand, L.: Predicting treatment response in depressed and non-depressed chronic pain patients. Pain *24*:343, 1986.

38. Doan, B.D., Wadden, N.P.: Relationships between depressive symptoms and descriptions of chronic pain. Pain *36*:75, 1989.

39. Wallerstein, N., Bernstein, E.: Empowerment education: Freire's ideas adapted to health education. Health Educ Q *15*:379, 1988.

40. Gal, R., Lazarus, R.S.: The role of activity in anticipating and confronting stressful situations. J Hum Stress *1*:4, 1975.

41. Morgan, W.P., Horstman, D.H.: Anxiety reduction following acute physical activity. Med Sci Sports *8*:62, 1976.

42. Brena, S.F.: Drugs and pain. Use and misuse. *In* Management of Patients with Chronic Pain (Edited by S.F. Brena and S.C. Chapman). New York, Spectrum Publications, 1983.

43. Brady, J.P., Cheatle, M.D., Ball, W.A.: A trial of L-tryptophan in chronic pain syndromes. Clin J Pain *3*:39, 1987.

44. Seltzer, S., Dewart, D., Pollack, R.L., Jackson, E.: The effects of dietary tryptophan in chronic maxillofacial pain and experimental pain tolerance. J Psychiatr Res *17*:181, 1982–83.

45. Seltzer, S., Stoch, R., Marcus, R., Jackson, E.: Alterations of human pain thresholds by nutritional manipulation and L-tryptophan supplementation. Pain *13*:385, 1982.

46. Tan, S.: Cognitive and cognitive-behavioral methods of pain control: a selective review. Pain *12*:20, 1982.

47. Soderberg, G.L.: Kinesiology: Application to Pathological Motion. Baltimore, Williams & Wilkins, 1986.

48. Panjabi, M.M., White, A.A.: Basic biomechanics of the spine. Neurosurgery, *7*:76, 1980.

49. Troup, J.D.G.: Biomechanics of the vertebral column. Physiotherapy, *65*:238, 1979.

50. Kapandji, I.A.: The Physiology of the Joints, Vol. 3. New York, Churchill Livingstone, 1979.

51. Jayasinghe, W.J., et al.: An EMG investigation of postural fatigue in low back pain—a preliminary study. Electromyogr Clin Neurophysiol *18*:191, 1980.

52. DeVries, H.A.: EMG fatigue curves in postural muscles. A possible etiology for idiopathic low back pain. Am J Phys Med *47*:175, 1968.

53. Parnianpour, M., Nordin, M., Frankel, V., Kahanovitz, N.: The triaxial coupling of torque generation of trunk muscles during isometric exertions and the effect of fatiguing isoinertial movements on the motor output and movement patterns. Presented at the International Society for the Study of the Lumbar Spine, Miami, Fl, April, 1988.

54. Westgaard, R.H., Aaras, A.: Postural muscle strain as a causal factor in the development of musculoskeletal illnesses. Applied Ergonomics *15*:162, 1984.

55. Nicolaisen, T., Jorgensen, K.: Trunk strength and back muscle endurance and low back trouble. Scand J Rehabil Med *17*:121, 1985.

56. Rosenstock, I.M., Strecher, V.J., Becker, M.H.: Social learning theory and the health belief model. Health Educ Q *15*:175, 1988.

57. Anderson, C.K., Chaffin, D.B.: A biomechanical evaluation of five lifting techniques. Applied Ergonomics *17*:2, 1986.

58. Hart, D.L., Stobbs, T.J., Jaraiedi, M.: Effects of lumbar posture on lifting. Spine *12*:138, 1987.

59. Adams, M.A., Dolan, P., Hutton, W.C.: Diurnal variations in the stresses on the lumbar spine. Spine *12*:130, 1987.

60. Tyrrell, A.R., Reilly, T., Troup, J.D.G.: Circadian variation in stature and the effects of spinal loading. Spine *10*:161, 1985.

61. Andersson, G.B.J., Ortengren, R., Nachemson, A.: Quantitative studies of back loads in lifting. Spine *1*:178, 1976.

62. Snook, S.H.: Approaches to the control of back pain in industry: job design, job placement and education/training. Spine: State of the Art Reviews *2*:45, 1987.

63. Troup, J.D.G.: Relation of lumbar spine disorders to heavy manual work and lifting. Lancet *1*:857, 1965.

64. Farfan, H.F.: The torsional injury of the lumbar spine. Spine *8*:53, 1983.

65. White, A.A., Panjabi, M.M.: Clinical Biomechanics of the Spine. Philadelphia, JB Lippincott, 1978.

66. Andersson, G.B.J., Murphy, R.W., Ortengren, R., Nachemson, A.L.: The influence of backrest inclination and lumbar support on lumbar lordosis. Spine *4*:52, 1979.

67. Magora, A.: Investigation of the relation between low back pain and occupation. 3. Physical requirements: sitting, standing and weight lifting. Ind Med Surg *41*:5, 1972.

68. Chaffin, D.B., Andersson, G.B.J.: Occupational Biomechanics. New York, John Wiley & Sons, 1984.

69. Salvendy, G.: Handbook of Human Factors. New York, John Wiley & Sons, 1987.

70. Sandover, J.: Dynamic loading as a possible source of low back disorders. Spine *8*:652, 1983.

71. Gyntelberg, F.: One year incidence of low back pain among male residents of Copenhagen age 40–59. Dan Med Bull *21*:30, 1974.

72. Hrubec, A., Nashbold, B.S.: Epidemiology of lumbar disc lesions in the military in World War II. Am J Epidemiol *102*:366, 1975.

73. Sedlak, K.: Low back pain. Perception and tolerance. Spine *10*:440, 1985.

74. McCaul, K.D., Malott, J.M.: Distraction and coping with pain. Psychol Bull *95*:516, 1984.

75. Wyke, B.: The neurology of low back pain. *In* The Lumbar Spine and Back Pain, 2nd Ed. Edited by M.I.V. Jayson, Turnbridge Wells, England, Pittman Publishing Company, 1980.

76. Beary, J.F., Benson, H.: A simple psychophysiologic technique which elicits the hypometabolic changes of the relaxation response. Psychosom Med *36*:115, 1974.

77. Hertling, D., Jones, D.: Relaxation. *In* Management of Common Musculoskeletal Disorders (Edited by R.M. Kessler and D. Hertling). Philadelphia, Harper & Row, 1983.

78. Beers, T.M., Karoly, P.: Cognitive strategies, expectancy, and coping style in the control of pain. J Consult Clin Psychol *47*:179, 1979.

79. Pawlicki, R.E., Wester, W.C.: Hypnosis. *In* Practical Management of Pain. Edited by P.P. Raj. Chicago, Year Book Medical Publishers, 1986.

80. Melzack, R., Jeans, M.E., Stratford, J.G., Monks, R.C.: Ice massage and TENS: comparison of treatment for back pain. Pain *9*:209, 1980.

81. Farber, S.D.: Neurorehabilitation. A Multisensory Approach. Philadelphia, WB Saunders, 1982.

82. Pollock, M., et al.: Effects of mode of training on cardiovascular function and body composition of adult men. Med Sci Sports *7*:139, 1975.

83. Scheuer, J., Tipton, C.M.: Cardiovascular adaptations to physical training. Annu Rev Physiol *39*:221, 1977.

84. Simonelli, C., Etton, R.P.: Cardiovascular and metabolic effects of exercise. Postgrad Med J *64*:71, 1978.

85. Urban, J.P.G., Holm, S., Maroudas, A., Nachemson, A.: Nutrition of intervertebral disk: effect of fluid flow on solute transport. Clin Orthop *170*:296, 1982.

86. Blair, S.N., Jacobs, D.R., Powell, K.E.: Relationships between exercise or physical activity and other health behaviors. Public Health Rep *100*:172, 1985.

87. Taylor, C.B., Sallis, J.F., Needle, R.: The relationship of physical activity and exercise to mental health. Public Health Rep *100*:195, 1985.

88. DeVries, H., Adams, G.M.: EMG comparison of single doses of exercise and meprobamate as to effects on muscular relaxation. Am J Phys Med *51*:130, 1972.

89. DeVries, H., Wiswell, R.A., Bulbulion, R., Moritan, T.: Tranquilizer affect of exercise. Am J Phys Med 60:57, 1981.

90. Baun, W.B., Bernack, E.J., Tsai, S.P.: A preliminary investigation: effects of a corporate fitness program on absenteeism and health care costs. J Occup Med 28:18, 1986.

91. Bowne, D.W., et al.: Reduced disability and health care costs in an industrial fitness program. J Occup Med 26:809, 1984.

92. Cox, M., Shepard, R.J., Corey, P.: Influence of an employee fitness program upon fitness, productivity and absenteeism. Ergonomics 24:795, 1981.

93. Shephard, R., Cox, M., Corey, P.: Fitness program participation: its effect on worker performance. J Occup Med 23:359, 1981.

94. Gibbs, J.O., et al.: Work site health promotion. Five year trend in employee health care costs. J Occup Med 27:826, 1985.

95. Janal, M.N., Colt, E.W.D., Clark, W.C., Gilusman, M.: Pain sensitivity, mood, and plasma endocrine levels in man following long-distance running. Pain 19:13, 1984.

96. Cady, L.D., et al.: Strength and fitness and subsequent back injuries in firefighters. J Occup Med 21:269, 1979.

97. Cady, L.D., Thomas, P.C., Karawasky, R.J.: Program for increasing health and physical fitness of fire fighters. J Occup Med 27:110, 1985.

98. Jackson, C.P.: Physical therapy for lumbar disc disease. Seminars in Spine Surgery 1:28, 1989.

99. Borenstein, D.G., Wiesel, S.W.: Low Back Pain. Medical Diagnosis and Comprehensive Management. Philadelphia, WB Saunders, 1989.

100. Jackson, C.P., Brown, M.D.: Analysis of current approaches and a practical guide to prescription of exercise. Clin Orthop 179:46, 1983.

101. Hanson, P.G., Giese, M.D., Corliss, R.J.: Clinical guidelines for exercise training. Postgrad Med J 67:120, 1980.

102. Pollock, M.L., et al.: Frequency of training as a determinant for improvement in cardiovascular function and body composition of middle aged men. Arch Phys Med Rehabil 56:141, 1975.

103. Johannessen, S., Holly, R.G., Lui, H., Amsterdam, E.A.: High frequency, moderate intensity training in sedentary middle aged women. Phys Sportsmed 14:99, 1986.

104. Biering-Sorensen, F.: A one year prospective study of low back trouble in a general population. The prognostic value of low back history and physical measurement. Dan Med Bull 31:362, 1984.

105. Whipple, B., Komisaruk, B.R.: Elevation of pain threshold by vaginal stimulation in women. Pain 21:357, 1985.

106. White, A.A.: Your Aching Back: A Doctor's Guide to Relief. New York, Bantam Books, 1983.

107. Simmons, J.W., Dennis, M.D., Rath, D.: The back school. A total back management program. Orthopaedics 7:1453, 1984.

108. Deyo, R.A., Diehl, A.K.: Predicting disability in patients with low back pain. Clin Res 34:814A, 1986.

109. Deyo, R.A., Tsui-Wu, Y.J.: Functional disability due to back pain. A population-based study indicating the importance of socioeconomic factors. Arthritis Rheum 30:1247, 1987.

110. Walsh, N.E., Dumitru, D.: The influence of compensation on recovery from low back pain. Spine State of the Art Reviews, 2:109, 1987.

111. Wilson, J.F.: Behavioral preparation for surgery: benefit or harm? J Behav Med 4:79, 1981.

112. Gage, N.L., Berliner, D.C.: Educational Psychology, 2nd Ed. Boston, Houghton Mifflin, 1979.

113. Deardoff, W.W.: Computerized health education: a comparison with traditional formats. Health Educ Q 13:61, 1986.

114. DiMatteo, M.R., DiNicola, P.D.: Achieving Patient Compliance: The Psychology of the Medical Practitioners Role. New York, Pergamon Press, 1982.

115. Holloway, R.L., Spivey, R.N., Zismer, D.K., Withington A.M.: Aptitude × treatment interactions: implications for patient education research. Health Educ Q 15:241, 1988.

116. Green, L.W.: Evaluation and measurement: some dilemmas for health educators. Am J Public Health 67:155, 1977.

117. Scott, L.E., Clum, G.A., Peoples, J.B.: Preoperative indicators of postoperative pain. Pain 15:283, 1983.

118. Sime, A.M.: Relationship of preoperative fear, type of coping and information received about surgery to recovery from surgery. J Pers Soc Psychol 34:716, 1976.

119. Deyo, R.A., Diehl, A.K.: Patient satisfaction with medical care for low back pain. Spine 11:28, 1986.

120. Barsky, A.J.: Hidden reasons why some patients visit doctors. Ann Intern Med 94:492, 1981.

121. Levine, P.H., Britten, A.F.: Supervised patient management of hemophilia: a study of 45 patients with Hemophilia A and B. Ann Intern Med 78:195, 1973.

122. Kaye, R.L., Hammond, A.H.: Understanding rheumatoid arthritis: evaluation of patient education programs. J Am Med Assoc 239:2466, 1978.

123. Miller, L.V., Goldstein, J.: More efficient care of diabetic patients in a county hospital setting. N Engl J Med 286:1388, 1972.

124. Healy, K.: Does preoperative instruction really make a difference? Am J Nurs 68:62, 1968.

125. Davis, K.E., Jackson, K.L., Kronfeld, J.J., Blair, S.N.: Determinants of participation in worksite health promotion activities. Health Educ Q 14:195, 1987.

126. Oldridge, N.B.: Compliance and exercise in primary and secondary prevention of coronary heart disease: a review. Prev Med 11:56, 1982.

127. Pederson, L.L.: Compliance with physician advice to quit smoking: a review of the literature. Prev Med 11:71, 1982.

128. Dishman, R.K.: Exercise compliance: a new view for public health. Phys Sportsmed 14:127, 1986.

129. Iverson, D.C., et al.: The promotion of physical activity in the United States population: the status of programs in medical, worksite, community and school settings. Public Health Rep 100:212, 1985.

130. Glossop, E.S., et al.: Patient compliance in back and neck patients. Physiotherapy, 68:225, 1982.

131. Zimmerman, R.S., Commor, C.: Health promotion in context: the effects of significant others on health behavior change. Health Educ Q 16:57, 1989.

132. Gatchel, R.J., Baum, A.: Introduction to Health Psychology. New York, Random House, 1983.

133. Mayer, T.G., Gatchel, R.J.: Functional Restoration for Spinal Disorders: The Sports Medicine Approach. Philadelphia, Lea & Febiger, 1988.

134. Evans, F.S.: The placebo response in pain reduction. In Advances in Neurology: International Symposium on Pain (Edited by J.J. Bonica). New York, Raven Press, 1974.

135. Jones, R.A.: Expectations and illness. In Interpersonal Issues in Health Care (Edited by H.J. Friedman and M.R. DiMatteo). New York, Academic Press, 1982.

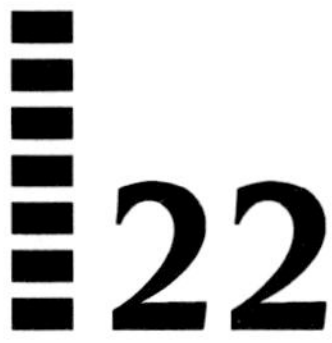

22

Stanley A. Herring

Sports Medicine Early Care

CONCEPTS

Sports Medicine continues to enjoy rising popularity among injured patients searching for treatment. In September, 1980, *The Physician and Sports Medicine* published its first directory of sports medicine treatment centers, listing 176 facilities.[1] By September, 1982, the directory had 410 entries. In 1988 more than 1000 independent sports medicine centers were operating,[2] and hospitals were increasingly opening their own on-site clinics. Eighteen million Americans suffer sports-related injuries and the cost of rehabilitation is estimated to be as much as 10 billion dollars annually.[2]

The dramatic growth of sports medicine may be a reflection of the injured athlete's search for specialized care. The sports participant, professional or recreational, often is significantly invested in his physical activity. An injury that prohibits participation is viewed as a real disability. Advice to simply rest or even to give up the particular sport leaves the patients unsatisfied. The patient wants not only relief of his discomfort, but also to return to his previous activity. The issue is not the treatment of symptoms; it is restoration of function.

The sports medicine community has responded to these patients. Early interventional care using diagnostic procedures coupled with supervised function-oriented rehabilitation has developed. There certainly have been abuses; unproven treatments and over-prescription of therapy by those more interested in business than in medicine. However, quality sports medicine does offer early accurate diagnosis and goal-directed rehabilitation. This combination may lead to safer, more expedient recovery for the athlete. An ongoing flexibility, strength, and training program may help to decrease recurrent injury. Without such a comprehensive program, rehabilitation may be inadequate as reflected by the remarkably high reinjury rate seen in sports.[3] Once injured, the athlete frequently reports recurrent problems in the same joint or limb after only a brief return to sports.[4]

The diagnosis and management of sports injuries can be divided into phases: the acute phase, the recovery phase, and the maintenance phase. Goals for each phase are predicated on prompt, appropriate diagnostic and treatment interventions (Table 22–1). Treatment has focused on peripheral joints, the mainstay of sports medicine. The most frequently reported injury in football (including medical illness) is knee injury.[5,6] Knee problems comprise a significant number of injuries in other collision sports, such as hockey and lacrosse, as well. Participation in contact sports such as basketball, soccer, and baseball, as well as endurance sports, also regularly results in knee problems. This joint serves as a relevant model for demonstrating a sports medicine approach to injury, detailing the phases of rehabilitation. A discussion of spinal pain follows this review of the knee.

Acute Phase of Rehabilitation—Knee

Large gains have been made in accurately diagnosing knee injuries. Physical examination techniques, aided and substantiated by arthroscopic examination, have produced increased diagnostic preciseness, particularly after trauma. Moving away from "sprained knee" or "runner's knee" to an exact diagnosis of the ligamentous, cartilaginous, bony or musculotendinous injury, has helped to structure logical intervention and rehabilitation. An accurate diagnosis is essential; without it appropriate treatment is almost impossible. Based on this accurate diagnosis, the acute phase of treatment offers appropriate medical and physical therapeutic measures to help decrease pain and rest the injured part. At the same time, steps are taken to protect the limb, and the body in general (the entire kinetic chain), from the effects of immobilization and decreased activity levels. Relative rest of the affected joint with substitute exercises for strength and cardiovascular status preservation are enacted. The athlete, coach, and family also are educated regarding the type of in-

Table 22–1
Injury Rehabilitation

Phases	Goals
Acute	Accurate diagnosis Pain relief Relative rest/protect kinetic chain Education
Recovery	Promote biologic healing Restoration of strength Restoration of flexibility Restoration of proprioception General fitness
Maintenance	Normal function of injured structure Development of task specific skills for return to activity

jury, plan for treatment, and realistic time frame for return to competition. These measures help to meet the goals of the acute phase of rehabilitation (Table 22–1).

Recovery Phase of Rehabilitation—Knee

As the recuperation process continues, the knee continues to undergo biologic healing. The athlete now may have little or no pain and knee-specific rehabilitation intensifies. The relative rest of the joint is decreased and selective strengthening, further flexibility, and proprioceptive retraining are introduced. General cardiovascular and strength conditioning is maintained and improved. However, the athlete does not return to usual sporting activity during the recovery phase of rehabilitation.

Maintenance Phase of Rehabilitation—Knee

A symptom-free knee still must be rehabilitated to meet the demands of a sporting activity. The knee should have normal function: full painless range of motion, equivalent strength and power as compared to the uninjured side, and kinesthetic or proprioceptive retraining. The athlete should have maintained or regained cardiovascular fitness, and should be able to demonstrate sports-specific skills before returning to participation. Also, appropriate protective equipment should be worn.

By rehabilitating sports injuries through the acute, recovery, and maintenance phases, the practitioner addresses functional deficits affecting athletic performance, not just the symptoms of an injury. Can acute cervical, thoracic, and lumbosacral injuries, athletic and otherwise, be treated using the same principles? Perhaps spine problems can be assessed

by appropriate aggressive diagnosis, short term palliative measures, and relative rest, while preserving overall fitness. Then flexibility, strengthening, and task-specific rehabilitation can be added. The treatment goal is not pain control but functional restoration and the patient, like the injured athlete, assumes a participatory role in the rehabilitation process.

DIAGNOSIS

The patient with new onset of spine pain should be subject to the same acute phase rehabilitation goals listed above. The paramount issue in initiating therapy is obtaining an *accurate diagnosis*. Not all spine pain is musculoskeletal. Careful history and physical examination, searching for gastrointestinal, genitourinary, rheumatologic, cardiac, pulmonary, and other nonorthopedic causes of spine pain are part of any assessment. Atraumatic constant pain suggests spinal tumor or infection. Progressive neurologic deficit can result from spinal tumor, infection, or massive disc protrusion. Most commonly, acute spine pain is given a nonspecific diagnosis. Nachemson states that only 10 to 20% of patients with lumbosacral pain can be given a precise pathomechanical diagnosis.[7] This information seems discouraging if the axiom of treatment based on accurate diagnosis is postulated as an integral part of acute phase rehabilitation.

Perhaps better diagnostic clarity is possible by understanding relevant anatomy and pathomechanics. Although absolute identification of the pain generator is not always possible, improved localization and identification of painful areas usually is. The supraspinous, intraspinous, and longitudinal ligaments, ligamentum flavum, fascial planes, facets and peripheral fibers of the annulus are all pain sensitive structures.[8,9] Muscles are pain sensitive and react to perimuscular sources of spine pain with spasm and guarding via the reflex arc at the level of the spinal cord. Muscles also receive input from other spinal cord levels, the brainstem, and the cerebral cortex. Local muscle injury or fatigue also may produce spasm.[10] Some or all of these pain sensitive structures can be sources of spine discomfort. Different structures may be symptomatic at different times during the course of a spine injury.

An understanding of the pathomechanics of lumbosacral spine degeneration underscores this concept. The landmark work of Kirkaldy-Willis demonstrates the stages of spine degeneration affecting both the anterior (discovertebral) and posterior (facet) structures (Fig. 22–1).[11,12] These anterior and posterior changes occur simultaneously and can pro-

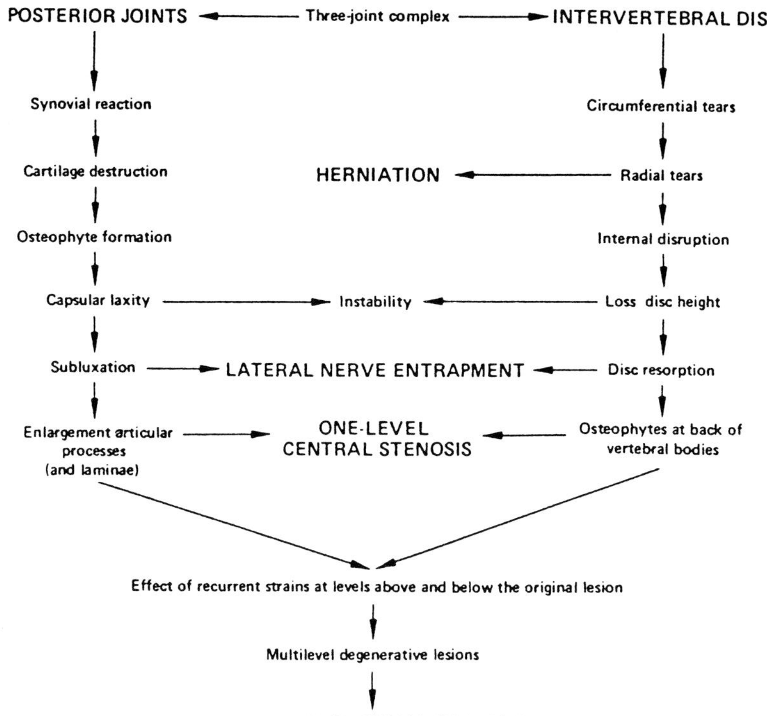

Figure 22–1. Stages of spine degeneration.

duce symptoms separately or together. Secondary fascial, ligamentous, and muscular changes accompany the stages of segmental degeneration and can themselves result in discomfort. Substantiating this concept of segmental injury are studies showing that repetitive torsional loads cause annular tears leading to disc degeneration.[13] Yet, the same torsional loading may shear the facet joints, injuring the synovium and capsule.[14] Facet degenerative changes follow.

Secondary soft tissue changes then occur leading to tightness, spasm, and shortening of these ligamentous, fascial, and muscular structures and contributing to the pain picture. Poor pelvic flexibility and lower extremity inflexibility also develops. These secondary changes and accompanying postural accommodations cause further segmental stiffness. This leads to an alteration of the normal loading patterns of the ligamentous system of the lumbar spine.[15] Poor flexibility of spinal segments, pelvis, and hips does not allow the thoracolumbar fascial and midline ligaments (supraspinous, intraspinous, ligamentum flavum, posterior longitudinal ligament, and facet joint capsule), to properly accept load with upright standing and flexion of the trunk.[15–17] These structures can normally dissipate force produced with flexion without creating torsional loads on the discovertebral joint or facet joint. With alteration of the normal ligamentous loading the paraspinal muscle increasingly is used to resist

flexion. The muscle has less biomechanical advantage and its contraction produces a greater compressive force on the disc and increases stress at the intervertebral joint.[16] This causes further acceleration of the discovertebral-posterior element degenerative process and a vicious cycle develops. Indeed not only do the discovertebral, posterior element, and soft tissue changes interact at one level, but adjacent levels can be affected. The spine is a coupled motion system.[18] Diagnostic testing must be interpreted in the context of this ongoing multilevel process. Imaging studies often show disc and facet changes in asymptomatic patients.[19,20] Radiographic findings must be correlated with clinical symptoms in order to make proper treatment decisions.

Clinically, the heavy laborer with acute spine pain may have a history and physical examination more suggestive of disc symptoms, whereas the gymnast may be more likely to have posterior element pain. The soft tissue pain component may be the most striking initial feature of both patients. The worker and the athlete may both have anterior and posterior segmental subclinical changes. The mechanism producing the acute injury is different in the two people and different pain sensitive structures are irritated and become symptomatic. The history and physical examination performed in the context of acute injury to a component or components of a spinal segment helps to specify the diagnosis to predominantly anterior element pain, posterior element pain, or soft tissue pain. The initial treatment may focus on disc, facet, or soft tissue, but all areas must be addressed during the phases of rehabilitation. This is true of injuries to the lumbosacral, thoracic, or cervical spine.

TREATMENT

The acute phase of rehabilitation begins with accurate diagnosis, as discussed above. This allows for appropriate selection of treatment methods to help meet the other goals of the acute phase of rehabilitation (Table 22–1). Not only is accurate diagnosis difficult, methods for treating acute back pain are controversial. Spine pain, like many other musculoskeletal problems, does not lend itself easily to critical study. Current literature does not demonstrate efficacy of several available treatments (Table 22–2) and significant research design problems exist (Table 22–3). The biggest stumbling block in determining treatment efficacy may be isolated treatments are attempted for spine pain without a precise diagnosis. When individual measures are tried in a setting of a multifactorial pain process, which is often episodic, determination of treatment effacacy can be confusing.

The sports medicine approach attempts to utilize and integrate a participatory treatment plan based on available sound knowledge. The previous chapters describe specific treatments in detail. Some of these measures will be discussed in the context of using therapeutic methods in a timely multifactorial manner to correct functional deficits. The rational choice of treatment and the timing of its use are

Table 22–2
Demonstrated Efficacy of Treatments for Acute Low Back Pain Patients

	Randomized Control Trial	Controlled Non-Randomized Trial	No Scientific Evidence
Bed rest	X		
Medications		X	
Back School	X		
Exercise			X*
Traction			X*
Manipulation			X*
Braces/Corsets			X
Massage			X
Cryotherapy			X
Thermotherapy			X
TENS			X
Laser			X

*Studies performed comparing this to other treatment in noncontrolled trial or equivocal findings reported.

(From Ohnmeiss, D., Stith, W., Gilbert, P., Rashbaum, R.: Treatment of acute back pain. *In* Lumbar Disc Disease. Spine State of the Art Reviews 3:69, 1989.)

Table 22–3
Spine Pain Research

Study Design Problems
No precise diagnosis
No description of the evaluation process
No appropriate control group
No long term functional followup
Incomplete patient demographic data
Incomplete description of treatment methods
Variable skill of treatment providers
Inadequate patient sample size

Adapted from Ohnmeiss, D., Stith, W., Gilbert, P., Rashbaum, R.: Treatment of acute back pain. *In* Lumbar Disc Disease. Spine State of the Art Reviews 3:69, 1989.

based on mechanism of injury and resultant dysfunction.

After accurate diagnosis has been established, *pain relief* is the next goal of the acute phase of rehabilitation. The patient is advised to rest in a comfortable position and is instructed in simple body mechanics. This allows sitting, standing, bathing, and other daily activities to be performed with as much comfort as possible, thus avoiding further irritation of the spine. The use of physical modalities is another way to help control spine pain. Cold treatment (cryotherapy) decreases spasm, pain, and capillary blood flow (swelling). The skin is cooled quickly, with the rate of muscle cooling directly proportionate to the thickness of overlying fat, taking anywhere from 10 to 30 minutes.[21,22] Ice or frozen gel may provide more consistent, longer duration cooling than chemical cold packs or refrigerants.[23] Heat (thermotherapy) also decreases spasm and pain but increases arterial and capillary blood flow. Superficial heating modalities, i.e., heating pads, hydrocator packs, heat lamps, and whirlpool penetrate to a depth of 2 cm or less. Any deeper response to these heating methods is by reflex pathways.[22] Cryotherapy is preferable for an acute injury; both superficial heat and ice control spasm and pain, but cold therapy also addresses acute inflammation. Deep heat, or diathermy (ultrasound, microwave, shortwave), is reserved for subacute or chronic injury.

Another physical modality, therapeutic electricity, has among its physiologic effects reduction of acute spasm, reduction of edema, and pain relief. It is usually administered as high voltage pulsed galvanic stimulation (HVGS). Electricity delivered as transcutaneous nerve stimulation (TENS) initially was used for chronic pain control. TENS may be have some effect on acute pain as well.[24,25] Electricity can help control acute spine pain but, as with any isolated measure, it may not be effective along.[26,27] It is a physical modality, as are heat and cold, to consider in combination with other treatments. One should prescribe these measures based upon the understanding of the biophysics of their actions.

In addition to physical modalities other methods help to relieve pain during the acute phase of rehabilitation. Medications frequently are prescribed for acute spine pain. Nonsteroidal anti-inflammatory drugs (NSAIDs) provide both an analgesic effect (in short-term small dosages) and an anti-inflammatory effect (in longer duration higher dosages). The duration of the analgesic effect of the NSAID may be different from that of the anti-inflammatory effect.[28] Patient response to the NSAID cannot be predicted based upon chemical class of medication or by the pharmacokinetics of the drug.[29] The true effectiveness of NSAIDs in acute spine pain is unknown because of the nature of the problem and poor study design.[26,27,30] NSAID prescription should be based upon the need to obtain analgesic effect or anti-inflammatory effect or both. Dosage and length of utilization can thus be determined. Changing to a different chemical class if the first NSAID is not effective may be reasonable. It may also be appropriate to begin with aspirin. Potential side effects should be remembered and reasonable patient warnings issued.

As noted, one effect of NSAIDs is analgesia, and other pure analgesics are used in acute spine pain cases. Non-narcotic analgesia can be obtained with acetaminophen. Patients who cannot tolerate the gastrointestinal side effects of the NSAID may benefit from acetaminophen. In addition, there is no cross tolerance between NSAIDs and acetaminophen.[10] Addition of acetaminophen to the patient's anti-inflammatory medication can help relieve pain. Stronger analgesics (narcotics) are available for short-term use in more severe acute spine pain. This medication should be given on a time contingent basis in adequate doses to produce analgesia. If employed in this fashion for a few days there is little chance of addiction.[31] There is no role for long term narcotic usage, and short term use does not substitute for the complete rehabilitation plan.

Muscle relaxants are prescribed for acute spine pain as well. Opinions differ regarding the site of action of these compounds. Some believe the muscle spindle is affected, whereas others think the action of these medications is sedation of the central nervous system.[10] Some of these agents (benzodiazepines) can be very addictive. Once again, few studies demonstrate efficacy.[26] The muscle relaxants can cause lethargy, making it difficult for the patient to participate in the other aspects of the rehabilitation plan.

One other medication should be mentioned. Corticosteroids have no direct analgesic effect; any pain relief is caused by the drug's anti-inflammatory action. Short-course oral corticosteroid treatment has been reported for acute spine pain.[32] Concern has been voiced about potential side effects (gastrointestinal irritation, hyperglycemia, hypertension, and infection). Corticosteroids also can be delivered via the epidural route. This method of administration is also controversial. Conflicting reports of efficacy and indications for utilization exist.[33-39] Once again, factors such as patient selection based on diagnosis, length of symptoms, and involvement in a total rehabilitation program often are not addressed in these studies. If meticulous technique is followed (including fluoroscopic guidance) and patient selection is based on appropriate symptoms (acute or subacute discogenic radiculopathy or central spinal stenosis with acute increase in symptoms), epidural steroid injection is indicated. The injection should be combined with a complete rehabilitation program. The discussion on the use of oral and epidural medications to control acute spine pain again demonstrates that review of available studies and literature shows unclear efficacy results. In the studies, the drugs were often given as the only treatment for a variety of diagnoses of spine pain. If these medications are used, prescription should be based on sound principles and a part of an overall treatment plan.

Instruction of proper and comfortable positioning, use of physical modalities, and prescription of medication help meet the goal of pain relief during the acute phase of rehabilitation. Another method used to help meet the goal of pain relief—active exercise—demonstrates an essential principle of the sports medicine approach to rehabilitation; participatory involvement by the patient. Initial exercises should be combined with the treatments listed above as soon as possible. Selection of particular exercises is based upon an understanding of the pathogenesis of spine pain as described previously. Most work with exercise for spine pain has been done with low back discomfort. If the patient's symptoms are predominantly discogenic, a trial of appropriately performed extension exercises may be appropriate. Whether anterior migration of the nuclear material results because of these exercises, or because neural tension is reduced, or both of these events occurs simultaneously, is not clear.[40-42] However, certain patients have significantly decreased discogenic radicular and lumbosacral symptoms with these extension exercises. Correction of lumbar shift is necessary before the initiation of these exercises. If the primary symptoms appear to originate from the posterior elements, extension exercises will increase symptoms. The exercises may also increase symptoms in cases of spinal stenosis. Flexion exercises decrease weightbearing stress on the facet joints[43] and are preferred in those cases of acute pain secondary to posterior element irritation. In contrast, flexion increases intradiscal pressure[44] and these exercises are not helpful for acute pain of a predominant discogenic nature.

One must be aware of several issues that have a major impact on the success of these exercise regimens. If muscle, ligamentous, or fascial tightness and shortening are present, the exercises may be painful and may not affect the relevant segments of the spine. Appropriate brief use of the physical modalities and medical measures discussed previously, combined with stretching techniques taught by a physical therapist, may be required before or in concert with the exercise regimen. Stiff spinal segments may be made more flexible by trained physical therapists utilizing soft tissue and articular mobilization techniques.[45] These techniques are only a part of the treatment plan and are used to make therapeutic exercise more effective and better tolerated. Mobilization and manipulation are generic terms; several different techniques exist. Distraction, nonthrust, or thrusting movements of joints can be provided. Physiologic explanations for pain relief are varied and unclear. There is no convincing evidence of actual realignment of vertebral bodies or reduction of disc herniation.[46,47] The utilization of mild to moderate segmental oscillatory joint movements and soft tissue stretching as a prelude or companion to active exercise may be helpful. No data exist to support the role of long-term mobilization or manipulation in spine pain. Such protracted passive treatment places the patient in a dependent role and can be counterproductive in attempts to move toward participatory function oriented care.

In cases of predominant discogenic symptoms, therapeutic exercises sometimes precede, or are supplemented with traction, another method to help meet the goal of pain relief. To achieve true distraction of vertebral bodies with the body in the horizontal position, a traction force of at least 25% (and probably greater) of body weight must be exerted.[10] Any reduction in disc protrusion appears to return rapidly after cessation of traction.[48,49] If horizontal traction is postulated to work by decreasing intradiscal pressure rather than true vertebral distraction, current research shows only small intradiscal pressure decreases.[50] Autotraction, traction utilizing a special frame anchoring the lower extremities and providing handles for the patient to pull, allows the patient to control the amount of traction and has had favorable reports.[51] However, others have actually shown increased intradiscal pressure with autotraction because of contraction of the thoracic musculature by the patient when placed in the

autotraction device.[52] Gravity assisted traction may cause 0.3 mm to 4.0 mm distraction of the vertebral bodies.

Effects on disc protrusion are unknown and potential side effects (e.g., increased blood pressure, increased heart rate, gastrointestinal reflex, and berry aneurysm rupture) exist.[53] Traction may provide pain relief by stretching muscle or other soft tissue structures or by enforcing rest. It should be used with the understanding that consistent disc reduction or decreased intradiscal pressure may not be achieved. Traction is passive treatment and, if employed, should be short-term and only as one part of the rehabilitation plan.

If the practitioner prescribes the appropriate combination of modalities, medications, initial therapeutic exercise, mobilization, and perhaps traction, the goal of pain relief during the acute phase of rehabilitation can be met. Part of this prescription entails having the patient find positions of comfort. Often, initially this involves bed rest. The area of bed rest focuses attention on another goal of the acute phase of rehabilitation, *relative rest while maintaining the rest of the kinetic chain.* Prolonged bed rest leads to significant deconditioning and has not been proven to be more effective in limiting back pain and disability than short-term bed rest.[54]

Long term bed rest has debilitating effects on muscle strength and flexibility, cardiovascular fitness and bone density,[55] as well as the specific negative effects of increased spinal segmental stiffness and decreased disc nutrition.[56] In addition, there is the absence of a participatory activity by the patient. It is reasonable to limit or modify the acute spine pain patient's activity, including periods of bed rest, during the day, but absolute bed rest for more than 2 to 3 days has no place. Relative rest of the painful spine helps protect the general cardiovascular and musculoskeletal function while providing initial symptomatic relief. This allows for reduction in the amount of total body reconditioning necessary during the recovery and maintenance phases of rehabilitation. Protecting the injured part while avoiding unnecessary side effects and allowing the patient to remain active in his treatment plan is an essential part of any functional rehabilitation program.

The remaining goal of the acute phase of rehabilitation is *education.* Just as it is beneficial for the athlete to understand his injury, the spine patient needs to be informed as well. This allows the patient to begin to develop perspective about the injury and may assuage fears and unrealistic concerns. It is reassuring to inform the acute low back pain sufferer that 40 to 50% of patients improve within one week,[57] and that number increases to 85 to 90% by 6 to 12 weeks.[58,59] Even 50% of the patients with sciatica recover within 1 month,[60] and 75% are improved within 6 months without surgery.[61] Often, it is helpful to explain this information to family members, friends, and employers, as well as to the patient. Back schools educate patients about the causes of back pain and teach patients ways to cope with their current discomfort. Armed with knowledge of anatomy, mechanism of injury, and proper body mechanics, the patients become less fearful. Such education programs have resulted in earlier return to work[58] and can be started in the acute phase of rehabilitation. The information provided by the physician and by the back school classes serves to diffuse the sense of helplessness often felt by the patient. Also, if the patient's recovery does not generally follow the above time tables, further testing and possible exploration of psychosocial issues can be undertaken.

RECOVERY PHASE

Education is an important component of the acute phase of rehabilitation. The patient has learned that his pain probably will not be long lasting. He must also understand, however, that absence of symptoms does not mean normal function. Pain may dissipate but spinal segmental stiffness, soft tissue changes, and lower extremity inflexibility may persist. The segmental changes described previously (Fig. 22–1) still must be addressed. Indeed, reinjury of the lumbar spine is common; recurrence rates as high as 70 to 90% have been reported.[62–64] Repeat episodes are more severe and last longer. One could postulate that either the patient returned to activity too rapidly or that the patient was inadequately rehabilitated, or both.

The acute phase of rehabilitation provides diagnostic accuracy, pain relief, relative rest, and education, but cannot address complete restoration of function. Cady[65] demonstrated that among firefighters, those with higher composite scores on strength, flexibility, and cardiovascular fitness tests were at less risk for back problems. He also showed that a fitness program reduced workers' compensation costs by 25%.[66] Mayer reported the rather profound loss of the trunk muscle strength in patients with back pain for 6 months or longer.[67] Equating back injury or reinjury to poor cardiovascular or strength conditioning is not completely straightforward, but adequate information exists to warrant intervention in these areas. This chapter focuses on early care for spine pain. However, some subacute therapies are outlined as part of the recovery and maintenance phases in order to emphasize a complete rehabilitation program.

During the recovery phase of rehabilitation initial exercise is progressed to more advanced activities as

symptoms dissipate. The focus of exercise is now not just on unloading the discovertebral joint with extension motions or decreasing facet joint irritation with flexion maneuvers, but now the acute discomfort has subsided allowing the patient to progress in exercise therapy. Increased physical activity improves disc nutrition[56] and collagen fiber growth in muscle, tendon, and ligament is stimulated by early tensile loading.[27,60] Therefore, *biologic healing* of the injured spine structures, a goal of the recovery phase (Table 22–1), can be promoted by exercise. Exercise also allows the patient to work toward another goal of the recovery phase, *restoration of strength*. Strength training of the spine and lower extremities is now introduced. Abdominal musculature attaches to the thoracolumbar fascia and, in concert with this fascia and the posterior midline spine ligaments, contraction of the abdominal musculature helps to decrease shear stress on the lumbar segments.[15,17] Strengthening of the rectus abdominis, abdominal obliques, and transversus abdominis helps improve this protective mechanism. The spinal extensors participate in maintaining upright posture. A particularly important muscle is the gluteus maximus. This muscle plays a key role in straightening the spine from the flexed position to the upright position.[16] Strengthening of the spine extensors in combination with abdominal (flexor) strengthening is necessary.

A balanced strengthening program is initiated using proper techniques to protect the spine from unnecessary loading and excessive range of motion. This concept is frequently referred to as "neutral spine" strengthening or stabilization. Implementation occurs after acute symptoms have dissipated and appropriate spine flexion and extension is tolerated without discomfort. Lower extremity strengthening is a component of the program as well. Quadriceps strengthening improves the patient's ability to squat comfortably rather than bend at the waist. This helps provide proper execution of body mechanics protecting the lumbar spine segments.

Proper posture is also encouraged, and this activity is partially related to muscle strength as well. An example is the cervical musculature which has a pivotal role in maintaining proper head position. Simply sliding the head forward 1 to 2 in. increases the pull of the posterior cervical musculature dramatically[69] and causes increased compressive shear on the cervical facet joints and posterior disc. Balanced strength of the anterior and posterior cervical musculature is important to help prevent this postural fault.

Strength training is initiated after the acute symptoms have dissipated but is ineffective alone; other goals of the recovery phase of rehabilitation must be met simultaneously. *Restoration of flexibility* is approached along with the strengthening program. Stiff spinal segments are initially addressed with proper modality and mobilization techniques. Self-directed stretching and mobilization programs for the spine continue to correct muscular, fascial, ligamentous and capsular tightness and shortening. The anatomic and biomechanical design of the spine results in certain ranges of motion and directions of motion occurring at particular segments. Cervical rotation receives its greatest normal contribution from C1-C2;[18] most lumbar flexion (75%) occurs at L5-S1.[10] If segmental spine stiffness prohibits the normal range of motion at a certain level, the motion will occur somewhere else in the coupled motion system of the spine. The accelerated degenerative changes at the level above or below a spinal fusion serve as a well known example. The ongoing patient-enacted spinal flexibility program attempts to regain proper segmental function resulting in more appropriate loading of the spine.

Restoration of flexibility is important not only for the spinal segments but also for the pelvis and lower extremity. Proper postural alignment requires normal flexibility and function of the lumbar spine, pelvis, and lower extremity.[10] Forward bending performed correctly involves linked lumbar spine and hip motion, lumbopelvic rhythm. This range of motion system produces adequate trunk flexion while properly loading the fascial and ligamentous structures of the spine. As discussed previously, this decreases shear of the disc.[16,17] Hamstring and gastrocsoleus flexibility are a necessary part of the lumbopelvic rhythm. In addition, the instruction of proper squatting, lifting, and other techniques during back school necessitates good lower extremity flexibility. Flexibility of the pelvis and lower extremity has an important contribution to segmental spine function and is necessary for the performance of proper body mechanics.

Interrelated with strengthening and flexibility training is *restoration of proprioception,* another goal of the recovery phase of rehabilitation. Early motion post-injury helps maintain or regain joint proprioception.[70] A complex network of nerves in the spine structures may be sensitive not only to pain but can transmit joint position information as well.[71] This input can be trained with repetitive exercises emphasizing proper form. The patient gains a kinesthetic sense, which maintain proper spine position (neutral spine) when doing strength and flexibility rehabilitation as well as during daily activities or sporting events.

During the recovery phase of rehabilitation the spine is protected and healing encouraged with instruction in strengthening and flexibility combined with proprioceptive retraining. Physical and occupational therapists with special background in spine care are necessary to provide direction and progression of this program. An understanding of the biomechanical basis of spine motion, as well as a familiarity with the actual flexibility, strengthening, and proprioceptive exercises, is essential.[72–74] While supervising exercise of the spine, therapists can also ensure that the patient continues a program to *maintain general cardiovascular and strength conditioning,* which is a final goal of the recovery phase of rehabilitation.

MAINTENANCE PHASE

A program of strength, flexibility, and proprioceptive retraining helps to further rehabilitate the spine during the recovery phase. These exercises are continued and further exercises added during the maintenance phase to try to assure normal function of the injured structures. If completely normal function is not possible the gains made in the areas listed above will help to protect the injured site as much as possible. The athlete then progresses to practicing motions required for an individual sport. This *development of task-specific skills necessary for return to activity* is the other goal of the maintenance phase of rehabilitation (Table 22–1). This supervised program is continued until all the necessary skills for full participation have been relearned and can be demonstrated. This same format has relevance to spine patients, who must use strength, flexibility, and proprioceptive ability, coupled with proper body mechanics, to avoid reinjury. Whether it is a work or recreational activity, the patient should be coached on proper execution of the movements required. Task-specific training is necessary. Mayer has proposed using exercises to simulate actual activities or motions of sport or work as an effective tool for spine rehabilitation.[75] The growing fields of work hardening and work readiness programs have developed along this concept. Detailed discussion of this area of post-injury therapy is not directly part of a chapter on acute care, but for complete functional recovery of an acute spine injury the maintenance phase goals must be met.

CONCLUSION

The field of sports medicine has developed to address the specific needs of the athletic population. Treatment has been based on the idea of returning the patient to participation and has resulted in prompt, supervised, participatory therapy. This model can be applied to acute spine problems. Goal-oriented treatment utilizing sound biomechanical, biophysical, physiologic, and pharmacologic principles and provided in an integrated fashion is necessary. Such programs may help not only to relieve symptoms but also to restore and maintain function of the spine.

REFERENCES

1. Hage, P.: Sports medicine clinics: are guidelines necessary? Phys Sports Med *10*:165, 1982.
2. Behar, R.: Medicines $10 billion bonanza. Forbes June 13, p. 107, 1988.
3. Robey, R., Blyth, C.: Athletic injuries; application of epidemiologic methods. JAMA *217*:184, 1971.
4. Lysens, R., et al.: The predictability of sports injuries. Sports Med *1*:6, 1984.
5. Canale, S., Cantler, E., Sisk, D., Freeman, B.: A chronicle of injuries of an American intercollegiate football team. Am J Sports Med *9*:384, 1981.
6. Shields, C., Zomar, V.: Analysis of professional football injuries. Contemp Orthop *4*:90, 1982.
7. Nachemson, A.: Advances in low-back pain. Clin Orthop *200*:266, 1985.
8. Hirsch, C., Ingelmark, B., Miller, M.: The anatomical basis for low back pain: studies on the presence of sensory nerve endings in ligamentous, capsular and intervertebral disc structures in the human lumbar spine. Acta Orthop Scand *33*:1, 1963.
9. Bogduk, N., Tyran, W., Wilson, A.: The innervation of the human intervertebral disc. J Anat *132*:39, 1981.
10. Borenstein, D., Wiesel, S.: Low Back Pain—Medical Diagnosis and Comprehensive Management. Philadelphia, W.B. Saunders, 1989.
11. Kirkaldy-Willis, W., Wedge, J., Yong-Hing, K., Reilly, J.: Pathology and pathogenesis of lumbar spondylosis and stenosis. Spine *3*:319, 1978.
12. Kirkaldy-Willis, W. (ed.): Managing Low Back Pain, 2nd Ed. New York, Churchill Livingstone, 1988.
13. Farfan, H., et al.: The effects of torsion on the lumbar intervertebral joints: the role of torsion in the production of disc degeneration. J Bone Joint Surg, *52A*:468, 1970.
14. Liu, Y., et al.: Torsional fatigue of the lumbar intervertebral joints. Spine *10*:894, 1985.
15. Gracovetsky, S., Farfan, H., Helleur, C.: The abdominal mechanism. Spine *10*:317, 1985.
16. Farfan, H.: Biomechanics of the lumbar spine. *In* Managing Low Back Pain, (Edited by W.H. Kirkaldy-Willis) 2nd Ed. New York, Churchill-Livingstone, 1988.
17. Bogduk, N., MacIntosh, J.: The applied anatomy of the thoracolumbar fascia. Spine *9*:164, 1984.
18. White, A., Pahjabi, M.: Clinical biomechanics of the spine. Philadelphia, J.B. Lippincott, 1978.
19. Wiesel, S., et al.: A study of computer-assisted tomography. The incidence of positive CAT scans in an asymptomatic group of patients. Spine *9*:549, 1984.
20. Gibson, M., et al.: Magnetic resonance imaging of adolescent disc herniation. J Bone Joint Surg *69B*:699, 1987.
21. Lehmann, J.: Therapeutic heat and cold. Clin Orthop *99*:207, 1974.
22. Lehmann, J., deLateur, B.: Diathermy and superficial heat and cold therapy. *In* Krusen's Handbook of Physical Medicine and Rehabilitation, (Edited by F.J. Kottle, G.K. Stillwell, and J.F. Lehmann). 3rd Ed. Philadelphia, W.B. Saunders, 1982.
23. McMasters, W., Liddle, S., Waugh, T.: Laboratory evaluation of various cold therapy modalities. Am J Sports Med *6*:291, 1978.
24. Roeser, W., et al.: The use of transcutaneous nerve stimulation for pain control in athletic medicine: A preliminary report. Am J Sports Med *4*:210, 1976.
25. Gersh, M.: Postoperative pain and transcutaneous electrical nerve stimulation. Phys Ther *58*:1463, 1978.
26. Deyo, R.: Conservative therapy for low back pain: distinguishing useful from useless therapy. JAMA *250*:1057, 1983.
27. Kellett, J.: Acute soft tissue injuries—a review of the literature. Med Sci Sports Exerc *18*:489, 1986.
28. Huskisson, E.: Non-narcotic analgesics. *In* Text Book of Pain, (Edited by P.D. Wall and R. Melzack). New York, Churchill-Livingstone, 1984.
29. Dahl, S.: Nonsteroidal anti-inflammatory agents: clinical pharmacology/adverse effects/usage guidelines. *In* Therapeutic Controversies in the Rheumatic Diseases, (Edited by R.F. Willkens and S.L. Dahl). Orlando, Grune & Stratton, 1987.
30. Quintet, R., Hadler, M.: Diagnosis and treatment of backache. Semin Rheum *8*:261, 1979.
31. Stimmel, B.: Pain, analgesia and addiction: an approach to the pharmacologic management of pain. Clin J Pain *1*:14, 1985.
32. Green, L.: Dexamethasone in the management of symptoms due to herniated lumbar disc. J Neurol Neurosurg Psychiatry, *38*:1211, 1975.
33. Cuckler, J., et al.: The use of epidural steroids in the treatment of lumbar radicular pain. J Bone Joint Surg, *67A*.63, 1985.
34. White, A., Derby, R., Wynne, G.: Epidural injection for the diagnosis and treatment of low back pain. Spine *5*:78, 1980.
35. Dilke, T., Burry, H., Grahame, R.: Extradural corticosteroid injection management of lumbar nerve root compression. Br Med J *2*:635, 1973.
36. Oudenhoven, R.: The role of laminectomy, facet rhizotomy and epidural steroids. Spine *4*:145, 1979.
37. White, A.: Injection techniques for the diagnosis and treatment of low back pain. Orthop Clin North Am *14*:553, 1983.
38. Brown, F.: Management of diskogenic pain using epidural and intrathecal steroids. Clin Orthop *129*:72, 1977.
39. Jeffries, B.: Epidural steroid injections. *In* Spinal Imaging: Diagnostic and Therapeutic Applications. Spine State of the Art Reviews, *25*:417, 1958.
40. McKenzie, R.: The Lumbar Spine, Mechanical Diagnosis and Therapy. Waikance, NZ, Spinal Publications, 1981.
41. Schnebel, B., Chourning, J., Davidson, R., Simmons, J.: A digitizing technique for the study of movement of intradiscal dye in response to flexion and extension of the lumbar spine. Spine *13*:309, 1988.
42. Schnebel, B., Watkins, R., Antonelli, D.: The role of spinal flexion and extension in changing nerve root compression in disc herniations. N Am Spine Soc, 1988.
43. Adams, M., Hutton, W.: The mechanical function of the lumbar apophyseal joints. Spine *8*:327, 1983.
44. Nachemson, A.: Disc pressure measurements. Spine *6*:93, 1981.
45. Van Hoesen, L.: Mobilization and manipulation techniques for the lumbar spine. *In* Modern Manual Therapy of the Vertebral Column (Edited by G.P. Grieve). New York, Churchill-Livingstone, 1986.
46. Frymoyer, J.: Back pain and sciatica. N Engl J Med *318*:291, 1988.
47. Jayson, M., et al.: Mobilization and manipulation for low back pain. Spine *6*:409, 1981.
48. Matthews, J.: Dynamic discography: a study of lumbar traction. Ann Phys Med *9*:275, 1968.
49. Gupta, R., Ramarao, S.: Epidurography in reduction of lumbar disc prolapse by traction. Arch Phys Med Rehabil *59*:372, 1978.
50. Nachemson, A., Elfstrom, G.: Intravital dynamic pressure measurements in lumbar discs: a study of common movements, maneuvers, and exercises. Scand J Rehabil Med (Suppl), *1*:1, 1970.

51. Ohnmeiss, D., Stith, W., Gilbert, P., Rashbaum, R.: Treatment of acute back pain. *In* Lumbar Disc Disease—Spine State of the Art Reviews, 3:69, 1989.
52. Andersson, G., Schultz, H., Nachemson, A.: Intervertebral disc pressures during traction. Scand Rehab Med (Suppl) *9*:88, 1983.
53. Gianakopoulos, G., et al.: Inversion devices: Their role in producing lumbar distraction. Arch Phys Med Rehab *66*:100, 1985.
54. Deyo, R., Diehl, A., Rosenthal, M.: How many days of bedrest for acute low back pain? A randomized clinical trial. N Engl J Med *315*:1064, 1986.
55. Bortz, W.: The disuse syndrome. West J Med *141*:691, 1984.
56. Urban, J., McMullin, J.: Swelling pressure of lumbar intervertebral discs: influence of age, spinal level, composition and degeneration. Spine *13*:179, 1988.
57. Fry, J.: Back pain and soft tissue rheumatism, advisory saervices colloquium proceedings. London, Advisory Services, Clinical and General, 1972.
58. Berquist-Ullman, M., Larsson, U.: Acute low back pain in industry: a controlled prospective study with special reference to therapy and vocational factors. Acta Orthop Scand (Suppl), *170*:1, 1977.
59. White, A.: Low back pain in men receiving workmen's compensation. Can Med Assoc J *95*:50, 1966.
60. Andersson, G., Svensson, H-O, Oden, A.: The intensity of work recovery in low back pain. Spine *8*:880, 1983.
61. Vanharanta, H.: Etiology, epidemiology, and natural history of lumbar disc disease. *In* Lumbar Disc Disease. Spine State of the Art Reviews, 3:1, 1989.
62. Dehlin, O., Hedenrund, B., Horal, J.: Back symptoms in nursing aides in a geriatric hospital. Scand J Rehabil *8*:47, 1976.
63. Hirsch, C., Jonsson, R., Lewin, T.: Low back symptoms in a Swedish female population. Clin Orthop *63*:171, 1969.
64. Horal, J.: The clinical appearance of low back disorders in the city of Gothenburg, Sweden. Acta Orthop Scand (Suppl) *118*:8, 1969.
65. Cady, L., et al.: Strength and fitness and subsequent back injuries in firefighters. Occup Med *4*:269, 1979.
66. Cady, L., Thomas, P., Karivasky, R.: Program for increasing health and physical fitness of firefighters. Occup Med *2*:111, 1985.
67. Mayer, T., Smith, S., Keeley, J., Mooney, V.: Quantification of lumbar function. Part 2: sagittal plane trunk strength in chronic low back pain patients. Spine *10*:765, 1985.
68. Oakes, B.: Acute soft tissue injuries: nature and management. Aust Fam Physician (Suppl) *10*:3, 1982.
69. Calliet, R.: Neck and Arm Pain. 2nd Ed. Philadelphia, F.A. Davis, 1981.
70. Leach, R.: The prevention and rehabilitation of soft tissue injuries. Int J Sports Med (Suppl) *3*:18, 1982.
71. Gracovetsky, S., Farfan, H.: The optimum spine. Spine *11*:543, 1986.
72. Gustavsen, R.: Training Therapy Prophylaxis and Rehabilitation. New York, Thieme, 1985.
73. Gunnari, H., Evjenth, O., Brady, M.: Sequence Exercise. Oslo, Dreyer, 1984.
74. Saal, J.: Sports-related lumbar spine injuries. In Rehabilitation of Sports Injuries Phys Med Rehabil State of the Art Reviews, *1*:613, 1987.
75. Mayer, T., Gatchel, R.: Functional Restoration for Spinal Disorders: The Sports Medicine Approach. Philadelphia, Lea & Febiger, 1988.

Timothy A. Garvey
Sam W. Wiesel

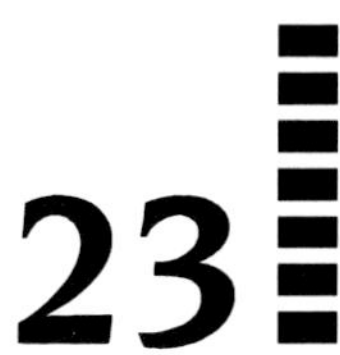

23

Surveillance Systems for Acutely Injured Patients

This chapter is concerned with the surveillance of the acutely injured patient with a painful spinal disorder. The concepts of why this is necessary in evaluating the quality of care, the outcome parameters that are used, and the role of industry are discussed. A review of the literature then is utilized to analyze the development and implementation of surveillance systems. We conclude with recommendations for surveillance.

CONCEPTS

Webster gives two definitions for surveillance: "1. Watch kept over a person, especially one who is suspect or prisoner. 2. Supervision or inspection."[1] Because many in the health care industry feel they are being held suspect, there is skepticism and contempt for implementing surveillance systems of any type. When reacquainted with the second interpretation, and when fully understanding that the mutual goal of the surveillance system and the individual practitioner is excellence in patient care, then careful analysis of how to monitor patient progress will be undertaken.

Quality Care

Why is there an interest in developing and implementing surveillance systems for patients with acute painful spinal disorders? Is it not enough for an individual patient to consult with a practitioner of his choice for diagnosis and followup care as needed? Unfortunately, the socioeconomic impact of the rapid increase in health care costs over the past two decades has brought the individual patient's problem out of his private practitioner's office, into the board rooms of employers, third-party payers, and

legislators. Fortunately, those involved in these developments should have the same goal, that is "quality care." With this emphasis on improved diagnosis, treatment, and outcome, the individual patient should benefit by ensurance of high standards for their care.

Given that "quality care" is the common goal of those caring for painful spinal disorders, the difficulty lies in selecting a definition. Because spinal care is generated by a broad spectrum of physicians and other health practitioners possessing a diversity of experience and educational backgrounds in varied practice environments and treating a multitude of patients with multiple potential diagnoses, patients with the same pathophysiologic process may receive different diagnoses and care from office to office, or even from the same physician. Therefore, a standardized set of diagnostic criteria and treatment regimens must be formulated.

It is well documented that systematic and regional differences exist among physicians in treatment and predilection for surgical options.[2] Few health care systems are capable of monitoring the care delivered, or the progress of an individual patient. As a result, the health care institutions, as well as the individual patients, are unable to assess the care that is given.

Objective Outcomes

The challenge in care of spinal disorders includes the lack of significant specific objective variables for measurement of damage. Much work is underway, and much has been accomplished in this area.[3–9] Mayer, et al., in 1985 won the Volvo Award in clinical sciences for work on the "Objective Assessment of Spine Function Following Industrial Injury."[3] The study was conducted on a group of chronic back pain patients and specifically collected functional capacity measures via various tests of physical function, as well as psychologic self-report measures, return to work data, and other parameters. Their findings suggested, "that quantitative functional capacity measures can give objective evidence of patient physical abilities and degree of effort, and can significantly guide the clinician in administering an effective treatment program."[3] Some type of objective measurement would thus seem useful in evaluating patients, particularly those who do not respond to nonoperative conservative care. These patients could be selected by a path of the surveillance system.

Subjective Outcomes

Although subjective reports of pain and dysfunction are modified by the patient's overall psychologic makeup,[10–12] as well as the potential effect of litigation or compensation, they still are the major measurement tools in the care and research of patients with painful spinal disorders. Work has been accomplished on demonstrating reliable and valid questionnaires of patier   satisfaction; on assessing the progress of the back pain patient via the development of a global subjective index that utilizes visual analogue scales; on utilization of pain drawings in monitoring care; and on the general psychosocial function of patients with low back pain.[13–19] It thus seems that quantifying the subjective response aides research on treatment, and can be factored into an automated surveillance system.

Industry

A major factor in the need to develop surveillance systems is the management of back pain in industry, where the goal of excellence in care is sometimes not met, and the potential for abuse of the Workers' Compensation system persists.[20–22] In a review on compensation for low back pain, Boden, et al., concluded that, "it is important to understand how the relationship of pain, impairment, and subsequent disability may be different in compensation low back patients, and that specially designed strategies for standardized evaluation and treatment of industrial low back pain have proven to be effective at delivering quality care, decreasing the cost of medical treatment, and minimizing the time of lost productivity."[23]

The area of injury prevention is a final area where systematic surveillance can be usefully implemented. Although contradictory data exists regarding the impact on reduction of incidence of low back

problems, the National Safety Council has endorsed implementation of programs for education and training in lifting methods.[20,24] Although Snook, et al., found back injury occurrence rate no different for those participating in a prevention program,[25] others, particularly in the health care setting, have reported positive results in back injury prevention.[26,27]

DIAGNOSIS-ANALYSIS

Algorithm Development

Analysis of the problem would lead to the development of monitoring systems that have the same goals as the treating physician: quality health care, appropriate health care, rapid functional return, and cost effectiveness.[28] The physician is concerned with efficient and precise use of diagnostic studies, minimizing the use of ineffectual surgery, and making therapy available at a reasonable cost to society.[29] To do so, as in the care of low back pain, a set of standards of care based on a consensus of current information acceptable to the majority of physicians must be generated.[30] An organized protocol is fashioned from these standards which, via a monitoring system (i.e., computerized algorithm), can prospectively survey a large patient population. This defines an algorithm for the particular problem, that is, an organized pattern of decision making thought processes that are useful in the care of patients with low back pain. This algorithm follows well delineated rules, which are established by a consensus of a broad segment of those who treat spine disorders, and assists in the optimal timing of diagnostic and therapeutic interventions. Then, by concurrently comparing the systems, examinations, diagnosis, treatment, and patient response for each patient to the accepted standards, the goal of excellence in care is achieved, and timely intervention can be made as needed.[30]

Computerized Surveillance—Medical

In 1978, Barnett, et al., reported on quality assurance through automated monitoring by a computer-based medical information system.[31] The system monitored positive cultures for beta hemolytic streptococcus in pharyngitis patients, and sent reminder notices if documentation of prescription of an appropriate antibiotic had not been made. They felt care was improved by monitoring possible deviation from standards, with timely and selective feedback to the provider, and that it was done in a cost effective fashion. This quality assurance was possible because the providers set standards and had their records audited against those standards by a computer-based medical information system.

Computerized Surveillance—Spinal Disorders

Strong evidence has been generated that an organized approach to examination, diagnosis, and treatment of industrial spine injuries, utilizing an algorithmic approach enhances quality of care.[28–30,32] A 1980 review of a public utility company, which revealed that low back injuries accounted for 45% of lost hours and that surgical care was selected more often than in noncompensation settings, was a stimulus to develop and study a treatment protocol in an industrial setting.[33]

The initial investigation applied diagnostic and treatment protocols to two groups of industrial workers.[32] An unbiased role was fashioned for the study physicians by not allowing him to participate in the patient's ongoing care. The clinical approach to each patient evaluated was consistent in that it was guided by a low back pain algorithm, shown in Fig. 23–1. The algorithm was derived from experience and data from both therapeutic triumphs and failures. Decisions in patient care thus were based on well delineated rules, rather than the occasionally haphazard treatment regimens that are generated when emotion or intuition intervenes. The fact that each back pain patient had application of a uniform approach was felt to be the significant factor. If a patient's care deviated from the set standards immediate intervention was instituted by contacting the treating physician for a full discussion of that patient. An acceptable program was usually worked out; if an agreement was not achieved, an independent medical opinion was sought from a third consultant. Surgery was performed only after thorough review of each patient and his myelogram. This approach was applied in "active" fashion to Group I, Potomac Electric Power Company (PEPCO), in that the monitoring physicians saw patients weekly or biweekly until they returned to work.

The second group (US Postal Service), was treated via "passive" surveillance. With each initial episode of back pain the patient was evaluated and a prediction made about the patient's ability to return to work. If the patient deviated from the predicted schedule or if surgery was proposed by the treating physician a repeat evaluation was performed.

Nearly 75% of PEPCO's 5380 employees are blue collar workers. The initial 2-year study was extended to a 5-year period (1981 to 1986).[30] By using a systematic approach, the actual number of low back cases decreased 56% (from 98 in the year preceding the study, to 42 in the final study year.) The average

number of work days lost decreased 54% (from 3640 the year preceding the study to 2118 in the final study year). The estimated cost savings averaged $430,000 per year, a dramatic two million dollars over the 5-year study. These savings were based on pre-inflation 1981 dollar estimates of wage-related costs and excluded the direct medical savings; accurate figures could not be generated for the year preceding the study.

The number of surgical procedures in the control year was nine, and it decreased to one or two for the next three years. The rate increased to the control value of nine in the final year of the study. Although this finding appears discouraging, the critical finding was that a greater percentage of patients who had surgery during the study years successfully returned to work. (This included job modification if their original position was considered heavy labor, e.g., lifting more than 75 pounds on a regular basis.)

The passive surveillance group in the initial study consisted of low back patients from the approximately 14,000 U.S. Postal Service employees in the Washington, D.C., area. A one-year study of the passive system, that is an initial evaluation and prediction of outcome, was documented. Results indicated a 41% decrease in the number of low back pain patients, a 60% decrease in days lost from work, and a 55% decrease in medical and compensation costs. One surgical procedure was performed the year prior to the study; one was performed in the year of the study. A second operation proposed in the year of the study was not felt to be indicated; hence it was cancelled and the patient returned to full duty.

This same systematic approach was prospectively applied in the industrial setting with the 5380 PEPCO employees undergoing care for cervical spine pain syndromes.[29] The protocol dealt with the wide spectrum of patients who have neck pain, with or without arm pain. The patients were followed in the active fashion. Results indicated a 54% decrease in the number of patients seen, a 65% decrease in the number of lost work days, and a 63% decrease in costs.

These studies demonstrate that good medicine leads to cost savings. The quality of care is ensured by adherence to a systematic protocol. The data prove that it is possible and practical to develop a computerized, quality-based protocol, and to use it as a concurrent monitoring system.

Exact cause of the large decreases obtained with the algorithmic approach is not fully appreciated. Because low back experts were monitoring care closely, workers may have realized that only those with legitimate problems would receive time off or light duty. The availability of light duty may have increased the savings. Light duty was made available to all recovering patients when appropriate.

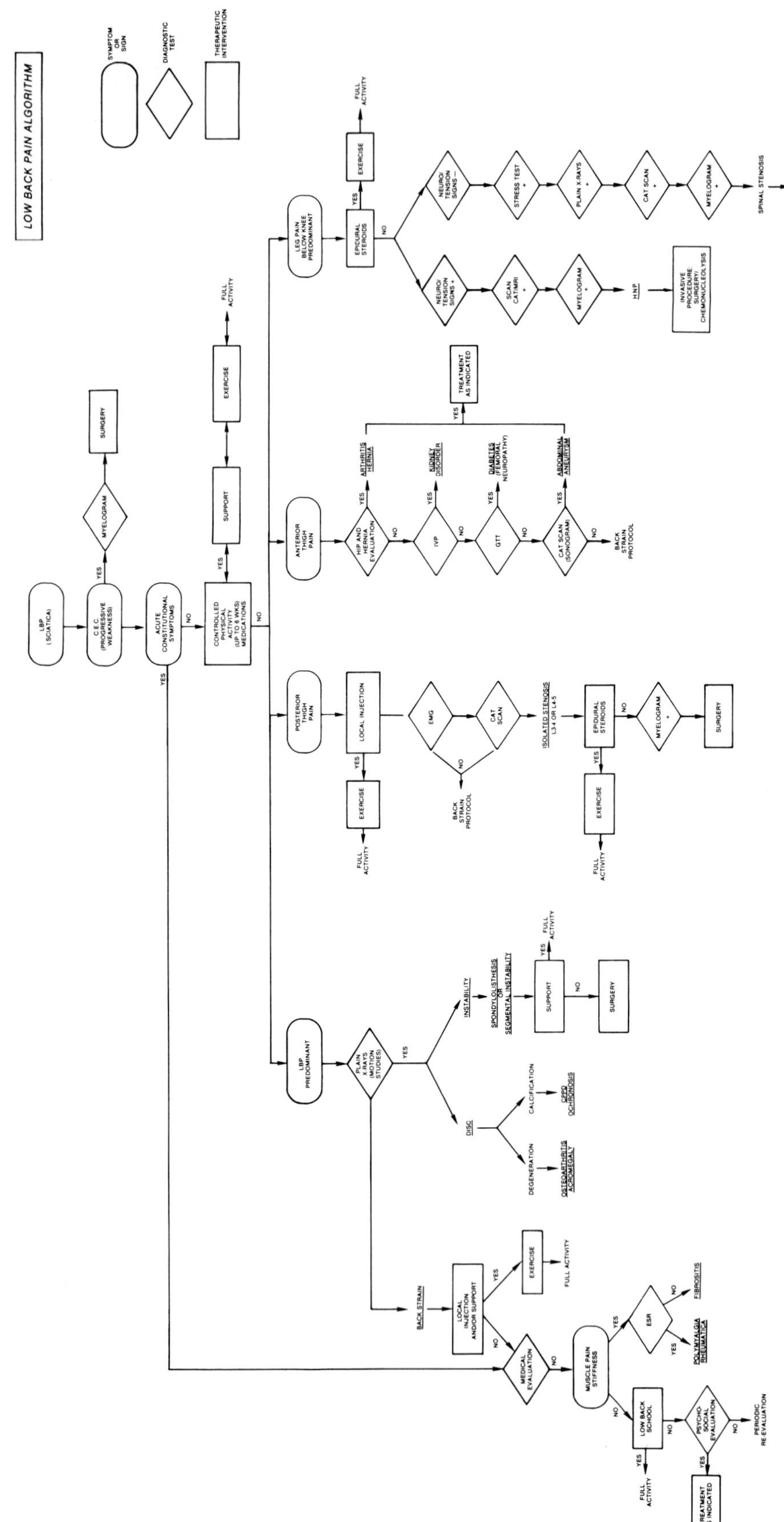

Figure 23–1. Low back pain algorithm. (From Kirkaldy-Willis, W.H., et al. Pathology and pathogenesis of lumbar spondylosis and stenosis. Spine 3:320, 1978.)

Records were not available regarding the opportunity for light duty in the year prior to the study. Recognition that surgical indications are limited and that surgery does not return workers to very heavy duty may have accounted for the decrease in the number of surgical procedures, particularly those procedures that did not allow a patient to return to work.

The response of physician and employee to these programs has been good. Because of the unbiased nature of the monitoring physicians, the treating physicians rarely felt threatened. The patients, realizing expert physicians were evaluating their care, were appreciative and conducted themselves accordingly.

TREATMENT

What Should We Do?

A major impetus has been to assure quality care for a large number of patients with similar problems. This is feasible with a computerized algorithmic approach. (The fact that there are cost savings in both time and money is a bonus). The system advised differs from those previously described in that it is driven by the basic medical information obtained from the history, physical examination, and radiographic findings. Computerization ensures that the data from these findings are consistent with the diagnosis made. Using the diagnosis as the starting point presumes the diagnosis to be correct and excludes evaluation of the consistency of information obtained.

Any algorithm generated, just as a patient with a painful spinal disorder, must be periodically re-evaluated. It must be modified to account for new data and advancing technology in diagnostic, therapeutic, and outcome paths. Because the algorithm is always evolving, the critical element is a systematic and standardized approach to each patient.

By utilizing a surveillance system, even the less demanding passive type, industry can deal with the problem of the large population of patients at multiple locations being treated by a broad spectrum of practitioners. Their goal of providing quality medical care is met via a standardized protocol and cost is acceptable (possibly decreased).

A noteworthy recommendation is made for periodic re-evaluation of patients who cannot be placed in a definitive diagnostic grouping. These patients are defined as having chronic low back pain of unknown cause. In a study of 5362 patients evaluated prospectively using a standardized approach, 2% (109) fell into this category.[34] Ten percent were found to have a major medical problem when re-evaluated by an independent rheumatologist. (Note that varied medical diagnoses, e.g., renal stones, gall stones, kidney disease, had been discerned previously in the low back clinic.) The remaining patients had new treatment plans, including detoxification, change of physicians, and arbitrary changes in therapy, which yielded 50% or greater reduction in subjective pain in approximately 75% of the group. The issue to note is not the care of chronic back pain patients, which is dealt with elsewhere in the text, but rather, the need for a physician to follow a patient, even with the lack of objective findings, as representing a small percentage who eventually reveal an underlying problem.

SUMMARY

A quality-based protocol can be successfully computerized and applied to a large group of patients as a concurrent monitoring system. Quality care is ensured by adherence to the protocol. The goals required of any health care system (early functional return, avoidance of unnecessary surgery, efficient and precise use of diagnostic studies, and cost effective care) are accomplished. Associated economic results may show decreases in the number of incidences each year, lost work days, and corporate costs. Future emphasis must remain on excellence and quality in medical care. This will lead to cost savings.

REFERENCES

1. Guralnik, D.B. (ed.): Webster's New World Dictionary, 2nd College Edition. Cleveland, Collins and Worud, 1974.
2. Eddy, D.M.: Variation in physician practice: the rule of uncertainty. Health Aff 3:76–89, 1984.
3. Mayer, T.G., et al.: Objective assessment of spine function following industrial injury: a prospective study with comparison group and one-year follow-up. Spine 10:482–493, 1985.
4. Mayer, T.G., et al.: Progressive isoinertial lifting evaluation: I. A standardized protocol and normative data base. Spine 13:993–997, 1988.
5. Mayer, T.G., et al.: Progressive isoinertial lifting evaluation: II. A comparison with isokinetic lifting in a disabled chronic low back pain industrial population. Spine 13:998–1002, 1988.
6. Mayer, T.G., et al.: Using physical measurements to assess low back pain. J Muscle Skel Med 2:44–59, 1985.
7. Davies, G., Gould, J.: Trunk testing using a prototype Cybex II isokinetic stabilization system. J Orthop Sports Phys Ther 3:164–170, 1982.
8. Hasue, M., Fujinara, M., Kikuchis: A new method of quantitative measurement of abdominal and back muscle strength. Spine 5:143–148, 1980.
9. Smith, S., et al.: Quantification of lumbar function. I. Isometric and multispeed isokinetic trunk strength measures in sagittal and spatial planes in normal subjects. Spine 10:757–764, 1985.

10. Beals, R.: Compensation and recovery from injury. West J Med *140*:233–237, 1984.
11. Dzioba, R., Doxey, R.: A prospective investigation into orthopedic and psychologic predictors of outcome of first lumbar surgery following industrial injury. Spine *9*:614–623, 1984.
12. Barsky, A.: Hidden reasons some patients visit doctors. Ann Intern Med *94*:492–498, 1981.
13. Deyo, R., Diehl, A.: Patient satisfaction with medical care for low-back pain. Spine *11*:28–30, 1986.
14. Deyo, R., Diehl, A.: Measuring physical and psychosocial function in patients with low-back pain. Spine *8*:635–642, 1983.
15. Million, R., et al.: Assessment of the progress of the back-pain patient. Spine *7*:204–212, 1982.
16. Ransford, A., Cairns, D., Mooney, V.: The pain drawing as an aid to the psychologic evaluation of patients with low back pain. Spine *1*:127–134, 1976.
17. Von Baeyer, C., et al.: Invalid use of pain drawings in psychological screening of back pain patients. Pain *16*:103–107, 1983.
18. Hildebrandt, J., et al.: The use of pain drawings in screening for psychological involvement in complaints of low-back pain. Spine *13*:681–685, 1988.
19. Margolis, R., Tait, R., Krause, S.: A rating system for use with patient pain drawings. Pain *24*:57–65, 1986.
20. Yu, T., et al.: Low-back pain in industry—an old problem revisited. J Occup Med *26*:517–524, 1984.
21. Spengler, D., et al.: Back injuries in industry: a retrospective study. I. Overview and cost analysis. Spine *11*:241–245, 1986.
22. Hadler, N.: Industrial rheumatology—the Australian and New Zealand experience with arm pain and backache in the workplace. Med J Aust *144*:191–195, 1986.
23. Boden, S., Lestini, W., Wiesel, S.: Compensation low back pain. Semin Spine Surg *1*:68–75, 1989.
24. Chaffin, D., Herin, G., Keyserling, W.: Pre-employment strength testing: an updated position. J Occup Med *20*:403–409, 1978.
25. Snook, S., Campanelli, R., Hart, J.: A study of three preventive approaches to low back injury. J Occup Med *20*:478–481, 1978.
26. Wood, D.: Design and evaluation of a back injury prevention program within a geriatric hospital. Spine *12*:77–82, 1987.
27. Videman, T., et al.: Patient-handling skill, back injuries, and back pain: an intervention study in nursing. Spine *14*:148–156, 1989.
28. Wiesel, S., Michelson, L.: Monitoring orthopedic patients using computerized algorithms. Orthop Clin N Am *17*:541–544, 1986.
29. Wiesel, S., Feffer, H., Rothman, R.: The development of a cervical spine algorithm and its prospective application to industrial patients. J Occup Med *27*:272–276, 1985.
30. Wiesel, S., Feffer, H., Rothman, R.: Low back pain: development and five-year prospective application of a computerized quality-based diagnostic and treatment protocol. J Spine Dis *1*:50–58, 1988.
31. Barnett, G., et al.: Quality assurance through automated monitoring and concurrent feedback using a computer-based medical information system. Medical Care *16*:962–970, 1978.
32. Wiesel, S., Feffer, H., Rothman, H.: Industrial low-back pain: a prospective evaluation of a standardized diagnostic and treatment protocol. Spine *9*:199–203, 1984.
33. Baur, W.: Scope of industrial low back pain. *In* Wiesel, S., Feffer, H., Rothman, R. (eds.): Industrial Low Back. Charlottesville, VA, The Michie Co., 1985.
34. Wiesel, S., Feffer, H., Borenstein, D.: Evaluation and outcome of low-back pain of unknown etiology. Spine *13*:679–680, 1988.

Subacute Spinal Disorders

24

The Subacute Patient: To Operate or Not to Operate—This is the Question

INTRODUCTION

One of the most difficult aspects of spinal care decision making is the timing for surgery. How do we identify that patient who will predictably respond well to surgery and who would not benefit from further nonoperative care? The recognition that early consideration of this question is necessary to ensure the best results was emphasized by the consensus report of the Quebec Task Force on spinal disorders.[1] In this report, 21 experts in the medical and economic aspects of back pain, noting the ill effects of delay, decided that presurgical diagnostic studies and multidisciplinary review should be considered after 7 weeks of treatment. This consensus emerged out of an extensive review of the literature, which notes that persistence of disability leads to less successful results and a greater potential for expensive long-term problems. The report also notes that active care is the most important preliminary approach before the 7-week decision making milestone. One must recognize the authorative character of this report compiled from 769 references by some of the most experienced experts of our time. This proposal for early extensive review is a potentially dangerous concept that must be viewed in the context of the natural course of the disease. Most medical evidence indicates that the disease is self-limiting and usually resolves itself any way. Thus, why consider operating so early? That probably is the most important economic question to be considered (Table 24–1).

What is the disease? Where does the back pain and leg pain come from? This discussion assumes that there are three sources of pain in activity-related spinal disorders. Obviously, this discussion does not apply to acute fractures, tumors, infections, and various metabolic arthropathies. This discussion applies to common back and leg pain, which make up about 40% of the musculoskeletal complaints for which patients seek medical attention. The three possible sources of pain are: (1) Injury to the supporting spinal soft tissues, i.e., muscle, tendon, and ligaments. (2) Injury and deterioration of the articular and skeletal structures, i.e., facet degeneration. (3) Injury to the disc.

In the context of decision making for surgery, we therefore must look at the rational treatment of these disorders. Such treatment must fail before consideration of surgery for this benign disease is warranted.

INJURY TO THE SOFT TISSUES

Let us first look at soft tissue injuries as a source of persistent back pain and a potential need for surgical care. Are any of the soft tissue injuries severe enough to warrant surgical care? If total disruption of ligamentus support to a motion segment has occurred, the general rules of musculoskeletal injuries should apply here. In other joints of the body, total disruption of the ligaments supporting the joint only occurs with traumatic dislocation or destruction by some external force, e.g., knife or bullet. Certainly, in the case of the spine, a total disruption would be

253

Table 24–1
Classification of Activity-Related Spinal Disorders as Presented by the Quebec Task Force.†

Classification	Presents With	Duration of Symptoms From Onset	Working Status at Time of Evaluation
1	Pain without radiation		
2	Pain + radiation to extremity, proximally	a (<7 days)	W (working)
3	Pain + radiation to extremity, distally*	b (7 days–7 weeks)	I (idle)
4	Pain + radiation to upper/lower limb neurologic signs	c (>7 weeks)	
5	Presumptive compression of a spinal nerve root on a simple roentgenogram (i.e., spinal instability or fracture)		
6	Compression of a spinal nerve root confirmed by specific imaging techniques (i.e., computerized axial tomography, myelography, or magnetic resonance imaging) other diagnostic techniques (e.g., electromyography, venography)		
7	Spinal stenosis		
8	Postsurgical status, 1–6 months after intervention		
9	Postsurgical status, >6 months after intervention 9.1 Asymptomatic 9.2 Symptomatic		
10	Chronic pain syndrome		W (working)
11	Other diagnoses		I (idle)

*Not applicable to the thoracic segment.

†The Quebec Task Force identified 7 weeks as the milestone at which a decision should be made regarding surgical treatment in the subacute patient who has failed to respond to nonsurgical treatment. (Adapted from Spitzer, W.O., et al.: Scientific approach to the assessment and management of activity related spinal disorders. Spine *12*(51):51–59, 1987.)

so traumatic that the diagnosis would be readily apparent both radiographically and clinically. One cannot dislocate his spine by bending over to pick up a lunch bucket. Usually, major trauma to the spine is associated with fractures, although it is possible to have a total soft tissue tear with dislocation and then relocation. This finding could readily be determined by using flexion extension x ray or distraction x rays. It is recognized that connective tissue repair in the spine is far less reliable than skeletal repair and, thus, if the rare event of dislocation followed by relocation was defined, serious consideration should be given to immediate surgical care with fusion. Even under these circumstances, the lumbar spine, because of its massive support structures, may not warrant surgical care (Fig. 24–1).

The majority of problems, however, are not due to massive injury, but rather minor tears secondary to overload, either acutely or from prolonged submaximal but cumulative activity. We know that muscles tear more readily in the eccentric mode (lengthening while under tension). There are no studies specifically focused on back muscles that give us information concerning muscle injury. We are aware that exercise induces muscle pain. Tests have shown that eccentric exercise may release a large quantity of soluble proteins per muscle, but the extent and time course of this release does not correlate with muscle pain.

Thus, discharge of proteins cannot be considered damage to the muscle.[2] Moreover, there is no evidence that exercise-related pain causes reflex activity. Painful muscles are electrically silent.[3] It is customary experience, however, that muscles are tender from overexertion. Is this a compartment syndrome? Studies specifically comparing eccentrically exercised muscles to control muscles indicate no pressure increase occurs in muscles such as the biceps.[2] There is no evidence that a compartment syndrome develops in the paraspinal muscles under normal circumstances. It is clear that on the occasion of attempted muscle biopsy, the procedure is painful until the fascia overlying the muscle is anesthetized. The muscle itself is not painful. Thus, it seems the majority of the pain comes from the fibrous tissue around the muscle, rather than the torn muscle.

Evidence points to connective tissue changes in the paraspinal muscles of people with chronic back problems, disc herniations, and surgery.[4] In these studies, thickening of the fibrous encapsulation of the muscles appeared in those with chronic inactivity related to the status of chronic disc syndrome. Multifidus muscle samples were used for biopsies. Thus, changes occur with inactivity and perhaps with neurologic embarrassment with partial denervation. This suggests that inactivity related to surgery is a negative factor that can impair recovery during long-term postoperative course. Here again, however, there was no evidence of specific tears within the muscle.

All current evidence suggests that when tears occur, they are not within midsubstance, but consistently at the myotendonus junction.[5] Thus, repair of

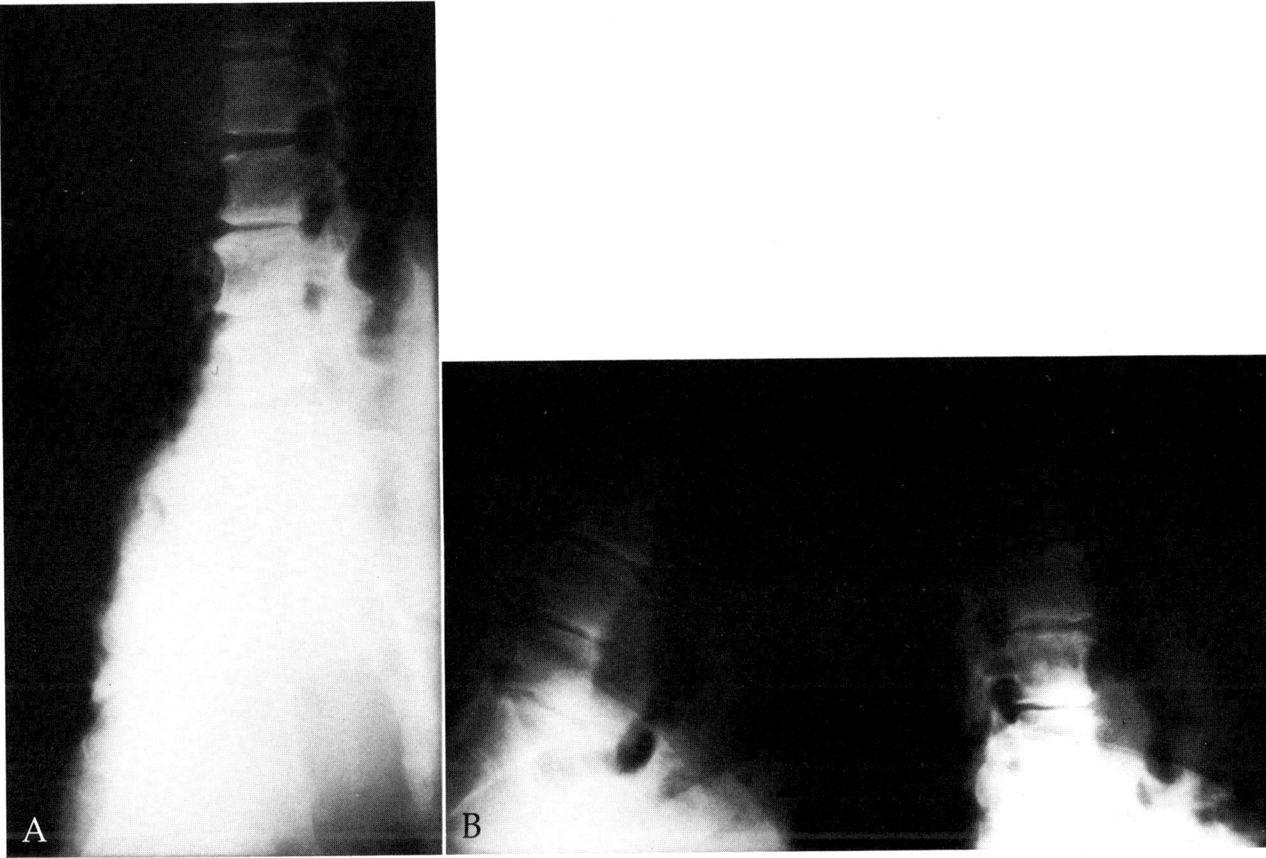

Figure 24–1. Two x rays demonstrate a significant traumatic displacement of the spine that healed spontaneously. The 45-year-old female patient pictured in the injury x ray **(A)**, and in the x ray taken 8 months after spontaneous repair **(B)**, had no pain complaints at 8 months. (Courtesy of Dr. Paul Martino, Long Beach, CA.)

overuse injuries must be focused at soft connective tissue rather than at the muscle itself. No surgical approach has been proposed for this type of injury.

There is a potential source of pain in the back arising from overload and overuse of the muscle. In the extremities, a compartment syndrome may develop because of increased intramuscular pressure. Indeed, this has been measured in the erector spinae muscles, and it is possible to increase the contraction pressure to 175 mm of mercury. This pressure, however, is unrelated to pain.[6] It has been difficult to find a clinical entity of compartment syndrome. In an extensive search for such an individual over a 4-year period, 12 patients could be categorized as potentially having a compartment syndrome. Pain was induced only by exercise; symptoms relieved at rest, and there were no neurologic deficits. In only one of these 12 patients was a persistent elevation of compartment pressure present. The discriminating characteristic of this one patient was that the elevated intracompartmental pressure did not return to normal after 20 minutes of rest. After a fasciaectomy of the erector spinae was performed, the muscle pressure returned to normal and the pain was relieved. But the other 11 patients with chronic low back pain had normal intramuscular pressures. Thus, pain caused by compartment syndrome is rare, but perhaps is a justification for surgery in the occasional patient with "injury" to the muscles.[7]

Another type of muscle soft tissue pain is known as fibromyalgia or fibrositis. Although this originally was thought to be a major source of persistent back pain, further experience has indicated considerable question regarding its structural sources. This disease is characterized by tiredness, stiffness, tender sites (known as trigger points), and an absence of positive diagnostic studies such as elevated sedimentation rate, radiographic changes, or EMG studies. The one objective finding is the presence of tender trigger points. Perhaps an additional finding is stiffness. There is no support, however, for the concept that these tender areas are secondary to structural injuries. In fact, the syndrome can be reproduced merely by sleep deprevation.[8] Moreover, the symptoms can be obliterated by fitness training.[9] In one study, individuals with the classic fibromyaglia syndrome, including trigger points, were randomly placed into two treatment groups. The first group performed stretching exercises and the second group was given aerobic training using a bicycle. Those with the aerobic (elevated pulse rate) training did twice as well as those with the stretching exercise. This would seem to confirm that the problem is a reflex abnormality and not secondary to structural changes within the soft tissues.

Attempts to identify characteristic soft tissue changes have been made by various investigators. It is true that biopsies performed on individuals with fibromyalgia syndrome show degenerating and regenerating "moth eaten" fibers and inflammatory infiltrates. However, biopsies of muscles in matched controls show the same findings.[10] This finding supports the view that fibromyalgia is not a structural abnormality, but rather a neural reflex problem or a result of deconditioning. Physical activity should be beneficial, and in various control studies, this turns out to be the only physical maneuver that is beneficial.[11]

If the muscles themselves are not the source of structural abnormality and are only the source of fleeting exercise pain, the persistent pain must result from the soft tissues and, therefore, from the tendon and bone attachments or the ligaments. We need, therefore, to turn to connective tissue research to identify potential sources of pain from these injuries. Unfortunately, no specific studies have been undertaken relative to spine connective tissue and we must look to other areas of connective tissue research to identify principles of injury and repair. The majority of this information emerges from sports medicine literature.

It is clear that because of the nature of strong connective tissue, slow repair must be expected. This tissue, with its necessarily poor blood supply and few cells, is designed to function as a tension-resistant material. Thus, on the occasion of incomplete tear, repair must be achieved by production of new collagen from the sparse cells with their poor blood supply. Much of the metabolic support must come from diffusion from surrounding soft tissues often totally absent of blood supply. Moreover, inactivity is a deterrent to repair because the random orientation of the proliferating collagen leaves a weakened structure (Fig. 24–2). Also, recovery at the surgical insertion site takes far longer than repair of the connective tissue itself. A general principle is that each day of delayed function requires 2 days of organized mechanical stress to repair the tissue back to its normal level. Also, immobilized ligament or tendon is half as strong as tissue that has been stressed (Fig. 24–3).

Thus, in summary, if the persistent pain is emerging from the soft connective tissues related to the spine (muscle, tendon, ligament), there is no support for treatment by continued inactivity. No scientific study suggests that continued use of rest or passive modalities, such as ultrasound, are beneficial in the treatment of these soft tissue injuries. Thus, when endeavoring to identify those patients with nonspecific back pain for whom surgical care might be appropriate, active exercise programs are the most rational approach in the decision making process. Even though pain may be increased initially due to stressing of noncompliant tissue, the persistence of pain on the basis of abnormal reflexes and limited end range is not a justification for surgical care. Spontaneous healing should be complete by 6 to 7 weeks, and thus is justification for that milestone identified in the Quebec consensus report.[1]

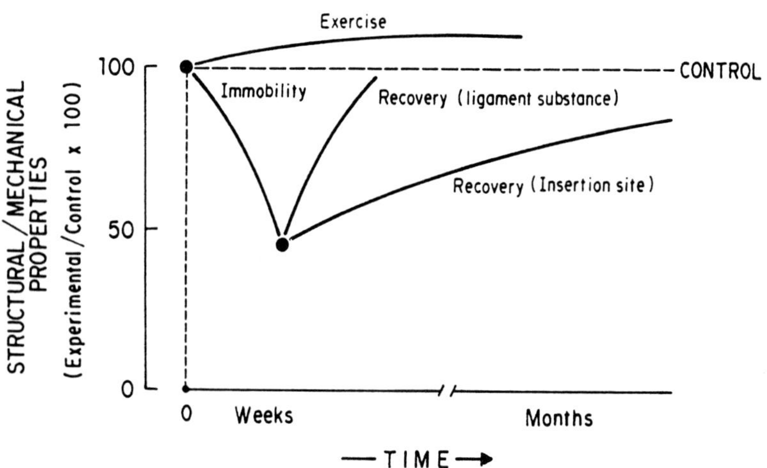

Figure 24–2. The effect of rest upon connective tissue. The time required for recovery at the insertion site is at least double the period of immobilization. (Adapted from Woo, S.L., Buckwalter, J.A.: Injury and repair of the musculoskeletal soft tissue. Am Acad Orthop Surg 5:171–207, 1988.)

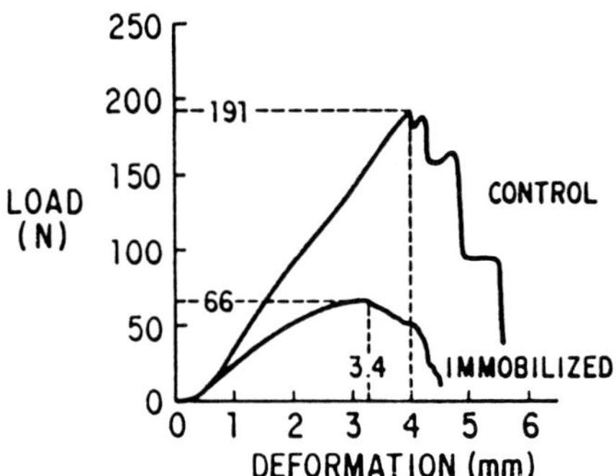

Figure 24–3. The strength of rested tissue deteriorates dramatically compared to normal tissue. In this medial collateral ligament of a rabbit knee that rested for 9 weeks, two thirds of the strength has been lost. (Adapted from Woo, S.L., Buckwalter, J.A.: Injury and repair of the musculoskeletal soft tissue. Am Acad Orthop Surg 5:171–207, 1988.)

INJURY AND DETERIORATION OF THE SPINAL JOINTS

Painful deterioration of the joints occurs elsewhere in the body and it is reasonable to expect that the same phenomenon occurs in the spine. To what degree are these degenerative or traumatic changes sources of persistent spine pain? In this discussion, we separate skeletal causes of nonspecific back pain from back pain with radiculopathy. Of course, back pain alone is more difficult to identify because of the lack of objective findings on physical examination and imaging studies. Some historic discussion is necessary.

Facet Joints

The concept of facet syndrome as a source of back pain was first proposed by Ghormley.[12] The disease entity he was describing, however, was radiculopathy secondary to nerve root pressure and thus sciatica. He did not consider the possibility of referred pain. Of course, his meaning is different than our current concept of the facet syndrome. The first clinician who suggested that the facet joints themselves serve as a major source of back pain was Goldthwait.[13] His focus on the facet joints is understandable. At that time, x ray studies of the spine had just become reliable enough to differentiate the abnormalities of these joints radiographically. However, once the disc became the central focus of interest for those interested in back pain, interest in the facet joints rapidly waned. Surgical solution inherent in understanding of disc disease made this a very attractive area of interest. It was not until 1941 that a major paper discussed the role of the articular facets in relation to low back pain.[14] Badgely pointed out what is still obvious today—that in a series of individuals with low back problems, less than 20% show any neurologic evidence of direct nerve irritation. Although he proposed many theories, he could not draw direct relationship between the radiographic pathologic changes and back pain with referred sciatica. Badgely had, however, for the first time proposed the concept that abnormalities within the facet joint could be a source of persistent pain. This was based on neuroanatomic dissections that identified the medial branch of the posterior primary ramus, which consistently innervated the capsule and periosteum of the joints.

A necessary concept to make the importance of these dissections understandable is the concept of referred pain. The dermatome distribution of innervation had been defined by Foerster in 1933.[15] It was apparent, however, that many pains were not distributed along these dermatome lines, and thus Kelgren made a great step forward by identifying the presence of referred pain.[16] Referral of the pain from skeletal structures of the back was specifically identified by Inman in the 1940s.[17] Recent dissections have shown a great overlap of innervation. Certainly, the complexity of the innervation to the spine is one reason for the great difficulty in assigning specific anatomic localization to pain descriptions by the patient. For each skeletal segment, three overlapping neurological segments supply innervation (Figs. 24–4, 24–5).[18] In addition, the somatic nervous system and the autonomic nervous system overlap considerably. Thus, it is reasonable that behavioral aspects such as anxiety and depression may affect the perception of pain.

The concept that facet joints could be a significant source of back pain was supported by the work of Steindler and Luck,[19] who injected local anesthetic percutaneously into the assumed area of the facet joint to relieve pain. They did not specifically identify the anatomic structure by x ray. Hirsch was able to recreate pain by injection of hypertonic saline into the facet joints.[20] These studies were not under radiographic control either. Radiographic localization was used in our studies to identify the role of the facets as pain sources in low back.[21] These studies demonstrated that noxious stimuli arising from the joint could be a source of pain even in pain free volunteers. Moreover, increasing the amount of noxious stimuli (increasing volume of hypertonic saline) slowly enlarged the distribution of the pain complaint. Thus, a small amount of hypertonic saline injected into the facet joint created only buttock pain, whereas increased volume (.2 ml to .8 ml) caused referral pain down the posterior thigh and into the

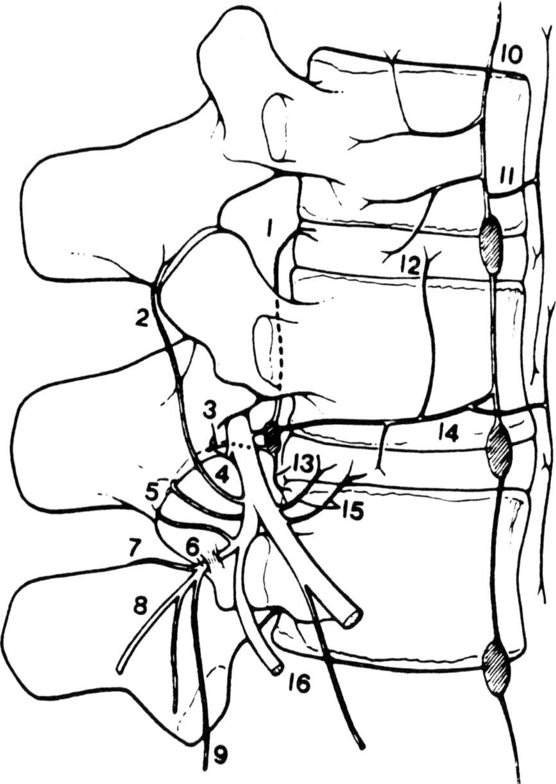

Figure 24–4. Innervation of the disc and posterior structures demonstrating the significant overlapping innervation. 1. Ascending branch of sinuvertebral nerve; 2. Ascending facet branch; 3. Sinuvertebral to facet; 4. Direct branch to facet; 5. Branches to multifidus; 6. Medial branch of posterior primary ramus; 7. Local facet branch; 8. Descending facet branch; 9. Branch to sacroiliac; 10. Sympathetic chain; 11. Branch under anterior longitudinal ligament; 12. Branches from grey ramus to disc; 13. Sinuvertebral to disc; 14. Grey ramus communicans; 15. Branches from anterior primary ramus to disc; 16. Lateral branch of posterior primary ramus. (Adapted from Paris, S.B.: Functional anatomy of the lumbar spine. Doctoral thesis, Union Graduate School, Atlanta, GA, 1983.)

calf. Interestingly, the pain created by this injection was of a delayed response, not the immediate response one has on the occasion of a pricked finger. Also, no skin sensory aberrations occurred with this pain, indicating that the pathways were not related to irritation of the anterior primary ramus or peripheral nerves. The concept that emerged from these studies was clear. Abnormalities in the facet joint could be a source of back pain. The amount of noxious stimuli could vary the amount of pain perceived. Because the delay in perception of pain, central nervous system processing has an important role in the perception of this type of pain.

One of the most important aspects of these injec-

tion studies was to confirm the reality of referred pain. It is possible to create pain in the buttock, as well as radiation of pain into the thigh and even occasionally in the calf, by irritating the facet joints. Thus, the presence of pain alone without evidence of irritation to the nerve roots need not be seen as an excuse to consider decompression of nerve roots. Leg pain can result from painful deterioration of the facet joints. Usually, this is more severe on one side than the other. Usually, efforts to improve range and nutrition to the articular surfaces by means of progressive repetitive exercises can resolve the problem before surgical consideration is necessary.

What can go wrong with the facet joints? The facet joints can deteriorate to the same degree as the other joints in our body or can fall apart secondary to injury and aging. The facet joints are true synovial joints with hyline cartilage, synovial lining, and joint capsule that encloses a joint space. Their function is to control the plane of mobility and limit rotation of the spine. Under normal circumstances, most of the axial load is borne by the vertebral bodies and discs; about 20% is borne by the facet joints, depending on degree of flexion or extension.[22] Eisenstein defined the histologic abnormality of the painful facet joint.[23] In a small group of patients whose source of pain had failed to be identified by numerous diagnostic criteria, but nonetheless had significant persistent pain, surgical excision of the facet joints with fusion was performed. The peculiar clinical features of these patients was pain at rest, somewhat relieved by motion. Histologic evaluation of the specimens demonstrated articular abnormalities that were reminiscent of abnormalities seen in Chondromalacia of the patella. In fact, Eisenstein coined the phrase chondromalacia of the facet in an attempt to define the disease.

It seems clear that mechanical phenomena can cause deterioration of the facet joint separate from the disc itself. In a series of cadaver dissections, Videman identified by discography and inspection that 20% of lumbar spines in elderly individuals have normal discs, but have degenerative changes of the facet joints (visible by x ray studies and direct inspection).[24] The question arises, however, as to which joints are painful and the source of referred pain. In the most precise study conducted, less than 20% of the individuals with nonspecific back pain had truly the facet as their source of pain.[25] In this study, to be classified as a facet syndrome, pain provocation could be achieved by either pain reproduction on radiographic insertion of the needle into the joint or by the injection of contrast material. Pain relief occurred following the injection of a small amount of local anesthesia after the aspiration of the contrast material. Additional patients had pain provocation but no pain relief, or had pain relief but no

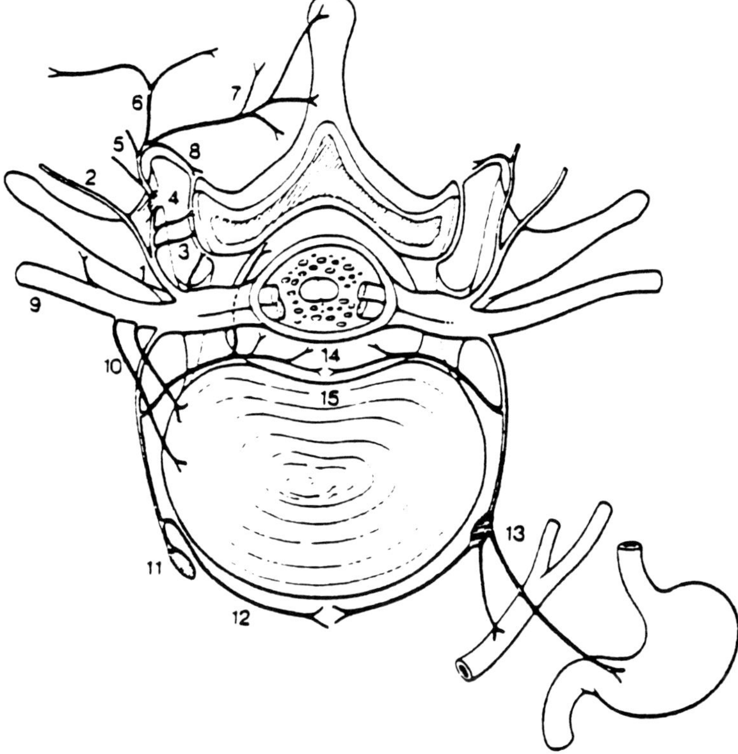

Figure 24–5. Axial view of innervation demonstrating the significant interlink with autonomic, anterior, and posterior innervation. 1. Posterior primary rami; 2. Lateral branch of the posterior primary rami to skin and muscles; 3. Muscular branches to multifidus and to facet capsule; 4. Medial branch posterior primary rami; 5. Branch to the posterior sacroiliac joint; 6. Muscular and cutaneous branches; 7. Muscular and ligamentous branches—large to multifidus; 8. Local branch to facet; 9. Anterior primary rami; 10. Branches to the disc from the anterior primary rami; 11. Sympathetic chain; 12. Recurrent grey rami communicans; 13. Branches to blood vessels and viscera; 14. Branches to dura; 15. Branches to posterior longitudinal ligament. (Adapted from Paris, S.B.: Functional anatomy of the lumbar spine. Doctoral thesis, Union Graduate School, Atlanta, GA, 1983.)

provocation. Only 18% of the 54 patients fell into the "pure" category. It is also possible that some of the pain relief may be caused by epidural flow of the local anesthetic. This has been demonstrated following arthrography using CT technique.[26] Most retrospective studies indicate only about a 20% long-term success rate in those with facet injections.

Probably the most disturbing aspect about the facet syndrome as a source of pain is the inability to define it clinically. In an extensive study of 454 patients with nonspecific low back pain, normal neurologic examinations, and no nerve root tension signs, discriminating symptom could not be found to identify the responders to injections.[27] In this study, 127 variables were monitored. Facet joint arthrograms were accomplished prior to intra-articular injection of local anesthetic and initial pain relief occurred in only 29% of the individuals. Individuals in the older age group with a prior history of low back pain and maximum pain on extension did correlate to a low degree with pain relief. The presence of tenderness or the presence of muscle spasm did not correlate with pain relief, and it was only extension after full forward flexion that correlated with pain relief. Rotation pain did not correlate. In this series, short term pain relief occurred in only 25% of the patients. Evaluation of the efficacy of steroids, which are normally used in patient injection, was not part of this study. The authors indicated that they also did a smaller controlled study involving random injection of saline or Lidocaine into the joints following arthrography. In this small group, there was no statistical difference in pain relief. This leads us, therefore, to a considerable dilemma regarding the role of facet joints in subacute pain. Their role can be identified by specific injections, however.

In summary, about 20% of the facet joints can deteriorate independent of abnormalities in the disc. Only about 20% of patients can be specifically identified as having pain caused by the facet joint and can have the pain obliterated by injection. There is no specific clinical syndrome that can identify these responders. Thus, the use of facet injections is appropriate to identify the 20% of people with nonspecific back pain who have pain-producing facet joints. It is occasionally necessary, however, to look at this small subgroup as the primary source of persistent back pain. Occasionally, these patients may need surgical care with excision and fusion as suggested by the Eisenstein study.[23]

Sacroiliac Joints

It is difficult to separate pain emerging from the sacroiliac joint from pain emerging from the facet joints. Overlapping innervation gives justification to assume that the pain perception from either of these sites would be similar. Clinically, there is significant support for the view that motion can be determined clinically and that abnormal motion is a source of pain.[28] Certainly, sacroiliac joint degeneration occurs with the passage of time. CT scans of patients over 55 years of age showed that 67% had degenerative changes in the synovial portion of the joint. Spurring was found in 34%, and bony bridging in about 20%.[29] However, radiographs demonstrate no major motion differences between normal and patients and those experiencing pain.[30] The only possible way pain emerging from the sacroiliac joints could be determined as the prime source of buttock, back and posterior thigh pain would be the radiographically controlled injection into the sacroiliac joint. Only one study has been presented to support this diagnostic and therapeutic program.[31]

Because of the great difficulty of diagnosing abnormal motion clinically and the potential for pain perceived as originating in the sacroiliac joint to really be originating from the facet joint or the disc itself, it is difficult to place the sacroiliac joints in the surgical decision making process. Certainly, the fusion of the sacroiliac joint, once strongly advocated as a method of pain control, now has long since grown out of style. Unless clearcut demonstration of abnormal motion or pain obliteration following local repeated x ray-controlled anesthetic injections can be offered, there is no justification for surgical care to sacroiliac abnormalities.

PAIN SECONDARY TO DEGENERATIVE FACET DISEASE WITH ASSOCIATED RADICULOPATHY

Pain from continuing degenerative changes at the lumbar spinal motion segment may be secondary to increasing deterioration of the facet joint with increasing reactive changes specific to the joint. The pain may also occur because of encroachment into the root canal, known as nerve root entrapment. This is distinct from the acute disc lesion. Decompression of the root canal surgically offers an opportunity to gain relief from persistent pain. As in all other cases of degenerative disease, there is a broad range of structural severity and symptoms. No study has shown a parallel between structural severity and radiographic findings and symptoms.

A study by Porter[32] gives useful information on the natural history of the nerve root entrapment problem. This may initially present as a subacute problem that does not go away after several weeks. A study of nerve root entrapment was conducted using 2360 patients who attended a back pain clinic in England. On a clinical basis, the diagnosis of root entrapment syndrome was made if the patient experienced single sided leg pain with distribution extending at least to the lower calf, which was more severe than back pain. Historically, usually the pain began months or years earlier as back and buttock pain and extended distally with the passage of time. In addition, contrasted to acute disc prolapse, the pain was unrelieved by bed rest. Frequent changing of position was usually beneficial. Also, in contrast to the typical acute disc syndrome, straight leg raising associated with the nerve root entrapment syndrome was usually equal to the uninvolved side, and it was usually no worse than 70°. In that this is a degenerative process, the patients in whom the clinical diagnosis was made were generally over 40 years of age. On a clinical basis, other diagnoses of these 2360 patients included acute lumbar disc, neurogenic claudication secondary to spinal stenosis, and degenerative back pain with no referral distal to the calf. A majority of the patients (56.1%) had back pain only and thus a nonspecific diagnosis was made (Table 24-2).

Distribution of patients with nerve root entrapment was 54% female and an average age of 51 years at the time of attendance at the clinic. Lack of extension was notable, with 88% showing significant restriction of motion and 25% having no extension at all. Despite the significant sensory complaints, 85% had normal reflexes, 82% had normal sensory perception, and 95% had normal muscle power. X rays of those with nerve root entrapment showed degenerative changes in 80% of the patients, with disc space reduction noted at the L5-S1 level in 56% of those patients. Size of the spinal canal based on ultrasound measurement was the same as in the general population.

Eighty-one percent of the patients required no specific treatment other than advice regarding home care and the natural history of the process. Pain was sufficient in 14% to require epidural injection. Surgical decompression was performed on 9.6% of the patients. Of the 24 patients treated with surgical de-

Table 24–2
Distribution of Clinical Syndromes in a Nonindustrial Clinic, Doncaster, England

Number of Patients	Nonspecific Back Pain	Pain Referred to Buttock	Nerve Root Entrapment	Disc Prolapse	Spinal Stenosis
2360	56.1%	18.2%	10.5%	8.7%	6.5%

Table of classification of low back problems in an English orthopaedic referral clinic.

compression, 18 felt that their condition was better and 6 indicated no changes after 12 months. Of the 90.4% who were not treated surgically, although most still had some leg pain, 90% were satisfied and sought no additional medical care. In fact, the problem seems to gradually resolve with time, and only 6% of those patients with clinical nerve root entrapment were over 65 years of age.

Thus, from this experience, some general guidelines can be identified. The degenerative process is a gradual progressive entity with varying degrees of severity inconsistently related to the passage of time. It tends to be a self-limited problem in many circumstances. Medical encouragement of balanced rest and physical activity is the major treatment. Some patients benefit from local infiltration with steroids (epidural block). This is the mainstay of initial treatment for this problem. The decision to operate is based on the fact that some patients, in spite of medical encouragement, medication, and the passage of time do not improve. Unfortunately, because of the chronicity of the problem, surgical decompression is not a total guarantee of leg pain relief. This problem may first surface subacutely.

Another aspect of the degenerative process is created by narrowing of the total spinal canal. This is known as spinal stenosis. Originally described by Verbiest,[33] it likewise is recognized by a distinctive clinical presentation. This, too, may appear as a subacute problem. These patients are quite specific about their leg complaints, which tend to be bilateral. The leg pains are aggravated by activity (in contrast to nerve root entrapment, which tends to be relieved by activity). Often, a short-distance walk creates unusual dysesthesias and other pains, which may seem bizarre. For that reason, the symptoms of spinal stenosis are reminiscent of those of vascular claudication, and often this disease is called pseudoclaudication. Like vascular claudication, it also occurs in older people with the majority of patients being slightly older than those with nerve root entrapment. It has been demonstrated in this group that the average size of the spinal canal is notably smaller than the population as a whole. This, of course, explains the pain complaints, in that chronic embarrassment of vascular supply to the cauda equina nerves creates pain on the occasion of increased metabolic demands of activity.[34] Here again, preliminary treatment with epidural injection often is beneficial. Ultimately, surgical decompression is necessary to relieve the symptoms. This is often one of the most difficult surgical decisions because often multiple levels of involvement are well depicted by imaging studies such as CT and CT/myelography. However, which of these levels are the cause of pain is usually not definable. Moreover, because of the

multiple levels of involvement, surgical decompression offers a significant threat to stability. It is in this particular area of care that internal fixation of the spine by pedicle screws and rod or plate connection has its best application.

PAIN ARISING FROM THE INJURED DISC

In the adult, under normal circumstances the disc is the largest avascular tissue in the body. Nutrition to the cells must occur by way of the blood vessels surrounding the annulus or through blood vessels penetrating the cartilage end plate. Solutes have been demonstrated to move into and through this avascular matrix by diffusion. Solutes can also be pumped in and out of the disc during movement. This transportation is the result of bulk flow or convection. The fluid exchange is minimal. Urban estimated that during walking, less than 0.01% of disc fluid is exchanged.[35] During the day, the net fluid lost from the discs measures 3 to 10%. It takes about 10 hours to achieve the total loss.[36] This, of course, returns at night during recumbency when the pressure in the disc decreased. Thus, we gain back about 1 to 2% of height when recumbent.[37] It takes about two hours to gain it all back. Certainly, the question of how fluid moves about the disc is important when one considers disc health and attempts to improve the repair process.

It has been demonstrated in dogs that, whether active or anesthetized, the diffusion of small particles such as radioactive sulfate^{35}S is the same. Under normal circumstances, therefore, the small solutes such as O_2 and glucose are transported by diffusion.[35] However, the significant difference in fluid movement during exercise could greatly affect the transportation rate of large molecules such as hormones and enzymes. The transportation of these large entities would be enhanced by "pumping." The tissue of the disc matrix can be thought of as a network of collagen fibers stuffed with proteoglycans that are inflated with water. The analogy to a group of balloons encapsulated by a fish net is not too far from the histochemical reality (Fig. 24–6). The greater the concentration of the proteoglycans and the greater the size of these proteoglycans, the smaller the pores available for diffusion of water and transport of solutes. Even moderate size solutes, such as glucose (200 molecular weight) are excluded from the 10 to 15% of the pores of the nucleus pulposus of a normal dog. With loss of proteoglycan, the pore size increases and serum proteins may be available in greater concentrations. And, indeed, higher concentrations of serum proteins have been

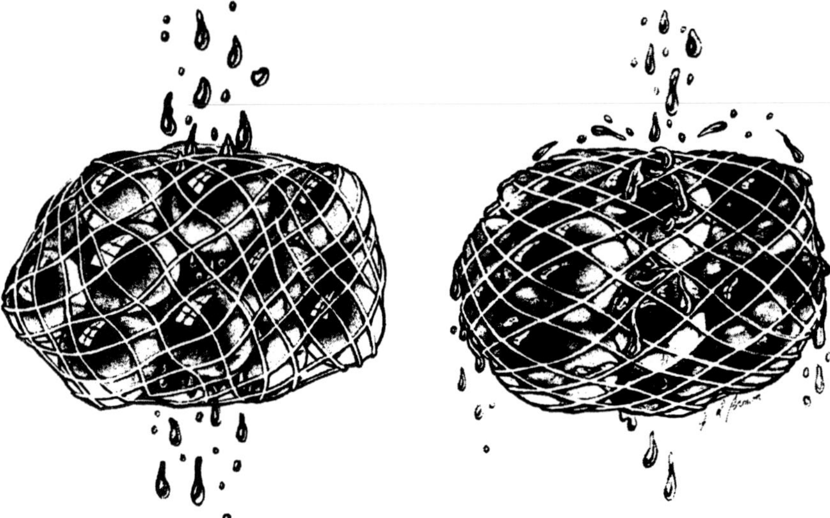

Figure **24–6.** The fishnet represents collagen fibers, which contain the water-filled balloons, representing the bound water held by the proteoglycans. If the proteoglycans become enlarged and trap more water some of the diffusion through the remaining porosity of the construct is limited, as characterized on the right.

reported in older degenerated discs. These discs, however, are from apparently nonsymptomatic people.[38]

Based on this understanding of normal physiology within the disc, the abnormalities that create the painful disc must be related in some manner to variations in disc nutrition and hydration. Certainly, the nutrition to the inner part of the disc must be diminished because of the distance from the blood supply. This is reflected by a significant increase in lactate concentration in the middle portion of the nucleus pulposus.[39] In spite of this, pH studies of normal and degenerative intervertebral discs show a pH near neutral. However, when the disc is symptomatic, the pH may be quite acid.[40] This acid pH is not consistently severe throughout the disc. Our own experiments have demonstrated that within the same disc, at nearly the same time, a variation of pH from 6.5 near the periphery to 6.2 near the middle (Fig. 24–7).[41] It is possible that an injured disc, for undefined reasons, has a greater concentration of proteoglycans or perhaps enlarged proteoglycans. We know that injured chondroblasts manufacture larger proteoglycans.[42]

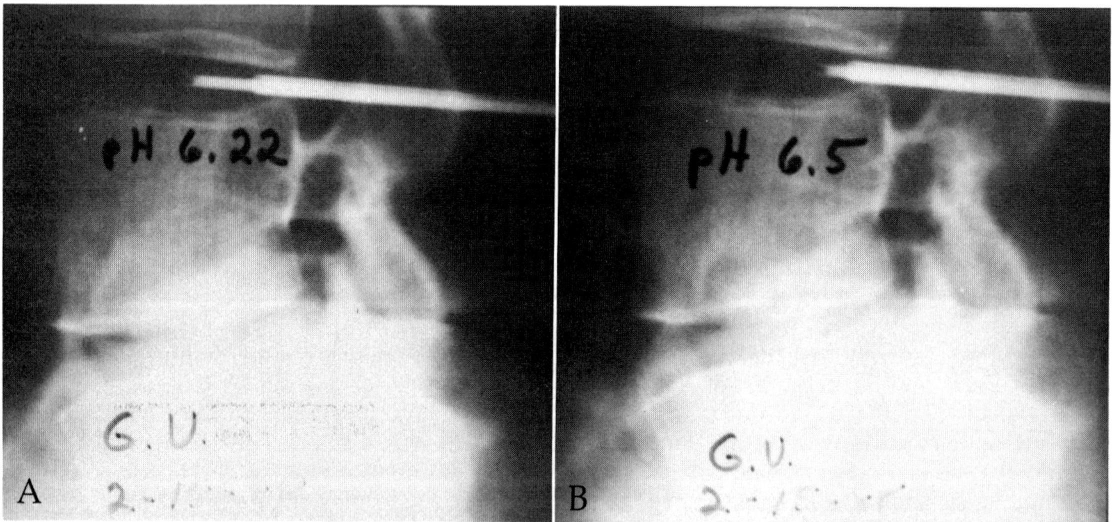

Figure **24–7. A.** pH measured in the center of a disc, which has herniated, causing painful radiculopathy. **B.** The same patient with pH measured closer to the periphery several seconds later. The discrepancy in pH measurement at sites so close to each other remains unexplained. Diminished fluid exchange is a possibility.

This gives justification for cyclic loading exercises in an effort to improve hydration of the disc and, hopefully, assist convection of larger molecules into the inner portion of the disc. We are aware that initial recumbency may decrease the gravity load and allow increased hydration of the disc to perhaps 1 to 2% increase in height over night. Traction does the same. However, this phenomenon happens over several hours and prolonged rest offers no greater benefit to increase hydration or transport of larger molecules. Thus, to achieve better nutrition of the disc, there is no justification for prolonged rest. As yet, no study has demonstrated that increased cyclic loading increases the hydration of the disc and widens the disc space. This phenomenon, however, does happen to the joints of exercised dogs.[43] Thus, it is reasonable to assume that similar phenomenon occurs within the human intervertebral disc.

Mechanism of Injury to the Disc

The disc is the most likely structure to be injured in the subacute patient complaining of back and leg pain following activity-related injuries. In the Quebec consensus report, division between acute and subacute was placed at one week. Realistically, division probably occurs a little later. This is an important differential, however, in that the majority of back complaints resolve spontaneously, without medical care other than perhaps symptomatic analgesics and short-term bed rest. In the classic study by Deyo, et al, concerning the efficacy of bed rest, less than 30 days was chosen as duration of acute pain. In this study, a week of bed rest delayed return to work significantly longer when compared to bed rest for less than 2 days.[44] In this group, the median duration of pain before the initiation of "treatment" was 9 days. The subacute patient is probably the individual whose complaints have lasted as long as 7 weeks. Spontaneous healing of the soft tissue injury is unlikely and concern about surgical correctability is reasonable at this time.[1]

In order to understand a candidate for surgical care of the disc, some understanding of the pathophysiology of disc deterioration is necessary. Unfortunately, we know little about the subacute stage. These individuals are seldom investigated by the only maneuver that really defines early disc deterioration—CT scan of a discogram. Only when neurologic deterioration is increasing is it ethical to proceed with imaging studies with the anticipation that surgery might be necessary in the subacute time span. Occasionally, disc rupture has been so significant that in the acute state, rapid neurologic deterio-

ration (cauda equina syndrome) occurs. This requires immediate surgical care. Even in the subacute state, evidence of neurologic deterioration with increasing weakness, increasing sensory loss, and progressive nerve root tension signs should suggest immediate investigation in search of objective evidence of structural abnormality. This is an unlikely natural history for disc disease. Currently, the MRI probably offers the most information from a single study. Myelography is seldom useful in the subacute setting and the CT scan offers the best delineation of skeletal structures. However, disc abnormalities are seen less well than with the MRI. Thus, what we know about early disc deterioration must be implied largely from pathologic studies, and perhaps also from information based on various treatment maneuvers (Fig. 24–8).

We are aware by pathologic dissections and discography studies that two modes of tear can occur within the disc. A peripheral tear may occur, apparently secondary to torsional overload.[45] Also, radial tears can occur that gradually progress to the periphery and then may communicate with a preexistent peripheral annular tear.[46] Whether these are painful has not been determined. In Park's study, the dissection of apparently healthy people following acute fatalities, chronic tears of the peripheral

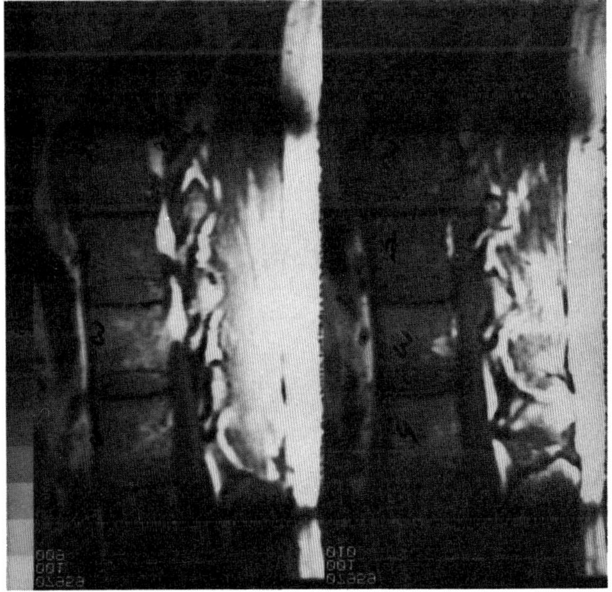

Figure 24–8. MRI demonstrating painful disc deterioration with a herniation at L5-S1. Loss of water is suggested by the gray appearance at the disc space L4-L5 and L5-S1 on the T2 weighted image (left). This patient responded well to a cyclic exercise program and became pain free (right). No change in contour of the disc was noted after treatment.

annulus were noted.[45] It has been demonstrated, however, that the character of the tear may correlate with symptoms. In a discography study that compared the nonsymmetrical radial tears with symmetrical degeneration, it was found that deep, but not generalized, tears of the annulus were more likely to be painful.[47] Also, pain may or may not occur in early tears.

What can be done to treat those in this early stage so that they can avoid surgery (Fig. 24–9)? Because it has been demonstrated in cadavers that nuclear material flow can occur with cyclic activity, it would seem reasonable to use this type of approach to effect the nuclear flow within the disc. This makes the assumption that flow of the nucleus to the periphery is a potential source of pain and reduction of the pressure of this flow would be an advantage.[48–50] To a certain extent, this concept has been tested clinically.[51] In a comparative study, the use of this type of cyclic exercise program has been demonstrated to be more effective than traction and back school.[52]

Thus, with an understanding of the sources of deterioration of the disc, no patient should be considered for surgical evaluation until disc health has been evaluated. Cyclic exercises, such as the McKenzie program, would seem to provide for early resolution of the disc abnormality. In the past, traction and other types of exercise programs have also been used in this preliminary stage.

One approach that offers symptomatic relief, as well as some diagnostic information, is an epidural injection. The role of epidural injections has been controversial in the past. Perhaps one reason is the variation in expectations from this approach. Because the deteriorating disc represents an ongoing problem, cure by any maneuver seems unrealistic. If the goal of treatment is short-term relief, appropriate exercise programs can be initated and the benefit of these programs can be developed. It is unrealistic, however, to expect that a few injections can solve a significant structural problem. Also, in the evaluation of efficacy, it is necessary to observe the patient for the duration of his pain. When a steroid is added to the epidural injection, one must expect some delay before the chemical influence of the steroid is available. A prospective blind study by Dilke demonstrated improvement may take up to a week to be notable.[53] In another prospective blind study, Snoek found no effect of epidural steroids; however, he only evaluated the patients 24 to 48 hours after injection.[54] In addition, some question exists regarding the consistent accuracy of injection. When epidural injections are performed on an outpatient basis, it is not appropriate to give sufficient concentration of local anesthesia that produce paralysis and sensory abnormalities following injection. If these occur, patients would have to remain at the hospital perhaps overnight—thus defeating the purpose of outpatient care. According to a study by White based on 2000 injections in the intraspinus root, it has been demonstrated that even in expert hands, about 20% of the time the injection is inaccurate and does not enter the epidural space.[55] Thus, the use of contrast medium at the time of injection with the availability of fluoroscopic localization offers a guarantee that appropriate localization of injection has occurred.

From a diagnostic as well as from a therapeutic standpoint, the epidural injection offers a mechanism to determine those who might be candidates for surgical care. It seems unlikely that an individual with significant symptomatic spinal canal disease would not have at least short-term relief from an appropriately localized epidural injection. Unless the findings are of profound and progressive disease, the epidural injection can serve as a very good predictor of an individual for whom surgical consideration should be made.

Of course, the problem concerning surgical consideration of the patient in the subacute phase is based on natural history. Probably the best descrip-

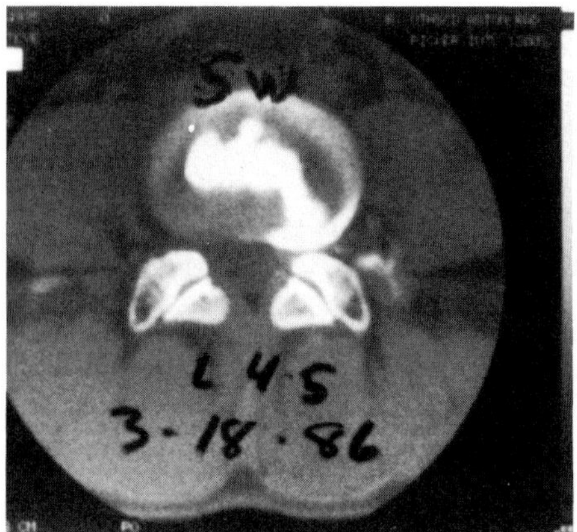
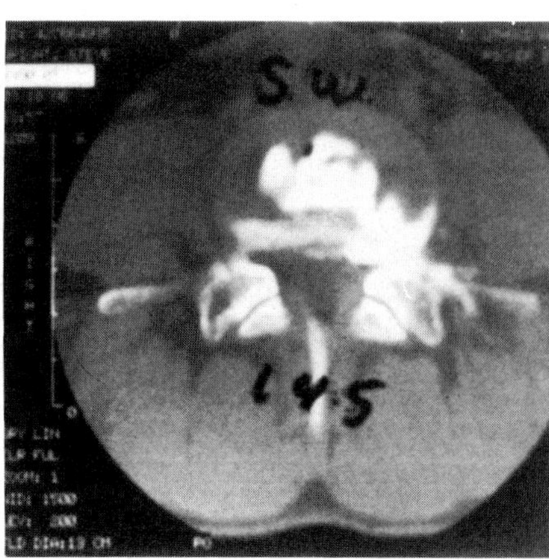

Figure 24–9. CAT scan of a discogram demonstrates the connection between a peripheral tear and a radial tear. Water-soluble nuclear material has apparently oozed to the periphery. This patient did not have radiculopathy, but did have significant leg pain. Should this be defined as referred leg pain?

tion of this natural history is from Henry Weber in a 10 year followup study.[56] In this study, patients with typical herniated disc syndrome were evaluated with myelography and demonstrated a correlation with the findings and the symptoms. They were alternately placed into a group of conservative care that utilized 2 weeks of progressive mobilization from bed rest, or operative care with excision of the disc. The disc surgery was successful in relieving the symptoms in the majority of patients, and in fact, in the group treated conservatively, 17 of 66 required surgical care because of increasing severity of pain. An interesting lesson from the study was, however, that although at a review one year later the results of surgery were better than nonsurgical care, at four years the results were only slightly better, and at ten years the patient complaints were essentially the same in both groups. The study documents the intuitive and clinical impression that surgical care only buys time in the continuing progress of a deteriorating disc. Injection techniques do a similar job of buying time, but at a much shorter dimension. In the Weber study, none of the patients treated conservatively were classed as a bad result at one-year followup (17 of the group, however, had to have surgery) and none of the surgically treated patients had a bad result. Nine of the remaining 49 in the conservative group had a poor result, whereas 5 of 60 in the operated group had a poor result. Certainly, these statistics justify that surgical care is reasonable for the right patient at the right time.

Discussion has been chiefly focused at the phenomenon of the herniated disc. Surgical care for this entity is well established. If after various studies, the diagnosis is specific and it has been demonstrated that resolution will not occur in spite of a vigorous nonoperative exercise program, early surgical care is appropriate. In a study from Finland, the natural history of those with surgery was reviewed as well.[57] In this study, the results were evaluated one month and six months postoperatively. The study is unique in that 98.7% of the lumbar disc surgery performed in Turku, Finland, over a two-year period (1980 to 1982) was reviewed. The study included 215 patients. (This computes to 36 operations per 100,000 population). The study gives a picture of the natural history postsurgical care. At the time of leaving the hospital, 97% estimated their condition to be much better than before surgery. One month after surgery, 62% estimated their condition to be much better, and at six months, 71% thought their condition was much better and 21% felt that they were somewhat better than preoperatively. Thus, at six months, 92% could be identified as significantly improved; 8% were considered as having a poor result. In this study, however, statistically, the patient was more likely to have an excellent result if the duration

off work was less than two months. This suggests that if a problem is so severe that it cannot be resolved by active effective care, early surgical care is warranted.

An additional lesson to be learned from this study, as well as many others, is that psychosocial factors play an important role in determining success or failure. This was a prospective study and various questions concerning social aspects were asked before undertaking surgery. In spite of good preoperative signs, symptoms, and radiographic correlation, the best correlation with failure was an indication on the part of the patient before surgery that he planned to retire after surgery. Other factors predicting a poor result were marital status (divorced or widowed) and lower level of education. Also, increasing age tended to predict a poorer result. These factors underlined the importance of vigorous early care, a focus on wellness and a healthy attitude, and the ability of appropriately defined surgical care to give excellent results.

ALTERNATIVE SOURCES OF PAIN IN THE SUBACUTE STAGE

Probably the most important differential in the subacute patient is the presence of a significant disease that can benefit from sophisticated evaluation and expert medical care and occasionally from surgery. Included in this category would be tumors, infections, and inflammatory or metabolic spine disease.

Of course, tumors are comparatively uncommon, but because of their devasting potential, they must constantly be kept in mind in evaluating somebody with persistent back or leg pain that has not resolved within several weeks. Primary tumors are seldom seen in the spine, but metastatic tumors are fairly common in older age groups. The metastatic tumors more often involve the bone and less often the epidural space. Thus, persistent gnawing pain may be expected in this disease category. In a consecutive series of studies from the University of Iowa, the mean age of patients with primary malignancy of the spine was 49, the mean age of patients with benign tumors was 21.[58] Although benign and malignant tumors may masquerade as a disc herniation, offering signs and symptoms typical of the herniated disc, probably the most consistent tip-off as to an alternative diagnosis is continued pain in spite of position and recumbency. Occasionally, a sacral tumor will also result in a change in bowel habits and gradual onset of perineal pain.[59]

The most common benign tumors are osteoid osteomas and osteoblastomas. These often give a clinical picture of dull but persistent pain. Frequently, however, the pain is dramatically resolved by aspirin. Frequently, lesions of the lamina or pedicle can cause persistent leg pain with even a positive straight leg raising test. Usually, a favorable result can be expected from surgical care of this type of lesion. In addition, benign intrathecal tumors involving the cauda equina can mimic disc disease. These are usually neurofibromas or meningiomas[60] (Fig. 24–10).

One of the most common spinal tumors is the chordoma. This serious tumor grows slowly, frequently has a predilection for the sacrum, and usually is so large by the time it is investigated it may be inoperative. Myeloma (plasmacytoma) is another malignant lesion that frequently is missed in the initial work up. As with most tumors, the sedimentation rate is elevated. Lesions of about 1 ml in diameter or larger can be seen in plain x rays as discreet punched out areas, and often are the first clue to this diagnosis.

Plain x rays are the cornerstone to tumor diagnosis. Thus, any patient with persistent back pain or neurologic deficit would benefit from x ray review. Neoplastic disease is best evaluated by bone scans. CT and MRI are also helpful in identifying the status of these lesions. Metastatic disease can often be differentiated from osteoporosis and metabolic disease in the MRI by the use of gadolinium injection. Awareness of the potential, of course, is the best defense.

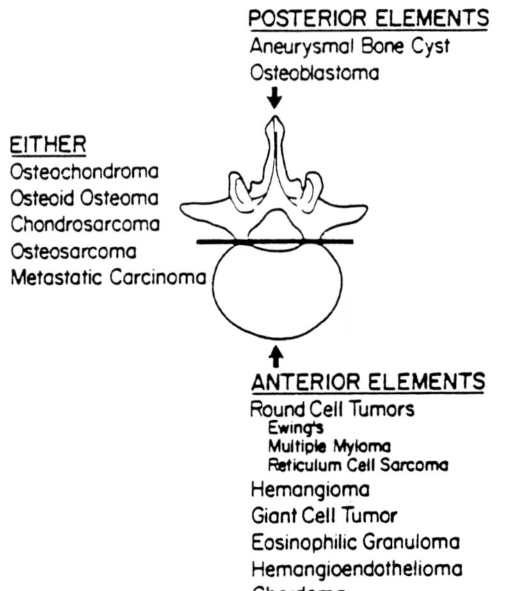

Figure 24–10. A wide array of lesions, both malignant and benign, may occur. The lesions are more likely to be benign in younger age groups. (Adapted from Andersson, G.B.J., McNeil, T.W.: Lumbar Spine Syndromes, Evaluation and Treatment. New York, Springer-Verlag, 1989.)

Spinal infection also is a source of pain masquerading as disc disease. Again, persistent pain of constant and perhaps increasing nature is not typical of pain arising from injury to the supporting spinal structures. Tuberculosis and fungal infections have a predilection to the spine. Even though the incidence of these diseases has been decreasing in the past decades, the growing number of AIDS patients with immune deficiencies creates a more susceptible environment and the incidence of these chronic spinal inflammatory diseases is now beginning to rise. Because of their low incidence, it is typical to experience a significant delay in the diagnosis of these diseases. Frequently, biopsy of suspicious lesions seen by x ray is the only mode of diagnosis. Of course, skin testing is available and is helpful in the diagnosis of tuberculosis and fungal diseases. Typically, the history of these diseases would be one of several months before ultimate diagnosis.

Vertebral osteomyelitis also presents an opportunity for misdiagnosis. The disease is not so rare that it should escape notice. In any patient who presents with severe back pain, unrelieved by rest, this must be a consideration. Often, there is a history of minor trauma that may delay the diagnosis. Frequently, the best test to identify the presence of pyogenic osteomyelitis is the elevated sedimentation rate. Occasionally, pain in the chest, hip, and abdomen may confuse the definition. Because of the nature of these infections, constitutional symptoms such as fever may be absent. This is especially notable in the elderly. In one series, the delay of diagnosis was two months from the onset of symptoms.[61] A usual tip-off in the clinical picture is the gradual onset of symptoms and, on physical examination, a well localized site of tenderness. Precise areas of acute tenderness are actually unusual in the subacute presentation of spinal disorders secondary to injuries. Radicular symptoms may also be present, but tend to occur later than the initial tenderness. Differential diagnosis usually lies between pathologic fracture, metastatic disease, and the the more chronic infections such as tuberculosis. The most common organism usually is Staphylococcus. If bacteriologic definition is not available by other means, open culture and drainage of the abscess is a surgical necessity. Usually, for bone infections intravenous therapy is necessary, occasionally with the use of implanted catheters. Excision of infected bone is feasible with replacement by bone graft and antibiotic intravenous therapy.

Disc space infections without any obvious source occur in childhood. These are extremely hard to identify and seldom is a bacteriologic diagnosis available. Usually in the adult, discitis is iatrogenic, such as after surgery, discography, and even caudal blocks.[62] The incidence of discitis following discography is probably about one in 1000. Usually following discography, the dominating organism is Staphylococcus epidermidis. Infections in the adult disc space obey strange rules. In the Fraser study, it was demonstrated that after 3 months of disc space contamination in an experimental model (sheep), no organisms could be found, but destruction of the disc continued. This was after injection of a few live bacteria into the disc space. Control injections with saline did not create destruction. In the adult, the best definition of the diagnosis emerges from bone scan and sedimentation rate. With MRI a clear definition of an adult discitis is available. In end plate erosions, narrowing of the disc space is seen in plain x rays and especially by tomography. Typically, an adequate cure may result from bed rest alone, with coverage of antibiotics. However, when abscess formation has been defined, surgical drainage is necessary.

Nonbacterial inflammatory disease of the spine is known as the spondyloarthropathies. A wide array of inflammatory diseases is covered by this heading. Ankylosing spondylitis, reactive arthritis, Reiter's syndrome, inflammatory bowel disease, and psoriatic arthritis all fall into this category. These diseases share a variety of clinical radiographic and genetic features.[63] Various other areas of involvement are typical of these diseases, including extra-articular foci urethritis, eye disease, gastrointestinal distress, and other joint complaints. Typically, these diseases strike the young adult, particularly males. Thus, they may easily masquerade as structural back problems. The most common is ankylosing spondylitis, in which low back pain and stiffness usually are early complaints. A prevalence of about one to two in 1000 can be expected.[64] Typically, the pain occurs in the early morning hours and stiffness lessons at the end of the day. Pain and stiffness thus increase with inactivity contrasted to the typical findings of the deteriorating disc. When the disease becomes progressive, spinal involvement may be first at the sacroiliac joints progressing upward along the spine with the cervical spine being involved last. Occasionally, other joints and the spine can be involved, but typically the disease involves only with spinal problems. The stiffness is often best monitored by a lack of chest expansion. Usually, the first objective changes are noticed in the sacroiliac joint. There is a high association of this disease with the antigen HLA-B27. A related disease is Reiter's syndrome, also with a high association to HLA-B27. Again, young male adults have a strong predilection. Sacroilitis is often associated with urethritis, arthritis in other joints, some skin lesions on the palms and soles and the most distinctive feature, conjunctivitis. Low back pain is thus a common association with this clinical disorder, but the radiographic abnormalities are not as common as with ankylosing

spondylitis. With inflammatory bowel disease, spinal involvement occurs less frequently, perhaps in 5 to 10% of those with the typical diseases—ulcerative colitis, regional enteritis, and Whipple's disease. The association with HLA-B27 is not as high as with ankylosing spondylitis and Reiter's syndrome, but usually at the level of about 50%. Psoriasis is associated with ankylosing spondylitis, but with a slightly different disease pattern. Stiffness is not as common and sacroiliac joint involvement is not as likely.[65] The best opportunity for definition of all of these diseases, therefore, is suspicion of presence. One should search for x ray evidence, especially at the sacroiliac joint. Seriologic studies including sedimentation rate and HLA B-27 are helpful. A bone scan is likewise helpful.

One other consideration for persistent spinal pain in the subacute time span is metabolic bone disease. Typically, this occurs in older patients, but the most common cause of osteopenia at its first clinical event is a compression fracture. This may be associated with such minimal trauma that the patient may not really be aware of it and merely complain of back pain. Significant back pain in older patients that persists for longer than a week deserves radiographic evaluation. Surgical care, of course, is seldom necessary for these compression fractures, which although painful in the early stages, gradually resolve to be inconsequential. Surgical care is indicated when there are several fractures that cause deformity with secondary strain. Once the source of the osteopenia has been clarified, appropriate therapy can be undertaken. Alternative diagnoses to the usual post-menopausal osteoporosis are osteomalacia, multiple myeloma, hyperparathyroidism, hyperthyroidism, and Cushing's disease. Actually, the definition of these various entities is best accomplished by a bone biopsy and histomorphometry. Interestingly, just as the basic theme for treatment of the activity-related disorders of the back is exercise, exercise is the major mechanism of treatment for osteoporosis. In addition, higher levels of calcium intake, Vitamin D, sodium fluoride, and estrogen for appropriate individuals, are an adjunct to treatment.

WHEN IS SURGERY INDICATED?

The subacute period of back pain is the ideal time for surgical decision making. Spontaneous healing has not occurred. Nor have chronicity based on deconditioning, habituation to pain, or permanent abnormalities secondary to scarring. What are the characteristics of a condition that requires surgical intervention?

Persistent and increasing pain suggests a disease process different from the deteriorating disc. As described above, this is usually secondary to infection or tumor and a definitive diagnosis is necessary. Occasionally, open biopsy is necessary; drainage of abscess is a possibility; and surgical reconstruction perhaps is necessary. These problems are rare.

Surgery for the deteriorating lumbar motion segment is chiefly focused at care of the herniated disc. In the subacute phase, surgical care for discogenic pain is unwarranted. Vigorous exercise programs focused at efforts to enhance metabolism of the disc have been emphasized. Spontaneous healing, change of lifestyle, and many other factors weave together to avoid the use of surgical care in the subacute time period for discogenic pain.

Nonetheless, if there is good evidence of a herniated disc with greater leg pain than back pain, imaging studies that correlate with these findings, and physical signs that validate the patient's complaint, early care for the herniated disc is appropriate. When the findings are not crisp, preliminary evaluation with facet joint injections to rule out these joints as a significant factor in the source of pain are appropriate. Although the facet joints are a major source of pain in only about 20% of the cases of nonspecific back and leg pain, the minimal risk of this diagnostic study makes it worth the effort in confusing cases. The same can be said for epidural injections. Certainly, if a disease process is within the spinal canal, an epidural injection should make a significant impact on this process. The effect may be fleeting, but the opportunity to proceed with an appropriately oriented exercise program is justified. If the individual has only brief relief from the epidural injection, and the findings are as identified above to corroborate a herniated disc, surgical care is appropriate.

Initially, surgery for herniated discs should merely remove the intrusion onto the nerve root with minimal destruction to supporting tissues. The use of fusion should not be expected. Single level, unilateral exposure is appropriate if traditional surgical care is undertaken. Microsurgery has less opportunity for soft tissue destruction. If the disc is extruded, surgical care is relatively simple and excellent results can be anticipated. If the disc is contained, relatively recent in onset, and well defined as the source of the patient's significant leg pain versus back pain, a percutaneous discectomy is a reasonable consideration. This procedure, conducted as an outpatient under local anesthesia, has similar risks and morbidity as a discogram study. Thus, there are few risks of significant complications following surgical procedure, other than a minimal risk of infection.

The most important aspect of this discussion is the recognition that early decisions are more cost-effective than delayed decisions. If the patient's pain complaints continue for 1 to 2 months, no improvement seems to be occurring in spite of the potential for spontaneous healing, and the patient has continuing distress in spite of an appropriate exercise program—surgery should be performed. One must recognize that this occurs in only a very small percentage of patients. The great majority of people, over 99%, should improve without the need for surgical care.

REFERENCES

1. Spitzer, W.O., et al.: Scientific approach to the assessment and management of activity related spinal disorders. Spine 12(S1):S1–59, 1987.
2. Jones, D.A., Newham, J., Obletter, G., Giamberaridino, M.A.: Nature of exercise-induced muscle pain. Adv Pain Res Ther 10:207–218, 1987.
3. Bobbert, M.F., Hollander, A.D., Huijing, P.A.: Factors in delayed onset of muscle soreness of man. Med Sci Sports Exercise 18:75–81, 1986.
4. Lehto, M., et al.: Connective tissue changes of the multifidus muscle in patients with lumbar disc herniation—an immunohistologic study of collagen types I and III and fibronection. Spine 14:302–309, 1989.
5. Woo, S.L., Buckwalter, J.A.: Injury and repair of the musculoskeletal soft tissue. Am Academy of Orthop. Surg., Chicago, pp. 171–207, 1988.
6. Styf, J.: Pressure in the erector spinae muscle during exercise. Spine 12:675–679, 1987.
7. Styf, J., Lysell, E.: Chronic compartment syndrome in the erector spinae muscle. Spine 12:680–682, 1987.
8. Moldofsky, H., Scaribrick, P., England, R., Smythe, H.: Musculoskeletal symptoms and non-REM sleep disturbance in patients with "fibrositis syndrome" and healthy patients. Psychosomatic Med 37:341–351, 1975.
9. McCain, G.A.: Role of physical fitness training in the fibrositis/fibromyalgia syndrome. Am J Med 81(S3A):73–77, 1986.
10. Bengstsson, A., Henriksson, K-G, Larsson, J.: Muscle biopsy in primary fibromyalgia. Scand J Rheumatol 15:1–6, 1986.
11. Simons, D.G.: Myofascial pain syndromes: where are we going? Arch Phys Med Rehabil 69:207–212, 1988.
12. Ghormley, R.K.: Low back pain with special reference to the articular facets, with presentation of an operative procedure. JAMA 101:1773–1775, 1933.
13. Goldthwait, J.E.: The lumbosacral articulation. An explanation of many cases of "lumbago, sciatica and paraplegic." Boston Med Surg J 164:356–372, 1911.
14. Badgley, C.E.: The articular facets in relationship to low back pain and sciatic radiation. J Bone Joint Surg 23A:481–496, 1941.
15. Kelgren, J.J.: Observation on referred pain arising from muscle. Clin Sci Mol Med 3:175–190, 1938.
16. Foerster: The dermatomes in man. Brain 56:1–39, 1933.
17. Inman, V.T., Saunders, J.B.: Referred pain from skeletal structures. J Nerv Ment Dis 99:660–667, 1944.
18. Paris, S.B.: Functional anatomy of the lumbar spine. Doctoral thesis. Union Graduate School, Atlanta, 1983.
19. Steindler, A., Luck, J.V.: Differential diagnosis of pain in the low back: allocation of the source of pain by procaine hydrochloride method. JAMA 110:106–113, 1938.
20. Hirsch, D., Inglemark, B., Miller, M.: The anatomical basis for low back pain. Acta Orthop Scand 33:1–17, 1963.
21. Mooney, V., Robertson, J.: The facet syndrome. Clin Orthop 115:149–156, 1976.

22. Lippett, A.B.: The facet joint in its role in spine pain. Spine *9*:746–750, 1984.
23. Eisenstein, S.M., Parry, C.R.: The lumbar facet arthrosis syndrome: clinical presentation and articular surface changes. J Bone Joint Surg *69B*:3–7, 1987.
24. Videman, T., Malmivaara, A., Mooney, V.: The value of the axial view in assessing discograms: An experimental study with cadavers. Spine *12*:299–305, 1987.
25. Moran, R., O'Connell, D., Walsh, M.G.: The diagnostic value of facet injections. Spine *13*:1407–1410, 1988.
26. Dory, M.: Anthrography of the lumbar facet joints. Radiology *140*:23–27, 1981.
27. Jackson, R.E., Jacobs, R.R., Montesano, P.X.: Facet joint injection in low back pain, a prospective statistical study. Spine *13*:966–971, 1988.
28. Don Tigny, R.L.: Function and pathomechanics of the sacroiliac joints: a review. Phys Ther *65*:35–44, 1985.
29. Yagan, R., Khan, M.A., Marmolya G.: Goal of abdominal CT, when available in patient's records, in the evaluation of degenerative changes of the sacroiliac joints. Spine *12*:1046–1051, 1988.
30. Walheim, G.G., Selvik, G.: Mobility of the pubic symphysis: in vivo measurements with an electromechanic method and a roentgen stereophotogrammetric method. Clin Orthop *191*:192–135, 1984.
31. Bernard, T.N., Kirkaldy-Willis, W.H.: Recognizing specific characteristics of nonspecific low back pain. Clin Orthop *217*:266–280, 1987.
32. Porter, R.W., Hibbert, C., Evans, C.: The natural history of root entrapment. Spine *9*:418–421, 1984.
33. Verbiest, H.: A radicular syndrome from developmental narrowing of the lumbar vertebral canal. J Bone Joint Surg *36B*:230, 1954.
34. Porter, R.W., Wicks, M., Hibbert, C.: The size of the lumbar spinal canal in the symptomatology of disc lesions. J Bone Joint Surg *60B*:485–487, 1987.
35. Urban, J.P.G., et al.: Nutrition of the intervertebral disc: Effect of fluid flow on solute transport. Clin Orthop *170*:296–302, 1982.
36. Eklund, J.A., Corlett, E.N.: Shrinkage as a measure of the effect of load on the spine. Spine *9*:189–194, 1984.
37. Pope, M.H., Klingenstierna, U.: Height changes due to autotraction. Clin Biomech *1*:191–195, 1986.
38. Holm, S.J., Urban, J.P.G.: The intervertebral disc: factors contributing to its nutrition and matrix turnover. *In* Biology and Health of Articular Structures (Edited by H.J. Helminen). Bristol, England, Wright, 1987.
39. Holm, S., Maroudas, A., Urban, J.P.G., Selstam, G., Nachemson, A.: Nutrition of the intervertebral disc. Connective Tissue Res *8*:101, 1981.
40. Diamant, B., Karlsson, J., Nachemson, A.: Correlation between lactate levels and pH in discs of patients with lumbar rhizopathies. Experientia, *24*:1195–1196, 1968.
41. Mooney, V.: A perspective on the future of low back research. Spine, State of the Art Reviews *3*:173–183, 1989.
42. Carney, S.L., Billingham, M.E., Muir, H., Sandy, S.D.: Structure of newly synthesized 35S-proteoglycan turnover products of cartilage cultures from dogs with experimental osteoarthritis. J Orthop Res *3*:140–147, 1985.
43. Kivaranta, I., et al.: Moderate running exercise augments glucose aminoglycans and thickness of articular cartilage in the knee joints of young beagle dogs. J Orthop Res *6(2)*:188–195, 1988.
44. Deyo, R.A., Diehl, A.K., Rosenthal, M.: How many days of bed rest for acute low back pain? A randomized clinical trial. N Engl J Med *315*:1064–1070, 1986.
45. Park, W.M., et al: Fissuring of the posterior annulus fibrosus in the lumbar spine. Br J Radiol *52*:382–387, 1979.
46. Hirsch, C., Schajowicz, F.: Studies on structural changes in the lumbar annulus fibrosus. Acta Orthop Scand *22*:184–231, 1952.
47. Sachs, B.L., et al: Dallas discogram description: a new classification of CT/discography in low back disorders. Spine *12*:287–291, 1987.
48. Adams, M.A., Hutton, W.C.: Gradual disc prolapse. Spine *10*:524–531, 1985.
49. Gill, K., et al: The effect of repeated extensions on the discographic dye patterns in cadaveric lumbar motion segments. Clin Biomech *2*:205–210, 1987.
50. Krag, M., et al: Internal displacements from in vitro loading of human spinal motion segments: Experimental results and finite element in model predictions. Presented at the meeting of the International Society for the Study of the Lumbar Spine, Dallas, TX, May, 1986.
51. Fredrickson, E., Murphy, K., Donelson, R.G.: McKenzie treatment of low back pain, a correlation of significant factors in determining prognosis. Orthop Trans *10,3*:534, 1986.
52. Vanharanta, H., Videman, T., Mooney, V.: McKenzie exercise, back trac and back school in lumbar syndrome. Orthop Trans *10,3*:534, 1986.
53. Dilke, T.F.W., Burry, H.C., Grahame, R.: Extradural corticosteroid injection in management of lumbar nerve root compression. Br Med J *2*:635–637, 1973.
54. Snoek, W., Weber, H., Jorgensen, B.: Double blind evaluation of extradural methyl-prednisolone for herniated lumbar discs. Acta Orthop Scand *48*:635–641, 1971.
55. White, A.H., Derby, R., Wynne, G.: Epidural injections for the diagnosis and treatment of low back pain. Spine *5*:78–86, 1980.
56. Weber, H.: Lumbar disc herniation: a controlled prospective study with ten years of observation. Spine *8*:131–140, 1983.
57. Hurme, M., Alaranta, H.: Factors predicting the result of surgery for lumbar intervertebral disc herniation. Spine *12*:933–938, 1987.
58. Weinstein, J.N., McLain, R.F.: Primary tumors of the spine. Spine *12*:843–851, 1987.
59. Sim, F.H., Dahlin, D.C., Stauffer, R.N., Laws, E.R.: Primary bone tumors simulating lumbar disc syndrome. Spine *2*:65–74, 1977.
60. Simeone, F.A., Lawner, P.M.: Intraspinal neoplasms. *In* The Spine (Edited by R.H. Rothman, F.A. Simone). Philadelphia, W.B. Saunders, pp. 1041–1054, 1982.
61. Griffiths, H.E.H., et al: Pyogenic infections of the spine. J Bone Joint Surg Br *53*:383–391, 1971.
62. Fraser, R.D., et al: Discitis following chemonucleolysis: An experimental study. Spine, *11*:679–687, 1986.
63. Jayson, M.I.V.: Spinal diseases and back pain. *In* P.A. Dieppe, et al.: Atlas of Clinical Rheumatology. Philadelphia, Lea & Febiger, pp. 13–17, 1986.
64. Bluestone, R.: Ankylosing spondylitis. *In* Arthritis and Allied Conditions, 10th Ed. Philadelphia, Lea & Febiger, pp. 819–840, 1985.
65. Habif, T.P.: Clinical dermatology. St. Louis, C.V. Mosby, 1985.
66. Andersson, G.B.J., McNeill, T.W.: Lumbar spine syndromes, evaluation and treatment. New York, Springer-Verlag, p. 164, 1989.

25

Tom G. Mayer

The Shift from Passive Modalities to Reactivation

Treatments for early stages of back pain have customarily evolved according to generalized approaches to pain prevalent in each locale, with little foundation in science.[1] Manipulation, temperature modulation, electrical stimulation, exercise, and education all have their adherents. Because of the natural history of spinal pain and the absence of objective markers of progress, and because spontaneous recovery so confounds outcomes, it is difficult, if not impossible, to organize truly valid prospective randomized studies during the early stages of the back pain process. However, if we consider the early development of spinal pain symptoms as emanating from a single anatomic source, certain approaches to the treatment of these conditions become evident. Even with a nontraumatic origin, symptoms caused by peripheral stimuli that persist beyond 6 to 8 weeks suggest an ongoing biomechanical or biochemical derangement originating from structural soft tissue dysfunction. As such, it may be worthwhile to review, once again, concepts of soft tissue healing.

THE MECHANISM OF SOFT TISSUE INJURY

Generally, initial phases of soft tissue injury are characterized, to some degree, by hemorrhage and edema. In the first few days, hemostasis is achieved and protective splinting or spasm may have occurred through injury reflex mechanisms that naturally immobilize and protect the injured area. Avoiding further harm and achieving a favorable environment for healing appear to be the basis of these protective mechanisms. Within a few days, cellular infiltration and enzymatic degradation occur, involving prostaglandins, bradykinins, and kallikreins. This is an intrinsic inflammatory process involving clearing of necrotic debris, and occurring primarily in an acidic environment.

A proliferative phase follows, with its timing and duration related to the quality of the blood supply in the area. Random deposition of collagen fibrils takes place initially. Subsequently, the collagen fibrils align along lines of stress and begin to assume certain (but not all) characteristics of the tissue being replaced. The location of the lines of stress appears to be related to the type of tissue formed, as well as its strength and physical characteristics, a process that might be termed the generalized Wolff's Law of Connective Tissue. Understandably, in the presence of a small degree of tissue injury with relatively good nutrition and low grade stresses, such as a mild sprain or strain, this healing process proceeds quickly. However, with more profound injuries, higher stress, larger areas of anatomic destruction, or poor nutrition, healing may be delayed. At the conclusion of the healing period, however, the injured area is left with a scar, visible or hidden, which will ultimately mature to fill the injured area, but lacks the resilience, strength, and durability of the original tissue. Given appropriate circumstances, both in early and late healing, the substitute fibrous scar, fibrocartilage, or bone might assume most of the mechanical and biochemical characteristics of the original tissue, but cannot achieve equivalence.[2,3]

In the spine, particularly the cervical and lumbar regions, expect this healing process to be relatively delayed compared to other parts of the body. Stresses are extremely high in these regions, with few other structures available to share or balance loads (akin to ribs in the thoracic spine). Hence, awkward postures, involuntary muscle splinting, and recumbent positions to relax hamstrings, abdominals, and iliopsoas may be chosen in the interest of tissue protection to promote healing. Almost any activity has potential to exacerbate symptoms, which may produce severe recurrent pain episodes that reinforce inactivity as an avoidance behavior.

Injury to the cervical and lumbar spine is not merely isolated to disc or facet derangement. It also involves a complex of joint muscles, fascia, and ligaments that represents the cervicothoracic or lumbopelvic functional unit. In the cervical area, paracervical, shoulder girdle, scapular, and upper thoracic structures are routinely involved, even in small, well localized cervical derangements. In the lumbar region, lumbar structures, as well as abdominal and hip musculature, representing the lumbopelvic functional unit, are associated with discrete soft tissue injuries. The vertebral structure itself requires the presence of short, strong, broad based muscles and ligaments, which, like the annulus fibrosis, can tolerate only limited strains or changes in length with application of loads. Supported by muscles with slips that extend over a variable number of vertebrae, and with coordination possibly substantially altered by the injury, these structures become subject to further biomechanical derangement with reimposition of high level stresses. As a consequence, a small primary injury of the low back may lead to secondary derangement and painful disorders in relatively more areas than injury to other parts of the musculoskeletal system.

Moreover, poor nutrition may be another adverse factor in spinal tissue healing. The intervertebral discs, the largest avascular structures in the body, can be expected to heal more slowly than tissues with a direct blood supply. Certain circumstances peculiar to the individual patient may act as nutritional determinants, such as diabetes, pulmonary disease, cardiovascular disease or cigarette smoking, shifting the healing balance even further "into the red."

What is a reasonable expectation for spinal soft tissue healing under these circumstances? Depending on some of the factors discussed above, a skin laceration can be expected to heal within 5 to 10 days. A sprain may heal within 2 to 4 weeks, and most fractures within 2 to 4 months. We can only speculate on healing rates in the spinal functional units because the specific injury is likely to be refractory to visual monitoring; however, 2 to 4 months should be sufficient for even severe derangements to have achieved primary healing. This time frame potentially accounts for the epidemiologic findings discussed earlier of spontaneous recovery within 3–4 months in the vast number of spine episodes. Do chronic patients, then, represent patients whose soft tissue injuries fail to heal? Or are there other hypotheses for organic causes of peripheral pain following soft tissue injury or sudden degeneration?

There are several existing models to explain such pain:

1. Chronic infection leading to an indolent ulceration or osteomyelitis. In these situations, the invading organism generally reaches symbiosis with its host, leading to alternating periods of quiescence and recrudescence. Such deep infections may be, at times, relatively free of symptoms or signs. In the spine, discitis is a known phenomenon probably associated with this type of condition.
2. Bone fractures may fail to unite and may be hypertrophic or atrophic. This may be painful, particularly if associated with gross motion or significant weightbearing (high stresses). Healing usually progresses for the balance of repair attempts; load-induced destruction leads to a fibrous ankylosis. Spinal conditions similar to this situation may include spondylolysis or pseudarthrosis following attempted spine fusion.
3. Post-traumatic arthritis. The facet joints are susceptible to cartilage degeneration, capsular laxity, disc degeneration-induced facet subluxation, and destructive changes consequent to localized injury or secondary biomechanical abberations. Facet arthritis or disc space narrowing is commonly noted on x ray examination, particularly in the older population. This provides evidence that such joint changes occur in spinal regions subjected to high loads and large ranges of motion.
4. Chronic musculoskeletal soft tissue disorders. Lateral epicondylitis, shoulder or knee tendonitises, and various bursitides generally are found in areas of high intermittent loading associated with unique localized biomechanical factors that increase stress. In these situations, a cycle of healing and reinjury may be stimulated by repetitive overload exacerbated by patients who respond to pain by oscillating between the extremes of excessive rest and excessive reloading. These conditions generally respond to anti-inflammatory medications or injections. This response is partial evidence that an enzymatic biochemical inflammatory cascade is associated with these conditions. Partial evidence for the conjecture that such inflammatory processes may take place internally within the degenerating "painful disc" also has been presented. This evidence is among the most intriguing yet offered for defining a pain source commonly associated with spinal disorders. However, no such disorders have been conclusively demonstrated to exist in the spine. It is similarly likely that such processes as facet dysfunction, iliolumbar ligament syndrome, and other "trigger" phenomena loosely termed fi-

bromyositis or fibromyalgia may potentially fall under this paradigm.[4]

Although these models for defining potential pain sources are attractive, little proof exists that they can account for the high number of chronic painful spinal conditions developing each year. Chronic infection is an unlikely event in the painful spine. It is often suspected, but rarely documented. Spondylolysis and low grade spondylolisthesis appear to be relatively common, particularly in certain ethnic groups, but are generally asymptomatic. Although these conditions are found frequently in the younger population, on x ray the older population shows a high incidence of "post-traumatic arthritis" of the facet joints and the intervertebral discs. Postulating that these changes are a cause for spinal pain is attractive, but flies in the face of considerable contradictory information. Such processes are accelerated by surgical intervention; however, the majority of patients undergoing such surgery experience relief from, not increase in, pain. Subjects over age 40 who have never had low back symptoms may demonstrate more than a 30% incidence of "herniated disc" on CT scan radiographic imaging.[5,6] Chronic soft tissue inflammation provides an attractive hypothesis, but is difficult to visualize or prove. Recently, serious question has even been raised concerning efficacy of injection treatment for facet joint syndrome.[7] The finding of the "painful disc" by discography, thought by many clinicians to be associated with several painful spinal conditions, may provide an attractive framework for future research.[8,9] However, the test has a strong subjective component and remains a controversial clinical tool at present.[10] Combined with findings of persistent acidic, inflammatory products in degenerated intervertebral disc nuclei, additional hypotheses for research can be expected to be pursued in the future.[4]

At the state-of-the-art of current understanding, we must conclude that there is little evidence for a chronically persistent lesion, resistent to healing, as a consistently stimulating peripheral "pain source." As such, recurrent biomechanical or biochemical processes must be presumed, but not proven, to be responsible for ongoing symptoms in the vast majority of patients who continue to have pain 2 to 4 months since symptom onset. Surgical trauma may add to the disease process, but should heal within 2 to 4 months postoperatively under the conditions discussed above.

Some basic scientific information specific to the spine is available to supplement our general knowledge. Disc nutrition is definitely improved by motion, probably because of a combination of improved oxygenation and a mechanical pumping mechanism using endplate diffusion.[11,12] Postoperative changes in experimental animals, as well as those resulting from immobilization, have been demonstrated.[13–16] In addition to intervertebral disc findings, the relationship between muscle, joint, bone, and ligament function and the beneficial effects of activity have strong basic scientific support.[2,17–21]

What is indisputable, however, is that the mechanics of the spine tend to produce an aversive response to activity within the affected individual. This leads, in time, to delayed maturation of collagen, muscle atrophy, deficits in joint lubrication, ligament atrophy, and bone loss.[19–23] Subsequently, muscular endurance and tone and cardiovascular aerobic capacity and mobility decline, followed by neuromuscular dysfunction with decreased proprioception, agility, and coordination. A vicious cycle of recurrent injury may occur more readily because of the decreased physical capacity and abnormal overload feedback mechanisms, termed the "Deconditioning Syndrome." As inactivity and recumbency lead to lower daily physical demands, including loss of responsibilities at work and in the home, physical capacity deficits spiral downwards. "Psychological Deconditioning" may follow as a natural consequence of physiologic incapacity.[24]

QUANTIFICATION OF SPINE FUNCTION

If we accept this view of the putative pain source in spinal disorders, certain approaches to diagnosis become evident. The individual with a painful spinal disorder naturally assumes a degree of protective disuse consequent to his or her injury. The extent of immobilization depends somewhat on the severity of injury, demands of daily life, and pain threshold and sensitivity. In the acute phases, acute tissue injury is thought to be the predominant pain source. As such, techniques to minimize pain and promote healing assume the highest priority. By contrast, patients with chronic spinal disorders not amenable to surgical intervention are thought to have soft tissues that heal with profound physical and mental deconditioning. Treatment is necessarily directed toward functional restoration rather than "curing" the pain source or promoting complete tissue healing. However, the *subacute patient* whose symptoms have persisted for 2 to 4 months may be in the "crossover period" wherein both passive modalities and reactivation therapy may be appropriate. As such, measurement of physical function may be an important adjunct to assist in decision making for treatment. In such circumstances, a basic understanding of principles of physical capacity measurement is necessary.

The recognition of the "Deconditioning Syndrome" as an important factor in spinal disability is rather recent.[2,18,25,26] Physiologic and psychologic deconditioning have been well understood as primary pathologic determinants of sports medicine rehabilitation for more than 25 years. Yet, prior to development of a variety of physical capacity measurements for the lumbopelvic and cervicothoracic functional units, these concepts were rarely applied to spinal pain. In retrospect, this appears to have resulted from the absence of visual feedback of the anatomic structures of the spine, with the concomitant necessity of relying solely on patient self-reports to guide treatment. Such habits are difficult to extinguish, and the transition to reliance on more objective measurement technology to steer spinal care is just beginning. Even as exercise treatment proliferates, valid measurement to guide the process lags behind. Clinicians, whose judgments have been based only on what they can see directly or what they are told, may continue to make subjective judgments of disability, support long-term passive rather than active care, and continue to apply inaccurate treatment principles. "If it hurts let it rest indefinitely" can only be supplanted when the physician and therapist rely upon objective testing.

The "Deconditioning Syndrome" is responsible for maintaining the organic component of disability in most patients with chronic painful spinal disorders. Increasing documentation of this relationship is available in the literature, specifically regarding measurement of range of motion, trunk strength in sagittal and axial planes, aerobic capacity, and functional task performance, such as lifting and bending.[24,27–39] Measurement of function has a variety of meanings, which are discussed in later chapters. The measurement of anatomic and physiologic capacity is distinguished in Table 25–1. Anatomic and physiologic measurements can take place in isolation and do not demand the task be performed within a certain time framework. On the other hand, functional measurements attempt to make statements about the subject's ability to perform "in the real world." Functional testing demands measurement of

both the *dynamic synthetic task* and the *time* taken to perform a single repetition. This introduces the concept of *efficiency* into functional measurements, which is not necessarily a characteristic of anatomic and physiologic measurements.

When looking at functional tasks performed by the spine, we are interested in the interconnection of multiple functional units. For example, when lifting, the spine serves as a "segmented crane" to allow movement from various heights and distances within a certain radius. After the load is placed into stable position, the "crane" can become a "forklift," carrying the object through the locomotor system. The lumbopelvic functional unit is the critical component in both of these important human physical demands (Figs. 25–1, 25–2).

Components of Physical Capacity Evaluation

In determining what to include in the evaluation of function, use of the most desirable assessment tools is only one part of the process. One must then find a technique for providing accurate and reliable information and standardizing the protocol. Both the testing device and the protocol must be safe, quick, and relatively easy to use. If a test meets the latter characteristics only, greater accuracy and reliability may be sacrificed by the clinical community. For example, a simple direct measure of cardiac output may be highly desirable, but in its absence, the use of easy pulse and blood pressure measures have been thought to be satisfactory for clinical use. In some cases, however, it is worthwhile to take the trouble to obtain more sophisticated measures to complement the simple ones.

The primary requirement to accurately evaluate physical capacity is a valid and relevant measurement method. Repeatability is a prerequisite for a valid measurement, but is not sufficient to guarantee validity. Additional tests must be applied to be certain that an accurate physical capacity measurement has been obtained. One important characteristic to assure validity is to ensure that the measurement device is accurate. We generally assume accuracy in weight scales or thermometers, but such accuracy may not be present in dynamometers or exercise bicycles displaying work rates or devices measuring trunk strength. As consumers, medical professionals should request data on the errors inherent in each device such as the dynamometer.

Once device validity has been established, protocols must be established. When measuring dynamic activities, unless the conditions of testing are virtually identical between subjects, valid comparisons cannot be made. The process of converting independent dynamic variables into dependent ones is very

Table 25–1
Distinction Between Anatomic and Functional Measurements

Measurement Type	Definition	Examples
1. Anatomic	Basic element of performance usually involving only a single functional unit.	Range of motion, Isolated functional unit strength
2. Functional	Measurement of ability to perform a synthetic task usually involving multiple functional units and also necessitating motion and time measurement.	Bicycle ergometry, Lifting tests

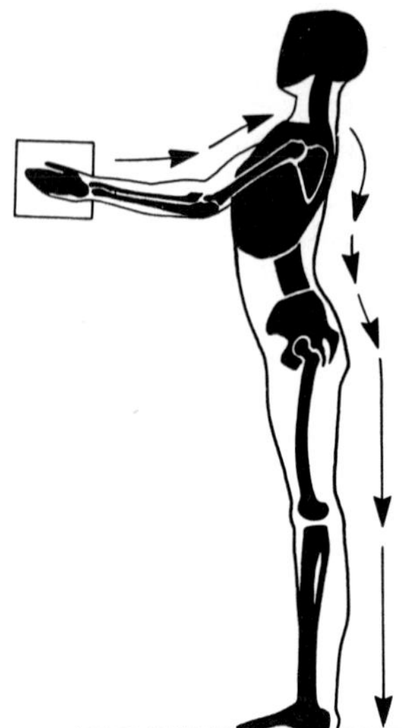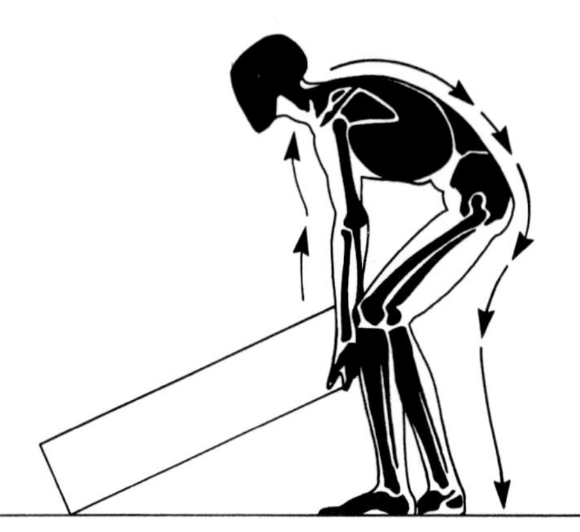

Figure 25–1. The "biomechanical chain" by which loads are transmitted from hands within a certain bodily radius to a stable foot/floor contact. (From Mayer, T.G., Gatchel, R.J.: Functional Restoration for Spinal Disorders: The Sports Medicine Approach. Philadelphia, Lea & Febiger, 1988.)

important in physical capacity measures, and the ultimate accuracy of clinical statements depends to a great extent on how well a given device and testing protocol accomplish this. For example, the principle of *isokinetic* strength testing converts the independent variables of acceleration and velocity into dependent ones, thus helping to improve test discrimination. The ability to convert independent variables to dependent variables is applicable to the development of normative databases, necessary in spinal physical capacity evaluation because of the lack of a

contralateral comparison side. Naturally, any normalizing factor used must diminish the variability of the primary measure before it can be employed.

Relevance is another important concept that refers to the closeness with which the test actually measures the quantity to be identified. For example, it was formerly thought that an isometric lifting test was a measure of trunk strength. However, the test is a static, whole-body measurement of function, whereas trunk strength is a dynamic process that requires an anatomic or physiologic measurement of a

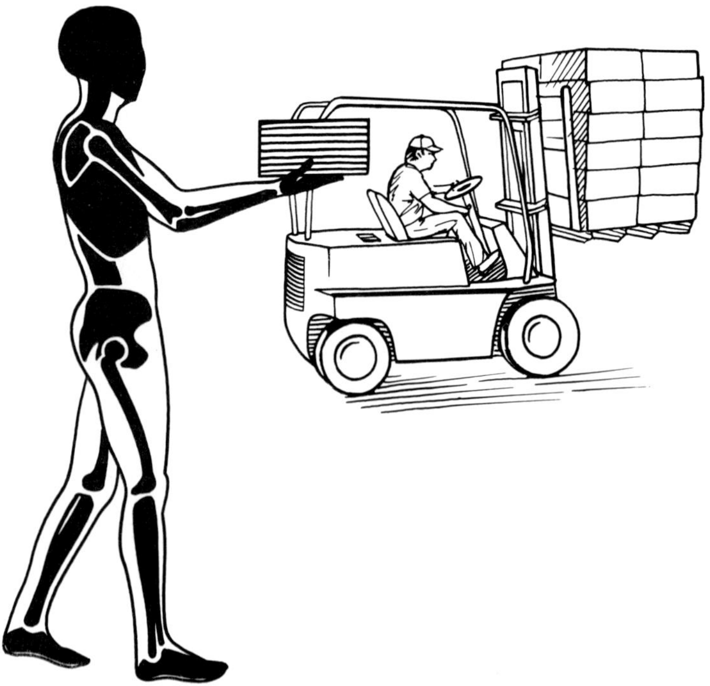

Figure 25–2. The human as "forklift," maintaining objects in a stable position by using the human locomotion system. (From Mayer, T.G., Gatchel, R.J.: Functional Restoration for Spinal Disorders: The Sports Medicine Approach. Philadelphia, Lea & Febiger, 1988.)

basic element of performance in a single functional unit. More generally, relevance applies to the relationship between the measurement and the basic element of performance to be described.

Measurement of physical capacity in the spine imposes test demands not usually encountered in the extremities. Because the spine is nonbilateral, the intraindividual controls, long utilized to measure physical capacity in the extremities, must be replaced by a large interindividual normative database. It also has become empirically evident that such databases must be specific for gender and age in order to decrease intersubject variability. Furthermore, population scatter in tests of muscular performance (i.e., trunk strength or shoulder strength) may be reduced if the tests are normalized to body weight and, in some instances, to a height variable.[24,33,40,41] Ultimately, databases may become large enough to relate anticipated physical capacities to the ergonomic demands of a specific job or daily activity level.

In developing such a database, it became obvious that because no interindividual controls exist; an effort factor must be identified for each test. Terminology may be confusing and the reader must understand that the limitations of effort infrequently result from conscious attempts by a subject to defraud the examiner and misrepresent his or her true abilities. Suboptimal effort usually results, at least on initial testing, from pain, fear of injury, neuromuscular inhibition, and involuntary splinting. Patients with spinal disorders usually have been conditioned by personal experience, as well as advice from friends and medical professionals that, "If it hurts, don't do it." We have already described the vicious cycle of overprotectiveness, leading to additional disuse and the resulting susceptibility to recurrent pain episodes caused by minimal additional trauma. Understandably, inactive patients also will have poor feedback of musculoskeletal performance, which makes it harder for them to monitor overload. Initial performance can therefore generally be expected to be suboptimal. After training, however, other factors such as motivation, training effect, stress, and ultimate neuromuscular capability become the limiting factors for test performance. The effort factor, together with a variety of psychological tests and patient self-report measures, identifies the cognitive and psychosocial barriers to function. It also identifies the degree of validity of the particular test, and the confidence that the clinician can put into the demonstrated physical capacity test scores. Low effort ratings imply the patient is at least capable of performing to the degree demonstrated in the test, but with education and training may be able to perform a great deal better with relatively little muscle hypertrophy.[42] Furthermore, the clinician's recogni-

tion of suboptimal effort also helps direct subsequent interventions to a greater emphasis on counseling for the psychosocial barriers.

The range of motion effort factor has been clearly delineated in other publications.[27,28,43] The aerobic fitness test can usually be calibrated for effort by use of a target heart rate (with notable exceptions, such as intercurrent cardiovascular disease or use of rate-limiting medications). Reaching the target heart rate in bicycle ergometry, upper body ergometry, or psychophysical lifting tests indicates that the patient has high motivation in achieving his or her ultimate work performance level.[40,41] From this point, the patient is usually able to continue reaching the target heart rate in subsequent tests as reconditioning proceeds to progressively higher work rates.

Dynamic strength testing (sagittal and axial trunk strength and isokinetic lifting) permits identification of another effort factor. It is related to the empirical observation that a maximum voluntary contraction is only truly reproducible through multiple trials. It has already been established in several studies that reproducibility of isometric lifting tasks (multiple functional units in a single dimension) leads to measurement precision of better than 10%. However, conscious efforts to produce suboptimal performance in similar dynamic tasks result in variances above 20%.[44,45] Though isometric testing may provide for comparison of peak forces, a dynamic test results in a curve that shows force or torque versus distance and allows for improved characterization of physical capacity through comparison of curve shape and work integral (area beneath the curve). In time, it should be possible to provide a normative database featuring acceptable variability between trials with regard to peak forces, curve shape, or work performance. In time, such research may lead to a truly quantified strength effort factor. At the present time, several computerized dynamic trunk strength measurement devices have computer programs to assess test variability.

It is probably reasonable to consider certain self-report and quantified psychosocial tests as a complement to physical capacity measures. Because the characteristic of the spinal disorders under consideration is pain, the patients' perception of pain, disability, and depression are important factors to compare to the physical and effort factors at each point in the evaluation. Clearly, these subjective perceptions have no objective validity. However, as quantified subjective measures[46–49] of patients' perceptions, the tests may be useful in comparing these perceptions within the same individual from one point in time to another. The factors considered in evaluating physical capacity measures are summarized in Table 25–2.

Table 25–2
Major Factors in Evaluating Physical Capacity Measurement Technology

Validity
Accuracy
Reproducibility/Reliability
Relevance for performance dimension being measured
Effort factor
Safety
Normative database

THE SUBACUTE PATIENT: PASSIVE MODALITIES VS. REACTIVATION

As discussed elsewhere in this book, numerous passive modalities can be applied to patients with painful spinal conditions. Passive modalities include all those things done to a patient, as opposed to those things a patient does himself. Surgical treatment, in the small percentage of cases in which it is necessary, is included within the passive modalities category. The goals of this type of treatment are minimization of pain and promotion of healing. Subgoals might include maintenance of comfort, decreasing inflammation, promoting improved tissue nutrition, decreasing tissue stresses and strains, and avoiding progressive tissue damage. In this way, the multitude of passive modalities already discussed may be appropriate for limited use.

During the 2 to 4 month subacute interval, progressive deconditioning occurs in response to the degree of immobilization, inactivity, and disuse incurred by the patient. Reactivation is the treatment method used to combat this progressive degradation of physical capacity. As the "Deconditioning Syndrome" begins to take effect, tissue healing results in lower levels of pain, neuromuscular inhibition, and splinting. Consequently, an inverse relationship exists between the two conditions during this critical point in time. Reactivation therapy implies a recognition of the dangers of progressive deconditioning and, if successful, impedes its development. Its primary components are exercise and education. Exercise may either be generalized or specifically tied to areas of developing physical deficits identified by quantitative testing.

Given our understanding of painful spinal disorders at this time, it should be apparent that the subacute patient does not require a sudden changeover from passive to active treatment. The subacute patient represents 20 to 30% of the patient population, and he may go on to a variety of outcomes based on the organic and inorganic issues in each case. The alternative outcomes include: (1) complete healing to asymptomatic status, (2) infrequent recurrences, (3) chronic episodic syndromes with intermittent disability, or (4) chronic disabling spinal pain and dysfunction. The goal of treatment during the subacute phase is to maximize the number of patients moving into the first two groups and minimize those falling into the latter two. If we hope to accomplish this, treatment must move gradually from passive modalities to reactivation, from emphasis on the patient as a dependent person to emphasis on the patient as an independent participant in re-achieving health and productivity. There are few disabling conditions with as much opportunity for patients to positively affect their own outcome. Therapies, both physical and psychomedical, must move gradually in this direction during this phase of treatment, guided by the hand of a skilled physician.

SUMMARY

The subacute phase of spinal disorders is a time of transition. Tissue injury or dysfunction may be improving spontaneously, even as negative deconditioning changes incapacitate the patient with longer-lasting impairments and disabilities. As these internal processes of healing and deconditioning are playing out, the patient's aversion to pain may promote damaging behaviors that fail to automatically extinguish themselves at the appropriate time. Reactivation therapy may then prove necessary to reprogram the human organism to independence and productivity. Nonspecific exercise and education programs may be useful and cost-effective. However, identification of deficits of physical capacity, patient effort, and quantified self-report may clarify baseline physical deficits and barriers to recovery of importance in future treatment. An understanding of basic measurement principles can assist the clinician in determining to what degree such methodologies may be necessary in dealing with these patients, and making the critical clinical judgment regarding when to move from purely passive modalities to a mixture of passive and active treatments.

REFERENCES

1. Deyo, R.: Conservative therapy for low back pain: distinguishing useful from useless therapy. JAMA 250:1057–1062, 1983.
2. Woo, S., Buckwalter, J.: Injury and Repair of the Musculoskeletal Soft Tissues. Park Ridge, IL, AAOS Symposium, 1988.

3. Wyke, B.: The neurology of low back pain. *In* The Lumbar Spine and Back Pain, 3rd ed. (Edited by M. Jayson). London, Churchill Livingstone, pp. 56–99, 1987.

4. Mooney, V.: The Disc. *In* New Prospectives on Low Back Pain (Edited by J. Frymoyer and S. Gordon). Park Ridge, IL, American Academy of Orthopedic Surgeons, 1989.

5. Bell, G., et al.: A study of computer-assisted tomography. II. Comparison of metrizamide myelography and computered tomography in the diagnosis of herniated lumbar disc and spinal stenosis. Spine *9*:552–556, 1984.

6. Wiesel, S., Tsourmas, N., Feffer, H., Citrin, C., Patronas, N.: A study of computer-assisted tomography. I: the incidence of positive CAT scans in an asymptomatic group of patients. Spine *9*:549–551, 1984.

7. Jackson, R., Jacobs, R., Montesano, P.: Facet joint injection in low back pain: a prospective statistical study. Spine *13*:966–971, 1988.

8. Vanharanta, H., et al.: Disc deterioration in low-back syndromes: a prospective, multi-center CT/discography study. Spine *13*:1349–1351, 1988.

9. Weinstein, J., Claverie, W., Gibson, S.: The pain of discography. Spine *13*:1344–1348, 1988.

10. Holt, E.: The question of lumbar discography. J Bone Joint Surg *50A*:720–726, 1968.

11. Urban, J., Maroudas, A.: The chemistry of the intervertebral disc in relation to its physiological function and requirements. Clin Rheumatol Dis *6*:51–76, 1980.

12. Holm, S., Nachemson, A.: Variations in the nutrition of the canine intervertebral disc induced by motion. Spine *8*:866–874, 1983.

13. Taylor, T., Ghosh, P., Braund, K., Sutherland, J., Sherwood, A.: The effect of spinal fusion on intervertebral disc composition: an experimental study. J Surg Res *21*:91–104, 1976.

14. Videman, T.: Connective tissue and immobilization: key factors in musculoskeletal degeneration. Clin Orthop *221*:26–32, 1987.

15. Cole, T., Burkhardt, D., Ghosh, P., Ryan, M., Taylor, T.: Effects of spinal fusion on the proteoglycans of the canine intervertebral disc. J Orthop Res *3*:277–291, 1985.

16. Holm, S., Nachemson, A.: Nutritional changes in the canine intervertebral disc after spinal fusion. Clin Orthop *169*:234–258, 1982.

17. Tipton, C., Vailas, A., Matthes, R.: Experimental studies on the influences of physical activity on ligaments, tendons and joints: a brief review. Acta Med Scand (Suppl) *711*:157–168, 1985.

18. Radin, E.: The role of muscles in protecting athletes from injury. Acta Med Scand (Suppl) *711*:143–147, 1985.

19. Akeson, W., Amiel, D., Woo, S.: Immobility effects on synovial joints: the pathomechanics of joint contracture. Biorheology *17*:95–100, 1980.

20. Gelberman, R., et al.: Flexor tendon repair. J Orthop Res *4*:119–128, 1986.

21. Rubin, C., Lanyon, L.: Osteoregulatory nature of mechanical stimuli: function as a determinant for adaptive remodeling in bone. J Orthop Res *5*:300–310, 1987.

22. Montgomery, J., Steadman, J.: Rehabilitation of the injured knee. Clin Sports Med *4*:333–343, 1985.

23. Salter, R., Field, P.: The effects of continuous compression on living articular cartilage: an experimental study. J Bone Joint Surg *43B*:376–386, 1961.

24. Mayer, T., Gatchel, R.: Functional Restoration for Spinal Disorders: The Sports Medicine Approach. Philadelphia, Lea & Febiger, 1988.

25. Bortz, W.: The disuse syndrome. West J Med *141*:691–694, 1984.

26. Akeson, W., Amiel, D., Abel, M., Garfin, S., Woo, S.: Effects of immobilization on joints. Clin Orthop *219*:28–37, 1987.

27. Keeley J, et al.: Quantification of lumbar function. 5. Reliabil-

ity range of motion measures in the sagittal plane and in vivo torso rotation measurement technique. Spine *11*:31–35, 1986.

28. Mayer, T., Kishino, N., Keeley, J., Mayer, S., Mooney, V.: Using physical measurements to assess low back pain. J Musculoskel Med *2*:44–59, 1985.

29. Mayer, T., Tencer, A., Kristofferson, S., Mooney, V.: Use of noninvasive techniques for quantification of spinal range-of-motion in normal subjects and chronic low-back dysfunction patients. Spine *9*:588–595, 1984.

30. Pearcy, M.: Measurement of back and spinal mobility. Clin Biomech *1*:44–51, 1986.

31. Davies, G., Gould, J.: Trunk testing using a prototype cybex II isokinetic stabilization system. J Orthop Sports Phys Ther *3*:164–170, 1982.

32. Mayer, T., Smith, S., Keeley, J., Mooney, V.: Quantification of lumbar function. 2. Sagittal plane trunk strength in chronic low back pain patients. Spine *10*:765–772, 1985.

33. Smith, S., Mayer, T., Gatchel, R., Becker, T.: Quantification of lumbar function. 1. Isometric and multispeed isokinetic trunk strength measures in sagittal and axial planes in normal subject patients. Spine *10*:757–764, 1985.

34. Mayer, T., et al.: Quantification of lumbar function. 3. Preliminary data on isokinetic torso rotation testing with myoelectric spectral analysis in normal and low back pain subjects. Spine *10*:912–920, 1985.

35. Thompson, N., Gould, J., Davies, G., Ross, D., Price, S.: Descriptive measures of isokinetic trunk testing. J Orthop Sports Phys Ther *7*:43–49, 1985.

36. Mayer, T.: Assessment of lumbar function. Clin Orthop *221*:99–109, 1987.

37. Chaffin, D., Herrin, G., Keyserling, W.: Pre-employment strength testing: an updated position. J Occup Med *20*:403–408, 1979.

38. Kishino, N., et al.: Quantification of lumbar function. Part 4. Isometric and isokinetic lifting simulation in normal subjects and low back dysfunction patients. Spine *10*:921–927, 1985.

39. Ayoub, M., Mital, A., Bakken, G., Asfour, S., Bethea, N.: Development of strength and capacity norms for manual materials handling activities: the state-of-the-art. Human Factors *22*:271–283, 1980.

40. Mayer, T., et al.: Progressive isoinertial lifting evaluation. I. A standardized protocol and normative database. Spine *13*:993–997, 1988.

41. Mayer, T., et al.: Progressive isoinertial lifting evaluation. II. A comparison with isokinetic lifting in a disabled chronic low-back pain industrial population. Spine *13*:998–1002, 1988.

42. Kohles, S., Barnes, D., Gatchel, R., Mayer, T.: Improved functional restoration of industrial injury CLBP patients. Spine (In Press).

43. American Medical Association Guides to the Evaluation of Permanent Impairment, 3rd ed. (Edited by A. Engelberg). Chicago, AMA Press, 1988.

44. Carlsoo, S.: With what degree of precision can voluntary static muscle force be repeated? Scand J Rehab Med *18*:1–3, 1986.

45. Hazard, R. Reid, S., Fenwick, J., Reeves, J: Isokinetic trunk and lifting strength measurements: variability as an indicator of effort. *Spine 13*:54–57, 1988.

46. Capra, P., Mayer, T., Gatchel, R.: Adding psychological scales to your back pain assessment. J Muscle Med *2*:41–52, 1985.

47. Mooney, V., Cairns, D., Robertson, J.: A system for evaluating and treating chronic back disability. West J Med *124*:370–376, 1976.

48. Beck, A.: Depression: clinical, experimental and theoretical aspects. New York, Harper & Row, 1967.

49. Million, R., et al.: Evaluation of low back pain and assessment of lumbar corsets with and without back supports. Ann Rheumatol Dis *40*:449–454, 1981.

26

Robert J. Gatchel

Early Development of Physical and Mental Deconditioning in Painful Spinal Disorders

The time course of low back pain often leads to perceptual distortion among medical observers. More than 90% of the time, back pain is a brief, time-limited condition for which the treatment chosen often appears irrelevant to the outcome. From the onset of symptoms, about half of the patients with acute low back pain are no longer disabled within 2 weeks, 70% have recovered in 1 month, and about 90% within 3 to 4 months. Yet, of those whose symptoms persist for more than 3 to 4 months, about 50 to 60% continue to be disabled at the end of the year, and the majority of these continue to be disabled even after 2 years. These individuals often go on to extensive medical treatment, compensation costs, and settlement awards that make their contribution to the problem disproportionate to that of the entire group suffering acute low back pain. In fact, 10% of the cases cost about 80% of the compensation money in a variety of industries.[1]

Mayer and Gatchel[1] have thoroughly discussed how sports medicine principles can be effectively applied in the treatment of spinal disorders. This chapter discusses the application of such principles to avoid the early development of physical and mental or psychological deconditioning, which can subsequently lead to chronic disability and the aforementioned dramatic costs. The longer the period of initial immobilization and inactivity, the greater the likelihood of developing various dysfunctional behaviors. These dysfunctional behaviors may be succeeded by further loss of physical capacity indices such as motion, strength, endurance, and agility. The longer the period of such inactivity, the greater the opportunity for disuse to create physical capacity deficits leading to decreased human performance, and ultimately to a variety of maladaptive psychosocial and affective concomitants such as depression, medication abuse, and disability habituation. Pain is usually an important parallel focus in the treatment of these disorders, but its direct relationship to changes in muscle or other mesothelial structures remains elusive. However, a major conceptual breakthrough in better understanding this association has been the recent recognition of the relationship between fitness and back pain.[1]

SPORTS MEDICINE PRINCIPLES AND THE DECONDITIONING SYNDROME

Physical Deconditioning

Sports medicine principles have been used not merely to treat the competitive athlete, but in a modified way to treat all individuals wishing to return to high levels of function after extremity injury. The following summary, previously presented by Mayer and Gatchel,[1] focuses on some of the basic principles of sports medicine rehabilitation that have been used in the extremities, primarily focusing on the knee. Many of these principles can be applied to the back.

In simplified terms, the initial phases of injury are

characterized by hemorrhage and edema. Within the first few days, cellular infiltration and enzymatic degradation occur, involving prostaglandins, bradykinins, and kallikreins. This inflammatory process involves clearing of necrotic substances. A proliferative phase follows, with its timing and duration related to the quality of the blood supply in the area; random deposition of collagen fibrils takes place initially. In subsequent phases, the collagen fibrils align along lines of stress (Wolff's Law of Mesothelial Tissues).

Quite understandably, a small amount of tissue injury with relatively good nutrition and low grade stresses, such as a wrist sprain or muscle contusion, proceeds through this process quickly. However, for the lumbar spine area extremely high stresses, large musculoligamentous structures, and poor blood supply (particularly involving the discs) probably make for considerably delayed healing. At the end of the healing process, however, the injured area is left with a scar, visible or hidden, which has matured to fill the injured area but lacks the resilience, strength, and durability of the original tissue. Such an asymmetric scar, produced either by injury, degeneration, or surgical trauma, may produce severe disturbances of biomechanical performance in the critical lumbar spine articulations.

A particular characteristic of the injured individual is to splint and protect the injured area. As noted in the previous chapter, this leads to a series of events that end in what has been termed the "deconditioning syndrome." "Mental deconditioning," discussed in the next section, follows as a natural consequence of physiological deconditioning.

Deconditioning is a progressive process related to disuse, the onset of which cannot be precisely documented. Some factors are clearly mechanical, such as maintaining static postures, wearing a brace, and prolonged or excessive bed rest. Others are more difficult to define, such as a painful peripheral stimulus that alters muscle tone through a set of neurologically mediated processes. Changes in the spinal reflex arc may reflect one such mechanism; higher centers may also be involved in the process. What is clear is that if the deconditioning process is not terminated, the process becomes a progressive cycle in which lower physical capacity predisposes to pain recurrence, which results in lower and lower levels of physical activity. The pain induced by increased activity may be perceived by the patient as a "new injury," leading to renewed efforts to find a solution through the medical care system. Mental passivity, dependence, and depression usually accompany the physical changes.

As Mayer noted in Chapter 1 of this text, inactivity and disuse leading to deconditioning can be modeled in both humans and experimental animals through immobilization studies. Research in this area has consistently demonstrated the negative effects of such immobilization on soft tissue homeostasis.[2,7] For example, healing tissue that is immobilized has a tendency to produce an amorphous, nonfunctional scar with low strength when it has been subjected to healing without adequate physiologic stress.

It should also be pointed out that the adverse effects of rest and disuse have been documented for every body system. For example, a review of the literature by Bortz[8] demonstrates that bedrest results in protein loss of approximately 8 grams per day and calcium loss of up to 1.54 grams per week. Inactivity also results in a great loss in cardiovascular functioning, including decreases in cardiac output and stroke volume, and increases in peripheral resistance and systolic blood pressure. Thus, the deconditioning effects are widespread and affect strength, flexibility, and endurance factors.

A recent study by Mayer, et al.,[9] present some intriguing results that further suggest the negative effects of deconditioning on spinal musculature. This study compared the computer tomography (CT) scan of muscle area/muscle density to isokinetic trunk strength for a group of spinal surgery patients 3 months postoperatively. Results demonstrated the trunk strength mean to be below 50% of gender-specific "normal" values obtained by evaluating a normative sample. Extensor strength was more significantly affected than flexor strength. Thus, significant postsurgery deficiencies in muscle strength were evidenced, as would be expected because of the deconditioning that would occur during recovery. The other interesting finding was that the single-cut CT scans performed at the time of isokinetic trunk strength assessment demonstrated psoas and erector spinal atrophy through a significant decrease in muscle density, with only a trend toward decreased cross-sectional area.

Figure 26–1 presents a typical CT scan slice from a normal comparison group subject from this study, taken at the inferior aspect of the L3 pedicle. The slice demonstrates normal findings for density and cross-sectional area of the erector, psoas, rectus abdominus, and oblique musculature. In contrast, Figure 26–2 depicts findings in a typical postoperative patient with a radiographic cut taken at the same level. In comparing these two figures, although all muscle groups show differences in density and cross-sectional area, (reflecting both anatomic size and physiologic atrophy differences), the most profound differences are noted in the erector spinae and rectus abdominus musculature.

Results of the study also indicated that a significant correlation exists between increased mechanical trunk strength performance and greater muscle den-

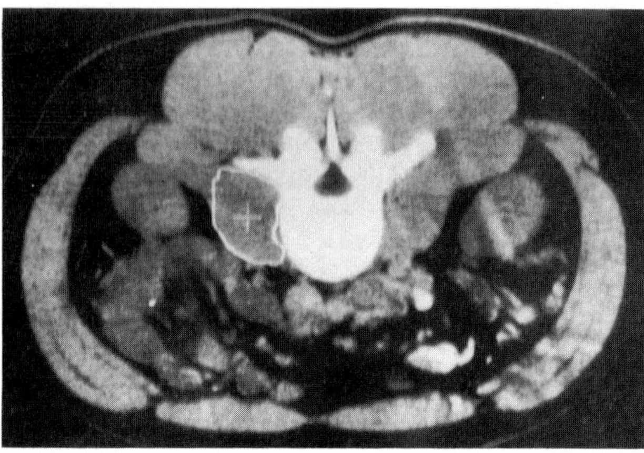

Figure 26–1. Single-cut CT scan of whole body taken at level of inferior aspect of L3 pedicle. (From Mayer, T.G., et al.: Comparison of CT scan muscle measurements and isokinetic trunk strength in postoperative patients. Spine 14:33–36, 1989.)

sity as seen on CT scan in the patient sample. Although it is still uncertain whether CT scanning density measurements can be used clinically to document muscle atrophy, these findings are intriguing because they suggest an association between disuse and deconditioning, trunk strength, and muscle atrophy. Future research will hopefully more clearly delineate these relationships.

Mental Deconditioning

Besides the physical deconditioning that can develop as a consequence of chronicity and disuse, a

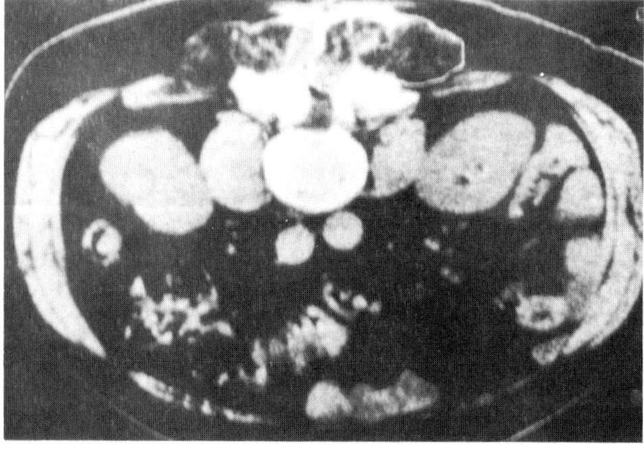

Figure 26–2. Single slice from CT scan taken at same level in study subject 3 months postoperatively. (From Mayer, T.G., et al.: Comparison of CT scan muscle measurements and isokinetic trunk strength in postoperative patients. Spine 14:33–36, 1989.)

collateral form of mental deconditioning also occurs. This refers to the development of a "layer" of behavioral and psychological problems that occur in response to the chronic pain and the patients' attempts to cope with it. These problems prevent the individual from maintaining a productive lifestyle. They prompt cessation or disuse of normal functioning, with all psychological resources being expended in an attempt to deal with the prolonged pain and disability. In a sense, there is an "atrophy" of normal functioning.

Fordyce and Steger[10] initially noted an important variable that differentiated acute from chronic pain—the type of anxiety experienced by the patient. In acute pain experiences, anxiety increases as pain intensity increases, which is then followed by a reduction in anxiety after treatment begins. A reduction in anxiety then generally results in a decrease in pain sensation. Thus, there is a cycle of pain reduction, followed by anxiety reduction, resulting in still more pain reduction, and so on. This cycle, however, is different for chronic pain patients. For these patients, the initial anxiety associated with the pain persists, and may eventually result in feelings of greater anxiety, despair, and helplessness because of the failure of the health system's attempts to alleviate it.

There is evidence to suggest that chronic pain patients develop specific psychological problems because of the failure of attempts to alleviate their pain that distinguish them from acute pain patients. For example, Sternach, Wolf, Murphy, and Akeson[11] compared the Minnesota Multiphasic Personality Inventory (MMPI) profiles of a group of acute low back pain patients (pain present for less than 6 months) to those of a group of chronic low back pain patients (more than 6 months). Results indicated significant differences between the two groups on the first three clinical scales (hypochrondiasis, depression, and hysteria). The combined elevation of these three scales is often referred to as the neurotic triad because it is commonly found in neurotic individuals who are experiencing a great deal of anxiety. These results indicate that during the early states of pain, no major psychological problems are produced by it. However, as the pain becomes chronic in nature, psychological changes begin to occur. These changes are most likely caused by the constant discomfort, despair, and preoccupation with the pain that comes to dominate the lives of these patients. As Sternbach[12] noted in his description of chronic-pain sufferers:

> Pain patients frequently say that they could stand their pain much better if they could only get a good night's sleep. They feel as though their resistance is weakened by their lack of sleep. They never feel

rested. They feel worn down, worn out, exhausted. They find themselves getting more and more irritable with their families, they have fewer and fewer friends, and fewer and fewer interests. Gradually as time goes on, the boundaries of their world seem to shrink. They become more and more preoccupied with the pain, less and less interested in the world around them. Their world begins to center around home, doctor's office, and pharmacy.

We found similar results from research conducted with chronic low back pain patients participating in a functional restoration program.[13] In this study, the first three clinical scales were significantly elevated before the start of the treatment program. However, at a 6-month followup after successful completion of this program, these scales were significantly *decreased* to normal levels. Thus, these results again suggest that the elevations of scores are most likely caused by the trauma and stress associated with the chronic pain condition and not by some stable psychological traits. When successfully treated, these elevations disappear. A graphic description of these results is presented in Chapter 36 of this text.

Thus, these results indicate that one of the consequences of dealing with chronic pain is the development of emotional reactions such as anxiety and dysphoria produced by the long-term "wearing down" effects and drain of psychological resources. This may produce a layer of behavioral and psychological problems over the original nociception or pain experience itself. It is generally accepted that chronic low back pain is a complex behavior that does not merely result from some specific structural cause.[1]

Indeed, Loeser[14,15] originally formulated a model outlining four dimensions associated with the concept of pain: nociception, pain, suffering, and pain behavior. *Nociception* refers to the actual physical units (chemical, mechanical, or thermal) that impact on specialized nerve fibers and signal the central nervous system that an aversive event has occurred.

Pain is the sensation arising as the result of perceived nociception. However, this definition is overly simplistic and less than certain because sometimes pain is perceived in the absence of nociception (e.g., phantom limb pain), or, conversely, when nociception occurs without being perceived (an individual being severely wounded without becoming immediately aware of the pain).

Nociception and pain act as signals to the central nervous system. In contrast, suffering and pain behavior are reactions to these signals that can be affected by past experiences as well as anticipation of future events. Specifically, according to Loeser, *suffering* refers to the emotional responses that are triggered by nociception or some other aversive event associated with it such as fear, threat, or loss. Because of a specific painful episode, the individual may lose his or her job and, as a consequence, develop anxiety and depression. *Pain behavior* refers to those things that individuals do when they are suffering or are in pain. For example, they may avoid exercise for fear of reinjury.

This biopsychosocial conceptual model of pain, which includes physical, psychological, and social elements, moves away from an overly simplistic physical disease model of pain, and replaces it with an alternative multidimensional model. It draws upon the biopsychosocial concept of illness originally proposed by Engel.[16] A similar model has been presented by Waddell[17] in discussing the treatment of chronic low back pain. Figure 26–3 presents these models.

To date, little empirical research has been conducted to evaluate these models or to assess the progression or development of this mental deconditioning process. Figure 26–4 presents my conceptual model proposing a number of stages that may be involved. The model is yet untested, but does present a number of testable hypotheses and important treatment implications. As can be seen, Stage 1 is emotional reactions such as fear, anxiety and worry, that result as a consequence of the perception of

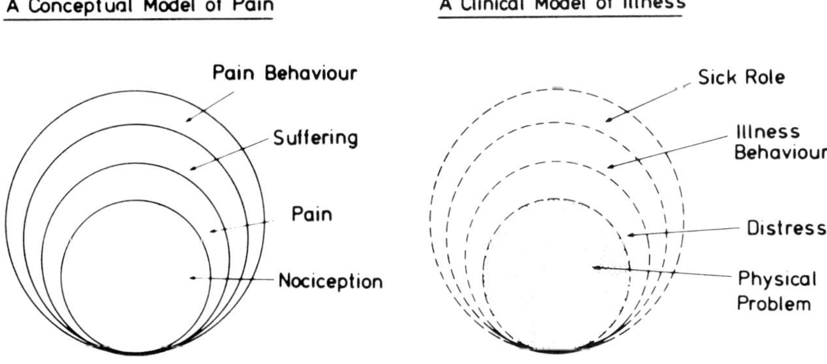

Figure 26–3. The biopsychosocial concept of illness (Engel, 1977 and Loeser, 1982) conceptual model of pain. (From Waddell, G.A.: A new clinical model for the treatment of low back pain. Spine 12:637, 1987.)

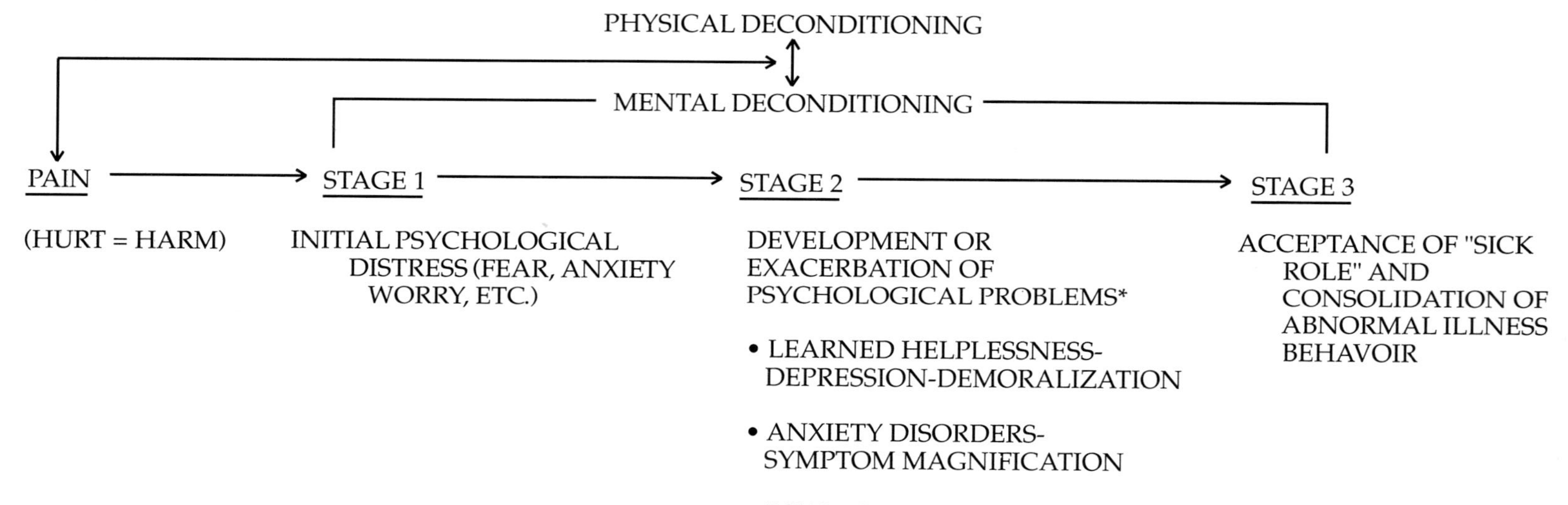

Figure 26—4. Progression of the mental deconditioning process, and its interaction with physical deconditioning.

pain. Pain or hurt is usually associated with harm, and there is a natural emotional reaction to the potential for the physical harm. If the pain persists past a reasonable acute period of time, this leads to the progression into Stage 2. This stage is associated with a wider array of behavioral and psychological reactions and problems, such as learned helplessness and depression, anger and distrust, and somatization, which are the result of suffering with the now chronic nature of the pain. It should be noted that the form these problems take primarily depends upon the *premorbid* or pre-existing personality and psychological characteristics of the individual, as well as current socioeconomic and environmental conditions. Thus, for an individual with a premorbid depressive personality who is seriously affected economically by loss of a job due to the pain and disability, depressive symptoms are greatly exacerbated during this stage. Similarly, an individual who had premorbid hypochrondriacal characteristics and who receives a great deal of secondary gain remaining disabled, will most likely display a great deal of somatization and symptom magnification.

Table 26–1 uses the example of depression to present the type of interactions that can occur between premorbid personality and psychological characteristics of an individual, socioeconomic variables (e.g., loss of income or job), and environmental factors. It should be noted that one of the major environmental factors is the presence or absence of social support, because social support has been shown to significantly buffer individuals from the impact of stress.[18] Other such environmental factors might be the secondary gain involved in being excused from normal responsibilities and obligations.

Obviously, this model does *not* propose that there is a pre-existing "pain personality," in keeping with a great deal of research that has not found any such consistent personality syndrome.[1] Rather, patients bring with them certain predisposing personality and psychological characteristics, i.e., they have a *diathesis* that is exacerbated by the stress of attempting to cope with the chronic pain. Basically, this is a diathesis-stress model. Indeed, the relationship between stress and exacerbation of mental health problems has been documented in the scientific literature.[19] This is not to say that predisposing factors make chronic low back pain a functional disorder and it is "all in the patient's head." The chronic problem represents a complex interaction between physical factors and psychosocioeconomic variables.

When one views the results of a National Institute of Mental Health epidemiologic study on the 1 month prevalence of various mental disorders in the general population,[20] it is not surprising that there are often psychiatric problems associated with these patients since the base rates for such problems in the general population are high. For example, statistics indicate that the prevalence rates for anxiety disorders and affective disorders are 7.3 and 5.1 percent of the population, respectively; symptoms of schizophrenia are 0.7 percent; and abuse of alcohol and drugs is about 3.8 percent. Thus, 15.4 percent of the population has some significant mental health disorder. Moreover, these prevalence statistics do not take into account the probably equally prevalent personality disorders such as antisocial, borderline, and paranoid personalities.

Returning to our discussion of Figure 26–4, as this "layer" of behavioral and psychological problems persists, it leads to the progression into Stage 3, which can be viewed as the acceptance or adoption of a sick role during which the patient is excused

Table 26–1
Proposed Interactions Between Premorbid Depressive Characteristics, Socioeconomic Problems, and Environmental Social Support in Determining the Expected Level of Depression in a Chronic Pain Patient.

(IF)	Premorbid Depressive Characteristics Present?	(+)	Socioeconomic Problems Present?	(+)	Environmental Social Support Present?	(THEN)	Expected Level of Depression
	Yes		Yes		No		High
	Yes		Yes		Yes		Moderate-High
	Yes		No		Yes		Moderate
	Yes		No		No		Moderate
	No		Yes		No		Moderate-High
	No		Yes		Yes		Moderate-Low
	No		No		Yes		Low
	No		No		No		Low

from normal responsibilities and social obligations. This may become a potent reinforcer for not becoming healthy. The medical and psychological disabilities (abnormal illness behaviors) are consolidated during this phase. Moreover, if compensation issues are still present, they can also serve as a disincentive for not becoming well again because compensation is a critical factor in the persistence of disability.[21]

Superimposed on these stages is the physical deconditioning syndrome discussed earlier. Usually, a two-way pathway exists between the physical deconditioning and mental deconditioning processes. For example, research has clearly demonstrated that physical deconditioning can feedback, negatively affecting the emotional well being and self esteem of individuals.[18] This can lead to further mental deconditioning. Conversely, negative emotional reactions such as depression can significantly feedback to physical functioning by, for example, decreasing the motivation to get involved in work or recreational activities and thereby further contributing to physical deconditioning.

Finally, these physical and mental deconditioning effects can also feedback to the initial pain perception process. For example, if the individual suddenly engages in an activity that produces some acute soreness or tenderness, it may be erroneously interpreted as harmful. This can then retrigger or reinforce the emotions and psychological problems associated with the other stages. Indeed, clinical researchers such as Fordyce[22] suggest that chronic pain patients must learn that hurt and harm are not the same. They must be re-educated to not accept the traditional dogma that pain is always a warning signal. Pain often accompanies the early stages of physical reconditioning and does not necessarily mean that some physical harm is being produced.

REVERSING THE DECONDITIONING SYNDROMES

Results such as those reviewed earlier revealing strength deficits in the postoperative patient may lead to improvements in rehabilitation and alter the results of a variety of surgical procedures. In general, the physiologic approach to the deconditioning syndrome, for both surgical and nonsurgical patients, involves exercise to address mobility, strength, endurance, and cardiovascular deficits. The exercises must then progress to involve simulation of customary physical activities to restore task-specific endurance, coordination, and agility through restoring neuromuscular inputs.[23] Obviously, the exercises must be focused at the specific functional units that have become deconditioned. Fi-

nally, mental reconditioning and a continued maintenance program must be initiated, including returning to the sport or work and activities of daily living characteristic of productivity. Effectively dealing with the psychological and behavioral problems that may develop during the different stages of mental deconditioning requires as much attention as dealing with the physical issues. One cannot deal with one without simultaneously dealing with the other.

Physical Reconditioning

Strength may be restored after injury in a variety of modes. Initially, soon after injury when continued immobilization may be necessary, isometric exercise may be the only type that can be performed by the patient. This involves exercising against a fixed resistance without accompanying joint motion. These exercises may be done in a cast or splint, but the method has many drawbacks. First, it is the most fatiguing and least effective type of exercise.[24] There is specificity of strength training to the length of the muscle fibers at the time of training, with rapid fall off in training efficiency at different muscle fiber lengths. Additionally, translation of endurance and agility from isometric training is limited to specific functional activities, though the exercises can be used during the early rest phases to maintain strength and produce relative resistance to muscle atrophy. There is also some suggestion of a benefit of electrical muscle stimulation in combination with isometric exercise, but some question of higher injury potential may be associated with overvigorous acceleration into a static pull.[25]

Dynamic muscle training, which has been shown to be the most efficient method of muscle training, can also be employed. It involves three basic modes: isotonic, isokinetic, and psychophysical (free weights).[26] *Isotonic* exercises are those in which the same force is applied throughout the dynamic range, and is often inappropriately used for exercises in which a changing lever arm actually alters the weight applied. This type of exercise is most appropriate to the variable resistance devices, utilizing a cam to maximize and equalize muscular demands throughout the dynamic range of motion.

By contrast, *isokinetic* devices require a sophisticated dynamometer, which limits the speed to a preset level. Thus, isokinetics maintain speed while allowing the production of torque around a central axis, thereby eliminating the effect of acceleration on energy production. These devices are generally accommodating to force application (providing injury protection), but also do not simulate the "real world" because of the compromises of the speed selection system. Unlike variable resistance devices, however, high speed training is possible to develop some specific agility and coordination goals.

Finally, psychophysical strength training using free weights, is limited to those positions in which weights can be attached to the body or held in the hands. The method is so termed because the subject self-selects the amount of weight that is acceptable. Although this is the closest to the "real world" strengthening, the maximum weight that can be handled is limited by the weakest portion of the dynamic range of motion and further compromised by limitations of the changing lever arm. However, if the exercise can be produced to simulate actual tasks or motions of the sport or work activity to which the patient is returning, this may be an effective training tool. Psychophysical and variable resistance lifting devices automatically provide concentric and eccentric contraction capability. This is more difficult and dangerous to provide in isokinetic devices, though computerized devices are being developed to produce these effects.

Secondary effects of a sports medicine program are also critically important. Training appears to have a specific beneficial effect on pain, and has been specifically demonstrated to prevent scarring and adhesions while improving cartilage nutrition.[3] This may be done initially through passive, and later through active, means.[2,5,27] Development of supernormal strength and endurance may be beneficial in protecting the damaged or unstable joint, particularly when complete return of normal architecture can no longer be anticipated.

Physical Progression Issues

The sports medicine approach involves a progression of physical activity in a graduated fashion. In Chapter 35 of this text, Mayer has succinctly summarized the important issues involved in such physical progression. How to provide this process to minimize pain complaints and also to provide sufficient tissue response to produce increased joint mobility and muscle strength and endurance, is the heart of the conundrum. These choices are generally made on an empirical basis, using information obtained from treating large numbers of patients. Specialists in the area of spinal disorders generally agree that pain cannot be "cured" in the majority of chronic cases. The complete cessation of pain is seldom a goal that should be presented to patients. Rather the adage "no pain, no gain" should be explicitly communicated to patients. They must move away from the misperception that hurt is always equated with harm.

As one might expect in the chronically disabled back pain patient, progression tends to be slow in the majority of patients unless they are cajoled by the therapist. However, in a minority of patients, a combination of impulsiveness and lack of coordination predisposes them to recurrent injury if they are not carefully monitored and kept within the limits of a graduated program. These "accident-prone" individuals are at the opposite end of the spectrum. The subacute work-motivated executive or professional person usually falls somewhere in between.

The critical aspect of progression is that it cannot be permitted to occur in a haphazard manner. The therapist, most important of all examiners, must recognize the limitations of relying on patient complaints and visual and palpatory skills alone in making judgments. The therapist must learn to place increasing reliance on objective functional capacity assessment technology for mobility, strength, and endurance, with tests being performed at multiple intervals throughout the treatment process. Furthermore, a generic program designed for all, like Williams' exercises, is inappropriate because the type and degree of deficits vary greatly from one patient to the next. Therefore, treatment programs must be individualized from the beginning, and modified as necessary based on the progression actually demonstrated by the patient.

As in other training regimens, progressive resistance above the subject's current capabilities may produce a painful episode that is interpreted by the patient as a new injury. In actuality, the patient has merely exceeded his or her pain threshold, which has generally been reduced to a low level by disuse, emotional distress, or medication. Such episodes are not merely common, they are nearly universal and must be dealt with promptly and effectively if the patient's confidence and willingness to participate in rehabilitation is to be maintained. Moreover, the need for education provided by the therapist to constantly validate the progression procedures in the patient's mind cannot be overemphasized.

The interrelationship between pain and progression is a fascinating one. Continued pain (the only perception the patient really has of back function) is often misinterpreted as a sign of failure to progress, leading the patient to become discouraged and decrease his adherence to training regimens. The physical therapist must be diligent in education on pain relief maneuvers consistent with the training, and also prepared to perform physical quantification tests as pain is increasing. By seeing progress on physical capacity in spite of pain, the patient is encouraged, develops a sense of mastery over fear and pain, and begins seeing himself or herself as more functional and on the road to recovery once again. Although the primary goal of rehabilitation is to re-

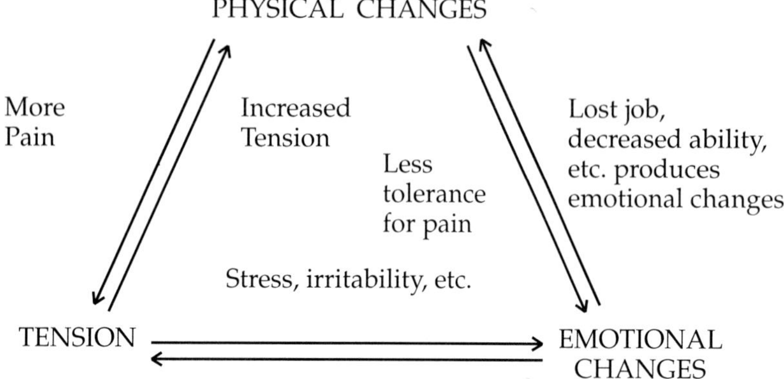

Figure **26–5.** The contribution of physical changes, emotional changes, and tension to the chronic pain process. (From Mayer, T.G., Gatchel, R.J.: Functional Restoration for Spinal Disorders: The Sports Medicine Approach. Philadelphia, Lea & Febiger, 1988.)

store function, the diminution of pain is a secondary goal that receives the therapist's highest priority. Because the patient is already well acquainted with the fact that pain can be relieved, albeit temporarily, by inactivity and passive modalities, it requires all of the therapist's skill to keep the patient's "eye on the ball" of functional restoration.

Mental Reconditioning

In addition to the above physical deconditioning effects, one must also be aware of many psychological factors that can contribute to an acute back pain episode becoming chronic. As discussed earlier in this chapter, a patient may progress through a number of stages (Fig. 26–4) as his or her pain and disability becomes more chronic. These may create formidable barriers to recovery if they are not effectively dealt with. As I review in Chapter 36 of this text, these barriers include psychological, functional, legal, social, and work-related issues that can significantly interfere with the patient's return to full functioning and a productive lifestyle. Psychologically, these barriers encompass traditional concepts such as secondary gain (e.g., the back episode may be allowing the individual to avoid an unpleasant job situation); symptom magnification (an increased sensitivity and concern about physical symptoms as a means of justifying continued disability); and resistance to change. At other times, real interfering circumstances may be used as smoke screens or excuses for sub-optimal performance and failure to adhere to the treatment regimen.

Treatment personnel must also be alert to potential secondary gains of continued disability, whether legal, financial, job-related, or familial. It is important that members of the treatment team are knowledgeable of all psychosocial issues while the patient is in rehabilitation. This knowledge allows staff members not only to better understand and serve the patient, but also to be more effective in problem-solving when the patient is not physically progressing as expected. Indeed, failure to progress physically generally represents psychosocial barriers to recovery, because the muscles and joints will not fail to respond if they are being exercised and trained as planned (unless rare denervation or ankylosis has occurred).

These barriers to recovery issues must be effectively assessed and brought to the attention of the entire treatment team. Steps can then be taken to understand their origins and avoid their interference with treatment goals. Again, in Chapter 36 of the text, I review various barriers to recovery, such as compliance and resistance issues, financial disincentives, symptom magnification, and general emotional reactions, such as depression, anger, entitlement, anxiety, and fear. It must be impressed upon the patient that psychological and emotional factors are invariably involved in the pain syndrome. Figure 26–5 presents a diagram that can be shown to patients to explain this relationship. Physical changes and their effects (such as inability to work, play, financial difficulties) can lead to emotional changes, such as anger, anxiety, depression, frustration, etc. These emotional changes, in turn, can lead to increased stress and tension, which exacerbates pain. The cycle can also work in the opposite direction, with physical changes and pain leading to increased tension, which produces additional stress and irritability, which leads to less tolerance for pain. Once the cycle is completed, it can begin at any new point in the cycle and start the whole process again.

RESEARCH ON PSYCHOSOCIAL PREDICTORS OF DISABILITY

An interesting and important question is why some patients progress through the deconditioning stages and assume the sick role more readily than others, and why they go on to experience chronic disability even though no significant organic cause can be found? Recent studies have been noteworthy for their attempts to identify psychosocial variables as possible predictors of costly back injuries in uninjured workers. Studies by Bigos and colleagues, for example, have identified job performance variables as possible predictors of costly back injuries in an uninjured industrial population.[28-30] Such predictors may be termed primary or preinjury predictors, in that they identify the percentage of an uninjured population likely to develop a low back pain incident. Secondary or prechronicity predictors identify those with an acute low back pain incident who are likely to develop chronic difficulties (5 to 10 percent of the injured population). Tertiary or chronic outcome predictors look at success and failure in the chronic patient. There is great research interest in isolating all three types of predictors.

Research has started to identify some important secondary predictors. For example, Frymoyer and Cats-Baril[31] presented a general multiattribute model devised by a panel of noted experts in this area. This model assigns relative weights to an array of variables thought to be involved in ultimate chronic low back pain-related disability. Such a model will hopefully provide a foundation for establishing secondary predictors. However, the model is yet to be tested and validated.

Polatin, et al.,[32] developed a psychosociomedical prediction model of success and failure in response to a comprehensive functional restoration program undertaken by workers who were chronically disabled with low back pain. A number of separate variables evaluated at the beginning of the treatment program were isolated and found to significantly predict those chronic low back pain patients who subsequently respond to a functional restoration program (Table 26–2). Such findings are encourag-

ing in demonstrating that the development of a tertiary prediction model is feasible. They again highlight the important role that various psychosocial factors, in combination with physical variables, can play in the development and progression of chronic spinal disorders.

PSYCHOPHYSIOLOGIC INHIBITION EFFECTS

Besides the psychosocial barriers to recovery discussed earlier, there are more subtle inhibitory factors that can significantly affect performance. Patients may enter a program with muscular deficits of varying degrees. Often, extremely low strength levels in patients are not a sign of severely advanced muscle atrophy in producing extreme loss of muscle bulk or fatty replacement. Rather, these deficits generally represent other factors, including neuromuscular inhibition, alteration of neural input to the muscle from higher centers, and conscious or unconscious fear of reinjury.

It is important for the therapist to keep in mind that changes brought about by factors other than structural loss of muscle bulk may be reversed quickly by training, and dramatic increases in measured trunk strength may be achieved during a short intensive training program. These changes are usually caused by enhanced cooperation and confidence rather than alteration in muscle bulk. Strength changes based on alteration of muscle size are harder to achieve and take considerably longer. Thus, some persistent physical capacity deficits following intensive training are the rule rather than the exception in chronically disabled back patients. It is critical that the patient continues to improve physical capacity through a home maintenance program of exercise. These programs may be assisted by a variety of home devices or regular attendance at a fitness center or health club, provided the appropriate variable resistance equipment is available. Ultimately, progressive change in muscle circumference may be demonstrable by single cut CT scans or magnetic resonance imaging.

A Study of Psychophysiological Inhibition Effects

A review of a study conducted at the Productive Rehabilitation Institute of Dallas for Ergonomics (PRIDE) illustrates the operation of inhibiting factors.[33] The purpose of this study was to evaluate the relative efficacy of a functional restoration treatment program at two distinct points in time. A group of chronic low back pain patients undergoing the comprehensive functional restoration during its first year of development (1983 to 1984) were compared with a

---

Table 26–2
Psychosociomedical Variables That Predict Chronic Low Back Pain Patients Who Responded Best to a Functional Restoration Program (Polatin, et al., 1989)

Lower back pain intensity ratings

Lower visual analog pain scores

Lower Beck depression inventory scores

Lower premorbid pessimism levels

Longer time at job before injury

Job still available after treatment

Reduced true lumbar flexion levels

Fewer operations

Sex of patient (model more predictive for male patients)

similar group of patients who completed the rehabilitation program in 1987. Such a comparison allowed an evaluation of the effect of the changes that occurred during the evolution of the treatment program, specifically, the expanded pre-program treatment phase emphasizing education and exposure to functional restoration principles, and a more aggressive rehabilitation and reconditioning philosophy, may have had on important physical capacity outcome criteria such as trunk strength and spinal range of motion.

The results of this study clearly demonstrated improved functional capacity performance for the 1983/1984 and 1987 groups of chronic low back pain patients following participation in functional restoration treatment. More important, however, the results indicated that the patients from the 1987 program achieved greater functional capacity levels than the earlier patients, both at program admission and at discharge.

Differences between these two groups at program admission were particularly noteworthy. The magnitude of these differences suggested severe deficiencies in spinal strength and range of motion in the 1983/1984 patient group at the time of program admission. Such deficiencies were significantly lower in the 1987 program graduates. It was speculated that the inclusion of an expanded pre-program treatment phase, which emphasized education and exposure to the treatment philosophy, may have "desensitized" patients to the treatment facility. This, in turn, may have produced an earlier decrease of inhibitory factors, both neuromuscular and psychological, that can negatively affect rehabilitation efforts. These higher functional capacity levels appear to reflect performance increments rather than actual strength gains in 1987 program patients, because strength gains of such magnitude are an unlikely consequence of a pre-program phase, which emphasizes education and mild flexibility exercises for 2 to 6 weeks. Indeed, desensitizing patients to the treatment environment and functional restoration philosophy most likely decreased inhibitory factors, such as fear of reinjury, that can impede reconditioning. Such inhibitory factors appear to contribute to the extreme deficiencies in functional capacity levels observed in early patients as much as muscle atrophy does. Of course, further research is necessary to more specifically isolate the relative contributions of these factors to decreased functional capacity levels.

The higher functional capacity levels in these patients at program discharge were also striking. A combination of two factors most likely explains these findings. The first was the decrease in inhibitory factors, believed to be related to pre-program phase training. When limiting factors such as pain and fear of reinjury are decreased, the patient appears to make greater performance efforts to achieve the maximum levels that they would be able to achieve without any new training or rehabilitation efforts. The second factor relates to increases in actual functional capacity levels resulting from training. As the treatment staff became more knowledgeable in the use of new functional capacity technology and as more normative data were collected to provide objective guidelines for therapists to use in "coaching" patients to certain strength and range of motion levels, the therapist became more aggressive in prompting patients to achieve higher levels of function over the course of the treatment program. In a sense, the treatment staff became "disinhibited" along with the patients, and became more aggressive in their treatment demands. Of course, this increased aggressiveness was carefully monitored and based upon objective and quantified data concerning safe levels of performance. The adherence to objective data, along with subjective or intuitive processes or judgments made by individual therapists, drove the rehabilitation effort. We have discussed at length elsewhere the critical importance of developing a normative database for physical capacity measures in order to effectively guide the reconditioning process.[1] It is also noteworthy that this more aggressive, but quantitatively guided, treatment philosophy did not result in increased aggravation of injuries.

The above results clearly demonstrate the operation of important inhibition effects that can significantly affect physical performance. Of course, a great deal of research is needed to isolate the specific underpinnings of such effects. However, such findings again illustrate the array of potential factors that can directly or indirectly affect physical performance.

SUMMARY

The method by which sports medicine principles can be effectively applied in the treatment of spinal disorders in order to avoid the early development of physical and mental deconditioning was discussed in this chapter. The longer the period of initial immobilization and inactivity, the greater the likelihood of developing various dysfunctional behaviors associated with physical capacity indices such as motion, strength, endurance, and agility. Physical reconditioning is important in order to avoid the development of these dysfunctional behaviors. Moreover, the development of mental deconditioning, and how it interacts with physical deconditioning, in the progression from an acute pain episode to a chronic stage was discussed. The greater the opportunity for disuse to create physical capacity deficits leading to decreased human performance, the greater the likelihood of a variety of psychosocial concomitants such as depression, medication abuse, and disability habituation. More subtle psychophysiological inhibitory factors, such as neuromuscular inhibition and fear of reinjury, can significantly affect rehabilitation performance.

REFERENCES

1. Mayer, T.G., Gatchel, R.J.: Functional Restoration for Spinal Disorders: The Sports Medicine Approach. Philadelphia, Lea & Febiger, 1988.
2. Akeson, W., Amiel, D., Woo, S.: Immobility effects on synovial joints. The pathomechanics of joint contracture. Biorheology 17:95–100, 1980.
3. Gelberman, R., et al.: Flexor tendon repair. J Orthop Res 4:119–128, 1986.
4. Montgomery, J., Steadman, J.: Rehabilitation of the injured knee. Clin Sports Med 4:333–343, 1985.
5. Salter, R., Field, P.: The effects of continuous compression on living articular cartilage. An experimental study. J Bone Joint Surg 43B:376–386, 1961.
6. Ruben, C.: Osteoregulatory Mechanism. Trans Annu Meet Am Acad Orthop Surg, New Orleans, 1985.
7. Woo, S., Buckwalter, J.: Injury and repair of the musculoskeletal soft tissues. Park Ridge, IL, AAOS Symposium, 1988.
8. Bortz, W.: The disuse syndrome (commentary). West J Med 141:691–694, 1984.
9. Mayer, T.G., et al.: Comparison of CT scan muscle measurements and isokinetic trunk strength in postoperative patients. Spine 14:33–36, 1989.
10. Fordyce, W.E., Steger, J.C.: Chronic pain. In Behavioral Medicine: Theory and Practice (Edited by O.F. Pomerleau and J.P. Brady). Baltimore, Williams & Wilkins, 1979.
11. Sternbach, R.A., Wolf, S.R., Murphy, R.W., Akeson, W.H.: Traits of pain patients: the low-back "loser". Psychosomatics 14:226–229, 1973.
12. Sternbach, R A · Pain Patients: Traits and Treatment. New York, Academic Press, 1974.
13. Barnes, D., Gatchel, R.J., Mayer, T.G., Barnett, J.: Changes in MMPI profile levels of chronic low back pain patients following successful treatment. J Spinal Dis. In press.
14. Loeser, J.D.: Concepts of pain. *In* Chronic Low Back Pain. (Edited by J. Stanton-Hicks & R. Boaz) New York, Raven Press, 1982.
15. Loeser, J.D.: Perspectives on pain. *In Proceedings of the First World Conference on Clinical Pharmacology and Therapeutics.* London, Macmillan, pp. 313–316, 1981.
16. Engel, G.L.: The need for a new medical model: a challenge for biomedicine. Science 196:129–136, 1977.
17. Waddell, G.: A new clinical model for the treatment of low-back pain. Spine 12:632–644, 1987.
18. Gatchel, R.J., Baum, A., Krantz, D.: Introduction to Health Psychology, 2nd Ed. New York, Random House, 1988.
19. Barrett, J.F., Rose, R.M., Klerman, G.L. (eds.): Stress and Mental Disorder. New York, Raven Press, 1979.
20. Regier, D.A., et al.: One-month prevalence of mental disorders in the United States. Arch Gen Psychiatry 45:977–980, 1988.
21. Beals, R.: Compensation and recovery from injury. West J Med 140:233–237, 1984.
22. Fordyce, W.E.: Pain and suffering: a reappraisal. Am Psychol 43:276–283, 1988.
23. Gould, J., Davis, G.: Orthopaedic and Sports Physical Therapy. St. Louis, C.V. Mosby, 1985.
24. Hoshizaki, T., Massey, B.: Relationships of muscular endurance among specific muscle groups for continuous and intermittent static contractions. Res Quart Exerc Sport 57:229–235, 1986.
25. Haggmark, T.: Comparison of isometric muscle training and electrical stimulation supplementing isometric muscle training in the recovery after major knee ligament surgery. Am J Sports Med 7:169–171, 1979.
26. Eriksson, E.: Sports injuries of knee ligaments: their diagnosis, treatment, rehabilitation and prevention. Med Sci Sports 8:133–144, 1976.
27. Noyes, F.: Functional properties of knee ligaments and alterations induced by immobilization. Clin Orthop 123:210–242, 1977.
28. Bigos, J.J., et al.: Back injuries in industry: a retrospective study. Spine 11, 241–256, 1986.
29. Bigos, S., et al.: Back injuries in industry: a retrospective study. III: Employee related factors. Spine 11:252–256, 1986.
30. Spengler, D., et al.: Back injuries in industry: a retrospective study. Spine 11:241–245, 1986.
31. Frymoyer, J., Cats-Baril, W.: Predictors of low back pain disability. Clin Orthop 221:89–98, 1987.
32. Polatin, P.B., et al.: A psychosociomedical prediction model of response to treatment by chronically disabled workers with low back pain. Spine 14:956–961, 1989.
33. Kohles, S., Barnes, D., Gatchel, R.J., Mayer, T.G.: Improved functional restoration of industrially injured chronic low back pain patients. *Spine,* 15:1321–1324, 1990.

27

Janice Keeley

Quantification of Function

Quantification of function or functional testing is the measurement by direct or indirect means of a dynamic aspect of bodily activity necessary in daily living. When using functional testing, it is important to differentiate between the phases of back pain. They are: (1) *the acute phase,* which extends from the day of injury to 8 weeks post-injury or post-surgery. This is a time for healing and gentle, guided exercise; (2) *the subacute phase* which extends from 6 weeks post-injury or post-surgery to 4 months. This is a time to progress from gentle exercise to more active physical training guided by quantification; (3) *the chronic phase,* which includes any injury past 4 months. The rehabilitation of the chronic patient requires a multidisciplinary approach using quantification to guide the team. Quantification is the key diagnostic test that determines specific treatment for the patient in the subacute and chronic phases. Without it, treatment is blind to progression and, because of the lack of visual feedback in the spine, are we led to progress by pain complaints only. This is like setting a fracture without an x ray.

Evidence suggests that a large number of postoperative patients, including those with relatively minimal symptoms, continue to have physical capacity deficits that may make them susceptible to recurrent injury.[1] In general, it appears that the more extensive the surgical procedure and the longer the time of disability, the greater the postoperative physical capacity deficits.

The methods used in the functional evaluation must be critical for it to be successful. Specifically, these measures must be valid (i.e., measuring accurately what they claim to measure), replicable, consistent, have a built-in effort factor, and have a normative database. The following review attempts to briefly cover current technology clinically most useful for this process.

RANGE OF MOTION MEASURES

Goniometric Measures

This measurement is taken with the patient standing vertically erect in a neutral position then bending forward.[2] One arm of the goniometer is kept in the vertical position while the other arm is aimed along the spine. At best, this method is a poor estimate. The flaws include: (1) the inability for hip motion to be separated from true lumbar spine motion, and (2) variability and reproducibility are questionable because the examiner must estimate the vertical or stationary placement of the first arm and no attempt is made to position the second arm at a standard point on the spine.

Fingertip-to-Floor

In this method, the distance between the floor and the fingertips is measured as the patient flexes forward. This is a simple test to perform, but is inherently inaccurate. The examiner is unable to separate spine motion from hip, shoulder, and elbow motion, which might affect this measurement. Because of variance in arm length, it is impossible to develop population standards for this measurement.

Tape Measure Method

Schober[3] first described the tape measure method, which has most recently been modified by MacRae and Wright.[4] When using this method a midline mark is drawn connecting the "dimples of venus." This is followed by two other marks, one 5 cm below and one 10 cm above the midline mark. The value used is in centimeters, which is the measured distraction greater than 15 cm when the patient flexes forward. This method gives some indication of spinal flexion, but does not give full information. The number of lumbar segments included in this measurement can vary from 2 to 5 segments, depending on the patient's height and the presence or absence of "dimples of venus." The dimples appear to be absent to visual inspection in 20 to 35% of subject populations. The height of the dimples also varies, which makes the midline mark vary. There is no effort factor in this method.

Flexicurves

The flexicurve uses a draftsman device that is made to conform to a patient's spine. The measurement is transferred to paper, where tangents are constructed to estimate the angular position of the spine.[5,6] The device appears cumbersome and calculations time consuming. However, the device dependably measures angular displacement of the spine and separates hip mobility from spine mobility.

Three-Dimensional Digitizer

The three-dimensional digitizer has recently become available and is known as the Metrocom (FARO, Medical Technologies, Inc., Montreal, CN). This digitizer has an electromechanical linkage with an angular displacement transducer at each joint in the system. This device is extremely accurate and reproducible in limb length measurements using IBM-PC software. Because the digitizer depends on absolute orientation and space relative to its fixed base, shifting of body position common in clinical practice produces significant error. Any additional difficulty in localizing anatomic landmarks in the course of running the digitizer tip down the spine compounds the error. These problems eventually may be overcome so that this unit is clinically accurate and relevant for measuring spine mobility.

Inclinometers

The use of inclinometers to measure spinal motion was first described by Asmussen,[7] and further developed by Loebl and Troup.[8] The fluid-filled inclinometers were initially used to measure posture and spinal mobility in flexion, including using a plumb line pointer. This method appears to have built-in variability, no effort factor, and fails to separate hip motion from spine motion. (The technique of separating hip motion from true lumbar spine motion using inclinometers[9] is described in more detail later in this chapter.)

Radiologic Range of Motion Measures

Radiologic evaluation can be used to assess spinal range of motion. Because of the concern about x ray exposure, this method may be better used for research purposes, possibly to identify segmental instability or to confirm findings of noninvasive techniques.[9]

Biplanar or stereoradiographs attempt to give a three-dimensional discrimination of motion[10] by using simultaneous x rays of the lumbar spine in a fixed position. Micromotion between exposures make x ray landmarks difficult to reproduce.

Vector stereography requires an electromechanical device that measures three-dimensionally by movement of a pointer over the spine, the position of which is constantly computed from a fixed base. There is variation because of movement artifact, sometimes requiring a stabilizing frame.

Optical Methods

There are a number of techniques using skin marking with photography for assessing spinal motion as well as complex computer-controlled video systems focusing on light emitting diodes or reflective markers.[11] The need for specialized expensive equipment and inconvenience may limit this method for general use, but may have future applicability.

PRIDE Range of Motion Tests

The technique used at Productive Rehabilitation Institute of Dallas for Ergonomics (PRIDE) involves either two hand-held inclinometers (Fig. 27–1) or a computerized device, EDI-320 (Fig. 27–2) (Cybex, Ronkonkoma, NY). This method allows hip motion to be separated from true spine motion and has a built-in effort factor to confirm test validity. This technique is described in the literature along with inter- and intra-rater reliability.[9,12]

When using the two hand-held inclinometers, the top inclinometer is placed at the T12-L1 interspace and the other on the sacrum. A neutral starting position reading is taken. The patient is then asked to flex forward with knees straight. An end range reading is taken. The patient then resumes the neutral starting position. The patient is asked to extend while placing hands on hips and keeping knees straight. An end range reading is taken. Coronal or side bending measurements can also be taken using this method. For the straight leg raising component of this measurement, the patient is supine and the examiner passively lifts the leg until the contralateral

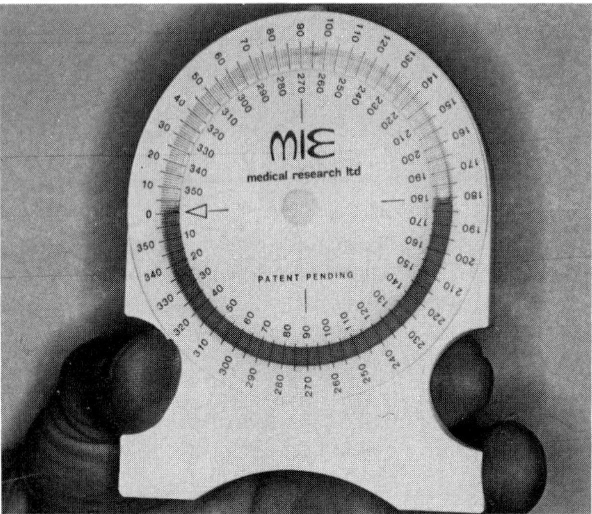

Figure 27–1. Fluid-filled inclinometer. (From Mayer, T.G., Gatchel, R.J.: Functional Restoration for Spinal Disorders: The Sports Medicine Approach. Philadelphia, Lea & Febiger, 1988.)

hip goes into extension or you see the pelvis begin to rotate.

To calculate true lumbar motion, the sacral reading is subtracted from the gross motion or the T12–L1 inclinometer reading in both flexion and extension measurements. To confirm test validity or effort factor, the comparison of the shortest straight

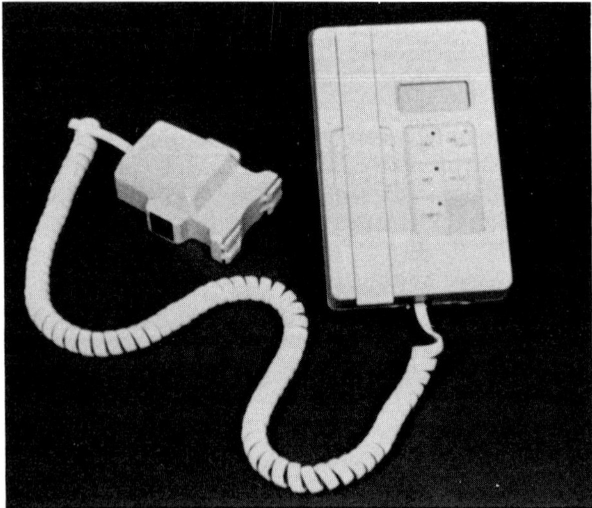

Figure 27–2. Computerized range of motion device (EDI-320). (Cybex, Inc., Ronkonkoma, NY.) (From Mayer, T.G., Gatchel, R.J.: Functional Restoration for Spinal Disorders: The Sports Medicine Approach. Philadelphia, Lea & Febiger, 1988.)

leg raise to the total of hip flexion and extension is made. Supine straight leg raising should be comparable to the hip component of spine mobility testing if given full effort because hip motion is limited by hamstring tightness and hip extension is limited by hip capsular and hip flexor tightness. If the straight leg raising component is considerably less than the hip component, either the patient has consciously restricted the leg raising on that side or the examiner did not lift the leg to the endpoint. If the straight leg raising is more than the hip component, which is more often the case, maximal bending was not performed by the patient. A small amount of difference may be accounted for by the fact that the hamstring extensibility may vary in supine and standing positions because of the hamstring contraction. When the difference between straight leg raise and hip mobility is large (more than 25°), the clinician should be alerted to suboptimal motivation. It is important to note, given suboptimal motivation, a distinction between spinal dysfunction and limitation due to pain perception or poor motivation with no organic soft tissue alteration can be made. This consistency check can be made by observing the spine/hip ratio component of movement (Fig. 27–3). In the normal subject, 62 to 70% of the initial motion is lumbar movement. As the lumbodorsal fascia and midline ligaments tighten, hip motion assumes the greater portion of motion until a crossover point is reached and the endpoint range of motion, both lumbar and hip, is achieved. Given this information, the treatment strategies can be geared more to specific physical activities or to counseling and education programs. This is the only spinal range of motion assessment to date that can provide all this information.

This measurement is taken using a computerized inclinometer, the EDI-320. This device has dual sensor inputs, permitting simultaneous calculations of motion from two separate points. When using this device, a neutral reading is taken at each of the measurement points (T12–L1 interspace and sacrum). Then readings are taken at each end range point. The computer does the calculations and gives a digital read-out on the monitor. This measurement can be taken for both sagittal and coronal motion. (Figs. 27–4 to 27–9).

TRUNK STRENGTH TESTING

Strength testing devices have a 40-year history, but the amount of research and interest has risen dramatically recently.[13–23] This emerging technology has provided a number of accurate assessment devices for measuring trunk strength. Because of the

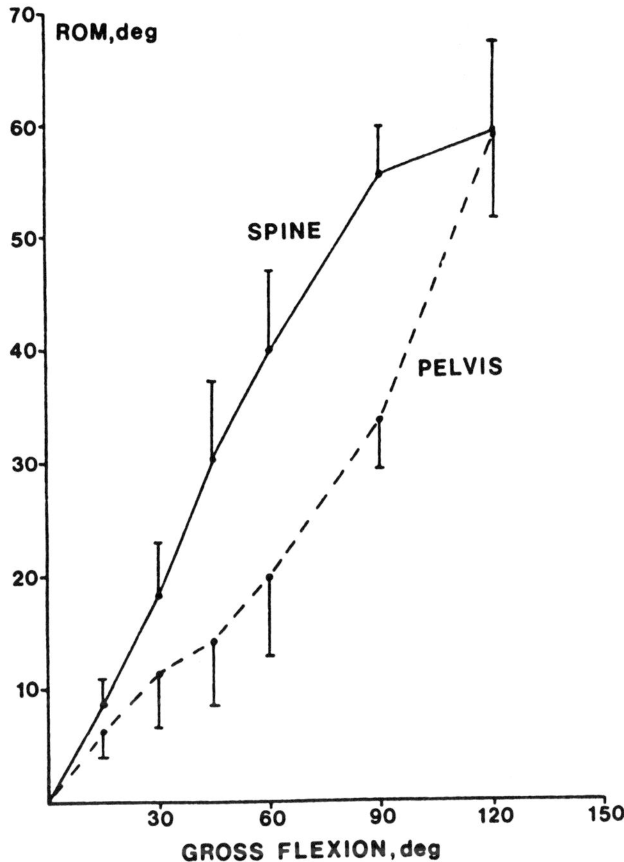

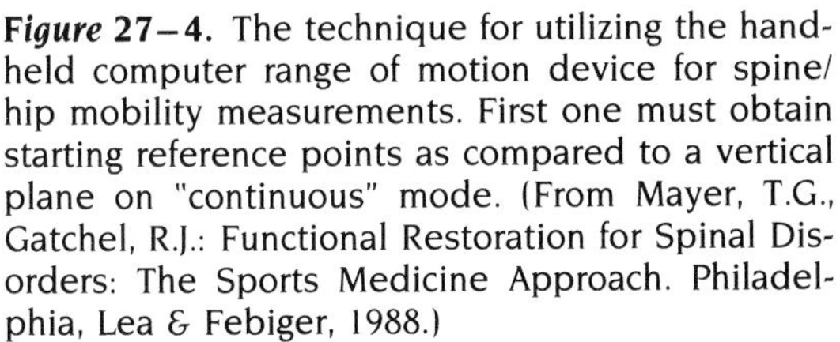

Figure 27–3. Spine/hip ratio in normal subjects. (From Mayer, T., Tencer, A., Kristofferson, S., Mooney, V.: Use of noninvasive techniques for quantification of spinal range of motion in normal subjects and chronic low back dysfunction patients. Spine 9:588, 1984.)

Figure 27–4. The technique for utilizing the hand-held computer range of motion device for spine/hip mobility measurements. First one must obtain starting reference points as compared to a vertical plane on "continuous" mode. (From Mayer, T.G., Gatchel, R.J.: Functional Restoration for Spinal Disorders: The Sports Medicine Approach. Philadelphia, Lea & Febiger, 1988.)

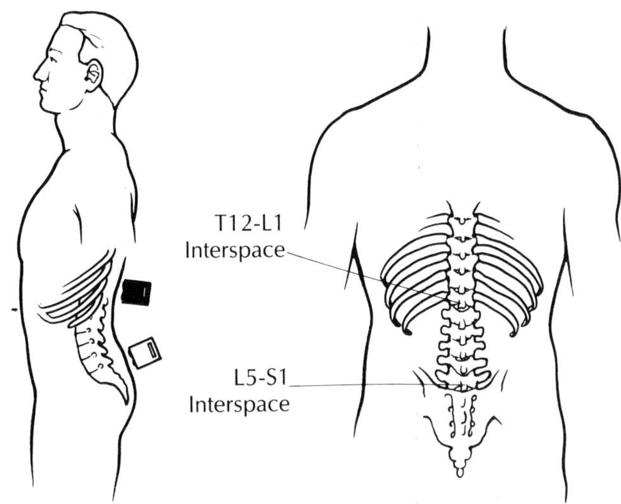

Figure 27–5. Palpate the T12-L1 interspace. Place the device over the interspace and place a skin mark opposite the upper edge of the device. Similarly, place the device over the sacrum, marking opposite the upper edge. (From Mayer, T.G., Gatchel, R.J.: Functional Restoration for Spinal Disorders: The Sports Medicine Approach. Philadelphia, Lea & Febiger, 1988.)

lack of visual feedback, mechanical devices supplement this objective examination for strength assessment. When comparing the trunk strength of normal subjects to that of chronic back pain patients, two critical points appear: (1) trunk muscle strength is an important component in functional capacity measures of the lumbar spine, and (2) because of the lack of visual feedback, mechanical devices are needed to directly measure trunk strength. Strength

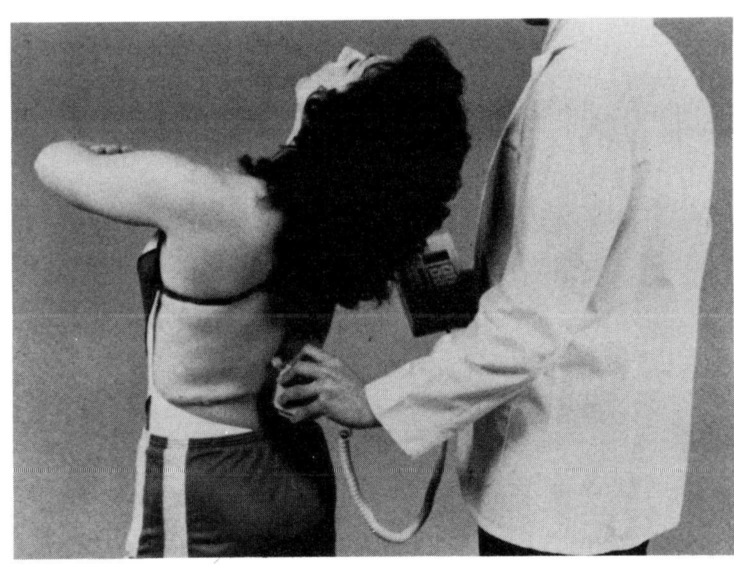

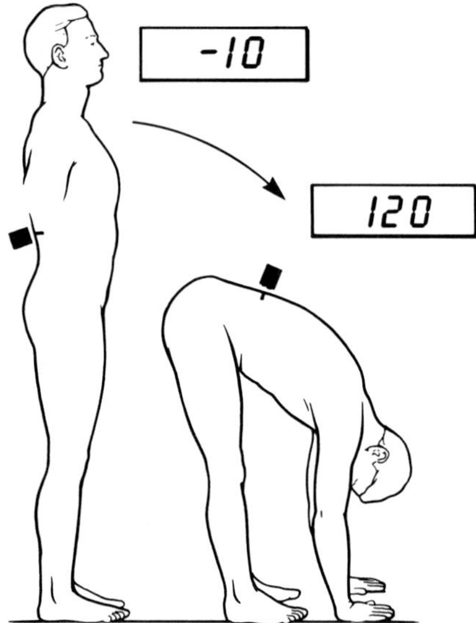

Figure 27–6. Press device to compound mode. Place the device on T12-L1 and press the activator. Return the device back on the sacrum and press the activator. Keeping the device on the sacrum, ask the patient to flex fully forward with knees straight. At terminal position, again trigger the activator. (From Mayer, T.G., Gatchel, R.J.: Functional Restoration for Spinal Disorders: The Sports Medicine Approach. Philadelphia, Lea & Febiger, 1988.)

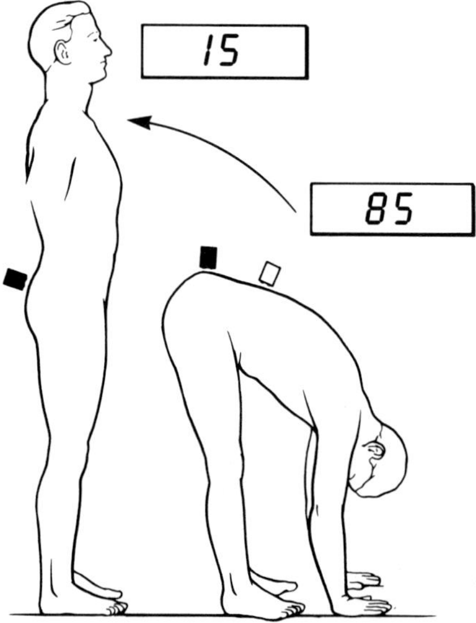

Figure 27–7. Immediately place the device opposite the original mark on T12-L1; trigger the activator and ask the patient to resume the erect position. Record hip and true spinal flexion readings. (From Mayer, T.G., Gatchel, R.J.: Functional Restoration for Spinal Disorders: The Sports Medicine Approach. Philadelphia, Lea & Febiger, 1988.)

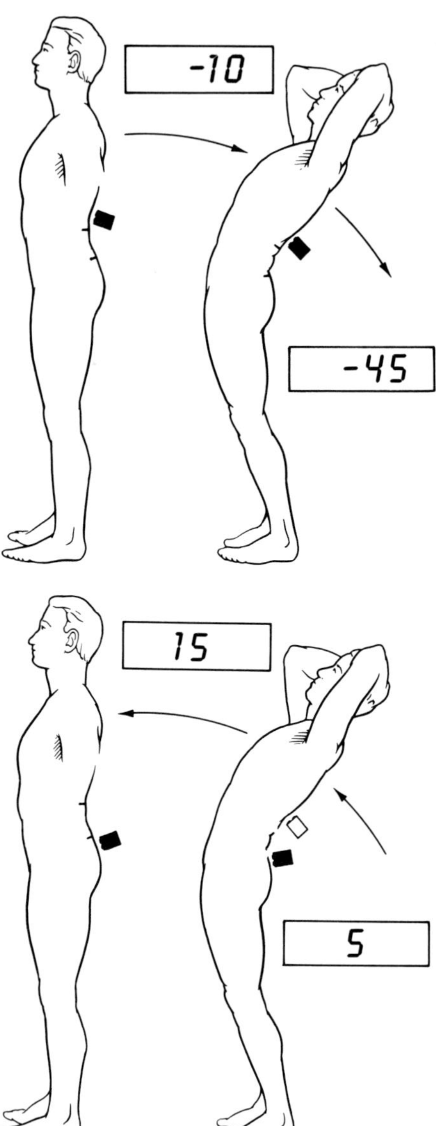

Figure 27–8. After making certain that the patient has returned to the starting reference points, repeat the sequence with the patient bending into extension in order to obtain hip and true spinal extension readings. (From Mayer, T.G., Gatchel, R.J.: Functional Restoration for Spinal Disorders: The Sports Medicine Approach. Philadelphia, Lea & Febiger, 1988.)

measures require subject motivation, therefore a validity check, or "effort factor," is also necessary.

Trunk strength measures refer to the measurements of the functional capacity of the lumbopelvic unit, and therefore appropriate isolation of the segment is necessary. The term strength is a term used loosely to connote a variety of muscular functions and values. Most of the various machines that measure trunk strength express the measurements in

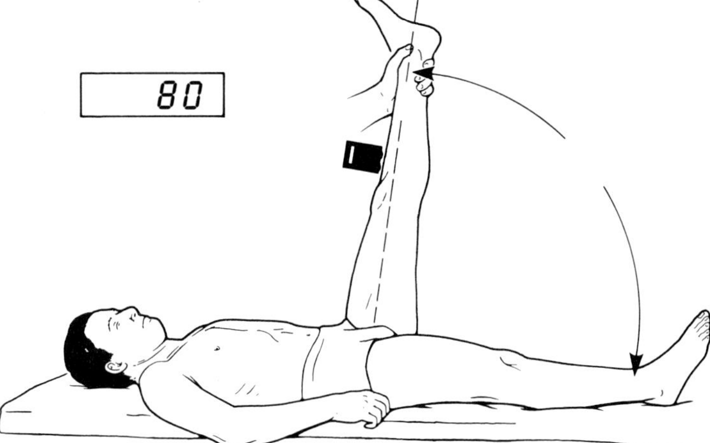

Figure 27–9. Supine straight leg raising using the inclinometer in its continuous or reference mode requires first triggering the activator with leg extended and reading maximum inclinometer with contralateral leg maintained straight, then performing the straight leg raise. (From Mayer, T.G., Gatchel, R.J.: Functional Restoration for Spinal Disorders: The Sports Medicine Approach. Philadelphia, Lea & Febiger, 1988.)

one of the following terms: (1) the ability to produce force or torque (force around an axis) either statically or dynamically, (2) the ability to produce work (force times distance traveled), or (3) the ability to produce power.

The methods used to acquire these measurements can be placed in three categories: (1) *Isometric technology* measures the maximal force a muscle can generate in a contraction with distance and velocity remaining zero. (2) *Isokinetic technology* measures the torque or force at a preselected fixed speed through a preselected distance or range of motion. Because the speed or velocity and distance are set, measurement of the accommodating variable resistance is possible. (3) *Isodynamic technology* measures the torque and position changes occurring around multiple centers. This is essentially an electronically monitored hydraulic system permitting no motion until a preselected minimum torque is produced after which the acceleration and velocity increase in proportion to the degree to which a torque exceeds the preset minimum. As torque varies, acceleration and velocity also vary independently.

Specific Commercially Available Trunk Strength Units

Cybex TEF (Trunk Extension Flexion) Unit

Cybex (Lumex Corp., Ronkonkoma, NY) has been involved in dynamic isolated joint testing since 1969.

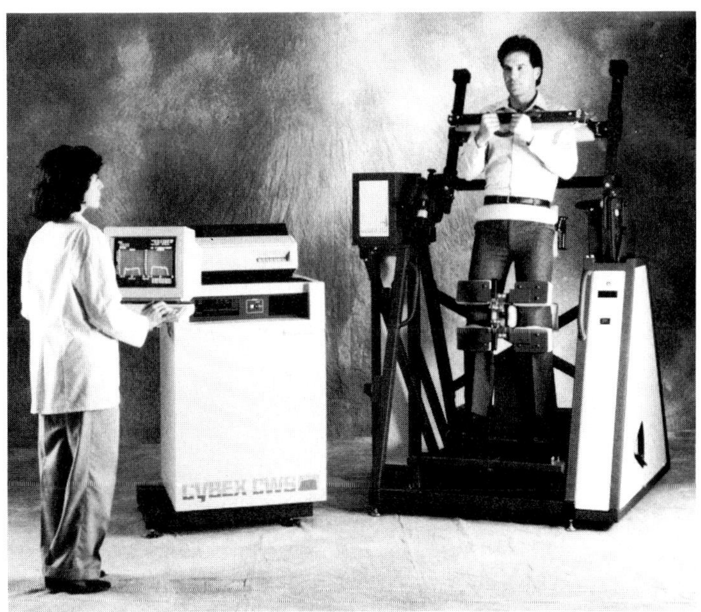

Figure 27–10. Cybex trunk extension flexion device. (Cybex, Inc., Ronkonkoma, NY.)

Realizing the need for a stabilized method of measuring the high torques produced by the trunk, they developed a series of prototypes (Fig. 27–10). Two commercial trunk strength machines resulted, measuring sagittal and axial plane motions. Both machines perform isometric and isokinetic dynamic tests. In the TEF, stabilization occurs across the chest between the scapulae and the sternum, at the pelvis across the pubis and iliac crest, and above and below slightly flexed knees. The axis of motion is set at the lumbosacral level. The test is begun in a "posturally neutral" position and allows a 120° arc of motion. Isometric measurements may be taken at any point along the range of motion; standard and custom multispeed isokinetic protocols also can be measured. Counterbalance and gravity correction procedures are available also. Each subject's original tested position can be retrieved on an individual computer disc for repeated tests. The machine records output in several parameters, including peak torque, acceleration time, angle of peak, work, power, and curve variability. Mechanical documentation of fatigue resistance, endurance, and recovery protocols is also possible.

The individual tests can be printed in numeric or graphic form. Graphic representations may be

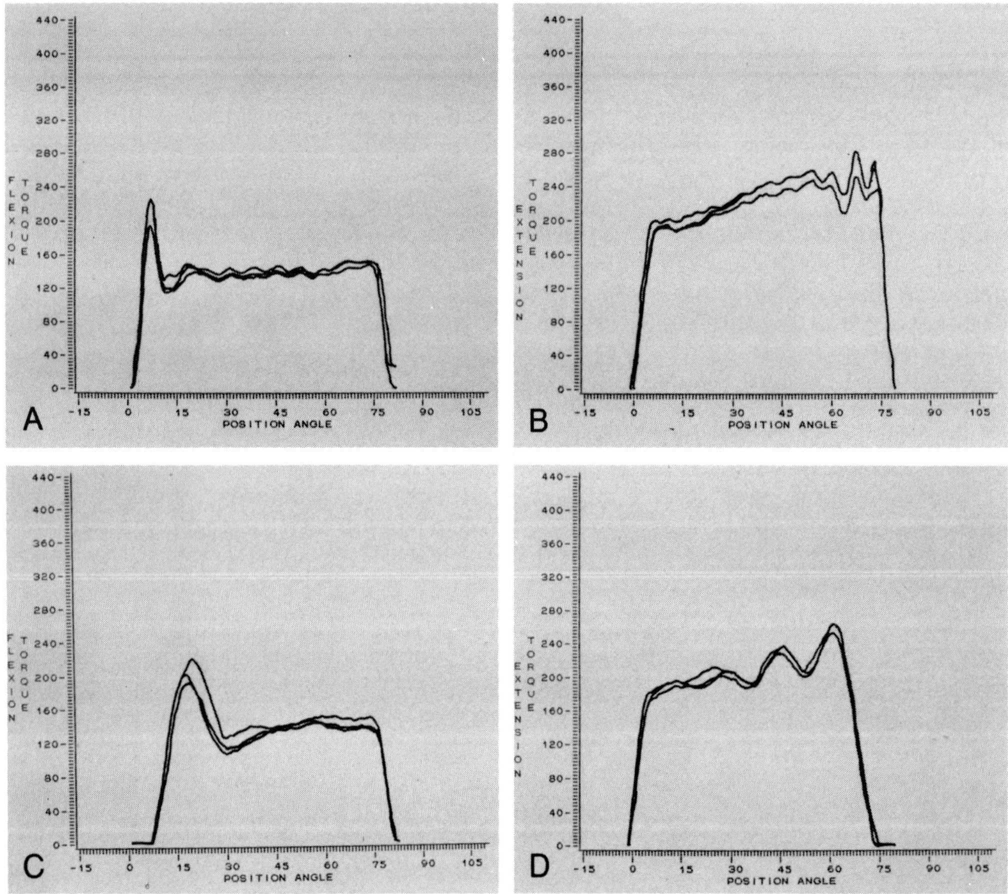

Figure 27–11. A series of computer curves demonstrating the three curves (APC, MPC, and BWPC) in flexion and extension. A through D show a normal spine at 60 and 150° per second. **A.** Flexion curve at 60° per second in a normal subject (read left to right). Note large impulse and "square wave" pattern. **B.** Extension curve at 60° per second in a normal subject (read right to left). Note torque is considerably higher than flexion curve with minimal "lag" prior to torque development. **C.** Flexion curve at 150° per second. Note slower development of torque and wider "impulse" oscillations; still maintaining minimum curve variability and "square wave" form. **D.** Extension curve at 150° per second. Note "high-speed dropoff" with some lag in torque development compared to extension at 60° per second. (From Mayer, T.G., Gatchel, R.J.: Functional Restoration for Spinal Disorders: The Sports Medicine Approach. Philadelphia, Lea & Febiger, 1988.)

printed as real time curves directly after the test, or as other curves plotted from the stored information, such as (1) Maximum points curve representing the maximum torque output at each degree in the range of motion of the total repetitions in that set. (2) Average points curve representing the average torque output at each degree in the range of motion. (3) Best work repetition curve. The actual repetition (real time curve) that produces the best work. An example of a typical curve from a normal subject at 60° per second is seen in Figure 27–11. The flexion curve, A, is read from left to right, and B is the extension curve, read from right to left. Note the "square wave" shape of the curve particularly through the end point. This shows that once a maximum torque has been reached, the muscular function was present to maintain the force through the entire range of motion. The initial slope of the increasing torque represents the amount of acceleration or explosiveness the subject exerts. Another consideration to take into account both graphically and numerically is the flexor/extensor ratio. Normally, this ratio should be between 1.2 and 1.4.[24] A reversed flexor/extensor ratio was found in a chronic back pain patient population.

Around the midpoint of rehabilitation, endurance and recovery protocols give the clinicians additional information. The *endurance protocol* compares work performed during the first 20% of the preselected repetitions with the last 20% of repetitions (Fig. 27–12). The *recovery protocol* compares the total work done in two identical fatiguing trials separated by a predetermined recovery period. With this additional information, comparisons of endurance and recovery can be made to a normative database. Specific databases can be developed for specific sports or job requirements. Normative testing has been published using the TEF prototype and has been compared with a group of chronic back pain patients.[25]

Cybex Torso Rotation Units

This isokinetic unit is similar to the Cybex TEF in all its functional concepts and operation but measures torsional strength instead of flexion and extension. The subject is seated in a hip abducted position, with the pelvis and the upper body stabilized. The torso rotation (TR) has an axially mounted dynamometer, allows a total of 120° of motion, and a speed of up to 200° per second (Fig. 27–13).

Characteristic databases have been published for a small group of normals (67) and patients (33).[26] EMG testing revealed that the highest RMS voltages that correspond to the highest force outputs was produced by the ipsilateral oblique to the direction of rotation. The contralateral oblique was approximately half the ipsilateral oblique's voltage, whereas a smaller voltage was produced by the contralateral erector spinae muscle and negligible voltage by the ipsilateral erector spinae muscle.

LIDO Back System

The LIDO Back System (Loredan, Inc., Davis, CA) tests isokinetically and isometrically in the sagittal plane (Fig. 27–14). The testing can be conducted in the standing or sitting positions. Stabilization points are at the knees, pelvis, and at a unique sliding

Figure 27–12. A. Decline in work output per repetition over the course of a fatiguing set of repetitions. (Represented separately for left rotation and right rotation.) **B.** Endurance protocol and recovery protocol. The comparison between the two pairs of lines represents recovery potential (second set vs. first set). These protocols are represented separately for flexion and extension. (From Mayer, T.G., Gatchel, R.J.: Functional Restoration for Spinal Disorders: The Sports Medicine Approach. Philadelphia, Lea & Febiger, 1988.)

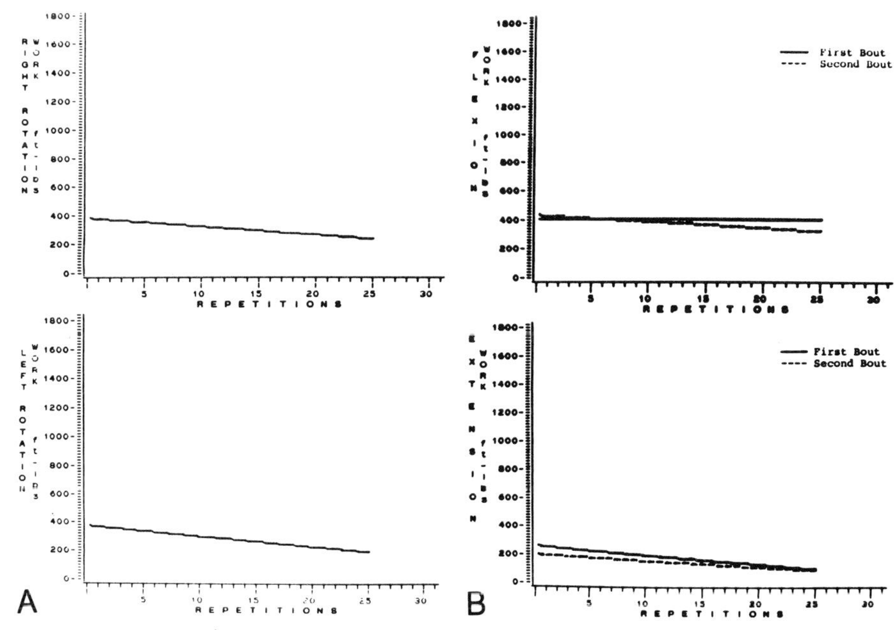

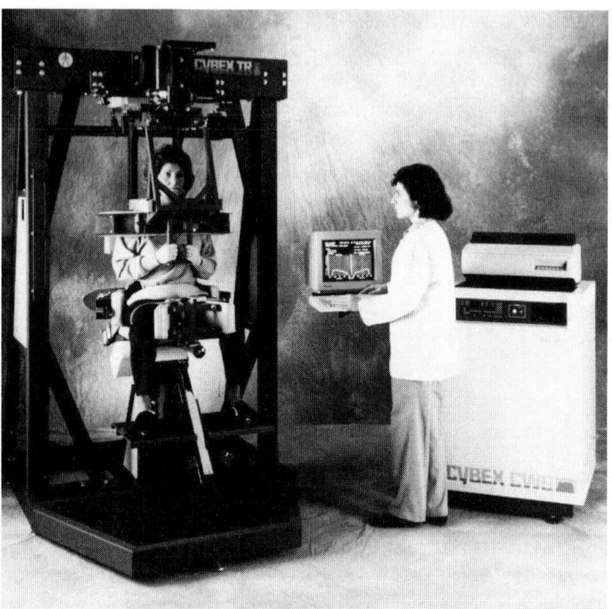

Figure 27–13. Cybex torso rotation device. (Cybex, Inc. Ronkonkoma, NY.)

chest carriage, which allows a greater amount of motion. The actual axis of motion is mounted in line with the lumbopelvic axis of rotation and an IBM PC computer is used to monitor the patient and calculate the range. The calculations can be viewed graphically and numerically as peak torque, acceleration, work, power, and range of motion. There is also an endurance protocol that calculates a fatigue index based on the amount of work done in each repetition. A coefficient of variation is a calculated measure of consistency of performance using a torque curve overlay of therapist-selected repetitions. No normative data has been published. Various sites around the USA are in the process of collecting normative data using a standard protocol.

Isotechnologies B-200

Isotechnologies B-200 (Isotechnologies, Hillsboro, NC) measures torque, angular position and angular velocity occurring about three axes of rotation (Fig. 27–15). This device can measure these values in all three axes simultaneously or a single axis can be isolated for sagittal or coronal measures. Testing can be performed in either sitting or standing positions. The subject is stabilized at the waist, hips, thighs, and upper trunk using a shoulder harness apparatus. The "isodynamic" technology is unique to these machines. It is basically an electronically monitored hydraulic system that permits no motion until a preselected minimal torque is produced, after which the

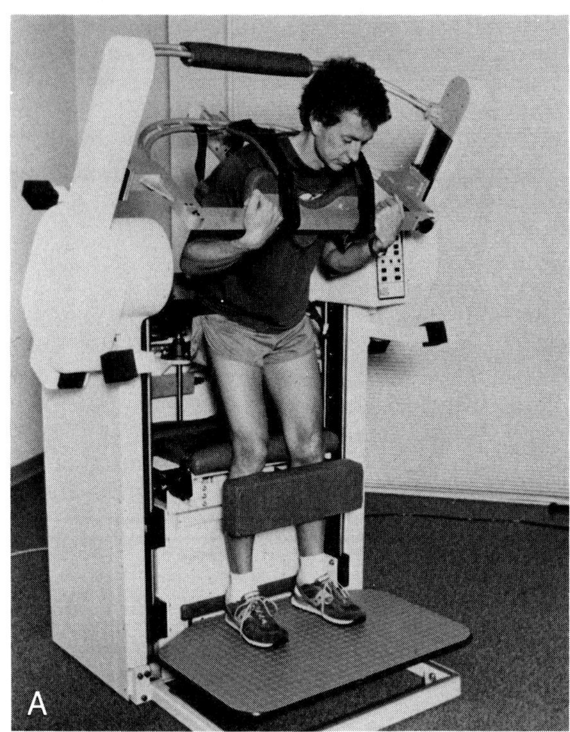

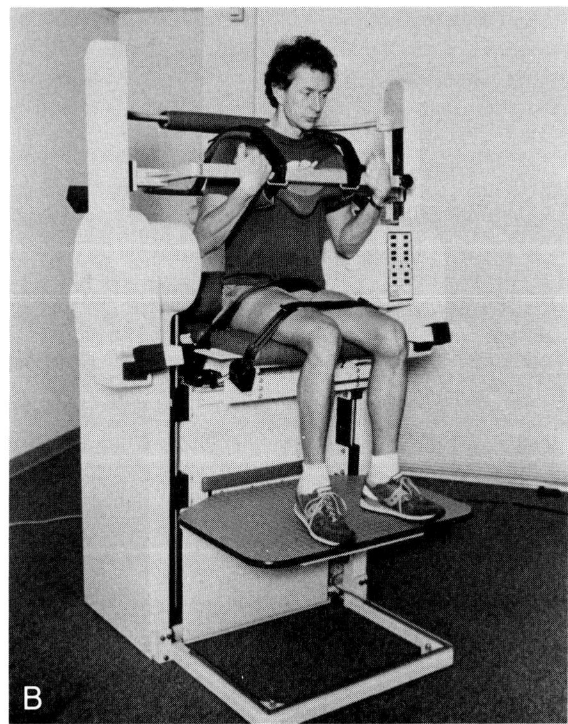

Figure 27–14A, B. Lido sagittal sitting/standing isokinetic strength testing device. (Loredan, Inc., Davis, CA.) (From Mayer, T.G., Gatchel, R.J.: Functional Restoration for Spinal Disorders: The Sports Medicine Approach. Philadelphia, Lea & Febiger, 1988.)

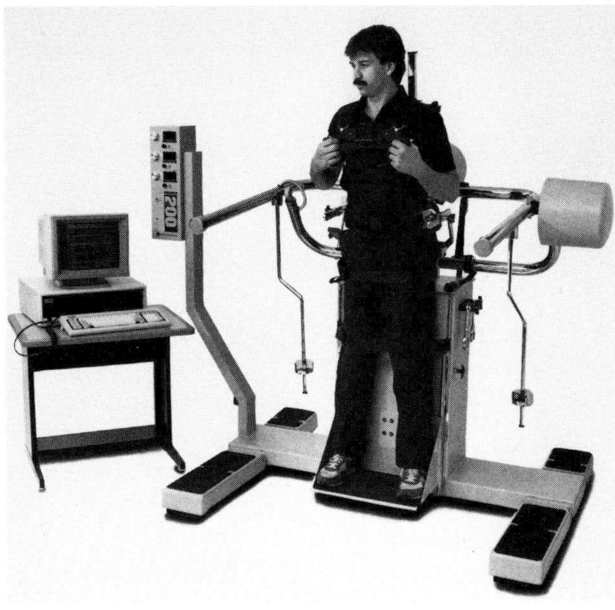

Figure 27–15. Isostation B-200. (Isotechnologies, Inc., Hillsborough, NC.)

acceleration and velocity are controlled by the degree to which the torque exceeds the preset minimum. As the torque varies, so does the acceleration and velocity, without control. The B-200 uses IBM PC or Apple computers for monitoring and calculations.

Currently, there are no published norms for the machine although data is being collected at a central data computation site. Isodynamic testing is not capable of isokinetic measurement. Although it offers flexibility and versatility, it sacrifices measurement accuracy in using poor anatomic stabilization and location of axis of rotation and by having no control of primary variables of velocity or resistance. As a training tool, this device appears to be a good choice, but as a testing device, questions remain about validity and consistency.

Kin-Com

The Kin-Com device (Chatteck Corporation, Chattanooga, TN) has a back testing attachment to its extremity dynamometer (Fig. 27–16). This machine allows for isometric and multispeed isokinetic measurement. An added option is measurement of eccentric as well as concentric strength by having a motor-driven force and resistance capability.

Testing is done in the seated position only, with stabilization at the pelvis using a belt and two rigid locking arms pressed against the pelvis. This rigid

seating device limits the amount of range of motion to be tested. This machine is capable of measuring flexion and extension separately only. Risk of injury during the eccentric mode has been reduced by using a computer-controlled "lockout feature" that halts the motion of the dynamometer arm when the subject breaks contact with the arm. A variable preload can be set to motivate a subject to exceed a certain level before motion can be initiated and eliminates the acceleration impulse "catching up to the speed" present on most isokinetic devices. A normative database is being developed on a research device in an academic setting.

Biodex Back Attachment

The Biodex Back Attachment (Biodex, Inc., Shirley, NY) is an attachment to an existing extremity system (Fig. 27–17). The attachment is a semireclining chair hinged in the lumbar spinal region, in which the subject is seated. The mobile dynamometer is disconnected from the extremity attachment and connected in line with the axis of rotation of the chair. Testing can be done in both isokinetic and isometric modes and is coupled to a computer which drives the dynamometer actively in both directions. Testing can be done both eccentrically and concentrically with built in safety stops.

The patient is positioned in a semireclined position with feet resting on footplates positioned so the knees are slightly flexed. Stabilization is attempted through upper thigh and pelvic belts, and a lumbosacral pad used to maintain postural pelvic tilt through the full sagittal flexion and extension mobility. The chest is stabilized by a harness consisting of two crossing belts anteriorly to stabilize the subject against the two extension pads posturally. The chair permits 80° of motion from flexion to hyperextension and can test up to 300° per second. The standard numerical and graphic values are calculated along with a mean peak torque and a fatigue ratio. A project to obtain normative data is currently underway in a large midwestern medical clinic.

Med-X

The Med-X lumbar extension testing and rehabilitation machine (MED-X, Ocala, FL) is relatively new to the market after many years of development (Fig. 27–18). This machine tests isometrically through a range of motion of 72°. The subject is placed in a seated position with stabilization at the thigh and uses a posterior pelvic pad designed to restrain the pelvis from moving. The subject is asked to grasp

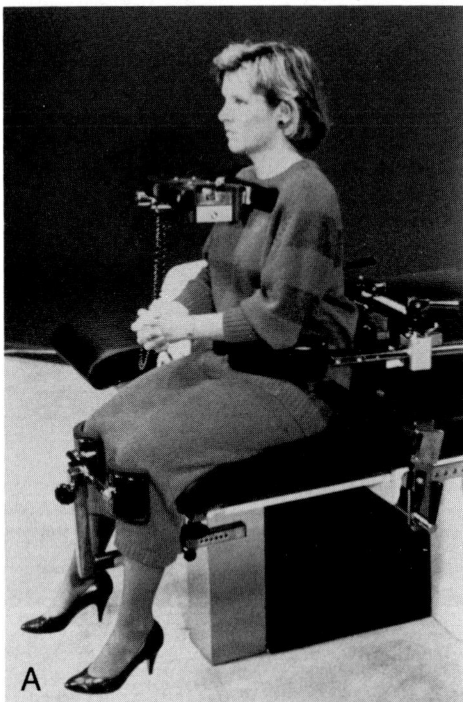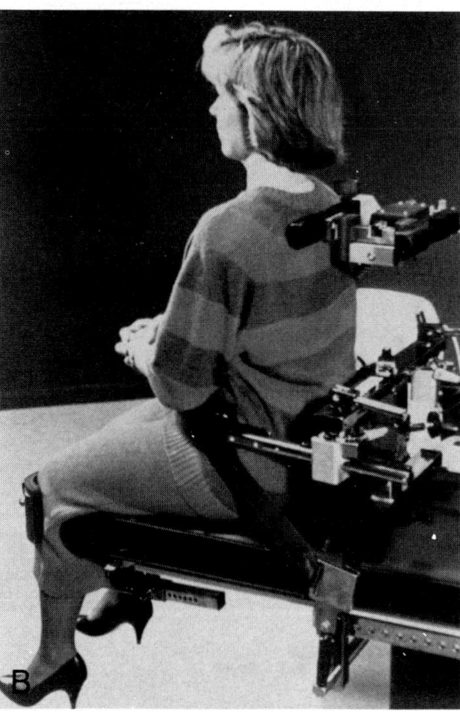

Figure 27–16. Kin-Com sitting sagittal strength testing device. (Chatteck Corp., Chattanooga, TN.) (From Mayer, T.G., Gatchel, R.J.: Functional Restoration for Spinal Disorders: The Sports Medicine Approach. Philadelphia, Lea & Febiger, 1988.)

handles to stabilize the arms and to keep the head on a cervical pad. Strength testing is done for lumbar extensors only. Isometric tests are done in multiple positions and can be displayed graphically. This machine can also train patients isotonically as it also has a weight stack. Values calculated include torque and range of motion along with a fatigue and recovery test.

MEASUREMENT OF FUNCTIONAL TASK PERFORMANCE

Testing and understanding of lifting mechanics has received attention for several reasons. Industry has identified lifting to be highly correlated with low back injury. It also is a full body activity that requires transfer of forces along the biomechanical chain from hands down to feet. This has led to both educational concepts of modifying lift techniques and mathematical models of lifting.[27,28] Study and analysis of lifting capacity has encompassed several different techniques including isoinertial tests,[29–33] isometric lift test,[34–36] and constrained isokinetic lifting.[37,38]

Isometric testing appears to be the most well established technique. It has been recognized in the National Institute of Occupational Safety and Health (NIOSH) Work Practices Guide for Manual Lifting as a way to identify workers who would be at a higher risk of injury. Isoinertial testing keeps the mass constant and velocity uncontrolled (or measured). Isoinertial lifting is basically an isotonic lift or psychophysical lift, in which the lifting capacity is determined by the subject's self-report of his or her maximum capability, usually to a point of discomfort or perception of impending injury if continued. Research and development of lifting and functional tasks devices is a new and expanding field.

Commercially Available Lift Testing Units

Cybex Liftask

The Cybex Liftask (Cybex, Ronkonkoma, NY) (Fig. 27–19) is an outgrowth of the same technology as the trunk strength units. It can test isometrically and multispeed isokinetically. It consists of a standing platform with foot placement grids and a lifting handle on a cable attached to the dynamometer. There is no joint stabilization thus allowing a wide selection of body positions and lifting styles. Computer-calculated values of measurement received in-

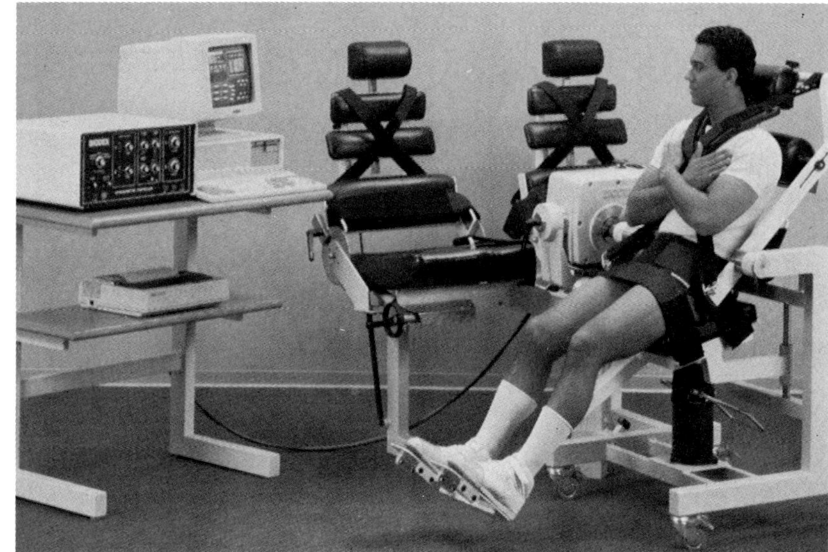

Figure 27–17. Biodex isokinetic dynamometer connects to semi-reclining back attachment for trunk flexion/extension measurements. (From Mayer, T.G., Gatchel, R.J.: Functional Restoration for Spinal Disorders: The Sports Medicine Approach. Philadelphia, Lea & Febiger, 1988.)

clude peak torque, average torque, work, power, and curve shape variability. These can be reviewed graphically or numerically. When designing a test protocol, you also have the option of doing an ergometric test or an anthropometric test. A normative database has been published.[37]

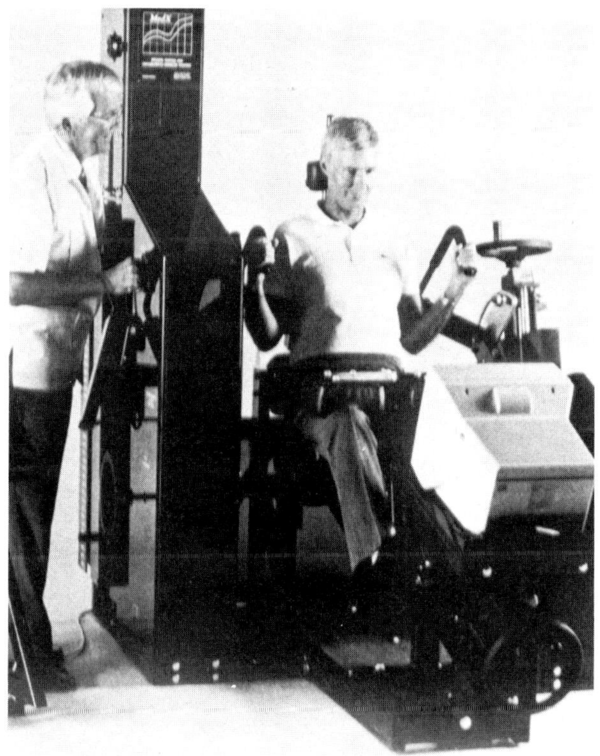

Figure 27–18. Med-X lumbar extension testing device. (Med-X Corp., Ocala, FL.)

Ergometrics Strength Testing Unit

Ergometrics strength testing unit (Ergometrics, Ann Arbor, MI) (Fig. 27–20) is a computerized isometric strength testing unit. This measures static lift capacity and is based on the biomechanical model for calculating percent strength impairment. Force curve values along with coefficient variation values are also calculated. Upper extremity attachments may be added for isometric strength test. A time motion control unit can be used with tool attachment to measure other functional tasks. As previously stated, isometric testing has been studied and has a large normative and industrial database.

LIDO Lift

The LIDO Lift (Loredan, Davis, CA) is new on the market with many added features (Fig. 27–21). This unit consists of a moveable arm to which various devices such as a box can be attached to and used for testing. This moveable arm allows movement from floor to shelves and walking a step or two. The modes of testing can be isometric, isokinetic, or gravity/inertia modeling. The data calculations require an IBM PC and include graphic and numeric values of torque, work, and measurement of consistency called coefficient variation (Fig. 27–22).

TASK PERFORMANCE TESTS

Because this is a new and growing area, many creative methods are used both individually and commercially to measure the ability to perform tasks.

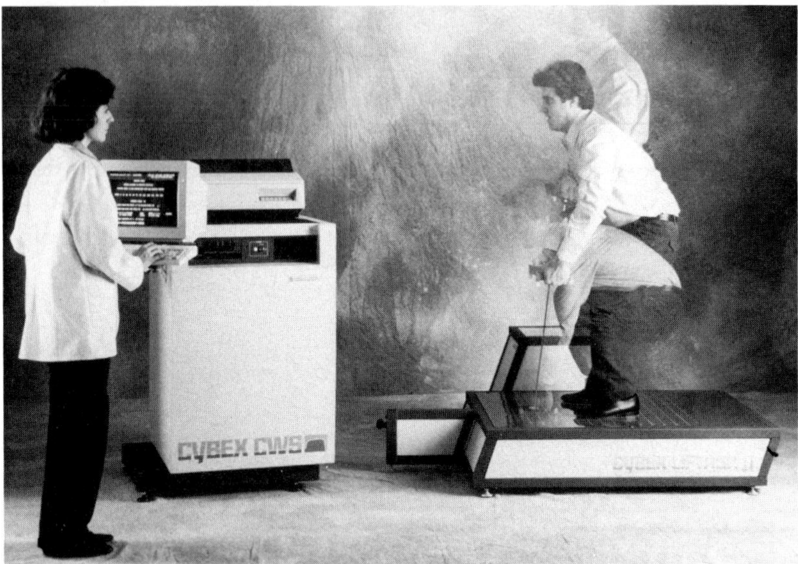

Figure 27–19. Cybex Liftask. (Cybex, Ronkonkoma, NY.)

The following is a brief synopsis of some of these methods.

Progressive Isoinertial Lifting Evaluation (PILE)

Progressive Isoinertial Lifting Evaluation (PILE) is a simple test that involves both psychophysical and progressive isoinertial components. The protocol involves the lifting of weights in a plastic box from floor to waist (0 to 30 in.) and waist to shoulder height (30 to 54 in.). Men begin with a 10-pound load and women begin with a 5-pound load. A rate

for four lifting movements in a twenty-second period is taken followed by a weight addition equal to the initial weight. Tests from floor to waist and waist to shoulder lifting are done separately. This sequence is maintained until one of the following endpoints is achieved: (1) *psychophysical endpoint*, voluntary test termination by the subject, (2) *aerobic endpoint*, achievement of a specific aerobic capacity goal, such as 85% of age-determined maximum heart rate or as other cardiac precautions dictate, or (3) *safety endpoint*, a predetermined "safe limit" of 45 to 55% of body weight. Results obtained from this easy-to-use protocol include maximum weights

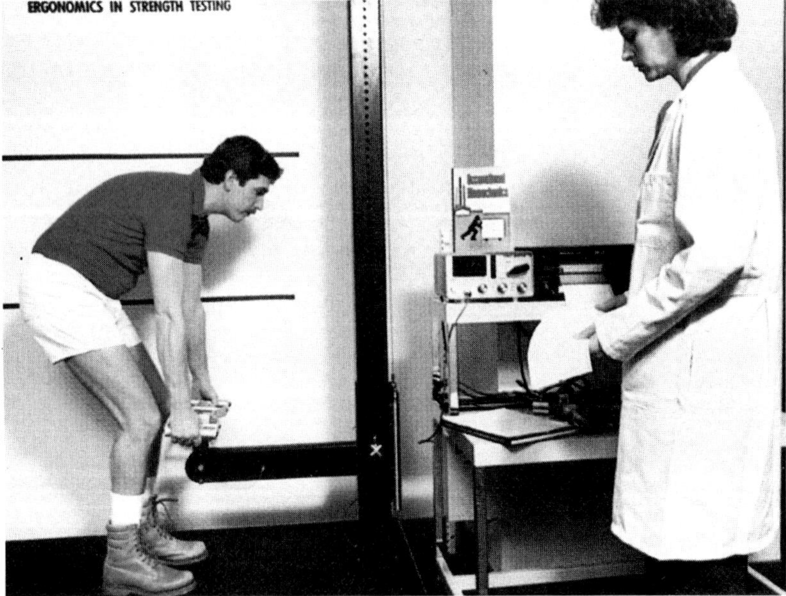

Figure 27–20. Ergometrics lifting device. (Ergometry, Inc., Ann Arbor, MI.)

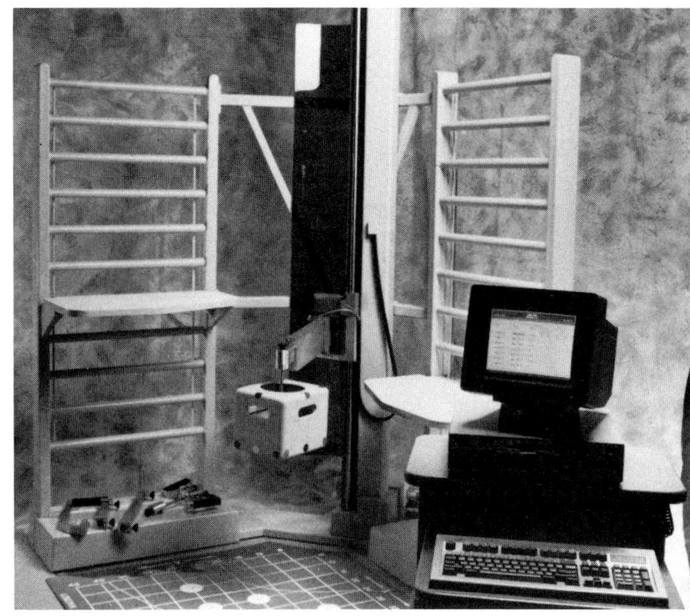

Figure 27–21. Lido lift device. (Loredan, Inc., Davis, CA.)

lifted floor to waist and waist to shoulder, endurance or total time, final heart rate, and work and power consumption.

WEST 2

The WEST 2 (Work Evaluation Systems Technology, Huntington Beach, CA) is a commercially available isoinertial lifting device (Fig. 27 23). It consists of a frame with projecting bolts with a bar that holds weights, which is lifted and "hooked" onto the bolts. This test involves lifting through preselected ranges and requires sufficient control of the weighted bar in order to hook it in place.

Functional Measurement Laboratory

The Functional Measurement Laboratory is a computer-assisted functional measurement laboratory

designed to test a large number of musculoskeletal and neurologic parameters. It was developed at the University of Texas Southwestern Medical Center at Dallas under grants from the National Institute of Disability Research and Rehabilitation (NIDRR). Parameters tested are balance, postural stability, reaction time, upper and lower extremity reaction time, speed, and coordination (Fig. 27–24).

A large normative database exists for comparisons.[46,47]

BTE

The BTE (Baltimore Therapeutic Equipment, Inc., Baltimore, MD) is a computer-assisted measurement system that measures hand and arm strength as they relate to tool use. This also has the potential to measure shoulder girdle or cervical function as it relates to tool usage. The computer is connected to a

WORK PER REPETITION TO BODY WEIGHT RATIO (%)		RANGE OF MOTION (degrees)	
flex	0%	flex	73°
ext	0%	ext	73°

ENDURANCE			
FATIGUE INDEX (%)		TOTAL WORK DONE (ft-lbs)	
flex	106%	flex	165
ext	102%	ext	369

Figure 27–22. Lido sagittal test results printout.

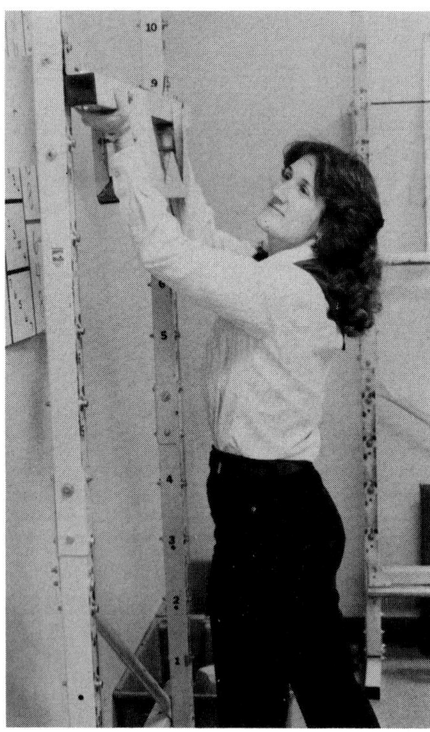

Figure **27–23.** Individual performing "lifting under load" isoinertial task on WEST 2 equipment. (WEST, Long Beach, CA.) (From Mayer, T.G., Gatchel, R.J.: Functional Restoration for Spinal Disorders: The Sports Medicine Approach. Philadelphia, Lea & Febiger, 1988.)

transducer allowing measurement of the torque produced by the tools, which are attached to the transducer. Sandbags can be attached to a set of pulleys and ropes for assessing lifting in a variety of positions.

Multiple Tasks Obstacle Course

PRIDE has designed an obstacle course that is used to measure actual physical tasks performance (Fig. 27–25). The obstacle course can be used to simulate various job demands of the workplace such as walking push-pull, squatting push-pull, twisting, bending (without lifting), crawling, and climbing. Resistance is set and controlled by a hydraulic mechanism. A normal database can be developed by testing the number of repetitions performed at each station during a fixed period of time. Pacing, conservation of energy, and agility can subjectively be assessed by therapists and objectively by measuring the subject's heart rate for effort.

AEROBIC CAPACITY TESTING

Much has been written concerning cardiovascular measures. These measures are linked to endurance both as extrinsic cardiovascular capacity and intrinsic muscle enzyme and muscle response to exercise demands. Cardiovascular capacity can be predicted by bicycle ergonometry to obtain physiologic information on work performance and oxygen consumption. Using standardized nomograms based on work rate and heart rate, predicted oxygen consumption data can be converted to a Vo_2max estimate and a fitness level by standard tables. There have been reports of linking poor cardiovascular fitness with increased risk of back pain,[48] and a study by Schmidt[49] indicated that chronic back pain patients have poorer physical performance levels in aerobic testing.

An upper body ergometer can be used to test the strength or endurance of the upper extremities and back functional unit. One testing procedure increases work rate at regular timed intervals and is completed when fatigue or the subject's target heart rate has been achieved. From current knowledge, this appears to be a test of upper body strength or endurance because the capacity to deliver blood to the upper extremities is limited by the size of the vessels, therefore preventing even high stress activities of the arms from placing a substantial load on the cardiopulmonary system.

CONSIDERATIONS IN EVALUATING QUANTIFICATION METHODS

The recent availability of these commercial devices makes it difficult for any clinician to have gained extensive experience with all the machines. Because the market is being flooded with new machines, the clinician will experience difficulty in distinguishing the accuracy of the marketing claims. To make matters more confusing, there are no generally accepted

Table 27–1
Critical Factors in Evaluating Physical Capacity Measurement Technology

Validity/Accuracy
Reproducibility/Reliability
Relevance
Effort factor
Normative database

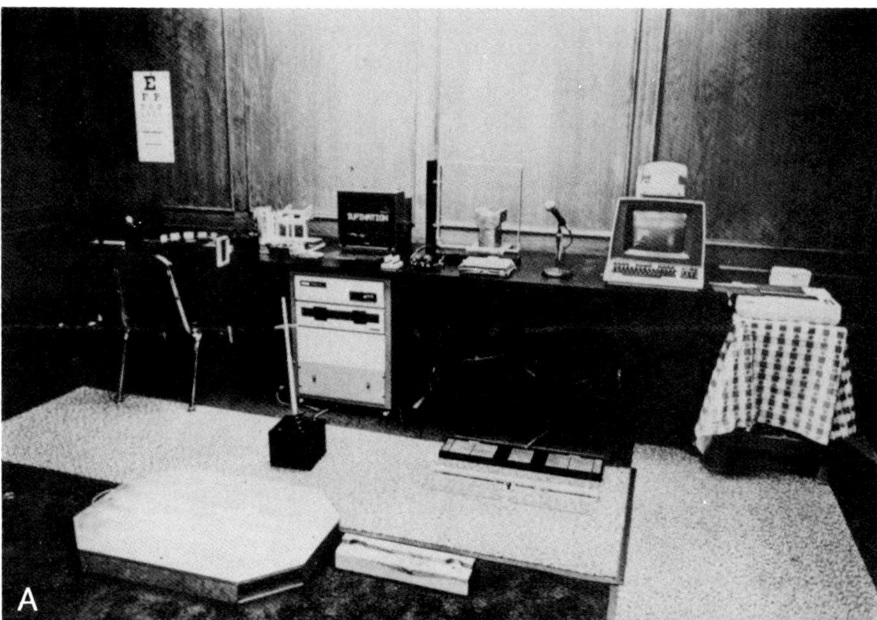

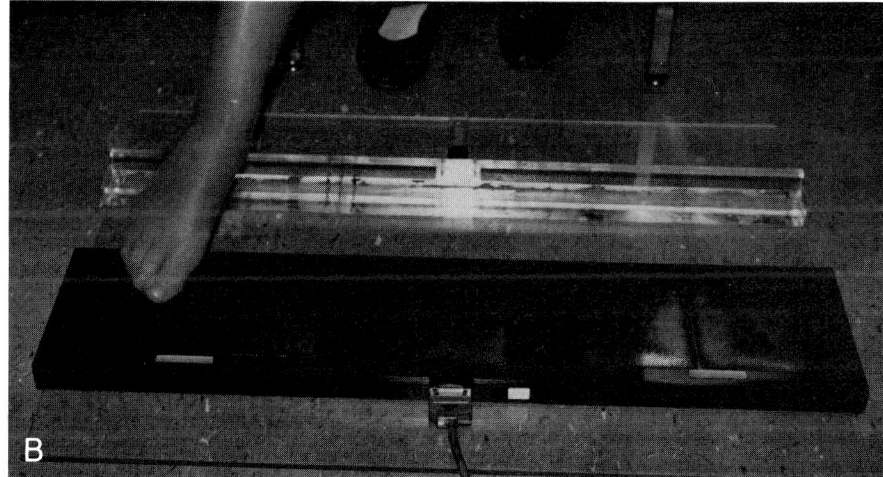

Figure 27–24. **A.** The function measurement laboratory at the Department of Physical Therapy, University of Texas Southwestern Medical Center at Dallas. **B.** Lower extremity reaction, speed, and coordination test board. (From Mayer, T.G., Gatchel, R.J.: Functional Restoration for Spinal Disorders: The Sports Medicine Approach. Philadelphia, Lea & Febiger, 1988.)

standards or protocols for strength testing to guide manufacturers or clinicians. At the present time, one manufacturer's machine information cannot be compared to another's, and in some cases cannot be compared to the same manufacturer's in another facility. Some questions that the clinician can ask when critically evaluating physical capacity measurement technology are (Table 27-1)[1]:

1. Is the test truly objective, with observations unaffected by effort or at least a mechanism used to identify or control effort?
2. Does the test accurately measure the specific function it proports to measure and in a reproducible manner?

3. Is the functional test relevant to the back disability process?
4. Does a large normal database exist against which statements concerning deviation from "normal" are meaningful?
5. Does the test have predictive value for injury or recurrence as shown in a prospective study?

The answers to these questions can help the clinician determine the usefulness of the physical capacity measures and assist in guiding rehabilitation. Because new devices are constantly appearing on the market, the astute clinician should use the above principles in an attempt to decide what is useful and what is not.

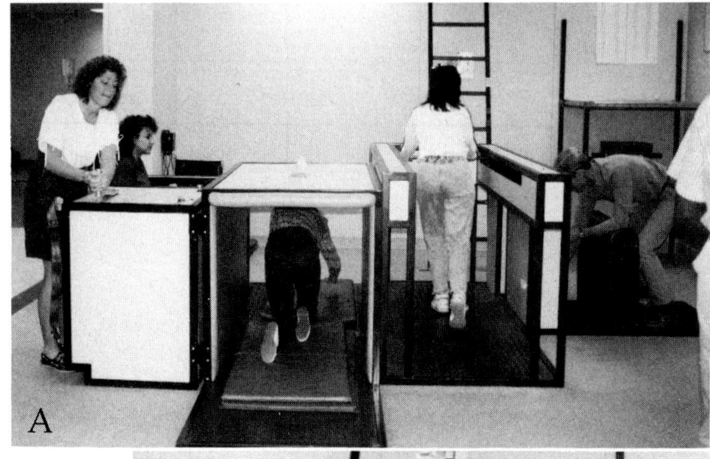

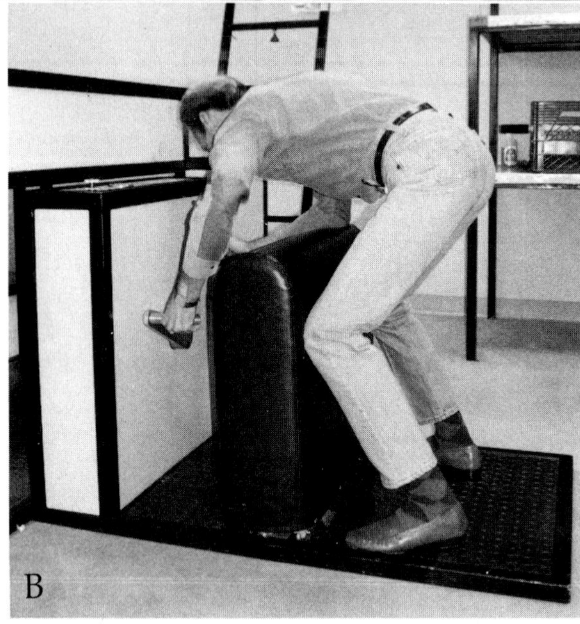

Figure 27–25A, B. Multiple task obstacle course simulating twisting, pushing, pulling, crawling, climbing, and bending.

CONCLUSION - SUMMARY

In summary, objective measurement of spinal function beginning with range of motion, progressing to trunk strength and functional capacity, is an important part of evaluating the need for rehabilitation and assessing its progress. Quantification assists the clinician in determining when and if a patient is ready to return to his sport or work instead of relying only on subjective information from the patient and "clinician experience." Through objectively guided active rehabilitation of the spine patient, we may enhance nutrition and healing of tissues. By achieving high levels of function and instruction on maintenance of this function, we can perhaps prevent further reinjury. By addressing spinal problems in an objective, active way in the subacute patient, we may also prevent some patients from lingering into the chronic phase of pain.

REFERENCES

1. Mayer, T., Terry, A., Smith, S., Gatchel, R., Mooney, V.: Quantitative postoperative deficits of physical capacity following spine surgery. *In* Orthopedic Transactions for Proceedings of Annual Meeting of American Academy of Orthopedic Surgeons. San Francisco, Jan. 24–28, 1987.
2. Joint Motion—Method of Measuring and Recording. Park Ridge, IL, AAOS 1965.
3. Schober, P.: Lendenwerelsaule and Kreuzschmergen. Munch Med Wschr *84*:336, 1937.
4. MacRae, I., Wright, V.: Measurements of back movement. Ann Rheum Dis *28*:584, 1969.
5. Anderson, J., Sweetman, B.: A Combined flexi-rule/hydrogoniometer for measurement of lumbar spine and its sagittal movement. Rheumatol Rehab *14*:173–179, 1975.
6. Burton, A.: Regional lumbar sagittal mobility: measurement of flexicurves. Clin Biomech *1*:20–26, 1986.
7. Asmussen, E., Huboll-Nielsen, K.: Posture, mobility and strength of the back in boys, 7–16 years of age. Acta Orthop Scand *28*:174, 1959.
8. Loebl, W.: Measurement of spinal posture and range in spinal movements. Ann Phys Med *9*:103, 1967.

9. Mayer, T., Tencer, A., Kristofferson, S., Mooney, V.: Use of noninvasive techniques for quantification of spinal range of motion in normal subjects and chronic low back dysfunction patients. Spine 9:588–595, 1984.

10. Seligman, J., Gertzbein, S., Tile, M., Kapasourit: Computer analysis of spinal segment motion

11. Thurston, A., Harris, G.: Normal kinematics of the lumbar spine and pelvis

12. Keeley, J., et al.: Quantification of lumbar function part 5: reliability of range of motion measures in the sagittal plane and in in vivo torso rotation measurement technique. Spine 11:31–35, 1986.

13. Andersson, B., Ortengren, R., Herberts, T.: Quantitative electromyography studies of back muscle activity related to posture and loading. Orthop Clin North Am 8:85–96, 1977.

14. Alston, W., Carlson, K., Feldman, D., Gumm, Z., Gerontinos, E.: A quantitative study of muscle fatigue in the chronic low back syndrome. J Am Geriatr Soc 14:419–423, 1966.

15. Cady, L., Bischoff, D., O'Connel, E., Thomas, P., Allan, J.: Strength and fitness and subsequent back injuries in fire fighters. J Occup Med 21:269–272, 1979.

16. Davies, G., Gould, J.: Trunk testing using a prototype Cybex II isokinetic stabilization system. J Orthop Sports Phys Ther 3:164–170, 1982.

17. Flint, M.: Effect of increasing back and abdominal muscle strength on low back pain. Res Quart 29:160–171, 1955.

18. Hasue, M., Fuguwara, M., Kikuchi, S.: A new method of quantitative measurement of abdominal and back muscle strength. Spine 5:143–148, 1980.

19. Langrana, N., Lee, C., Alexander, H., Maycott, C.: Quantitative assessment of back strength using isokinetic testing. Spine 9:287–290, 1984.

20. Mayer, L., Greenberg, B.: Measurements of the strength of trunk muscles. J Bone Joint Surgery 24:842–856, 1942.

21. McNeill, T.W., Warwick, D., Andersson, C., Schultz, A.: Trunk strength in attempted flexion, extension, and lateral bending in healthy subjects and patients with low back disorders. Spine 5:529–538, 1980.

22. Suzuki, N., Endo, S.: A quantitative study of trunk muscle strength and fatigability in the low back pain syndrome. Spine 8:69–74, 1983.

23. Thorstensson, A., Nilsson, J.: Trunk muscle strength during constant and velocity movement. Scand J Rehabil Med 14:61–68, 1982.

24. Smith, S., Mayer, T., Gatchel, R., Becker, T.: Quantification of lumbar function part 1: isometric and multispeed isokinetic trunk strength measures in sagittal and axial planes in normal subjects. Spine 10:757–764, 1985.

25. Mayer, T., Smith, S., Keeley, J., Mooney, V.: Quantification of lumbar function part 2: sagittal plane trunk strength in chronic low back patients. Spine 10:765–772, 1985.

26. Mayer, T., et al.: Quantification of lumbar function part 3: preliminary data on isokinetic torso rotation testing with myoelectric spectral analysis in normal and low back pain subjects. Spine 10:912–920, 1985.

27. Chaffin, D., Andersson, G.: Occupational Biomechanics. New York, John Wiley & Sons, 1984.

28. Pope, M., Frymoyer, J., Andersson, G., Occupational Low Back Pain. New York, Praeger Scientific, 1984.

29. Snook, S., Companelli, R., Hart, J.: A study of three preventive approaches to low back injury. J Occup Med 20:278–481, 1978.

30. Snook, S., Irvine, C.: Maximum acceptable weight of lift. Am J Indust Hyg 9:322–329, 1967.

31. Kroemer, K.: An isoinertial technique to assess individual lifting capability: human factors 25:493–506, 1983.

32. Ayoub, M., Mital, A., Bakken, L., Asfour, S., Bethea, N.: Development of strength and capacity norms for manual materials handling activities: the state-of-the-art. Hum Factors 22:271–283, 1980.

33. Asfour, S., Ayoub, M., Mital, A.: Effects of an endurance and strength training program on lifting capability of male. Ergon 27:283–290, 1984.

34. Chaffin, D., Herrin, G., Keyserling, W.: Pre-employment strength testing: an updated position. J Occup Med 20:403–408, 1978.

35. Keyserling, W., Herrin, G., Chaffin, D.: Isometric strength testing as a means of controlling medical incidents on strenuous jobs. J Occup Med 22:332–336, 1980.

36. Harber, P., Soohoo, K.: Static ergonomics strength testing in evaluating occupational back pain. J Occup Med 26:77–82, 1984.

37. Kishino, N., et al.: Quantification of lumbar function part 4: isometric and isokinetic simulation in normal subjects and low back dysfunction patients. Spine 10:921–927, 1985.

38. Mital, A., Channaveeraiah, C., Fard, H., Khaledi, H.: Reliability of repetitive dynamic strengths as a screening tool for manual lifting tasks. Clin Biomech 1:125–129, 1986.

39. Arnold, J., et al.: Validation and utility of a strength test for selecting steelworkers. J Appl Psychol 67:588–604, 1982.

40. Chaffin, B.: Human strength capability and low back pain. J Occup Med 16:248–254, 1974.

41. Jackson, A., Osburn, H., Laughery, K.: Validity of isometric strength tests for predicting performance in physically demanding tasks. Proc Annu Meet Hum Factors Soc. San Antonio, TX, October 22–26, pp. 451–454, 1984.

42. Kamon, E., Kiser, D., Pytel, J.: Dynamic and static lifting capacity and muscular strength of steelmill workers. Am Ind Hyg Assoc J 43:853–857, 1982.

43. Pytel, J., Kamon, E.: Dynamic strength test as a predictor for maximal and acceptable lifting. Ergonomics 24:663–672, 1981.

44. Reilly, R., Zedeck, S., Tenopry, M.: Validity and fairness of physical ability tests for predicting performance in craft jobs. J Appl Psych 64:262–274, 1979.

45. Schultz A., et al.: Analysis and measurement of lumbar loads in tasks involving bends and twists. J Biomech 15:669–675, 1982.

46. Kondraske, G.: Towards a standard clinical measure of postural stability (Edited by G. Kondraske and C. Robinson). *In* Proc 8th Annu Conf IEEE Eng Med Biol Soc 3:1579–1582, 1986.

47. Kondraske, G., Potvin, A., Tourellatte, W., Syndulko, K.: A computer-based system for automated quantification of neurologic function. IEEE Trans Biomed Eng 31:401–414, 1984.

48. Cady, L., Bischoff, D., O'Connell, M., Thomas, P., Allan, J.: Strength and fitness and subsequent back injuries in firefighters. J Occup Med 21:269–272, 1979.

49. Schmidt, A.: Cognitive factors in the performance level of chronic low back pain patients. J Psychosom Res 29:183–189, 1985.

Preoperative Care and Education

The aphorisms of Hippocrates are one early example of medical education. Typically students and members of the profession were the intended audience. No attempt was made to educate the patient. More than 2000 years later in many parts of the world, this approach remains unchanged. Patients rarely question their physicians and accept the decision for surgery without understanding what the operation is designed to achieve or even why it is necessary.[1]

With the rise of consumerism in the West during the latter half of the 20th century, the situation is changing. Consumer advocates have appeared in all aspects of our society and medicine is no exception. Popular books preach self-help. Television exposés document the shortcomings of the medical profession and expose the fallacies of current treatment. Disputes, once conducted out of public view by learned men of medicine, are now scrutinized in the public press and become the topics of everyday conversation.[2] In a modern society, even Hippocrates would have been called upon to provide prospective clinical trials to defend his use of conflagration rather than advanced chemotherapy. The impact of this interest is clearly visible. The popularity of operations as ubiquitous as tonsillectomy or hysterectomy has withered under the heat of professional skepticism in a public arena.

A patient's decision to accept chymopapain or suction discectomy in lieu of conventional spinal surgery may depend more on public perception than upon scientific information.[3,4] Modern medicine is a victim of its own success. New concepts and state of the art techniques continue to raise patient expectations. Medical entrepreneurs provide the public with varying combinations of science and showmanship, marketing and medical care.[5]

It is against this background of intense consumer pressure, unyielding demands for medical candor, and a panoply of technology that we must assess contemporary preoperative care and education. The medical message in our increasingly concerned and litigious society is strangely at odds with itself. We strive to provide our patients with the latest, often contradictory, information while defending the continuity and competence of our earlier methods; to progress and yet never change.[6] The elimination of prolonged bed rest and the introduction of posture training and exercise in the preoperative routine are typical examples.[7-10] What was right then is wrong now, and yet, preserving the patient's confidence demands that trust in the message remains intact. Delivering effective preoperative education is a greater challenge than many surgeons face.

The patient facing surgery is under considerable pressure. Decisions must be made that will change the quality or even the quantity of life. Choosing options intelligently depends upon an adequate level of knowledge, and knowledge depends upon education. How much the patient finally understands is the measure of the educational effort; who teaches, who listens, and what is taught. The outcome may also depend on when and where the message is delivered. But first, we have to determine why the health care professions should gain the expertise and take the time to educate patients. Until clinicians recognize why they must become involved, they will not make the effort.

WHY

The obvious goal of preoperative care and education is to improve the surgical result.[11] Yet even this apparently self-evident statement is open to question. Until now, there has been little evidence that increased patient understanding actually correlates with an improved outcome. Recent studies, however, indicate that patient comprehension is a signif-

308

Table 28–1
Why

Why?	Why Not?
Improve results	Incorrectly precipitate surgery
Reduce apprehension	Incorrectly postpone surgery
Limit malpractice	Incorrectly eliminate surgery
Promote compliance	

icant factor in the restoration of function and return to work.[12,13]

Although it has been difficult to establish the abstract principle that better education means a better result, there are concrete ways in which greater patient understanding improves outcome. Aligning preoperative expectations with the realistic surgical goals not only promotes patient satisfaction but greatly reduces the risk of malpractice litigation. Patients who understand the intended outcome of the surgery beforehand and who are aware of the operative limitations and potential risks are more likely to accept a final suboptimal result without complaint.[14] Failure to provide adequate education before surgery may leave an unbridgeable gap between expectation and reality. Excusing a minor complication after it develops has a far different psychological impact than predicting the same complication before it occurs.[15] Patients can be remarkably sanguine about postoperative problems when they know what to expect. The same knowledge makes them better able to distinguish trivial situations from those that demand prompt medical attention.[16]

Fear of the unknown increases apprehension and pain. Reassurance before surgery is more effective than reassurance when the patient is already experiencing postoperative pain.[17] Anticipating the patient's concerns not only reduces unnecessary apprehension but strengthens confidence in the surgeon's knowledge and indirectly in the surgeon's skill.

Postoperative rehabilitation often means overcoming the patient's natural reluctance to increase activity. Preoperative care and education that includes training in the postoperative routine can improve and accelerate compliance.[18] By including the patient as an active member of the health care team, responsibility for the preoperative preparation, postoperative recovery, and ultimate surgical outcome can be shared more equitably.

There are less obvious functions for preoperative education. Although the information providing facts and options based on an impartial assessment of the diagnosis and the available treatments is usually regarded by the doctor and the patient as irrefutable,

this is not necessarily the case.[19] Preoperative education is a powerful tool to direct patient behavior and can be used to influence the patient's decisions regarding acceptable management. Formalized education carries a greater impact than casual doctor-patient communication. An institutionalized program places weight on opinions that may or may not hold scientific validity.

Depending upon its emphasis, preoperative teaching can accelerate or even precipitate a surgical decision. Given information that there is no alternative but surgery and that any delay will seriously compromise the chance of success, few patients would opt for long-term conservative care. Conversely, emphasis on adequate presurgical training, physical conditioning, dietary control, weight loss, or the cessation of smoking, may delay surgery for many months.

Promoting nonsurgical options may eliminate the operation altogether. Preoperative care and education can become nonoperative care and education.[20] The power of a well delivered negative message is enough to frighten some patients away from a particular surgical technique or even from a particular surgeon judged unsuitable by the preoperative teacher. Ultimately, this type of education may lead the patient to refuse all surgery and choose instead some form of alternate therapy.

Why should health care professionals take the time and trouble to develop educational skills? Because it offers one of the most efficient methods of altering outcome and, if used appropriately, of improving the surgical result. Furthermore, if we do not guide the education of our own patients, someone else will.

WHO

One of the fundamental principles of effective education is to focus on learner learning rather than on

Table 28–2
WHO

Talks	Listens
Physician/Surgeon	Patients
Physician Assistant	Peer Group
Nursing Staff	General Public
Physical Therapist	Legislators
Occupational Therapist	Third Party Carriers
Exercise Therapist	
Patients	

teacher teaching.[21] What is retained and, more significantly, what changes occur in student behavior are the most accurate measures of an educational program.[22] The choice of content, however, depends upon the interests and background of the teacher. In preoperative care and education, we must look at both participants.

Who Talks

Doctor

It is fitting that the surgeon participates in the preoperative instruction. The most basic form of education before surgery is to answer a patient's questions. Explaining the decision to operate, outlining the preoperative requirements, and discussing the pertinent technical aspects of the procedure are done best by someone with direct involvement and responsibility. It is most appropriate for a member of the surgical team to warn the patient about possible risks and complications.[23]

This aspect of preoperative education is usually carried out individually. Each patient has his or her own set of questions and unique array of fears. Allow adequate time for an open, nonthreatening discussion with ample opportunity for repetition and review. The patient's failure to comprehend a few basic points can lead to a misunderstanding of the entire procedure or intended outcome.

Physician's Assistant

Interns, house officers, clinical fellows, and physician's assistants may act as surrogate surgeons in the educational process. However, although the information may be the same it is more difficult for this group to allay a patient's apprehension. Even the teacher's ignorance of some irrelevant technical information may destroy the listener's confidence and bring into question the validity of the entire presentation. Patients need to be assured that the speaker has a depth of knowledge and experience sufficient to address every contingency. At the same time, the nonsurgeon instructor must avoid raising expectations that cannot be met, or detailing complications that cannot occur. Close communication between the surgeon and his assistants is essential. To avoid intimidating the audience and still maintain control, the young lecturers must develop the ability to convey a sense of authority in a conversational style.

Nursing Staff

Many hospitals provide a formal orientation to acquaint patients with the hospital routines and eliminate much of the mystery and fear surrounding the patient's time in the institution.[24] An effective preoperative program conducted by the nursing service and involving health care professionals not only reduces patient anxiety but improves the surgical outcome through enhanced patient cooperation.[25]

Topics covered during the nursing presentations to the preoperative patient may touch upon the specifics of the surgical procedure but should not include information or concerns best addressed by the surgeon or the surgical team.

Physical Therapist

The physical therapist can play a major role in the preoperative care and education of patients considered for spinal surgery. The patient and professional

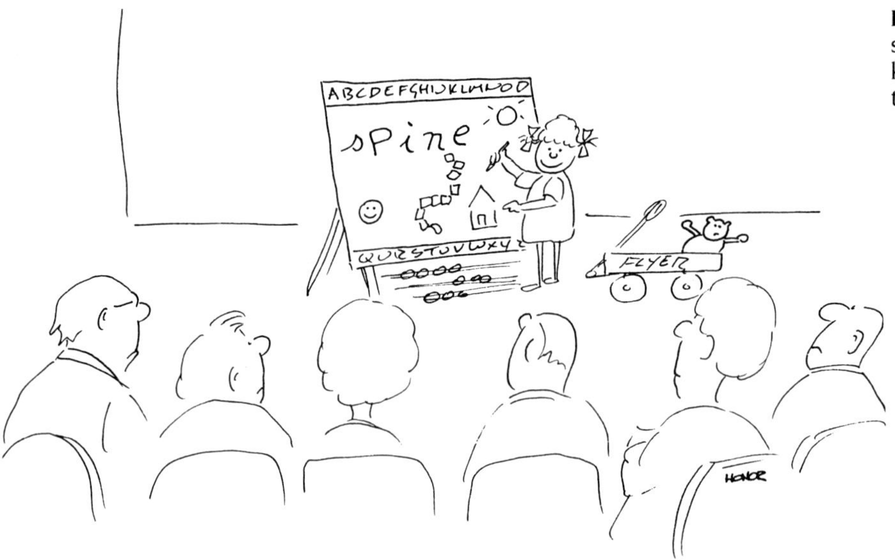

Figure 28–1. Patients need to be assured that the speaker has a depth of knowledge and experience sufficient to address every contingency.

staff often view the operation as an isolated event bearing little relevance to the preoperative treatment or indeed to the entire preoperative period. One goal of education is to ensure that the patient recognizes that surgery is only one, admittedly large, step in a continuing course of treatment. Nowhere is this idea more easily presented than in a program of active preoperative physical therapy.

Like their patients, many surgeons fail to recognize the importance of continuing back care and exercise in both the pre- and postoperative periods.[26] Once surgery has been decided upon, many doctors advise their patients to discontinue further active treatment as it is now perceived to have no additional value. A more appropriate approach would be the concept of a training period preceding the "main event." Patients should be encouraged to take an active role in preparing for surgery through weight loss, cessation of smoking, and regular exercise.

Occupational Therapist

Because the goal of surgery is usually functional restoration and because the return of normal function implies a return to regular employment, the occupational therapist has a place in preoperative care and education. Although the surgically treated spine may be capable of normal activity, the spine itself can no longer be considered normal. Modifications in the workplace, new methods of performing routine tasks, or the need for retraining are issues that involve the occupational therapist. Realistic postoperative expectations and a willingness to continue active rehabilitation after surgery both make the patient a better surgical candidate.

Exercise Therapist

The role of the exercise therapist or trainer overlaps that of the physical or occupational therapist. Providing and supervising an appropriate exercise program requires a great deal of time. Enlisting the aid of exercise specialists can extend the influence of the therapist in the preoperative routine. Because these trainers are not directly associated with the operation, their approach to the patient's problems may differ from that of the more conventional health care team. Added insight, fresh alternatives, and vigorous encouragement help the patient maintain an active role. In some circumstances, an aggressive preoperative training program can lead to such clinical improvement that the operation itself may no longer be required.

Other Patients

Whether the surgeon likes it or not, much of the information about an impending operation comes to the patient through the peer group. The credibility of personal experience gives this source great impact. Selecting patients to share their experiences and offer their own insights presents a point of view that may not be available from the health care professionals.[27] This type of preoperative instruction is best done in a classroom setting in small group discussion. Obviously patients invited to speak must be chosen carefully both for their skill in communication and for the positive aspects of their memories.

Who Listens

Patients and Peers

Preoperative education is obviously directed at the preoperative patient. But the individual about to undergo surgery is not the only one listening to what is said. Friends and relatives often become involved and may require even more information and reassurance than the patient. For this reason it is important to include discussions about the effect of surgery on the patient's activities at home, at work, and in the community. Gaining the support of friends and family members during the postoperative period begins with good preoperative education.

Public

When patient education is provided in an open forum, the general public becomes an audience as well. Many back education programs allow and even invite unlimited participation. Questions about spinal surgery are common and everyone, it seems, has a surgical horror story to tell. Disseminating accurate information about the role, the benefits, the results, and the limitations of surgery can create a more accurate public perception and make it easier to educate the individual.

Third Party

The ramifications of a preoperative educational program can extend far beyond the patient and his peers. Legislators and third party carriers have demonstrated a growing interest in preoperative descriptions of proposed surgery and the definition of an accepted standard of care.[28] Society's willingness to accept and pay for a specific spinal procedure depends on the understanding of those charged with making the administrative and financial decisions, and their understanding, in turn, depends upon effective education.

Those who listen do so with varying degrees of interest. Personal involvement is a superb motivator but anxiety and fear can reduce comprehension.[29] The individual most directly involved may be prevented from assimilating the information. Educating those who provide support for the patient can be valuable.

Each listener listens with a special purpose and harbors particular preconceptions. Those with no more than a general interest may find the information of little immediate value. Others will be looking to confirm or refute a specific proposition or justify a fiscal position. Back education in general and preoperative instruction in particular must contain a positive message that defies misinterpretation. Regardless of the speaker's personal perspective, tailoring content to the needs of the listener is the ultimate goal.

WHERE

At first, the choice of locale for preoperative care and education seems almost irrelevant. In reality, the location affects the educational approach, the emphasis of the message, the degree of retention, and even the purpose of the effort.

Medical Office

The office setting is ideally suited for detailed medical explanations and personal counseling. It is a venue that enhances the image of medical authority and adds weight to the individual physician's opinion. This location is ideal for a medical dissertation to ensure the patient's acceptance of a proposed surgical procedure.

Although the time honored doctor-patient relationship appears to flourish in an office setting, the medical establishment is also a source of anxiety and mistrust for many people. Intimidation can prevent the free exchange of ideas and may lead to a significant lack of "learner learning." In the isolation of the office, a medical practitioner may appear to voice only a personal opinion, an opinion that may conflict with facts the patient has obtained from other sources. Recognizing the doctor's authority in this location the patient may be unwilling or unable to reject unacceptable information.

The space and time constraints of the medical office dictate that preoperative education in this setting is almost always an individual conversation or, at most, a small group discussion. The opportunity for a more elaborate presentation or more detailed explanation is not available.

The intimacy that is one of the benefits of this type of preoperative care is also one of its dangers. The surgeon with a vested interest in a specific procedure or technique will find it easier to persuade

Table 28–3
WHERE

MEDICAL OFFICE	
Pro	**Con**
Increase Authority	Intimidating
Personal & Private	Limited Resources
	Professional Bias

CLINIC	
Pro	**Con**
Convenient	Distracting
Inexpensive	Intimidating
Staff Support	Public

HOSPITAL	
Pro	**Con**
Emotional Impact	Intimidating
High Motivation	Surgical Emphasis
Extensive Resources	Reduce Physician Participation

SPECIAL FACILITY	
Pro	**Con**
Educational Aids	Expensive
Positive Atmosphere	Nonsurgical Emphasis
Peer Support	Institutional Bias
Exercise & Training	
Increase Authority	

the awestruck individual than to confront the skepticism of a larger audience.

Outpatient Clinic

The clinic setting is often both a convenient and inexpensive site for preoperative care and education. While maintaining a high level of medical contact within a conventional medical setting, the treating physician or surgeon also gains support from medical students, residents, and clinic staff. The impact of one medical opinion can be reinforced by other apparently impartial sources.

The proximity of other staff, one of the advantages of a clinic location, can also detract from dis-

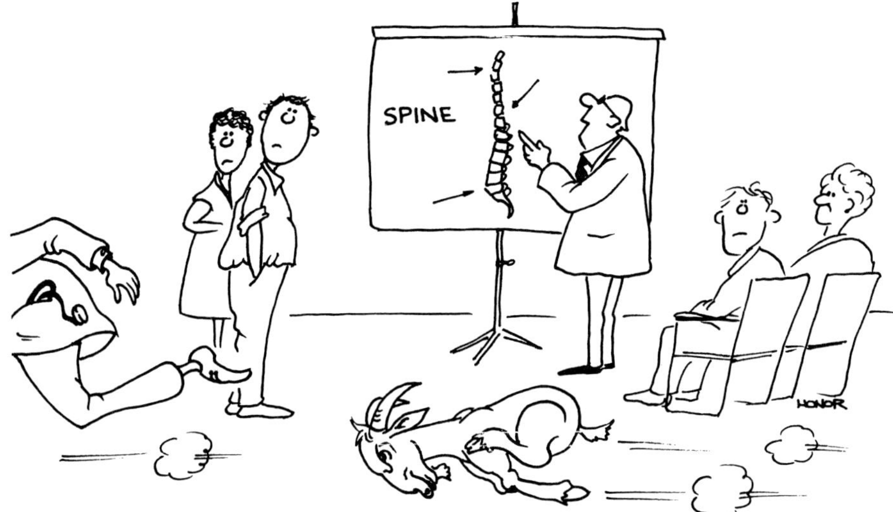

Figure **28–2.** The distraction of routine clinic operation and the proximity of patients uninvolved in preoperative preparation may prove distracting.

seminating preoperative information. Easy patient contact may not equate with adequate patient education. For example, embarrassing personal matters may never be broached in the more public forum. Like the medical office, a busy outpatient clinic may possess time and space limitations that reduce the effectiveness of the program. The distraction of routine clinic operation and the proximity of patients uninvolved in preoperative preparation may prove distracting. The clinic is also part of the accepted medical model. Although this has the advantage of establishing authority, it can also be detrimental to the development of patient self-reliance and self-determination. Counseling the preoperative candidate in a medical setting tends to eliminate nonmedical options and can reinforce passive patterns of behavior.

Hospital

The proximity to the location of the proposed operation makes the hospital preoperative program effective. The patient's initial visits to the hospital have impact and focus attention. By creating a formal program, the hospital can offer both time and space for preoperative care and education.[30] The teaching responsibilities can be delegated to the nursing staff or other hospital employees with particular areas of expertise. This wider involvement adds credibility and addresses additional concerns that may be overlooked in a more circumscribed medical presentation. Bringing together small groups of preoperative patients adds the element of group dynamics and makes use of positive peer pressure.

Again one limitation of the hospital locale is the persuasive medical atmosphere. Patients receiving preoperative instruction in this location are clearly committed to an operative course. The potential to develop a program that eliminates the need for surgery is gone. Furthermore, education tends to focus on the practical aspects of the impending procedure with little or no discussion of alternative treatments. Yet even with these narrowed objectives, the intimidation of the hospital setting can reduce the patient's retention of information.[31]

The availability of auxiliary teachers within the hospital can lead, not to a more cohesive approach, but to an abdication by the surgeon of his educational responsibilities. Time pressure, schedule conflicts, and the inconvenience of traveling to a different location become insurmountable obstacles to the physician's participation in the preoperative program.

Special Facilities

The use of a "back school" as the site for preoperative care and education offers many advantages.[32] At an educational facility, patients have access to classrooms and teaching aids that clarify the message. The ambiance of these locations reflects a positive outlook and emphasizes the need for self-help and self-reliance.[33]

Varying the size and composition of the classes allows patients to exchange information with others in a similar situation, with those who have already undergone an operative procedure and with patients responding to conservative care. Under careful direction, the available small group dynamics can motivate and reassure. Many back schools have developed affiliated exercise and training programs.

Physical conditioning in the preoperative period improves patient morale, enhances the physical response to surgery, and sets a pattern for postoperative rehabilitation.[34] Preoperative physical training can even produce sufficient clinical improvement to justify postponement or cancellation of the operation.

Maintaining a back school requires space and administrative effort.[35] The creation of a special facility to be used solely as a preoperative training center is impractical and unnecessarily expensive. Even when an established back school exists, this approach is not entirely satisfactory. The classroom is the wrong place to discuss individual patient problems of little relevance to the rest of the group. The back school's heavy emphasis on education, self-help, and exercise may deter patients from accepting an operation that is, in fact, their best treatment option. Unless the surgeon provides medical input or is intimately involved in training the back school staff, irrelevant differences of opinion or variations in the style of presentation may appear as significant areas of controversy that can undermine patient confidence and reduce the acceptability of treatment.

The school format is open to abuse. The opinion of an individual surgeon, no matter how intimidating it may be in the confines of a medical office, is still only one person's point of view. In back school, a dramatically presented message gains authority from the institution, which implies universal acceptance. The temptation is always present, and easily rationalized, to introduce a biased judgment or a vested interest as an impartial fact.

WHEN

To qualify as preoperative care and education, treatment and training must take place before surgery. But the length of time between the instruction and the operation has a direct effect upon the message.

Some Time Before

Patients for whom the prospect of surgery lies well in the future are less interested in the specifics of the procedure and more concerned with the possibility of avoiding an operation altogether. The information they require pertains more to the general nature of their spinal problem, its natural history, and the role surgery might take in improving the outcome. Attention is given to the practical physical means by which the patient can improve back care and reduce discomfort and less emphasis is placed on the psychological aspects of treatment. In this

Table 28–4
When

Some Time Before
General Information
Nonsurgical Options
Total Treatment Plan
Promote Teamwork
Just Before
Adjust Expectations
Surgical Details
Pre and Postoperative Planning
Patient Responsibilities
Not Before
Reassurance
Realistic Options
Active Participation
Lifestyle Modification
Exercise

group the overall level of interest may not be as high as it is in patients for whom surgery is imminent, however neither is their retention reduced by excessive anxiety.

At this time it is important to present surgery as part of the complete treatment program rather than as an isolated event. Instead of accepting someone else's decision, the patient should come to his or her own conclusion that surgery is necessary. Allowing a patient to explore alternatives, even when these prove unsuccessful, promotes active participation, increases confidence in the surgical option and creates a sense of teamwork that will last through the operative period and beyond.

Postoperative exercises are best learned and practiced before the overwhelming distraction of postoperative pain.

Just Before

When surgery is on the immediate horizon, there is an obvious need to ensure that the patient's expectations match those of the surgical team. Obtaining an informed consent, for example, is one byproduct of adequate preoperative education. As the time of surgery approaches, patients focus more on

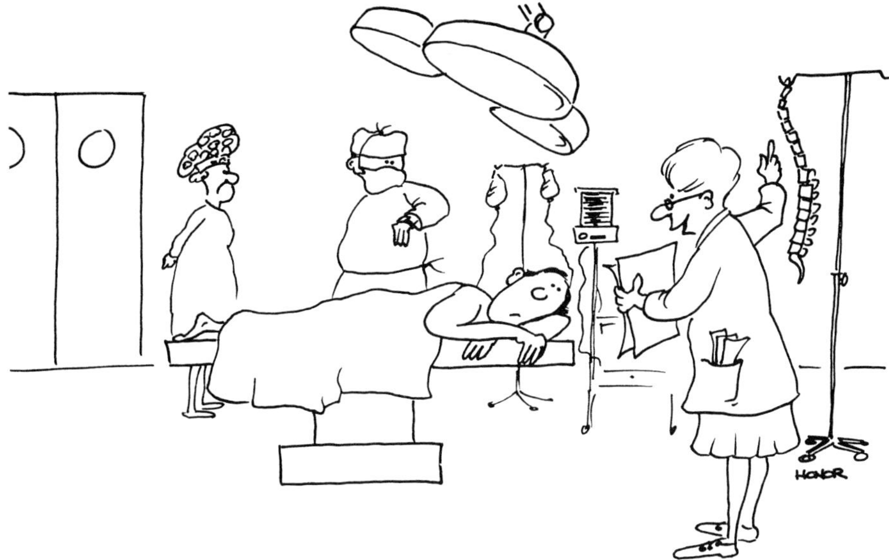

Figure 28–3. As the time of surgery approaches, patients focus more on the details of the pre- and postoperative period.

the details of the pre- and postoperative period. Teaching should review pertinent parts of the procedure, potential complications and, most important, the patient's responsibilities.[36] The time for prevention or alternative treatment is past and patients must be reassured that they are correct in their decision to accept surgery.[37]

Not Before

The success of conservative care is measured in the amount of functional recovery. The goal should be a patient who, having received and complied with the instruction, no longer requires the surgical procedure. Unfortunately with some surgeons, conservative management is seen only as a holding pattern to be maintained until it is time to operate. The balance is a delicate one; convincing patients to work diligently to prevent an operation without eliminating the acceptance of surgery should it become necessary.

Patients without a surgical option can regard their back problem as incurable. The prestige of modern medicine and the strength of the popular misconceptions cause some patients who are denied surgery to fail to appreciate the generally benign natural history of back pain and the importance of simple self-help routines. The situation is aggravated by a surgeon who focuses more on the procedure than on the patient. The phrase, "I can't help you," does not, as the patient fears, imply that the situation is hopeless, but rather that the doctor has determined surgical intervention is not the solution.[38] For non-operative patients a program of back care and education restores perspective and defines a practical approach to recovery. Like patients facing surgery, those receiving nonsurgical care must play an active role in the recovery process.

WHAT

Ultimately, the content of the message has the greatest influence on the preoperative program. But almost as important are the style of presentation, its comprehensibility, and its emphasis.

The language used must be the patient's. There is no place for technical jargon. Translating medical diagnoses and procedures into simple terms is more difficult than many physicians realize, but a message conveyed in words that frighten or confuse is of no value and may be detrimental. The word "arthritis" is an excellent example. To the medical practitioner, it is only a descriptive term describing joint inflammation and used in a variety of contexts with a range of diagnoses. The word itself carries no diagnostic significance and therefore no prognostic value. To the average patient, arthritis defines a progressive illness afflicting most joints of the body and leading to permanent deformity and loss of function. For most, the term conjures up an image of severe late stage rheumatoid disease. The casual use of the word arthritis to describe benign inflammatory changes within the spinal apophyseal joints during a discussion of the common sources of back pain completely reverses the intended reassuring image.

The use of medical terminology is only one possible mistake. The old adage goes, "It's not what you say, it's the way that you say it." The lecturer's enthusiasm or apparent skepticism makes an enormous difference. In describing a new and unproven

Table 28–5
What

BASICS

   Anatomy

   Physiology

   Pathology

   Surgical Logic

   Emotional Impact

TECHNIQUES

   Pre & Postoperative Routines

   Role & Rationale of Surgery

   Patient Participation

OPTIONS

   Nonsurgical Alternatives

STYLE

   Informal

   Understandable

   Convincing

   Comprehensive

surgical technique, for instance, the phrases "this potentially useful technique" and "this highly experimental technique" may both be true, but the message conveyed to the listener is quite different.

Even the style of presentation has an effect. Formal instruction may enhance the image of authority, but it stifles feedback and conversation. An informal discussion is usually more appropriate. Creating the impression that both the lecturer and the audience are involved in the planning and decision making process goes a long way to reassure the patient about the wisdom of his or her decision to accept surgery.

Basics

An understanding of simple anatomy and physiology is essential to the patient's comprehension of most spinal procedures. It is a challenge to convey this information in a fashion that average patients can understand. If patients appear slow and uncomprehending because of a lack of knowledge of the terminology or a scientific background, translating the information into an accessible form can have dramatic results. Most spinal procedures are simple in concept and the correct decision to operate em-

ploys straightforward logic.[39] When the surgeon finds it impossible to describe this decision making process to the patient in clear definitive steps, it is wiser to question the validity of the surgeon's logic than the intelligence of the listener.

Because technical detail is unimportant in the early stages of preoperative education and because a decision to operate is rarely made on the basis of available technique alone, the primary level of education should be set at a basic level. For the average patient, it is more helpful to learn that discs do not actually slip out from between the bones of the spine than to hear a discussion on the biomechanical properties of a new surgical implant. A knowledge of simple functional anatomy makes it possible to grasp the purpose of the proposed operation without comprehension of the surgical detail.

Understanding the emotional impact of surgery is as fundamental as understanding the physical problem. The role of fear and anxiety in the amplification of pain must be thoroughly discussed.[40] When a painful experience is anticipated and explained, most patients accept it. Predicting the problem before it occurs demonstrates the doctor's competence. Offering sympathy after the fact is no substitute.

Perhaps the most important emotional issue to be discussed before surgery is the concept that an operation treats mechanical derangements—it does not directly treat pain. The presence of a chronic pain state with the intensity of the symptoms bearing little relationship to the physical abnormalities in the spine is a strong contraindication to surgery. Recognizing the problem in the preoperative period and taking remedial action benefits both the patient and the surgeon.

Techniques

As surgery becomes imminent, many patients develop considerable curiosity regarding the technical aspects of the procedure. Inherent in their questioning is the need to understand how the physical act of surgery will resolve their specific spinal problem. Once again, the surgeon must be able to explain the logic which led to the operative decision or to the choice of a particular procedure.

In addition to operative detail, the technical description should focus on the patient's role, not only in the preoperative period, but also during the time in the hospital and in the postoperative phase. The final outcome is best presented as a risk/benefit equation allowing the patient the opportunity to understand both what can be gained and what may be lost. Unfortunately, this may also be the first time the surgeon draws a concise comparison between the natural history of the disease and the surgical probabilities.

Options

Once surgery has been agreed upon it is difficult to remember that other options always exist.[41] Preoperative care and education must include a review of these alternatives. Furthermore, the alternatives must be presented honestly and with the same amount of conviction given to the operative choice.[42] Patients and surgeons primed for a major technical tour de force may have little enthusiasm for discussing basic lifestyle modification or routine exercise. But surgery is rarely the only answer. Before surgery is judged the best option, the other less glamorous but less dangerous approaches must be fairly considered.

Explaining the positive sides of a procedure is easy. Outlining the negative aspects must be done with care. Far from providing reassurance, a poorly conceived preoperative program can threaten or at least discomfort both the patient and the surgeon.

The outcome and the value of preoperative care and education ultimately depend upon the motivation of those involved as well as the skill of the teacher, the receptiveness of the listener, the quality of the message, and an appropriate choice of location and timing.

REFERENCES

1. Rosenthal, E.: Out of Africa. Discover *10*(8):37, 1989.
2. Mooney, V.: Where is the pain coming from? Spine *12*(8):754, 1987.
3. Davis, G.W., Onik, G.: Clinical experience with automated percutaneous lumbar discectomy. Clin Orthop *283*:98, 1989.
4. McCulloch, J.A.: Ruptured lumbar discs (herniated nucleus pulposis). *In* Current Therapy in Sports Medicine-2 (Edited by J.S. Torg, R.P. Welsh, and R.J. Shephard). Toronto, B.C. Decker, 1990.
5. Gortner, S.R., Hudes, M., Zyzanski, S.J.: The appraisal of values in the choice of treatment. Nursing Research, *33*:319, 1984.
6. Dandy, W.E.: Loose cartilage from intervertebral disc simulating tumor of the spinal cord. Arch Surg *19*:660, 1929.
7. Deyo, R.A.: Conservative therapy for low back pain. JAMA *250*(8):1057, 1983.
8. Spitzer, W.O., et al.: Scientific approach to the assessment and management of activity-related spinal disorders. Spine *12*(7S):S24, 1987.
9. Deyo, R.A., Diehl, A.K., Rosenthall, M.: How many days of bedrest for acute low back pain? N Engl J Med *315*:1064, 1986.
10. Jackson, C.P., Brown, M.D.: Analysis of current approaches and a practical guide to prescription of exercise. Clin Orthop *179*:46, 1983.
11. Linde, B.J., Janz, N.M.: Effect of a teaching program on knowledge and compliance of cardiac patients. Nurs Res *25*(5):282, 1979.
12. Hall, H., Iceton, J.A.: Back school, an overview with specific reference to the Canadian Back Education Units. Clin Orthop *179*:10, 1983.
13. Lacroix, J.M., et al.: Low back pain: factors of value in predicting outcome. Spine, *15*:495–499, 1990.
14. Johnson, J.E.: Effects of structuring patients' expectations on their reactions to threatening events. Nurs Res *21*:499, 1972.
15. Sime, A.M.: Relationship of preoperative fear, type of coping, and information received about surgery to recovery. J Pers Soc Psychol *34*:716, 1976.
16. Anderson, E.A.: Preoperative preparation for cardiac surgery facilitates recovery, reduces psychological distress, and reduces the incidence of acute postoperative hypertension. J Consult Clin Psychol *55*(4):513, 1987.
17. Egbert, L.D., Battit, G.E., Welch, C.E., Bartlett, M.K.: Reduction of postoperative pain by encouragement and instruction of patients. N Engl J Med *270*:825, 1964.
18. Edwinson, M., Arnbjörnsson, E., Ekman, R.: Psychologic preparation program for children undergoing acute appendectomy. Pediatrics *82*(1):30, 1988.
19. Newcombe, R.G.: Towards a reduction in publication bias. Br Med Bull *295*:656, 1987.
20. Mooney, V.: Alternate approaches for patients beyond the help of surgery. Orthop Clin North Am *6*:331, 1975.
21. Bugelski, B.R.: The Psychology of Learning Applied to Teaching. New York, Bobbs-Merrill, 1971.
22. Caplan, R.M., Solomon, L.M.: Instructional objectives in dermatology. Arch Derm *104*:345, 1971.
23. Egbert, L.D., Battit, G.E., Turndorf, H., Beecher, H.K.: The value of the preoperative visit by an anesthetist. JAMA *185*:553, 1963.
24. Redman, B.K.: The process of patient teaching in nursing. St. Louis, C.V. Mosby, 1968.
25. Healy, K.M.: Does preoperative instruction make a difference? Am J Nurs *68*(1):62, 1968.
26. Jackson, C.P., Brown, M.D.: Is there a role for exercise in the treatment of patients with low back pain? Clin Orthop *179*:39, 1983.
27. Hall, H., Hunt, M., Tennant, H.: Talking Back in Class. Toronto, The Canadian Back Institute, 1983.
28. Blankstein, A., et al.: Disc space infection and vertebral osteomyelitis as a complication of percutaneous lateral discectomy. Clin Orthop *225*:234, 1987.
29. Orr, D.: Reducing presurgical anxiety. Canadian Operating Room Nursing Journal *51*(2):29, 1986.
30. McClurg, E.: Developing an effective patient teaching program. AORN Journal *34*(3):474, 1981.
31. Chansky, E.R.: Reducing patients' anxiety: techniques for dealing with crisis. AORN Journal *40*(3):375, 1984.
32. Jackson, C.P., Klugerman, M.: How to start a back school. JOSPT *10*(1):1, 1988.
33. Moffett, J.A.K., Chase, S.M., Porter, I., Ennis, J.R.: A controlled prospective study to evaluate the effectiveness of the back school in the relief of chronic low back pain. Spine *11*:121, 1986.
34. Jackson, C.P.: Therapeutic exercises for low back patients. Presented at the Challenge of the Lumbar Spine, New York, October, 1987.
35. Matmiller, A.W.: The California Back School. Physiotherapy *66*(4):118, 1980.
36. Tagliacozzo, D.L., Mauksch, H.D.: The patient's view of the patient's role. *In* Patients, Physicians and Illness (Edited by E.G. Jaco). London, Collier-Macmillan, 1972.
37. Ramsay, M.A.E.: A survey of preoperative fear. Anesthesia *27*:396, 1972.
38. Hall, H.: The Back Doctor. New York, McGraw-Hill, 1980.
39. Hall, H.: More Advice from the Back Doctor. Toronto, McClelland and Stewart, 1987.
40. Bacal, S., Lacroix, J.M.: Illness schemata in multisymptomatic patients. Can Physiologist *28*(2a):17, 1987.
41. Hall, H.: Conservative back care. *In* Current Therapy in Sports Medicine—2. (Edited by J.S. Torg, R.P. Welsh, and R.J. Shephard). Toronto, B.C. Decker, 1990.
42. Hall, H.: Better Backs in 30 Days. Toronto, McClelland and Stewart-Bantam, 1989.

Jeffrey A. Saal
Joel S. Saal

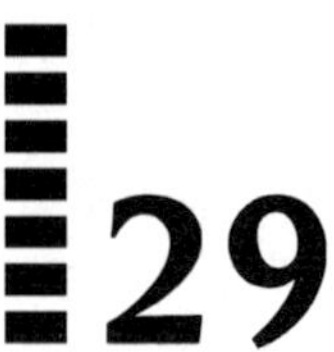

Postoperative Rehabilitation and Training

INTRODUCTION

Rehabilitation of the postoperative patient is a comprehensive process, the primary goal of which is to optimize function. The focus of the rehabilitation program must be on improving function and the quality of life rather than on primarily treating pain. Although some patients become pain free following the postoperative period, this period is frequently marked by new symptoms of back pain or by the persistence of the patient's all too familiar preoperative symptom of leg pain. Residual structural abnormalities and a progression of degenerative changes at the operative segment and adjacent levels may surface as sources of pain in the early or late postoperative period.[1] In more complex cases of multilevel disease, there may be some residual pain, with resolution of only part of the preoperative complaints. The primary purposes of a postoperative rehabilitation program should be to expedite and maximize return to function, limit the accelerating progression of degenerative changes, and prevent further injury. The program should teach patients to assume control of their lumbar dysfunction rather than allow their pain to dictate their lives. It is important to establish realistic goals for each individual at the outset of the program, with modification of those goals at intervals of progress assessment. Evaluating each patient's goals individually will set exit criteria for treatment. Because cure is rarely accomplished in the treatment of any medical condition, successful treatment should be judged by the degree of functional improvement attained.

Factors to Consider in the Postoperative Patient

A number of negative metabolic factors noted in the postoperative patient must be addressed. Post-operative discectomy patients will have suffered significant losses in truncal muscular strength and endurance.[2] Surgical intervention often results in a loss of total body iron and protein and other nutrients. In addition, bed rest causes aerobic deconditioning and loss of mineral matrix from the skeleton.[3-6] Finally, preoperative diseases and symptoms cause losses in spinal range of motion and muscle contracture.[7] All of these factors must be addressed in the postoperative rehabilitation program.

There is limited information available on postoperative rehabilitation research.[2,8-12] The results of one of these studies,[2] a single, controlled, randomized trial of postoperative rehabilitation versus normal care in discectomy patients, would suggest that the level of preoperative disability is a more important predictor of disability outcome than the type of postoperative care received. However, this study's short observation period and the insensitivity of the outcome measurement used limits the scope of the application of this conclusion. Thus, it is valid to hypothesize that a well designed postoperative rehabilitation program should be able to reverse the disability more rapidly than an unguided and self paced return to activity regime.

The major factors to consider prior to planning a postoperative program are the type of surgery, the length and degree of preoperative debility, the surgical complications encountered, residual pathology, and patient motivation. Underlying medical conditions, such as cardiovascular disease and diabetes, must also be accounted for. Age as an independent variable probably will not significantly affect the outcome.[13] Ideally, prior to surgery, the patient will have already undergone back school education and dynamic muscular stabilization training. If, however, significant preoperative debility limited the preoperative training program, then the training process must begin immediately in the postoperative period.

Therefore, the postoperative treatment program must really begin at a preoperative stage. The stronger, more flexible and better trained the patient is the shorter the postoperative recovery period. Surgery should be considered part of a rehabilitation continuum. The patient should be exercise-trained up to the time of surgery, and no postoperative delay should ensue prior to starting the postoperative phase. Obviously, postoperative success depends on an accurate and precise postoperative diagnosis. If a painful disorder, such as nerve root canal stenosis is left unaltered, the preoperative radicular pain cannot be expected to improve. A therapeutic plan for residual pain is also important and is discussed later in this chapter.

Dynamic Muscular Stabilization Training

Training for dynamic muscular stabilization should be the focal point of a patient's exercise program. Stabilization as program focus is motivated by the following observations. Repetitive flexion and torsional stress to the lumbar intervertebral discs and facet joints lead to advanced degenerative changes through microtrauma of the lumbar segments.[14–18] Gradual disc prolapse secondary to fatiguing of the annular fibers is another important factor of repetitive microtrauma.[15] Stabilization eliminates this repetitive microtrauma to the lumbar motion segments, thereby limiting the injury that has occurred and allowing healing to take place. Stabilization is accomplished through coordinated use of the trunk and proximal extremity musculature in order to limit microtraumatic motions during activity. This musculature also absorbs external forces otherwise directly transmitted to the motion segment. In this manner, stabilization may alter the natural history of the degenerative cascade.

In the postoperative spine, it is important to allow the annulus to heal, thereby guarding against reherniation of nuclear material.[19,20] Additionally, proper muscular stabilization allows fusions to heal by limiting excessive motion, a task that bracing is unable to accomplish. Theoretically, fusion mass loading and muscle contraction increase fusion mass incorporation and maturation by increasing the piezoelectric activity of the newly forming bone matrix.[21] The mechanical consequences of discectomy allow for decreased mechanical stiffness of the segment, and increased creep at a given level of applied force. If indeed dynamic muscular stabilization training is able to impede the degenerative cascade[1] this should slow the development of postoperative stenosis and disc breakdown at adjacent levels.

Muscle fusion is the implementation of the musculature to brace the spine and protect the motion segments against repetitive microtrauma and excessively high single occurrence loads. The abdominal mechanism, a coupling of the midline ligament with the dorsolumbar fascia, combined with a slight reduction in the lumbar lordosis can eliminate shear stress to the lumbar intervertebral segments.[22,23] The abdominal musculature has the unique ability to flex the lumbar spine through its action on the superficial portion of the dorsolumbar fascia. This musculature can also extend the lumbar spine through its action on the deep portions of the fascia that form the alar interspinal ligaments.[22–24] The action of the abdominal musculature corsets the lumbar region when working in concert with the latissimus dorsi, a muscle which also acts upon the dorsolumbar fascia. The abdominal musculature is the only muscle group able to protect the spine from torsional stresses. The spinal extensor muscles exert a force vector that is too close to the midline to accomplish this task.[22,23]

These biomechanic and pathophysiologic descriptions arise from the hypothesis that for its own protection, the intervertebral joint has the capacity to react to its internal stress. It has the capacity to control the force exerted upon it by an applied load. The idea is that a feedback mechanism monitoring the forces at the intervertebral joint can modify muscular activity in such a way as to minimize stress at the joint and, therefore, reduce the risk of injury. Muscular activity can adaptively control this internal stress it modifies by spinal geometry. The forces induced by these muscles and their activity can also be monitored and controlled by a potential feedback mechanism. By lowering the level of equalized stress to a minimum, the risk of injury to the lumbar spine can be lowered.

The existence of a well developed network of nerve fibers connecting receptor systems located in places such as periosteum and annulus has been identified.[22,25] This system is not only important in pain transmission but may also be important in kinesthetic feedback for joint positioning. Disruption of these structures, the proprioceptive fibers and the thoracolumbar fascia, occurs during surgical exposure and removal of bone. Afterward, the feedback loop must be retrained to use existing pathways.

Considering the degrees of freedom of axial rotation that are allowable in each intervertebral segment at different degrees of lordosis, one can see the importance of controlling lordosis during flexion or extension. Lordosis is controlled by a dynamic assessment and adjustment of the lumbosacral angle and by combined use of the spine extensors and flexors. Control of lordosis is an essential component of a lumbar spine rehabilitation program. Thus, balanced muscular function and flexibility ultimately control the stresses applied to the lumbar intervertebral segments.

It should be pointed out that the annulus of the intervertebral disc appears to be almost entirely responsible for the load transmission of the intervertebral segment. Removal of the nucleus does not greatly affect joint response. Therefore, repetitive loads applied to the lumbar intervertebral joint fall upon the posterolateral fibers of the annulus, leading to progressive tearing, fatigue, and potential disc prolapse.[14,15] Load transmission to the facet joints occurs through repetitive extension maneuvers. It has been well demonstrated that narrowing of the intervertebral disc also increases load transmission to the facet joints.[14] The combination of a degenerative segment combined with repetitive extension and rotation loads to the lumbar intervertebral joints can lead to progressive joint failure. The principles of neutral spine positioning and dynamic control of lumbar lordosis help to protect this portion of the motion segment.

In summary, muscle fusion involves the cocontraction of the abdominal muscles to maintain a corseting effect to the lumbar spine using the midline ligament and thoracolumbar fascia, coupled with proper pelvic positioning. The reduction of translational stress to the intervertebral segments by spinal extensor muscles is important during activity, and the extensors must be trained to balance shear stress to the intervertebral segments. The multifidus muscle appears to be the most active in this regard[22,23] and is also the most difficult to strengthen because of its short segmental nature. The gluteus maximus may indeed be the most important extensor muscle controlling the lumbar spine's lifting power.[22] The postoperative training program should be directed at improving the endurance, power, and coordination of all these muscle groups. Figures 29–1 to 29–8 present examples of such training exercises.

POSTOPERATIVE REHABILITATION PROGRAM—SPINECARE MEDICAL GROUP

In-Hospital Phase

Following is an explanation of the postoperative rehabilitation program used by SpineCare Medical Group in the treatment of our patients. The in-hospital phase of the program includes the following:

1. Hamstring stretches
2. Knee-to-chest stretches
3. Two-flights-of-stairs walk prior to discharge

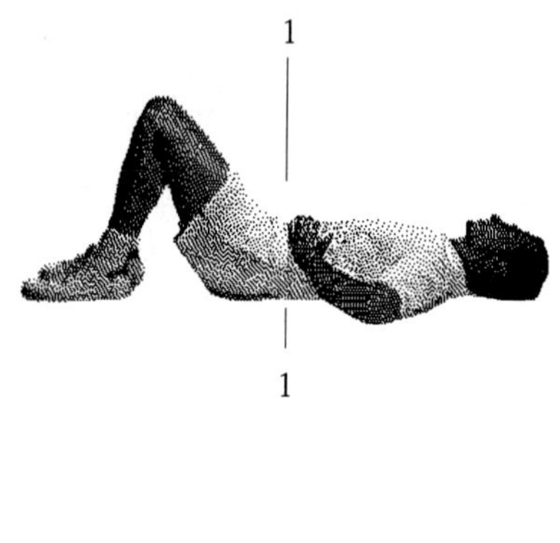

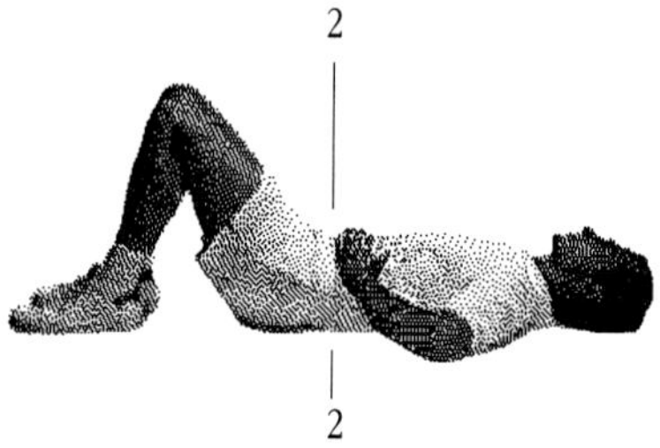

Figure 29–1. Isometric abdominal bracing. *Purpose*: To strengthen your abdominal muscles. 1. Lie on your back with your knees bent. 2. Contract your abdominal muscles. Continue to breathe while contracting them.

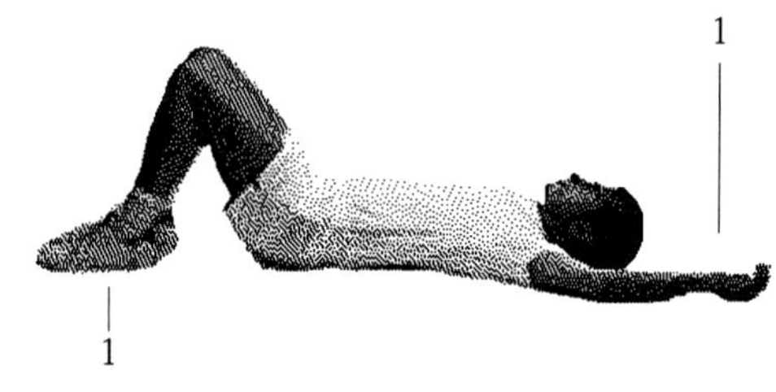

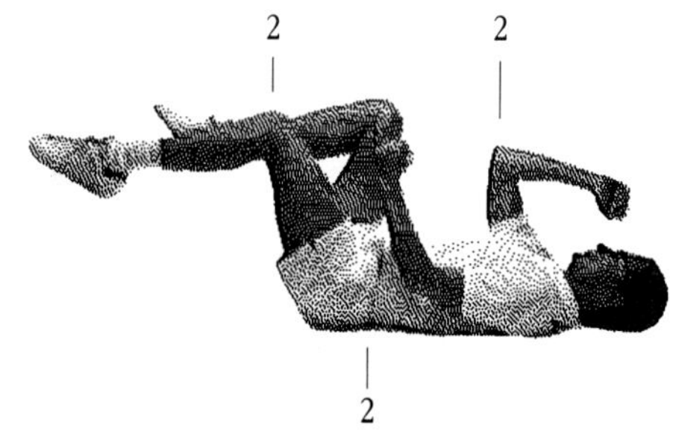

Figure 29–2. Dynamic abdominal bracing. *Purpose*: To strengthen your abdominal muscles. 1. Lie on your back with knees bent, one arm above your head, and one arm at your side. 2. Raise your legs off the floor with knees bent. Pump your arms and legs.

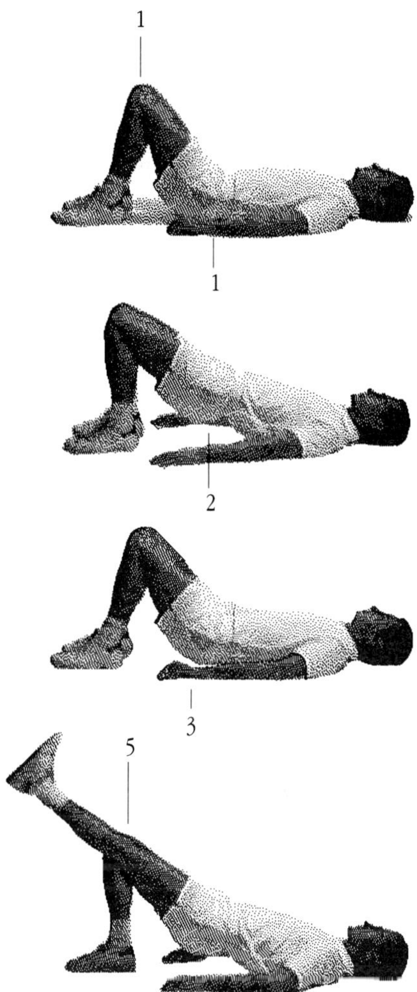

Figure 29–3. Bridging. *Purpose*: To strengthen your abdominal, buttocks, and low back muscles. 1. Lie on your back with knees bent. 2. Raise your hips and back from the floor. Hold this neutral bridge position. 3. Lower yourself to within one inch off the floor. Repeat the exercise. *With Leg Extension*: 4. Perform steps 1 and 2 above. 5. From the neutral bridge position, slowly straighten your left leg from the knee. Hold this position. Lower your left leg. Then extend your right leg.

4. Abdominal bracing
5. Activities-of-daily-living stabilization training

Patients are taught to stretch their hamstrings while lying in a supine position using a belt or bed sheet for assistance and are cautioned not to stretch to the point that radicular symptoms flare. Strict adherence to neutral spine stabilization is reinforced during this phase. Limitation of any flexion during stabilization is important, and excessive flexion is the most common mistake patients make. Flexion exercises have the benefit of stretching the dorsolumbar fascia.[24] However, flexion must be used

cautiously because of the rises in intradiscal pressure that result and because of the heightened stress that is placed on the posterior annulus.[15] Flexion when sitting is the most hazardous because of the acute rise in intradiscal pressure that results. Additionally, lumbar flexion exercises performed with the legs fully extended cause the greatest degree of flexion of the lower spinal segments and exposes the posterior annulus to potentially injurious forces. Therefore, if flexion exercises are to be done, they must be performed in spine-safe positions. These positions unload the spinal segment, but still allow a flexion stretch to occur.

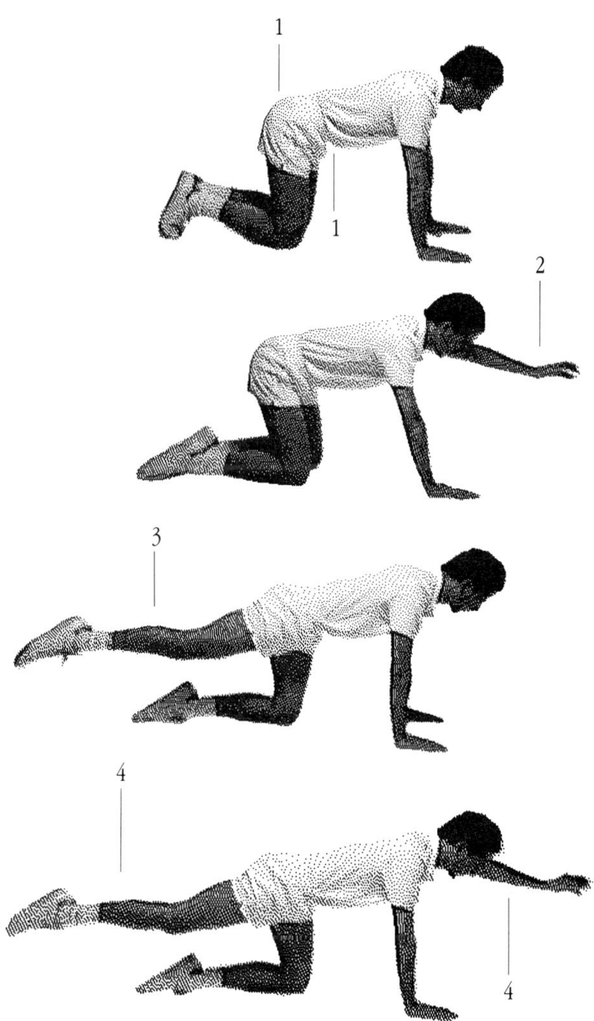

Figure 29–4. Quadriped arm and leg. *Purpose*: To strengthen your abdominal, buttocks, and back muscles. 1. Get down on your hands and knees. Tighten your stomach and buttocks muscles. 2. Raise your arms alternately. 3. Raise your legs alternately. 4. Alternately raise your opposite arms and legs.

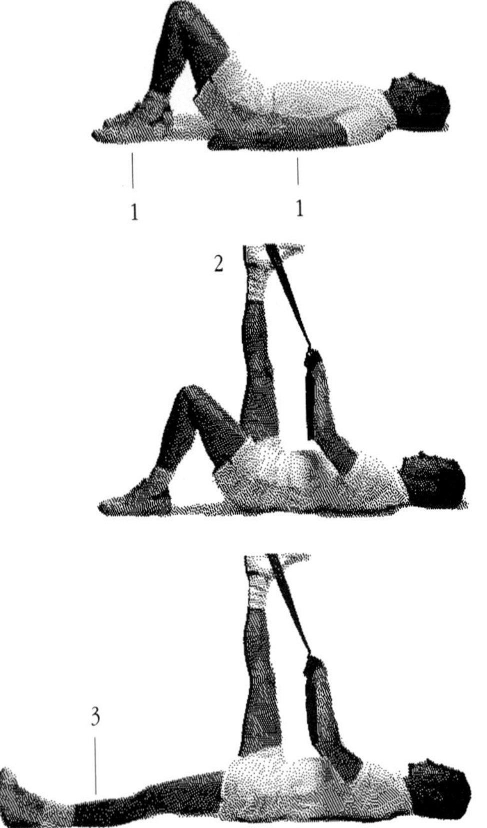

Figure 29–5. Hamstring stretch. *Purpose*: To stretch the muscles of the back of your thighs. 1. Lie on your back with your knees bent. 2. Loop a long strap under the sole of your right foot. Straighten your right leg, then pull it toward you until you feel a stretch at the back of your thigh. 3. Slowly extend your left leg, keeping it on the floor. Repeat with the other leg.

Post-Hospital Phase

After being discharged from the hospital, patients are instructed to increase their walking capacity up to one mile per day. Obviously, some elderly and more debilitated patients may not be able to meet this goal. Patients are expected to continue the exercises they were taught during the 2-week period after surgery, the in-hospital phase.

At 2 weeks, after an office evaluation by one of the nonoperative team members, usually a physiatrist, the patient is placed in a supervised physical reconditioning program that meets three times a week. During this phase, the exercise program proceeds from basic level exercises to exercises that progressively challenge the muscular and cardiovascular system. A home program is prescribed for the patient to practice when not in the supervised sessions. The home program closely follows the supervised regimen, and is undertaken on all days that lack a supervised session.

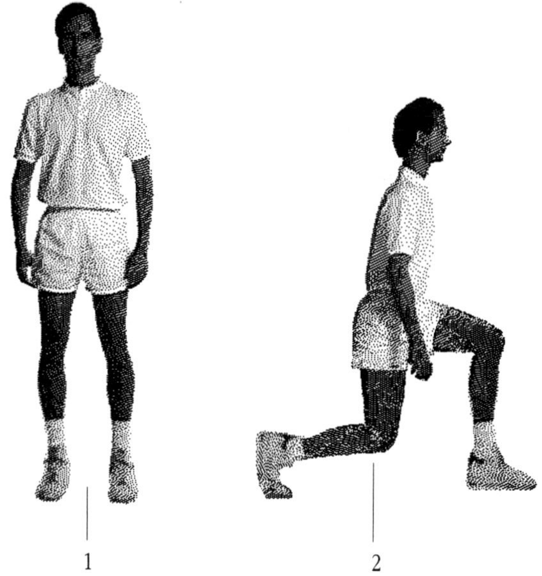

Figure 29–6. Forward lunge. *Purpose*: To strengthen your thigh and buttocks muscles. 1. Stand with your feet, shoulder width apart, knees slightly bent. 2. Lunge forward with your left leg. Your right knee should almost touch the floor. Return to your original standing position. Repeat the exercise with the opposite leg.

Pain Relieving Modalities

Pain relieving modalities such as transcutaneous nerve stimulation and pulsed alternating electrical muscle stimulation together with ice can be useful to reduce postoperative pain.[12] Spinal immobilization with a corset or semirigid brace may be useful for patients who are not yet strong enough to use their own musculature to stabilize the spine. Studies of these devices have demonstrated the corset's inability to immobilize the lower lumbar spinal segments.[26] Thus, caution must be exercised when prescribing these appliances because they may lead to trunk flexor and extensor muscle weakness if over used. Patients must be instructed to remove the orthotic device at least once daily to exercise the trunk musculature. Patients who have become dependent upon the appliance must be weaned from it slowly while progressively strengthening their supporting musculature to replace the corset. Our patients are not routinely given a brace after fusion.

Epidural cortisone injections may be useful for controlling persistent disabling radicular pain, but they are usually reserved for the period after the first six weeks following surgery. Epidural cortico-

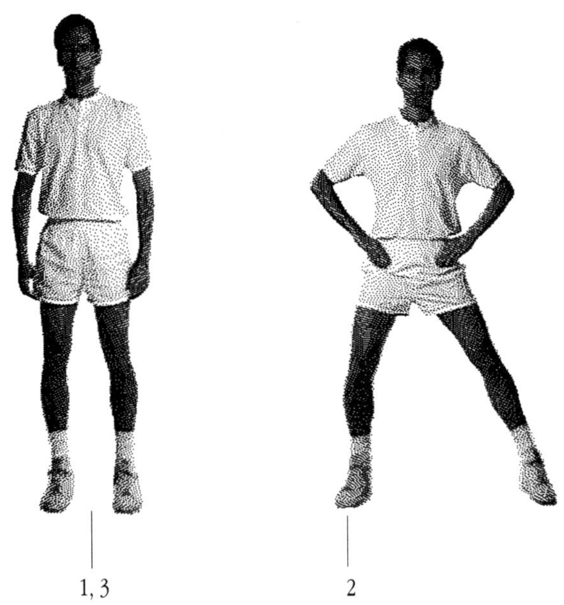

Figure 29–7. Sideways lunge. *Purpose*: To strengthen your thigh and buttocks muscles. 1. Stand with your feet shoulder width apart, knees slightly bent. Contract your abdominal muscles. 2. Lunge sideways with one leg. 3. Return to your original standing position. Repeat the exercise with the opposite leg.

steroids are most beneficial for patients with more leg pain than back pain and for those who manifest dural tension signs on physical examination. These injections are purely facilitators to a rehabilitation program, not a treatment in their own right.

Intra-articular lumbar facet injections under fluoroscopic guidance place corticosteroids into inflamed facet capsules. These injections are sometimes necessary for a patient having persistent mechanical symptoms that cannot be controlled by the stabilization training. They are also reserved for the later phases of the postoperative program. Anti-inflammatory medication in the early phases of treatment may be appropriate. The report of high levels of phospholipase A2 activity in herniated discs supports the contention that inflammation plays a role in symptomatic disc herniation.[27] The analgesic effect of the nonsteroidal anti-inflammatory drugs (NSAIDs) as well as their ability to act as prostaglandin synthetase inhibitors mean that these medications have a role in the treatment of lumbar pain syndromes. Oral corticosteroids can be useful in the treatment of radicular pain. The exact dosage and optimal time frame are unclear, but their efficacy has been satisfactorily established.[28]

The use of opiate analgesics is often necessary in the initial week after surgery. The proper use of positioning, rest, ice, transcutaneous nerve stimula-

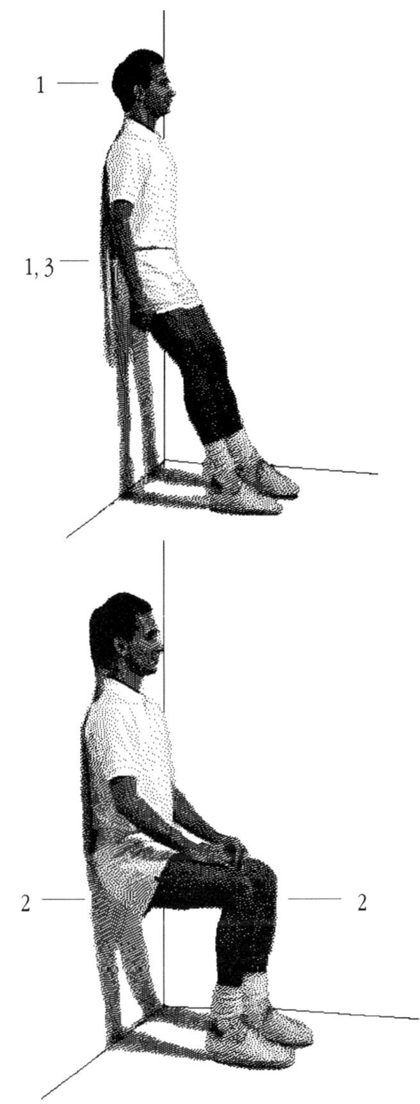

Figure 29–8. Wall slide. *Purpose*: To strengthen your thigh muscles. 1. Lean against the wall. 2. Slide down the wall to a position that your leg muscles will tolerate. Do not bend your knees more than 90 degrees. 3. Return to starting position.

tion, and NSAIDs usually precludes the need for opiate analgesics. During the initial weeks, pain is the guide for exercise progression. An increase in radicular pain is cause for program re-evaluation. If patients can use their musculature to stabilize their spine during activities, that should control their pain. Therefore, an increase in pain is usually caused by poor technique or inadequate muscular strength and endurance. The increase in pain can usually be controlled by a careful review of the exercise and the patient's body mechanics technique. A retailoring of the exercise and activity program then allows an increase in activities parallel to the patient's increase in muscular strength and endurance.

Postoperative fusion patients usually have an increase of symptoms until the fusion mass is sufficiently solid to withstand the normal biomechanical stresses of daily life. The use of a body jacket or corset for these patients may control their symptoms until the fusion is solid.[29] There is no evidence, however, that bracing promotes successful or earlier fusion. On the other hand, weight bearing activity has been demonstrated to increase bone mineral mass,[30] and therefore should be encouraged.

Communication of Basic Precautions and Exercise Training

The patient and the therapist are instructed in basic precautions during the postoperative period, which are described below. For discectomy patients, no flexion or torsion is permitted for 8 to 12 weeks. For posterior-lateral fusion patients, no flexion, extension, or torsion is permitted for 12 weeks. For anterior fusion cases, no flexion, extension, or torsion is permitted for 16 to 24 weeks.

Manual treatment in the form of joint mobilization is restricted from the surgical segments for 3 months in discectomy patients. The adjacent segments and the cervicothoracic spine may be mobilized earlier if the restricted motion is creating pain or if patients are having difficulty performing the exercise program. Soft tissue mobilization of the scar and lower extremities may also begin early in the program. The healing surgical wound resolves into scar tissue and can often be a source of pain. Local treatment with scar mobilization can be valuable to promote soft, pliable, and painless scar formation. Occasionally cutaneous neuromata may need a series of injections with local anesthetic to control local dysesthetic pain, which can often become quite disabling.

The key element in the exercise training phase is to attain adequate dynamic control of lumbar spine forces to eliminate repetitive injury to the intervertebral discs, facet joints, and related structures. Stabilization exercise routines are divided into basic and advanced levels.

Prior to strengthening exercises, soft tissue flexibility and joint range of motion is addressed. Flexibility training focuses on the musculotendinous units of the hamstrings, quadriceps, Iliopsoas, rectus femoris, external and internal hip rotators, and gastrocsoleus. Strict attention is paid to maintenance of neutral spine posture while stretching exercises are performed. They are carried out on a daily basis, following warm up, and are repeated after the exercise program. Some interesting work regarding diurnal variations and stresses on the lumbar spine notes changes in lumbar disc and ligament extensibility as the day progresses.[31] These changes are based upon creep of the soft tissue structures, leading to increased range of motion. Adams, et. al., point out that bending and lifting activities early in the morning when applied to nonextensible ligamentous and annulus fibers cause the disc to accumulate fatigue damage more easily than those same activities performed later in the day. The same holds true for flexibility of the structures that eliminate this repetitive fatigue stress to the intervertebral joint. The muscles that attach to the pelvis should be thought of as guy wires that can effectively change the position and symmetry of the pelvis. Considering that the pelvis is the platform that the lumbar spine rests on, pelvic positioning is the key to postural control of the lumbar spine. Therefore, adequate hamstring, quadriceps, iliopsoas, gastrocsoleus, hip rotator, and iliotibial band flexibility is important. A note should also be made for the necessity of flexible neural elements as well. Excessive epidural or perineural scar formation can tether the nerve root and may lead to pain. Carefully stretching the nerve roots, for example, by hamstring stretching for the L5 and S1 nerve roots and quadriceps stretching for the upper lumbar nerve roots, can increase flexibility.

The training program should be structured according to a patient's physical capacity for occupational and recreational activities. A weight training program need not be geared solely toward the truncal musculature, but should be taken a step further, becoming a total fitness program. Aerobic and anaerobic training should be incorporated into the total fitness program. Aerobic conditioning should have begun early in the program in the form of walking. As soon as patients can tolerate the sitting position, they should be taught to stabilize their spines while riding a stationary bicycle. Those patients wanting to return to running should be supervised while running on a treadmill, and, if needed, their technique should be videotaped. Swimming should be encouraged for those patients interested in it, but should not be uniformly recommended for all patients. Training levels should be tailored to the patient's age, medical history, and level of aerobic conditioning according to previously established American College of Sports Medicine guidelines.

DYNAMIC MUSCULAR LUMBAR STABILIZATION TECHNIQUES

The Basic Level Program

The basic level program has been classified by some as a neurodevelopmental stage of postural control starting from supine and prone lying, then advancing to kneeling, standing, and movement of position transition. Meticulous technique should be required in the performance of these exercises. Therefore, a skilled and experienced physical therapist or exercise trainer should work with the patient in a painstaking manner. Initially, the exercises should be performed during one-on-one instruction. Then, after satisfactorily completing the basic stages, patients may begin exercising in a class. Each of the exercises is designed to develop isolated and cocontraction muscle patterns that stabilize the lumbar spine in its neutral position.

Neutral position must be defined for each individual. Neutral spine does not necessarily mean zero degrees of lordosis, but rather the most comfortable position for the individual based on the biomechanical principles discussed earlier in the chapter. This modification of lordosis, controlled by the abdominal muscles, is the position in which patients find most relief from their back and radicular symptoms. The therapist must carefully monitor the patient for optimal positioning while the patient exercises and progresses through each level of the program. Care must be taken to ensure proper form and a slow speed at which exercise repetitions are performed. The neurophysiologic principle of central pathway irradiation secondary to increased amplitude of effort must be continually kept in mind. Volitional forceful effort results in spreading of the neural impulses (irradiation) yielding an uncoordinated movement that may include eccentric loading.

Engram motor programming is the goal. An engram can be defined as a neurophysiological phenomenon that contains the motor information necessary to perform a complex movement. The individual components of a complex motor act are stored together as a unit forming an engram. This data, which is stored in the motor cortex, is retrievable without the need for conscious control. A voluntary complex motor act can be converted to an engram by continued, effortless, precise repetition. Therefore, precise repetition and monitoring of an exercise is important in the process of retraining.

Graduation From the Basic Level Program

Demonstration of proper form and technique is a requirement for the individual to graduate from the basic level. The same principles are then applied to the weight training portion of the program. The patient is taught how to get on and off weight training equipment while continuing to adhere to stabilization principles. Care should be exercised when changing the weight stack resistance pin on the machines as well as when lifting and racking free weights. The patient is then taught how to use resistance equipment including free weights, pulleys, and single station weight machines using cocontraction of the lower abdominal musculature to maintain optimal anteverted pelvic positioning while flattening the lower back against a back support maintaining a stabilized neutral spine. The specific strengthening program is tailored to the individual. Decisions for advancement of the program are based upon functional progress rather than pain level. Patients progress through the dynamic muscular lumbar stabilization program as follows:

1. Identifying the back's neutral position in sitting and standing positions.
2. Performing supine pelvic bracing, after which patients progress to dynamic abdominal bracing.
3. Performing prone gluteal squeezes, after which patients progress to unilateral leg lifts, then bilateral arm and leg lifts, and eventually to trunk raises.
4. Performing a bridging progression:
   a. In the basic position.
   b. Having one leg raised.
   c. Stepping.
   d. Balancing on a gym ball.
5. Performing quadruped exercises with alternating arm and leg movements.
6. Kneeling stabilization during:
   a. Double knee exercises.
   b. Single knee exercises.
   c. Lunges.
7. Wall slide quadriceps strengthening.
8. Position transition with postural control.

Abdominal muscle strengthening is initiated with simple curl ups, followed by dynamic abdominal bracing, an exercise that uses alternate arm and leg movements while lying supine and contracting the abdominal musculature and holding the spine in a neutral position. Further progression includes diagonal curl ups and diagonal curl ups performed on an inclined board. Once the patient is able to carry out 3 sets of 15 repetitions, the exercise is advanced. Finally, lower abdominal muscle strengthening is emphasized with straight leg lowering exercises.

The basic gym program includes the following:

1. Latissimus pull downs.
2. Angled leg presses.
3. Lunges with and without weight.
4. General upper body resistance exercises, including biceps curls, triceps push downs, and bench presses.
5. Upper extremity pulley exercises to stress postural control.

Obviously, not all patients should undergo a vigorous gym training program. But patients who desire to return to athletics or to physical labor must undergo this phase of the program. The muscle groups exercised by these techniques correspond to the muscles necessary for truncal spine stabilization. In addition, upper body muscle development is needed to ensure adequate strength for lifting and pushing.

Specialized and Advanced Programs

Rehabilitation of the athlete who has undergone lumbar spine surgery requires a highly specialized and advanced program.[32] For example, the training program for football linemen incorporates the same principles already discussed. However, in this particular program the tasks of the athlete are broken down into individual components. This includes stance positioning, back pedaling while pass blocking, as well as pulling and dive positions for run-play blocking. A great deal of emphasis is placed on adequate knee flexion and strong abdominal muscles that cocontract with the gluteus maximus to attain the forward pelvic tilt, thereby eliminating excessive lordosis of the lumbar spine during axial loading. The player is taught how to take a blow and use a contraction of his abdominal muscles to stabilize the spine. The player is also taught how to fall and roll with abdominal contraction. The motivated football player finds this type of positioning comfortable, efficient, and powerful. One-on-one drills are designed to reinforce stabilization principles while the player is being pushed and pulled. It is critical that these skills are brought to the engram level of motor programming, so that the sport can be played with spine stabilization techniques as components of the athletic technique.

During the sports specific training programs, athletes work through the basic level of exercises, then through advanced level training. Following this, they go on to the sports-specific training. The sports-specific training begins with hands on, one-on-one mat work advancing from isolated to compound movements. Video taped exercise sessions and video taped performance of specific athletic techniques are valuable coaching and training aids. The principles mentioned regarding athletic spine training can be applied to virtually all sports. Working carefully with individual coaches is imperative prior to designing any training programs. The team approach must always be kept in mind in the rehabilitation of an individual with complicated back problems.

The nature of many sports includes torque applied to the lumbar spine, making it impossible to totally eliminate rotational stresses. The goal is to try to minimize torque, controlling it in those situations when control can be exercised. The majority of athletic lumbar spine injuries actually occurs in the weight room, secondary to repetitive microtrauma and before the athlete ever sets foot on the playing field or gymnasium floor.

The time frame for a return to normal athletics for the discectomy patient is 8 to 12 weeks. A return to sedentary work can be expected in 3 to 4 weeks. The return to heavy labor more closely parallels the return to athletic activities. However, the time frame for return to work of a patient receiving worker's compensation may depend on motivational issues. It is in this subgroup of patients that objectification of function is critically important.

Patients having undergone posterior fusion require 16 to 18 weeks to return to athletics and 12 to 14 weeks to return to work. Patients having undergone anterior fusion require 6 to 10 months to return to athletics and 3 to 6 months to return to work. Obviously, patients who have undergone fusions may not be able to return to heavy labor and must undergo vocational retraining and reassignment.

Postoperative Goal Setting

Postoperative treatment must meet reasonable time and cost criteria. Early and accurate goal setting is imperative. An understanding of the patient's occupation, recreational desires, and functional level help guide the setting of goals. Once patients reach a plateau in their functional improvement that is unaffected by alterations in their program of physical therapy, that supervised program should be discontinued. The patient should be placed in an independent exercise program as soon as possible. The goal of treatment should be to strive for patient independence rather than to foster a dependent relationship. Drug dependency is not the only possible development to guard against. Patients may also develop a dependency to physical therapy and manipulative treatment. Therefore, active exercise programs should be encouraged, and passive treatment discouraged.

If patients are unable to improve their functional status following surgery, several questions should be considered. Does the residual disorder require additional surgery? Are mitigating emotional and psychological factors delaying or blocking recovery? Does residual structural disease exist, which is not amenable to further surgical correction? These questions usually arise after 6 months have passed during the postoperative period. Occasionally, it becomes obvious that the persistent symptoms result from remaining disorders such as nerve root canal stenosis that may need to addressed within the first 6 months to ensure a successful outcome. A word of caution is in order here. The diagnostic workup of the failed surgical patient is more complex than the workup of the virgin spine. Rushing back into a second or third operation without precise confirmation of residual pain generators and psychological factors may lead to more failure.

SUMMARY

Postoperative rehabilitation includes back education training, physical conditioning, and dynamic lumbar muscular stabilization. It is a comprehensive process that is based on biomechanical aspects of lumbar spine function and pathophysiology. These components are the same for all patients; however, each program must be individualized to meet the diverse vocational and recreational needs of a particular patient.

REFERENCES

1. Yong-King, K., Kirkaldy-Willis, W.H.: The pathophysiology of degenerative disease of the lumbar spine. Orthop Clin North Am 14:1983.
2. Kahanovitz, N., Viola, K., Gallagher, M.: Long term strength assessment of postoperative discectomy patients. Spine 14(4):402–404, 1989.
3. Booth, F.W.: Time course of muscular atrophy during immobilization of hind limbs in rats. J Appl Physiol 43:656–661, 1977.
4. Booth, F.W., Seider, M.J.: Effects of disuse by limb immobilization on different muscle fiber types. *In* Plasticity of Muscle (Edited by Pette). New York, de Gruyter, 1980.
5. Muller, E.A.: Influence of training and of inactivity on muscle strength. Arch Phys Med. Rehabil 51:449–462, 1970.
6. Saltin, B., et. al.: Response to exercise after bed rest and after training. Circulation 38:1–55, 1968.
7. Mellin, G.: Physical therapy for chronic low back pain: correlations between spinal mobility and treatment outcome. Scand J Rehabil Med 17:163–166, 1985.
8. Alaranta, H., et. al.: Rehabilitation after surgery for lumbar disc herniation: results of a randomized clinical trial. Int J Rehabil Res 9(3):247–257, 1986.
9. Findeklee, R., Büttner, K.:. Stationäre Rehabilitationsmabnahmen in der Frühphase nach Bandscheibenoperation als wirksame Alternative zur ambulanten Nachsorge. Rehabil 27:112–116, 1988.
10. Mooney, V.: Surgery and postsurgical management of the patient with low back pain. Phys Ther 59(8):1000–1007, 1979.
11. Postacchini, F., Montanaro, A.: Early mobilisation and functional re-education in the post operative treatment of prolapsed lumbar disc. Italian J Orthop Traumatol 4(2):231–236, 1978.
12. Schuster, G.D., Infante, M.C.: Pain relief after low back surgery: the efficacy of transcutaneous electrical nerve stimulation. Pain 8:299–302, 1980.
13. Hurme, M., et. al.: Factors predicting the results of surgery for lumbar intervertebral disc herniation. Spine 12:933–938, 1987.
14. Adams, M.A., Hutton, W.C.: The mechanical function of the lumbar apophyseal joints. Spine 8(3):327–330, 1983.
15. Adams, M.A., Hutton W.C.: Gradual disc prolapse. Spine 10(6):524–531, 1985.
16. Farfan, H.F.: Effects of torsion on the intervertebral joints. Can J Surg 12:336, 1969.
17. Farfan, H.F.: Muscular mechanism of the lumbar spine and the position of power and efficiency. Orthop Clin North Am 6:135–144, 1975.
18. Adams, M.A., Hutton, W.C.: Mechanics of the intervertebral disc. *In* The Biology of the Intervertebral Disc (Edited by P. Ghosh). Boca Raton, CRC, 1988.
19. Brinckmann, P.: Injury of the annulus fibrosus and disc protrusions: An in vitro investigation on human lumbar discs. Spine 11(2):149–153, 1986.
20. Hampton, D., Laros, G., McCarron, R., Franks D.: Healing potential of the annulus fibrosus. Spine 14(4):398–402, 1989.
21. Cruess, R.L.: Healing of bone, tendon, and ligament. *In* Fractures in Adults (Edited by C.A. Rockwood and Green). Philadelphia, J.B. Lippincott, 1975.
22. Gracovetsky, S., Farfan, H.: The optimum spine. Spine 11(6):543–573, 1986.
23. Gracovetsky, S., Farfan, H., Helleur C.: The abdominal mechanism. Spine 10(4):317–324, 1985.
24. Bogduk, N., MacIntosh, J.E.: The applied anatomy of the thoracolumbar fascia. Spine 9(2):164–170, 1984.
25. Bogduk, N.: The innervation of the intervertebral disc. *In* The Biology of the Intervertebral Disc (Edited by P. Ghosh). Boca Raton, CRC Press, 1988.
26. Lantz, S.A., Schultz A.B.: Lumbar spine orthosis wearing. Spine 11(8):834–842, 1986.
27. Saal, J.S.: Biochemical evidence of inflammation in discogenic lumbar radiculopathy: analysis of phospholipase A2 activity in human herniated disc. Presented at The International Society for the Study of the Lumbar Spine, Tokyo, May, 1989.
28. Ghosh, P.: Influence of drugs, hormones and other agents on the metabolism of the sequelae of its degeneration. *In* The Biology of the Intervertebral Disc (Edited by P. Ghosh). Boca Raton, CRC Press, 1988.
29. Keim, H.A.: The technique of the bilateral-lateral lumbar spine fusion. *In* Lumbar Spine Surgery, Techniques and Complications (Edited by A.H. White, R.H. Rothman, and C.D. Ray). St. Louis, C.V. Mosby, 1987.
30. Lanyon, L.E., O'Connor, J.A.: Adaptation of bone artificially loaded at high and low physiological strain rates. J Physiol 303(36P):1980.
31. Adams, M.A., Dolan, P., Hutton, W.C.: Diurnal variations in the stresses on the lumbar spine. Spine 12(2):130–137, 1987.
32. Saal, J.A., Saal, J.S.: Nonoperative treatment of herniated lumbar intervertebral disc with radiculopathy: an outcome study. Spine 14(4):1989.

30

Susan J. Isernhagen

Functional Capacity Evaluation and Work Hardening Perspectives

WHY ARE WE INTERESTED?

A humanistic dilemma has become a financial dilemma. The lack of accountability in the return to work of an injured worker has produced problems for the injured worker and significant dollar losses for industry. Because the injured worker causes the dilemma, the medical community comes to assist in solving the problem. Workers' compensation costs have gotten well out of hand in most states in the United States and in most industrialized countries. Although the medical professions were slow to realize the delay in returning injured workers to employment, the financial implications were not lost on industry and workers' compensation systems.[1]

This new found awareness has resulted in changes in the medical professional's viewpoint on injured workers. No longer are clinicians content only with diagnosis and treatment; now they are interested in the outcomes of their services.

- Is the injured worker healed or rehabilitated enough to return to work?
- Will work stresses result in reinjury? Are we clear, concise, and objective in our evaluations of the worker?
- Are we facilitating communication between employers, insurance companies, and workers compensation systems?

These and other questions are not only necessary to ask, but also worthwhile to solve. Taking the injured worker through the evaluation of capacities and through work re-entry is a satisfying use of our professional skills. In addition, the outcome is satisfactory for the injured worker who gets better and

more thorough service, for the employer who is made part of the process, and for the insurance companies and workers compensation systems that incur lower costs.

Therefore, functional capacity evaluation and work hardening, which became nationally recognized in the 1980s, are progressing into more advanced levels of work. These programs have proved to be beneficial and their continued use in work injury management is virtually assured.[2–7]

ANALYZING THE FLOW OF WORK INJURY MANAGEMENT

In order to see where functional capacity assessment and work hardening programs fall on the continuum of work injury management, one must first look at the sequence of events surrounding each injury.

1. An individual is injured at work. This could be a cumulative injury, the effects of which are felt over time, or a sudden injury caused by a single traumatic event.
2. The injury is recognized by the worker and reported to the management at the work site.
3. The case is disposed through decision making.
   a. The worker may be referred to a medical professional on site, such as an occupational health nurse or company physician.
   b. The worker may be referred to a physician outside the plant.
   c. In severe injuries, a hospital emergency room may be required.

4. After the initial medical intervention is chosen, the injured worker receives the required attention.
5. A decision regarding immediate care and possible return to work is made. If the injury is severe enough to cause the worker to lose time at work, he likely will be at home during the duration of the healing process. Medical treatment or intervention may be conducted during this time.
6. As time passes, the medical professional in charge of managing the work injury continually reevaluates the worker to determine whether a return to work is appropriate. At the point when the worker has plateaued, the return to work decision falls in the following categories:
   a. Return to work with no restrictions
   b. Return to work with restricted duties
   c. Restorative program indicated prior to return to work
   d. Return to work is not indicated

The Decision to Return to Work

In the past, the decisions regarding return to work were made by a general physician with little pressure from outside agencies to promote early and full return to work. The physician, who traditionally had been a patient advocate, was often placed in the middle between a patient with positive or negative feelings regarding return to work and an employer requiring a sound worker. Ambiguous releases to work or slow releases to work were often the result.

To make the doctor's statement allowing the worker to return to the workplace more helpful, many state workers' compensation systems and insurance companies developed a list of functional information that must be collected prior to sending the injured worker back to the work site. Table 30–1 is a form compiled from these generic work tasks. The list includes items related to functions performed on many jobs and identifies critical factors in the injured workers' return to work. Some categories, such as lifting, carrying, pushing, and pulling, need definition in maximum capacity and in endurance. Other categories include movement and positional work. For these categories, it is necessary to note the maximum time during an 8-hour day that the task is performed.

Although the list of items in this form is generally correct, one can see that the format in which it is written is unclear. For example, in lifting, weight in pounds is required, but the type of lift is not defined. This could lead to erroneous reporting or interpretation, as each of type of lift requires different muscle use and has different maximum effort capac-

ities. Also, the form is general enough that "guesstimates" often were promoted. These forms, however unclear, were nevertheless a great improvement over the lack of structure that was formerly seen in return to work judgments.

In the mid 1980s, when the workers' compensation system began to put increased pressure on physicians to release the worker to work more quickly and more specifically, frustration was evident. The more specific the release form, the greater the dilemma the physician faced. It was not possible to truly judge activity that would relate to 8 hours a day and 40 hours a week from a patient office visit. Physicians did not have enough time with their patients to evaluate them fully and were somewhat reluctant to base their judgment solely on the patient's word or brief observation. The medical and legal implications of subjective information also became a factor.

Enter the Rehabilitation Process

Because physical and occupational therapists had shown expertise in physical and functional evaluation in the rehabilitation field, the next step was to integrate these concepts into work injury management. Just as in traditional rehabilitation, work injury evaluation must be made on an individual level. The concepts used for work injury evaluation followed those activities of daily living (ADL) evaluation, only they focused on work activity instead of home activity. Generalizations are not made; each work function must be tested individually.

For example, the diagnosis for three individuals might be L4 and L5 bulging disc, yet the three individuals may have different functional capacities. The diagnosis is not enough to account for individual differences, such as age, gender, tolerance to discomfort, overall strength and endurance, tightness, functional movement patterns, motivation, and general health.

Beyond the individual differences also are the differences in physical demands of work sites. Even if the three people had identical diagnosis, symptoms, and functional levels, their ability to return to work would not be the same because of the differences in their jobs. If one is a mail carrier, one a truck driver, and one an office administrator, the ability for each to return to work would be very different because different physical capacities are needed.

Therefore, the essence of the situation of return to work depends upon two main factors:

1. The functional capacity of the injured worker.
2. The critical demands of the job.

PATIENT: ____

I estimate this person is able to:

	Never	Occasionally (1–33%)	Frequently (34–66%)	Continuously (67–100%)
1. LIFT:				
a. up to 10 lb.	_______	_______	_______	_______
b. 11–25 lb.	_______	_______	_______	_______
c. 26–35 lb.	_______	_______	_______	_______
d. 36–50 lb.	_______	_______	_______	_______
e. 51–75 lb.	_______	_______	_______	_______
f. 76–100 lb.	_______	_______	_______	_______
2. CARRY:				
a. up to 10 lb.	_______	_______	_______	_______
b. 11–25 lb.	_______	_______	_______	_______
c. 26–34 lb.	_______	_______	_______	_______
d. 36–50 lb.	_______	_______	_______	_______
e. 51–75 lb.	_______	_______	_______	_______
f. 76–100 lb.	_______	_______	_______	_______
3. CAN THE PERSON PERFORM THE FOLLOWING TASKS:				
Push/Pull—Seated	_______	_______	_______	_______
Push/Pull—Standing	_______	_______	_______	_______
Bend	_______	_______	_______	_______
Squat	_______	_______	_______	_______
Crawl	_______	_______	_______	_______
Climb	_______	_______	_______	_______
Reach above shoulder level	_______	_______	_______	_______

4. CIRCLE THE NUMBER OF HOURS FOR EACH ACTIVITY:
   Note: Does not have to total 8 hours.

										Continuously	With Rests
Sit	1	2	3	4	5	6	7	8	(hrs)	_______	_______
Stand	1	2	3	4	5	6	7	8	(hrs)	_______	_______
Walk	1	2	3	4	5	6	7	8	(hrs)	_______	_______
Sit/Stand	1	2	3	4	5	6	7	8	(hrs)	_______	_______

5. CAN PERSON USE HANDS FOR REPETITIVE ACTION SUCH AS:

	Simple Grasping	Firm Grasp	Fine Manipulating
Right	Yes _______ No _______	Yes _______ No _______	Yes _______ No _______
Left	Yes _______ No _______	Yes _______ No _______	Yes _______ No _______

6. CAN PERSON USE FEET FOR REPETITIVE MOVEMENTS, AS IN OPERATING FOOT CONTROLS?

Right	Left	Both
Yes _______ No _______	Yes _______ No _______	Yes _______ No _______

7. ANY RESTRICTIONS OF ACTIVITIES INVOLVED?

8. CAN PERSON NOW RETURN TO FORMER JOB?

Yes _______ No _______

Table 30–1 (continued)

CAN PERSON RETURN TO OTHER WORK ACCORDING TO RESTRICTIONS DEFINED ABOVE?

Yes ________   No ________

IF NOT, GIVE ESTIMATED DATE FOR RETURN TO WORK ___________

Work part-time?   ________ hrs./day   Work full-time?   Yes ________   No ________
Disability rating   _____________ % (if applicable)

9. COMMENTS: ____

____

____

____

____

____

________________________________	______________________________
Physician	Date

THE PROGRESSIVE FUNCTIONAL CAPACITY EVALUATION

How to Analyze a Client's Functional Capacity

Test the Body

Two primary methods of evaluating a person's ability to return to work have been used in the past years. The first is the functional capacity evaluation, which assesses *the body's physical ability to perform physical work tasks*. This evaluation follows the form shown in Table 30–1, which has been specifically developed for identifying work capabilities and limitations. Because the list is specific, testing also must be specific. Effective evaluation techniques and protocols have developed that allow for confidence in the functional evaluation process.

The first step is to functionally define the method of testing. The second step is to ensure standardization of testing procedures. The standardization of the test avoids rater bias, and the referring party understands that testing is conducted in the same manner on each injured worker. This standardization also allows for accurate retesting.

Because of the specific list of functional work tasks required by workers compensation systems and because of the subsequent development of accurate test methods for assignment of these tasks, the evaluation described here is one that tests body capabilities for performance.

The results of the body evaluation are much like the results of a stress test of a person who has had a cardiac incident. The person is stressed to the cardiac limit so the limit may be identified to prevent an overstress or injury situation. The ability of the client to perform safely at submaximal levels is also valuable information. Likewise, functional capacity assessments are designed to be a musculoskeletal stress test, identifying physical work maximums and safe functional activity levels.

Once the basic information on the body's functional abilities is known, then the results can be interpreted and extrapolated to different types of work situations. In the functional capacity evaluation tests, the comprehensive components give an excellent overview of the body's work competency.

Test of Work: The Work Capacity Evaluation

A second evaluation method is not body-specific, but rather work-specific. This is the work tolerance test or *work capacity evaluation*. In this test, a specific job is identified that the referrer primarily wants information on the worker's ability to perform. This is not a functional capacity evaluation, but rather an individually designed test for specific outcomes. For example, a truck driver may be given a test that evaluates driving abilities, vibration tolerance, loading and unloading, and visual acuity. This test would evaluate the basic critical demands of the truck driving job. If the worker is not able to perform the tasks in truck driving job description, the physician is left without good information regarding other work aptitudes. Therefore, if a work capacity evaluation shows that a person can go to work, it is valuable in the return to work process. If discrepancies exist between the person's abilities and the tasks listed in the job description, however, the work capacity evaluation does not give good correlative information regarding many other work tasks. Therefore, the functional capacity evaluation is a stronger tool for overall work functional capacity but is specific to the worker, not the work.

What Components are Necessary to Analyze Return to Work Options?

Table 30–2 is an updated functional capacity form that evaluates all items on the old form, but is more defined and allows for important comments and recommendations. It is worth noting that individual parts of the body (i.e., back, neck, hands, and knees) are used many times in a variety of ways so that correlation comparisons may be made about overall ability of, and overall stress to, a weak area.

What Does the Physician Expect?

The physician wishes to have specific information on the following questions:

1. Is this injured worker physically able to do a specific type of work?
2. Must any safety precautions be taken at work to prevent reinjury?
3. Do physical problems make longevity in a particular occupation hazardous?

Qualitative Functional Capacity Evaluation (FCE) Components

In addition to the work activities listed in Tables 30–1 and 30–2, other factors that the physician, employer, and insurance company should consider as critical to work performance are:

- Strength: The maximum strength for specific work tasks must be identified. Heavy manual materials handling may be required on the job. Therefore, a critical level of strength must correspond with the demands.

- Endurance: Because work is performed during an 8-hour day and 40-hour week (at least), endurance is also a factor. This endurance may be of a muscular nature, as activity must be able to be sustained at submaximal levels over a full day. Endurance also falls into the area of aerobic conditioning, as the metabolic and physiologic demands of work must be met also.
- Coordination: Many work injuries are caused by lack of ability to coordinate at critical moments. Balance is also a safety factor in handling loads or in body positioning.
- Pace: Many types of work require that a certain pace be met either because of machine requirements or because of a productivity level. Each worker has an individual pace set internally. Some people are rapid workers, some are moderate, and some are slow. In addition, the work injury may have changed the worker's internal pacing ability. Pace must be compared to job requirements.
- Safety: Working safely is also a critical aspect of medical evaluation. The employer will be interested in the safety practices of a particular worker. The worker also needs to internally recognize safe work levels and practices and to recognize when safety is in question.

DEVELOPMENT OF THE KINESIOPHYSICAL MODEL

What is Behind the Label?

Today, the potential evaluator hears of many testing techniques that are labeled functional capacity tests. What do they really assess?

1. Isometric: Force is applied to an immovable object so that the force measured is that of muscles, which produce tension but do not actually produce movement at a joint. Therefore, isometric testing only measures unidimensional force exerted on a fixed object, without producing information on the quality of movement, coordination, joint function, or muscle function at different positions. Isometric testing as a measure of functional capacity evaluation is supported by numerous studies, many coming from the work on static strength testing done at the University of Michigan and included in the *Guide to Manual Materials Handling*, developed by NIOSH.[8]
2. Isokinetic and isoinertial: Both measure muscle group motions produced with restricted move-

ment and stabilization patterns. Emphasis is on force or speed. Movements are dynamic but not necessarily functional. Certain muscle groups and joints are stressed, but the patterns of movement do not directly correlate with work functional actions. Isokinetic and isoinertial equipment, although expensive, can assist researchers and professionals who are interested in quantification of selected aspects of function.

3. Dynamic: This infers that motion occurs both within the muscle and at all related joints. Movement, pattern, and speed are not restricted. Dynamic testing can be any desired activity. Dynamic testing is a method traditionally used by rehabilitation professionals who desire to see the actual functional activity in order to perform a realistic evaluation. Objective observations can be made regarding speed, coordination, direction, quality of motion, quantity of motion, and functional outcomes.

Table 30–2
FCE Form

____
Client

____
Date

Item	Percent of 8-hour Day					Restrictions	Recommendations
	0	*1–5*	*6–33*	*34–66*	*67–100*		
WEIGHT CAPACITY IN LBS.							
Floor to waist lift							
Waist to overhead lift							
Horizontal lift							
Push							
Pull							
Right carry							
Left carry							
Front carry							
Right hand grip							
Left hand grip							
FLEXIBILITY/POSITIONAL							
Elevated work							
Forward bending/sitting							
Forward bending/standing							

Copyright 1989, Isernhagen Work Systems, Duluth, MN

Table 30–2 (continued)

Item						Restrictions	Recommendations
	\multicolumn{5}{Percent of 8-hour Day}						
	0	1–5	6–33	34–66	67–100		
Rotation sitting							
Rotation standing							
Crawl							
Kneel							
Crouch—deep static							
Repetitive Squat							
STATIC WORK							
Sitting tolerance							
Standing tolerance							
AMBULATION							
Walking							
Stair climbing							
Step ladder climbing							
Balance							
COORDINATION							
R. upper extremity							
L. upper extremity							

_______________________________   _______________________________
             Evaluator   Date

All three approaches to functional capacity evaluation have inherent strengths and weaknesses. However, if functional capacity evaluation is designed to give accurate information on true functional activities, dynamic testing is the most logical choice. It can be designed to simulate work movement most closely and can, therefore, stress the body (muscles, joints, circulation) in the same manner as the actual demands of work.

Types of Dynamic Testing

Psychophysical vs. Kinesiophysical Testing

When functional capacity evaluation was first considered, the psychophysical approach had a history of use in research that led to its consideration for work testing. The purposes were to determine lifting limits in a relatively uninjured and highly motivated population. It was found overall that uninjured motivated people could have a certain degree of accuracy in determining their maximum limits and also the amount they could tolerate in handling during the day. It is logical then, that the psychophysical testing was first considered for functional capacity testing.

However, patients who are injured at work have a vested interest in the outcome of the evaluation (under motivation or over motivation). In many cases, the injured workers are suspected of giving incorrect information. Therefore, to use the client or the injured worker as the determinant of the physical abilities may be unsuitable in many instances.

In order to avoid putting the injured worker in control of the test, the kinesiophysical approach is used. Kinesiophysical is defined as the use of physical movement to determine abilities. Inherent in this approach is kinesiological principles, including muscle and joint function in relationship to strength, endurance, speed, coordination, and safety. This approach is similar to other rehabilitation evaluative approaches in that the skilled therapist is in control of the testing.

The patient is known to have a potentially physically handicapping condition and the therapist or evaluator must use expertise in determining the patient's safety and competency for return to work. In return-to-work testing, medical objectivity becomes extremely important in avoiding adversarial relationships, which can be prevalent. It is much easier for an employer, insurance company, or a patient to believe medical-based testing rather than the subjective report of testing. Therefore, the kinesiophysical approach has been used and will continue to be used in functional capacity evaluations.

Attributes of the Kinesiophysical Approach

The Qualities of Effort

During any physical activity, sets of muscles are used in sequence. When activity is light, only the primary muscles needed to sustain the movements are used. When a movement becomes heavy or an individual becomes fatigued, accessory muscles automatically contract to assist the prime movers. The activation of these accessory muscles is involuntary and normal. They contribute to the movement more strongly as stresses increase. The objective observation of the activation of accessory muscles is a strong indicator of high or maximum effort. Other indications apparent to the trained therapist would be changes in body mechanics, balance, postural accommodations, or quality of movement. In addition, the therapist can evaluate coordination, symptomatic accommodations, and the relationship between strength and endurance.

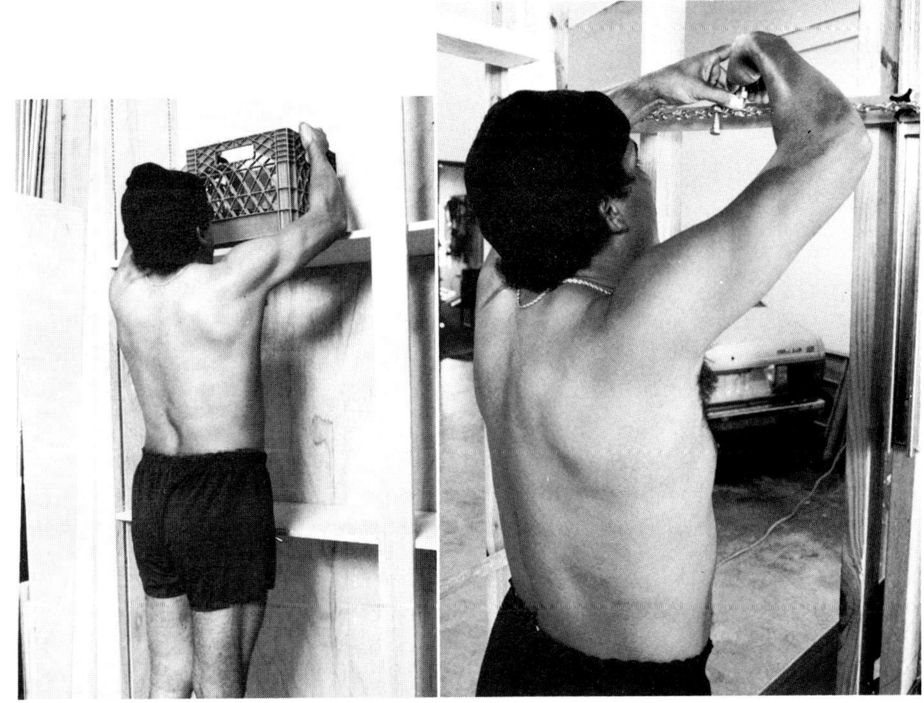

Figures 30–1, 30–2. Two functional capacity tests that allow evaluation of a similar activity for two different purposes. Overhead lifting, pictured in Figure 30–1, tests manual materials handling. Figure 30–2 shows the same position and muscle use in a sustained unloaded endurance capacity. The kinesiophysical approach is concerned not only with strength and endurance, but also with neck extension, low back extension, wrist position, and heart rate.

The Highest Functional Level

Because the therapist is able to identify changes in accessory muscles and movement patterns as heavier objects are used, the maximum function can be verified. A patient approaches a maximum effort gradually, and the evaluator can identify early indications of fatigue, coordination changes, and progression of body mechanics. The evaluator can then be primed to recognize when maximum function has been reached. The objective documentation of signs that occur with maximum function assists all parties in identifying the effort and safety level of each patient in each activity and gives credibility to the verification of maximum effort. In a similar manner, the absence of indicators of maximum effort can also be identified. The therapist is able to objectively differentiate an artificial end to activity from a true maximum effort.

The Ethical Approach to Safety

The kinesiophysical approach also stresses safety. Professionals who work with patients are ethically bound to make sure that no harm comes to the patient while in his care. This ethical consideration is equally important in work-injured clients.

In order to assure safety in testing procedures, there must first be safety standards. It is the responsibility of each medical practitioner or facility to determine what constitutes safe procedures. For example, most clinics that specialize in injured worker rehabilitation have standards on lifting techniques. The standards may be presented in the form of booklets, a back school, or safety posters. If safe body mechanics are indicated in these teachings, it is up to each professional doing testing to make sure safe lifting occurs during the evaluation process. In addition, therapists doing the testing must be alert for any contraindications relating to heart rate, blood pressure, joint symptoms, and neurological signs.

The "Why" Behind Functional Limitations

The importance of the kinesiophysical approach becomes even more clear when physical findings are correlated with functional limitations. The reason behind each work deficiency is noted based on kinesiophysical observations.

For example, three workers who are not able to lift more than 20 lbs from the floor to waist may have the same maximum (20 lbs) but there may be a different physical cause for each maximum. In the first case, the weight limitation might be caused by a degenerative knee condition. In the second case, it could be a result of low back instability. In the third instance, biceps weakness may be the factor. Knowledge of the physical limitation is critical in determining recommendations for remediation of the problem or recommendation of job modifications. If weakness is the cause, the worker can be strengthened. If permanent losses are the cause, the work must be modified, not the worker.

Summary

The kinesiophysical approach is the testing method of choice for functional capacity evaluation. Its strong points are:

1. It allows the evaluator, not the worker, to be in charge of the testing situation.
2. The maximum objective strength of the client can be determined.
3. Tolerance level can be determined for activities, position, and repetition.
4. Safe procedures are used to ensure that no injuries occur during the testing situation and to reinforce safe work behaviors in the client.
5. Functional limitations are linked with their underlying physical causes.
6. Clients who use only submaximal effort in a testing situation can be identified.
7. A specific objective report with recommendations can be generated from the objective observations and testing methods.

See Table 30–3 for a comparison of the testing methods discussed.

CONSTRUCTION OF FUNCTIONAL CAPACITY EVALUATION

Definitions

Functional: Meaningful, useful. In this context, functional indicates purposeful activity that is an actual work movement. Functional implies a definable movement with a beginning, an end, and a result that can be measured.

Capacity: Maximum ability, capability. Capacity indicates existing abilities for activities, including the maximum function that can be used.

Evaluation: Systematic approach, including observation, reasoning, and conclusion. Going beyond monitoring and recording, the evaluation process implies an outcome statement that is explanatory, as well as an objective measurement of the activity.

Table 30–3
A Comparison of Philosophies Using Drivers' Testing as an Example

Evaluations of an individual's capacity are measured in many different formats. Although each method has strength, some are not compatible with functional outcomes. To clarify the capability measured by various forms of testing and to measure function, the following example was designed:

ISOMETRIC
The driver is able to produce 70 lb of force bilaterally in hand grip and 160 lb of push force with the right leg. The steering wheel force description indicates 30 lb is needed and brake pedal indicates 60 lb. The driver is capable of driving and passes the test.

HIGH-TECH EQUIPMENT
In a fixed driver seat simulator, the driver can produce reproducible torque on a steering wheel and reproducible extension torque on a pedal. Torque curves exceed the minimum standard. Time and motion are also judged to be adequate. The driver is capable of driving and passes the test.

SUBJECT CONTROL—PSYCHOPHYSICAL
A driver drives through a standard course in a standard car, using any lanes and any speed desired. Potential accidents or unsafe conditions are allowed, as the driver would most likely do this in normal driving anyway. The examiner merely records the driver's observations, such as, "I can drive this speed well. I turn corners comfortably." At the end of the testing, the examiner notes: "The driver passes, as he went through testing and felt comfortable at a normal level," or, in the case of a driver who does not want to drive, "This driver is not capable of driving because of statements of discomfort in his back—not able to return to driving."

EVALUATOR CONTROL—KINESIOPHYSICAL
A driver drives through a standard course in a standard car, using lanes and speed as determined as safe and documented in drivers manual literature. If unsafe speed or procedures are noted, the examiner asks for a correction and allows the test to proceed if safety is attained. If dangerous driving is noted, the test is stopped, the driver is informed of problems, and unsafe driving is not allowed to continue. If safe functional driving is noted throughout the test, the driver passes.

If the examiner is a physical therapist, occupational therapist, or physician with musculoskeletal evaluation skills, there also would be a record of:

—Highest ability level of safe speed.
—Qualitative and quantitative description of abilities in turning, parking, and stopping.
—Documentation of the physical problems behind insufficiencies, such as "cervical tightness prevents turning head when backing up, causing deficient safety in backing car. Loss of extension strength in left quadriceps prevents adequate use of clutch."

Once deficiencies and physical limitations are known, modifications can be suggested, such as use of additional mirrors for reversing or physical restoration and clutch simulator program to increase quadriceps strength and clutch action.

Parameters of Functional Capacity Evaluation

Purpose

The purpose of the test is to stress the person's physical abilities to the maximum in order to produce objective documentation regarding work and activities of daily living. The FCE describes the full function of the injured worker in the 29 identified work tasks. Limitations also are described in order to prevent further reinjury. In the process of functional evaluation, injured workers are educated in their own abilities and limitations to facilitate a more productive role in their return to activity.

Relationship With Other Professionals Involved in the Return-to-Work Evaluation

Functional evaluation information should interface with medical and physical information collected in the work injury management spectrum. Functional evaluation should use diagnostic and prognostic information from physicians, as well as incorporate information from ergonomic job assessment, vocational and rehabilitation counselors, and employers. After the evaluation, the information should be written in terms that are understandable to all the referral sources and potentially interested professionals.

Those who will receive functional capacity evaluation reports include: physician, employer, rehabilitation or vocational counselor, insurance companies, workers' compensation system, attorney, and the injured worker.

Physical Pretest Examination

Before an FCE is performed, the therapist reviews pertinent medical records. The first activity when the worker is evaluated is a musculoskeletal assessment screening to objectively measure motion, strength, and symptoms. Once completed, the therapist is able to note the potential physical limitations.

Two-Day Testing

The FCE takes 4 to 6 hours. The most accurate format requires the evaluation to be performed over two days. This promotes the ability to retest critical items, such as lifting, and also to evaluate the response of the individual to the first day of testing.

Repeat testing on the second day adds a dimension that one-day testing does not have. The second day allows the evaluator to see the injured worker at least twice, reducing the possibility that the worker had an unusually good or unusually bad day the first day of the test. In addition, a most important value lies in the ability for the evaluator to observe the effect of the first day's testing on the injured worker. Signs and symptoms may occur on the second day as a result of the first day's testing. These are objectively evaluated for intensity and functional changes. They may be a normal occurrence after heavy activity or may be a physical change in condition. In all cases, the results gained on the second day will be the ones used for the functional assessment, as they will be more realistic of conferenced daily activity similar to work.

Completing the Picture

The overall evaluation of the 29 work tasks is greater than the sum of each individual task. A whole body work summary can be made as a result of each of the specific work tests and their effect on the worker.

A summary report that pulls together the information on the quantity of work activities from the FCE report, the quality of movement and behavior of the client, and the definitive comparison between functional capacities and the critical demands of the job is then generated. If no job description is available, then the therapist will make a conclusion regarding the strengths and weaknesses of work activities.

After the comparisons are made, recommendations logically follow regarding physical ability to return to work, further intervention that can facilitate return to work, or other options.

1. Return to work. When the functional capacity evaluation shows a match between physical abilities and the critical demands of the job, a return to work is indicated. The physician or employer is able to allow a return to work based on the physical match.
2. Worker modification to facilitate return to work. If the worker has physical limitations that prevent an immediate return to work, one recommendation might be to improve the condition of the worker. This is possible when the physical abilities are amenable to treatment and a restoration program can be cost effective. In most comprehensive rehabilitative formats, the title of this format is called "work hardening." The functional evaluation itself can delineate specifically the goals and objectives of the work hardening program, as a result of the limitations and work function that have been identified.
3. Work site or work modification prior to return to work. When work hardening would not be cost effective or when the physical problems are not amenable to physical treatment (such as degenerative joint changes, debilitating syndromes, or cardiovascular insufficiencies), the most logical return to work method may be to implement a work modification. In this case, the work could be made easier by changing the positions of objects on the frequency of repetition, or by alternating work activities, or by using adaptive tools. In most cases, the injured worker is capable in many areas and only needs modification in specific tasks.
4. Patient unable to return to work in present situation. When the physical condition of a patient does not approximate the physical demands of the job, the process of returning the injured worker to the former occupation ends. In this case, the rehabilitation consultants or vocational counselors evaluate the worker's remaining physical capabilities and residual vocational abilities. A disability settlement using FCE information may be part of the process. Further retraining and reactivation for return to other types of work based on FCE could be a logical choice. See Table 30–4 for a case report on this outcome.

WORK HARDENING

Progression From FCE to Work Hardening

The work hardening rehabilitation program bridges the gap for an injured worker whose functional capacities do not meet the critical demands of the job. Medical practitioners accept work hardening as an extension of rehabilitation that is used for other injured patients. The rehabilitation principles of the team approach, the focus toward function, and the whole body approach are typical of both traditional rehabilitation and work hardening.

Reimbursers for work injuries also recognize that prolonged workers' compensation costs are detrimental to productivity and to industries' budgets. A significant amount of money is lost because of work injuries, and this is a major factor in a state's ability

Table 30–4
Case Study 1 Functional Capacity Evaluation: Summary Report

NAME: Jessica Client

TEST DATES: June 30, and July 1, 1989

ADDRESS: 4444 Aura Avenue, Duluth, MN 55000

DATE OF BIRTH: 08/03/47

PHYSICIAN: Dennis Dean, MD

REFERRAL SOURCE: Laura Black, Rehabilitation Consultant

DIAGNOSIS: Low Back Injury, 08/19/87

DESCRIPTION OF TESTS: Ms. Client participated in all functional capacity evaluation tests. In the optional category, she took the walking and standing tolerance evaluations.

CONSISTENCY OF PERFORMANCE: Within each test item, the client demonstrated consistent performance for the repetitions or time limit tested. However, there was a noted improvement in performance on the second day of testing. She performed with some self-limitations on the first day, but by the second day of testing, stated she felt much more comfortable in understanding her true capabilities. The performance on the second day is consistent with performance should she return to work or increase daily activities at home. These scores are documented on FCE Form.

Her performance is consistent with a patient who has been self-limited because of fear of reinjury. The second day's performance indicated she had overcome the fear and is able to perform at a higher functional level.

OBJECTIVE OBSERVATIONS:

Cooperation: Although the client was cooperative for the two days of testing, she was more eager to participate on the second day. The items that caused her the greatest fear were the lifting tasks. But when they were repeated in the testing, she did not appear fearful and was pleased with her scores.

Safety: Although she moves with a slow, guarded movement, all her motions are safe. She used good body mechanics throughout the testing.

Quality of Movement: She exhibited smooth motions and had excellent hand coordination. Balance testing stressed her, but she slowed her pace to ensure adequate balance during this type of testing. All other movements were coordinated.

Outstanding Physical Features: Decreased trunk motion was typical in her activities. Although this did not prevent good functional scores on test items, it is a feature that should be investigated further for remediation.

Physical Return-to-Work Options Explored: Her rehabilitation consultant, Laura Black, stated that Ms. Client could rejoin the Simms Nursing Home as a staff member in either an RN position or a night supervisor position. Therefore, this test addressed capacities needed for both positions.

Work Strengths Compared to Job Description: Because the job description of unit RN requires a significant number of patient transfers, Ms. Client would not meet the lifting requirements for this job description.

The night supervisor position would not require patient transfers, and would mainly consist of recordkeeping, light patient care, and passing medications. Functional actions involved are sitting, standing, walking, moderate flexing during light duty care, and supervisory and counseling activities that could be carried out in a self-selected position.

Limitations, re: Job Description: If supervisory nurse job description is adhered to, there should be no physical restrictions. It will be necessary, however, that self-pacing and frequent change of positions are allowed. Client needs to alternate sitting, standing, and walking so no one activity is done for prolonged period. She fully understands her ability to self-pace and change positions and should be able to accomplish this at work.

If lifting is required, she will be limited to the pounds of lifting indicated in the FCE form. This eliminates patient transfers but not pushing wheel chairs.

Recommendations:
1. Functional capacities match job description of nurse night supervisor. Precautioning areas exist in heavy activities, bending, prolonged positioning, and overall endurance. Return to work process can continue.
2. Because of physical constraint in trunk mobility and strength and in low endurance levels, a program of rehabilitation is indicated. This could precede full time work or coincide with part time return to work.

Recommendations: Reconditioning or work hardening to increase trunk flexibility, trunk stability, bending tolerance, and overall tolerance to working an 8-hour day.

Jessica Client
Client

June 30, and June 1, 1989
Date

FCE *Form*

Item	0	1–5	6–33	34–66	67–100	Restrictions	Recommendations
		Percent of 8-hour Day					
WEIGHT CAPACITY IN LBS.							
Floor to waist lift		15	0	0	0	Hip stabilizer & quadriceps weakness limitation.	Cannot be performed repetitiously.
Waist to overhead lift		25	10	0	0	Back extension limitation.	Should not reach higher than eye level.
Horizontal lift		30	15	0	0		
Push		40	15	10	0		Should move slowly.
Pull		50	15	10	0		Should move slowly.
Right carry		15	0	0	0	Trunk stabilizers weak.	
Left carry		10	0	0	0	Trunk stabilizers weak.	
Front carry		35	25	10	0	Guarded trunk position.	Should walk slowly.
Right hand grip		55	30	10	0		
Left hand grip		50	30	10	0		
FLEXIBILITY/POSITIONAL							
Elevated work		X				Back extension limitation	Must self-limit any reaching.
Forward bending/sitting			X			Flexes at hips; keeps back ext.	Should alternate positions.
Forward bending/standing		X				Increased symptoms and inability to maintain.	Must stand and bend only for brief periods of time.

Item		Percent of 8-hour Day				Restrictions	Recommendations
Item	*0*	*1–5*	*6–33*	*34–66*	*67–100*	*Restrictions*	*Recommendations*
Rotation sitting		X				Limitation in trunk motion.	Should use a swivel chair.
Rotation standing			X				Should pivot at feet.
Crawl		X				Weak back extensors.	Limit or avoid crawling.
Kneel		X					
Crouch—deep static	X					Unstable at hips, poor balance.	Should not crouch.
Repetitive squat		X				Hip stabilizers and quadriceps weakness.	Minimize squatting.
STATIC WORK							
Sitting tolerance				X			Should alternate positions.
Standing tolerance				X			Should alternate positions.
AMBULATION							
Walking			X			Deconditioning prevents speed.	Capacity moderate, but should walk slowly.
Stair climbing		X				Hip and quadriceps weakness.	Should self-pace and use rail for support.
Step ladder climbing		X				Hip and quadriceps weakness.	Should self-pace and use ladder for support.
Balance					X	Weak hip stabilizers.	Even surfaces—no difficulty. Uneven surface—requires caution.
COORDINATION							
R. upper extremity					X		Excellent aptitude.
L. upper extremity					X		Excellent aptitude.

____
Evaluator

____
Date

to maintain business and the ability of individual business to be successful.

Injured workers themselves who participate in work hardening are usually interested in rehabilitation rather than litigation. They can become willing partners in the work hardening process when specific positive reasons for a better quality of life are understood.

Definition and Description

Work hardening is the rehabilitation of an injured worker with the goal of attaining a physical level of competence that allows a return to work. It is implemented after the patient has medically stabilized, after physical deficiencies that interfere with work have been identified, and after specific goals have been set for the restoration process.[9]

The aspects of work hardening that set it apart from traditional treatment modes are:

1. Goal specific: The return to function and general strength may be early objectives, but the successful return to work is the ultimate goal of this treatment system.
2. Job directed: A functional job description should be used to assist in goal setting.[10] In addition to preparing physical attributes for the return to work, work-related activity is incorporated in the treatment to simulate realism in occupational situations. Levels of work categories may also be used.[11]
3. Program intensive: A professionally supervised work hardening program maximizes the time during the day and the days of treatment in a week and, concurrently, minimizes the total length of stay in the program. The program intensity both encourages faster progress and decreases the time off work and the associated costs.

Components of Work Hardening

Physical Reconditioning

Behind each limitation of an injured worker is a physical inability to perform a certain task. This may be in the form of loss of muscle strength, loss of endurance, decreased aerobic capacity, decreased mobility, or inability to coordinate properly. As in all medical situations, the underlying cause of the problem must be eliminated before the actual functional problem can be alleviated.

Reconditioning prepares the body to do work ac-

tivities. If work motions are done prior to strengthening or reconditioning, the client may be forced to use substitution patterns or poor body mechanics in order to perform a task. For example, if weak quadriceps are the limiting factor behind inability to lift from the floor, then repetitious practice of lifting will only accentuate the dysfunctional body mechanics. More damage than good may be done. Instead, the quadriceps strength and endurance must be addressed and improved before a safe functional lift is possible. At that point, lifting work simulation becomes a component of the work hardening program.

Improvement in physical conditioning is not an end in itself in work hardening. The purpose is to prepare a physical base for safe and functional work tasks. Therefore, reconditioning in isolation, although restorative and measurable, must be associated with the specific work task involved.

Work Simulation

Work simulation is designed by referring to the actual job description. When deficiencies in specific work activities are measurable, the goals of work hardening are to restore lost work ability. At this time, a specific work task evaluation should be added. The work simulation must be specific to the job (Figures 30-3 and 30-4).

The work hardening therapist studies the actual specifics of the work, designs the work simulation to reproduce the job functions, and trains the worker. The work simulation includes practice in body mechanics, progression of activity levels, and expansion of the work simulation until it approximates at least the amount of activity that is done on a job on a daily basis.

To improve work simulation, actual tools or conditions of the job must be set up. A carpenter, for example, could use the tools of the trade. Industries also are open to lending equipment and tools used on the job because this facilitates the safe and effective return of their worker.

Aerobic Conditioning

Underlying the ability to do sustained work over an 8-hour day and a 40-hour work week is the necessity for metabolic efficiency of the body. A patient who has been off work and is deconditioned may not have the capacity to sustain activity over time, even though he has the ability to do brief tasks.

Merely doing repetitive tasks without stressing the heart or lungs does not facilitate an increase in the conditioning level of the worker. The work hardening patient will be discouraged if the work tasks

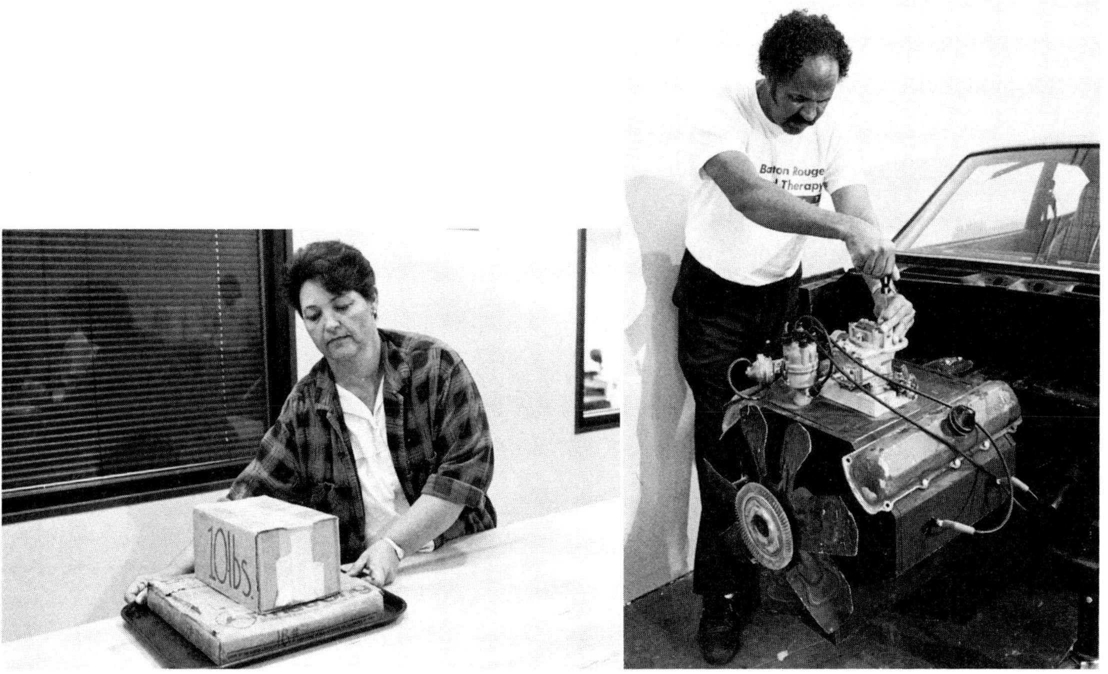

Figures 30–3, 30–4. Work hardening tasks are developed to work on a common goal through different activities. In both pictures trunk strength, stability, and positional tolerances are being developed. Figure 30–3 shows a patient strengthening trunk muscles, practicing weight shifts, and building endurance in upper extremities by simulating her job using cafeteria trays. Figure 30–4 demonstrates activity designed to build tolerance to flexed posture work for patient with low back injury. This posture is alternated with extension for sustained work.

are difficult and produce breathlessness, exertion, or general fatigue.

The work hardening client should be aerobically improved, at least to the point that his job demands. However, to give them the edge on fitness and health, greater aerobic conditioning is recommended. This gives the work hardening client a reserve of conditioning to provide a safety edge.

Education

The individual's recognition of his own abilities and limitations is critical in order to maintain safety at the work site. It is important that the worker understands what his capabilities are and when he must refrain from an activity at work. The first line of defense against reinjury is a knowledgeable worker.

Body mechanics is a habit, rather than a learned skill. We use our bodies in subconscious patterns. Therefore, if good body mechanics are to be consistent, practice is the only sure method. Work hardening is a repetitious activity, and a good opportunity to reinforce proper and safe body movements through continued practice day by day. This will make an impact on habitual patterns.

Another form of education in work hardening is formalized classes. These should be conducted in a group setting and be led by a professional with expertise in the subject matter. Pertinent classes in work hardening are:

1. Body mechanics and back school information. The review of body movement and the structures involved enhances the knowledge in safety concerns and reinforces concepts taught in work hardening.
2. Return to work skills. This often missed subject includes interviewing skills, communication with potential or current employers, communication with coworkers, and preparation of vocational goals.
3. Psychosocial groups for workers who have difficulties over and above physical problems. Topics may include workers compensation dilemmas, poor relationships with work supervisors, the effect of family and societal problems on the individual, and the effect of positive or negative attitudes.

Program Dynamics

Admittance Conference

An initial conference to discuss the goals and direction of work hardening is necessary prior to program implementation. Included are the injured worker, the employer, the rehabilitation or vocational consultant, a representative of the insurance company, and the physician. At this time, work hardening goals are thoroughly discussed for appropriations and agreement. By understanding the goals and directions at the beginning, expectations of the work hardening program and the return to work possibilities will be realistic.

Work hardening programs are most effective when conducted five days a week, 4 to 8 hours per day programs. The schedule is worklike in that attendance is mandatory, and punctuality and responsibility are critical. Table 30–5 gives some examples of work hardening tasks. They are explicit, allowing the client to progress without daily re-evaluation, and giving the therapist options that can be used for many clients.

Self-Responsibilities

A condition for success of work hardening is compliance of the client to the rules and procedures for

Table 30–5
Work Hardening Weekly Report

Week of	Objective	Exercise or Work Simulation Station	Monday Goal	Monday Actual	Tuesday Goal	Tuesday Actual	Wednesday Goal	Wednesday Actual	Thursday Goal	Thursday Actual	Friday Goal	Friday Actual
Mar 4–7 1988	Increase aerobic capacity	Ride Airdyne bicycle at 2.0 setting	5 min	X	6 min	X	7 min	6½	8 min	7	9 min	7½
	Increase right & left quadriceps & hamstring strength	Cybex Standard workout #3 protocols	Day 1	X	Day 2	X	Day 3	X	Day 4	X	Day 5	X
	Lift from floor using upright back posture	Work station- 12 x 12 boxes Simulation protocol #1	10#	X	12#	X	13#	12#	14#	12#	15#	13#
	Increase push-pull poundage & distance	Push-pull sled Route B	50# 900 ft.	X	50# 1000 ft.	X	60# 1000 ft.	X	60# 1100 ft.	X	70# 1100 ft.	X
	Increase tolerance for working at loading dock	Loading dock work simulation	40 min.	X	45 min	X	50 min.	X	55 min.		60 min.	X

the work hardening program. It is more like a work situation than a treatment situation. Therefore, the patient takes responsibility for his daily routine, monitors his body mechanics and safety, and adheres to the time schedules, just as he would at work. Although the work hardening staff make a strong attempt to encourage compliance, the decision for compliance rests on the individual. The therapist assumes a facilitative rather than a treatment role.

Interim Reports

Interim reports are sent regularly, documenting the patient's progress toward work goals. If any readjustment in goals or deadlines is needed, these interim reports provide the objective evidence.

A premature medical dismissal from work hardening may happen if goals cannot be met or if the problems are not amenable to physical treatment. This may not have been apparent at the inception of work hardening and may only become clear after consistent activity does not produce results. A second type of premature discharge could happen if progress is not made because of a noncompliant attitude. In this case, the evidence is documented, a conference is held, and the client may be asked to leave work hardening. This is much like being fired.

Discharge Reports

This report is the most critical, as it must clearly establish outcome of the program and work capability of the patient. It should be written in physical terms and in work terms with a clear message. The format should be:

Brief review of work hardening program (day length, duration).
Review of initial goals and accomplishment of goals.
Work abilities compared to job or job level.
Work limitations.
Further need for physical intervention (if any).
Work modification suggestions (if any).
Updated FCE form for workers' compensation and insurance company.
Summary and conclusion.

FUTURE PERSPECTIVES

Both functional capacity assessment and work hardening are programs long overdue. They bridge the gap between work injury and return to work for workers. When utilized early and appropriately in the return to work process, they have the potential not only to substantially reduce long-term costs, but to diminish the waste of human health and talent that comes with chronic injury.

The challenge for us in the future will be to:

- Introduce more effective quantification in both functional assessment and work hardening.
- Continue reliability studies in functional assessment.
- Enlarge and publish outcome studies in work hardening.
- Define, refine, and teach the concepts inherent in these programs to ensure their continued use for the injured worker and in the work injury management system.

REFERENCES

1. Haddad, G.H.: Analysis of 2932 workers compensation back injury cases: the impact on the cost to the system; Spine *12*(8):765–769, 1987.
2. Lett, C., McCabe, N., Tramposh, A., Tate-Henderson, S.: Work hardening. *In* Work Injury: Management and Prevention (Edited by S.J. Isernhagen). Rockville, MD, Aspen Publishers, Inc., 1988.
3. Isernhagen, S.: Functional Capacity Evaluation. *In* Work Injury: Management and Prevention. Rockville, MD, Aspen Publishers, Inc., 1988.
4. Matheson, L.: Work Capacity Evaluation. Employment Rehabilitation Institute of California, Anaheim, CA, pp. 1–20, 1987.
5. Mayer, T., et al.: Objective assessment of spine function following industrial injury: a prospective study with comparison group and one-year follow-up. Spine *10*:482–493, 1985.
6. Schultz-Johnson, K.: Evaluating the workers functional capacities for repetitive work. Semin Occup Med *2*(1):21–40, 1987.
7. Wilson, S., Mejia, D.: Work hardening: back disabilities take on a new dimension. Top Acute Care Trauma Rehabil *2*(4):73–83, 1988.
8. National Institute for Occupational Safety and Health: Work Practices Guide for Manual Lifting. Pub 81–122, Dept of Health and Human Services, Niosh, Cincinnati, OH 45226, pp. 121–125, March 81.
9. Isernhagen, S.: Work hardening case study. *In* Physical Therapy. Philadelphia, J.B. Lippincott, 1988.
10. Isernhagen, S.: Functional job descriptions. Semin Occup Med *2*(1):50–55, 1987.
11. US Department of Labor: Dictionary of Occupational Titles, 4th Ed. US Government Printing Office, Washington, DC, 20402, 1977.

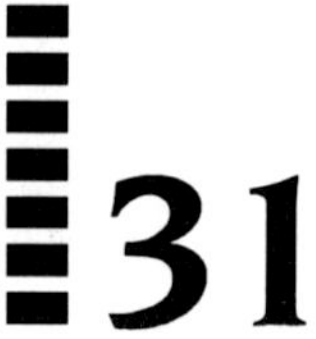

31

Leonard N. Matheson

Integrated Work Hardening

CONCEPTS: WHY ARE WE INTERESTED?

Although progress has been made to avoid the occurrence of chronic disability after a painful spinal injury, much work remains. This is especially true in the vocational rehabilitation of individuals who are chronically disabled because of a painful spinal disorder. Much of this is a result of the fact that painful spinal disorders are neither life threatening nor visibly disfiguring. Because the medical consequences of painful spinal disorders are less dramatic than those of other disabling disorders, they have not received as much attention from the medical rehabilitation community. For many of the same reasons, the vocational rehabilitation community has only recently begun to address the difficult issues posed by individuals who suffer from painful spinal disorders. For example, the Commission on Accreditation of Rehabilitation Facilities has, in its 22 years, developed accreditation criteria for 19 service delivery models. It is only within the last few years that service delivery models, which include substantial numbers of people who suffer from painful spinal disorders (chronic pain programs and work hardening programs), have been developed. This lack of formal program identification is paralleled in university training curricula for both medical and vocational rehabilitation professionals. Attention given to painful spinal disorders in curricula for physicians, occupational therapists, physical therapists, rehabilitation counselors, and vocational evaluators has been scanty in comparison to education for disorders that are more visible and dramatic.

Vocational Consequences of Painful Spinal Disorders

Whether or not the vocational consequences of painful spinal disorders have been given appropriate attention, they are substantial. Among employed adults, painful spinal disorder is the most frequent cause of chronic disability. For example, out of 1136 disabled adults who were referred to the Employment and Rehabilitation Institute of California for rehabilitation services from 1984 through 1988, 58% had spinal disorders. At the time of injury, these individuals had been out of work for substantially longer than injured workers disabled from other causes. As a group, these disabled workers had a mean time lag of 21.4 months from date of injury to date of referral, and individuals with spinal disorders averaged 31 months, compared with 21 months for individuals with upper extremity injuries, and 14 months for individuals with lower extremity disorders.

What is the mechanism of occupational disability for individuals with painful spinal disorders? Because painful spinal disorders produce global dysfunction, they tend to result in a broader range of functional limitations and greater impact on the vocationally relevant resources that an injured worker has developed up to the time of his disability. If we conceptualize a worker as possessing a gradually increasing fund of "employability resources" that increases his value to an employer, the impact of various types of disabling conditions can be considered in terms of the residual transferable skills that continue to be available once a chronic disability state is achieved. If we consider these resources in terms of the system developed by the United States Department of Labor, we can develop scenarios that help to depict the effect of a painful spinal disorder in terms of subsequent labor market access. For example, consider a 45-year-old individual with a 10th grade education who has the work history shown in Table 31–1.

If we identify the occupations in the American economy that continue to be available to this person through the use of the Vertek Occupation Assessment System (OASYS), we find that 453 occupations can be identified that provide a reasonable match to the employability resources that he has developed. If we "disable" this individual because of one or an-

346

Table 31–1
*Example of the Work History of a 45-Year-Old Individual
with a 10th Grade Education*

Dot Code	Occupational Title	Months Employed
905.663–014	Truck Driver, Heavy	120
620.281–018	Auto Maintenance Equipment Operator	60
600.281–022	Machine Builder	48
620.261–010	Automobile Mechanic	48
914.667–010	Loader 1	60

Table 31–2
*Example of the Work History of a 45-Year-Old Individual
with a 4-Year College Education*

Dot Code	Occupational Title	Months Employed
003.061–010	Electrical Engineer	96
003.281–101	Drafter, Electrical	60
726.131–010	Electronic Computer Subassembler	48
726.381–010	Electronics Inspector I	60

other condition, restricting him with functional limitations based on the biomechanical limits inherent in various diagnoses, we find that fewer occupations are available and that the number of occupations available is related to the disabling condition and its unique functional limitations. Figure 31–1 illustrates these relationships.

As can be seen, the global nature of spinal disorders brings about a loss of labor market access that is substantially greater than would be found with the other disorders. Is this effect less substantial with an individual who has a higher level of education? Let us see. For another example, we can consider the case of a 45-year-old individual with a four-year college education and a degree in engineering. The individual's work history is dipicted in Table 30–2.

An OASYS[1] analysis indicates that 131 occupations are available to this person. If we apply the same functional limitations as with the first example, we find the loss of labor market access depicted to those shown in Figure 31–2.

As can be seen, the functional consequences of the lumbar spinal disorder are less substantial in vocational terms for the individual with this work and educational history. However, "pure" functional limitations based on biomechanical function are only part of the story. What are the other consequences of disabling pain, in addition to the biomechanical dysfunction we have ascribed to the injured workers in the cases above? It can be shown that the vocational consequences of pain are closely related to educational level, and consequently to labor market access. That is, more highly educated people who suffer from painful spinal disorders lose more in terms of labor market access than will individuals with less education. This is because the painful disorders cause problems with attention and concentration that have greater impact on the educated indi-

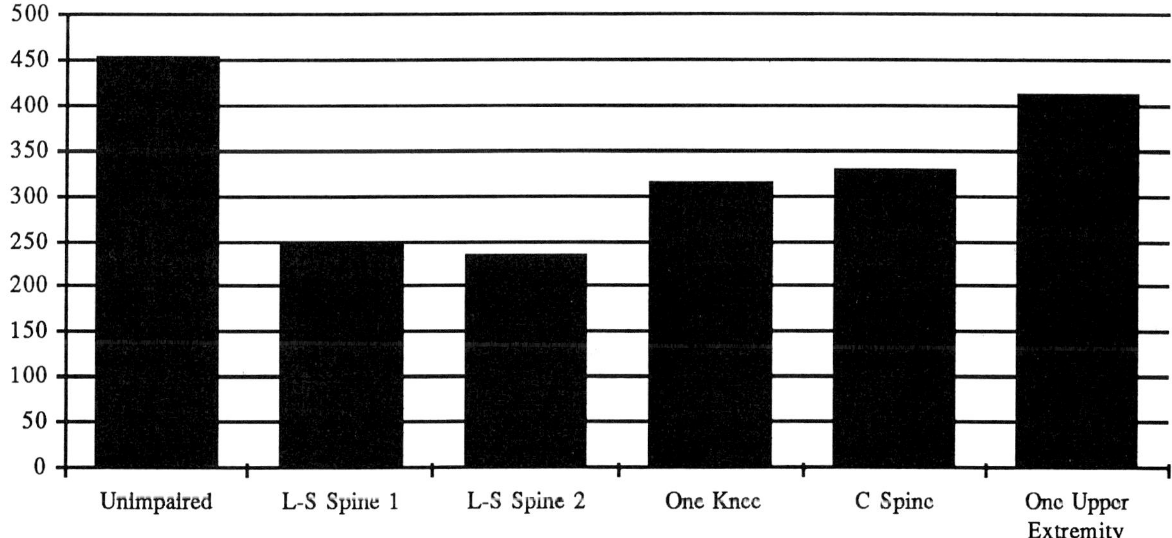

Figure 31–1. Relationships between number of available occupations (y-axis) and type of disabling condition (x-axis).

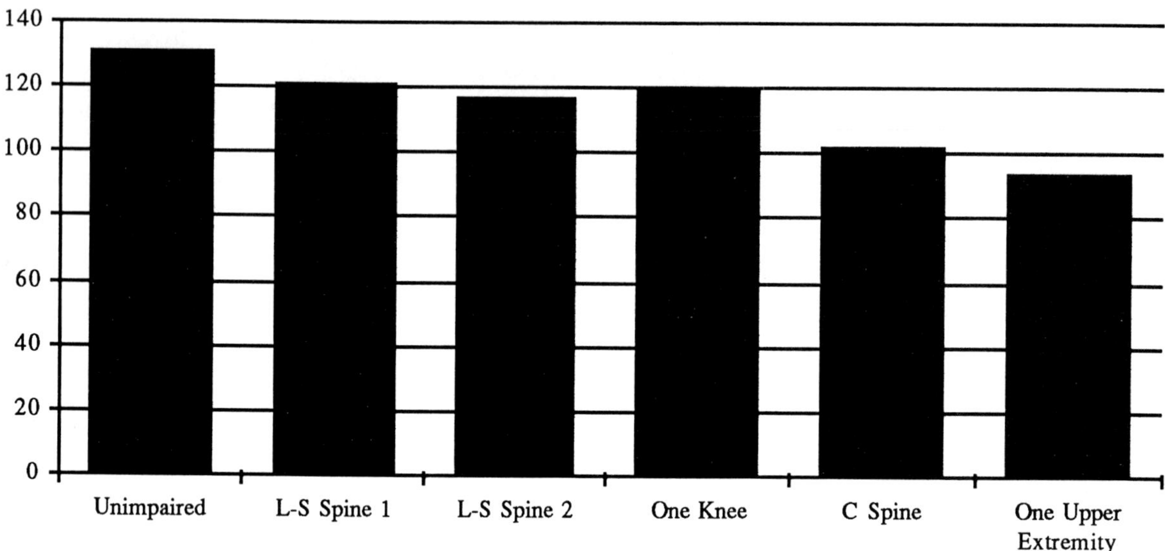

Figure 31–2. The number of occupations available to this person (Table 31-2) on the basis of functional limitations.

vidual's transferable skills than on the less educated person's transferable skills. The comparison between the two examples previously presented is extended to include pain as an additional disabling condition in Figure 31–3.

Because painful spinal disorders result in important vocational consequences and because often these preclude an individual's ability to return to his previous employment, vocational rehabilitation is necessary. Additionally, the vocational consequences of painful spinal disorders present serious challenges to the medical rehabilitator in terms of lost or misdirected motivation that stem from the adverse effect of the painful spinal disorder on the patient's vocational status. Certainly, a coordinated approach to these problems that integrates the contributions of all health care and rehabilitation providers is needed.

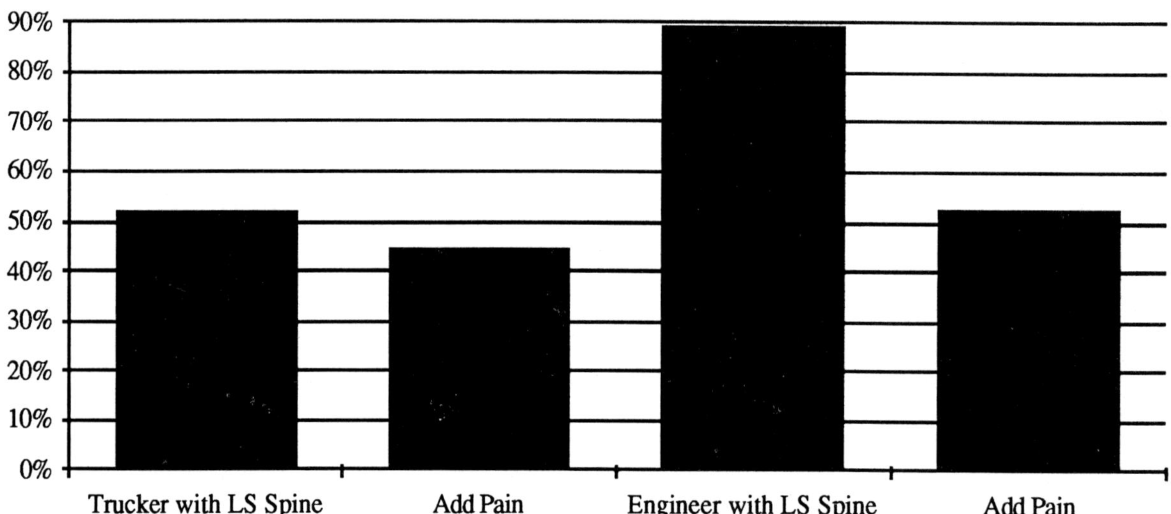

Figure 31–3. Loss of occupational access based on biomechanical limitations with and without pain.

Three Concurrent Domains of Function

As we evaluate and treat the individual with a painful spinal disorder, we must consider three domains of function: the biomechanical, psychophysical, and cardiovascular or metabolic. It is important to recognize that, although each performance measure reflects the injured worker's most limiting domain, all domains contribute to his performance.

Biomechanical

These are the demands placed on the worker by the work tasks that challenge the injured worker's anatomic and musculoskeletal levers and fulcrums. Skeletal muscles produce torque at the various biomechanical linkages in the body. In the biomechanical model,[2–4] the stresses on the musculoskeletal system during lifting are measured isometrically with maximum strength tests. A two-dimensional static model has been developed by these researchers to allow estimates of the forces at various joints, including compressive and shear forces at the L5/S1 disc interspace. Single plane isokinetic techniques have been developed to determine spinal and extremity capacity through assessment of dynamic muscle strength.[5] Promising multiplane isoinertial techniques have been developed to measure strength and fatigue tolerance,[6] although the application of these findings to determine work capacity has yet to be undertaken.

Psychophysical

These are the demands placed on the worker by the work tasks that challenge the injured worker's self-perceptions, fears, and built-in work function themes and limits. This is often the most limiting domain for most low back injured workers who suffer painful spinal disorders. The psychophysical model[7–9] predicts lifting capacities for several lifting ranges and sizes of objects with a degree of reliability that exceeds the static biomechanical model with characteristically lower achieved maximum force values. Comparison of these results with isokinetic and isoinertial models is scanty but promising.

Cardiovascular or Metabolic

These are the demands placed on the worker by the work tasks that challenge the injured worker's cardiac, respiratory, and metabolic systems. This domain limits the worker in tasks that require prolonged, sustained work. For the injured worker who has remained off work for more than 3 months and has not maintained a level of activity that approxi-

mates his previous work demands, the cardiovascular or metabolic domain will present significant limitations. Similarly, the injured worker who has become depressed will experience problems within this domain that exhibit themselves as malaise and fatigue. Cardiovascular or metabolic models, usually based on measurement of oxygen consumption during prolonged lifting tasks, have been offered by Erb[10] and Genaidy & Asfour.[11]

Although the presenting issue may clearly be identified to exist in one domain, all three domains are needed to perform work. Given the patient's particular strengths and weaknesses, the most limiting domain may or may not coincide with the domain that is the intended focus of study.

Stages of Recovery from Painful Spinal Disorders

Evaluation and treatment of painful spinal disorders is most easily understood within the context of the "Stage Model of Industrial Rehabilitation,"[12] which provides an organized framework within which to consider the issues that are encountered (Table 31–3). The Stage Model encompasses eight stages, beginning at the point at which the disorder is identified and extending through the restoration and rehabilitation process to the point at which earning capacity is determined. Each stage has one

Table 31–3
Stage Model of Industrial Rehabilitation

Stage	Area Assessed	Measured by or in Terms of . . .
One	Pathology	Studies of tissue and bone.
Two	Impairment	Anatomy, physiology, psyche.
Three	Functional limitation	Symptoms and limitations.
Four	Occupational disability	Role consequences of functional limitations.
Five	Vocational feasibility	Acceptability of the patient as an employee in the most general sense.
Six	Employability	Ability to become employed.
Seven	Vocational handicap	Ability to perform a particular job.
Eight	Earning capacity	Income measured over expected worklife.

unique area that is addressed. Each area involves evaluation or treatment, measured in terms of particular types of information collected by different team members.

Although each stage is important, the stages of functional limitation, occupational disability, feasibility for competitive employment, and employability are integral to the vocational rehabilitation of individuals chronically disabled with painful spinal disorders.

Functional Limitation

As noted in the earlier examples, painful spinal disorders result in a global dysfunction that has both biomechanical and cognitive components. The biomechanical components limit the person in terms of his ability to bring strength to the job task, as well as his ability to stoop, kneel, crouch, climb, lift, and carry. The cognitive components relate to his ability to maintain adequate error control and concentration and to deal with complex cognitive tasks. Although the musculoskeletal limitations that stem from a painful spinal disorder are usually quantified in terms of biomechanical function, the biomechanical limitations are often much greater than the musculoskeletal impairment would bring about. The magnification of the biomechanical consequences of the musculoskeletal impairment is based in the psychophysical domain, although it is certainly expressed and measured in the biomechanical domain. Limitations that stem from motivational issues and learned adaptive behavior magnify the functional consequences of the painful spinal disorder. In terms of motivational issues, the connotative meaning of pain to the individual is fear associated with the original injury, prospects for reinjury, and pending losses, and the need that can be met as a consequence of the injury work together in various combinations to increase the limiting effect of the original painful spinal disorder. In terms of learned adaptive response, the symptom magnification syndrome[12] is a learned behavioral response pattern that functions to control the individual's environment, in place of volitional control, initiated by the individual who suffers from a painful spinal disorder. Although this behavior is adaptive within a narrow scope and for a brief duration, it often persists so that its incidence in a population of chronically disabled is substantial.[13]

Occupational Disability

Based on residual functional capacity, occupational disability must be considered in terms of both the competence of the individual for the job and the potential for reinjury because of occupational de-

mands. This has led to a bifurcated process in which the safety of the injured worker is assumed to be defined by the physician-imposed work restrictions, whereas the competency issues are assessed by an occupational therapist, physical therapist, or vocational evaluator in terms of the functional match between the individual's abilities and the job's critical functional demands. It is important to note that occupational disability can result from insufficiency in terms of either set of issues: the safety issues addressed by the physician or the competency issues addressed by the allied health professionals. The difficulty with painful spinal disorders, in contrast to other disorders in which pain does not always denote reinjury, is that the individual must learn to "work with his pain" or perform productive activity at the same time that pain is present.

This raises two problems that are difficult to resolve. The first issue is "where to draw the line?" with regard to how much pain is acceptable before the risk of reinjury becomes sufficiently real to modify activity. The second problem has to do with the effect of pain on productivity. Individuals with high levels of pain frequently work more slowly, take extra breaks from work, must leave the workplace early, produce more errors because of problems with concentration, and are less tolerant of interpersonal problems than other workers who are not experiencing substantial levels of pain. Thus, although work tasks can still be accomplished by many individuals with painful spinal disorders, being able to assume the customary worker role involves much more. In fact, experience has shown that many individuals are able to perform usual and customary work tasks but are unable to resume the worker role because of more general issues that are subsumed under the next stage in the process that relates to vocational feasibility.

Feasibility for Competitive Employment

Feasibility for competitive employment is defined as the acceptability of the patient as an employee to an employer. We are concerned with the work behavior of the employee-to-be. Vocational feasibility is compromised by the painful spinal disorder because of the generalization of the individual's learned response to pain. That is, as the individual experiences symptoms and interacts with the environment, symptom-based behaviors are reinforced. These behaviors supplant the productivity-based behaviors for which the individual has been reinforced as a worker. Gradually, the individual with a painful spinal disorder abdicates the worker role and assumes the patient role. The social, vocational, familial, and personal roles that were based on a perception of the individual as a productive and responsible participant are strongly colored by a perception of the individual with a painful spinal disorder as one who is less responsible for productivity than others. In rehabilitation, this is a transitional stage in that the individual is no longer considered a "patient" and is now identified as a "worker." This is the first stage in which the individual is formally assessed in terms of worker behaviors that can be grouped into three major areas:[12]

1. General productivity–The worker's ability to perform work tasks with sufficient speed, endurance, quality, and consistency to allow the employer to profit from his employment.
2. Safety in the workplace–The worker's ability to perform the job tasks within the work environment in a manner that is safe to himself and his fellow workers.
3. Interpersonal behavior–The worker's ability to get along with others, accept direction from a supervisor, and adjust to different supervisory styles.

The concept of feasibility as an external touchstone allows the treatment team to bring part of the reality of the individual's eventual context of living into the clinical environment to be used as part of the rehabilitation process. The interpretation of the individual's behavior in terms of his acceptability as an employee can begin to orient the individual (and his family) toward eventual return to work as a goal. There may be no better opportunity to begin to learn appropriate employer-relevant behavior than in the supportive atmosphere of the hospital or rehabilitation center. In addition to its importance as a transition stage as the individual moves from the patient role into the worker role, feasibility is an important communication link between the individual and the treating professional, superior to the traditional communication link, i.e., symptoms. Because treatment professionals interpret the patient's behavior in terms of symptoms, the patient communicates through the use of symptom displays and reports. Although the use of symptoms as a communication link between patient and health care practitioner has stood the test of time, an alternative approach is to consider the patient's behavior in terms of feasibility for competitive employment. Feasibility for competitive employment can actually be superior to symptoms as a communication link for four reasons:

1. It is the context of the employer. The factors that we consider within feasibility are those factors that are easily understood by any employer. Similarly, the patient who has been an employee un-

derstands the measures that are being used to conduct the evaluation.
2. It is a multidimensional factor. Through the application of the concept of feasibility, it is possible to identify specific feasibility issues and develop specific strategies to remedy the feasibility problems.
3. It is verifiable. Feasibility can be validated through cross reference to observable behaviors. Agreed upon standards of feasibility have been developed; symptoms are not verifiable.
4. It has a positive orientation to results. As the patient is considered in terms of feasibility, he is assisted to achieve improved attendance, workplace tolerance, and productivity. Productivity is reinforced in the social environment and contributes to the growth of the person and his perception of his options. By comparison, when the patient is considered in terms of symptoms, the focus is on the avoidance of pain or other symptoms. Avoidance behavior that is reinforced can become the predominant behavioral style of the individual with painful spinal disorder, generalizing to all aspects of his life and social environment. Additionally, although pain behavior and the patient's reports of symptoms can be difficult to extinguish, competing behaviors that are productivity-oriented can be strongly reinforced. This will result in a loss of the patient's focus on symptoms and a subsequent refocus on productivity.

Employability

Defined as the patient's ability to become employed within a particular labor market, this is distinct from the feasibility stage in that the latter is concerned with the general acceptability of the patient as an employee without regard to a specific occupation, whereas employability is concerned with the ability of a person to become employed within a particular occupation. Employability considers the worker's physical work tolerances, general educational development, aptitudes, temperament, interests, and geographic location. It can be statistically calculated as the proportion of jobs in a particular labor market that are accessible to the low back patient given the constellation of these factors that the patient presents to the labor market.[14] In this sense, employability can be thought of as the probability that a patient will become employed. As illustrated in Figures 30–1 to 30–3, employability is directly affected by painful spinal disorders, both by the functional limitations that are a consequence of the disorder and by the effects of the disorder on the patient's feasibility for competitive employment.

Clearly, painful spinal disorders bring about important changes at each of the rehabilitation stages and result in vocational, personal, and financial consequences for the injured worker. In addition, to the degree that the problem of painful spinal disorders affects the workforce, it strikes at the heart of society's ability to prosper and grow.

DIAGNOSIS: HOW DO WE IDENTIFY AND ANALYZE THE PROBLEM?

Evaluation Guidelines

The evaluation process that is used with painful spinal disorder has two primary components, Work Tolerance Screening,[15] and Specific Vocational Exploration.[12] Although each component is presented separately below, it is important to bear in mind the criteria for the selection, administration, and interpretation of evaluation procedures that have been developed by the American Psychological Association[16] and the National Institute of Occupational Safety and Health.[17] Every procedure used for the evaluation of a disabled worker must meet the following five criteria:

Safety

The evaluation equipment, procedures, and environment must not expose the patient to undue risk of reinjury. The evaluation of a disabled worker within the litigious medicolegal system requires more than the usual degree of care and professional acumen and the rigorous adherence to procedures that are accepted standards of community practice.

Reliability

Reliability is the degree to which the worker's performance is consistent over time, between different raters, or across different parts of the same test. This is an especially troublesome factor with individuals who suffer from a painful spinal disorder in that it is not possible to assume that the patient has "tried his best" or performed at a level that will be consistent. Given the litigious context within which the back injured person is evaluated and treated, challenges to the reliability of the measure of performance can be expected.

Validity

Validity is the extent to which the performance measure is related to some true criterion. That is, how closely does the worker's performance in the evaluation task approximate his performance when subsequently faced with the job demand? The content validity of a measure is a professional judgement regarding the degree to which the test measures the job's demands and is based on a thorough job analysis.

Practicality

The task must be reasonably easy to administer and reasonably priced. Equipment expense must be balanced against cost of administration. The evaluation must be accepted by the patient so that full participation is quickly achieved. Evaluation results must be quickly available, readily understood, and defendable.

Utility

Utility is the ability to apply the findings to the problem at hand. It is often defined as "ability to predict future injury" or "ability to predict future work performance."

Work Tolerance Screening

Work tolerance screening focuses on the patient's functional limitations and residual functional capacity. Both issues can be addressed during the work tolerance screening, depending on the skill of the evaluator. The goal of the work tolerance screening is to develop a model of the functional competence of the patient along with guidelines for prophylactic work restrictions to minimize the likelihood of reinjury.

Work Tolerance Screening Battery

The Employment and Rehabilitation Institute of California (E.R.I.C.) Work Tolerance Screening Battery[15] is a collection of tests that are commercially available and on which safety and reliability studies exist. The test battery has been in use since 1980. In that time, the author has participated in more than 2000 evaluations with this test battery. The test battery also has been in use throughout the United States and Canada. Because it is not proprietary nor controlled in any way, it is not possible to ascertain the number of evaluations that have been conducted in other settings, but it is estimated to be tens of thousands. The test battery begins with low physical demands and gradually increases. In addition to maximizing safety, this graduated approach to evaluation maximizes efficiency because evaluation tasks that are beyond the individual's capability can be identified prior to administration. It is not unusual for a patient to be unable to complete all the tests in the battery. What is more, some of the more demanding tests in the battery have levels of demand that are beyond many patients' capability. Each evaluation instrument is provided by its publisher with its own instruction manual and normative data.

Health Screening

Prior to administration of the test battery, screening for health status is conducted through the use of a structured intake interview and the *Cornell Medical Index Health Questionnaire*.[18] The intake interview is comprised of questions that are designed to collect information concerning the patient's demographics, use of medications, goals, general health, reported functional tolerances, and symptoms. The interview is also designed to screen for gross psychological dysfunction and the symptom magnification syndrome. The *CMI* is useful for identifying other health care issues that are outside of the focus of the presenting impairment. In addition, the *CMI* is useful for screening for psychological adjustment problems and emotional distress.

Perception of Function Card Sorts

An important part of the evaluation of the patient concerns his perception of his own functional limitations. Information about the patient's perception of disability is collected in the intake interview and through the use of one or more of the activity sort procedures, including the WEST Tool Sort,[19] Loma Linda Activity Sort,[20] and Spinal Function Sort.[21] In these procedures, the patient sorts cards on which there are drawings of tasks from a card deck in terms of the patient's perception of his or her own ability to perform the task. Sample cards from the Spinal Function Sort are presented in Figure 31–4.

Through the use of computer-assisted factor analysis,[13] a profile of the underlying demands inherent in each of the cards presented to the patient provides information about the individual's "work function themes," the unconscious rules that guide participation in work activity. Individuals who suffer from painful spinal disorders generally demonstrate work function themes that are constricted and reflect a generalized avoidance behavior beyond that which is tied to the strictly biomechanical limitations of the musculoskeletal impairment.

Maximum Voluntary Effort Test Battery

Maximum voluntary effort (MVE) testing[22] is an important part of every work tolerance screening. Various approaches to maximum voluntary effort testing have been developed. Those that are in use on a regular basis at E.R.I.C. include the JAMAR Five-Span Test, a five-handle test with the BTE Work Simulator, and the WEST 4 Torquing Test. The protocol for each of these tests is presented elsewhere.[13] In brief, this involves three test trials at

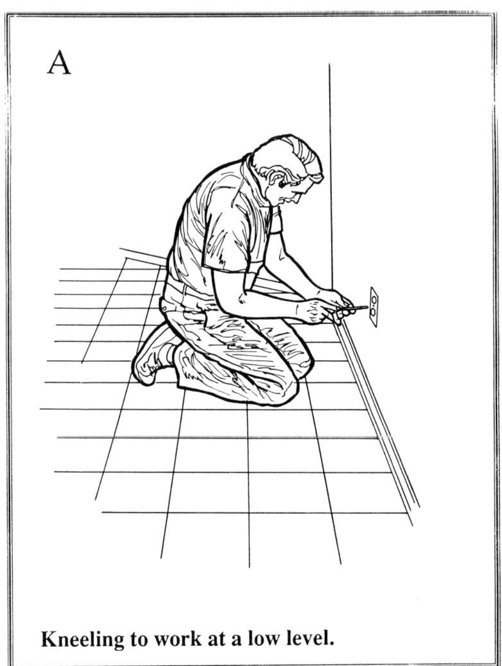

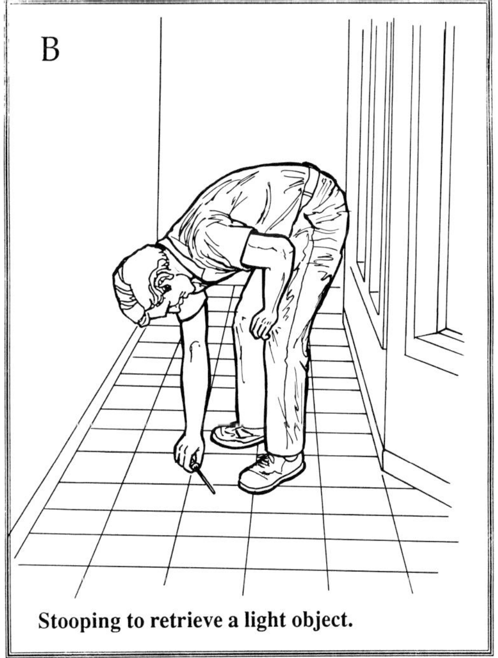

Figure 3–4A, B. Sample cards from the Spinal Function Sort test.

each position or direction. The trials are spaced to avoid problems with fatigue. A coefficient of variation is calculated for each of three trials. The obtained coefficient of variation is compared against an expected coefficient of variation. If the obtained coefficient of variation exceeds the expected coefficient of variation, the presumption is that the patient put forth less than full effort. Although formal decision rules are under development, this method has been used successfully at E.R.I.C. since 1985. It appears to have good sensitivity but only modest specificity. That is, a positive result often leads to an admission on the part of the patient that he was putting forth less than full effort, whereas a negative result does not always mean that the individual is putting forth full effort. Recent research[23,24] has provided standards against which to measure performance. One or another of the MVE tests is administered to every patient with a painful spinal disorder in order to formally screen for full effort. In addition, data are collected with each of the instruments in the work tolerance screening test battery in a manner that allows identification of less than full effort. This vigilance and the willingness of the evaluator "to take a stand" and confront the individual with objective data that indicate less than full effort results in improved effectiveness and an earned reputation for integrity and evaluative skill.

Employee Aptitude Survey #9[25]

This is a paper and pencil test that is used to evaluate manual speed and accuracy (or coordinated response speed). The standard test administration requires the evaluee to make rapid and accurate pencil dots in a series of "Os" over a five minute testing period. The evaluator records the number of trials completed at the end of each of the five one-minute periods without interrupting the patient. This allows the test to provide additional information about the potential decrement or increment in function that may be caused by disuse, deconditioning, or other more directly impairment-related functional problems.

Crawford Small Parts Dexterity Test[26]

The patient's unilateral and bilateral coordination with small tools is evaluated with this instrument. In Part I, the patient uses tweezers in the dominant hand to place a small pin in each of 36 holes and then place a pop rivet collar on each pin. Part II requires the patient to use a small screwdriver bilaterally to spin a small machine screw into each of 36 threaded holes. In each of the two parts, the 36 holes are arranged into 6 rows of 6 holes each. An additional line of 6 holes is provided as a practice

trial. Sitting, neck flexion, sustained horizontal reaching, sustained dominant hand palmar pinch, and repetitive fine fingering are assessed. The evaluator records the worker's time to complete each row without interrupting the worker. Increased duration from row to row may be indicative of pain, fatigue, or breakdown of concentration. Decreased duration may result from learning or a warmup effect. This test is customarily administered with the patient seated. In selected cases in which sitting tolerance or tolerance of neck flexion is severely impaired, the test can be performed by the seated patient at an elevated or slanted worksurface or standing at a counter. Forearm support supplied by armrests may improve performance when tolerance of sustained horizontal reaching with the upper extremities is low.

VALPAR 4 Upper Extremity Range of Motion[27]

This is a work sample that measures fine to medium dexterity and parts handling. It examines the worker's ability to rapidly manipulate small to medium sized parts in a closed area that obscures vision and requires the use of a variety of upper extremity positions, some of which are awkward. Using one hand at a time, the evaluee removes hex nuts from a tray and spins them onto the ends of ¼ in. and ¾ in. bolts protruding into a 14 in. cube by reaching through a 5 in. hole in the front of the cube. He then removes the nuts from the inside of the cube and replaces them in the tray. Dominant versus nondominant performance is observed. Sitting or standing, horizontal reaching across the midline, rapid fingering using primarily the thumb and radial fingers, forearm supination and shoulder external rotation, forearm pronation and shoulder internal rotation, wrist flexion, and ulnar deviation are evaluated. The VALPAR 4 is designed to be administrated with the patient in a standing position. The manual specifies that if the individual's disability prevents him from standing during administration, the work sample can be completed in a sitting position. However, working when sitting tends to produce more lumbar torque with reaching across the midline. If the patient has a severe intolerance of minimal twisting motions of the spine, this test is best administered when standing. A padded standing mat makes standing more easily tolerated. The work height may be adjusted to minimize trunk flexion.

VALPAR 8 Simulated Assembly[28]

This is a work sample that presents a bilateral, highly repetitive three-part assembly process for a duration of 20 minutes. The worker removes plastic discs and a small metal post from bins at approximately waist level. The post is inserted into a hole on a moving wheel that is approximately chest height. The discs are then fit over the post. Sitting or standing, sustained horizontal reaching, repetitive forearm supination and pronation, repetitive fingering and handling are evaluated. The VALPAR 8 is designed to be administered with the worker in a standing position, but can be conducted with the worker in a sitting position if he has difficulty standing. A padded standing mat, as well as adjustment in the work height to minimize spinal flexion, will facilitate comfortable standing. Without interruption of the worker's work, the number of assemblies completed every five minutes over a twenty-minute span is recorded. Most patients are able to maintain or increase speed over the course of this test. A decrease of 5% per period is considered significant. Patients who have moderate to severe pain disorders of the cervical or lumbar spine may be unable to complete this task because of intolerance of sustained reaching because this places increased stress on the postural extensor muscles of the back. Severely deconditioned individuals may experience aching, burning, or cramping in these same postural muscles, usually of the middle to upper back, because of fatigue and strain of weak muscle groups.

Minnesota Rate of Manipulation[29]

A measure of manual speed and dexterity, this test is comprised of a series of five tasks that require sustained eye-hand coordination with unilateral and bilateral tasks. During each subtest, the subject retrieves, manipulates, and places brightly colored plastic discs according to a standardized pattern. Standing, repetitive fingering, repetitive light palmar pinch, sustained horizontal reaching within 12 in. of the body, repetitive horizontal reaching beyond 12 in. of the body, and repetitive forearm supination and pronation are evaluated. The manual specifies that the worker should stand at a testing table between 28 and 32 in. in height. Patients who cannot stand or who have limited standing tolerance can be tested in a sitting position with the modification noted in the report. However, working when sitting produces lumbar torque when the patient reaches across the midline. This aggravates most pain disorders of the lumbar spine. A padded standing mat or a short sitting or walking break between subtests helps make standing more tolerable. Individuals who are very tall and those with severe intolerance of lumbar or cervical flexion benefit from having the testing table raised. One must document all position changes or workstation modifications. The MROM is a good evaluation tool to screen for intolerance of repetitive or sustained horizontal reaching within or beyond 12 in. from the body.

BTE Work Simulator[30]

Consisting of an electronically-controlled variable resistance brake head from which a shaft protrudes, the assembly can be set in any one of five vertical-to-horizontal positions, depending on the desired simulation. By slipping one of the many different BTE attachments onto the shaft and adjusting the resistance via the control panel, the evaluator is able to simulate a selected work demand at a controlled effort level. The control panel also receives feedback from the shaft assembly and provides a reading of the amount of force exerted. In addition to a measure of maximum voluntary effort, the Work Simulator is used to measure dynamic pushing and pulling strength. Standing, grip, isometric torquing, forearm supination and pronation, elbow flexion and extension, stabilization using the trunk, and stabilization using the lower extremities can be measured.

WEST Brief Tool Use Test[31]

Using the WEST 1 or WEST 2 frame, the patient installs a bolt, two washers, and a nut, beginning at waist height and continuing on a graduated basis to full extension overhead before returning to waist height and moving downward to floor level. Two installations are made at 10 to 14 levels, depending on the height of the worker. The worker uses a nut driver and wrench to complete the installation. Subsequently, the worker uses the nut driver and wrench to begin the removal process, which begins at waist level and continues upward to full extension overhead before returning to waist level and moving down to the floor or the lowest extent of the person's reach. The patient's performance is timed on a level-by-level basis. As the worker nears the end of his functional tolerance, a slowing of response will be noted. This test is used to establish the individual's ability to perform repetitive tool-handling tasks at various levels involving various ranges of motion and postural strategies.

WEST Standard Evaluation[32]

The WEST 2 is used to determine the worker's lifting and lowering tolerance. Standing, vertical and horizontal reaching with load, crouching, and kneeling or stooping with load are measured. This evaluation task can be graded to range from 5 pounds to 100 pounds. Prescreening is used prior to the graded evaluation of range of motion under load. The patient briefly lifts and lowers a graded series of weights that is resting at a height that allows him to lift and lower with the spine in an upright position. In this way, the worker's probable maximum load is determined prior to the graded evaluation of lifting and lowering through the full range of motion. The WSE was developed by the author and has been tested for safety on thousands of patients. When a significant symptomatic response occurs during the WSE, stop the evaluation and observe the patient when he is resting or performing a lighter activity. If symptoms resolve at this time, continue the evaluation. If symptoms do not resolve or become worse, discontinue testing and resume the following day, after symptoms have improved. If the cause of the significant symptomatic response has been determined, eliminate this factor from subsequent testing. The WSE is generally not appropriate for individuals whose lifting capacity is less than 10 pounds.

Specific Vocational Exploration

This process addresses the injured worker's aptitudinal resources, his vocational interests, and his work temperament. The goal of this process is to develop a model of the injured worker's employability resources and to compare this model to the job market so that several occupations can be identified that provide a "best fit" to the injured worker's assets.

The specific vocational exploration process begins with an evaluation of the individual's residual transferable skills based on work history, training, and education. Transferable skills are the skills that remain after the effects of the chronic disability have been considered. At E.R.I.C., the OASYS system is used to perform a computerized transferable skills analysis.

The next step in the specific vocational exploration process is to evaluate general educational development, including ability to reason and perform numeric tasks along with the individual's ability to read and understand spoken language. In addition, nine of the eleven aptitude factors found in the United States Department of Labor's system for classifying the aptitudinal demands of occupations are evaluated. The following tests are used.

Raven's Standard Progressive Matrices

This is a 60-item paper and pencil nonverbal test that measures reasoning ability. In each problem the worker is presented with a pattern or figure design that has a part missing. The worker's task is to select one of six possible parts to complete the pattern.

Wechsler Revised Adult Intelligence Scale[33]

This is the predominant test of general intelligence in use in the United States today. This individually administered test is composed of eleven subtests, divided into two major divisions, verbal and performance. The WAIS-R was developed in 1981, with a standardization sample based on the 1970 census consisting of subjects grouped by socioeconomic status, sex, and occupation in proportions similar to those found in the United States population as a whole. Norms are presented over nine age groups, from 16 years through 74 years.

The Wechsler Memory Scale[34]

This is a brief seven subtest scale that assesses gross memory function. In one brief study at Rancho Los Amigos Hospital, the author used the Wechsler Memory Scale to identify memory difficulties in 23% of the patients referred for work capacity evaluation. This is noteworthy because none of the patients presented with history of head injury or brain damage. In subsequent contact, the evaluator uncovered histories of forgotten (often childhood) head injury or unreported substance abuse (usually alcohol) that may have contributed to impaired memory function.

Gates-MacGinitie Reading Tests[35]

This is a multiple item paper and pencil test that measures reading achievement in the areas of speed, vocabulary, and reading comprehension. Six different levels of test difficulty allow appropriate evaluation of individuals in grades one through twelve.

Adult Basic Learning Examination[36]

A multiple item paper and pencil measure of vocabulary, reading comprehension, spelling, arithmetic computation, and arithmetic problem solving.

Employee Aptitude Survey Test 2[37]

This is a 75 item paper and pencil multiple choice test arranged in three parts (integers, decimals and percentages, and fractions) of 25 items each. This test measures basic arithmetic skill.

Personnel Test for Industry—Numerical[38]

A multiple item paper and pencil test of mathematical competence, this test evaluates the ability to solve "word problems" that are common in the industrial environment.

16 *Personality Factors Questionnaire*[39]

This is a paper and pencil test of 105 to 187 items depending upon which of the five forms is used. This test measures 16 primary personality traits. Properly interpreted, the 16 PF can predict such items as probable length of employee tenure, tolerance for routine, and work efficiency. Occupational profile data based on 11,000 cases are available.

Career Assessment Inventory[40]

A 300 item paper and pencil test that measures Holland's six general occupational types, 22 basic occupational interest scales, and 91 specific occupational scales.

Self-Directed Search[41]

A multiple item paper and pencil self-guided assessment of Holland's six general occupational types. It also provides a look at the patients perception of employability resources.

Data collected in the specific vocational exploration process are used to present a profile of the worker that is matched against profiles of occupations maintained in a computerized database. As of this writing, more than 90 occupational matching systems are available in the United States. The author has investigated most of these and has purchased and uses the following on a regular basis.

OASYS Job Match Analysis—A highly sophisticated relational database and expert system resident on an MS DOS system that contains all of the occupational titles, descriptions, and statistical profiles for the U.S. Dictionary of Occupational Titles.[42]

TREATMENT: HOW DO WE REMEDY THE PROBLEMS WE IDENTIFY?

Integrated Work Hardening

In the mid 1970s work hardening as a treatment concept was developed at Rancho Los Amigos Hospital in Downey, California. This concept involves the use of graded work simulation as physical and emotional conditioning tasks in which the patient would be involved to achieve rehabilitation. In 1988, the Commission on Accreditation of Rehabilitation Facilities convened a committee of experts to develop guidelines for accreditation of work hardening programs. This committee defined work hardening as:

> Work hardening programs, which are interdisciplinary in nature, use conditioning tasks that are graded to progressively improve the biomechanical, neuromuscular, cardiovascular/metabolic and psychosocial functions of the individual in conjunction with real or simulated work activities. Work hardening provides a transition between acute care and return to work while addressing the issues of productivity, safety, physical tolerances, and worker behaviors. Work hardening is a highly structured, goal oriented, individualized treatment program designed to maximize the individual's ability to return to work.

This definition and its attendant standards are now used throughout the United States for accreditation of rehabilitation facilities that offer work hardening as a treatment program. The prevalence of chronic disability because of painful spinal disorders is such that these individuals constitute the model disability group found in work hardening programs.

In recent years, the concept of "integrated work hardening" has been put forth[43] as an important extension of the work hardening concept. In this approach, individuals receive testing and counseling to explore vocational options in the course of a work hardening program that provides the physical and emotional fitness necessary to return to work. As a consequence of this approach, the individual completes the work hardening program and is prepared to go into a specific occupation or is prepared to participate in training for a specific occupation.

Treatment Context

The development of a sense of competence, behaviorally defined in terms of vocational feasibility, provides the context within which integrated work hardening is conducted. Vocational feasibility focuses on the worker trait behaviors exhibited by the individual with a painful spinal disorder. Issues of productivity, safety, and interpersonal relations are addressed in the integrated work hardening program through the program's structure and activities.

Temporal Demands of Work

The development of a sense of competence in integrated work hardening is based on mastery of the work environment. Integrated work hardening involves the patient in a rehabilitation program 5 days per week and usually requires 4 to 6 weeks to complete. Early in the program, the patient attends from 9:00 A.M. until 12:00 noon each day. As the program progresses, this expands to 9:00 A.M. to 3:00 P.M., usually within 5 days. Near the end of the program, the patient attends at 8:00 A.M. and remains involved in work activities until 4:30 P.M.* The usual coffee and lunch breaks are taken. The rationale for less than a full day of involvement up to the last several days of the program is that the work hardening benefits can be adequately attained with less expense on a partial day program. Additionally, if the individual is being adequately challenged, he will generally be unable to work a full day. From the patient's perspective, this progression is seen to be an important challenge. "I really felt like I was accomplishing something when I finally got up to a full day" is frequently heard near the end of the work hardening program. Another report that is often made by patients as they ready themselves to exit from the work hardening program is, "If I'm working this hard for a full day, I might as well get paid."

Environmental Demands of Work

The physical environment within which integrated work hardening is conducted is of paramount importance.[44] As an example, the E.R.I.C. Center in Anaheim presents two milieux, one that simulates an industrial setting and one that simulates an office setting. The industrial setting includes concrete floors, minimal temperature control, and substantial ambient noise. The office setting exposes the patient to professional level office equipment including computer keyboards and video display terminals used at work desks, much like the desk one would find at a typical place of employment.

Procedural Demands of Work

In addition to simulating the physical and temporal structure of a work environment, the procedural structure of the program must simulate the work environment. The patient's day begins by selecting his time card from the time card rack, "punching in" on the time clock, and reviewing his clipboard on which his individual daily schedule is laid out in quarter-hour increments. The following behavioral demands must be met:

1. Safety. Follow rules and instructions. Do not exceed work restrictions. Use proper body mechanics.
2. Interpersonal behavior. Accept supervisors' directions. Get along with fellow workers.
3. Attendance. Daily, Monday through Friday.
4. Workplace tolerance. Start each morning on time.

Take only scheduled breaks and return on time. Remain in the workplace for a full work day.
5. Productivity. Work at the maximum pace that will allow next day attendance, completion of the scheduled workday, and sustained activity without an unscheduled break from work.

These demands are consistent with the expectations of employers in the competitive labor market. Prioritization of factors is central to the evaluation process.

Program Staffing

The work hardening program's professional staff consists of a core team including a physical therapist, occupational therapist, psychologist, and vocational specialist, each professionally certified. Although these professionals do not have to be full-time staff, each must be readily available to the integrated work hardening program. The core team designs and manages each patient's program. The professional staff is assisted by technicians, usually not more than a one staff professional to four technicians. Technicians are responsible for the direct supervision of the patients, usually one technician to five patients.

Equipment

Equipment used in work hardening programs includes work simulation tasks and apparatus that are used for physical conditioning. Programs that do not offer both work simulation tasks and physical conditioning equipment will not be able to provide an adequate range of services. The basic criteria of all such equipment is that they are safe, reliable, valid, practical, and useful. In terms of safety, the equipment must have a demand that is able to be measured and controlled by the professional and must be gradable in terms of duration, frequency, and load. That is, the task must be able to be increased along these gradients as the patient demonstrates the ability to handle increased load. In terms of reliability, the equipment used in work hardening must have a demand that can be replicated, performance that can be measured, and a reasonable expectation that the patient's performance can be replicated. In terms of validity, the equipment must sample critical content of the target job's demands or the demands of a job cluster. The better the sampling of such critical job demands, the higher the validity. In terms of practicality, this equipment must have a daily cost (capital and staff) that is less than or equal to 15% of the daily service fee and a daily cost of dedicated floor space that is less than or equal to 10% of the daily

---

*Service fees are graded accordingly.

service fee. For those tasks which have consumables, the daily cost of equipment *and* supplies must be less than or equal to 15% of the daily service fee. In terms of the usefulness or utility of the equipment, it must be able to bring about improvement in the target domain at whatever stage of the rehabilitation process the patient is performing.

Integrated Work Hardening Process

The integrated work hardening process begins with application of the work tolerance screening battery and the specific vocational exploration battery. After baseline information is collected, the work hardening program begins to assist the individual with a painful spinal disorder to increase functional capacity and productivity. As this process unfolds, information from the specific vocational exploration battery is used to begin to identify occupational options toward which the patient begins to orient. The integrated work hardening process can be thought of as having three stages.

STAGE 1: EVALUATION

At this stage the work tolerance screening and specific vocational exploration batteries are administered. Information about baseline functional tolerances as well as aptitudes, interests, and goals are collected. This usually requires 3 to 5 days of active involvement.

STAGE 2: CAREER DEVELOPMENT

The information from the specific vocational exploration process is combined with the functional model developed in work tolerance screening to begin to identify occupations towards which the patient is to become oriented. Because the functional limitations to a large degree determine the range of options available, this process continues up to the point at which a clear picture about the probable work capacity level is reached. Once this is achieved, the individual is encouraged to identify a specific vocational goal, which becomes the basis of the next stage in the integrated work hardening process.

STAGE 3: CONSOLIDATION

Once a particular vocational goal has been identified, the individual begins to participate in work simulation tasks and formal conditioning tasks that are designed to achieve a level of function that assures competence on the job and provides a reasonable margin of safety and confidence that a reinjury

can be avoided. A specially constructed work simulation can be developed to focus on specific job task and worksite demands.

Structured Intake Interview

After appropriate screening for adequacy of medical evaluation (disease and impairment must be adequately evaluated before referral), the process begins with an intake interview conducted with the program manager or senior clinician, the patient, and usually the physician. If the physician is unavailable to participate in the intake interview, the program manager should represent the goals and expectations of the physician. The interview is a structured process that has been described elsewhere.[13] It provides an opportunity for the program manager to gather information about the patient's current status in terms of his functional limitations, use of medications, goals, expectations, and symptoms. Information from the interview is used to complete a formal written document that is often called an "Individualized Work Adjustment Plan" (IWAP). The IWAP lists the work hardening targets that will be addressed during the program, along with some of the intervention tasks. Although this document will be modified as further information about the patient is gathered, usually it is sufficient to initiate the program. The IWAP is maintained in a central card file, easily accessible to all team members. It also is used as a primary document for assuring that the integrated work hardening process is "on course" when reviewed at daily staffing rounds.

Work Simulation Project Tracks

Competence in work tasks is developed as the patient produces tangible output in work simulation project tracks that are meaningful. For example, woodworking is a project track in which many patients are involved at E.R.I.C. There are 12 projects in this track, beginning with a low skill project that requires from 60 to 120 minutes to complete without the use of power tools, up to intermediate skill projects that require the use of hand and power tools and take 12 to 15 hours to complete. Symptom control development that is used to develop functional capacity is practiced within the context of this work simulation project track. Because the work is meaningful and challenging, the cognitive demands of the task compete with the learned cognitive response to the symptoms in a way that causes the response to the symptoms to be modified to be less disabling. The key is to involve the patient in a task that is meaningful and graded so that the challenge is appropriate. Given an appropriate challenge, competence and improved self-confidence will be a natural consequence of mastery of the task.

Functional Capacity Development

Functional capacity development progresses in the three work function domains simultaneously. All domains, the biomechanical, psychophysical, and metabolic-cardiovascular, must be addressed in a coordinated fashion in the work hardening program so that the development of one of the domains does not limit the development of the others.

In the psychophysical domain, functional capacity development depends largely on the involvement of the individual with the painful spinal disorder in work simulation project tracks over several days. Project tracks are selected for the individual based on the appropriateness of the project in terms of the individual's goals and aspirations. To the degree that the project is meaningful, involvement will lead to an improved sense of self-confidence, competence, and ego development. During involvement with project tracks, symptom control strategies are used to assist the individual with a painful spinal disorder to learn that it is possible to "negotiate" with his symptoms and thereby improve psychophysical functional capacity. The sense of lost control over one's body and social and vocational activities that is experienced by individuals with painful spinal disorders can be somewhat attenuated through the appropriate utilization of symptom control strategies. More to the point, to the degree that the patient can integrate the strategies adaptively to learn to negotiate with his symptoms and maintain productivity, the secondary disabling effects of pain will be minimized. Strategies that are in use at E.R.I.C. include.

POSTURAL EDUCATION

Through the use of training aids, information about the proper use of the spine can be provided to individuals with painful spinal disorders. Application of this information is encouraged in subsequent work simulation tasks.

WORK PACING

As the individual is involved in work simulation tasks, the pace of activity is monitored and modulated. The patient learns that control of work pace is a fundamental means to control symptoms and maintain productivity. The balance between the need to maintain an acceptable work pace from the employer's standpoint and an acceptable work pace in terms of the symptom response that the patient experiences is a basic conflict that is best handled in the sheltered environment of a work hardening program.

POSTURAL CONTROL

Although proper postural alignment may not be possible at the work site, it is often necessary to begin the patient's involvement in work simulation tasks at a work station that is optimally designed in terms of postural demands. An elevated work surface that allows the patient to be involved in work tasks with minimized spinal flexion is often necessary. The use of a standing mat can assist the development of prolonged standing tolerance. If an appropriate work stool is made available at this work station, the patient may be able to continue work activity without a break by moving from a sitting to a standing position as needed.

BIOFEEDBACK

Symptom control can be assisted through the use of various mechanisms to provide feedback about proper musculoskeletal use. The application of duct tape to the patient's skin along the spine extending from the shoulders to the sacral area provides immediate feedback about changes in spinal flexion. The use of the Back Box Lift Angle Sensor,[45] a battery-powered signaling device that uses a mercury switch to sense gravity, can provide an immediate reminder about movement out of a vertical position. The Back Box can be adjusted so that various degrees of movement from vertical are acceptable. EMG biofeedback that is provided an on in vivo basis with a portable unit is also useful in assisting individuals with painful spinal disorders to appropriately negotiate with symptoms. Use of in vivo EMG biofeedback may need to be preceded by training with biofeedback in a controlled setting that promotes relaxation and the operant conditioning that subsequently will be utilized at the work station.

VIDEOTAPE RECORDING

Throughout the process, information is collected about the patient's performance through the use of passive videotape recording. In use by the author for more than 12 years and in use constantly at the E.R.I.C. clinic, this has proved to be an important and necessary component of the process. Videotape records of the individual's sitting and standing tolerances, involvement in various activities, use of proper body mechanics, and adherence to daily schedule are readily available through a review of the daily videotapes. Two videotape cameras survey approximately 80% of the floor space in the E.R.I.C. clinic and maintain an ongoing record of all of the day's activities. A library of 20 videotapes is maintained and recycled. That is, every 20th day, the same videotape is used so that the information previously recorded is no longer available. This, coupled with the assurance provided to the patient that videotape records are used only for evaluation and treatment purposes, has allowed this practice to continue without any serious challenge. The few people who have objected to the use of passive videotape recording have been excluded from the program. Given the straightforward nature with which this is presented (the equipment is readily observable throughout the clinic), less than one in 500 individuals have raised a serious objection.

In the biomechanical domain, integrated work hardening focuses on the musculoskeletal system's ability to perform tasks requiring strength and flexibility. In addition to involvement in work simulation project tracks, development of functional capacity is formally addressed each day in conditioning tasks. In the E.R.I.C. program, a combination of constant isotonic resistance on the B.T.E. Work Simulator, accommodating resistance on the Tru-Trac Floor Platform and Wall Unit,[46] and dynamic lifting with the WEST Lifting Frame are used to develop biomechanical musculoskeletal strength and flexibility. Validation of gains achieved, as well as interpretation of the utility of these gains, is obtained through serial testing with selected components of the work tolerance screening battery.

In the metabolic and cardiovascular domain, development of functional capacity begins with aerobic conditioning using a bicycle ergometer or exercise treadmill. Exercise activities gradually progress to 30 minutes each day. In addition, depending on the physical demand level of the targeted job, the patient will be involved in work simulation project tracks and other formal conditioning activities with equivalent MET levels, following the five levels of strength demands developed by the U.S. Department of Labor.[47] This is supplemented with ratings of typical energy expenditure based on MET equivalencies of work metabolic rate over basal metabolic rate, defined as the rate of energy expenditure requiring an oxygen consumption of 3.5 ml/O_2/kg body weight/minute.[10,12] These are:

SEDENTARY WORK

This is defined as exerting up to 10 pounds of force occasionally or a negligible amount of force frequently or constantly to lift, carry, push, pull, or otherwise move objects, including the human body. Sedentary work involves sitting most of the time, but may involve walking or standing for brief periods of time. Jobs are sedentary if walking and standing are required only occasionally and all other sedentary criteria are met. Typical energy expenditure of 1.5 to 2.1 METS.

LIGHT WORK

This is defined as exerting up to 20 pounds of force occasionally, or up to 10 pounds of force frequently, or a negligible amount of force constantly to move objects. Physical demand requirements are in excess of those for sedentary work. Light work usually requires walking or standing to a significant degree. However, if the use of arm or leg controls requires exertion of forces greater than that for sedentary work and the worker sits most of the time, the job is rated for light work. Typical energy expenditure of 2.2 to 3.5 METS.

MEDIUM WORK

This is defined as exerting up to 50 pounds of force occasionally or up to 20 pounds of force frequently, or up to 10 pounds of force constantly to move objects. Typical energy expenditure of 3.5 to 6.4 METS.

HEAVY WORK

This is defined as exerting up to 100 pounds of force occasionally, or 50 pounds of force frequently, or up to 20 pounds of force constantly to move objects. Typical energy expenditure of 6.0 to 6.4 METS.

VERY HEAVY WORK

This is defined as exerting in excess of 100 pounds of force occasionally, or in excess of 50 pounds of force frequently, or in excess of 20 pounds of force constantly to move objects. Typical energy expenditure of 6.4 to 12.0 METS.

In this system, "occasionally," "frequently" and "constantly" describe activities or conditions that exist up to ⅓ of the time, from ⅓ to ⅔ of the time, and for ⅔ or more of the time, respectively. This is graphically displayed in Table 31–4.[12,48]

Results

Individuals are admitted to the Integrated Work Hardening Program at E.R.I.C. as a "last chance" in the rehabilitation process. Of those individuals who have already been found to be "qualified injured workers" and are determined by their physicians to be "permanent and stationary," the mean time from date of injury to date of referral has been 37 months.

Table 31–4
Physical Demand Characteristics of Work

Physical Demand Level	Occasional 0–33% of the Workday	Frequent 34–66% of the Workday	Constant 67–100% of the Workday	Typical Energy Required
Sedentary	10 lbs.	Negligible	Negligible	1.5–2.1 METS
Light	20 lbs.	10 lbs. and/or Walk/Stand/Push/Pull of Arm/Leg controls	Negligible and/or Push/Pull of Arm/Leg controls while seated	2.2–3.5 METS
Medium	50 lbs.	20 lbs.	10 lbs.	3.6–6.3 METS
Heavy	100 lbs.	50 lbs.	20 lbs.	6.4–7.5 METS
Very heavy	Over 100 lbs.	Over 50 lbs.	Over 20 lbs.	Over 7.5 METS

Although a growing number of referrals are received prior to the permanent and stationary finding while the physician remains actively involved, these individuals are involved in a process of "functional restoration"[38] rather than in integrated work hardening. Individuals who are no longer in active treatment and who have been found to be qualified injured workers are presumed to be unable to return to previous employment and require the vocational exploration components of integrated work hardening. The majority of these individuals are referred to the program by rehabilitation counselors with preauthorization provided by the workers' compensation insurance carrier or self-insured employer.

In a study conducted at the Employment and Rehabilitation Institute of California based on 312 referrals for work hardening service, approximately 15% of the people who were referred to the E.R.I.C. work hardening program were not accepted. Principle reasons for nonacceptance were the need for prework hardening services such as basic physical therapy, occupational therapy, or drug detoxification, and mismatch between the type of work simulations needed by the person referred and those available in the program. Approximately 68% of the people who entered the work hardening program were feasible for competitive employment at discharge. Additionally, most of those who completed all three stages of the program were able to be considered feasible for competitive employment. A statistic that is important to insurance claims personnel is that approximately 20% of the people who entered the program did not complete Stage One *and* subsequent withdrawals were more modest. That is, if one makes it through Stage One, it is highly likely that he will complete the program and become feasible for competitive employment. Of those people who began formal vocational rehabilitation programs after leaving the work hardening program, approximately 12% were closed prior to plan implementation for various reasons, including declination of further services. Of those who completed formal vocational rehabilitation, 82% returned to work.

REFERENCES

1. Rosenoff, J., Gibson, G.: OASYS Software Program. Belleview, WA, Vertek, Inc.
2. Chaffin, D.B., Herrin, G.D., Keyserling, W.M.: Preemployment strength testing. An updated position. J Occup Med 20(6):403–408, 1978.
3. Keyserling, W.M., Herrin, G.D., Chaffin, D.B.: Isometric strength testing as a means of controlling medical incidents on strenuous jobs. J Occup Med 22(5):332–336, 1980.
4. Harber, P., SooHoo, K.: Static ergonomic strength testing in evaluating occupational back pain. J Occup Med 26(12): 877–884, 1984.
5. Kishino, N.D., et al.: Quantification of lumbar function. Part 4: Isometric and isokinetic lifting simulation in normal subjects and low-back dysfunctional patients. Spine 10(10): 921–927, 1985.
6. Parnianpour, M., Nordin, M., Frankel, V.H., Kahanovitz, N.: The triaxial coupling of torque generation of trunk muscle during isometric exertions and the effect of fatiguing isoinertial movements on the motor output and movement patterns. Bull Back Res Spring:1, 1988.
7. Snook, S.H.: A study of three preventive approaches to low back injury. J Occup Med 20(7):478–481, 1978.
8. Ciriello, V.M., Snook, S.H.: A study of size, distance, height, and frequency effects on manual handling tasks. Hum Factors 25(5):473–483, 1983.
9. Snook, S.H.: Psychophysical considerations in permissible loads. Ergonomics 28(1):327–333, 1985.
10. Erb, B.D.: Applying work physiology to occupational medicine. Occup Health Saf June, 1981.
11. Genaidy, A.M., Asfour, S.S.: Review and evaluation of physiological cost prediction models for manual materials handling. Hum Factors 29(4):465–476, 1987.
12. Matheson, L.N.: Work capacity evaluation. Trabuco Canyon, CA, Rehabilitation Institute of Southern California, 1982.
13. Matheson, L.N.: Symptom magnification casebook. Anaheim, CA, Employment and Rehabilitation Institute of California, 1987.
14. Vander Vegt, D., Summit, W., Field, T.: Labor market access. Athens, GA, VDARE Service Bureau, 1981.
15. Matheson, L.N., Ogden, D.: Work tolerance screening. Trabuco Canyon, CA, Rehabilitation Institute of Southern California, p. 128, 1983.

16. The Committee to Develop Standards for Educational and Psychological Testing: Standards for educational and psychological testing. Washington, D.C., American Psychological Association, Inc., p. 100, 1985.
17. National Institute of Occupational Safety and Health: Work practices guide for manual lifting. Cincinnati, Ohio, U.S. Department of Human Services, Division of Biomedical and Behavioral Science, 1981.
18. Cornell Medical Index Health Questionnaire: New York, Cornell University Medical College, 1972.
19. WEST Tool Sort: Huntington Beach, CA, Work Evaluation Systems Technology, 1982.
20. Loma Linda University Medical Center Activities Sort: Huntington Beach, CA, Work Evaluation Systems Technology, 1987.
21. Spinal Function Sort: Rancho Santa Margarita, CA, PACT, 1989.
22. Matheson, L.N.: Maximum Voluntary Effort Software. Anaheim, CA, RMA & Associates, 1988.
23. Matheson, L.N., Carlton, R., Niemeyer, L.O.: Grip strength in a disabled sample: reliability and normative standards. Ind Rehabil Quart *1*(3):9, 17–23, 1988.
24. Niemeyer, L.O., Matheson, L.N., Carlton, R.S.: Testing consistency of effort. BTE Work Simulator. Ind Rehabil Quart *2*(1):5, 12, 1989.
25. Employee Aptitude Survey Test #9: San Diego, CA, Edits, 1970.
26. Crawford Small Parts Dexterity Test: Cleveland, The Psychological Corporation, 1961.
27. VALPAR 4: Tucson, AZ, Valpar International Corporation.
28. VALPAR 8: Tucson, AZ, Valpar International Corporation.
29. Minnesota Rate of Manipulation: Circle Pines, MN, American Guidance Service, Inc., 1969.
30. BTE Work Simulator: Hanover, MD, Baltimore Therapeutic Equipment (BTE), 1989.
31. WEST Brief Tool Use: Huntington Beach, CA, Work Evaluation Systems Technology, 1989.
32. WEST Standard Evaluation: Huntington Beach, CA, Work Evaluation Systems Technology, 1989.
33. Wechsler, D.: Wechsler Adult Intelligence Scale—Revised. Cleveland, The Psychological Corporation, 1972.
34. Wechsler, D.: The Wechsler Memory Scale. Cleveland, The Psychological Corporation, 1972.
35. Gates, A.I., MacGinitie, W.H.: Gates-MacGinitie Reading Tests. Iowa City, IA, The Riverside Publishing Company, 1964.
36. Karlsen, B., Madden, R., Gardener, E.F.: Adult Basic Learning Examination. Cleveland, The Psychological Corporation, 1967.
37. Employee Aptitude Survey Test #2: San Diego, CA, Edits, 1980.
38. Doppelt, J.E.: Personnel tests for industry-numerical test. Cleveland, The Psychological Corporation, 1969.
39. Sixteen Personality Factors Questionnaire: Champaign, IL, Institute for Personality and Ability Testing, Inc. (IPAT), 1979.
40. Johansson, C.B.: Career Assessment Inventory. Minneapolis, National Computer Systems, Inc., 1984.
41. Holland, J.L.: The Self-Directed Search. Odessa, FL, Psychological Assessment Resources, Inc., 1985.
42. Dictionary of Occupational Titles, 4th Ed., Supp. Washington, DC, U.S. Department of Labor, Division of Planning and Operations, Employment and Training Administration, 1986.
43. Matheson, L.N.: Integrated work hardening in vocational rehabilitation: an emerging model. Vocational Evaluation and Work Adjustment Bulletin, *Summer*:71–76, 1988.
44. Ellexson, M.: Environmental enhancements for work hardening. Ind Rehabil Quart *1*(1):14–15, 1988.
45. Creative Specialists. Cloquet, MN, 1988.
46. Tru-Trac Therapy Products, Inc. Temecula, CA, 1988.
47. Rules and Regulations. Equal Employment Opportunity Commission, Civil Service Commission, Department of Justice, Department of Labor. Federal Register Aug 25; *43*(166):38290–38307, 1978.
48. Matheson, L.N.: Industrial Rehabilitation Resource Book. Anaheim, CA, Employment and Rehabilitation Institute of California, 1989.
49. Mayer TG, et al.: A prospective two-year study of functional restoration in industrial low back injury. JAMA *258*(13):1763–1767, 1987.

32

Arthur H. White

Structural Diagnostic Testing

INTRODUCTION

Structural diagnostic testing is a means of answering the following question: Where is the pain coming from? Previous chapters in this book have described pain in relation to the psychologic processes that affect it. This chapter begins by assuming the existence of a structural peripheral pain generator that can be identified and corrected surgically. If any question exists in the surgeon's or diagnostician's mind that psychologic factors might obscure further diagnostic testing, those factors should be dealt with first. *Central* pain, which is pain resulting from psychologic causes, can be identified and distinguished from *peripheral* pain, that which results from structural causes, by means of the history and physical examination, psychologic interviews and psychologic testing, as well as through the use of more objective physical procedures, such as an indwelling epidural block or a Brevital evaluation.

Upon assuming a significant peripheral pain generator, a spinal diagnostician should first make a diagnosis from the history and physical examination. Mechanisms of injury and factors that aggravate or relieve spinal injury are likely to fit specific patterns that can be evaluated during the history and physical examination. For example, disc injuries, such as annulus tears that occur with flexion and loading, are aggravated by flexion and relieved by repeated extension. On the other hand, spinal stenosis is aggravated by lumbar extension and, usually, by walking. Thus, a diagnosis is likely to be 90% accurate from the history and physical examination alone.

Remaining diagnostic tests should be confirmatory. With a surgical failure rate of 10 to 30% for low back pain, frequently linked to inaccurate diagnosis, the diagnostician must use all the tools possible to confirm a preliminary diagnosis in a case that seems equivocal. Tests used to confirm a spinal diagnosis include imaging, electrodiagnostics, diagnostic blocks, and miscellaneous tests for specific disease processes such as infection, arthritis, neoplasm, and metabolic diseases. However, mechanical structural disease arising from the degenerative cascade may not produce significant changes in laboratory studies. Furthermore, diagnostic tests should not be used casually. They are expensive and some carry significant risks. The diagnostician should perform sufficient tests, however, to confirm a diagnosis with certainty before embarking on surgery, an even more expensive and dangerous an endeavor.

The following is a reasonable algorithm for diagnosis and treatment planning that accounts for economy, potential danger and discomfort to the patient, precise medical management, and reasonable time frames to avoid leading a patient into syndromes of psychologic disability: Any given incidence of back pain that is not spontaneously resolving within 6 days should be evaluated by a clinician knowledgeable about spinal problems. A history and physical examination should identify the underlying cause and recommend a treatment plan that brings resolution to the problem within 6 weeks. This scenario applys to 90% of the cases of back pain. The remaining percent of the occurrences of back pain that do not resolve in 6 weeks need further diagnostic measures to identify structural abnormalities for which surgical attention might be necessary. A few cases may be so severe that structural diagnostic measures may be required within a few days of the occurrence because of neurological loss or severe pain.

As the spinal column ages, more than one area (facet or disc) usually is abnormal. The structures involved, as well as the role of each structure in the disabling condition, should be identified. In a complex multidisciplinary setting, a Brevital evaluation, psychologic testing, and indwelling injection techniques may be used to determine the degree to which a given patient's condition is *central* and the degree to which the condition is *peripheral*. Each structure of the spine may then be evaluated using a variety of diagnostic tools. X rays or scans of the spinal elements may be taken, the neurological structures may be evaluated with electrodiagnostic testing, and identification of the pain generator may be undertaken by producing and relieving the pain consistently using diagnostic blocks or discograms. Thus, the diagnosis may be verified in at least five different ways: historically, through physical examination, through imaging, electrodiagnostic testing, or pain provocation.

Although a clinician may master all of these diagnostic procedures, it is most common to rely on subspecialists to perform some of these tests. All clinicians should be capable of handling a history and physical examination, and should be able to interpret x rays and scans. Although radiologists most often interpret x rays and scans, these tests should also be read by a clinician who can integrate the patient's clinical information with the visual information.

It is difficult for clinicians to remain up to date about the most current findings and issues in allied disciplines. However, clinicians should read extensively, go to spinal conferences, and visit medical and research centers. It is important to maintain good connections with subspecialists in the community in order to exchange information about the availability and efficacy of diagnostic tools.

THE PLAIN X RAY

With the recent increase in the use of computerized tomography (CT scans) and magnetic resonance imaging (MRI) for diagnosis, plain x rays have become less important. Two decades ago, plain x rays were virtually all that was available and every patient with significant back pain received at least anterior, posterior and lateral views, and frequently oblique views of his back. With a more sophisticated understanding of spinal biomechanics, flexion, extension, and lateral bending views were occasionally

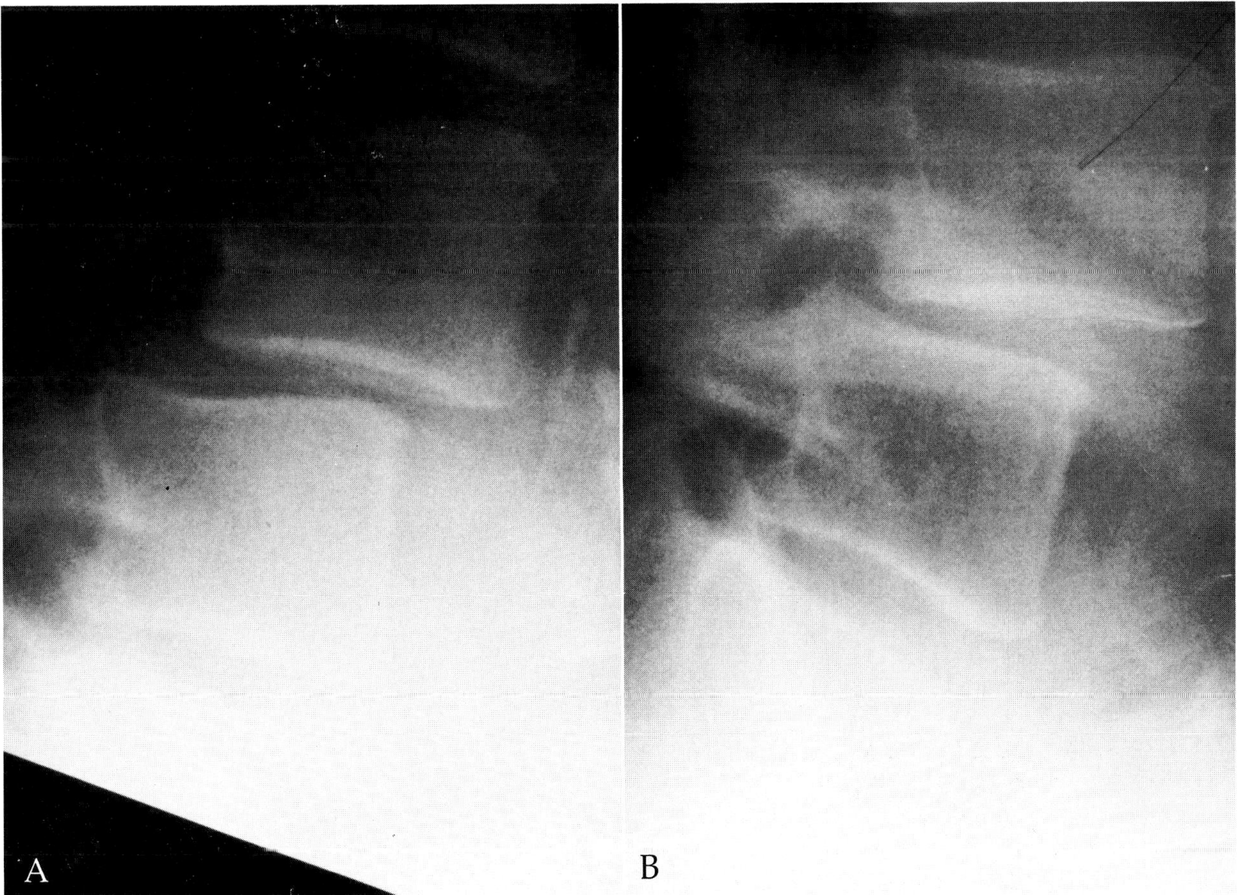

Figure 32–1. Flexion **(A)** and extension **(B)** views. These views demonstrate decreased disc height, rocking at L4-L5 level, along with an anterolysthesis.

used to track the motion of the various spinal segments (Fig. 32–1).[1] Apart from these applications, plain x rays have been used primarily to screen for tumor, fracture, arthritis, and infection (Fig. 32–2). X rays are not precise. Up to 40% of bone structure must be lost before plain x rays reveal spinal abnormality. When there is a strong clinical suspicion of abnormality, a CT scan is a much more accurate method of defining it. However, for situations such as scoliosis plain films are valuable for visualizing the overall configuration of the bony spinal column. Many other imaged abnormalities may correlate with the clinical picture, such as multilevel degenerative changes, spondylolysis, tropism, and unilateral sacralization. However, none have been proven significant. (Fig. 32–3).[2]

In summary, the value of plain x rays for the clinician in the diagnosis of low back pain is minimal. Aside from tumor, infection, and fracture, x-rays taken by the clinician early in an evaluation of a low back pain patient may not disclose abnormalities that have a significant correlation to the underlying clinical picture. For this reason, in our practice, we establish a working diagnosis based on the history and physical examination alone and begin a trial of treatment. If a patient does not respond rapidly and appropriately, we select an imaging procedure we feel is most likely to give us a maximum amount of information about the specific case and the current working diagnosis. For example, in a 30-year-old patient given a working diagnosis of a herniated disc, we ask for an MRI because it is the best procedure to visualize a herniated disc and the neurological structures at its interface. In an older individual, given a working diagnosis of spinal stenosis, we request a CT scan because it is a more appropriate imaging technique for demonstrating the bony configuration of the central canal lateral recesses and intervertebral foramen.

THE BONE SCAN

Before the advent of MRI and CT scans, the bone scan was the only test that could show bone destruction before it could be captured by plain x rays. The bone scan still remains a valuable tool for screening the entire bony skeleton for osteoblastic activity, a condition produced mainly by tumor, infection, and trauma. However, the CT scan and MR image cannot evaluate an entire skeleton. Furthermore, it may be arthritis that causes the low grade osteoblastic activity. When infection is strongly suspected, a gallium scan is suggested.

When good CT and MR imaging is not available, the clinician must be more astute. After initial history, physical examination, and plain x rays, if a clinician is uncertain of the diagnosis and preliminary treatment has not been successful, a bone scan is appropriate. With mediocre or inferior MR imaging and CT scans, a clinician must be extremely careful of false negatives. Small herniated discs and bone spurs may be missed because scanning is done only of the disc spaces and the scan slices are 5 mm or more apart.

Because of its cost, a clinician is well advised to postpone CT scans or MR imaging until later in the diagnostic evaluation. Only severe anomalies are likely to be disclosed by a mediocre scan, so the clinician should attempt to make the diagnosis without it. A better decision might be to send the patient some distance away for an excellent scan rather than waste money on an easily available mediocre scan that yields little significant information.

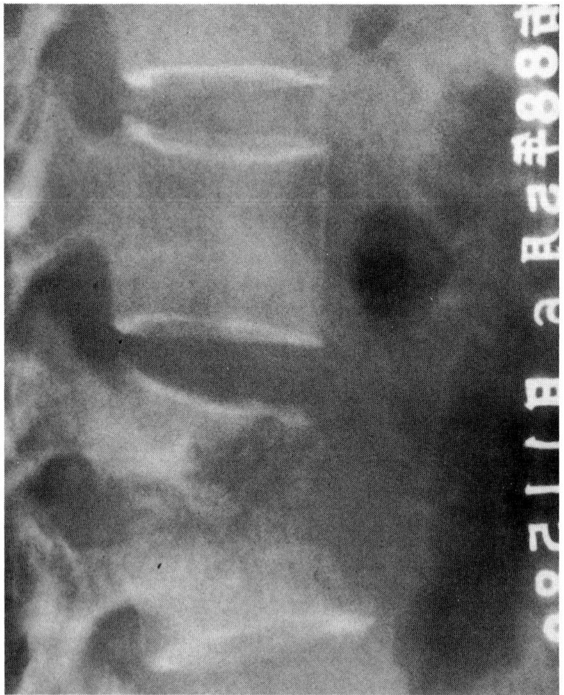

Figure 32–2. Plain radiograph. This image demonstrates tuberculous spondylitis with destruction of disc and adjacent vertebrae.

MYELOGRAPHY

The myelogram has been the standard of care in diagnosis for spinal disorders for many decades (Fig. 32–4). In some communities, it is still the standard.

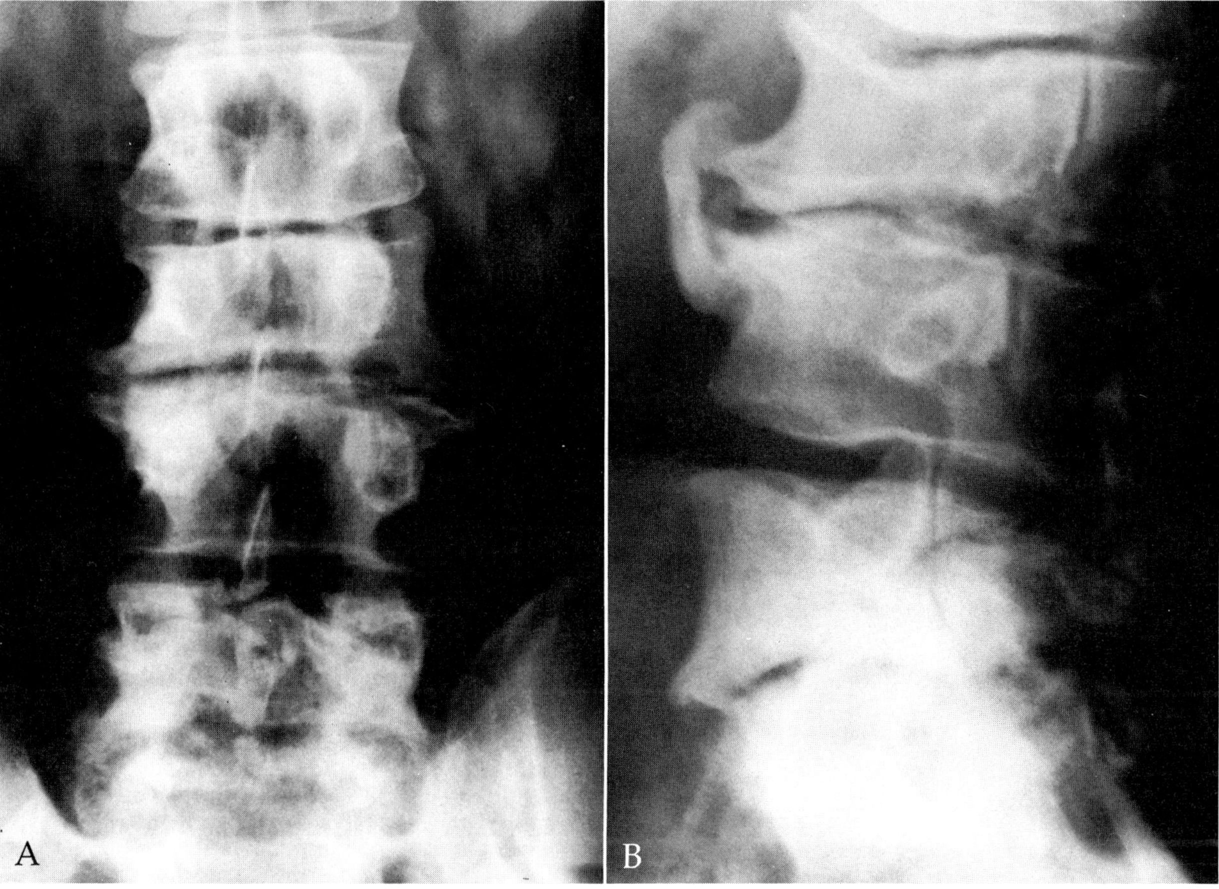

Figure 32–3. Plain radiographs. These films demonstrate severe multilevel degenerative changes in an asymptomatic world class athlete.

When good MRI and CT scans are available, myelograms are seldom used unless tumor, arachnoiditis, or pseudomeningocele are suspected. In other areas, if scanning is good but not excellent, the CT myelogram frequently is still used (Fig. 32–5). With the newly available water soluble myelographic contrast material, the problems of arachnoiditis are virtually nil. Furthermore, allergic and chemical reactions to the contrast are rare with low dose myelographic CT scans, and smaller needles result in infrequent spinal headaches. Myelograms do not depict foraminal spinal stenosis. This has been one of the major problems in spinal diagnosis and treatment over the last half century. Patients have been proclaimed normal because their myelogram was normal when, in fact, they have significant spinal stenosis. Patients have been operated on for herniated discs on the basis of myelography without the secondary spinal stenosis being appreciated. Because both herniated discs and spinal stenosis can be depicted better on CT and MRI scans, the myelogram is becoming unneces-

sary. Furthermore, intrathecal needles and foreign substances do have their complications and should not be used unnecessarily.

SCANS

The least invasive, least painful, and most informative tests are the scanning procedures. If a clinician does not have a wide variety of scanning techniques available, he should probably use the technique with the highest quality. Assuming that the clinician does have scanning modalities of equal caliber, some guidelines should be followed for choosing an MRI scan over a CT scan. No radiation is associated with an MR image, and it does define soft tissues such as discs and nerves, which may be the source of significant pain in younger patients. A CT scan defines bone better than an MRI and may be more valuable in evaluating older patients with spinal stenosis. Scans, in general, depict more ab-

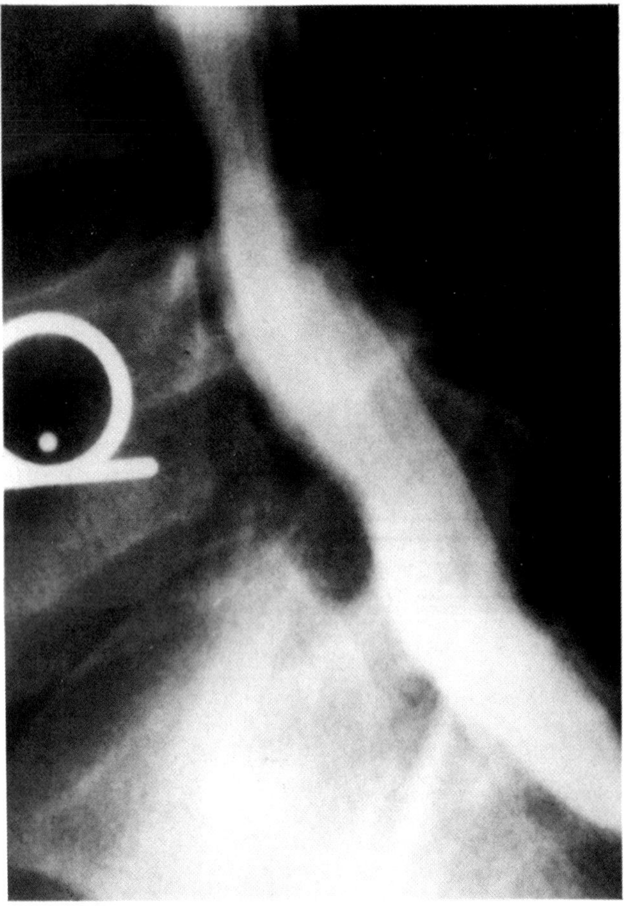

Figure 32–4. Myelogram—lateral film. Anterior extradural defect at the L5-S1 level at surgery was proven to be a disc extrusion.

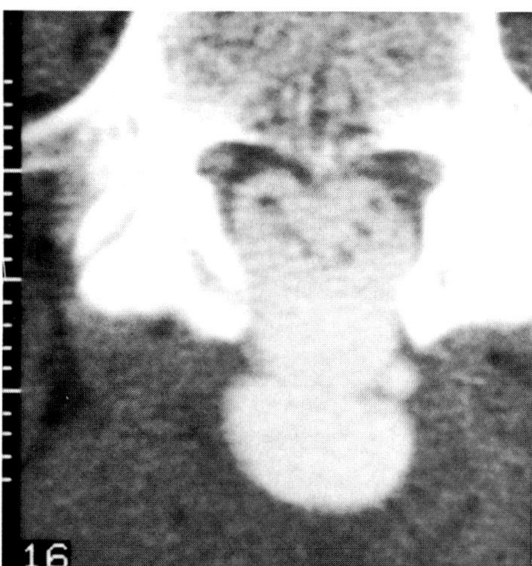

Figure 32–5. CT myelogram—axial view. Postoperative pseudomeningocele extending posteriorly through the laminar defect.

normalities than are actually symptomatic. Therefore, it is imperative that clinicians closely correlate their working diagnoses and their patients' signs and symptoms with the findings and suggested diagnoses of the scan procedures.

Two problems are encountered when describing the clinical usefulness of CT and MRI scans: assessing their range of availability and keeping abreast of the rapid changes imaging technology is undergoing. At best, a clinician will have available to him excellent MRI and CT scanning. Excellent CT means that the equipment should offer multiplanar reformatting (Fig. 32–6). Technically, one should be able to scan at increments as small as 1.5 mm. One should be able to screen the entire area in question, and it should be possible to rescan suspicious areas more precisely if necessary. Both soft tissue and bone windows should be provided for imaging appropriate detail in the tissue under review. MR imaging at its best is even more complex than CT scan-

ning (Fig. 32–7). There are more technical kinds of imaging available depending on what tissue is being viewed. Classically, there are T1 and T2 weighted images that allow interpretations of the degree of hydration of intervertebral discs (Fig. 32–8). There are innumerable other options, however, that the well trained radiologist can choose from to observe infections, tumors, and hematomas.

MR images can be valuable when compared to CT scans. An MRI scan can evaluate the entire lumbar spine in a single scanning session, whereas CT scans evaluate only three or four segments at a time. Furthermore, MR images do not produce radiation that might affect the patient, whereas CT scans produce considerable radiation, although it is confined to the area being scanned.

MR images display soft tissues better than CT scans and provide information about the degree of hydration and degeneration of the intervertebral disc. CT scans present bone more precisely and are better for defining spinal stenosis (Figs. 32–9 and 32–10) and small calcifications and bone spurs that might be missed on MR images.

Both CT and MRI scans can be faulted in one respect, namely that they present too many structural abnormalities. Most patients, especially the elderly, may have many abnormalities, but most of those abnormalities are not painful or clinically significant at the time of the evaluation. The clinician may be thrown off the diagnostic track by the scans he reviews that present all the abnormalities in detail. Therefore, MRI and CT scans should not be used as the primary or sole diagnostic procedure.[2] If unsuspected abnormalities are disclosed, they should be critically evaluated to see if they fit the current clinical picture and the clinician's working diagnosis. Additional diagnostic tests should be conducted to confirm or exclude any abnormalities so presented.

Once good images are obtained, a clinician has either confirmed his working diagnosis or identified abnormalities that might explain why the patient has not improved adequately. A new direction in the treatment of the patient may now be taken. If addi-

tional, more precisely directed, conservative care helps the patient return to normal within a reasonable period of time, no further diagnostic testing is indicated. If, however, there is no improvement or if surgery is anticipated, further diagnostic tests must be performed to confirm or more clearly define the patient's spinal abnormalities.

Looking to the future, MRI scans may become so effective that they may be able to define stenosis as well as CT scans do. If so, an MR image will be the

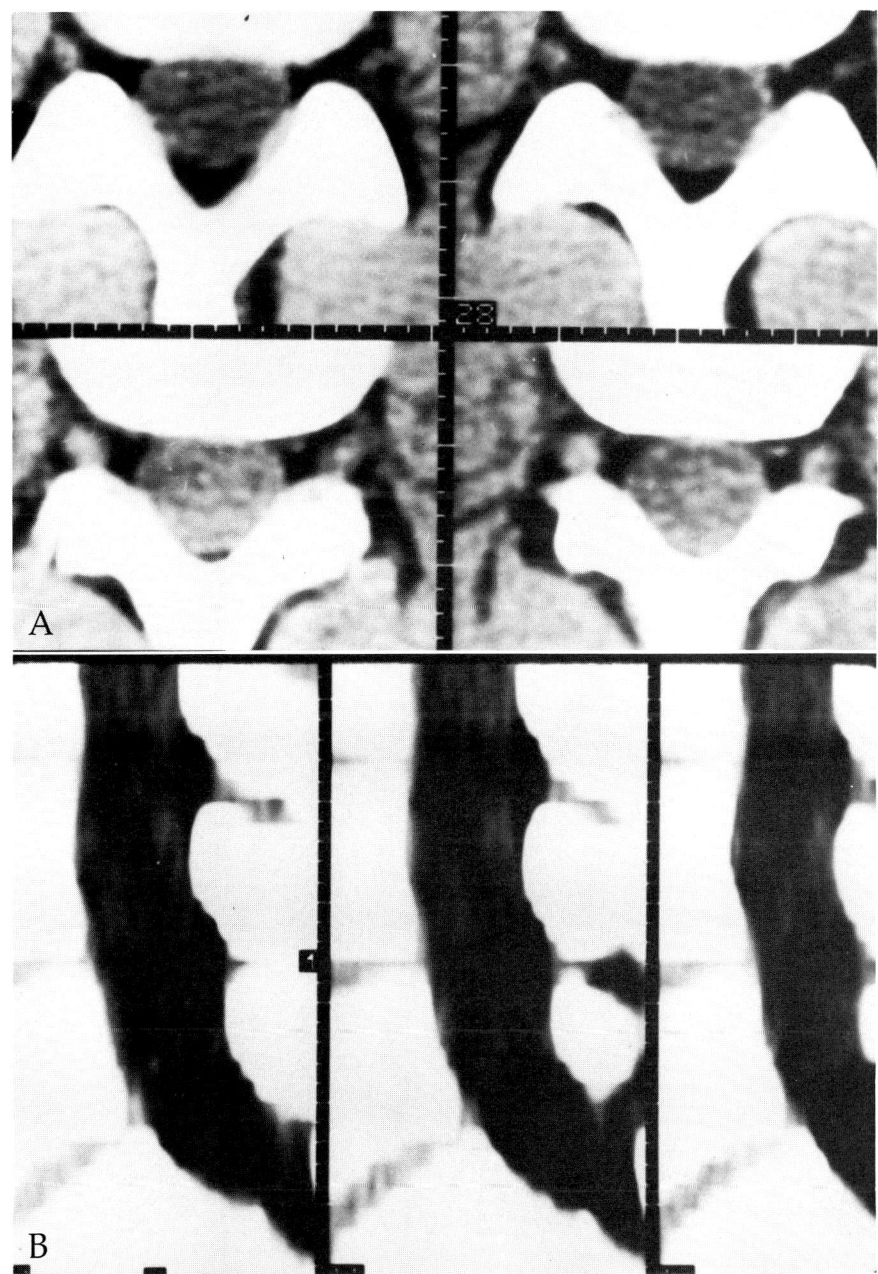

Figure 32–6. High resolution multiplanar CT—axial and saggital images. These images were photographed to optionally evaluate soft tissue **(A,B)** and osseous **(C,D)** structures.

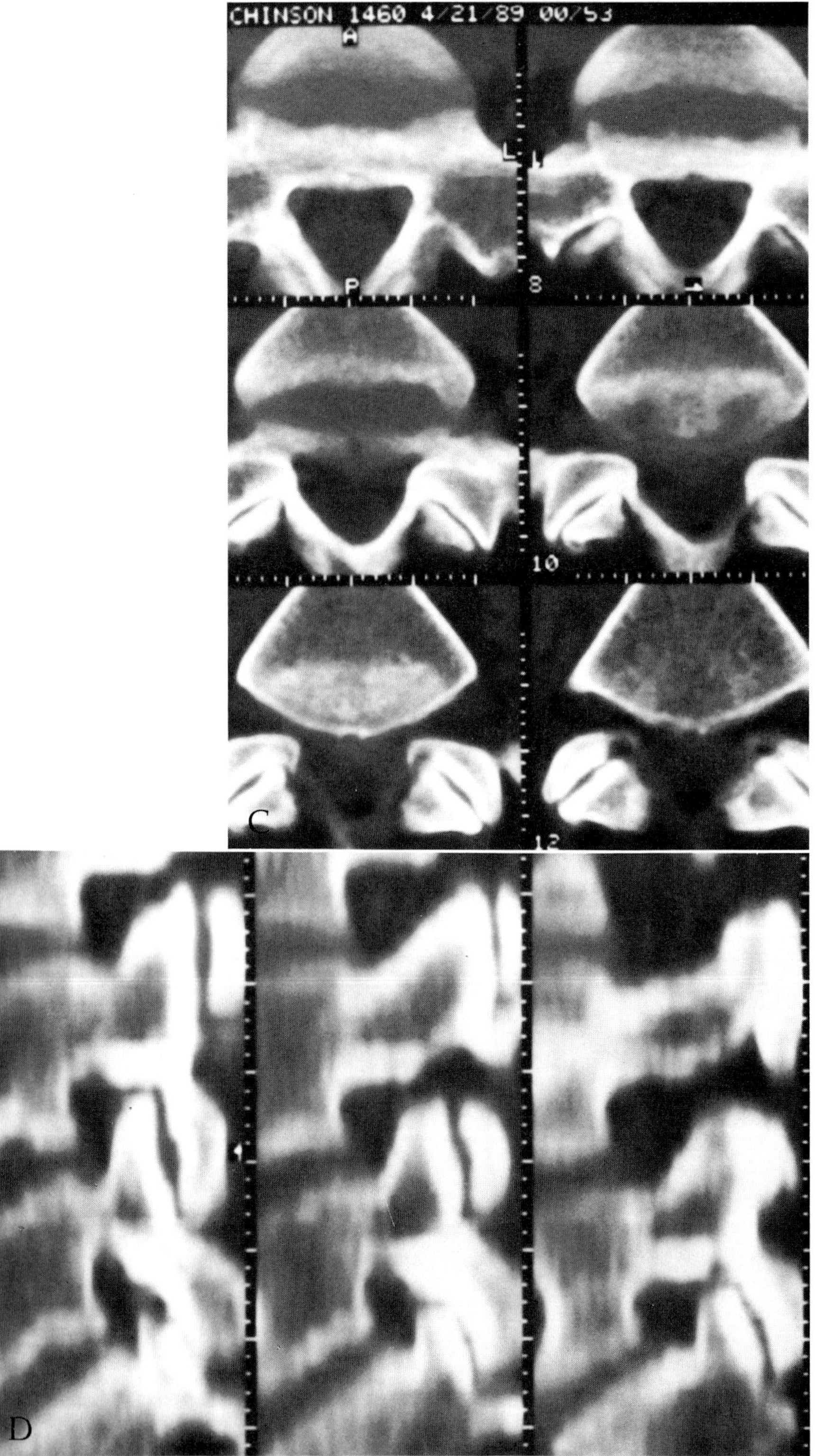

Figure 32–6 *(continued).*

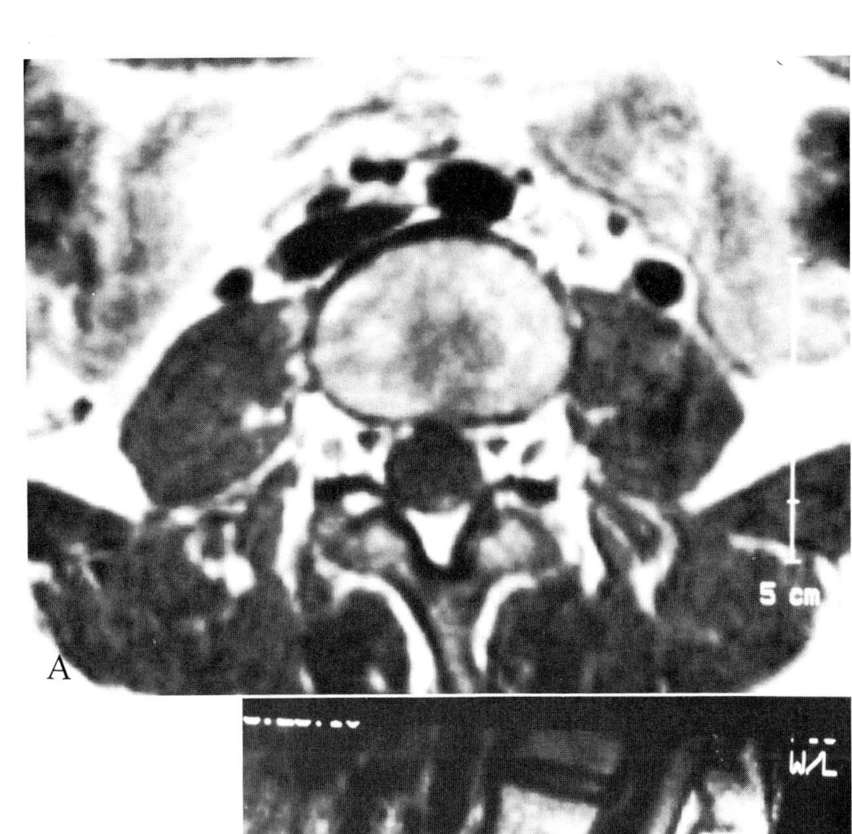

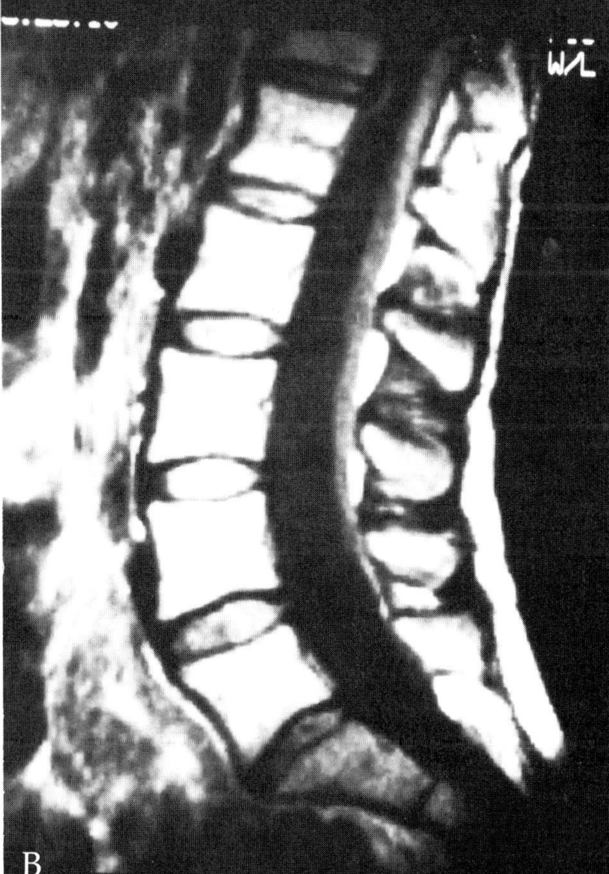

Figure 32–7. Standard MRI evaluation: selected images. **A.** Axial sequence (T1 weighted). Level of the intervertebral nerve root canals—normal anatomy. **B.** Saggital sequence (T1 weighted). Midline image demonstrating normal vertebrae, discs, thecal sac, and conus medullaris.

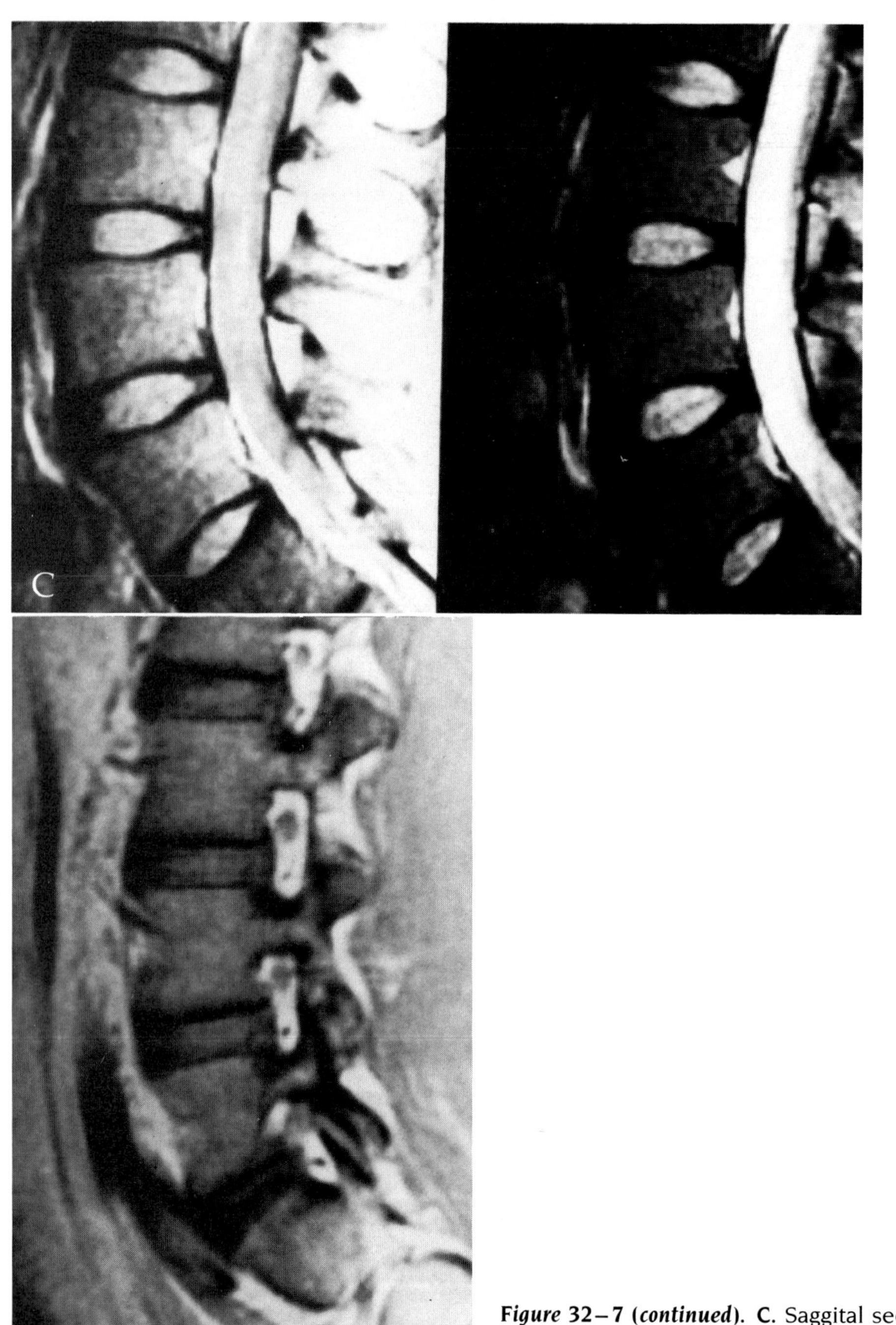

Figure 32–7 (continued). **C.** Saggital sequence—proton density (I) T2 weighted (II). CSF myelographic effect and normal disc hydration. **D.** Saggital sequence (proton density) parasaggital image. Normal vertebral and intervertebral canal anatomy.

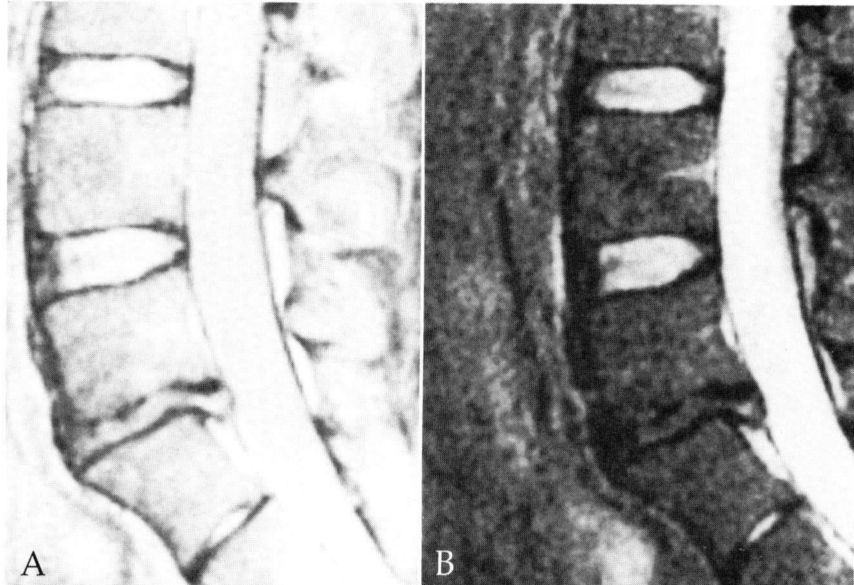

Figure 32–8. Saggital MR images. Proton density **(A)** amd T2 weighted **(B)** midline images demonstrating disc herniation at the L5-S1 level and associated disc dessication. Normal disc morphology and hydration is identified at the L3-L4 and L4-L5 levels.

only tool needed until the next, enhanced diagnostic modality is developed.

SUMMARY: WHAT A CLINICIAN SHOULD KNOW ABOUT RADIOLOGIC IMAGING

1. Order imaging to confirm a diagnosis, not to make one.
2. Plain x rays have little value in diagnosing most kinds of structural problems related to low back pain.
3. Gadolinium enhanced MRI is an excellent technique for differentiating scar tissue from recurrent herniated discs in a case of failed spine surgery syndrome.
4. CT discograms can also be good for differentiating scar tissue from recurrent herniated discs. In addition, with discography, it is possible to evaluate the patient's pain response upon injection.
5. Scans do not indicate where the pain is coming from.
6. An MRI may be negative, yet a discogram and discoCT scan of the same problem may be significantly abnormal.
7. When a clinical picture is not explained by scanning, i.e., when the working diagnosis is not confirmed by scanning, it is not necessary to immediately change or exclude the working diagnosis. Other types of scanning and diagnostic testing may confirm the working diagnosis. MR images miss early internal disc disruption, early facet degeneration, spondylolysis, and small bone spurs. CT scans miss desiccated discs, instability, arachnoiditis, and soft tissue lesions.

ELECTRODIAGNOSTICS

Electrodiagnostic testing is one of the most specialized areas a physiatrist or neurologist is asked to handle. Because physiatrists and neurologists are highly qualified clinicians, it is important to use them as such and not view them merely as technicians. Not only are physiatrists technically proficient at electrodiagnostic testing, but they also have specialized knowledge about rehabilitation, one of the most valuable tools in the treatment of sports medicine and spinal surgery patients.

If neurological involvement is suspected, electromyography (EMG) or SSEP will give electrophysiologic evidence without invasive danger. Electrodiagnostic testing may provide valuable physiologic information when surgery is being considered. The information obtained from EMG and SSEP studies should be correlated with the gross structural data obtained from MRI or CT scans and other radiological studies.

The electrophysiologic information is valuable in characterizing the type and chronicity of a lesion to spinal nerves. Not all structural lesions visualized cause nerve damage. In a patient with multiple structural lesions, electrodiagnostic data can be useful in localizing the injured spinal nerve.

Electromyography (EMG) can also discriminate between neurologically acute or chronic lesions. As the electrophysiologic findings become more subtle, suggesting a more chronic process, it is more difficult to use EMG data in clinical decision making. When electrodiagnostics are significantly positive, they weigh heavily in diagnostic decision making and in disability rating.[2] A negative EMG can be sig-

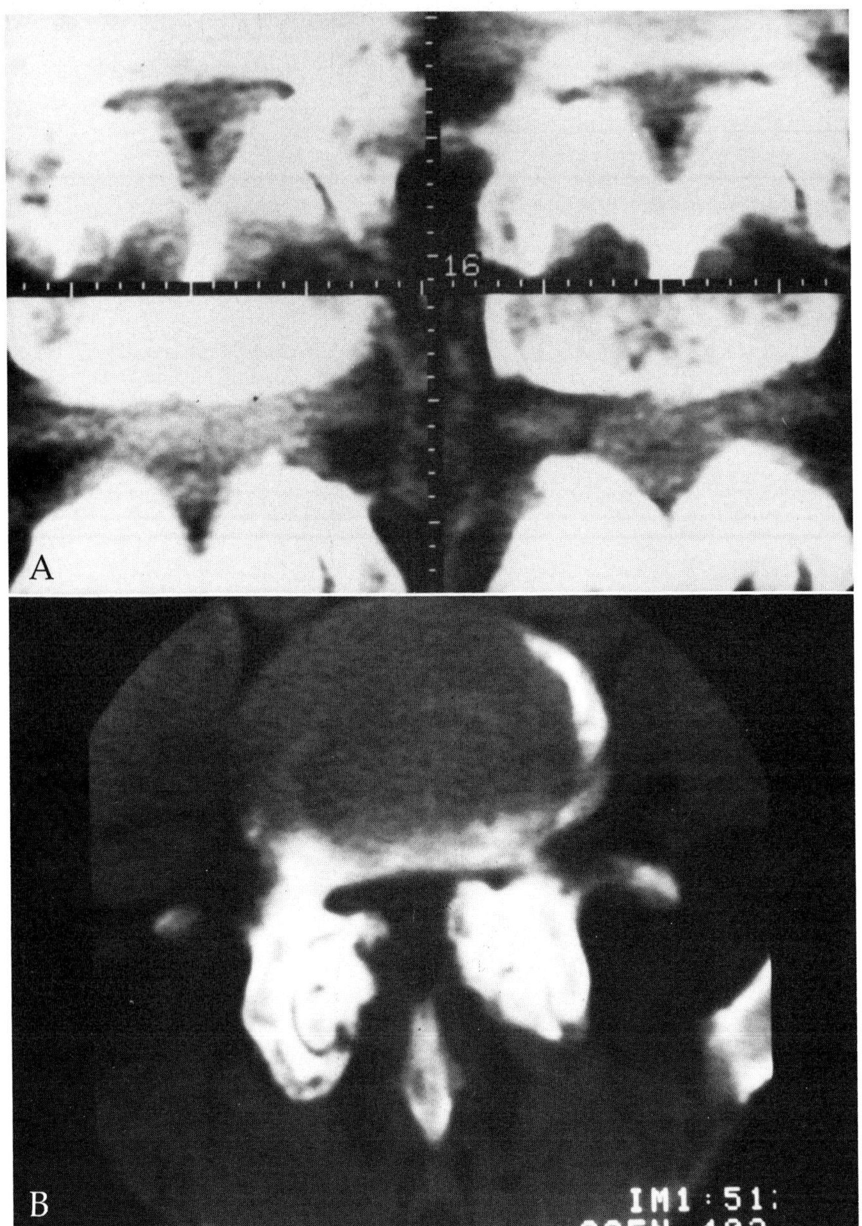

Figure 32–9. Axial CT images. The importance of high resolution soft tissue **(A)** and bone **(B)** images to demonstrate the exact cause of severe central canal stenosis.

nificant when the clinician is faced with a patient who seems to have major weaknesses or neurological involvement. A negative EMG in such a case indicates that the patient's major neurological involvement is either very old, very new (within two weeks), or psychologically provoked (hysteria, malingering).

Clinicians usually refer patients for electrodiagnostic testing and the clinician should have excellent communication with the individual who performs the testing. A short report is not acceptable for a clinician who needs the details about the chronicity, severity, and clinical implications of the patient's ab-

normalities. Clinicians handling electrodiagnostic testing themselves should answer whatever questions they may have about a patient. However, when clinicians refer the study to a subspecialist who does not follow through with complete communication of the results, they lose much of the clinical value of the diagnostic test.

PSYCHOLOGIC TESTING

There has been a barrage of psychologic tests for pain patients over the past few years. The MMPI has

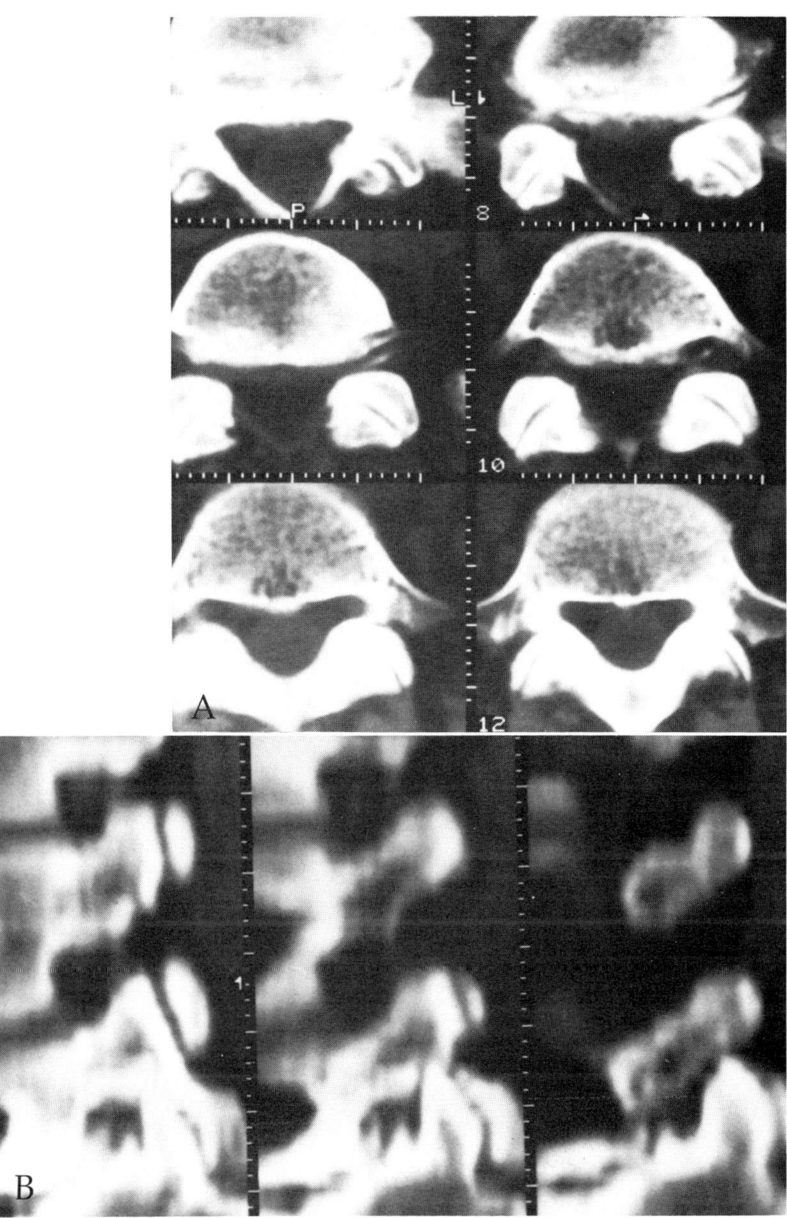

Figure 32–10. Multiplanar CT for stenosis evaluation—selected images. The importance of high resolution saggital reformatted images in bone **(B)** and soft tissue **(C)** format demonstrating severe stenosis of the left L5-S1 intervertebral canal, which is difficult to detect on the standard axial images **(A).**

been the standard for decades, but current investigation shows that a disjunction now exists between the population on which the MMPI was based and the present population. This disjunction, perhaps resulting from the complexity of our current society, probably makes the MMPI considerably less valuable than some of the more recently developed, more easily administered psychologic tests.

However, for psychologic assessment no psychologic test can be as helpful and instructive as an in-depth interview conducted by a well trained psychiatrist familiar with the psychologic demands of spine pain. Just as the patient's history is one of the more important aspects of structural diagnostic test-ing, the psychologic interview is one of the most important aspects of psychiatric diagnosis. Forms for screening a patient's history are valuable for a physical diagnosis, and psychologic questionnaires may provide helpful clues for a psychological assessment of a patient. For the more severe types of psychiatric disturbance, psychologic testing can be an important adjunct to a psychiatric interview. However, for screening a relatively normal population to identify the occasional patient with personality or maladaption difficulties, there is no better evaluation than a psychiatric interview. Filling out a form describing a history of back pain is not nearly as effective and valuable as an interview that allows a candid and in-

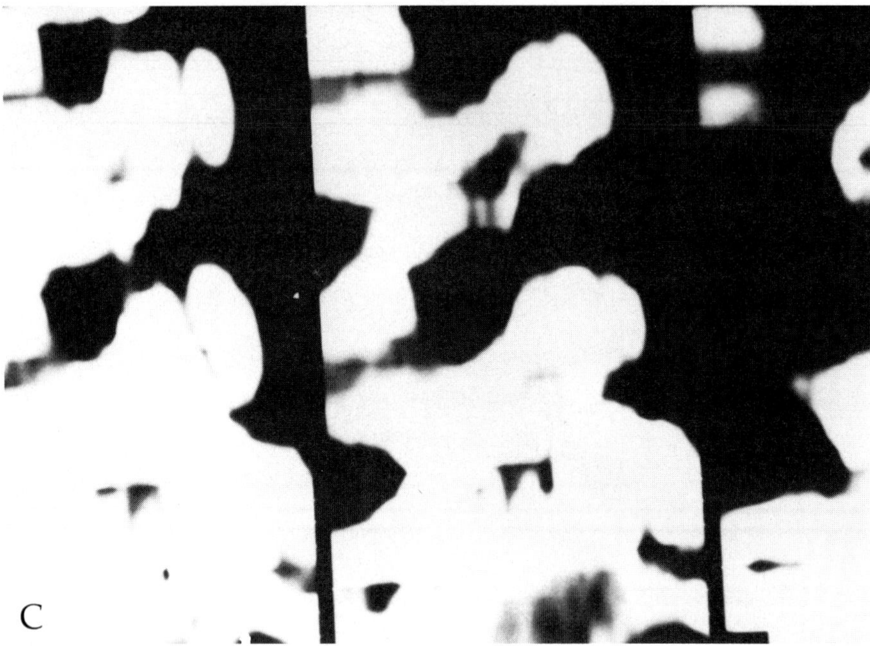

C

Figure 32–10 (continued).

depth picture of the psychologic background and current environment of the patient.

Certain screening questions that give some idea of the presence or potential for development of significant psychologic disturbance may be included in an initial questionnaire. A few examples of important screening information follow:

- The presence or history of alcohol dependency in the patient or in one or both parents.
- A history of physical or sexual abuse as a child or adolescent.
- The presence of three or more of the following disturbances: weight loss or gain, sleep disturbance, altered mood, emotional lability, feelings of worthlessness, thoughts of suicide, and fatigue or loss of energy.

BLOCKS

Diagnostic blocks, although less sensitive and accurate than diagnostic imaging and electrodiagnostics, are certainly a valuable tool for evaluating patients in yet another way. These blocks confirm structural abnormality by producing and relieving pain. During blocking procedures, placebo response must be taken into consideration. At any time during blocking procedures, a placebo block may be given to evaluate a patient's placebo response. We routinely give a placebo injection when performing indwelling epidural blocks (Fig. 32–11). The first injection is usually executed with saline and patients are tested for perceived pain relief. If they have significant pain relief with saline, then the blocks are not undertaken. If a patient is not a placebo responder, we give a generalized epidural injection of 1% Xylocaine and re-evaluate the patient. An epidural injection may affect many structural areas, multiple disc levels, and nerve roots. Therefore, although it does not yield specific information, from its results the clinician can determine whether a generalized injection is capable of reducing or eliminating a patient's pain for a short period of time. Then, a steroid preparation is injected to give the patient some long-range relief, during which time the patient's training may be accelerated. At a later time, more selective blocks, e.g., selective nerve root blocks or facet blocks, are administered, which help to localize specific lesions such as spinal stenosis or facet arthritis (Fig. 32–12).

When the entire clinical picture points to a single structural abnormality, the likelihood of a higher success rate for surgery is obvious. For example, unilateral leg pain in an L5 distribution with a positive EMG, herniated disc at the L4-L5 level on scan, and relief with an epidural block and selective nerve root block of L5 is a precise verification of a diagnosis. That type of structural abnormality would probably respond satisfactorily to surgery if all conservative measures failed. Some clinicians might settle for just the history and physical examination, with an image that confirmed the working diagnosis. Frequently, however, imaging is imprecise or reveals multiple areas of potential abnormality. Conducting further diagnostic tests might narrow down the pos-

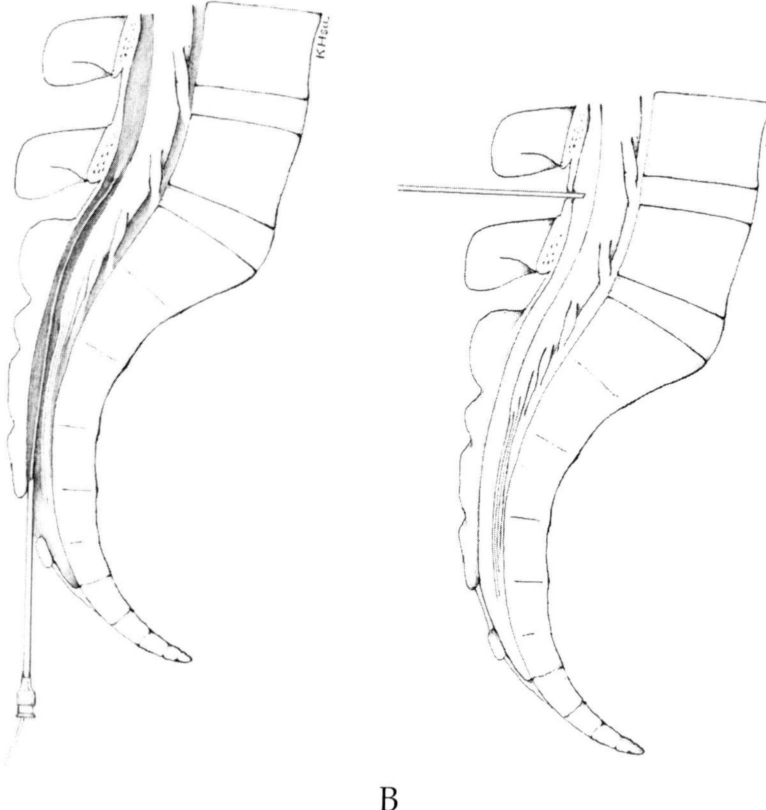

Figure 32–11. A. Indwelling epidural. **A**
B. Translumbar epidural injection. **B**

sible sources of a patient's disabling condition and increase the likelihood of surgical success.

DISCOGRAMS

Discograms have a definite place in the methodology of the spinal diagnostician (Fig. 32–13). They have had a bad reputation because they have been abused by surgeons in the past, who have done unnecessary spinal surgery on the basis of a discogram alone. High incidences of positive discograms in asymptomatic populations do exist.[3] A patient with a degenerative disc may have a positive discogram but may not necessarily be a candidate for surgery because most individuals over the age of 40 have degenerate discs and do not need surgery.

Annular injections can create significant pain in the face of an otherwise normal disc. However, the North American Spine Society has released a positional statement that acknowledges the respect that a significant number of investigators have for discography as a means of accurately obtaining information about the disc itself. In addition, they present guidelines for appropriate interpretation of discograms that address the previous objections to the use of discography.[4]

Surgeons have advocated for decades[5] that discograms should be performed prior to a fusion of the lumbar spine. It is well accepted that performing a fusion adjacent to a degenerative segment is highly likely to increase the symptoms and degeneration of that segment.

There are times when the discogram may be the final and most convincing piece of diagnostic information in clarifying an otherwise complex and difficult case. A discogram should be one of the last tests performed because of its invasiveness. Infections can occur with discograms, and neurologic, vascular and bowel damage can also result from them. Surgery, of course, has much greater dangers and complications. If a patient is on the way to surgery with an unclear diagnosis, which a discogram could help clarify, it might well be indicated.

In order to avoid overuse of the discogram, it is a good rule of thumb to have exhausted all other reasonable diagnostic procedures and conservative measures before resorting to a discogram. Discograms can be valuable in the following situations:

1. In the case of a severely disabled patient who is being considered for surgery with multiple level disc disease demonstrated by scans. Prior to surgery, a discogram can help define the multilevel

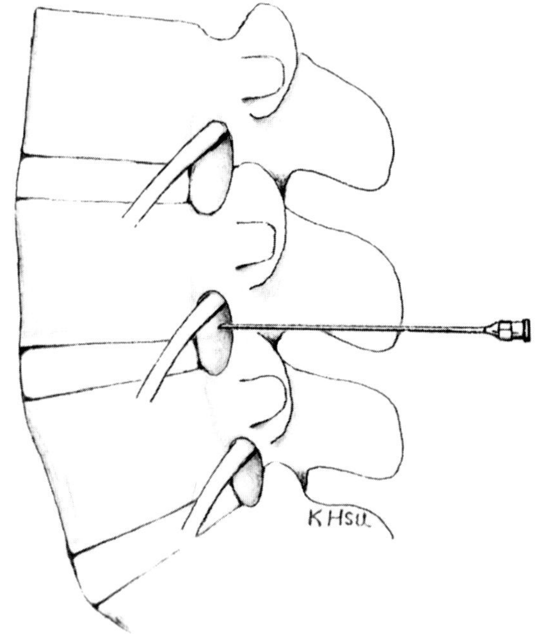

Figure 32–12. Selective nerve root block.

disc abnormalities that are painful and that most exactly reproduce the patient's usual pain.
2. Prior to surgery, a discogram can verify that a lumbar level adjacent to a proposed fusion is normal and can support a fusion.
3. In the rare case of internal disc disruption, or another discogenic syndrome that has a strong, consistent history and failure of conservative care, the scanning procedures will be relatively normal, as will be myelograms, bone scans, and

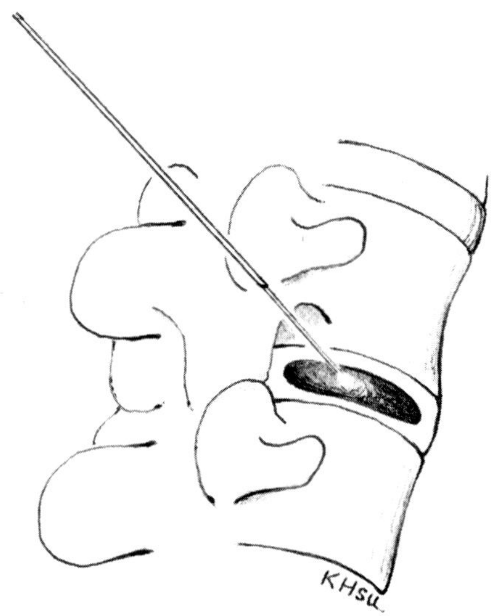

Figure 32–13. Discogram.

EMG. It is a good idea to have psychologic studies performed on this type of patient.

If the psychologic profile merits it, or if inconsistencies exist in the physical examination or response to treatment, a second opinion or multidisciplinary evaluation may be appropriate. When no inconsistencies exist and psychologic evaluation is normal, a discogram of several levels is indicated. Normal lumbar levels should be examined first, as a control procedure to assess the patient's pain tolerance and for comparison with the L4-L5 and L5-S1 discs, one of which may exactly reproduce the patient's pain to a severe degree. Such a response is a fairly strong indication that the disc so injected is the symptomatic one and might benefit from surgery. If the pain provoked during the discogram injection is not exactly like the patient's usual pain and is not severe, one would be less inclined to consider surgery.

In classic internal disc disruption, the concordant severe pain reproduction is created with a small volume of contrast liquid injected (less than 1 ml). When performing discograms, the volume injected should be noted. Most discs will accept approximately 2 ml of contrast liquid. Thus, the endpoint should be recorded. When a disc has a tear in the annulus that allows the contrast liquid to leak out, many units can be injected and such a disc should be reported as having no endpoint. After injecting three or four units with no endpoint, the discographer should stop injecting. Discs with small or slow leaks should be recorded as a soft endpoint.

There are strong advocates and opponents of discography. This has partly come from the abuses of discography and because of an article published by Holt[3] several decades ago. The Holt study is no longer representative of the way discography is performed. Holt's study has recently been repeated by James Weinstein[6] with different results. Before one uses discography as a major diagnostic tool, a clinical diagnostician should have a good understanding of the uses and abuses of discography.

MEDICAL EVALUATION IN RELATION TO STRUCTURAL DIAGNOSIS

For the purposes of this chapter, specific structural abnormalities are identified, which are to be treated by particular physical means, namely, surgery, therapy, manipulation, and injection. There are certain medical diseases that can cause or aggravate back pain and not present as a specific structural or anatomical abnormality; for example, osteoporosis, peripheral neuropathy, ankylosing spondylitis, and other forms of systemic arthritic diseases. These disorders are diagnosed primarily through laboratory testing, not structural diagnostic testing. The clinician specializing in spinal diagnosis should be aware of these medical possibilities, just as he should be aware of the effects of the psychologic state of a patient who has low back pain. He may not do psychologic testing himself nor may he do laboratory testing. However, he should work with subspecialists who look into all the medical possibilities to ensure a better success rate for treatment of back pain.

Osteoporosis may be diagnosed by a dual photon densimeter or a specific CT scan for bone density. However, this does not tell the clinician the underlying cause for the osteoporosis, nor does it suggest the medical treatment required. A specialist in metabolic bone disease should be consulted to determine serum and urine calcium and total endocrinological status. Peripheral neuropathy can be diagnosed by electrodiagnostic testing, but the source of the peripheral neuropathy requires a medical evaluation for diabetes, toxins, and other medical conditions that can lead to peripheral neuropathy.

Arthritis can be diagnosed by some basic laboratory studies, such as sedimentation rate, HLA-B27 antigen, and rheumatoid factor. The exact diagnosis and its management is generally turned over to a rheumatologist.

SUMMARY

In summary, surgery for lumbar spine pain or low back pain with radiating leg pain has a notoriously unsuccessful track record. Anything that can be done to increase the success of this type of surgery is worthwhile. A little extra time and expense for additional tests confirming a diagnosis and eliminating other possibilities could increase the surgical success rate by as much as 30%.

All subspecialists of the spinal field have their specific biases and wear certain blinders. Spinal surgeons all too often think that their tools can fix all ailments of the spine. Nonsurgical diagnosticians may be a bit more skeptical and cautious. More tests and more conservative care within a reasonable time frame of 1 to 3 months from the time of injury might well lead to higher success rates for spinal surgery for those patients who have received better supported specific diagnoses and who are better prepared for surgery.

Studies have shown[7] that time alone may cure herniated discs for which surgery has been indicated. Somewhere between 64 to 80% of patients who are being considered for surgical intervention for herniated discs return to normal activities in one year. According to these studies, by 4 years, 90% of such patients have returned to normal activities. Other studies[8] have shown that aggressive conservative care (aside from time alone) return as many as 92% of patients with herniated discs to normal activities in a few months. A surgeon, therefore, needs to be selective of the patients on which he chooses to operate. If he can select those patients who will not return to normal through the cure of time alone, he will be doing a great service to a small percentage of spinally disabled individuals. However, if he operates on all comers, he will be doing a disservice to many patients who could have avoided surgery and the risks it generates.

REFERENCES

1. Weisz, G.: Value of computerized tomography in diagnosing diseases of the lumbar spine. Med J Aust *1*:216–219, 1982.
2. Clark, W.L., et al.: Back impairment and disability determination. Another attempt at objective reliable rating. Spine *13*(3):332–341, 1988.
3. Holt Jr., E.P.: The question of lumbar discography. J Bone Joint Surg *50A*:720–725, 1968.
4. NASS: Position Statement on Discography. Spine *13*(12):1343, 1988.
5. Wiltse, L.: Personal communication.
6. Weinstein, J.: The Pain of Discography. Spine *13*(12):1344–1348, 1988.
7. Weber, H.: Lumbar disc herniation: a controlled prospective study with ten years of observation. Spine *8*:131–140, 1983.
8. Saal, J.A., Saal, J.S.: Nonoperative treatment of herniated lumbar intervertebral disc with radiculopathy: an outcome study. Spine *14*(4):431–437, 1989.

Part VI

The Place for Surgical Treatment

Steven R. Garfin
Harry N. Herkowitz

33

Surgical Management of Low Back Pain Disorders

INTRODUCTION

This chapter provides an overview of the surgical treatment of low back disorders. The emphasis is on degenerative disc disease. The first few sections deal with the issues related to lumbar laminotomy and laminectomy for disc herniation. This includes a discussion of laminectomy, microdiscectomy, chemonucleolysis, and percutaneous nucleotomy, as the authors see the roles for these various treatment options. This is followed by a section on the surgical treatment of spinal stenosis and the controversies related to fusion when operating on patients with this disorder. Though these cases constitute the majority of surgery that is performed on the lumbar spine, we also include our indications for fusion for low back pain, including spondylolisthesis, disc degeneration, and lumbar instability. For completeness, a brief discussion of the primary instrumentation systems that are currently available and used in the treatment of low back disorders is included. Finally, we conclude with a discussion of causes for back pain other than degenerative disc disease: tumors, infections, spondyloarthropathies, and other medical conditions.

LUMBAR LAMINECTOMY FOR DISC HERNIATION

Patient selection is crucial in contributing to a successful outcome. The axiom that, "we operate on patients, not diagnostic studies" certainly holds true for patients with low back disorders. Hitzelberger demonstrated a 24% false positive rate for lumbar disc herniation in asymptomatic patients undergoing myelography for evaluation of a posterior fossa tumor.[34] Wiesel demonstrated a 19% false positive rate for lumbar disc herniation in asymptomatic volunteers under the age of 40, and a 30% false positive rate for magnetic resonance imaging (MRI) in a similar group.[91] Patients with sciatica predominating over back pain with positive straight leg raise (SLR) contralateral SLR with neurologic deficit (reflex loss or weakness), and a contrast study consistent with the clinical findings, constitute the "ideal" operative profile.

There are two situations, however, in which surgery should not be considered elective. The first is progressive neurologic deficit. The second is cauda equina syndrome, fortunately a rare occurrence. Spangfort reported a 1.2% incidence of cauda equina in his series of 2500 cases; and an overall incidence of this syndrome in 2.5% of patients with lumbar disc herniation. The L4-L5 level is most commonly involved.[73] Kostiuk, et al., reported on 31 patients (17 male and 14 female, mean age 40 years) with cauda equina syndrome caused by central disc herniation. They found that the classic presentation of bilateral sciatica, saddle dysesthesia, motor weakness in the lower extremities, and bladder or bowel dysfunction did not occur in the majority of their patients. Seventeen of the 31 patients had unilateral sciatica. Those patients with bilateral sciatica and saddle dysesthesia also had decreased anal spincter tone and perianal sensory loss. All patients developed urinary retention prior to surgery. Eight had sexual dysfunction. The onset of symptoms and signs was rapid in 10 patients and gradual in 17 patients. The L5-S1 level was most frequently involved, followed by L4-L5. Motor recovery occurred fully in the majority of cases. However, bladder function fared poorer in those with an acute onset. The authors recommended that surgery be performed as soon as possible to maximize recovery.[43]

Assuming that the patient does not have a cauda equina syndrome or progressive weakness, the question of when surgery should be performed must be addressed. Weber prospectively studied surgical and conservatively treated patients with lumbar disc herniations. At one year, 92% of the surgical group improved, whereas only 60% of the nonoperatively treated group demonstrated improvement. At the end of 4 years, however, the surgery group remained at 90%, and the conservative group reported 85% satisfactory results.[88] These results indicate the advantage of early surgery, and that a gradual improvement will occur in the conservative group over years. Hakelius reported similar findings in his retrospective review of over 500 patients with lumbar disc herniation. In his study, the conservatively treated group reported, after 7 years, more low back pain, more restricted sport activity, and more time off work than the surgical group.[29] In reviewing the studies of Hakelius and Weber, it appears that the results of surgery are not negatively influenced by a waiting period of three months before recommending surgery. It should also be emphasized that in Weber's 10-year followup, the improvement in muscle weakness, extensor hallucis longus (EHL), sensory dysfunction, or reflex loss was not statistically improved in the surgery group over the conservative group.

In general, back surgery for leg pain, if the patient is selected properly, is highly successful. Hirsch and Nachemson evaluated the surgical findings and correlated them with the preoperative clinical and radiological evaluation. The group that demonstrated the greatest number of disc herniations and the highest degree of success were those patients who had positive neurologic findings, positive tension sign, and a myelogram consistent with the clinical exam.[33] This study pioneered in defining the patient population that would most benefit from a laminectomy. Their success rate of 90% (208 out of 232 patients improved) represents the standard against which other series have been judged. Weber, reporting his long-term results following lumbar discectomy, found that 4-year followup results decline only slightly from the 1-year results (90% vs. 92%, respectively).[88] A recent report summarizing the Pennsylvania Hospital surgical experience for disc herniation and spinal stenosis demonstrated a 93% success rate for patients with a herniated lumbar disc.[24] Although surgery for a herniated lumbar disc is performed primarily for leg pain, 88% of patients had improvement in their back pain.

RECURRENT DISC HERNIATION

The reported incidence of recurrent disc herniation ranges from 3 to 6%.[8,23,24] Frymoyer, et al., reported on 22 patients undergoing a second laminectomy following an initial disc excision. Ten of the 22 patients (45%) were found to have a recurrent disc herniation at the same level, whereas 5 of 22 patients (22%) had a recurrent disc herniation at a different level. Seven patients underwent another operation for bony instability. In addition, the majority of re-operations occurred in the first 5 years.[23]

Cauchoix, et al., noted that of 49 patients requiring re-operation for recurrent disc herniation, 34 were at the same level (69%). Of those at the same level, 28 (57%) were on the same side, whereas 6 (12%) were on the opposite side. Fifteen (31%) were at a different level.[8] Garfin, et al., reporting on the Pennsylvania Hospital experience of 274 patients undergoing laminectomy for disc herniation and spinal stenosis listed the re-operation rate as 6%, with recurrent disc herniation at the same level being the most common finding.[24]

DISC EXCISION WITH FUSION

Long-term studies have verified the excellent results obtained with discectomy alone in those patients whose primary diagnosis is lumbar disc herniation.[87] Despite this, reports surface periodically expounding the virtues of concomitant fusion.[84] Gurdjian, et al., reported on 10-year followup of over 1000 patients operated on for lumbar disc herniation. They compared those patients undergoing discectomy with a similar group undergoing discectomy and fusion. Satisfactory results were obtained in 76% without fusion, as opposed to 72% with fusion.[28] Lamont, et al., reported on long-term results (7 to 10 years) of 125 patients undergoing discectomy with and without fusion. Satisfactory results were obtained in 83% of the nonfusion group and 85% of the fusion group. In addition, they found strong correlation with the extent of disc disease and the final result.[44] Those patients with disc extrusion did significantly better than those with only a degenerative disc (79% vs. 43% irrespective of whether or not a fusion was performed), reinforcing the principle set forth by Spangfort that the greater the disease the better the result.[73]

Recently, Vaughan, et al., reported on 85 patients undergoing disc excision at L4-L5.[84] Fifty-two patients underwent disc excision alone and 33 patients had discs excised and posterolateral fusions performed. They demonstrated satisfactory results in 85% of the fusion group, and 39% in the nonfusion patients. The 39% satisfactory result is suspect in light of the results obtained by other authors for single level disc excision. Further analysis reveals that of 15 patients who had workers' compensation in the nonfusion group, 14 had a poor result as opposed to 2 of the 6 patients in the fusion group. Second, the cause of poor results in the nonfusion group was a result of progressive degenerative disc disease in the majority of patients. A review of the authors' technique found that they advocate a complete discectomy with curetting of both end plates. Biomechanically, this has been shown to lead to significantly greater motion at the surgical site than partial discectomy.[27] In addition, a comparison of radiographic changes 10 years after discectomy, with and without fusion, found no correlation between the clinical result and plain radiograph appearance, leading one to search for other causes of poor results.[22]

It is clear from the review of the literature and our experience that the vast majority of patients undergoing disc excision do not require fusion. There are, however, several situations in which bilateral lateral fusion should be considered along with discectomy. They are: (1) significant low back pain along with disc degeneration and spondylosis; (2) complete laminectomy with bilateral partial facetectomies for central disc herniation; and (3) recurrent disc herniation at the same level when significant removal of facet is required.

MICROSURGERY

The microsurgical approach to the removal of herniated disc has received considerable press in the lay literature. True microdiscectomy suggests that minimal to no bone from the lamina is removed and the "disc removal" is done through a surgical microscope. By exposing the interlaminar space through a small skin incision (1 in.) and resecting the ligamentum flavum, proponents of this technique claim that adequate exposure of the nerve root occurs to visualize the disc herniation and remove it. Zahrani reported on 60 patients undergoing microdiscectomy with an average followup of 33 months.[94] Fifty-one patients had CT scan only preoperatively. Followup was by phone or office visit with no physical examination. The authors reported a 93% success rate. However, complications were reported in 5 patients (8%): 1 dural tear, 4 wound infections, and 1 disc space infection. Williams, in reviewing 903 patients undergoing microlumbar discectomy, reported a 14.2% re-operation rate with recurrent disc herniation at the same level most common, followed by disc ruptures at a different level.[92] The 14.2% re-operation rate is significantly higher than other surgical series on lumbar disc herniation.[24,33]

A number of technical problems that can occur when removing a disc herniation without any bone resection are well known to any spine surgeon. In many cases of disc herniation, extruded fragments may migrate proximal or distal to the disc space. In addition, adhesions between the nerve root and disc often make it difficult to mobilize the nerve root in order to expose the herniated disc. In order to prevent excessive traction on the nerve root and avoid a "battered root," it is essential that the root be exposed at its lateral border. This may require significant bone removal before the root can be safely mobilized.

In reality, microdiscectomy, as we use it, refers to a small incision with adequate bone removal, including a portion of the superior and inferior lamina, that may require a partial facetectomy. Advocates of the microscope claim that one of the main advantages is the intense light source it provides. The use of a headlight, occasionally supplemented by a lighted Taylor retractor, provides more than adequate light.

In summary, microdiscectomy without adequate bone removal does not provide enough nerve root exposure to allow satisfactory nerve root decompression in most instances. Microdiscectomy, as it refers to small incision (1 to 2 in.) with adequate bone removal to clearly visualize the nerve root and the compressive disease, is the preferred method for surgical removal of a herniated lumbar disc.

SPINAL STENOSIS

Spinal stenosis, unlike a herniated lumbar disc, is a "global" degeneration of one or more lumbar segments, usually affecting an older age group. The initial treatment, however, is similar to a herniated disc. The usual modalities of physical therapy, rest, anti-inflammatory medication, and corsets should or can be tried. In many instances, the passage of time, with or without other modalities, lessens the patients symptoms. The question that must be answered in those patients who do not improve is, "How long can I wait before recommending surgery?" Johnsson, et al., studied three groups of patients with myelographically proven spinal stenosis.[39] Group I (conservative treatment) consisted of 19 patients. Group II consisted of 30 surgical patients without complete myelographic blocks; Group III was composed of 30 surgical patients with total occlusion of the dural sac. The mean duration of followup was 29, 41, and 43 months, respectively. Of those patients not operated on (Group I), 11 showed improvement (58%), 7 showed no change (37%) and 1 patient got worse. Those patients without a complete myelographic block who were operated on noted improvement in 19 (63%), and no change in 11 (36%). No patient deteriorated as a result of the surgery. Of the 14 patients with complete block who were operated on, 9 (64%) improved, 4 (29%) were unchanged, and 1 was more debilitated than before the surgery.

Walking capacity, a common indication for surgery, was evaluated in the three groups. In the nonoperated patients improvement was noted in 8 (42%), unchanged in 6 (32%), and worse in 5 (26%). In the group without a complete block who were operated on, 15 (50%) improved, 8 (27%) were unchanged, and 7 (23%) were worse. For the group with complete blockage undergoing surgery, 11 (79%) were improved and 3 (21%) had reduced walking capacity.

The authors also compared the postoperative results with the duration of symptoms in the different groups. Although better results were noted in those patients with a shorter duration of symptoms, (mean = 28 ± 22 months − improved, 38 ± 42 months − not improved), this was not statistically significant. Thus, it appears from this study that a significant number of patients with spinal stenosis who are treated conservatively do not deteriorate over time and, in fact, over 50% improve clinically.

What is a reasonable period of time to wait before recommending surgery? Johnsson, et al., feel that 2 to 3 years of observation is reasonable. In our practices, if the patient has not shown improvement after six months of conservative treatment, we consider surgery because it is unlikely that further time will significantly benefit the patient. Our indications for surgery in the patient with documented spinal stenosis are:

1. Significant limitation of walking ability because of neurogenic claudication or leg pain.
2. Progressive neurologic dysfunction.
3. Restriction of lifestyle that is unacceptable to patient.

A successful outcome following decompressive laminectomy has been reported to occur in 60 to 90% of all cases.[24,37,60,65,74,79] As in surgery for a herniated lumbar disc, relief of leg pain is the primary goal of a decompressive laminectomy for spinal stenosis.

Complications occurring with this procedure include infection, dural tear, pulmonary emboli, hematoma causing cauda equina compression, and postoperative slipping (iatrogenic spondylolisthesis). These complications are rare and in most instances avoidable. Postoperative slipping appears to be the most common problem occurring with decompressive laminectomy. Therefore, some consideration for fusion with the operation should be made.

The criteria for spinal fusion in conjunction with decompression have been previously outlined by Wiltse, et al.[93] They are: (1) 60 years of age or less, with degenerative spondylolisthesis when total facetectomy has been performed, (2) 55 years of age or less with degenerative spondylolisthesis, (3) less than 50 years of age with isthmic spondylolisthesis. It is difficult, however, to base a decision solely on the patient's age because many other factors must be considered.

The incidence of postoperative slip after decompression for degenerative spinal stenosis ranges from 2 to 20% in published series.[38,46,56,67,75] Patients with degenerative spondylolisthesis have a higher percentage of postoperative slippage. The factors that may influence postoperative slippage in degenerative spinal stenosis and spondylolisthesis include the extent of the decompression, the amount of slip present preoperatively, the sex of the individual, the severity of spondylosis of the anterior column, the number of levels decompressed, abnormal frontal or lateral plane alignment, and finally, penetration of a disc space at the time of decompression.

Johnsson reported on 45 patients who had undergone decompression for spinal stenosis, 25 for degenerative stenosis, and 26 for degenerative spondylolisthesis.[38] The mean age was 64 years with a mean followup of 46 months. Of the degenerative spondylolisthesis group, 65% (13 out of 20) slipped postoperatively, as compared to 20% (5 out of 25) in the degenerative stenosis group. However, of the 13 with degenerative spondylolisthesis that slipped, 7 were classified as a good result, whereas the 5 postoperative slips for degenerative stenosis were all poor results. One reason for this may be related to the better adaptability of the nerve roots to slippage in patients with a pre-existing spondylolisthesis. In a followup study, Johnsson reported a higher incidence of slippage and poor results in patients with excessive mobility documented on preoperative flexion-extension myelograms.

Rosenberg reported a 10% incidence of postoperative slip after decompression for degenerative spondylolisthesis.[68] There was no correlation between slippage and surgical outcome. Lombardi, et al., compared wide decompression, midline decompression, and decompression and fusion in 49 patients undergoing surgery for degenerative spondylolisthesis.[47] The best results were in those patients undergoing decompression and fusion. The factors contributing to the development of the postoperative slip were preoperative disc heights greater than 6 mm and the extent of facet decompression. In addition, postoperative slip greater than 50% of the vertebral body width was associated with a poor result.

Feffer, et al., reported on 19 patients undergoing surgery for degenerative spondylolisthesis.[17] Eight patients underwent decompression only, and 11 patients had decompression and bilateral fusion. The group with fusion had a better overall outcome. In addition, 4 out of the 11 patients who had decompression only developed postoperative slipping. This, however, was not correlated to symptomatic results.

Brown and Lockwood reported postoperative slipping in 14% (7 out of 51) of patients undergoing decompression for degenerative spondylolisthesis.[7] They felt this correlated with a poor result and, therefore, have recommended fusion along with decompression in degenerative spondylolisthesis.

Dall and Rowe compared 6 patients undergoing laminectomy and complete facetectomy to 11 patients with laminectomy and foraminotomy for degenerative spondylolisthesis.[13] No fusion was performed. Those patients receiving facetectomies had the better outcome. In addition, slipping occurred up to 3 mm in both groups.

The surgical management of scoliosis in combination with spinal stenosis was reported by Epstein.[18] Of the 12 patients in whom decompression was performed, 5 excellent results were obtained in single-level decompressions, whereas multiple-level decompression resulted in satisfactory results in 5 patients and fair and poor results in one patient.

The problems associated with the published series have been a lack of uniform grading for results and lack of uniform criteria for instability.

The following trends appear in the literature as predictors of postoperative instability.

1. The larger the preoperative slip, the greater the risk of postoperative slippage.
2. Postoperative slip does not necessarily correlate with development of symptoms.
3. Decompression across disc space of normal height may lead to postoperative slip.
4. Excision of over 50% of both facets at the same level increases the risk of slip.
5. Increasing the levels of decompression increases the risk of slip.
6. Penetration of the disc space at a decompressed level increases the risk of slip.
7. Females are at a higher risk than males for development of postoperative slip.

One hundred and twenty-five patients who had decompression for myelographically confirmed spinal stenosis were retrospectively reviewed from one of Herkowitz' series.[32] The ages ranged from 34 to 91 years (mean = 64 years). There were 77 females and 48 males. The followup was 2.1 to 7 years (mean − 3.9 years). Fifty-eight patients had degenerative stenosis, 41 had degenerative spondylolisthesis, and 26 had degenerative scoliosis. Decompression was performed at 5 levels in 12 patients, 4

Table 33–1
Results of Study of Decompression for Myelographically-Confirmed Spinal Stenosis

Type	Results		
	Excellent-Good	*Poor*	*E-G%*
Degenerative stenosis	50	8	84%
Spondylolisthesis	32	9	78%
Scoliosis	19	7	73%

levels in 17 patients, 3 levels in 50 patients, 2 levels in 29 patients, and 1 level in 17 patients. The results are presented in Table 33–1.

Those factors more often associated with a poor result in degenerative stenosis were multiple level decompression (three or more) with disruption of the facets, minimal anterior column degeneration, and prior surgery at the same levels. Age was not a factor.

For patients with degenerative spondylolisthesis those factors that tended to lead to a poor result were a progressive slip preoperatively, bilateral facet disruption, normal disc height, loss of lordosis, and prior surgery at the same levels. Age was not a factor.

For patients with degenerative scoliosis those factors associated with a poor result were larger curve (excellent to good results with a 13° curve, poor results with a 36° curve), documented curve progression, and decompression within the apex or along the length of the curve along with minimal anterior column degeneration. Age was not a significant factor. Based on these results a patient profile was developed to determine those patients who would benefit from a spinal fusion at the time of decompression.

INDICATIONS FOR FUSION AFTER DECOMPRESSIVE LUMBAR SURGERY

Fusion is indicated if the following conditions are present after the patient has undergone decompressive lumbar surgery:

Spinal Stenosis

1. Multiple-level decompression (three or more) with minimal anterior column degeneration.
2. Surgical disruption of over 50% of each facet joint at the same level.
3. Prior decompression at the same level.

Degenerative Spondylolisthesis

1. Documented preoperative progressive slip.
2. Minimal anterior column degeneration at the level of decompression.
3. High lumbosacral angle.
4. Sacralization of L5 (L4-L5 spondylolisthesis).
5. Surgical disruption of over 50% of each facet joint at the same level.
6. Prior decompression at the same level.
7. Penetration of the disc space at the time of decompression.

Degenerative Scoliosis with Spinal Stenosis

1. Larger curve (mean = 36°).
2. Decompression within the apex of the curve.
3. Lateral spondylolisthesis.
4. Decompression along the length of the curve with minimal anterior column degeneration.
5. Curve progression prior to surgery.

THE SURGICAL TECHNIQUE FOR LAMINECTOMY PREOPERATIVE EVALUATION

Perhaps more important than technique, is the preoperative evaluation. The decision to operate should be based on a consistent pain, that is explainable by objective signs and that can be corroborated by appropriate radiographic studies. For the most part, leg pain, which is related to a degenerative or herniated disc or to spinal stenosis, should be radicular in nature. Spinal stenosis, however, may produce atypical leg pain, which may vary over time and may not be purely dermatomic in distribution. CT scans, myelograms, and magnetic resonance scans (at this time complementary to CT scans) are critical in determining the level of involvement and confirming the diagnosis. Additionally, a detailed medical evaluation should be performed on each patient to ensure that no other possible cause exists for the pain, as well as to prepare the patient for surgery. If fusion is recommended, evidence of instability or deformity should be observed radiographically.

Positioning

Positioning for posterior spine surgery is important to help decrease bleeding, and thereby aid visualization at surgery. In general, we use a kneeling position with the abdomen free and noncompressed (Figure 33-1). This helps decrease intra-abdominal and inferior vena cava pressure, and also decrease the amount of blood in the epidural vascular system. Therefore, when the nerve roots are decompressed and explored, the epidural vascular network does not bleed as freely, hemostasis is easier to obtain, and the operation is not compromised by lack of visualization because of excessive bleeding. The kneeling position does place the spine in some degree of extension. However, with the decompression performed in this position, the result is more likely to be adequate when the patient is flexed or in a neutral position.

Standard Laminectomy

A standard laminectomy is performed through a midline posterior incision down the fascia (Figure 33-2). The fascia then can be stripped subperiosteally to the facet joints. For a single level disc herniation, the approach need only be performed on one side. For spinal stenosis or a large central disc, the subperiosteal dissection should be performed bilaterally. Hemostasis, using electrocoagulation, should be performed at each tissue level beginning at the subcutaneous tissues down to the interlaminar spaces. The surgical levels should then be identified anatomically or radiographically. The appropriate interlaminar spaces should be debrided of soft tissue using curettes and rongeurs. Again, hemostasis is essential. The ligamentum flavum, spanning the interlaminar space, can be separated from the inferior aspect of the cephalic lamina with a small curet. The ligamentum flavum can then be teased off distally and sharply excised. The dura should be protected with a small elevator when sharply excising the ligamentum flavum. For a single-level discectomy, the laminotomy should be widened to visualize the lateral aspect of the involved nerve root using rongeurs and Kerrison punches. At this point, the proximal and distal aspects of the root can be packed off with small cottonoide, and the root retracted medially. This gives good exposure to the disc space and the protruded and free disc fragments. It is important to emphasize that the laminotomy should extend lateral to the nerve root, to avoid inadvertent injury to the nerve root because the surgeon is trying to "limit" the bony resection.

For decompression for spinal stenosis, bilateral laminectomies are required. The laminectomies should extend across all levels of compromise observed on myelogram, CT scan, or MRI scan. The laminectomies should be performed using rongeurs and Kerrison punches, completing the midline canal

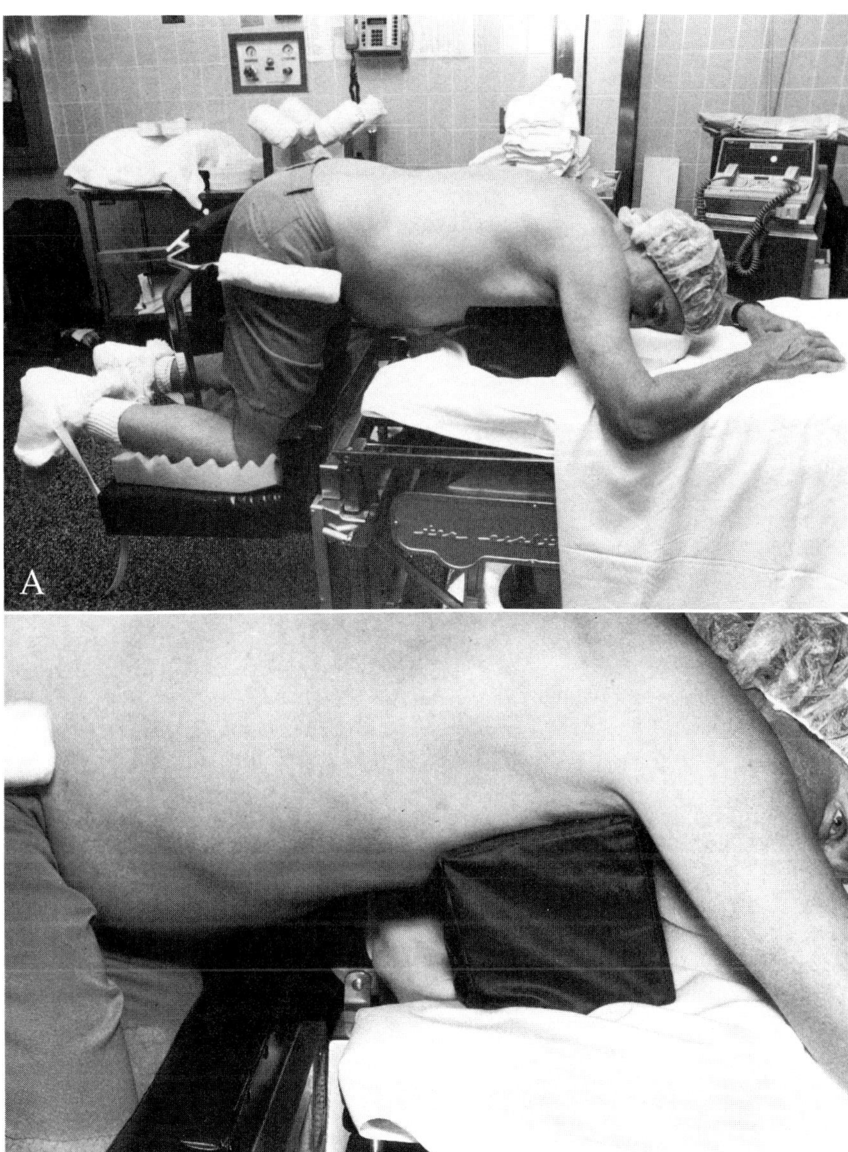

Figure 33–1. A model positioned on an Andrews frame. (From Amundson, G.A., Garfin, S.R.: Minimizing blood loss during spine surgery. In, Complications of Spine Surgery. (Garfin, S.R., Editor) Baltimore, Williams & Wilkins, 1989. **A.** The model is in the kneeling position. His chest and knees are supported. His abdomen is free. **B.** A close-up showing that the abdomen is free, without evidence of compression. The body is supported by a chest pillow and by the knees. In this picture the head is to the right and the chest is on the black chest support.

decompression from distal to proximal, and then working laterally. Finally, each nerve root should be explored to ensure that it is free in tension and compression. A Frazer elevator should pass easily anterior and posterior to the nerve root and out of the foramen. If evidence of residual compression exists, more bone or disc should be removed and the foraminotomy extended until the root is totally free.

Throughout the procedure 3.5 loupe magnification and headlights should be worn to improve visualization and help identify the nerve root, the disc margins and the epidural vessels. In the epidural space hemostasis should be obtained with bipolar electro-

coagulation. If necessary, Gelfoam* (absorbable gelatin sponge), Surgicel† (oxidized regenerated cellulose), and Avitene‡ (microfibrillar collagen hemostat) can be used to help control bleeding. Drains are routinely used in the wound and pulled at 24 to 48 hours. The drains are used to minimize the risk of a postoperative cauda equina syndrome developing from a postoperative hematoma.

---

*Upjohn Co., Kalamazoo, MI, 49001.
†Alcon Laboratories, Fort Worth, TX, 76134.
‡Johnson & Johnson, New Brunswick, NJ, 08903.

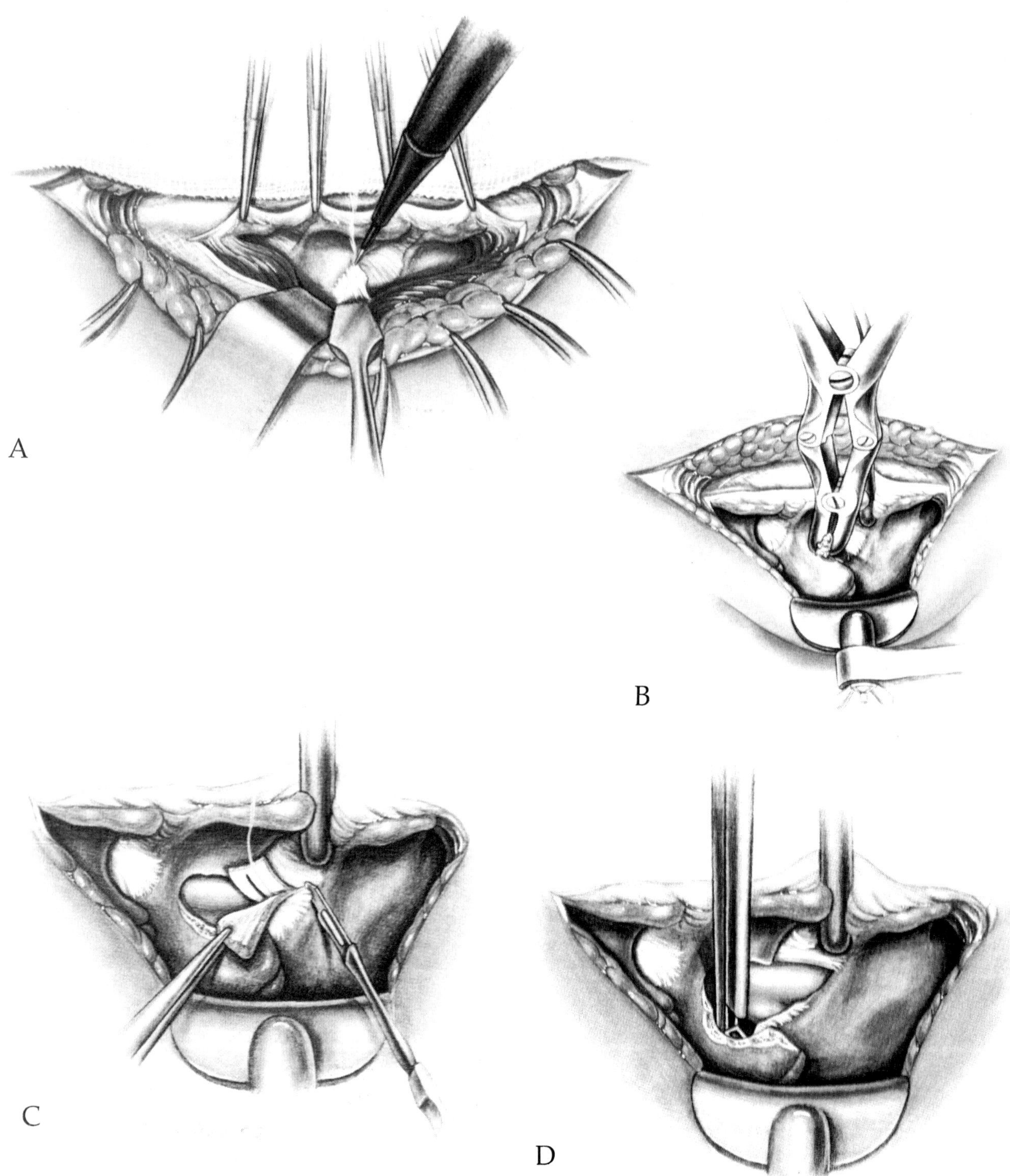

Figure 33–2. **A.** The soft tissue and lamina are stripped subperiosteally over the involved lamina and intra-lamina areas. **B.** A curette and rongeur are used to debride the interlaminar space and completely expose the lamina and intervening ligamentum flavum. **C.** The superior aspect of the ligamentum flavum is exposed by removing a small amount of the overlapping lamina, if necessary. It is then sharply excised as shown here. **D.** After visualizing the dura and identifying the nerve root, more bone and tissue may be removed laterally with a Kerrison punch.

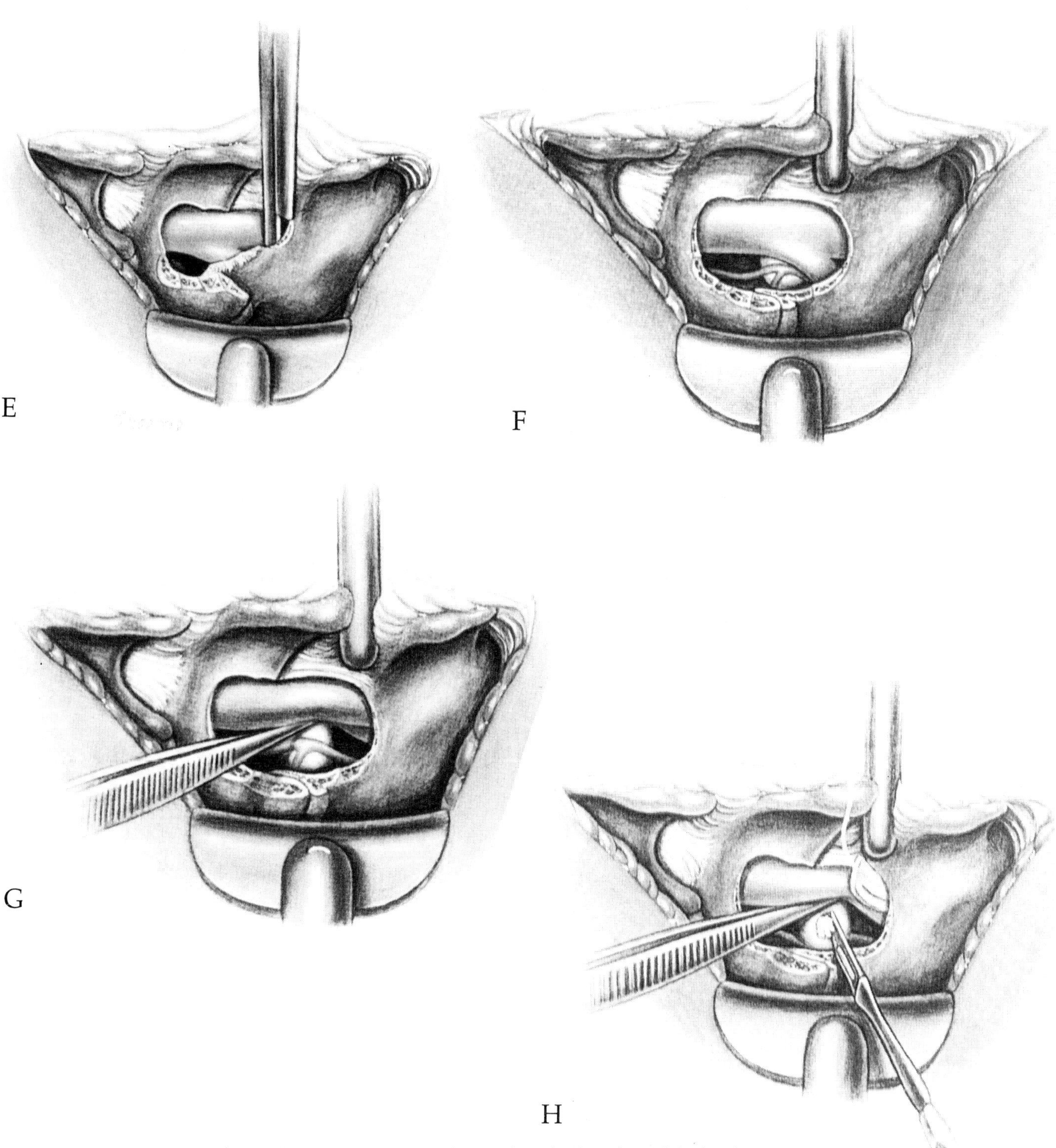

Figure 33–2 (continued). E. The bony opening is then widened inferiorly and further laterally until the lateral aspect of the nerve root is well identified. **F.** At this point, with loupe magnification, the lateral aspect of the nerve root and underlying disc hernation can usually be seen, as well as the epidural veins, which course in this area. In this artist's depiction, which is under the shoulder of the exposed nerve root. **G.** The nerve root and dura of the cauda equina can then be retracted medially (shown with forceps in this case) to better expose the disc and protect the neural elements. **H.** With adequate protection and visualization, a knife can be used to incise the posterior longitudinal ligament and annulus.

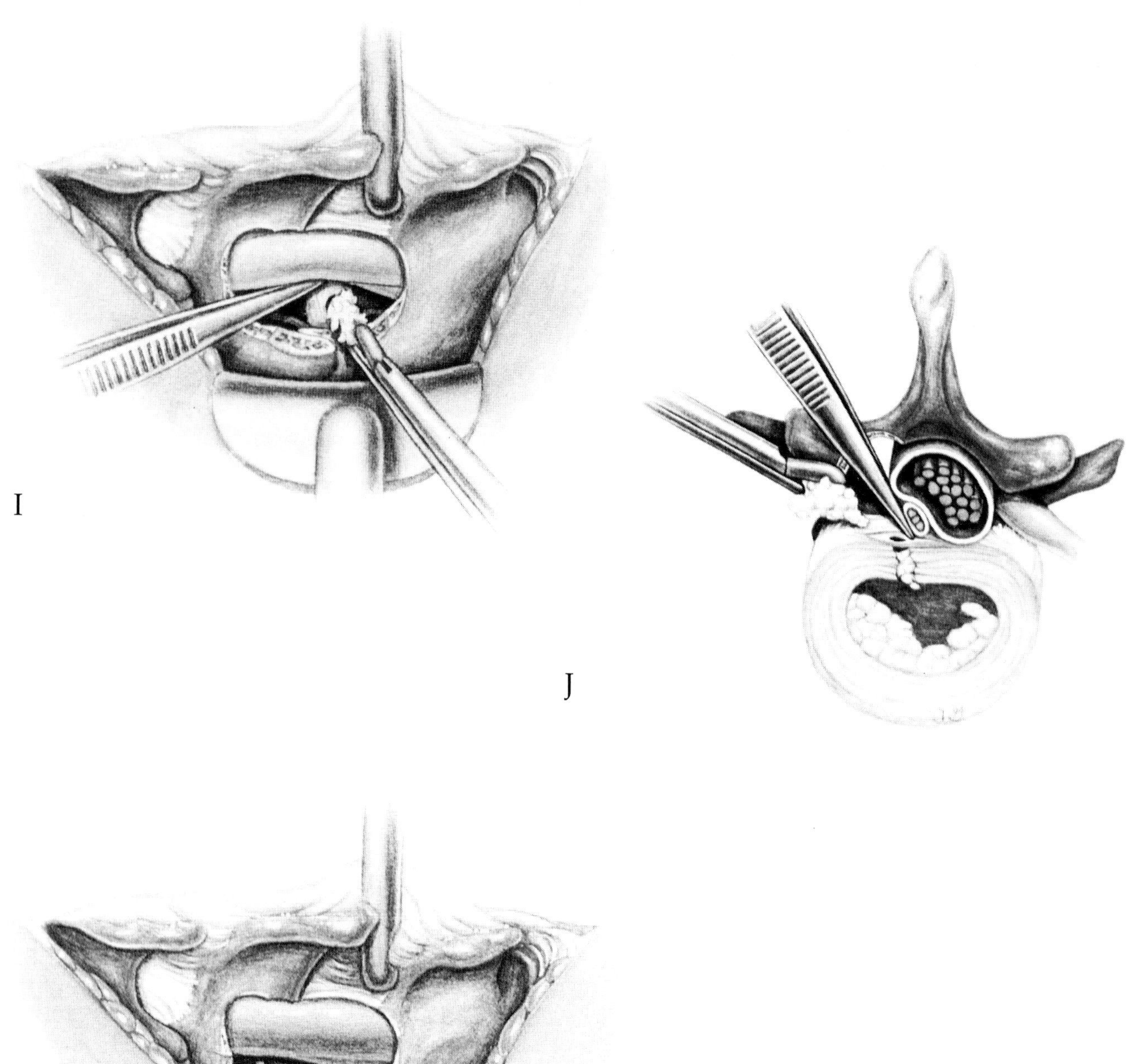

Figure 33–2 (continued). I. The free disc fragment or protruded disc material can then be removed with a pituitary rongeur. **J.** As shown in this artist's conception, with protection of the root medially, the pituitary is used to remove free fragments and can enter the disc space if necessary. **K.** At the completion of the diskectomy, the nerve root should be free in tension and compression and lie undeviated in the canal. (From Fager, C.A.: Atlas of Spinal Surgery. Philadelphia, Lea & Febiger, 1989.)

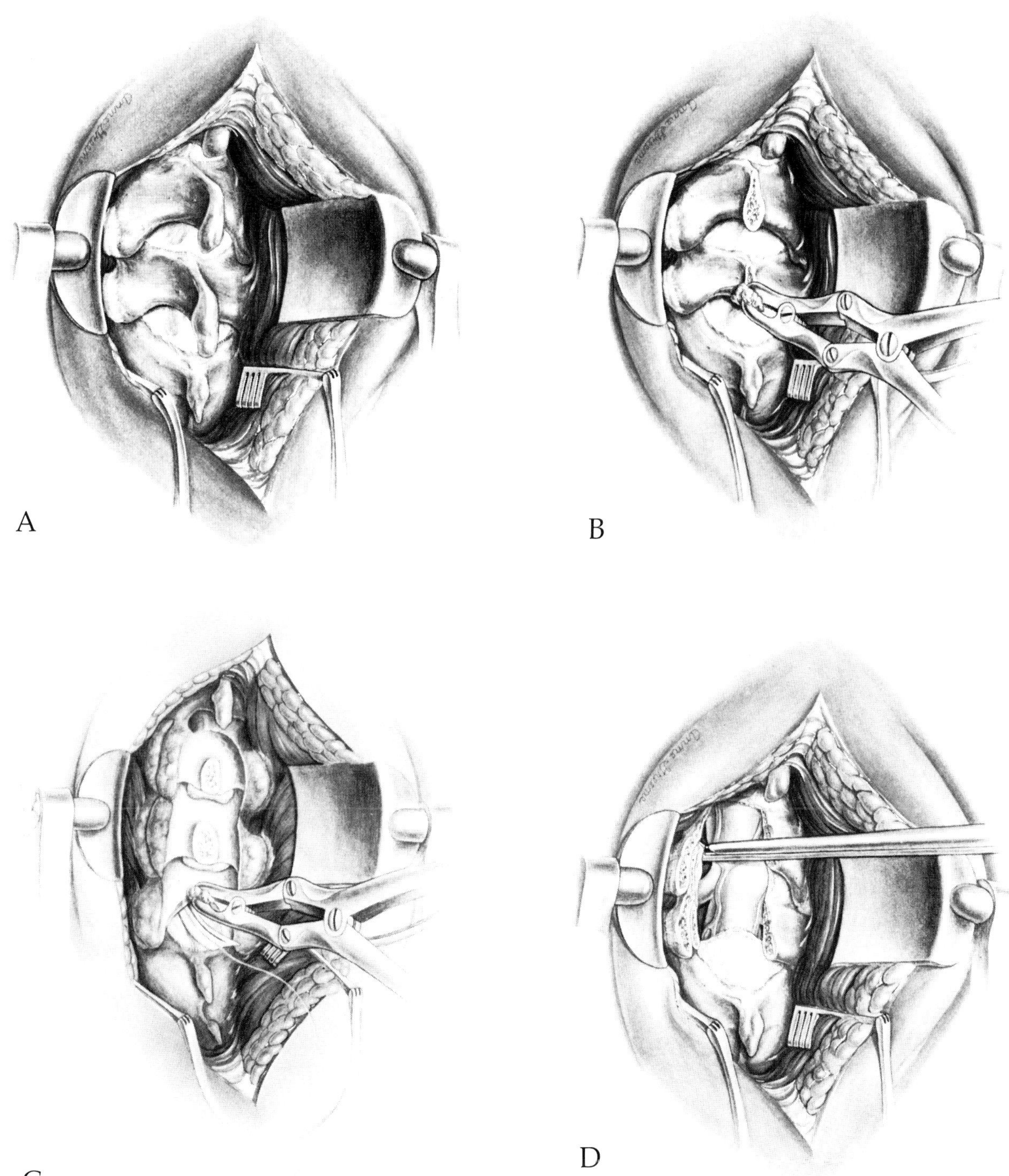

Figure 33–3. A. Subperiosteal stripping should be bilateral, exposing laterally to all lamina and facets involved. The lamina and interlaminar spaces should be debrided of all soft tissue. **B.** The spinous processes that will be included in the laminectomy can be removed with a bone cutter and rongeur. **C.** The ligamentum flavum is then separated from the overlying lamina and laminectomies initiated with a rongeur. **D.** The laminectomy can then be widened with Kerrison punches and curettes to expose the involved nerve roots (as shown here). If there are large epidural vessels, they should be cauterized. In this artist's conception, epidural veins are shown posterior to the nerve root which can be seen just to the right of the Kerrison.

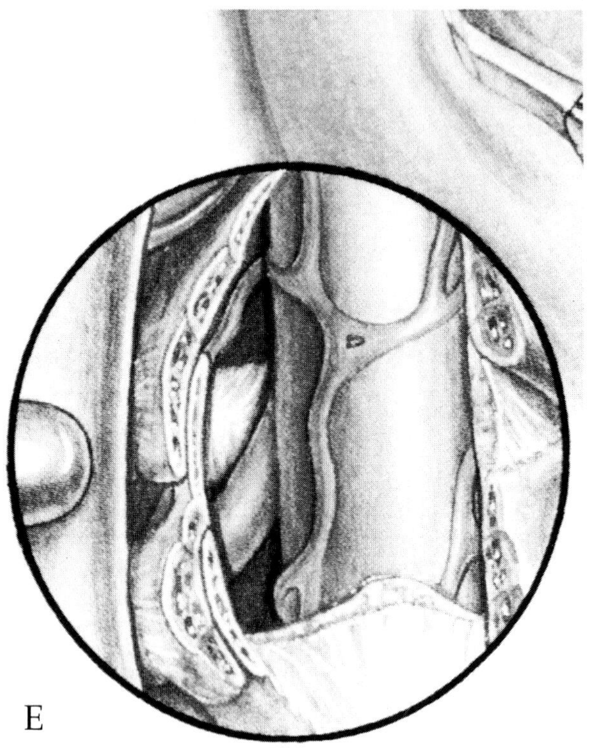

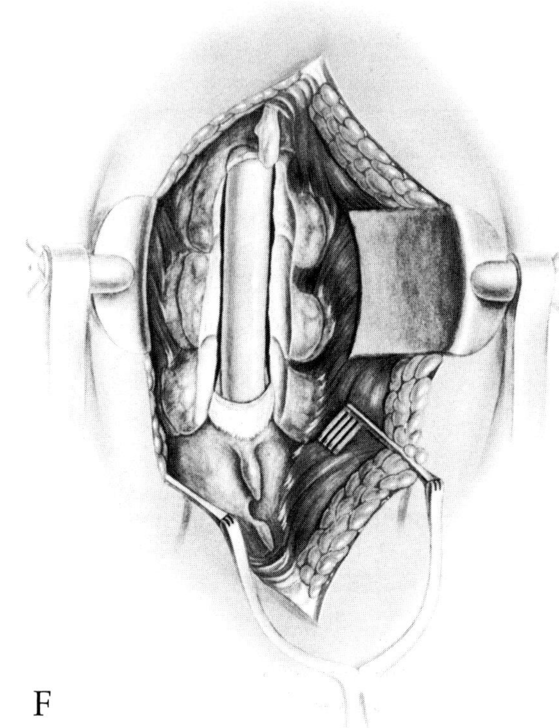

Figure 33–3 (continued). E. At the completion of the decompression, the cauda equina and nerve roots involved should be well exposed. Each disc space should also be explored to assure there are no disc herniations which were compounding the symptoms. **F.** At the completion of the case, the dura should be well exposed. It then can be covered with an interpositional material which may help decrease epidural scarring. (From Fager, C.A.: Atlas of Spinal Surgery. Philadelphia, Lea & Febiger, 1989.)

Postoperative Management

In general, we mobilize the patients early. Assuming no complications or dural tears, the patient can be allowed out of bed the next day. We ask patients to minimize sitting for a week, other than bathroom privileges, and avoid driving a car for 3 to 4 weeks. Aerobic exercise is encouraged at 2 to 3 weeks, but twisting activities, such as golf or tennis, are best avoided for 3 months. These general guidelines are empirically derived. However, by following these broad recommendations, we have noted a less than average incidence of failed back syndrome, recurrent leg, and recurrent back pains.

CHEMONUCLEOLYSIS

No form of invasive treatment for the herniated disc has been as controversial as chymopapain. It had been used on over 16,000 patients from 1969 to 1975 before it was withdrawn following a double blind study demonstrating no significant difference in result between chymopapain and placebo. Further studies in the early 1980s using a refined form of chymopapain reported statistically significant improved results over a placebo.[7] Following this, the FDA released chymopapain for clinical use in 1982. Since then it has continued to spark considerable controversy. The use of chymopapain has diminished considerably since 1982. According to a recent manufacturer's survey, the estimated number of procedures performed in 1987 was 3631, as opposed to over 16,000 cases from 1982 to 1985.[9] The reasons for the sharp decline are related to several factors. First, published reports show the superiority of surgery over chymopapain injection.[84,94] Second, an ongoing study by Weber comparing the natural history of sciatica with the results of chymopapain injection demonstrates no significant alteration of the natural history following chymopapain injection.[59] Third, the decline of chymopapain use is related to the occurrence of anaphylaxis and unpredictable neurologic complications.

Allergic reactions vary from itching and urticaria to death from anaphylactic shock. The incidence of death caused by chymopapain injection is reported to be 1:30,000. Prior to refinements in detection of individuals sensitive to chymopapain and the use of local, as opposed to general, anesthesia, the incidence was 1:5000.[30] The incidence of anaphylaxis from 1983 to 1987 was 0.4% in Caucasians, 0.9% in blacks, and 0.4% in hispanics. Black females have the highest percentage (1.7%) of allergic reactions.[9]

More than any other factor, the neurologic problems associated with chymopapain have led to its decreased popularity. From 1982 to 1985, 57 neurologic problems were reported in over 116,000 procedures, for an incidence of 0.05%. For 1986, 5 cases were reported from over 8200 patients (0.06%), and in 1987, 1 case out of 3600 patients was reported, for an incidence of 0.03%. Despite refinements in technique, no statistical difference has occurred in the incidence of neurological problems since 1982. Smith laboratories, the supplier of Chymodiactin wrote, "Data indicate that the incidence of serious neurological experiences is lower than previously reported, but the reduction is not statistically significant. However, in those cases recently reported, substantial improvement or recovery has occurred more frequently than in the past."[9] Agre has reviewed the neurologic complications following chymopapain injection.[1] They included cerebral hemorrhage, seizures, paraparesis, paraplegia, subarachnoid hemorrhage, Guillian Barre syndrome, and quadriplegia. Of the 28 patients reported with paraparesis or paraplegia, 11 had intrathecal injection of chymopapain. Chymopapain has been shown to induce neural injury when it comes in direct contact with nervous tissue, leading to subarachnoid hemorrhage. Epidural leakage from the disc space may occur in up to 25% of cases according to Wiltse, et al.[59] It is not necessary to inject the enzyme directly into the subarachnoid space to have the chymopapain interact with nervous tissue.

In the United States, 6 cases of acute transverse myelitis have been reported. This syndrome is characterized by a delayed onset of paraplegia, occurring slowly 2 to 5 weeks after injection. The incidence of transverse myelitis following chymopapain injection is greater than that occurring in the general population from other causes.[9]

The cause of transverse myelitis following chymopapain injection may be related to a delayed sensitivity reaction, immune complex disease, or arterial thrombosis. However, it must be emphasized that these are theories and the true cause is unknown.

The risks of neurologic injury are diminished if: (1) discography is not used at the time of chemonucleolysis, (2) local rather than general anesthesia is used, and (3) multiple injections are not performed. Although it is apparent that many of the cases of neurologic injury can be explained by inadvertent injection of chymopapain into the subarachnoid space, there remains a significant number of patients for which the cause has not been determined. The physician must, therefore, weigh the perceived benefits of chymopapain against the risks and complications, including neurologic injury, in deciding the appropriate definitive care for the patient with a herniated lumbar disc.[53]

PERCUTANEOUS DISCECTOMY

The latest invasive modality for the treatment of a lumbar disc herniation is percutaneous discectomy. This procedure uses a localizing probe followed by a cannula, which holds the nucleotome probe. The nucleotome probe simultaneously cuts and sucks nuclear material from the disc space into a special canister. Percutaneous discectomy is performed under local anesthesia and is an out-patient procedure. The success of this procedure is based on decompression of the disc space by producing a hole in the annulus with the cutting probe and then evacuating nuclear material with the cutting-suction probe. Kambin and Brager measured intradiscal pressure on 10 patients before and after percutaneous discectomy. The mean preoperative pressure was 191 mm Hg, which dropped to a mean of 19.4 mm Hg following percutaneous discectomy.[40]

Disc herniations are classified into three types. A protruded disc implies bulging with an intact annulus. An extruded disc implies that the annulus is disrupted but the posterior longitudinal ligament remains intact. A sequestered disc fragment migrates through the posterior longitudinal ligament away from the disc space.[74] Proponents of percutaneous discectomy advise that its use be limited to disc protrusion only.[52] The majority of surgical discectomies, however, are for extruded or sequestered disc ruptures. Most lumbar disc protrusions have a self-limited clinical course and, rarely require surgical intervention. Percutaneous discectomy must be evaluated against the natural history of a herniated disc to determine its true effectiveness, rather than against surgical series, which include a majority of extruded or sequestered disc ruptures.

Another factor that must be evaluated is the cause of sciatica. It is well known that the size of the herniation is not the sole cause for the pain associated with a herniated disc. Patients with large disc herniations may have a self-limited course without pain recurrence, whereas a small disc herniation may cause intense pain and neurologic dysfunction leading to surgical intervention. Chemical factors as well as mechanical factors must be considered. A chemical radiculitis occurring from breakdown products of the herniated disc or from an autoimmune reaction between the herniated disc and adjacent tissues may also produce the pain associated with a herniated lumbar disc.[25] Adhesions between the nerve root and the disc that cause a traction phenomenon also may contribute to the development of the pain. Percutaneous discectomy cannot completely address these factors because only indirect decompression is performed. Advocates of this procedure claim its simple technique leads to a low complication rate while providing satisfactory results.

Blankstein, et al., reported a case of staphyloccus discitis and osteomyelitis following percutaneous discectomy. Their concern was that organisms introduced into the disc space have no means of drainage because of the small hole made in the annulus and the lack of vascularity to the disc space.[3] Potential risk of nerve root penetration exists when the trocar is not inserted parallel to the disc space and when it is not inserted far enough posterolaterally from the midline. Although local anesthesia allows the patient to respond to an inadvertent needle injection into the root, the damage may have already been done.[40] Another concern of needle insertion is at the L5-S1 interspace where bowel may overlap the desired needle tract. Preoperative CT scans may detect this. However, patient positioning may change the location of the abdominal contents leading to a false scan reading.

The reported incidence of two-level disc herniation is less than 5%.[24] The published series of the results of percutaneous discectomy report up to a 40% incidence of two-level aspirations.[14] Because the disc pressure changes are altered dramatically by insertion of the trocar into the annulus, one can speculate that such pressure changes may lead to premature disc degeneration. Only with longer followup studies can this be determined.

At present, we are evaluating percutaneous discectomy under conditions of central disc protrusion with predominant symptoms, and signs of sciatica not responsive to conservative treatment, and disc protrusion superimposed on narrow spinal canal. The basis for differentiating a *protrusion* from an *extruded* or *sequestered* disc is:

1. Dural sac compression less than 50% of the total dural sac diameter on myelogram or MRI at the level of the disc space.
2. Disc material *not* present on more than three consecutive CT scan slices.
3. Disc material present on CT scan or MRI at level of the disc space only.

The presence of these factors indicates a protrusion, rather than an extruded or sequestered disc, in most cases.

SPINAL FUSION FOR LOW BACK PAIN

Numerous techniques exist for lumbar fusion, including anterior fusion, posterior fusion, posterolateral fusion, posterior lumbar interbody fusion, and fusion with instrumentation. Unfortunately, the types of fusion described are not accompanied by clear indications for fusing an individual with low back pain. The following discussion focuses on the indications for fusion in disc degeneration, spondylolisthesis, and lumbar instability.

Disc Degeneration

Vernon-Roberts and Pirie have clearly shown in specimens of the lumbar spine the normal degenerative process that the lumbar disc undergoes. In addition, disc degeneration in their specimens was often a self-limiting process without progression to further spondylotic changes.[83] Seligman, et al., have shown that in early disc degeneration, the axis of movement is erratic, but as disc degeneration progresses the axis of movement approaches normal, indicating a reduction in motion.[70] Several studies comparing plain lumbar radiographs in normal subjects and those with low back pain found *no* statistical difference in the incidence of disc degeneration.[21,81]

Surgical series reporting results of fusion for low back pain caused by disc degeneration have demonstrated uniformly poor results. Sorenson performed anterior interbody fusion on 98 patients with incapacitating low back pain. Of 95 patients followed 3 to 8 years, 34% reported no pain, 32% reported periodical pain, and 31% described constant pain.[72]

Flynn and Hogue reported on 50 patients undergoing anterior lumbar fusion for low back pain.[19] The results were successful in 52% and unsuccessful in 48%. Successful union occurred in 50% of the patients with good results, indicating that bone union is not necessary for a successful result. Of 7 patients with a primary diagnosis of degenerative disc disease, 2 had good results. Jackson, et al., reporting on long-term results after posterolateral fusion for low back pain, noted only 60% good results for patients fused for a degenerative lumbar disc.[37] Therefore, it appears that regardless of the technique used, results of fusion for a degenerative disc are less than satisfactory.

Spondylolisthesis

Saraste reported a long-term study (20 years) on 255 patients with spondylolysis and spondylolisthesis.[70] In adolescents, progression of the slip occurred with a mean of 2.5 mm; in the adults it was 5 mm. Spondylolisthesis at L4 progressed farther than that occurring at L5. Disc degeneration was present in 20% of the patients at the initial diagnosis. At followup, 50% of L5 spondylolisthesis and 70% of L4 spondylolisthesis were noted to have disc degeneration. Patients with a 25% slip or greater had an increased incidence of disc degeneration. During the observation period, 91% experienced low back pain, with 73% categorizing it as chronic. Disabling pain was reported by 13% of patients. Sciatica was reported in 55%, usually of an intermittent nature. The results of the study demonstrate a higher incidence of low back symptoms than seen in the general population. The risk factors for the development of low back symptoms in patients with spondylolisthesis were 25% slip or greater spondylolisthesis, low lumbar index for an L5 spondylolysis, L4 spondylolysis (listhesis), and early disc degeneration. This study did not address the influence of surgery on this condition.

Harris and Weinstein compared 11 patients treated nonoperatively to 21 patients treated by in situ posterior lumbar fusion for grade III (50 to 75%) and grade IV (75% or greater) spondylolisthesis.[31] The results in the nonoperative group, with an average 18 year followup, were 4 asymptomatic patients (36%), 6 patients with mild symptoms (55%), and 1 patient with significant symptoms. In the surgical group, comprised of 21 patients, with an average 24 year followup, 12 were asymptomatic (57%), 8 had mild symptoms (38%), and 1 patient had significant symptoms. This study points out the satisfactory results of nonoperative treatment for severe spondylolisthesis. In addition, in situ fusion for persistent pain or neurologic dysfunction provides good long-term results.

The results of anterior fusion for spondylolisthesis have been reported by Thomasen.[80] One hundred and twenty patients fused for spondylolisthesis, with the majority having a less-than-50% slip, were followed for 2 to 20 years. Significant improvement in low back pain and radicular pain was noted. Flynn noted similar results in a series of 16 patients with low grade spondylolisthesis reporting an 87% success rate with anterior fusion.[19]

Jackson, et al., noted successful results in 94% of patients undergoing posterolateral fusion for isthmic and dysplastic spondylolisthesis.[36]

Bilateral-Lateral Fusion

The most common fusions are those performed lateral to the facets of the transverse processes. The stripping, performed with an electric knife and sharp periosteal elevators, is continued to the lateral tips of the transverse processes. The transverse processes and lateral aspect of the facets should be decorticated. The capsules and cartilage of the facet joints also should be decorticated to subchondral bone. The facets can then be packed with cancellous bone graft.

Cortical-cancellous and cancellous strips and chips of bone should be removed from the iliac crest (if allograft is not used) and placed over the decorticated transverse processes. Regularly encountered blood vessels which course cephalad and caudal to each transverse process, along the facets, should be anticipated and coagulated, otherwise they can lead to brisk bleeding. Postoperatively, for the most part, a one- or two-level primary fusion does not need strict postoperative immobilization. Refusions should be treated postoperatively with a rigid lumbosacral orthosis.

Posterior Lumbar Interbody Fusion (PLIF)

The most commonly used fusion is the bilateral-lateral fusion, as described above. However, some surgeons prefer a posterior lumbar interbody fusion, because of its potential biomechanical superiority. The technique, however, is somewhat more complicated than that for the bilateral-lateral fusion. The procedure is performed following a complete laminectomy. The nerve roots and cauda equina are retracted, and the disc completely excised using osteotomes, curets, and burrs. Rectangles of cortical-cancellous pieces of bone are then placed from posterior to anterior across into the disc space, bridging the inferior aspect of one vertebra to the superior aspect of the subjacent one. In general, four rectangles of cortical-cancellous bone are required to completely fill and support the intervertebral space. Theoretically, this procedure helps "open" the neural foramen by maintaining "disc space" height. Additionally, it provides some mechanical stability to the anterior vertebral column. Technically, however, the risks of PLIF are higher than those for a standard fusion or laminectomy because of the amount of retraction of the cauda equina required. Additionally, the graft can retropulse into the cauda equina and lead to neurologic deficit. The union rate is the same for PLIF as for bilateral fusions.

Anterior Lumbar Interbody Fusion (ALIF)

To circumvent the risks and technical problems of inserting an interbody graft through a posterior laminectomy some surgeons prefer an anterior lumbar interbody fusion. This, in general, is performed through a retroperitoneal approach. The segmental vessels need not be ligated. The disc space and end plates are decorticated with an osteotome using direct visualization. There is significantly less risk to the neural elements and the dura is not retracted. The bone graft in the intervertebral space is inserted with direct visualization. ALIF, however, requires experience with the retroperitoneal approach, and detailed knowledge of the anatomy and risks associated with this technique.

Posterior Instrumentation

The Harrington rod is the standard instrument that has been used in association with spine fusions for the last 2 to 3 decades. However, there is a high incidence of hook cutout if the inferior aspect of the rod is in L5 or the sacrum. It cannot be used following multiple level laminectomies. When used, it is difficult to recreate the lumbar lordosis that is believed to be important in decreasing long-term back problems. Though a useful tool in the treatment of fractures and deformities, the Harrington rod has limited use in degenerative disc disease or spondylolisthesis.

Knodt rods have been used by some surgeons to supplement fusions in the lumbar spine. They insert from lamina to lamina, and are usually used for posterior distraction. The concept is to open the neuroforamen posteriorly while the fusion is solidifying. Unfortunately, this leads to a flat back deformity (loss of lumbar lordosis), which may cause other back-related complaints. Additionally, Knodt rods are often inserted under the S1 lamina, which is a weak structure and frequently cannot support the instrumentation.

Segmental instrumentation was introduced by Luque using smooth rods and sublaminar wires. This technique allows contouring of the rod and maintenance of lumbar lordosis. The rods can be fixed into the ilium and to the posterior elements of the lumbar spine. If lamina are not present, wires can be passed through drill holes or through pedicles placed around the facets. However, this is technically difficult and structurally not as sound as sublaminar wires. This technique entails a risk of neurologic damage by passing curved wires sublaminally, or adjacent to each nerve root. In the proper setting and with skilled surgeons, however, this is a useful technique. Because of newer instruments this form of sublaminar wire fixation is used less frequently. However, the concept of segmental fixation is important and, historically at least, can be related to this instrumentation system.

Cotrel-Dubousset (C-D) instrumentation is essentially a rod-hook and pedicle screw system. Its major advantage is that multiple hooks can be fixed to a knurled rod. This allows for segmental fixation by many hooks. The risks of passing sublaminar wires are decreased, but there is a significant amount of instrumentation required to successfully master this technique and stabilize the spine or correct deformities.

Currently, pedicle screw systems are being evaluated for use in the lumbar spine. A number of systems are under investigation. All involve placement of screws into the pedicle (from posterior to anterior), and then fixing the screws to a rod, plate, or other means of internal fixation. The pedicles are entered just lateral to the facet joint and medial to the transverse process. The posterior aspect of the pedicle can be visualized by burring away the cortical bone overlying the cancellous center. Using small curets and probes the pedicle can be entered from posterior to anterior under radiographic control. Deviation out of the pedicle can lead to injury of nerve roots, cauda equina, or anterior vessels, or to fracture of the pedicle or bone and loss of fixation. Though the degree of fixation exceeds that of any other form of spine internal fixation, it has not led to a documented increase in the fusion rate nor an increase in the success rate of treating back pain related to degenerative disc disease. These tools do, however, allow great control of each spinal motion segment. At this time, however, it is not clear which pedicle screw systems are required in disorders of the lumbar spine or when they are required, other than for fractures in the lower lumbar spine.

CONDITIONS OTHER THAN DEGENERATIVE DISC DISEASE THAT CAUSE LOW BACK PAIN

The majority of patients with low back pain have pain related to degenerative disc disease or musculoskeletal strains or sprains. However, some may have disabling, though non-life-threatening, diseases such as spondyloarthropathy, whereas a few may have more life-threatening conditions such as vertebral osteomyelitis or tumors. Additionally, some patients have pain referred to the spine from nonspinal sites or diseases such as peptic ulcers, retroperitoneal tumors, abdominal aortic aneurysms, and hematopoietic disorders. Most of the conditions listed here occur in less than 5% of patients with low back pain, but are the more important ones to diagnose or rule out, before standard treatment protocols for low back pain are initiated. For the purpose of this chapter, because the primary focus is on low back pain related to degenerative disc disease, we only review the pertinent history, physical examination, and treatment options.

Infection

Lumbosacral infections can occur in the postoperative setting initiated from a discitis or postoperative wound infection. Alternatively, osteomyelitis or discitis can occur "spontaneously" from hematogenous spread. The latter frequently occurs in intravenous drug users or patients with debilitating medical disorders such as diabetes, leukemia, and renal disease, and in other immunologically compromised individuals. Typically, the pain is constant and less mechanical in nature than degenerative disc disease. It tends to awaken the patient at night. He may have systemic signs such as fever, chills, or other stigmata of systemic illness.

Early in the course of the disease the radiographs may be normal or may demonstrate only mild narrowing of a disc space or irregularity of an end plate. In general, infections tend to cross a disc space and involve two contiguous vertebral bodies. A bone scan may be useful, particularly early, when the radiographs are still negative. CAT scans show multiple levels of lytic destruction, usually in two adjacent vertebral bodies. Frequently, islands of bone remain between lytic areas, which helps distinguish infection from the lytic destruction seen with tumors. Additionally, the CT scan may show surrounding soft tissue edema or an abscess adjacent to the vertebra. Magnetic Resonance Images (MRI) may be helpful in the diagnosis, particularly to demonstrate areas of surrounding edema and early changes within the disc space and end plates. In the laboratory the sedimentation rate may be elevated and the white count and differential may suggest infection. Negative studies, however, are frequently seen in the presence of a spine infection.

The treatment depends on isolating the organism. The work-up should include blood cultures and a needle biopsy of the involved vertebra and disc space. If the involvement is early and the collapse relatively minimal, specific parenteral antibiotic treatment and immobilization with bed rest or a body jacket are indicated. Parenteral antibiotics should be continued for 6 weeks, and some consid-

eration for continuation of prolonged oral antibiotics should be made. If the sedimentation rate or white count do not improve, or if there is a progressive collapse of the vertebra, anterior surgical debridement and fusion should be undertaken. On the other hand, if at presentation the destruction of the vertebra and deformity are significant, a primary surgical debridement and fusion should be performed (if the patient can tolerate the anterior procedure). This should be followed by 6 weeks of parental antibiotics and, if appropriate antibiotics are available, oral antibiotics until bone union is evident. The white count and sedimentation rate should be followed throughout the course of treatment to ensure the infection is under control.

If surgical debridement is undertaken, it should be aggressive and relatively complete. A retroperitoneal approach is useful, debriding as much of the involved vertebrae as technically possible. The bone graft (a strut of allograft or autograft) should be keyed into relatively normal vertebral bodies above and below the area of infection. The surgical results with this technique are good. The bone graft incorporates rapidly and does not appear to be destroyed by the infection. We routinely follow the anterior procedure with posterior compression instrumentation and fusion. Mobilization of the patient wearing an external orthotic is then safe. A Hickman or Brovice catheter should be considered early in the treatment, because the parenteral antibiotics have to be maintained for a minimum of 6 weeks.

Tumors

Tumors do occur in the lumbosacral spine. They can be primary, or metastatic, benign or malignant. The patient usually presents with persistent, if not increasing, low back pain. The pain is often present and, perhaps, worse at night. It may decrease with bed rest. Patients may have symptoms and signs of systemic involvement such as cachexia, weight loss, cough, urinary dysfunction, or abdominal pain. Tumor, unlike infection, tends not to cross disc spaces. Radiographically, a vertebra may have lytic destruction and collapse, although the disc space is relatively well maintained. For most tumors, the bone scan shows increased activity (although it may be normal in myeloma). A CAT scan reveals diffuse lytic destruction throughout the vertebra, and may demonstrate epidural extension. The work-up should include evaluation of any systemic signs of malignancy, with a detailed general medical evaluation (including prostate exam), chest radiographs, liver function tests, complete blood count with white count, sedimentation rate, and serum protein electrophoresis. If the tests do not demonstrate a primary tumor location, needle biopsy of the involved vertebra should be performed. If there is mainly bone destruction, without retropulsion of bone or significant neurologic compromise, and the tumor is radiosensitive (e.g., myeloma, plasmacytoma, or pulmonary), radiation therapy is the preferred and primary treatment. If, however, the spinal cord is involved and the bone is retropulsed, surgical debridement should be considered. If the life expectancy of the patient is greater than two to three years and radiation therapy and chemotherapy can be delayed, bone grafting should be performed along with the debulking and tumor excision. If the life expectancy is less than two to three years, but greater than two to three months, the debrided vertebral space should be strutted with Knodt rods and polymethylmethacrylate or a similar construct with polymethylmethacrylate. (Anterior surgical debridement should not be performed if the patient only has one to two months to live.) This gives immediate stability, and there is no contraindication to postoperative radiation or chemotherapy because no bony union is required.

Benign tumors should be surgically excised and the vertebra bone grafted if stability is compromised. Certain tumors with known recurrences, such as giant cell tumor, may benefit from postoperative radiation therapy, but this should be delayed until some evidence of bone graft incorporation is observed radiographically. Laminectomy (unless the tumor is in the lamina or posterior epidural space) has little or no role in the treatment of tumors of a vertebral body. The primary approach should be anteriorly, where the pathologic process is located.

Spondyloarthropathy

Spondyloarthropathies that affect the lumbosacral spine are primarily seronegative. The patients tend to have mechanically related back pain, but not exclusively. Their pain tends not to improve in 6 to 8 weeks, unlike low back pain related to degenerative disc disorders or musculoligamentous strains or sprains. They frequently have other joint involvement. On physical examination they demonstrate limited range of motion of their spine. With flexion there may be decreased motion and separation between the lumbar and sacral spinous processes (Schoberg's Test). Radiographically, in more advanced cases, a squaring of the vertebral bodies occurs. Marginal or nonmarginal syndesmophytes may be noted. In the early stages, however, the first signs may be erosions and other evidence of involvement of the sacroiliac joints. Therefore, in persistent low back pain, with no evidence of tumor or

infection, a routine radiograph including an anteroposterior (AP) pelvis examination to evaluate the sacroiliac joints should be performed. HLA-B27 will be positive in 95% of individuals with seronegative spondyloarthritis. However, 5 to 10% of the normal population have positive HLA-B27s, and 5% of seronegative spondyloarthropathy patients have a negative HLA-B27 study. Though a marker, it is not diagnostic. The diagnosis of spondyloarthropathy depends on the history, physical examination, and radiographs showing evidence of S1 joint involvement, ligamentous calcification, or squaring and alternations of the vertebral bodies.

Other Causes of Low Back Pain

There are, of course, a number of other causes of low back pain. In persistent back pain, which is present beyond the expected time for recovery, particularly in individuals without litigation, medical, legal, or psychosocial concerns, one should consider other conditions as a cause for persistent low back pain. Peptic ulcer disease, aortic aneurysms, colitis, retroperitoneal or pelvic tumors, infections, subphrenic abscesses, and genitourinary disorders (prostatic, ovarian, or uterine), to list a few, should be considered. In general, screening laboratory studies to include complete blood count with differential, erythrocyte sedimentation rate, a routine chemistry panel, serum protein electrophoresis, and urinalysis should be performed on all individuals with persistent low back pain that cannot easily be explained. Psychosocial factors (narcotic dependence, disability, workers' compensation, and litigation) can also lead to persistent low back disorders. However, the latter, though present, should not be assumed to be the reason for intractable back pain, until other diagnoses are excluded following a detailed general medical evaluation. The best means to rule out the above listed medical disorders are: (1) an awareness of the potential causes of low back pain, (2) a detailed history, (3) a intensive general medical evaluation, with attention to abdominal and genitourinary disorders, and (4) appropriate laboratory and radiographic screening.

REFERENCES

1. Agre, K., et al.: Chymodiactin post-marketing surveillance. Spine 9:479–485, 1984.
2. Arnoldi, C.C., et al.: Lumbar spinal stenosis and nerve root entrapment syndromes: definition and classification. Clin Orthop 115:4, 1976.
3. Blankstein, A., et al.: Disc space infection and vertebral osteomyelitis as a complication of percutaneous lateral discectomy. Clin Orthop 225:234–237, 1987.

4. Boccanera, L., Laus, M.: Cauda equina syndrome following lumbar spinal stenosis surgery. Spine *12*(7):712–715, 1987.
5. Brown, M.D.: Paraplegia following chymopapain injection. A case report (letter). J Bone Joint Surg *67*A(3):504, 1985.
6. Brown, M., Currier, B.: Chemonucleolysis. *In* Lumbar Disc Disease. Chicago, International Society for the Study of the Lumbar Spine, 1989.
7. Brown, M., Lockwood, S.: Degenerative spondylolisthesis. *In* Academy of Orthopaedic Surgeons: Instructional Course Lecture. *28*:162–169, 1983.
8. Cauchoix, J., Ficat, C., Girard, B.: Repeat surgery after disc excision. Spine *3*(3):256–289, 1978.
9. Chemonucleolysis Update. Product literature by Boots-Flint, Inc., 1988.
10. Crawshaw, C., et al.: A comparison of surgery and chemonucleolysis in the treatment of sciatica: a prospective randomized trial. Spine *9*:195, 1984.
11. Crock, H.V.: Anterior lumbar interbody fusion. Clin Orthop *165*:157–163, 1982.
12. Dabezies, E., et al.: Safety and efficacy of chymopapain in the treatment of sciatica due to a herniated nucleus pulposus. Spine *13*(5):561–565, 1988.
13. Dall, B., Rowe, D.: Degenerative spondylolisthesis: its surgical management. Spine *10*(7):668–672, 1985.
14. Davis, G., Onik, G.: Clinical experience with automated percutaneous lumbar discectomy. Clin Orthop, in press.
15. Ejeskar, A., et al.: Surgery versus chemonucleolysis for herniated lumbar discs: a prospective study with random assignment. Clin Orthop *174*:236, 1983.
16. Epstein, N.E., et al.: Degenerative spondylolisthesis with an intact neural arch: a review of 60 cases with an analysis of clinical findings and development of surgical management. Neurosurgery *13*:555–561, 1983.
17. Feffer, H., Wiesel, S., Cuckler, J., Rothman, R.H.: Degenerative spondylolisthesis: to fuse or not to fuse. Spine *10*(3):287–289, 1985.
18. Fitzgerald, J.A.W.: Degenerative spondylolisthesis. J Bone Joint Surg *58*(B):184–192, 1976.
19. Flynn, J., Hogue, M.: Anterior fusion of the lumbar spine. J Bone Joint Surg *61*(A):1142–1150, 1979.
20. Friberg, O.: Lumbar instability. Spine *12*(2):119–129, 1987.
21. Frymoyer, J., et al.: Spine radiographs in patients with low back pain. J Bone Joint Surg *66*(A):1048–1055, 1984.
22. Frymoyer, J., et al.: A comparison of radiographic findings in fusion and non-fusion patients ten or more years following lumbar disc surgery. Spine *4*(5):435–439, 1979.
23. Frymoyer, J., et al.: Failed lumbar disc surgery requiring second operation. Spine *3*(1):7–11, 1978.
24. Garfin, S., Glover, M., Booth, R., Simeone, F., Rothman, R.H.: Laminectomy: a review of the Pennsylvania Hospital experience. J Spinal Dis *1*(2):133–161, 1988.
25. Garfin, S., Herkowitz, H.: Disc disease—does it exist? *In* Lumbar Disc Disease. International Society for the Study of the Lumbar Spine, Chicago, 1989.
26. Gertzbein, S., et al.: Centrode patterns and segmental instability in degenerative disc disease. Spine *10*:257–261, 1985.
27. Goel, V., et al.: Kinematics of the whole lumbar spine: effect of discectomy. Spine *10*(6):543–554, 1985.
28. Gurdjian, E., et al.: Herniated lumbar intervertebral discs—an analysis of 1176 operated cases. J Trauma *1*:158, 1961.
29. Hakelius, A.: Prognosis in sciatica: a clinical follow-up of surgical and non-surgical treatment. Acta Orthop Scand (Suppl) *129*:1–76, 1970.
30. Hall, B.B., McCulloch, J.A.: Anaphlactic reactions following the intradiscal injection of chymopapain under local anesthesia. J Bone Joint Surg *65*(9):1215–1219, 1983.
31. Harris, I., Weinstein, S.: Long term follow-up of patients with grade III and IV spondylolisthesis. J Bone Joint Surg *69*A(7):960–966, 1987.
32. Herkowitz, H.N.: The Role of Fusion in Decompressive Surgery of the Lumbar Spine. Presented at the Spine Study Group 6th Symposium, Palm Springs, CA, Nov., 1988.
33. Hirsch, C., Nachemson, A.: The reliability of lumbar disc surgery. Clin Orthop *29*:189–195, 1963.
34. Hitselberger, W., Witten, R.: Abnormal myelograms in asymptomatic patients. J Neurosurg *28*:204, 1968.
35. Hopp, E., Tsou, P.: Post-decompression lumbar instability. Clin Orthop *227*:143–151, 1988.
36. Jackson, R.K., Boston, D.A., Edge, A.J.: Lateral mass fusion: a prospective study of a consecutive series with long term follow-up. Spine *10*:828–832, 1985.
37. Johnsson, K., Wilner, S., Pettersson, H.: Analysis of operated cases with lumbar spinal stenosis. Acta Orthop Scand *52*:427, 1981.
38. Johnsson, K., Wilner, S.,: Post-operative instability after decompression for lumbar spine stenosis. Spine *11*(2):63, 1986.
39. Johnsson, K., Uden, A., Rosen, I.: The effect of decompression on the natural course of spinal stenosis—a comparison of operated and non-operated patients. (Submitted for publication.)
40. Kambin, P., Brager, M.: Percutaneous posterolateral discectomy. Clin Orthop *223*:145–154, 1987.
41. Kirkaldy-Willis, W., Wedge, J., Yong-Hing, K., Reilley, J.: Pathology and pathogenesis of lumbar spondylosis and stenosis. Spine *3*:319–327, 1978.
42. Kiuiluoto, O., et al.: Posterolateral spine fusion. Acta Orthop Scand *56*:152–154, 1985.
43. Kostiuk, J., et al.: Cauda equina syndrome and lumbar disc herniation. J Bone Joint Surg *68*A(3):386–391, 1986.
44. Lamont, R., Morawa, L., Pederson, H.: Comparison of disc excision and spinal fusion for lumbar disc ruptures. Clin Orthop *121*:212–216, 1976.
45. Leavitt, F., Garron, D.C., Whister, W.W., D'Angelo, C.M.: A comparison of surgery and chemonucleolysis in the treatment of sciatica: a prospective randomized trial. Spine *9*:195–198, 1980.
46. Lee, C.K.: Lumbar spine instability (listhesis) after extensive posterior spinal decompression. Spine *8*:429–433, 1983.
47. Lombardi, J.S., Wiltse, L., Reynolds, J., Widell, E., Spencer, C.: Treatment of degenerative spondylolisthesis. Spine *10*(9):821–827, 1985.
48. MacNab, I.: Spondylolisthesis with an intact neural arch: the so-called "pseudo" spondylolisthesis. J Bone Joint Surg *45*B:39–59, 1963.
49. Maroon, J., Onik, G.: Percutaneous automated discectomy. J Neurosurg *66*:143–146, 1987.
50. McCulloch, J.A.: Chemonucleolysis. J Bone Joint Surg *59*B:45–52, 1977.
51. McCulloch, J.A.: Chemonucleolysis: experience with 2,000 cases. Clin Orthop *146*:128–135, 1980.
52. Morris, J.: Percutaneous discectomy. Orthopedics *11*(10):1483–1487, 1988.
53. Mulawka, S.M., Weslowski, D.P., Herkowitz, H.N.: Chemonucleolysis: the relationship of the physical findings, discography, and myelography to the clinical result. Spine *11*(4):391–396, 1986.
54. Nachemson, A.: The role of spine fusion. Spine *6*:306–307, 1981.
55. Nachemson, A.: Advances in low back pain. Clin Orthop *200*:266–276, 1985.
56. Nachemson, A.: Lumbar spine instability. Spine *10*(3):290–291, 1985.
57. Nachemson, A.: Fusion for low back pain and sciatica. Acta Orthop Scand *56*:285–286, 1985.
58. Nachemson, A., LaRocca, H.: Editorial. Spine *12*(5):427–429, 1987.

59. Nachemson, A., Rydeuik, B.: Chemonucleolysis for sciatica: a critical review. Acta Orthop Scand 59:56–62, 1988.
60. Nasca, R.: Surgical management of lumbar spinal stenosis. Spine 12(8):809–816, 1987.
61. Newman, P.H.: Surgical treatment for spondylolisthesis in the adult. Clin Orthop 117:106–111, 1976.
62. Newman, P.H.: Stenosis of the lumbar spine in spondylolisthesis. Clin Orthop 115:116–121, 1976.
63. O'Brien, J.P.: The role of fusion for chronic low back pain. Orthop Clin North Am 14(3):639–647, 1983.
64. Onik, G., et al.: Automated percutaneous discectomy: initial patient experience. Radiology 162:129–132, 1987.
65. Paine, K.: Results of decompression for lumbar spinal stenosis. Clin Orthop 115:96–100, 1976.
66. Posner, I., White, A., Edward W., Hayes, W.: Biomechanical analysis of the clinical stability of the lumbar and lumbosacral spine. Spine 7(4):374–390, 1982.
67. Reynolds, J.B., Wiltse, L.L.: Surgical treatment of degenerative spondylolisthesis. Spine 4:148–149, 1979.
68. Rosenberg, N.J.: Degenerative spondylolisthesis. J Bone Joint Surg 57A:467–474, 1975.
69. Rothman, R.H., Simeone, F., Bernini, P.: Lumbar disc disease. In The Spine, Philadelphia, W.B. Saunders, 1982.
70. Saraste, H.: Long term clinical and radiological follow-up of spondylosis and spondylolisthesis. J Pediatr Orthop 7(6):631–638, 1987.
71. Seligman, J., Gertzbein, S., Tile, M., Kapasouri, A.: Computer analysis of spinal segment motion in degenerative disc disease with and without axial loading. Spine 9:566–573, 1984.
72. Sorenson, K.: Anterior interbody fusion for incapacitating disc degeneration and spondylolisthesis. Acta Orthop Scand 49:269–277, 1978.
73. Spangfort, E.V.: The lumbar disc herniation: a computer aided analysis of 2504 operations. Acta Orthop Scand (Suppl) 142:61–77, 1972.
74. Spengler, D.: Lumbar discectomy: results with limited disc excision and selective foraminotomy. Spine 7(6):604–607, 1982.
75. Spengler, D.: Degenerative stenosis of the lumbar spine: current concepts review. J Bone Joint Surg 69A(2):305–308, 1987.
76. Splithoff, C.A.: Lumbosacral junction roentgenographic comparison of patients with and without backache. JAMA 152:1610–1613, 1953.
77. Surin, V., Hedelin, E., Smith, L.: Degenerative lumbar spinal stenosis. Acta Orthop Scand 53:79–85, 1982.
78. Szypryt, E., et al.: The long term effect of chemonucleolysis on the intervertebral disc as assessed by magnetic resonance imaging. Spine 12(7):707–711, 1987.
79. Tile, M., et al.: Spinal stenosis: results of treatment. Clin Orthop 115:104–108, 1976.
80. Thomason, E.: Intercorporal lumbar spondylodesis. Acta Orthop Scand 56:287–293, 1985.
81. Torgerson, W., Dotter, W.: Comparative roentgenographic study of the asymptomatic and symptomatic lumbar spine. J Bone Joint Surg 58A:850–853, 1976.
82. Tria, A., et al.: Laminectomy with and without spinal fusion. Clin Orthop 224:134–137, 1987.
83. Vernon-Roberts, B., Pirie, C.J.: Degenerative changes in the intervertebral discs of the lumbar spine and their sequelae. Rheum Rehabil 16:13–21, 1977.
84. Vaughn, P., et al.: Results of L4-L5 disc excision alone versus disc excision and fusion. Spine 13(6):690–695, 1988.
85. Watters, W., Mirkovic, S., Boss, J.: Treatment of the isolated lumbar intervertebral disc herniation: microdiscectomy vs. chemonucleolysis. Spine 13(3):360–362, 1988.
86. Watts, C.: Complications of chemonucleolysis for lumbar disc disease. Neurosurgery 1(1):2–5, 1977.
87. Weber, H.: Lumbar disc herniation: a prospective study of prognostic factors including a controlled trial. J Oslo City Hosp 28:36, 1978.
88. Weber, H.: Lumbar disc herniation: a controlled, prospective study with ten years of observation. Spine 8:131, 1983.
89. Weinstein, J.N., Lehmann, T.R., Hejna, W., McNeill, T., Spratt, K.: Chemonucleolysis versus open discectomy: a ten year follow-up study. Clin Orthop 206:50–55, 1986.
90. White, A.A., et al.: Spinal stability: evaluation and treatment. In American Academy of Orthopaedic Surgeons: Instructional Course Lectures 30:457. St. Louis, C.V. Mosby, 1981.
91. Wiesel, S.W., et al.: A study of computer assisted tomography: Part I. The incidence of positive CAT scans in an asymptomatic group of patients. Spine 9:549, 1984.
92. Williams, R.: Microlumbar discectomy. Spine 11(8):851–852, 1986.
93. Wiltse, L., et al.: The treatment of spinal stenosis. Clin Orthop 115:83–91, 1976.
94. Zahrani, F.: Microlumbar discectomy. Spine 13(3):358–359, 1988.
95. Zeiger, H.E., Jr.: Comparison of chemonucleolysis and microsurgical discectomy for the treatment of herniated lumbar disc. Spine 12:796–799, 1987.

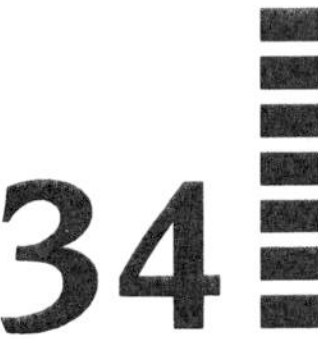

34

Vert Mooney

Surgical Decision Making: A System Based on Classification and Symptom Chronology

Surgical decision making for painful spinal disorders, of course, must have a rationale and conceptual framework to justify the risks and expense of surgery. This chapter, as many others in this book, focuses on activity-related back problems. This section does not discuss surgical need for acute trauma, tumors, infections, and inflammatory disorders. Nor does it discuss the timing for care of ideopathic and adolescent scoliosis. With these exclusions, therefore, two major categories remain for discussion. The first is problems related to spondylolishesis, and the second is problems related to the deteriorating spine secondary to cumulative injury and degeneration.

NONDEGENERATIVE SPONDYLOLYSIS AND LISTHESIS

Spondylolisthesis fits nicely into the activity-related disorders. The classification of Wiltse, et al., summarizes the variations available with this entity (Table 34–1).[1] For the purpose of our discussion, the most important distinction is the recognition that the threat to stability, and thus the potential for persistent pain, is caused by a combination of traumatic and developmental characteristics.

This classification for spondylolisthesis was presented in 1976.[2] This classification recognized that a type of spondylolisthesis occurs soon after birth that is secondary to lack of development of the support-

ing joints at the L5-S1 and is called dysplastic. This is seen on x rays.

The second type of spondylolisthesis is called isthmic. It is the more familiar type seen in adolescents. In this type of spondylolisthesis, abnormalities occur at the pars interarticularis, the bony connection between superior and inferior articular facets. These abnormalities are secondary to trauma, perhaps superimposed on boney structures that are slightly predisposed to failure. Radiographically, a defect in the pars is noted. This is apparently secondary to a fatigue fracture that has failed to heal, and thus the bony defect fills with fibrous tissue. This fracture may heal with fibrous tissue and become stable, causing no pain. The second subgroup of the isthmic type demonstrates an elongation of the pars interarticularis. Under these circumstances, the healing potential of the bone has not been exceeded although a slip has occurred, usually of L5 upon S1, thus requiring the pars to be elongated. The third subgroup is secondary to an acute fracture. The instability may not have been manifest yet and there may not be a slit forward. Nonetheless, x rays may show a bony defect and certainly several weeks later the bone scan demonstrates increased bone uptake, suggesting attempted repair. In fact, it is possible to have a fracture caused by overload (stress fracture) that heals with rest and allows return to normal activity.

Decision making regarding the need for surgical care in youthful spondylolysis and spondylolisthesis is often complex. As indicated above, the causes of

Table 34–1
Classifications

I. Dysplastic	Congenital abnormality of the upper sacrum or arch of L5.
II. Isthmic	Lesion of the pars interarticularis. a. Lytic fatigue fracture of the pars b. Elongated but intact pars c. Acute fracture
III. Degenerative	Progressive intersegmental instability.
IV. Traumatic	Fracture or dislocation of the facet joint to allow forward displacement.
V. Pathological	Loss of stability secondary to pathologic destruction of facets or pars interarticularis.

Clasification of various spondylosis and spondylolisthesis according to Wiltse, et al.[2]

spondylolisthesis and spondylolysis are a combination of inherited predisposition and trauma. An example of the inherited predisposition is the higher incidence of this disease in various populations, such as Eskimos.[3] On the other hand, the incidence of spondylolysis and listhesis is greater in various athletes, such as American football linemen and young female gymnasts, who require significant hyperextension to perform.[4] When symptomatic adolescents are seen with the radiographic abnormality of a defect of the pars interarticularis, it is important to avoid the athletic endeavor that caused the problem. In addition, abdominal muscle strengthening should be initiated. Under these circumstances, approximately 50% of adolescent spondylolysis cases resolve before the end of the active teenage years.[5]

Certain skeletal aspects require consideration that may encourage early surgery. For this particular entity, radiographic studies should always be accomplished in the standing, weightbearing position. This tends to accentuate any slip characteristic. Because of the age group being treated, radiographic studies should be kept at the minimum. The slip is defined as a percentage of the superior vertebral body upon the inferior vertebral body forward displacement, usually at L5 and S1. Greater than 50% slip in the adolescents is a significant predisposing factor suggesting significant instability, potentially requiring surgery. Another significant radiographic finding is the sagittal rotation, which is a description of the relationship between the sacrum and L5. A line extended inferiorly from the anterior border of L5 bisects a line extended inferiorly from the posterior border of S1. Greater instability occurs as the pelvis rotates backward while the spine rotates forward, as exemplified by the sagittal rotation (Fig. 34–1A).[1] If an adolescent complains of significant back pain and the x rays show no significant abnor-

malities, a bone scan is necessary to assure that a stress fracture has not occurred. On the other hand, if the x rays demonstrate a pars defect that shows sclerotic changes, especially when seen on tomograms, it is unlikely healing will take place spontaneously, and even the use of a brace for a prolonged period of time probably will not solve the problem. Nonetheless, avoiding the inciting activity may be sufficient to allow the patient to become nonsymptomatic as the years progress. Another radiographic characteristic that would suggest instability and potential need for surgery is rounding of the front of the sacrum, especially if there is a fair degree of sagittal rotation. This suggests that anterior support from the sacrum to the L5 vertebrae is not available. This is especially significant in the younger individual. Females have a greater risk because of the inherent laxity of their tissues in the adolescent era.

Also, patients who have a dysplastic spinabifida seem to be more unstable secondary to diminished posterior support. Actually, the phenomenon of the absence of posterior structures is a safety mechanism that allows a significant forward slip without compression of the spinal canal. On the other hand, when normal posterior elements exist, extreme hyperextension such as on the occasion of surgical care, may indeed cause compression to the nerve roots and paralysis.

If instability persists in spite of conservative care and loss of lordosis is evidenced radiologically by increased pelvic rotation, instability of the superior aspect, and a hot bone scan with associated back pain, surgical care may be necessary. If the bone scan is not active and none of the predisposing radiographic characteristics mentioned above are present, yet the pain remains, what is the possible cause of the pain? In these circumstances, an MRI may show disc changes at or above the involved level. Rarely is it possible to have a herniated disc associated with a spondylolisthesis. It is also possible to have normal appearing discs associated with a spondylolisthesis. The spondylolisthesis and spondylolysis may become stable with a fibrous healing process and one must look for other sources of pain. This must be questioned before an attack on "instability" is undertaken.

The question of instability raises the problem of where the source of pain in adolescent spondylolisthesis is located. Typically, the patient presents with significant hamstring spasm with associated loss of lumbar lordosis and a noncosmetic flat back. Positive straight leg raising is usually associated with a hamstring spasm and often this may be confused with a suggestion of neurologic deficit or at least nerve root tethering. It is thought that perhaps the hamstring spasm is secondary to irritation to the L5

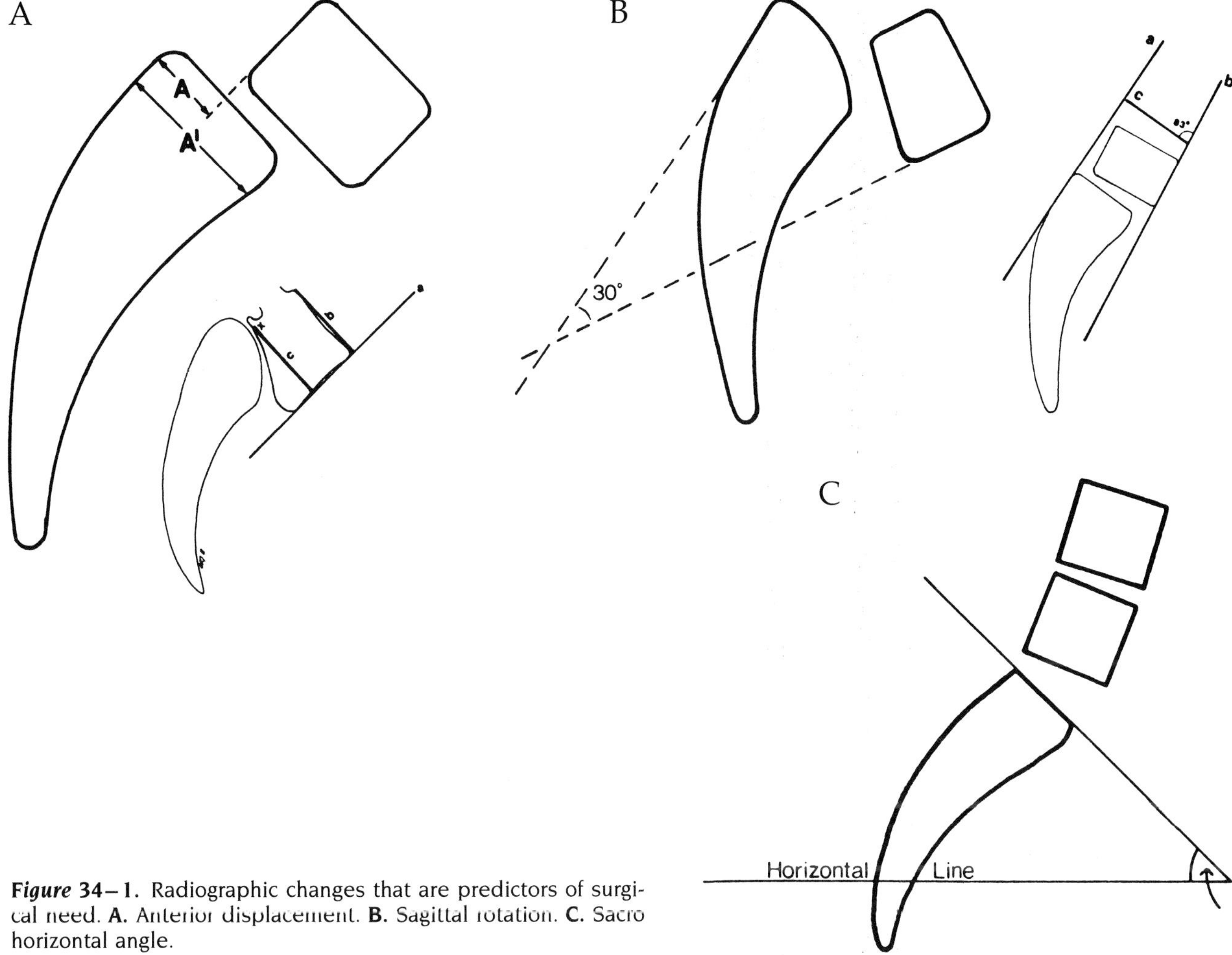

Figure 34–1. Radiographic changes that are predictors of surgical need. **A.** Anterior displacement. **B.** Sagittal rotation. **C.** Sacro horizontal angle.

nerve root or merely an attempt of either body to stabilize the L5–S1 articulation by rotating the pelvis posteriorly. It is clear, however, that once solid fusion has occurred, the hamstring spasm seems to diminish and flexibility of the hips and back returns to normal. It is certainly the fusion that creates this phenomenon and not just the decompression itself. The loss of hamstring spasm usually occurs 6 to 7 months after surgery. It is possible to have nerve root irritation associated with spondylolisthesis. This may be the L5 nerve root that exits at the level of the slip or the S1 nerve root that is tethered over the ledge of the posterior sacrum. A significant controversy exists regarding whether it is necessary to decompress L5 to relieve the irritation. This, likewise, might be considered a justification for the reduction of the slip by surgical approach. Experience suggests, however, that stabilization of the segment is sufficient to relieve the irritation at L5.[6,7] In the case of the S1 nerve root, however, decompression may not occur with the stabilization of the segment. Un-

der these circumstances, the nerve root may need to be decompressed by removal of the inferior articular process after stabilization has occurred.

When we turn to the adult with spondylolisthesis, the problem of deciding whether to operate becomes more complex. Our literature does not clarify the issue of who becomes more painful—adults or adolescents. For instance, in a Swedish population Saraste found a high instance of disability caused by spondylolisthesis.[8] On the other hand, we know that perhaps 40% of normal adults have significant back pain at some time and, therefore, it is hard to assign the back pain purely to spondylolisthesis. In a long-term study of children with known spondylolysis, only 4 of 30 developed significant back pain[9] and in pre-employment x ray studies, incidence of back pain is not increased in those who radiographically demonstrate spondylolysis and spondylolisthesis versus those who do not.[10] Probably it is the degree of slip that makes the difference because, in Saraste's study, those with greater than

25% slip had a greater incidence of back pain over 20 years.

In summary, it is important to evaluate the chronology of pain in the adolescent, especially the athlete. This is a different problem than recent onset of pain in the mature individual with x ray evidence of spondylolysis or even listhesis. Possible change in lifestyle, greater potential for healing, and tolerance of braces, are possible solutions for the adolescent with spondylolisthesis. Currently, we do not have a good predictor of those who become painful when the slip angle is not severe and the sagittal rotation is not significant. Those who fail conservative treatment of rest, bracing, and exercises probably warrant surgical care because the success rate of this particular procedure is the most predicable of all fusion procedures.

In the young adult, however, the questions become more complicated. Because we are not secure about the natural history of spondylolysis and spondylolisthesis, predictors about the future are limited. Frequently, a question arises on a pre-employment examination regarding whether the individual should be hired when radiographic evidence of a defect of the pars is noted. No good evidence exists to prove that a minor slip or mere spondylolysis will progress to be painful. Whether back pain is secondary to instability at the abnormal skeletal location or to other factors cannot be defined. This patient may indeed have purely degenerative back disease and should fall into a different classification of when making a decision.

SURGICAL CARE FOR SPONDYLOLISTHESIS

In spondylolisthesis of adolescence, the decision about whether to operate is based on a different set of factors than for adult spondylolisthesis. Essentially three types of surgical procedures are available. First, is to remove the offending loose bone posteriorly. This is known as the Gill procedure. The only time this might be beneficial is when the segment anteriorly has fused spontaneously, essentially in an adult. This procecure is only useful because it reduces the irritation to the L5 nerve root created by the proliferative repair reaction, but does not resolve the problem of instability. It is rarely used alone today. In fact, the use of the Gill procedure may increase the degree of spondylolisthesis.

The second kind of operation is an in situ fusion. Under these circumstances, one attempts to fuse L5 to the sacrum and L4 to L5, if necessary, by the posterior lateral approach. In this procedure, bone graft is laid across the transverse process and onto the alae of the sacrum. This may be accomplished either by a posterior approach or a posterior lateral approach using a muscle splitting incision.[11] This gives a high level of success, especially in the adolescent because of the inherent good blood supply and healing potential. Also, occasionally the transverse process is so small that it is difficult to fuse the L5 to the sacrum and inclusion of the level above is necessary. Two levels should be fused if the sacrum superior end plate is tilted significantly (>55°) from the horizontal, thus creating severe lordosis and greater instability. This is known as the sacral horizontal angle (Fig. 34–2). Thus, inherent instability potential is called an excessive sacral horizontal angle. In this measurement, which is accomplished using a standing x ray, a line is drawn across the superior end plate of the vertebrae that is slipped and drawn to the horizontal level. Experience has indicated that an angle greater than 55° is unstable and should require fusion of the segment above. This is a more reliable measure of potential instability than the percentage of slip.

The third method of care for spondylolisthesis is reduction of the forward slip and internal fixation with wire, rods, screws, and plates. This is still in its developmental phase and considerable controversy exists regarding the role of reduction and fixation devices.

Evidence is emerging that the longer the duration of stability in the segments below, the greater the potential for failure at the above segments that are not stabilized. Thus, a two-level fusion in an adolescent may lead to a high level of failure at the 3-4 level in later years. Moreover, the stiffer the stabilization of the fusion site, the greater the potential for failure of the mobile segments above. This may occur within several years after the surgical care. The use of internal fixation for adolescents is seldom an appropriate method of care. Probably the most appropriate use of internal fixation is the chronic problem in which the bone scan is no longer hot.

In the chronology of spondylolysis and spondylolisthesis in the adolescent and the young adult we can see the perfect model for mechanical instability. There seems to be a predisposition to the injury; however, it usually is a result of acute or overload trauma. For unpredictable reasons, sometimes the slip increases with the passage of time. When caught early, the slip and the instability can be retarded and even healed by allowing the spontaneous healing of this stress fracture, which we call spondylolysis. Predictors of the progression of disease are based on the angulation of the sacrum and the L5 vertebral body. Surgical care with fusion is highly successful, even if reduction has not been achieved. Reduction is a technical potential that remains in the exploratory stage. The potential for suc-

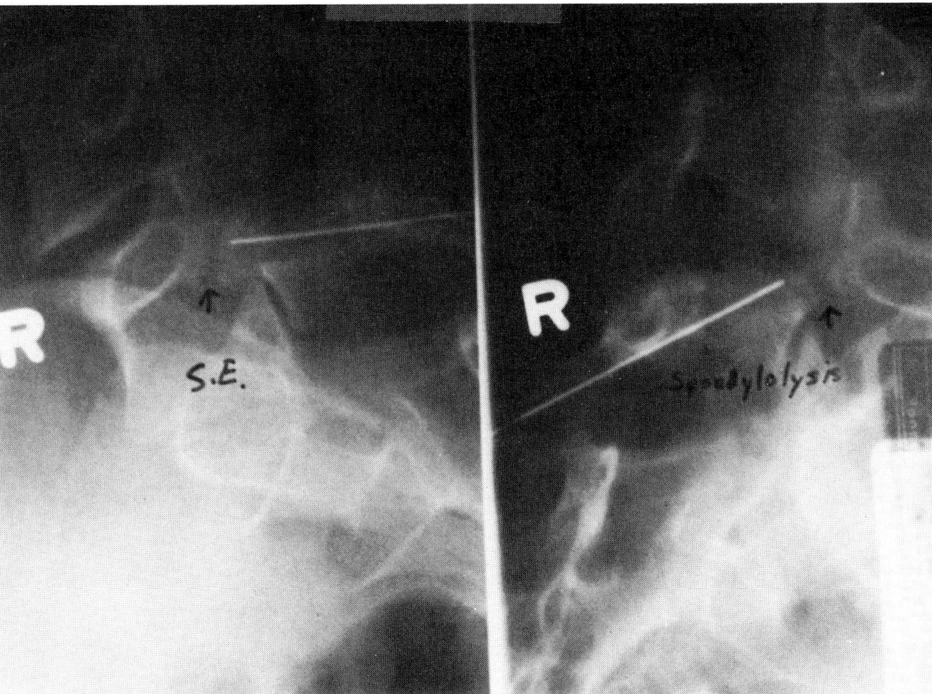

Figure 34–2. Spondylotic defect. Symptomatic status may be confirmed in this older individual by radiographically controlled injection into the defect.

cessful fusion is high based on the positive metabolic characteristics of youth; thus, internal fixation is not necessary. Because the fusion is performed with native bone, with the biomechanical characteristics typical of this bone, the mechanical setting is responsive to the stresses of function and deterioration of the segment above is not an expected natural history. Finally, prediction of the future after the young adult phase is not clear. We have no evidence to indicate that an asymptomatic individual with spondylolysis or spondylolisthesis when discovered in early adulthood is at greater risk for back problems than the population as a whole.

CHRONOLOGY AND SYMPTOMS OF THE DETERIORATING SPINE

The chronology of deterioration has been best described by Kirkaldy-Willis in his description of the cascade of degenerative changes (Fig. 34–3)[12]. This conceptual scheme recognizes the participation of the two major supporting components—the intervertebral disc and the posterior facet joints. It displays the concept that deterioration of one aspect of the supporting structures usually leads to gradual deterioration of the other. Let us first focus on the deterioration of the disc. A historic review of the development of our concept of the herniated disc is valuable.

A herniated disc is an abnormality wherein disc tissue protrudes into the spinal canal and creates noxious stimuli to the nervous system. These stimuli are created by chemical or mechanical irritation of the nerve roots or other innervated structures within the spinal canal. The disc "prolapse," therefore, is essentially a soft tissue phenomenon and should not be confused with pain created by degenerative disease of the facet joints, internal deterioration of the discs, soft tissue tears at other areas of the spine, or systemic problems such as arthropathies, infections, and osteoporosis. Because the disc problem represents a soft tissue injury to living tissue, there is considerable potential to treat the problem earlier before it has become so irreversible that surgery is necessary. Discussion of whether to operate is essentially based on a discussion of failed nonsurgical care.

The Cause of Herniated Discs

In the 1930s, when the concept of disc herniation emerged as a source of sciatica and lumbago, it was a conceptual breakthrough to recognize that soft tissue found at surgery to be protruding into the spinal canal was not a tumor but rather abnormally located disc tissue. The insight occurred when it was apparent that the microscopic anatomic structure of the tissue removed was similar to that of the interverte-

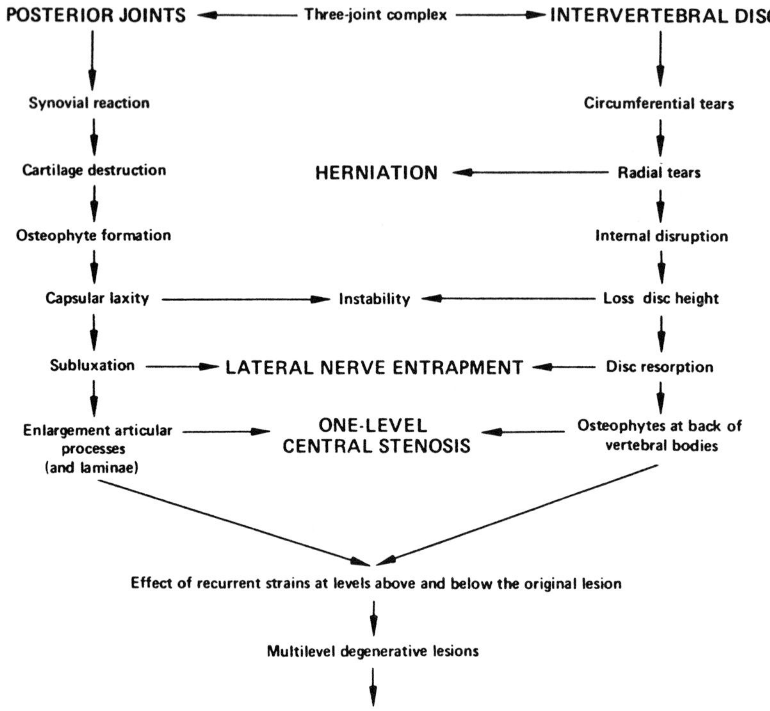

Figure **34–3.** The degenerative cascade according to Kirkaldy-Willis.[12]

bral nucleus.[13] Thus, the framework of understanding easily emerged that the nucleus and a portion of associated encapsulating tissue, the annulus, moved to the periphery. Why this happened in only a few people remains unknown. This conceptual framework is far too simplistic, however. Lipson has demonstrated with sophisticated tissue typing studies that the majority of the protruding tissue is actually repair tissue, and not native to the internal aspects of the disc.[14] In addition, the surgical excision of apparently offending material, which had been defined earlier by imaging studies, does not remove it completely and it persists even after successful surgical care.[13] Thus, we do not seem to really understand the mechanical aspects of the problem yet.

One is tempted to assign the ruptured disc phenomenon as a characteristic of the aging process. But the facts do not seem to support this simplistic view. Even though degenerative changes in the spine, initially seen histologically and later represented radiographically, increase in linear fashion with increasing age, these significant degenerative abnormalities occur at about the same pace that other connective tissues begin to show aging characteristics. Wrinkles of the skin and gray hair are the ever present examples. These changes are most clearly manifest in people in their 50s and 60s. The peak occurrence of herniated discs, however, is in people two decades younger. Herniated discs can occur in adolescents who have no characteristics of

degenerative disease in their connective tissue. The process of aging is essentially a loss of water bound to the soft tissues. However, the typical herniated discs appears normal on x rays. Normal x rays means that the disc heights are normal. Disc herniations occur, however, usually in discs that have less water, as defined by the MRI T-2 weighted image. It is not clear yet whether this implies loss of water or that water is bound in a different manner.

To a large extent, our lack of understanding of early events before a frank disc herniation occurs is secondary to the inability of current imaging techniques to identify what occurs inside the disc. The only method that can identify the processes that occur within the disc is a CT scan of a lumbar discogram (injection of water soluble contrast into disc). The axial view, available only by CT, accurately defines the relationship between the nucleus and the periphery. This invasive procedure is usually not done or warranted on an ethical basis prior to the presentation of a clinical syndrome typical of significant disc disease that may require surgery.

We must assume that the disc herniation occurs in an injured disc. No one has presented information to demonstrate that a completely normal disc can herniate. On a mechanical basis, it seems clear that the injury can occur either by a compression overload or a torsional overload. Farfan, et al., on the basis of cadaver studies and engineering principles, hypothesized that a peripheral tear of the annulus at the outer edge of the vertebral body would be most likely in the case of torsional overload.[15] In fact, Parke, et al., confirmed this event by noting peripheral annular tears in two fresh young cadavers who had normal intervertebral discograms.[16] Thus, the peripheral annular tear would seem to be one link in the chain of events that leads to the prolapsed disc. The circumferential annular tear at the peripheral vertebral body annulus interface can connect with annular radial tears starting from deep within the annulus. This has been noted by investigators studying correlation between lumbar discography in patients and cadavers.[17]

But even if there has been a tear of the annulus, how does that explain the usually posterior displacement of nuclear material? There seems to be no study in the living individual to demonstrate flow of nuclear material. Cadaver studies, however, quite clearly show that posterior herniation and rupture of the annulus can be created by cyclic loaded hyperflexion forces.[18] Interestingly, this event of gradual disc prolapse caused by nuclear material moving posteriorly through, or creating tears of, the inner annulus occurred more likely in the lower lumbar spine in young cadavers. This is similar to the typical clinical presentation. Older discs with pre-existing degenerative changes appear to be more stable and do not have the same potential for flow of nuclear material.[19] Another demonstration of the potential for nuclear flow was presented by Krag, et al., who studied displacement of metal pellets in cadaver discs on the occasion of cyclic flexion loading. Under these circumstances, the pellets, again with repeated flexion, displaced posteriorly.[20] These are demonstrations of the biomechanical events that occur simultaneous to disc herniation.

But why is the disc herniation painful in some individuals and not in others? Unfortunately, there have been few imaging studies on normal individuals, but whenever they are accomplished 20 to 25% of the population demonstrate abnormalities of the disc that would be read as pathologic conditions if the individual were symptomatic. It is not clear why one individual has disc prolapse to such a degree that the nerve root is irritated and another individual, with apparently similar life history of physical events, demonstrates no sciatica secondary to nerve root irritation. One explanation for the differences between the painful disc and the degenerating disc may be the greater hydrogen ion content in the painful disc. It has been demonstrated that the pH in the symptomatic disc is acid, whereas in the degenerative but nonsymptomatic disc, the pH is near normal.[21] This is a surprising finding. It is normal to have elevated lactate acid concentrations in the middle of the disc at some distance from the end plate and its blood supply (Fig. 34–4). In our studies,

painless degenerative discs had a slightly lower pH than normal physiologic tissue (7.1 vs. 7.2). However, this is not the case in symptomatic discs, which have been consistently below neutral when measured on the occasion of percutaneous discectomies. Also, pH in the nucleus of the symptomatic disc is not homogeneous in what would be expected to be a consistent aqueous medium (Fig. 34–5). If we assume that injured or "sick" disc proteoglycans are larger and hold more water, the model proposed by Broom would explain why diffusion is diminished in the symptomatic disc, and thus exchange of metabolites retarded.[22] This model justifies increased cyclic activity to the disc when disc injury has occurred and abnormal proteoglycans are being manufactured. Thus, flexion-extension exercises are justified purely for the benefit of enhancing metabolic exchange by way of improving water diffusion within the disc. This concept also explains why prolonged bed rest with its limited potential for vigorous attempts at fluid exchange is no more effective than brief bed rest. In a randomized study by Deyo of individuals with back pain for several weeks,[23] those patients treated with less than two days of rest were happier with their treatment and got back to work sooner than those patients treated with at least seven days of bed rest. Emerging information seems to indicate that cyclic motion offers the greatest potential for metabolic exchange, and thus the potential to return to normal homeostatic function for the soft tissues.[24]

As stated earlier, the decision to consider surgical care for the ruptured disc most of the time can be based on failure of a treatment program that was oriented to disc health. The natural history of a symptomatic disc herniation usually includes several weeks, months, or years of intermittent back pain before the more prominent leg pain becomes a factor. Our current understanding of the pathophysiology does not allow a clinician to predict which disc presenting early as an intermittent back problem will suddenly herniate and offer the classic symptom complex of an acute disc hernia. Thus, an appropriate method of evaluation is essentially to track response to treatment. Rational treatment of disc disease can offer an opportunity to reduce the incidence of symptomatic ruptured discs. This discussion, however, is irrelevant when the clinical presentation is one of progressive neurologic deficit or cauda equina syndrome. This requires immediate imaging investigation and probably prompt surgical care. This probably occurs in less than one in 1000 patients and the great majority of people with symptomatic ruptured discs or preruptures can be evaluated at a slower pace.

Because it is believed that improved hydration of the disc is an advantage, would traction be benefi-

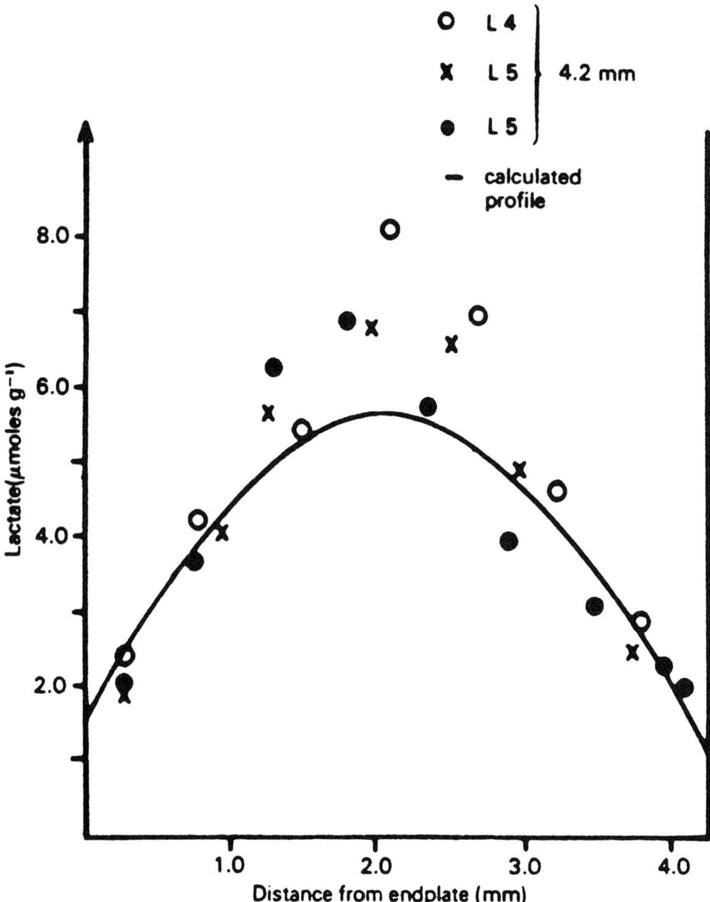

Figure 34–4. Normal diminished metabolic exchange in the intervertebral disc measured in dogs shows an increased level of lactate in the center of the disc. Usually this does not correlate with an acid pH. (Adapted from Holm S., et al.: Nutrition of the intervertebral disc: solute transport and metabolism. Connect Tissue Res 8:101–119, 1981.)

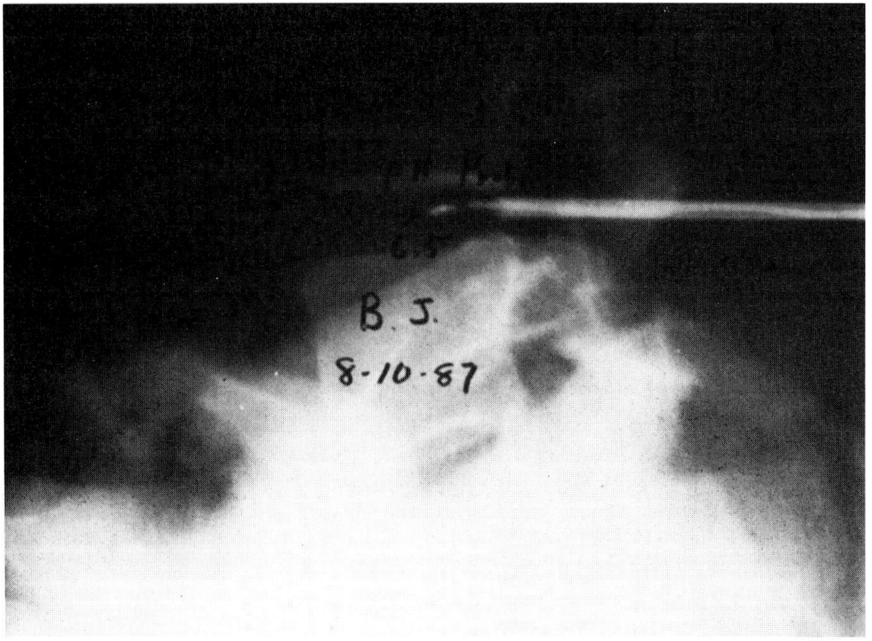

Figure 34–5. The pH is acid in the center of this disc, which is symptomatic and herniated.

cial? Traction is a well established, nonsurgical care that can be accomplished by several modes. In the traditional method, attachment to the pelvis is achieved by a fabric girdle that transfers the distraction force of various size weights to the body while the patient is recumbent. Unfortunately, it takes about 25% of body weight to achieve any distraction force under the circumstance and this is too uncomfortable to tolerate. Smaller forces are generally used, but on this basis, little benefit can be expected other than maintaining the patient in a supine position.[25] Bed traction in the past has been used as an excuse for hospitalization; however, economic pressures have now largely wiped away this method of care.

Several other forms of traction have emerged that use body weight as the countertraction; thus greater dimensions of distraction force are available. One method, known as 90-90 traction, uses the upper body as the weight and flexes the hips and knees 90° with a sling under the buttocks that just raises the body off of the ground by way of weights attached to the sling. In this manner, significant force to straighten the lumbar spine is achieved. This is about one half body weight.[26] An alternative method using body weight has been suggested by Burton[27] that involves suspending the patient in a nearly erect position by means of a corset wrapped around the rib cage leaving the lower body suspended. The individual rests on a tilt table so that gradually greater distraction forces can be created as the individual is tilted into the nearly erect position. The reverse, known as inversion traction, was proposed by Sheffield in 1964.[28] Inversion traction achieves upside down suspension of the patient by means of special boots that allow the patient to dangle freely in an inverted position. Numerous variations on this scheme have been proposed. Unfortunately, little is really proven regarding the efficacy of these various treatments. In a prospective study by Weber, autotraction, which is a self-propelled type of traction, was compared to other passive traction systems and no clear benefit of one versus the other was offered.[29] In summary, traction has been demonstrated to be successful, especially for short-term use. It provides the opportunity to reduce interdiscal pressure and has the potential for relocating the disc material. Overall, it is a safe method, worthy of use in conjunction with exercise programs that are focused on continued efforts toward disc health, best achieved by repetitive motion.

One study has specifically focused on the role of cyclic exercises as a selector for surgery. In these circumstances, the exercises were frequent extension exercises as advocated by McKenzie.[30] The focus of these exercises is to move the leg pain to a more cen-

tral location. This phenomenon itself suggests that biochemical events are associated with the frequent extension exercise—perhaps a change in the pH level. In the first study, 105 patients with symptoms of herniated disc were treated with a conservative 6-week program of bed rest and passive care. All had leg pain. Seventy-five percent of those operated on had either an extruded disc fragment or significantly herniated disc.[31]

SURGICAL CARE FOR THE HERNIATED DISC

The herniated disc is a relatively benign problem and surgical care should pose no risk of additional disability. Proper surgical technique is, therefore, critical. One must recognize that the goal of this operation is to relieve sciatica, not necessarily back pain. Surgical treatment, moreover, should not exacerbate back pain. Spangfort has made a significant contribution in identifying expectations from surgical presentation and surgical care.[32] In the chronology of disc deterioration, this is an early middle age disease that affects the lumbosacral junction first. As is demonstrated by the distribution of disc operations of 4–5 between 5–1, after the age of 45, the 4–5 level is far more likely to be the area of involvement (Figs. 34–6, 34–7). Spangfort also demonstrated that although most patients were relieved of sciatica following disc surgery, 30% still had back pain. This study was based on 2504 patients after disc excisions. Failure to relieve the sciatica was directly proportional to the degree of herniation. Thus, patients with extruded discs had a 90% success rate for relief of sciatica, whereas those with a minimally bulging disc, sciatica was relieved in only 38%.

Currently, the options for excision of a disc range

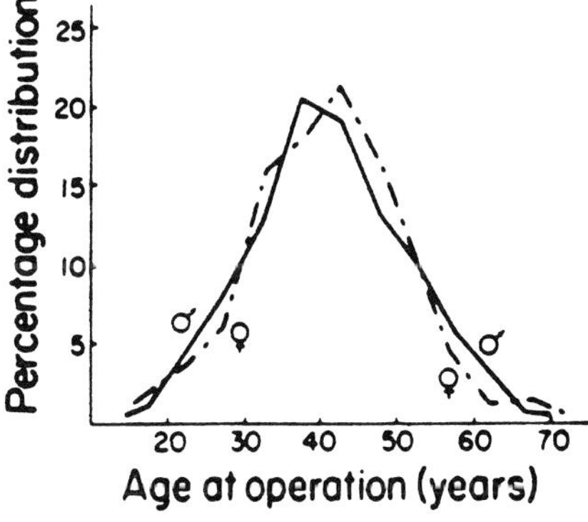

Figure 34–6. The incidence of disc herniation requiring surgery is most frequent in people in their mid 40s.

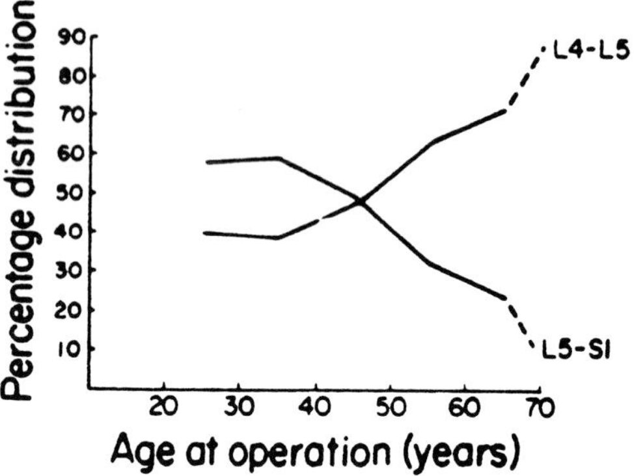

Figure 34–7. Age and level of surgery as defined by Spangfort. (Adapted from Spangfort, E.V.: The lumbar disc herniation: A computer-aided analysis of 2504 operations. Acta Orthop Surg 142(S):1, 1972.)

from the standard laminotomy to microsurgery, to percutaneous discectomy, to chymopapain injection. The methods progress from significant disc tissue removal to a discrete approach. There has been considerable progress in the mechanism by which discs are removed. Surgery in the 1930s was a massive approach that removed most of the bony elements posteriorly and approached the disc by incising the dura both front and back. Later, the approach became smaller and the understanding became clear that the disc could be visualized by retracting the dura and nerve root medially.[33] Nonetheless, because surgical decision making depended upon clinical findings and the imaging studies were so inaccurate, two-level explorations were advocated in the 1930s and even until recent times.[34] As time passed, it became evident that results did not depend upon the amount of disc material excised, rather than potential for decompression. Thus by 1982, Spengler could advocate a limited disc excision.[35]

Another step forward in the "discrete care" of ruptured discs was first advocated by Williams who coined the phrase, "microdiscectomy."[36] This approach was initially created merely to result in a tiny scar, but with improved and appropriately designed equipment, it became apparent that this was a excellent way to treat the herniated disc. Success rate is reported to be 95%.[37] This approach to surgical excision of the disc is discrete because it minimizes soft tissue trauma, avoids coagulation of the muscle, uses no rongeuring of the lamina or facet, and preserves some of the ligamentum flavum and extradural fat. In spite of the small approach, the incidence of recurrences is small (3.9%) with most of those occurring only after significant subsequent trauma. Williams believes the incidence of spontaneous recurrent disc herniations after microdiscectomy is about 1% in a 13.7 year study of 945 patients.[37]

There are problems in initially learning the technique as well as extra costs necessary to compensate for this additional skill. Inpatient time, however, is usually less than 2 days.

An even more discrete approach was reported first by Hijikata.[38] This requires a 5 mm cannula, which is inserted against the lateral annulus percutaneous with x ray control. Kambin used a similar approach with specially designed rongeurs to achieve a greater than 80% success from a posterior lateral approach.[39] An alternative to the 5 mm cannula was proposed by Jacobson and reported by Friedman.[40] This procedure, however, used a larger cannula, the size of a chest tube (10 mm), and a more lateral approach. General anesthesia was required and thus the potential for injury to nerves and blood vessels has been reported. This procedure is no longer performed.

Onik, a radiologist, recognized the similarity between the vitreous material of the eye and the nucleus of the disc, and suggested the use of the tool used by the opthalmologists to remove the material from the eye. The redesigned system for the disc used a 2 mm somewhat flexible nucleotome, allowing for minimal intrusion into the disc. The first operations of this type were performed in 1984. To prevent the potential for nerve injury, local anesthesia is used.[41]

All the percutaneous methods have the advantage of a posterior lateral approach, which avoids the potential of scarring within the spinal canal. They have the disadvantage of being unable to retract into the disc space material that has already extruded into the spinal canal. Actually, whether any of the disc material can be removed from the periphery is questionable. However, a success rate of about 75% has been reported from a multicenter study.[42] This rate is not as high as the success rate reported with open surgical care, rather it is about what has been expected from chymopapain in the past. Apparently, the lower success rate is caused by the inability to achieve mechanical decompression at the periphery in those patients who have trapped fragments. Most researchers report, however, that after failure of suction discectomy, surgical excision of the disc offers an excellent result. The procedure is less expensive than open surgery because the initial cost of the procedure is less and it is accomplished as an outpatient.

Chemonucleolysis

In 1959, the concept of chemical dissolution of the nucleus was suggested by Carl Hirsch.[43] In 1964, the concept was put into practice by Dr. Lyman Smith.[44]

When injected intradiscally, the action of chymopapain is limited to the nucleus pulposus, and has no effect on the annulus fibrosis.[45] Chymopapain rapidly hydrolizes the noncollagenosis peptides and proteins of the proteoglycans. These large molecules are responsible for the water retaining capacity of the disc. The hydrolysis of chymopapain is a rapid action that may reduce interdiscal pressure. No studies are available to identify before and after injection interdiscal pressures. An alternative theory is that the introduction of the alkaline substance, chymopapain, and other agents within the commercial preparation may neutralize free hydrogen ions. It may be that the increase in intradiscal pH from acid to neutral can explain the temporary symptomatic improvement. This is similar to the explanation for the efficacy of intradiscal cortisone.[46] Narrowing of the disc space is routine after the injection, but usually the disc reconstitutes itself. No long-term adverse results have been reported from this change in disc height in the form of degenerative changes.[47] In support of the view that there may be other events occurring chemically, the study by Fraser demonstrated chymopapain superior to a saline injection in relief of radicular low back pain. At 6 weeks, 73% of the patients receiving chymopapain reported their symptoms relieved, whereas in the placebo group only 37% were relieved. At 6 months, these changes had increased to 80% success with chymopapain and 50% with the saline treatment.[48] We need to know why the saline worked at all.

Most articles by advocates of the procedure suggest that success of the procedure at about 80% should be expected from open surgical procedure.[49] An interesting finding reported more recently is that the size of the herniation probably has an important bearing on the efficacy of chymopapain. Herniations greater than half of the spinal canal, or those that are obviously extruded and remote from the intervertebral disc space, are unlikely to have a successful result. Smaller herniations which are not extruded have an excellent potential for a success rate over 90%.[50]

In spite of the potentials for successful care and the lack of potential to create spinal canal scarring, chymopapain has fallen into disrepute secondary to unexplained complications. The rates of complications were relatively small, with a .06% rate of neurologic complication, but a mortality rate of .02% in the initial experience with the newer chymopapain used in the early 1980s.* These rates are less than for open surgery. But some of these complications were unexplained and apparently not based on poor in

jection technique. Because of this, considerable fear of litigation has brought a discontinuation to the routine use of chymopapain. Another adverse effect was an initial increase in back pain following chymopapain use. This no doubt was secondary to a significant structural change occurring in the disc space at the time of injection. More recently, however, a few surgeons with extensive experience in chymopapain continue to use it and find it effective. Wiltse indicates that ⅕ of the original suggested dosage can achieve excellent results and advocates the use of the material in lower concentration.[51]

One of the problems about a procedure that is as simple as placing a needle within a disc space is that a significant potential exists for overuse. Norton emphasized this in a study of Oregon's workmens' compensation system. This study is an expression of community practice.[52] Twenty-nine surgeons performed 61 chymopapain procedures, as well as 44 surgical discectomies for a workers' compensation insurance company. In this population group of 115 workers, because of the high incidence of failures from injections, 72% had an unsatisfactory result and a large number of complications resulted. Many required surgical care after the injection. The average cost per claim for the unsatisfactory result was double that of satisfactory results ($42,000 versus $21,000). This was considerably more total cost for surgical care. Thus, because of the high failure rate of patients treated with chymopapain and the need for surgery after failure of the treatment, the cost of caring for a patient by chymopapain was greater than the cost of the standard surgical approach. This has led many insurance companies to be wary about innovations that are thought to be less costly at the beginning. As usual, the criticism of a procedure that is relatively simple is that the criteria for use of the treatment is broadened to a greater degree than the ideal as presented by the advocates of the procedure. The advocates of the procedure obviously wish to demonstrate efficacy in a significant degree and thus are careful about the selection, so that ultimately they can report favorable statistics. However, in groups of clinicians who do not plan to publish their results and who are working in the community and not necessarily under the gaze of large institutions, overuse of any procedure is possible. This apparently explains the poor results reported by Norton.

In summary concerning the treatment of the herniated disc, creating less damage and destruction is the goal of surgical care. Often, a balance must be reached between expense, risks, and potential for morbidity of a laminotomy versus the lesser success from a percutaneous approach. The larger the herniation, the more likely a classic surgical approach will be successful, but with moderate herniation, excel-

---

*Periodic adverse experience report to the FDA on Chemodiactin: 110,000 VS patients. Fling Laboratories, Inc., Deerfield, IL, 1986.

lent results can be expected from the safe percutaneous approach.

INTERNAL DISRUPTION AND THE PAINFUL DISC

A disc may herniate to the point of internal tearing that allows a gradual progression of nuclear material to the periphery. However, it is also possible for the disc to have torn without progression of the nuclear material to the periphery. This is known as internal disruption and brings into question pain arising purely from the disc with no potential for irritating the nerve roots. This is probably a preliminary phenomenon to a greater degree of degeneration. The incidence of back pain is related to the incidence of annular tears, as is portrayed in the extensive study by Hirsch and Schajowicz (Fig. 34–8).[53]

One of the most controversial aspects of spine care and spine surgery is the source of the pain. Some of the aspects are easily understood, such as instability secondary to skeletal defects such as spondylolisthesis. On the other hand, we know the presence of degenerative changes does not necessar-

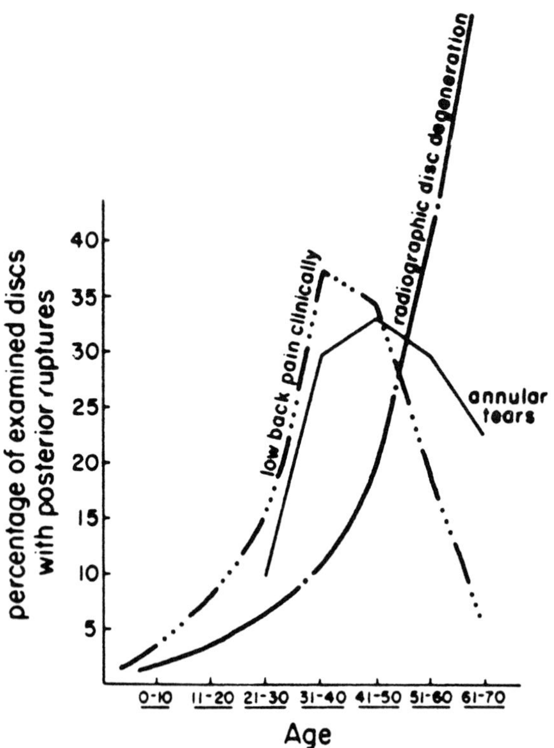

Figure 34–8. The delay of radiographic changes compared to the clinical incidence of back pain. Also, the incidence of annular tears seen by discography in the study by Hirsch and Schajowicz.

ily equal the presence of painful instability. No specific study correlates radiographic changes with back pain or even abnormal motion with symptomatic individuals. Certainly, instability can occur from a mechanical basis, but in most chronic back pain, we cannot identify this.

It has long been demonstrated that discs can be painful. Discography, first described by Lindbloom in 1948, identified the difference between duplicating the same pain described by the symptomatic patient and other pains.[54] The presence of nerve fibers in the intervertebral discs has been well demonstrated. Nerve fibers protrude at least into the outer third of the intervertebral disc.[55] The nerve endings found in the various areas of the annulus fibrosis are not different from nerve terminations described elsewhere in the soft tissues. The nerves derived from the lumbar sinuvertebral nerves of Luschka innervate the posterior longitudinal ligament as well as the posterior annulus. There is considerable overlap of these nerves so that one skeletal segment is supplied by at least the three neurologic segmental levels. Three types of branches have been found to innervate the lateral surfaces of the intervertebral disc. One branch emerges from the ventral primary rami and two branches arise from the rami communicantes, which is derived from the autonomic system. Thus, there is every reason to believe that discs can be painful. It was apparently first demonstrated by Steindler that injection of procaine into the painful disc could abolish back pain.[56] The pain that Steindler spoke of, however, was largely sciatic pain. Falconer, in 1948, induced back pain by pressing on the intervertebral disc doing operations under local anesthesia.[57] No one is really clear why the pain in some discs is significant whereas other discs are not painful. However, it is believed that the organization of the disc is significant. Using CT scan discography, one could demonstrate that discs with more generalized disruption involving all aspects of the discs were less likely to be the source of the patient's specific pain complaint than discs with a nonsymmetric tear into the annulus. This radial tear does not necessarily have to communicate with a peripheral tear to be painful.[58] Still it is not clear what the mediator of that pain might be. Pain could be reproduced by injection of water soluable contrast into the disc (discogram). The pain report was either no pain, slight pain, different pain, or same pain. Only 1.5% of radiographically normal discs in this study were a source of symptomatic pain. In a prospective study comparing symptomatic patients with volunteers, patients had pain at least at one level on occasion of discography, whereas none of the healthy volunteers had pain on occasion of discography.[59] This refutes an older study by Holt,[60] which was performed on "volunteer" prisoners with crude techniques by today's standards. In that study, disc pain was produced in those with normal appearing discography.

An explanation for the pain must reside somewhere in the area of chemical irritation. It has been demonstrated in dogs that changes occur in chemical mediators in the dorsal root ganglions in the segments with degenerative discs versus those with normal discs.[61] Another explanation has been proposed by Mooney.[42] In this concept, the abnormality of the disc is believed to be secondary to limitation of the diffusion of free water. This limitation is secondary to the concept that bound water takes up more space. This would offer a reasonable explanation of why the acid pH that is apparently secondary to build up of waste products that have not been flushed away by fluid exchange is associated with symptomatic discs. It is recognized that acid pH is a stimulus to free end pain fibers to create a noxious stimuli and, thus, pain perception.

Whatever the explanation, there does seem to be an entity of discogenic pain that is not related to mechanical instability.[62] The clinical entity was first described by Crock.[63] In this entity, typically the patient had a history of a significant traumatic event, but the routine studies were normal. The pain was extremely disabling and sometimes spread to other systems in the form of headaches, nausea, and weight loss associated with the back symptoms. The only definition of these particular patients that Crock postulated was an internal disc disruption monitored by discography with note of pain response. The extent to which this syndrome is prevalent in the population remains extremely controversial. A study by Donelson[64] in a group of 87 patients who were treated with extension exercises for back and leg pains found several to require surgical care because of failure of the exercise program. Only one of the 87 was found to have a syndrome typical of disc disruption, as described by Crock.

Great concern exists regarding the potential overuse of discography as a source of explanation for back pain and, thus, the need for surgical care. In Crock's original experience, the only maneuver available to resolve the problem was replacement of the painful disc material by bone graft (anterior lumbar interbody fusion). The early philosophy did not emphasize disc nutrition and health. We now think that physical activity and frequent motion may have been beneficial to the disc and thus reduce the numbers of patients requiring surgical care. Nonetheless, it is clear that in some patients, discs can remain persistently painful, in spite of an effective exercise program. Also, it has been demonstrated that discs may become painful underlying an apparent solid fusion. In those circumstances, surgical care with removal of the disc is necessary and has resulted in successful pain relief after solid fusion of the ante-

rior interbody graft. One question remains, and that is when is it necessary to proceed with the use of an invasive procedure such as discography. Will the arrival of the MRI, which can demonstrate subtle changes within the disc itself, replace the use of discograms? Probably not. MRI abnormalities do not correlate with symptomatic discs most of the time. Also, it is possible to have normal magnetic resonance imaging but have painful discs as identified by discography and their radiographic appearance.[65] Studies in a group of 18 patients with normal MRIs and a CT discography revealed clinical pain reproducing peripheral annular tears.[1] Thus, for the present, there seems to be a role for discography.

In summary, clinical pain reproducing discs can be defined by discography. The presence of a painful disc, however, does not necessarily equal the need for surgical care. Donelson's series is most illustrative in that it represents a series of a general orthopaedic surgeons review of a consecutive series of patients referred for consultation because of persistent back and leg pain.[64] His series demonstrated that most patients can have their problems resolved by an appropriate exercise program. Few, in spite of extreme efforts and enthusiasm, will not have back pain resolved and in these situations surgical care is necessary. This is indeed a small number. Usually, an appropriate exercise program can be initiated early. If it is, it usually is not necessary to consider surgery for discogenic pain. The study by Choler demonstrates that in a large series of industrial injuries, if active exercise programs were initiated early, none went on to have persistent discogenic pain (Fig. 34–9).[66]

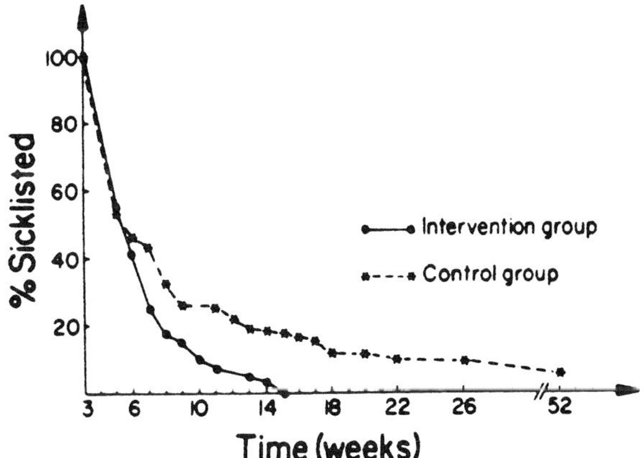

Figure 34–9. In a large group of patients with industrial back pain, early intervention was shown to eliminate the need for surgical care of discogenic pain. (Adapted from Choler, U., Larsson, R., Nachemson, A., Peterson, L.-E.: Back pain—attempt at a structured treatment program for patients with low back pain. Spri Report 188. Spri, Stockholm (In Swedish), 1985.)

With the presence of MRI, we now have a better ability to understand what goes on inside of the disc. Our focus at posterior herniations was largely driven by the potential for surgical care. However, with the axial view seen on MRI as well as the lateral view, herniations at other locations are more easily noted. In a recent study of 145 positive MRI studies, 30% of the peripheral disc extrusions were anterior; 56% were posterior; 14% were central, i.e., extrusion into the vertebral body itself. In a subgroup of this study, all had more severe low back pain than lower extremity pain. The majority of pain complaints were central rather than localized either to the left or right.[62]

THE PLACE FOR SURGERY

In spite of excellent results reported in recent series, does a strong case exist for the long-term benefit of surgical care? In a recent study from Switzerland, experience in long-term followup of neurosurgically treated lumbar disc surgery was reported.[67] In this study of 371 patients, 70% still complained of back pain, 23% complained of severe pain, 45% had residual sciatica, 35% were still seeking medical care, and 14% were receiving disability. One might think this was caused by poor selection. However, the series was divided between those who had excellent operative criteria and those who did not. The operative criteria were: (1) radicular radiation, (2) antalgic posture, (3) positive straight leg raising under 45°, (4) positive cross straight leg raising under 60°, (5) hypalgesia in a dermatomal distribution, (6) muscle weakness in the peripheral extremities, and (7) depressed or absent deep tendon reflexes. In this group, no difference existed in success between those who met all the criteria and a second group who did not meet the criteria. This is startling because between those with classic disc herniations and those with softer evidence for nerve root imitation no difference existed in residual symptoms, need for further medical treatment, recurrences, change of profession, and incapacity for work. The only predictor of success that differentiated the groups was time off work before and after care. Those with sick leave greater than 4 months prior to surgery did far worse than those with less sick leave. This study did not have the advantage of the best imaging equipment, such as current MRI, and perhaps this improves the predictor value. Nonetheless, when the study was analyzed further, predictors such as MMPI and psychosocial abnormalities were more useful in identifying the successful long-term result. The fact that surgical care in itself cannot offer a long-term solution was earlier emphasized by an excellent randomized prospective

study by Weber.[68] In this study, 126 patients were randomized into a surgery and nonsurgical group. It is true that some of the patients had so much distress they had to leave the nonsurgical group to be treated surgically. Although at 1-year followup better results were reported in the group that underwent surgery; at 4-year and 10-year followup, no difference could be identified between the clinical characteristics of either group.

In summary, disc deterioration is demonstrated by circumferential tears and radial tears. Currently, we do not have information regarding the type of tear that occurs first or is more significant. These tears occur at the early phase of deterioration, which Kirkaldy-Willis calls dysfunction. It is clear that in some cases gradual progression occurs, however, which leads to herniation. This disease process in the disc may be independent of deterioration of the facet joints with the gradual progression into instability and later potential for nerve root compression. The fact that disc deterioration may be independent of synovial and facet deterioration was pointed out by Videman, et al., in cadaver dissections. In this study, 20% of cadavers that had normal discograms had degenerative changes in the facet joint.[69] Currently, we do not have a clear understanding how to prevent articular deterioration and degenerative changes in joints. For that matter, it is not clear why some significant degenerative changes are not painful and other relatively minor changes are painful. This is the underlying dilemma in understanding for whom surgery is most appropriate.

Let us return to the Kirkaldy-Willis' disease cascade from the standpoint of the disc. Because of the decision making process regarding surgical need, we must try to define when disc deterioration has occurred to such a degree that irreversible changes have developed and pain is unacceptable. Imaging the diseased structure is important. The current imaging techniques alone even MRI, do not allow us to separate the incidence or occurrence of radial tears from circumferential tears in the disc. Only a CT scan of a discogram (injection of radio-opaque contrast medium into the disc) can determine radial tears. Circumferential tears are only evident from discograms that show the water-soluble contrast material "staining" the vertebral body annulus interface at the disc periphery, indicating a connection between these kinds of tears (Fig. 34–10). We know that not many of these tears are symptomatic. But there is some suggestion that in the earlier deterioration process, the nonsymmetrical radial tear is more likely to be a source of pain than more generalized radial and circumferential tears typical of a degenerating disc.[58] In fact, some evidence now exists that what we once thought was a rather sudden event defined as a ruptured disc is merely the end stage of

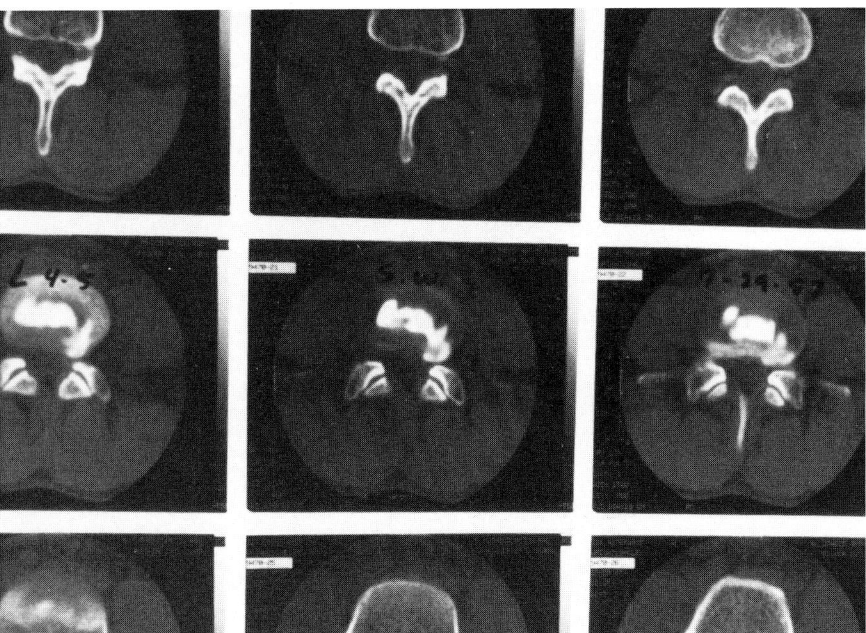

Figure 34–10. A series of computer tomography cuts of a discogram demonstrating the connection of a radial tear with an anular tear at the L4–5 level.

a proliferative healing process. Lipson has shown that the material removed in the so-called herniated disc at the time of surgery for classic ruptured disc is really repair collagen and was not native to the disc itself.[14] This information, however, justifies the expectation that we might achieve soft tissue repair before surgery is necessary.

Currently, we know of no mechanism that will enhance soft tissue repair more than disc nutrition improvement by exchange of fluid by way of motion of the spine. Progressive mechanical stresses also tend to align repair collagen in response to these stresses. Thus, one principle in decision making is that no candidate for decompression of intervertebral disc should have disc surgery until an attempt at cyclic activity to improve repair process has been made. This, of course, assumes that neurologic function is not deteriorating. Such a case would, indeed, require surgical care.

POSTERIOR JOINTS

Simultaneous and perhaps independent of disc deterioration, deterioration of the facet joints occurs. The end stage of this phenomenon has been defined as facet syndrome. There is no clinical picture typical of a facet syndrome, but nonetheless, at the end stage, we are aware that the facet joints deteriorate, instability develops, and the patient presents with proliferative changes that have the potential for nerve root irritation and diminished stability. Currently, we have no way of evaluating the early

phases of facet joint deterioration. Synovial reaction and cartilage destruction are not visualized until abnormal stresses cause bone proliferation and osteophyte formation. Before osteophytes form a symptomatic deteriorating facet joint can only be identified by specific injection of local anesthetic into the joint. If we assume that reactive inflammation occurs at the joint, the addition of steroids should be beneficial.

The potential for the posterior structures to cause pain independent of nerve root irritation was described in the early 40s, first by Badgley.[70] He believed the deterioration of the facets could become painful but erronesously thought it was secondary to lack of symmetry in the joints. Further radiographic studies have not supported this. Inherent in the understanding of this phenomenon is the concept of referred pain, introduced in the late 30s by Kelgren.[71] The concept of pain from the deteriorating facet lay dormant until it was rekindled by Rees in Australia in 1971.[72] Although he proposed a preposterous theory that percutaneous denervation was feasible, and he reported an outlandish success rate, nonetheless, based on the recognized innervation of the facet joints, their potential as a source of pain was clinically apparent. Thus denervation of the joint to control pain would seem reasonable.

The denervation concept was developed by Shealy, who could create dramatic loss of pain using a percutaneous radio frequency thermal destruction tool.[73] A simpler maneuver to reduce reactive inflammation by the injection of steroids was advocated shortly thereafter.[74] Because this is symptomatic treatment for a continuing problem, it is unrealistic to expect that either denervation or steroids can resolve the problem. Perhaps 20% of individuals have long-term benefit from these approaches. Their main value is from a diagnostic standpoint as a means of identifying the chief source of pain. The problem does not become surgically important until deterioration of the facet joint has proceeded to create instability or neurologic embarrassment because of stenotic effects (Fig. 34–11).

Degenerative changes within the spinal canal may cause nerve root irritation to a sufficient degree that decompression is considered. The pathophysiology of degenerative nerve root entrapment is apparently somewhat different than that of nerve root irritation secondary to a herniated disc.

Clinical characteristics of this syndrome are similar to those of the herniated disc syndrome. Back pain usually is not as severe as leg pain. However, con-

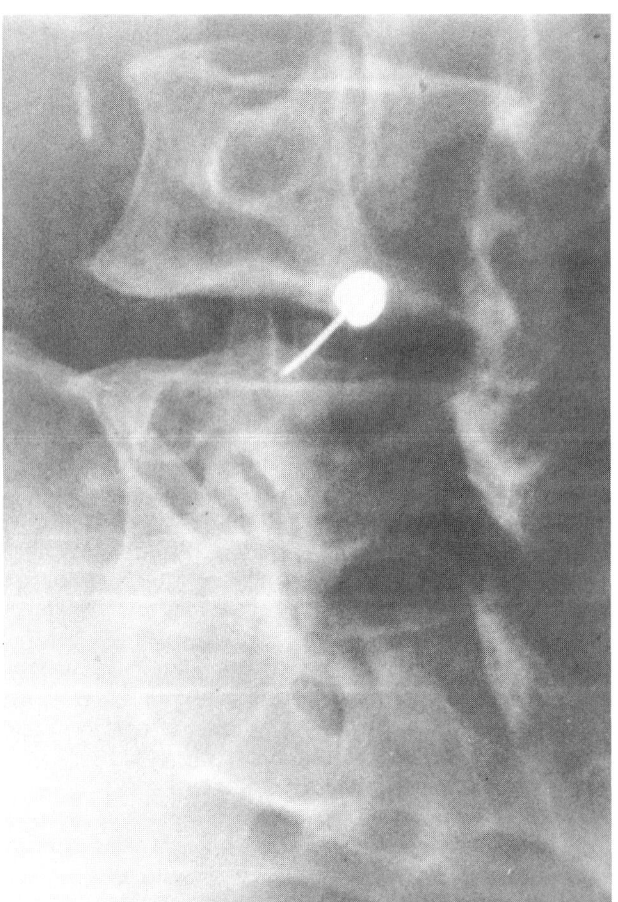

Figure 34–11. A facet joint injection at L4–L5 to identify a symptomatic level. L5–S1 has obvious degenerative changes, and although L4–L5 has reactive changes at the vertebral body, none are noted at the facet joint. Short term relief is expected at the symptomatic joint.

trasted to the herniated disc syndrome, leg pain usually is not relieved by rest. Also, contrasted to disc herniation, only minimal nerve root tension signs exist and straight leg raising is usually better than 70°. The explanation for this finding is the gradual development of the syndrome. The majority of patients are over 40 years of age and the degenerative changes have occurred over years. One of the best epidemiologic studies of this phenomenon was presented by Porter.[75] Out of 2360 patients seen in an English back pain clinic, 11% met the criteria of degenerative nerve root entrapment identified above (249). In contrast, 8.7% of the patients had a symptomatic disc herniation and 6.5% had neurogenic claudication secondary to central stenosis of the spinal canal. Eighteen percent had back pain with referred pain into the legs but not radiculopathy (pain with dermatome distribution).

Another major finding with nerve root entrapment is the limitation to extension. For instance, 84% of the population in Porter's group could bend forward sufficiently to touch below their knees, but 88% had limitation to spinal extension and 25% of the individuals with nerve root entrapment syndrome had no extension at all. Back pain usually was a persistent problem with a prior history averaging seven years. Radiographically, most of the patients demonstrated degenerative changes in the facet joints and half of them had disc space narrowing. Total spinal canal dimensions, however, were normal for the population as a the whole. Appropriate treatment for most was education, a discussion of exercises, and avoidance of excessive stress. Fourteen percent received an epidural injection but in many this was not permanently successful, 9.6% of the patients required surgical decompression. In this conservatively treated English population, the most of the 24 patients who were surgically treated had relief of the root pain, but 6 of the 24 were no better at 1-year followup. Ninety percent of the entire entrapment group were sufficiently satisfied that no other medical attention was sought.

These statistics emphasize the relatively benign and overall relatively infrequent presentation of nerve root entrapment secondary to degenerative spine disease. Nonetheless in those few who do not benefit from either steroid infiltration or educational exercises, surgical improvement can be expected.

SPINAL STENOSIS

An alternative source of encroachment to the nerve roots is known as spinal stenosis. In this syndrome, the spinal canal itself is smaller than average. It was first reported to surgical clinicians in 1954 by Vebiest, a neurosurgeon from Belgium.[76] The syndrome associated with this abnormality is also known as pseudoclaudication. The reason for this, of course, is the similarity in symptom complaint to the symptom secondary to ischemia of musculature caused by great vessel disease. There are significant contrasts, however. In pseudoclaudication, the ischemia is to the nerves within the spinal canal rather than to the muscles. The structure, therefore, occurs in the spinal canal. Because metabolic demand to the nerves increases with activity, it is similar to activity-induced pain caused by claudication secondary to arterial blockage in the peripheral vascular system. In the pseudoclaudication syndrome, however, the pain is improved by rest in a forward flexed position. This enlarges the spinal canal. Frequently, the pain is worse when walking downhill, which requires an increase in lordosis (and thus a slight decrease in spinal canal size) to maintain the upright posture of the head. In pseudoclaudication, bicycle riding is often well tolerated, whereas walking is not. This is not the case for true claudication of peripheral vascular disease.

The syndrome of central spinal stenosis avoided medical recognition for many years because of the somewhat bizarre complaints of the patients. It necessarily is a dynamically induced complaint. It only occurs after activity such as walking and thus when the patient is seen in the physician's office, no abnormality can be defined. No neurologic changes are seen. The patient's definition of the problem often includes bizarre characterizations not complying to normal neuroanatomic distribution. Now with our understanding of the phenomenon of a tight spinal canal, the explanation for these bizarre complaints is due to the somewhat random ischemia created by vascular blockage along the spinal nerves. Thus, a patchy distribution of complaints is reasonable. The description of symptoms may be so bizarre that occasionally the disease process is confused with peripheral neuropathy secondary to diabetes and alcoholism. Of course, central stenosis can overlap lateral entrapment so that characterizations of both complaints may occur within the same patient.

The anatomic definition of the problem is best seen with a CT scan or an axial MRI view. Because the problem is related to the spinal canal size, encroachment can best be seen in the axial view. Here a myelogram often still is beneficial to identify the distribution of the nerves within the dura sac as related to the array of degenerative changes. Frequently, many degenerative changes occur and it is often difficult to identify exactly which are the major source of symptoms (Fig. 34–12).

Surgical decompression for nerve root entrapment and central spinal stenosis is necessary if conservative care has failed. The patient probably will benefit from short-term epidural treatment. The surgical care can be accomplished purely as a decompression, but stabilization may be necessary if too much bone is removed.

DEGENERATIVE SPONDYLOLISTHESIS

Another expression of instability is known as degenerative spondylolisthesis. This is a different disease than spondylolisthesis of adolescence.

It is more common at L4–L5 levels and frequently occurs in women over the age of 40. Because this entity is a type of spinal stenosis, not only narrowing the spinal canal, but also decreasing the size of the nerve root foramen, decompression is necessary. Earlier it was believed that decompression was sufficient to resolve the problem, but emerging experience has deomonstrated that the instability created by the decompression often is sufficient to create symptoms known as a "tired back." Thus, the addition of a fusion on the occasion of the decompression offers a significant advantage.[77] Initially, the fusion was merely a posterior lateral fusion but now with the emerging enthusiasm and comfort with pedicle screws immediate stabilization is more easily accomplished by this procedure (Fig. 34–13).

The radiographic appearance of degenerative spondylolisthesis does not necessarily require surgical care. Frequently, the source of pain is painful overload of the facet joints caused by the incompetent disc. Local steroid infiltration into the facet joints may be sufficient to reduce this pain and allow the patient to return to a more normal physical activity level. Although this does not cure the problem, it must be recognized that many nonsymptomatic patients have x rays showing severe degenerative changes of the back, especially with forward slip at the L4–L5 level. Normal flexibility and strength often can be achieved by the relief of pain temporarily by injection and, therefore, this should be encouraged before surgical procedure is undertaken. Also, spinal canal invasion by proliferative changes secondary to degeneration may be a source of irritation. However, instillation of steroids by means of the epidural route may reduce these pain complaints likewise and allow the patient to become more active. Thus, trial at epidural injection should be undertaken as well.

Both of these treatments should be accomplished in association with a guided exercise program. Nonetheless, if these two maneuvers fail and the pain is persistent, interfering with the patient's life style, surgical decompression and associated fusion is a rewarding procedure. Success rate with this approach is nearly that which might be expected with the fusion for the adolescence spondylolisthesis. More important, the success seems to improve with

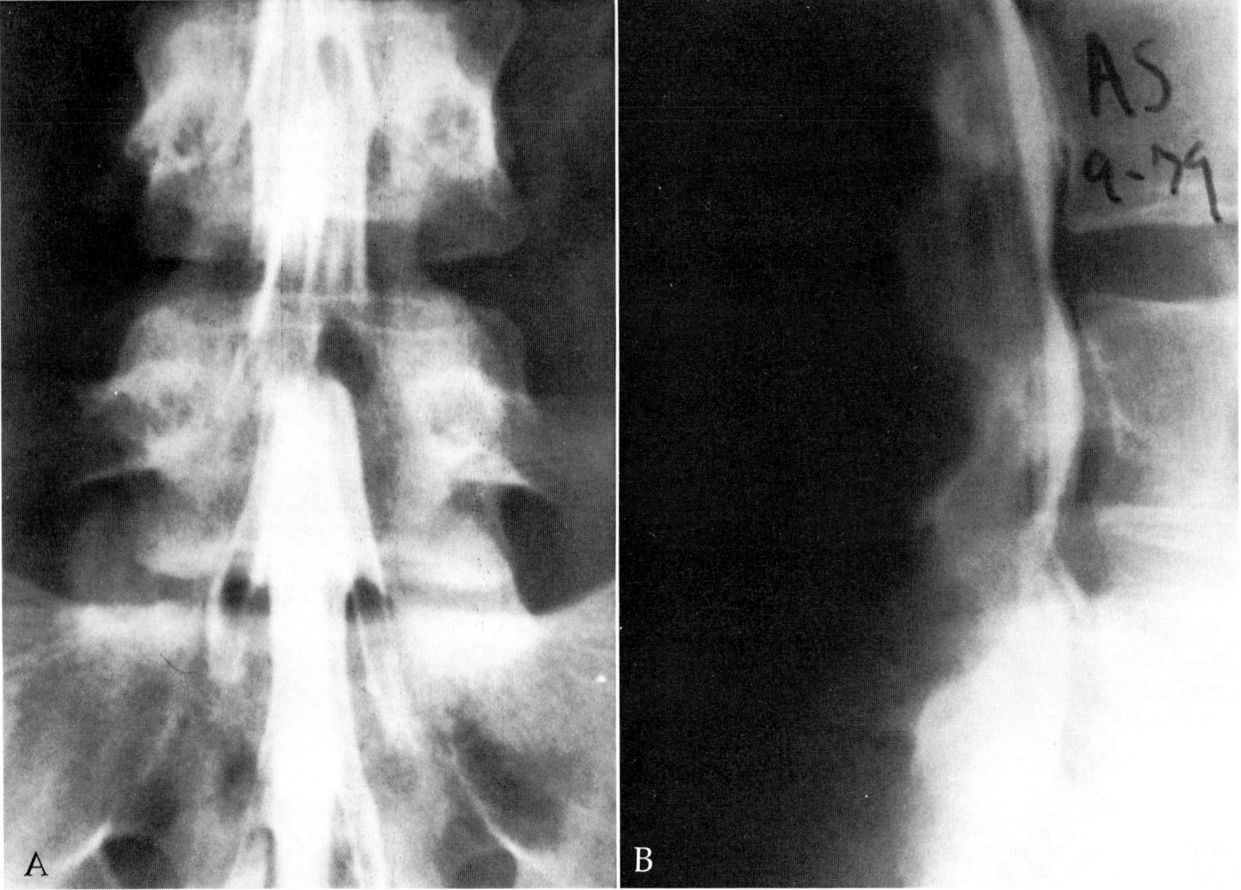

Figure 34-12A, B. Extreme narrowing at the L4–L5 level is noted secondary to a bulging disc as well as reactive changes at the facet joints.

the passage of time. Experience has shown that decompression alone leaves a weak back and the individual generally plateaus in terms of success at the end of a year. However, in the case of the added fusion to the spondylolisthesis, improvement continues after fusion has been solid, and some individuals indicate they feel as fit as they ever were.

DEGENERATIVE SCOLIOSIS

Degenerative scoliosis has a similar cause as degenerative spondylolisthesis. Failure of the motion segment soft tissue connection results in displacement of one vertebral body on the other. The displacement is controlled somewhat by the orientation of facet joints so that degenerative spondylolisthesis occurs readily. However, with nonsymmetric settling of the disc spaces, curvature of the spine develops in the anteroposterior perspective. This scoliosis may stabilize or gradually progress. Currently, there are no predictors of causes or rate of progression. Nonetheless, with increasing distortion of alignment, the stress forces become magnified on the degenerative joints. These gradually fail and allow increasing curvature. Frequently, pain relief is available by various anti-inflammatory maneuvers. Injection into the spinal canal by epidural root or into the facet joints with radiographic control of the steroid injection often reduces the pain considerably for a period of time.

However, if the patient's lifestyle is so invaded by the diminished function caused by increased pain and motor control, surgical care is necessary. Surgical care under these circumstances is often one of the most difficult decisions to make. If the pain is essentially secondary to nerve root entrapment, decompression of nerve roots is available without significant destabilization of the joint. However, when significant back pain is the basic cause of the problem, obliteration of the stresses, especially to the facet joints, is necessary. This is the role of fusion.

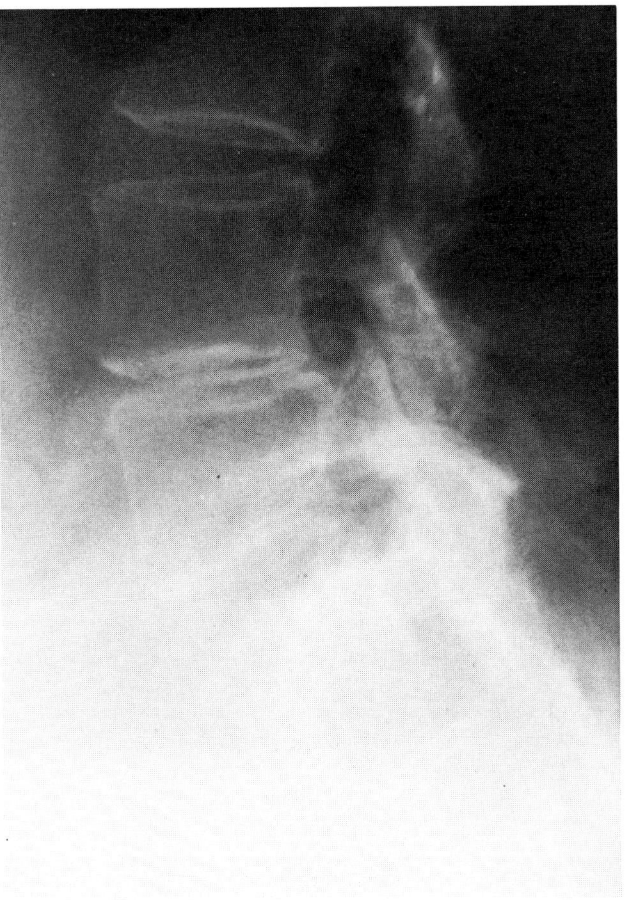

Figure 34–13. Degenerative spondylolisthesis, early in the process. Minimal forward displacement is noted, but narrowing of the disc space is readily identified at the atypical L4–L5 level.

The maneuver of surgical care under these circumstances requires stabilization either after correction of the alignment or by fusion in situ. Correction of alignment is something of a problem because considerable scarring leads to significant tethering of nerve roots, which may be distorted by the realignment. Also, stress to the anterior tissues, including the great vessels, may occur. The problem of stabilization of joints in situ, however, requires specialized internal fixation equipment that is sufficiently flexible on the occasion of implantation to allow curvature as one segment with pedicle screws connected to the next. Apparently, the Wiltse system is the only one that is available to accomplish this maneuver.

This, of course, finally brings us to the question of spinal fusion. When is it appropriate? To a certain extent, the application of spinal fusion is based upon the success of the technique. The development of our philosophy in this area may help to understand the status of spinal fusion today.

METHODS TO ACHIEVE SPINAL FUSION: HISTORIC DEVELOPMENT

The concept of spinal fusion was introduced in 1911. At that time, two basic principals were confirmed. First, deterioration of spinal alignment could be stopped by a fusion.[78] Second, and equally import was the concept that bone graft could be used to fill areas in the spine where nature had only provided soft tissue and the body could heal the graft to native tissue.[79] These were essentially posterior approaches and became the standard method of fusion for the next 50 years. Alternative methods were sought to improve the success rate. In the spine, the largest interfacing bone surface is between the vertebral bodies. Thus, a surgical approach for anterior interbody fusion was proposed first in 1933.[80] The same maneuver—interbody fusion—was proposed from the posterior aspect in 1945.[81] An alternative to the posterior fusion was to use the transverse processes, accomplished by Watkins in 1953.[82]

The final stage in the development of spine fusion was the use of internal fixation. Initially, this was performed just with screws across the facet joint, as proposed by King.[83] This method was tricky and not generally accepted. There are several other opportunities to achieve temporary stability of the spine using internal fixation. The French in the late 1960s first used the concept of internal fixation by connection of screws placed into the pedicles. The idea of placing screws down the pedicle from a posterior approach was first proposed by Jude and applied clinically by Roy-Camille, and later revised by Rene' Louis. The history of this development is summarized by a symposium edited by Leon Wiltse in 1986.[84] Other methods of internal fixation include the use of wires attached to lamina and tightened to a metal bar. This was first proposed by Luque in 1973 as reported in 1982.[85] A specific application of the concept to the lumbar spine using a rectangle with wires to the lamina of the sacrum and low lumbar areas was reported by Dove.[86] A technique for stabilization of the lumbar spine using hooks was advocated by Knodt in 1964.[87]

The modern American era of pedicle fixation was first reported in 1986 by Steffee, et al.[88] Now several systems of pedicle screws and various connector systems are used. Finally, another approach to fusion for low back problems uses nearly all the principals described. This is a simultaneous combined anterior interbody and posterior lateral fusion for multilevel diseases of the low back using internal fixation.[89] This is a procedure essentially designed for failed previous surgery and multilevel disease. It requires, however, an experienced team of surgeons in order to complete the operation in a reasonable period of time.

What principles guide the surgeon to make the appropriate choice from this wide array of surgical approaches to fusion of the lumbar spine? The procedure must be safe and accomplished without excessive complications. In general, the disease being treated is benign and the addition of greater morbidity secondary to the surgical procedure is not warranted. Another consideration of additional morbidity is the subject of bone graft. The massive amount of bone graft necessary to achieve bony union between segments that are naturally mobile is an important consideration. In the earlier history of spine fusions, essentially the only source of bone graft was donor from the patient, usually from the iliac crest. The donor site often becomes a new source of pain. More recently, the use of frozen grafts from cadavers has been advocated. This has the advantage of an availability of a wide array of size, shapes, and characteristics such as cortical bone versus cancellous. Experience suggests that at least for the interbody aspect, allograft (cadaver graft) is as effective as autogenous graft in achieving union.[90] This is not the case for posterior lateral fusions.

A goal of surgical fusion is to minimize complications secondary to the complexity of the procedure. In the most recent review of experience with pedicle screw and plate fixation by a group of surgeons who were not the developers or advocates of the procedure was reported in 1989. Complications arose 27% of 124 consecutive patients studied from 1985 to January 1987. Neurologic deficits occurred in 6% secondary to errors in pedicle fixation. It should be pointed out, however, that after the first 50 cases, there was only one neurologic deficit. As all surgeons report, a significant learning curve exists for this new type of surgery. The wound infections, however, were minimal, with only 1.6% incidence. The rest of the complications were relatively minor.[91]

To confirm the safety of this method, another study presented at the annual meeting of the Academy of Orthopaedic Surgeons presented 200 cases of pedicle screw fixation. These operations were performed without a wound infection and, in this group, only three patients suffered transient nerve root deficits secondary to pedicle fixation.[92] In this group, of those patients who had no prior surgery, 80% experienced excellent relief and 13% demonstrated moderate improvement. On the other hand, those who had failed to improve following previous surgery demonstrated only 35% excellent results and 35% moderate results.

Unfortunately these studies all used short fol-lowups because of the relative recent arrival of the procedure. Opportunities for failure yet exists. Clinical deterioration of the motion segment above the fusion is a reasonable concern. With the older experience using posterior lateral fusion, this incidence of failure above the fusion is about 6%.[93] However, more recent information compared the incidence of breakdown above the fusion in patients with and without internal fixation (in this case, a varying rigid fixation including Knodt rods). Those with internal fixation had a mean of 5.3 years before deterioration occurred, whereas those without instrumentation had onset of symptoms at a mean of about 10 years (2 to 28 years). It has been pointed out that posterior lateral fusion provides the least stiffness of the adjacent unfused segments, whereas an interbody fusion provides the largest increase in stiffness.[94] Thus, there is reason to be concerned about the long-term effect of rigid stabilization on the tissues above a fusion mass.

With these potential problems, why do we perform internal fixation for lumbar spine fusion? Clinical experience suggests that postoperatively the patients who underwent internal fixation have a more comfortable course. This, of course, is similar to the experience of patients being treated with closed reduction versus open reduction internal fixation for fractures. The best older series for success with a posterior lateral fusion is about 80%,[95] whereas the success rate to achieve fusion by other maneuvers is higher. Using internal fixation, it is difficult to truly identify whether a fusion has occurred from a posterior approach. Only the eventual fatigue of screws or loosening of hardware will demonstrate this. For an anterior interbody fusion series, however, success rate may be as high as 95%.[96] It therefore comes down to the higher rate of fusion associated with earlier mobilization, and less hospitalization necessary with the use of internal fixation. Also, the use of internal fixation allows correction of a deformity.

The natural history of a deteriorating motion segment is difficult to predict. Figure 34–14 demonstrates lateral x rays of a 52-year-old female with significant back pain who was advised to have surgical care. Figure 34–14A shows the surgeon's suggested location for the bone grafts. The patient decided to proceed without surgery. The follow up x ray taken 8 years later shows further narrowing of disc space and displacement. This time the patient returned seeking further medical advice. She remains fully active in a sedentary job. She believed that exercises might be beneficial to her intermittent chronic backache and thus was placed on the program. Her only complaint was significant back pain. The width of the patient's spinal canal and neuroforamen have been kept her from progressing into the need for surgical care.

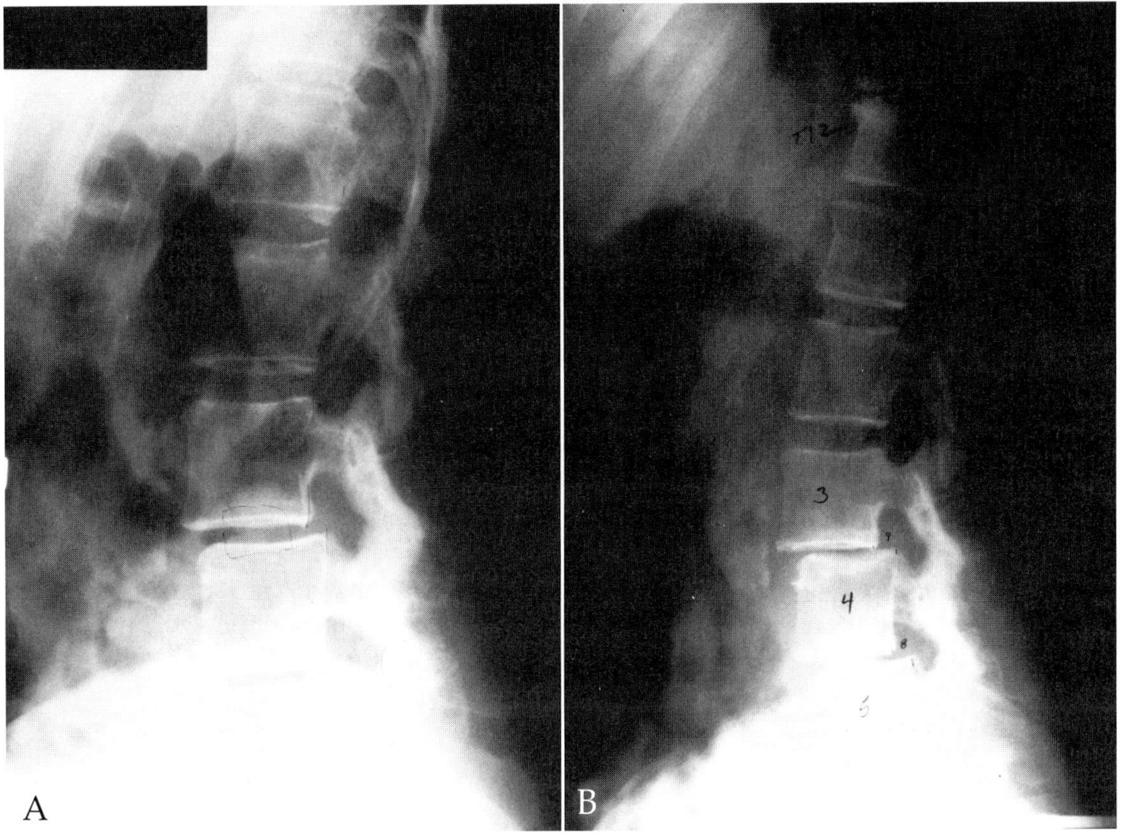

Figure 34–14. A. Degenerative spondylolisthesis at two levels with the surgeon's suggested fusion locations penciled in at the intervertebral space and at the posterior facets. Surgery was not performed. **B.** Progression 8 years later when the patient appeared requesting physical therapy for her tired back.

FAILED SURGERY

One last element should be discussed under the heading of decision making for surgical care. This is related to the causes and solution of failed first operations.

The number of patients with failed first operations may have many causes. First, more surgery is performed for lumbar spine problems per capita in the USA than in any other country. Perhaps double the number of operations are performed in the USA compared to Sweden, Finland and England. Thus, the mathematical potential for failed surgery is greater. In addition, the type of failed spinal surgery is changing significantly because of changing treatment methods.

The most common cause for spine surgery is removal of the disc. When a disc has protruded to such an extent that a nonoperative care program cannot resolve the problem, surgery is justified. Because the operation treats the disease of disc deterioration and does not cure the disease by removal of the protruding material, it is reasonable to expect recurrence. Statistics from slightly older literature suggest that recurrence is in the realm of 10 to 12%.[97–99] To a certain extent, these statistics are on account of the customary method of surgical care at that time. By traditional teaching, the surgical plan was to remove all loose material within the disc space. Often, the surgeon scraped the end plates of the vertebral bodies to gain more loose disc material. In fact, the search for loose disc material deep within the intervertebral space (usually before the days of improved surgical illumination and optical magnification) occasionally lead to intrusion into the abdominal cavity with injury to the great vessels and, occasionally, even fatalities secondary to uncontrolled hemorrhage. More recently, however, surgical removal with minimal exposure, attempting only to excise the protruding tissue, has led to a smaller recurrence rate. The use of microsurgery wherein excellent illumination is available and the use of operating microscopes allow the surgery to be accomplished through very small incision sites, apparently leading to a lower recurrence rate. Williams, the pioneer of this type of surgery, indicates recurrence to be about 2% in his study.[100] Even surgeons using a standard surgical approach, in which only the protruding fragment is removed, report a lower recurrence rate. In a report of discectomies, recurrence rate was 6 out of 93 in a consecutive series.[101]

Probably a more common cause of failure is surgery performed on inappropriate disorder. Because surgical care for disc excision is accomplished for mainly sciatica, but often back pain, the relief of these two components is an important aspect. In probably the largest post-surgical review, Spangfort analyzed the results of 2504 lumbar disc excisions in Sweden. Failure to relieve sciatica was directly proportional to the degree of herniation noted in surgery. Among patients with extruded discs, the most extreme protrusion of disc material, 90% reported complete relief of sciatica with surgery. Whereas when only a minimal bulging disc was identified, only 38% had relief of sciatica with removal of the disc. This confirms that a mechanical-chemical relationship exists between disc protrusion and potential for pain relief.[32] Thirty percent of the patients who were relieved of sciatica still had back pain. Improvement in imaging techniques now currently available to us should change this statistics. The older statistics reported by Spangfort were largely based on a preoperative work-up of clinical findings supported by oil based myelography. Oil-based contrast material did not offer the definition of nerve root orientation that current water-soluable myelography allows. The use of oil-based contrast material created its own problems. It has been implicated as the major cause of arachnoiditis (scarring of nerve roots within the spinal canal).[102] The use of water-soluble contrast material has not been reported to be a source of arachnoiditis. Currently, with our superior systems of investigation, the status of the disc can be more clearly identified by innocuous MRI.

Another reason for past failure should likewise be diminishing. In the study by Burton and Kirkaldy-Willis, about 57% of the problems of failure were secondary to lateral spinal stenosis. This entity is not easily identified by myelography. Symptoms of lateral spinal stenosis (nerve root entrapment) often do correlate with abnormalities in the plain x rays, but degenerative changes of lumbar spine x rays in the older age group are so nonspecific that it is difficult to make the diagnosis from normal x rays. Now the CT scan makes it possible to clearly identify narrowing within the neuroforamen under the facet joints.[103] Thus, the failure of recognition of narrowing laterally in the past has made up for over half of the problems but the incidence should be improved with better imaging. Surgical decompression can be

accomplished but, because of the gradual chronicity of the problem, it is not always successful.[75] Chronic scarring about the nerve roots resulting after years of impingment cannot always be relieved by decompression. Also, decompression of the nerve root canal may require the removal of so much bone that the system is destabilized. This brings into question the need for surgical care in the form of additional fusion surgery. The fusion surgery now is usually accomplished with the addition of internal fixation. As mentioned elsewhere, the surgical experience with pedicle screw fixation is so new that experience has not defined exactly those patients who require surgical stabilization. In fact, this often cannot be predicted until the occasion of surgical care.

Central stenosis secondary to congenitally small dimensions of the spinal canal or induced by proliferative overgrowth above pre-existing fusion accounts for about 10% of the failures.[97] This incidence, however, will increase with the increased use of rigid internal fixation to achieve stabilization for lumbar fusion. Breakdown of the segment above must be expected in an increasing percentage of patients. The breakdown will be greater in younger patients and in those who underwent a greater number of segments fusions.

The role of spinal scarring is difficult to assess. As indicated above, lumbosacral adhesive arachnoiditis occurs because of scarring within the dural sac. In this disease, the nerve roots begin to clump around the periphery and become adherent to the dura. This may be secondary to hemorrhage, inflammation, and reaction from contrast material.[102] Its occurrence rate in a large series of 800 failed back operations was about 10%. Surgical relief of this condition is extremely difficult. Any approach that attempts to remove scar surgically must contend with the physiologic fact that scar replaces scar. Thus, although short-term relief from excision of scar usually occurs, long-term relief for this type of problem seldom is possible.

The only maneuver that seems to offer some potential for success is the use of chronic electrical stimulation. This stimulation is achieved by the implantation of electrodes within the central nervous system, which are then stimulated by electrical pulses usually by way of an implanted neurostimulator. Usually, temporary stimulation is accomplished by various percutaneous insertions of electrodes to evaluate whether efficacy is possible. Reports from this type of treatment are widely varied, but average about 50%, which gradually deteriorates over time.[104]

Epidural fibrosis is another problem. This occurs secondary to scarring after surgery or trauma in the extradural space. Here again, surgery cannot be accomplished without the potential for more scar. It remains a large question, however, as to what role scar plays in the generation of pain. This has seldom been investigated carefully. When an operation is performed for failed back surgery, scar is noted and it is assumed that its presence contributes to the pain problem. Usually, no reason exists to investigate successful surgery, and thus we have no understanding of the presence of scar when there is no pain.

However, such a study has been accomplished.[105] In this study, CT scans were done preoperatively as well as 1 week and 7 weeks after successful surgery. In 85% of these successful cases, major changes occurred in the spinal canal with complete occlusion of the extradural space on the operated side as evidenced by by scan density material, which persisted into the seventh week. This material apparently was scar and will remain indefinitely.

This report confirms the clinical reality that all scar is not painful. Nonetheless, in the large Burton study, the presence of epidural fibrosis was thought to be the source of persistent pain in 7% of those with failed previous surgery. The solution for the formation of scar has been the implantation of fat grafts, which can obliterate scar formation in the post-surgical state. In these circumstances, the "dead space" posterior to the dural sac and nerve roots is filled with fat that has been grafted from the buttocks or surrounding subcutaneous tissue. Unfortunately, this approach does not resolve the problem of scar forming anterior to the dural sac with proliferation into the posterior spinal canal from surgical sites in the disc. This probably is the more significant location of scar formation because later it can harden to firm induration or even calcify.[106] At the present time, there seems to be no clear understanding of the role of epidural fibrosis as the source of pain. The amount of epidural fibrosis that is seen at autopsy in individuals having no significant pain complaints in a radicular orientation suggests that factors other than purely the presence of scar itself must exist to cause persistent pain.

Failed back surgery may result from failed diagnosis.[107] This was perhaps more common in an era before the sophisticated diagnostic tools that are available to us. Now with the bone scan, presence of tumor or infection is highly unlikely to escape preoperative diagnosis. With the presence of the MRI, even tumors within the spinal canal can be identified. Various metabolic studies can rule out inflammation such as ankylosing spondylitis. Infection should be easily identified because of a clinical picture of persistent pain in spite of position and time, as well as definition from the bone scan. The one area that cannot easily be identified by any specific

test is abnormal illness behavior. The problem with this diagnosis is that its presence probably is linked to the persistence of pain and thus it is hard to identify which is the cart and which is the horse.

In summary, there are various structural sources exist for failed spinal surgery. In a long-term followup of failed surgery for patients seen at least 10 years after the first operation, the incidence of sources was varied.[93] If the patients had previously had fusion surgery, about half of those had pseudoarthrosis as the source of pain. In fact, one had additional slip forward. Recurrent discs occurred in a few, even under a solid fusion. In those patients who had not undergone previous spine surgery, disc recurrence at a different level was half as common as the disc recurrence itself at the old operative site. About a third who failed previous disc surgery 10 years later had developed some sort of segmental instability with persistent back pain.[93]

SUMMARY

The decision making process can be subgrouped into four different categories based on a failure of the repair process. The failure can be basically that of skeletal formation and repair. This is essentially a problem of growth and adolescence. Second, is a failure of disc repair. This is a problem of the middle years. Apparently, the disc develops senescence earliest of all tissues and has the least potential for repair. The third is failure of connective tissue repair. This is a manifestation of the older age group, progressively more severe as associated with aging itself. The problems are related to overgrowth and reactive changes of both hard and soft tissues. Finally, there is the failure of surgical care in the past. This may be based on failure of natural healing potential as well as iatrogenic factors.

Table 34–2 demonstrates decision making of spondylolisthesis and spondylolysis. Appropriately chosen, an excellent result can be expected because of the great potential for healing manifested in youth. Early identification and close followup is helpful in avoiding the severe slips that can become surgical nightmares. Although reduction of the slip is tempting, controversy still exists regarding its value. A definitive answer is not yet available. In the hands of the most skilled surgeons with the most appropriate equipment apparently this is a justifiable maneuver.

Table 34–3 depicts the decision making process in the failure of disc repair. In the previous paragraphs, considerable focus on the pathophysiology of disc failure has been emphasized. This is the area in which early prophylactic care might offer some

Failure of Skeletal Formation and Repair

Problem	Predictor	Plan
Spondylolysis—Failure of stress fracture repair.	Persistent pain after months rest and a cooling bone scan.	Posterior lateral fusion.
Spondylolisthesis—Progressive forward slipping of cephalod vertebral body.	Greater than 50% slip with increasing sagittal posterior rotation of the sacrum. Anterior rounding of the superior surface of the caudal vertebral body.	Usually fusion in situ posteriorly. Reduction is tricky. Fixation seldom necessary.

Table 34–3
Failure of Disc Repair

Problem	Predictor	Plan
Herniation—Nuclear material and annulus invade the spinal canal with nerve root irritation.	Failure of active exercise program. Persistent neural deficits with imaging correlation. Early surgery.	Removal of offending material only with as little additional tissue as possible. Approach may be posterior, microsurgical, or intradiscal.
Internal disc disruption—Pain from the disc annulus secondary to chemical irritation.	Spectacular pain reproduction on discography at usually 1 level. Failure of active program. Significant lifestyle change has occurred.	Interbody fusion. Front and back approach is necessary with stabilization for 2 levels or more.

Table 34–4
Failure of Connective Tissue Repair

Problem	Predictor	Plan
Central stenosis—Developmental small canal made worse by degeneration.	Bilateral dysaethesias limiting walking or standing. General involvement seen best by myelography.	Laminectomy at involved levels. Fusion may not be needed in the aged with facet preservation.
Foraminal stenosis—Degenerative overgrowth of facet, annulus, and end plate.	Radiculopathy lateralized and definable at segmental levels. CAT scan the best tool.	Surgical decompression. Fusion with fixation if >one-third of facet removed.
Degenerative instability—Loss of alignment because of disc and facet incompetence.	Progressive curvature or slip seen by plain x rays with associated incapacitating back pain.	Fusion with fixation front and back probably with pedicle screws.

Table 34–5
Failure of Surgical Repair

Problem	Predictor	Plan
Pseudarthrosis—Lack of fusion following previous surgery.	Smoker, too much early postoperative motion, lack of fixation.	Confirm motion and refuse with fixation.
Recurrent disc—New disc herniation at previous site. Question of role of scar.	Pain free interval after last surgery. CAT scan discogram best tool. MRI with gadolinium also.	Repeat resection of disc and fuse if young or at the L4–L5 level. Percutaneous suction may be useful.
Spinal scarring with intradural and extradural scar.	No pain free interval. arachnoiditis seen by myelogram.	Fusion and bony decompression seldom helps. Behavioral care seems best. Occasionally electrical stimulation.
Incomplete decompression—Failure to remove sources of nerve root irritation.	Better imaging studies. Nerve root injection.	Discrete additional decompression when possible. Fusion probably necessary.

benefit to avoid surgery. The literature emphasizes that when appropriate surgery should be performed, it should be done early to avoid additional spinal canal scarring. Discrete surgery is the most appropriate maneuver. Controversy still exists about the reality of pain arising from the disc itself. There seems no reason to avoid the conclusion that it happens. The problem revolves around the potential to resolve this pain by either an exercise program or by disc replacement with bone graft. This issue is not yet solved. The majority of discogenic back pain problems, however, can be resolved with an active exercise program.

Table 34–4 depicts failure of connective tissue repair. The proliferative changes can effect the nerve roots in the central canal and those in the lateral canals. With growing incompetence of the connective tissue react to repair, true instability can be manifest. It is in this particular area that technical advances in surgical stabilization of the lumbar spine have made their greatest impact. Without the pedicle screw systems, in the past it was impossible to stabilize the severe degenerative spondylolisthesis and scoliosis. We still are a long way off from a total disc replacement, the ultimate answer. Nonetheless, spine stabilization and fusion can offer a great potential for benefit in the aged population.

Table 34–5 demonstrates failures of surgical repair. Many of the factors leading to failure are technical and can only be resolved with greater experience, training, and equipment. The skills required to be an expert spinal surgeon are becoming less widespread as demands of experience and technique grow. The fact that this complex operation does not always result in a happy ending is demonstrated by the large number of surgical failures. The solution to these failures is better selection of a correctable problem, surgeon, technique, and patient.

Decision making regarding surgical care for the painful back is one of the most complex issues in all of surgery. Failure to operate seldom leads to disaster, but alternatively persistent pain lingering from a correctible spinal problem may destroy an otherwise effective life. Unwise surgery may create a disaster. Are the risks worth it? Usually they are. Greater understanding will continue to improve the odds that the quality of life can be improved in those few patients out of the many thousands with back problems who benefit from surgery.

REFERENCES

1. Wiltse, L.L., Winter, R.B.: Terminology and measurement of spondylolisthesis. J Bone Joint Surg *65*A:768–778, 1983.
2. Wiltse, L.L., Newman, P.H., MacNab, I.: Classification of spondylolysis and spondylolisthesis. Clin Orthop *117*:23–29, 1976.
3. Kettlekamp, D.B., Wright, D.G.: Spondylolysis in the Alaskan Eskimo. J Bone Joint Surg *53*A:563–566, 1971.
4. Jackson, D.W., Wiltse, L.L., Cirincione, R.J.: Spondylosis in the female gynmast. Clin Orthop *117*:68–73, 1976.
5. Hensinger, R.N.: Spondylolysis and spondylolisthesis in children. AAOS Instructional Course Lectures, *32*:132. St. Louis, C.V. Mosby, 1983.
6. Harris, I.E., Weinstein, S.L.: Long-term follow up of patients with Grade III and IV spondylolisthesis. Treatment with and without posterior fusion. J Bone Joint Surg *69*A:960–969, 1987.
7. Johnson, J.R., Kirwan, E.O.: The long term results of fusion in situ for severe spondylolisthesis. J Bone Joint Surg *65*B:43–46, 1983.
8. Saraste, H.: Long term clinical and radiological follow up of spondylosis and spondylolisthesis. J Pediatric Orthop *7*:631–638, 1987.
9. Fredrickson, B., Baker, D., McHolick, W.J.: The natural history of spondylosis and spondylolisthesis. J Bone Joint Surg *66*A:699–707, 1984.
10. LaRocca, H., MacNab, I.: Value of pre-employment radiographic assessment of the lumbar spine. Can Med Assoc J *101*:383, 1969.
11. Wiltse, L.L., et al.: The paraspinal sacrospinalis splitting approach to the lumbar spine. J Bone Joint Surg *44*A:532–569, 1962.
12. Kirkaldy-Willis, W.H., Wedge, J.H., Yong Hing, K., Reilly, J.: Pathology and pathogenesis of lumbar spondylosis and stenosis. Spine *4*:319–328. 1978.
13. Mixter, W.J., Barr, J.S.: Rupture of the intervertebral discs with involvement of the spinal canal. N Eng J Med *211*:210–214, 1934.
14. Lipson, S.J.: Metaplastic proliferative fibrocartilage as an alternative concept to herniated intervertebral disc. Spine *13*:1055–1059, 1988.
15. Farfan, H.F., Cossette, J.W., Robertson, J.H., Wells, R.B., Kraus, H.: The effects of torsion on the lumbar intervertebral joints. The role of torsion in the production of disc degeneration. J Bone Joint Surg *52*A:468–471, 1970.
16. Parke, W.M., McCall, M.B., O'Brien, J.P., Webb, J.K.: Fissuring of the posterior annulus fibrosis in the lumbar spine. Br J Radiol *52*:382–390, 1979.
17. Hirsch, C.: An attempt to diagnose the level of disc lesion clinically by disc puncture. Acta Orthop Scand *18*:132–135, 1948.
18. Adams, M.A., Hutton, W.C.: Prolapse intervertebral disc: hyperflexion injuries. Spine *7*:135, 1982.
19. Adams, M.A., Hutton, W.C.: Gradual disc prolapse. Spine *10*:524, 1985.
20. Krag, M., Seroussi, R., Wilder, D., Byrne, K., Traush, I.: Internal displacements from an in vitro loading of human spinal motion segments: experimental results in finite element model predictions. Spine *12*:1001–1007, 1987.
21. Mooney, V.: A perspective on the future of low back research. Spine, State of the Art Reviews, *3*:173–183, 1989.
22. Broom, N.D., Marra, D.L.: New structural concepts of cartilage demonstrated with a physical model. Connect Tissue Res *14*:1–8, 1985.
23. Deyo, R.A., Diehl, A.K., Rosenthal, M.: How many days of bed rest for acute low back pain? A randomized clinical trial. N Eng J Med *315*:1064, 1986.
24. Vanharanta, H., Videman, T., Mooney, V.: McKenzie exercise, back trac and back school in lumbar syndrome. Orthop Trans *10*(3):534, 1986.
25. Quinet, R.J., Hadler, N.M.: Diagnosis and treatment of back ache. Semin Arthritis Reum *8*:261, 1979.
26. Lancourt, J.E.: Traction techniques for low back pain. J Musculoskel Med *3*:44, 1986.
27. Burton, C.V. The gravity lumbar reduction therapy program. J Musculoskel Med *3*:12, 1986.

28. Sheffield, F.J.: Adaption of tilt table for lumbar traction. Arch Phys Med Rehabil 45:469, 1964.
29. Weber, H., Ljunggren, A.E., Walker, L.: Traction therapy in patients with herniated lumbar intervertebral disc. J Oslo City Hosp 34:61, 1984.
30. McKenzie, R.A.: The Lumbar Spine, Mechanical Diagnosis in Therapy. Waikanae, New Zealand, Spinal Publications, 1981.
31. Kopp, J.R., et al.: The use of extension in the evaluation and treatment of patients with acute herniated nucleus pulposus. Clin Orthop 202:211–214, 1986.
32. Spangfort, E.V.: The lumbar disc herniation: A computer-aided analysis of 2504 operations. Acta Orthop Scand 142(S):1, 1972.
33. Love, J.G.: Removal of protruded intervertebral disc without laminectomy. Mayo Clin Proc 14:800–804, 1939.
34. Semmes, R.E.: Diagnosis of the ruptured intervertebral disc without contrast myelography and comment upon recent experience with modified hemilaminectomy for their removal. Yale Biologic Med., 11:433–439, 1939.
35. Spengler, D.M.: Lumbar discectomy: results with limited disc excision and selective foramenotomy. Spine 7:604–607, 1982.
36. Williams, R.W.: Microlumbar discectomy: a conservative approach to the virgin herniated lumbar disc. Spine 3:174–178, 1978.
37. Williams, R.W.: Microlumbar discectomy: a 12 year statistical review. Spine 11:851–852, 1986.
38. Hijikata, S., Yamaghishi, M., Nakayama, T.: Percutaneous discectomy: a new treatment method for lumbar disc herniation. J Toaden Hosp 5:22, 1975.
39. Kambin, P., Gellman, H.: Percutaneous lateral discectomy of the lumbar spine, a preliminary report. Clin Orthop 174:127–129, 1983.
40. Friedman, C.: Percutaneous discectomy, an alternative to chemonucleolysis. Neurosurg 13:542–544, 1983.
41. Onik, G.M., et al.: Percutaneous lumbar discectomy using an aspiration probe: initial patient experience. Radiology, 162:129, 1987.
42. Mooney, V.: Percutaneous discectomy: Spine, State of the Art Reviews 3:103–112, 1989.
43. Hirsch, C.: Studies on the pathology of low back pain. J Bone Joint Surg 41B:237–243, 1959.
44. Smith, L.: Enzyme dissolution of a nucleus pulposes in humans. JAMA 197:137–140, 1964.
45. Stern, I.J., Smith, L.: Dissolution of chymopapain in vitro of tissue from normal and prolapsed intervertebral discs. Clin Orthop 50:269–271, 1967.
46. Sutton, C.J.: Chemonucleolysis in lumbar spine surgery. In Lumbar Spine Surgery (Edited by J.C. Cauthen). Williams & Wilkins, Baltimore, 1988.
47. Flanagan, N.M., Chung, B.U.: Retinographic changes in 188 patients 10 to 20 years after discography in chemonucleolysis. Spine 11:444–448, 1986.
48. Fraser, R.D.: Chymopapain for the treatment of intervertebral disc herniation. Spine 7:608–712, 1982.
49. Javid, M.: Efficacy of chymopapain chemonucleolysis. A long-term review of 105 patients. J Neurosurg 62:662–666, 1985.
50. Postacchini, F., Lamni, R., Massobrio, M.: Chemonucleolysis versus surgery in lumbar disc herniations: correlations of the results of pre-operative clinical pattern and size of herniation. Spine 12:87–96, 1987.
51. Wiltse, L.L.: Personal communication, 1989.
52. Norton, W.L.: Chemonucleolysis versus surgical discectomy—a comparison of costs and results in workmen's compensation claimants. Spine 11:440–443, 1986.
53. Hirsch, C., Schajowicz, F.: Studies on structural changes in the lumbar annulus fibrosis. Acta Orthop Scand 22:184–231, 1952.
54. Lindbloom, K.: Diagnostic puncture of intervertebral discs in sciatica. Acta Orthop Scand 17:231–234, 1948.
55. Bogduk, N., Tynan, W., Wilson, A.S.: The nerve supply of the human lumbar intervertebral disc. J Anatomy 132:39–56, 1981.
56. Steindler, A.: Lectures on the interpretation of pain in orthopaedic practice. Toronto, Charles C Thomas, 1959.
57. Falconer, M.A., McGeorge, M., Begg, A.C.: Observations on the cause and mechanism of symptom production in sciatica and low back pain. J Neurosurg Psych 11:12–15, 1948.
58. Sachs, B.L., et al.: Dallas discogram description: a new classification of CT/discography in low back disorders. Spine 12:287–294, 1987.
59. Walsh, T.R., et al.: Lumbar discography, a controlled perspective of normal volunteers to determine the false positive rates. Presented at the AAOS annual meeting, Las Vegas, Feb., 1989.
60. Holt, E.P.: The question of lumbar discography. J Bone Joint Surg 50A:720–796, 1968.
61. Weinstein, J., Claverie, W.C., Gibson, S.: The pain of discograph. Spine 13:1344–1348, 1988.
62. Jinkins, J.R., Wittemore, A.R., Bradley, H.G.: The anatomic bases of vertebrogenic and the autonomic syndrome associated with lumbar disc extrusion. Am J Neuro-Radiol 10:219–231, 1981.
63. Crock, H.V.: A reappraisal of intervertebral disc lesions. Med J Australia 1:983–990, 1970.
64. Donelson, R.: Centralization phenomenon: its usefulness in evaluating and treating sciatica. Orthop Trans 10:533, 1986.
65. Zuckerman, J., et al.: Normal magnetic resonance imaging with abnormal discography. Spine 13:1355–1359, 1988.
66. Choler, U., Larsson, R., Nachemson, A., Peterson, L-E: Back pain—attempt at a structured treatment program for patients with low back pain. Spri Report 188. Spri, Stockholm (in Swedish), 1985.
67. Dvorak, J., Gauchat, M-H, Balach, L.: The outcome of surgery for lumbar disc herniation. A four to seventeen year follow up with emphasis on sommatic aspects. Spine 13:1418–1419, 1988.
68. Weber, H.: Lumbar disc herniation: a controlled prospective study with ten years of observations. Spine 8:131–140, 1983.
69. Videman, T., Malmivaara, A., Mooney, V.: The value of axial view in assessing discograms: an experimental study with cadavers. Spine 12:299–305, 1987.
70. Badgley, C.E.: The articular facets in relationship to low back pain and sciatic radiation. J Bone Joint Surg 23A:481–496, 1941.
71. Kelgren, J.J.: Observation on referred pain arising from muscle. Clin Sci Mol Med 3:175–190, 1938.
72. Rees, W.E.S.: Multiple bilateral subcutaneous rhizolysis of segmental nerves in the treatment of the intervertebral disc syndrome. Ann Gen Practice 26:126–127, 1971.
73. Shealy, C.N.: Percutaneous radiofrequency denervation of spinal facets and treatment for chronic back pain and sciatica. J Neurosurg 43:448–451, 1975.
74. Mooney, V., Robertson, J.: The facet syndrome. Clin Orthop 115:149–156, 1976.
75. Porter, R.W., Hibbert, C., Evans, C.: The natural history of root entrapment syndrome. Spine 9:418–421, 1984.
76. Vebiest, H.: A radicular syndrome from development stenosis of the lumbar vertebral canal. J Bone Joint Surg 37B:576–583, 1954.
77. Lombardi, J., Wiltse, L.L., Reynolds, J., Widell, E.H., Spencer, C.W.: Treatment of degenerative spondylolisthesis. Spine 10:821–829, 1985.
78. Hibbs, R.A.: An operation for progressive spinal deformities. NY Med J 93:1013–1015, 1911.
79. Albee, R.H. Transplantation of a portion of the tibia into the spine for Potts disease. JAMA 57:885–886, 1911.

80. Burns, B.H.: An operation for spondylolisthesis. Lancet, *1*:1233–1236, 1933.

81. Cloward, R.B.: New treatment of ruptured intervertebral disc. Presented at the annual meeting of the Hawaii Territorial Medical Association, 1945.

82. Watkins, M.B.: Posterior lateral fusion of the lumbar and lumbosacral spine. J Bone Joint Surg *35*A:1014–1018, 1953.

83. King, D.: Internal fixation for lumbo-sacral fusion. J Bone Joint Surg *30*A:560–565, 1948.

84. Wiltse, L.L.: Internal fixation of the lumbar spine. Clin Orthop *203*:2–219, 1986.

85. Luque, E.R.: Segmental Spinal instrumentation. Clin Orthop *206*: 126–134, 1986.

86. Dove, J.: Internal fixation lumbar spine—the Hartshill rectangle. Clin Orthop *203*:135–140, 1986.

87. Knodt, H., Larrick, R.B.: Distraction fusion of the spine. Ohio Med *60*:12, 1964.

88. Steffee, A.D., Biscup, R.S., Sitkowski, D.J.: Segmental spine plates with pedicle screw fixation—a new internal fixation device for disorders of the lumbar and thoraco-lumbar spine. Clin Orthop *203*:45–54, 1986.

89. O'Brien, J.P., et al.: Simultaneous combined anterior and posterior fusion, a surgical solution for failed spinal surgery with a brief review of the first 150 patients. Clin Orthop *203*:191–196, 1986.

90. Loguidice, V.A., et al.: Anterior lumbar interbody fusion. Spine *13*:366–369, 1988.

91. West, J.L., Ogilbie, J.W., Bradford, D.S.: Complications of the variable screw plate pedicle screw fixation. Presented at the AAOS annual meeting, Las Vegas, Feb., 1989.

92. Davne, S.H., Myers, D.L.: Lumbar spinal fusion for degenerative and disc disease using transpedicular plate fixation. Presented at the AAOS annual meeting, Las Vegas, Feb., 1989.

93. Frymoyer, J.W., Hanley, E.: Disc excision and spine fusion in the management of lumbar disc disease. Minimum 10 year follow up. Spine *3*:1–5, 1978.

94. Lee, C.K., Noshiral, A.W.: Lumbosacral spinal fusion. Spine *9*:574–581, 1984.

95. Stauffer, R.N., Coventry, M.: Posterior lateral lumbar spine fusion. J Bone Joint Surg *54*A:195–204, 1972.

96. Inoue, S., Watanabe, T., Hirose, A.: Anterior discectomy and interbody fusion for lumbar disc herniation. Clin Orthop *183*:22–31, 1984.

97. Burton, C.V., Kirkaldy-Willis, W.H., Yong-Hing, K., Heithoff, K.H.: Causes of failure of surgery in the lumbar spine. Clin Orthop *157*:191–199, 1981.

98. Weir, B.K.A., Jacobs, G.A.: Reoperation rate following lumbar discectomy. Spine *5*:366–370, 1980.

99. Frymoyer, J.W., Matteri, R.E., Hanley, E.N., Kuhlmann, D., Howe, J.: Failed lumbar spine disc surgery. Spine *3*:7–11, 1978.

100. Williams, R.W.: Microlumbar discectomy: A surgical alternative for initial disc herniation. *In* Lumbar Spine Surgery (Edited by J.C. Cauthen). Baltimore, Williams & Wilkins, 1988.

101. Shapiro, D.E., Hanley, E.N.: Lumbar disc surgery in appropriately selected patients: results and factors influencing them. Presented at the AAOS annual meeting, Las Vegas, Feb., 1989.

102. Burton, C.V., Wiltse, L.L.: Editorial and Symposium on lumbar arachnoiditis: nomenclature etiology and pathology. Spine *3*:23–92, 1978.

103. Modic, M.T., Masaryk, T.J., Ross, J.S., Carter, J.R.: Imaging of degenerative disc disease. Radiol *168*:177–186, 1988.

104. Ray, C.D.: Implantation of spinal cord stimulators for relief of chronic and severe pain. *In* Lumbar Spine Surgery (Edited by J.C. Cauthen). Baltimore, Williams & Wilkins, 1988.

105. Montaldi, S., Fankhauser, H., Schnyder, B., deTribolet, N.: Computed tomography of the post-operative intervertebral disc and lumbar spinal canal: investigation of 25 patients after successful operation for lumbar disc herniation. Neurosurg *22*:1014–1022, 1988.

106. Burton, C.V.: Full thickness autogenous fat grafts in the prevention of epidural fibrosis. Contemp Neurosurg *5*:1–16, 1984.

107. O'Brien, J.P.: The role of fusion for chronic low back pain. Ortho Clin North Am *14*:639–649, 1983.

108. Holm, S., et al.: Nutrition of the intervertebral disc: solute transport and metabolism. Connect Tissue Res *8*:101–119, 1981.

Part VII

Rehabilitation of the Patient with Chronic Spinal Disorders

Tom G. Mayer

Rehabilitation vs. Conservative Care: Patient Selection Criteria

DEFINITIONS: REHABILITATION VS. CONSERVATIVE CARE

Although *conservative care* is a generic term used here for nonoperative treatment, it also has a more specific meaning. Treatment that is rendered during the early phases of painful spinal disorders, when soft tissue healing may not have reached its ultimate endpoint, may involve this type of care. Similarly, care provided during the postoperative period, at least until soft tissue healing from surgical trauma has taken place, is also included. Conservative care may be passive, active, or both, and may be integrated into an interdisciplinary program, or be unidisciplinary depending on the needs of the situation. It generally provides the simplest, least expensive care options available for an individual clinical problem. This is necessary because sufficient medical resources must be available to provide such treatment for large numbers of affected individuals entering the medical care system with painful spinal disorders.

By contrast, *rehabilitation* also has specific identifying markers. Its time interval is near the conclusion of treatment, as the final medical care provided, following soft tissue healing. Whether soft tissue injury arose from degeneration, "injury" or surgical trauma is not consequential. Such care is, of necessity, interdisciplinary, with a team approach designed to be able to provide all necessary physical, psychosocial, and vocational interventions called for in a specific clinical situation. Physician guidance is necessary for final re-review and affirmation that all appropriate medical options have been tried and that impairment and disability and physical capacity have been properly determined at maximum medical recovery. Although rehabilitation treatment may take place over two or three sessions in an outpatient environment (which is almost always suitable for conservative care), rehabilitation programs, particularly if necessary after prolonged total disability, are usually provided in comprehensive programs. These programs, to be discussed in subsequent chapters, have been termed either pain clinic programs or functional restoration programs. Distinctions between the specific definitions of conservative care and rehabilitation are indicated in Table 35–1.

Rehabilitation has focused on early investigations into psychosocial concomitants of long-term disability, leading to recognition of the relationships between illness behavior and operant conditioning models. This information also led to potential for behavior modification interventions.[1–6] Unfortunately, controversy has arisen about effectiveness of rehabilitation methodology in painful spinal disorders for a variety of reasons. Patients have often objected to the intervention into psychosocial issues as peripheral to the pain bringing them to the physician. "The pain is in my back, not in my head, doc" or some variation is frequently stated. Lack of quantitative measures of physical capacity also prevented a standardized approach to the physical problems, and prevented patient adherence to specific physical training methods. Similarly, this deficiency prevented effort evaluation. Societal outcomes related to overcoming disability were generally ignored (as they were by other health professionals treating this group of patients). Finally, other participants in the disability system found rehabilitation to be either superfluous or threatening to the indemnity process.

Recently, application of sports medicine principles to the problem, availability of technology for quantification of spinal function, improved standardization

433

Table 35–1
Specific Characteristics of Conservative Care Differentiated From Rehabilitation.

Category	Conservative Care	Rehabilitation
Time interval	Less than 6 mos. total disability; indefinite partial disability.	More than 4 mos. total disability; more than 6 to 8 months partial disability.
Pathophysiology	Postinjury or postoperative soft tissue incomplete; may involve preoperative or prerehabilitation trial.	Soft tissue healing has reached maximum healing improvement.
Modalities	Reactivation is goal; use of passive or active therapies.	Functional restoration is goal; active therapies only.
Diagnostics	Assessment may be incomplete; additional surgery possible.	Assessment complete; surgery ruled out; quantitative physical approach customary.
Care professionals	Uni- or interdisciplinary; 2 to 4 outpatient visits.	Interdisciplinary only; comprehensive treatment customary.
End point	May accompany or precede invasive treatment, or reach maximum medical improvement.	Maximum medical improvement should conclude treatment accompanied by impairment and disability evaluation, physical capacity assessment, and vocational assessment.

of impairment and disability evaluation, and standardization of physical and psychosocial treatment approaches have brought renewed interest in the rehabilitation process.[7–9] While considerable disagreement remains concerning specific essentials of rehabilitation programs, they are beginning to achieve general acceptance as the "end of the line" of treatment for these disorders.

As we have already noted, important barriers to restoring function may be inherent in the involvement of a disability system in the customary doctor-patient relationship. A generation of employers have grown up convinced that the high incidence of recurrent back problems in the previously injured population, and the frequently ambiguous circumstances of back injury, make these patients of dubious value for re-employment. This thinking is magnified by insurance companies, attorneys, and state workers' compensation boards who, lacking objective criteria for determining disability, are inevitably disagreeing over financial compensation to be granted to back claimants. The view of the patient as a claimant projects major distortions into the medical process, requiring special demands for documentation of injury, physical harm, loss of work capacity, and impairment level.[10–12] Unfortunately, but understandably, a hostile, adverse atmosphere is created.

Elsewhere in this book, the complex financial and social costs of disability have been discussed in detail. Moreover, we have also considered the basics of conservative care, structural diagnostic testing, and surgical treatment of the large majority of painful spinal disorders. However, this leaves a relatively large group of about 30% of patients who have recurrent or episodic back pain after initial episodes. More importantly, it leaves a small percentage of chronic back pain patients (but very large numbers in industrialized societies) who become the most seriously disabled, unproductive, and psychologically crippled, demanding constant access to the medical care system. It is this group of patients for whom the rehabilitation option should identify an ultimate solution (though probably not a cure) to their quest.

MAJOR COMPONENTS OF REHABILITATION TREATMENT

Rehabilitation programs for patients with chronic spinal disorders require an interdisciplinary team approach using physical and occupational therapy, psychology, nursing, and vocational specialists. It is guided by a supervising physician who is trained in at least one of the major areas of specialty required in spine rehabilitation. This may involve orthopedic or neurosurgical experience, or a nonsurgical psychiatric, rehabilitation, or sports medicine background. The physician must have an understanding of neurologic and musculoskeletal disorders, and must clearly recognize the difference between previous passive intervention and the patient's active participation in restoring function. He or she must be prepared to evaluate structural diagnostic tests to determine need for additional surgical treatment, and to communicate readily with a surgeon involved in care, to optimize combined surgical and rehabilitation alternatives. The physician must also understand issues of disability evaluation and management, and be prepared to participate in medical or legal proceedings surrounding indemnity issues. Nursing personnel must be capable of functioning as physician assistants, providing counseling on medical matters, patient education, medication control, communication with outside agencies, and examinations for minor intercurrent illnesses and pain flares.

Physical therapists provide a vital service to this program. They are concerned with mobilizing and strengthening the injured part of the body. Their focus on the "weak link" functional unit affected by the spinal disorder involves them in guiding a sequential reconditioning program. Moreover, they must be expert in dealing with the minor overuse problems accompanying rebuilding of a severely deconditioned anatomic area. In functional restoration programs, their role is clearly defined as they treat and educate based on quantification of physical capacity using technology that specifically guides the treatment program and provides a useful body of patient information and documentation (Table 35–2).

Occupational therapists and vocational specialists also play an important role in this program. They have two main roles. The first is to provide training in real world task performance, either synthetic or actual. This may involve some creativity in developing tasks and taking motion-time measurements. In physiological terms, they are helping to resynchronize or coordinate the injured weak link functional unit with other whole body functional units in improving the ability to perform specific tasks. These may be generic, such as lifting, bending, twisting, squatting, and climbing. Alternatively, they may include more complex activities that represent true work simulations involving specific tasks like

Table 35–2
Cardinal Purposes of Assessment

Identify correctable deficits in physical capacity.

Identify psychosocioeconomic barriers to functional restoration.

Establish level of patient effort.

Guide physician and therapists in establishing treatment goals.

Document patient progress to feedback information to patient and clinicians.

Provide reassurance to patients to participate in reconditioning that may occasionally require working through pain.

Document patient physical capacity, work tolerance, and motivation to overcome structural lesions upon completion of rehabilitation.

---

plumbing, carpentry, or wiring. A diversity of activities simulating tasks of a physical nature are used. Improving positional tolerance for sitting and standing are additional major training goals. The second major role of these professionals is to become involved in the socioeconomic consequences of disability, and the various societal outcomes that must be dealt with to promote the patient's recovery, such as employment and litigation.

Psychologists involved in functional restoration programs also have a dual role. First, they have a general crisis intervention obligation, which they must coordinate with the occupational therapist to help the patients deal with the termination of total disability, as well as the economic, vocational, and family changes associated with an anticipated alteration in status. Second, they must help other team members recognize the barriers to functional recovery in an individual patient, and help the patients and staff deal with these barriers. We have found that a cognitive-behavioral treatment orientation is appropriate and effective for functional restoration rehabilitation programs. This orientation emphasizes the importance of simultaneously dealing with thoughts, feelings, and overt behaviors in correcting maladaptive psychosocial performance.

Under medical supervision, the psychologists may also provide valuable assistance in dealing with medication issues, such as educating patients concerning habituating drugs and withdrawal. They may monitor medication effectiveness when used in treatment for depression, anxiety neurosis, or psychosis. Counseling for specific individual problems identified through psychological testing or interviews is a critical part of their role. Long-term psychotherapy, however, is inappropriate in this type of a goal-oriented rehabilitation effort. Certainly, getting to the root cause of maladaptive behaviors is a laudable goal, but the cost and lack of objective measures of success for long-term psychotherapy makes these techniques adjunctive for only a small percentage of patients undergoing functional restoration. If patients were working in gainful employment prior to appearance of spine-related disability, functional restoration primarily seeks to return them to the previous level of functioning. Hopefully, educated to an interest in exploring the causes of maladaptive behaviors, the needy patient will choose to seek prolonged psychological treatment on his or her own.

There are other important "players" involved in the rehabilitation process. As emphasized earlier, low back disability is not just a disease, but a manifestation of a complex system. The resolution of disability also involves employers, attorneys, physicians, unions, insurance companies, and governmental agencies. All of these groups may have fixed perceptions and deeply rooted resistance to change. These groups must be educated concerning the problems of disability management and the multiple accompanying problems that range from the loss of productivity to the financial drain on society. Once aware of the problems, these groups will, in time, be able to accept the crucial role of rehabilitation in the ultimate solution to the patients' difficulties.

All industrialized societies have a variety of financial social systems set aside to compensate individuals for injury, illness or lost wages. From the relatively low reporting rate of back disability in emerging third world countries, which have limited compensation systems, we can deduce that financial benefits for lost time may play a role in a worker's decision to miss work after an injury. However, the literature is ambiguous regarding its role in maintaining disability. The involvement of the disability system forces the rehabilitation team to consider the critical aspects of impairment evaluation, physical capacity assessment, and vocational assessment. Inherent in this process is the determination of the healing period, causation, and maximum medical improvement to a permanent and stationary status. All of these terms should be familiar to the specialist in rehabilitating patients with chronic painful spinal disorders.

Traditional pain clinic programs have often been content to alter patients' self-report of pain complaints. Physical treatment has generally been adjunctive only. The last several years has seen a variety of work hardening programs appear separately to provide more vigorous physical training recognized as necessary for the re-emergence of patient physical competence. Although the term reactivation is used in conservative care to underline the need for recovery of activity tolerance and avoidance of deconditioning, restoration is more appropriate for referring to the chronic situation. This need for restoration emerges because few patients become totally disabled for prolonged periods of time with painful spinal disorders without a combination of physical and psychosocial contributors to the problem. As such, these wounded individuals require the more aggressive, interdisciplinary and quantified team approach compatible with the severity of their conditions. Functional restoration rehabilitation follows the model set for extremity musculoskeletal rehabilitation, the primary goal of which is the return of the patient to the highest possible level of physical capacity and productivity. Extensive evaluation now documents the ability of such programs to significantly influence important societal issues such as return to work, settlement of litigation, additional medical cost, recurrent injury, functional capacity deficits, and pain reduction.[8,9]

POTENTIAL ISSUES FOR PATIENTS ENTERING SPINAL REHABILITATION

Physical Issues

There are a number of important physical issues that need to be addressed in spine rehabilitation. Although these problems usually are most apparent to physicians and physical therapists, the other disciplines also encounter them and often must address them.

Uncorrectable Structural Disorders

The patient prepared for rehabilitation should have undergone all appropriate invasive treatment and initial or repeat structural diagnostic tests to assure the physician that no additional surgical treatment is necessary. Unfortunately, surgical care of spinal disorders is not an exact science, so the evaluation of surgical "necessity" may be a dynamic process. It may hinge, in part, on a patient's failure to progress with conservative care. Different surgeons and radiologists may have alternative points of view on treatment options given the same set of circumstances. Conversely, a patient may be motivated by changing circumstances to seek additional medical opinions of more or less aggressive nature depending on his present attitude toward maintenance of disability. These searches will inevitably be phrased in terms of increasing pain. As such, as much communication as possible should take place between health professionals prior to commencement of functional restoration to clarify the need for invasive treatment.

Specialists in the area of spinal disorders recognize that pain cannot be cured in most chronic cases. Complete cessation of pain is seldom a goal presented to patients by reputable physicians and surgeons. Scar tissue is an anticipated concomitant of injury, surgical intervention, or degeneration, and can be expected to impede ideal biomechanical and biochemical recovery of function. Joint stiffness, adhesions, and muscle injury, accompanied by neural entrapment, may lead to some absolute limits on recovery potential. It cannot be emphasized strongly enough that the patient, the surgeon, and the rehabilitation team must be persuaded that all reasonable structural testing and surgical options have been considered before embarking on a rehabilitation program.

The Deconditioning Syndrome

Deconditioning is a progressive process originating from disuse, inactivity, pain, or fear of injury. Effects include stiff hypomobile joints, muscle atrophy, loss of endurance, inhibition of neural outflow, and loss of cardiovascular fitness. Atrophic muscles are more irritable and subject to overload, leading to recurrent spasm or pain episodes. These symptoms may be misinterpreted by an anxious patient as new injuries, inspiring him to additional inactivity, which perpetuates the disuse phenomenon.

Physical Progression Issues

In the past, continued pain and disability in the back-injured patient was treated by passive means only. However, the use of bedrest after a sufficient healing period only amplifies the secondary deconditioning problem. Traction, heat, massage, ultrasound or lasers, and psychologic techniques are unlikely to provide prolonged benefit, and may actually predispose to deleterious changes in connective tissues. Such treatments tend to teach the patient to become more dependent on medical professionals, rather than to actively engage in individual responsibility for personal health. This adds to the patient's feeling of helplessness and hopelessness while putting unrealistic expectations on health professionals that never can be met.

In order to address these issues, gradual physical progression of the patient to normal, or even supernormal, functional capacity is necessary. The quantitative methods now available to measure basic elements of performance, such as mobility and strength, have made this system possible. Not only does quantification allow for strenuous, yet safe, conditioning, but it gives objective feedback to the patient and therapist alike. As in other forms of sports medicine rehabilitation, the training regimen often results in temporary pain flares. Among many patients, this may initially be perceived as injury, and may heighten their fears about reconditioning. Continued pain often may be misinterpreted as a sign of failure to progress, leading to discouragement and decreased adherence to treatment protocols. Objective quantification helps overcome these hindrances, encouraging the patient to develop a sense of mastery over fear and pain. Although the primary goal of treatment is to restore function and secondarily to ameliorate pain, the vast majority of patients experience significant pain reduction once they have achieved their anticipated level of mobility, strength, and endurance in the spinal functional unit.[13]

Stages of Progression

The spine is a single link in the body's biomechanical chain. It is used in most full-body tasks to transmit loads from hands to foot or floor. In the initial stages of rehabilitation, the main goal is to increase the patient's flexibility and mobility, particularly the injured weak link functional unit. Through stretching and range of motion exercises, the patient is able to mobilize scar, tight muscles, and contracted connective tissues. A full range of motion is essential to attain maximum benefit from the subsequent strengthening exercises.

Based on initial functional capacity (determined by a quantitative functional evaluation), the patient enters a progressive resistive strengthening program. The purpose of this program is to increase overall physical strength and endurance in all body functional units, but particularly in the weak link areas. The beginning exercise level and rate of progression are based on several factors, including initial physical capacity, effort, age, gender, customary activity level, height, and weight. Simultaneously, the patient is engaged in activities designed to increase cardiovascular endurance. Moreover, as strength increases, coordination, and agility training are emphasized. These exercises build on the foundation of strength and flexibility initially established, assisting the patient in returning to the functional positions and activities encountered in daily living. Finally, throughout all of these steps, the patient trains in synthetic tasks as well as overall body fitness.

Failure to Progress

Failure to progress physically represents psychosocial barriers to recovery, rather than structural incapacity, in the majority of cases. For a given level of structural damage, scar tissue, or instability, the muscles, joints, ligaments, and nerves respond to higher levels of performance if exercised in a standardized protocol in the absence of systemic disease or toxic drugs. Quantitative data may represent objective evidence that nonphysiologic influences are impeding progress. As such, they may be used by all members of the treatment team to educate the patient about how to progress in spite of barriers to recovery. Additionally, they provide documentation of the patient's effort to achieve higher levels of physical performance. The data also document compliance with medical treatments designed to help the patient, assisting the physician in formulating his or her view of the patient's contribution to reducing disability. The disability system is likely to be more sympathetic to a claimant who has done more to help himself, than to one who seeks to look as bad as possible.

Barriers to Recovery

Barriers to recovery can include psychologic, socioeconomic, or work-related issues that interfere with a smooth return to a functional and productive lifestyle. This concept encompasses, but is not limited to, traditional concepts of secondary gain, symptom magnification, and psychologic resistance. Financial and work-related disincentives may also play a role as barriers. The patient's response to the barriers may be conscious, unconscious, or a combination of both. The barriers may range from intervening life events that impede treatment (e.g., transportation problems, lack of child care), to more subtle emotional issues (e.g., depression, anger at the work place), to conscious attempts to manipulate the system (although uncommon). At other times, real problems may be used as smoke screens or excuses for suboptimal performance and failure to adhere to the treatment regimen, with the patient playing a passive victim role. All staff members on the rehabilitation team must be alert to potential secondary gains of continued disability whether legal, financial, family, or job-related. It is incumbent on members of the treatment team to be knowledgeable of all psychosocial issues in general, as well as those specific to the individual patient. This knowledge allows staff members not only to better understand and serve the patient, but also to be more effective in problem solving when the patient is not progressing as expected.

Occasionally, a painful spinal disorder may hide a serious characterologic disorder or psychosis. Many professionals have only limited training in identifying or dealing with such patients. Early identification of these patients is important, and therefore psychiatric consultation with a trained professional astute in cognitive and behavioral training may be invaluable. For some of these patients, skilled use of medication may change an intractable patient into a manageable one (Table 35–3).

Pain Issues

Pain complaints are subjective phenomena. They represent a central, cognitive interpretation of multi-

Table 35–3
Issues in Spinal Rehabilitation

---

1. Physical Issues
   Unresolved structural disease and scar.
   The deconditioning syndrome.
   Physical progression.
   Stages of progression.
   Failure to progress.
2. Barriers to Recovery
3. Pain Issues
   Pain vs. function.
   Hurt is not equivalent to harm.
   Addressing pain issues with the patient.
4. Medication Issues

---

ple events such as peripheral stimuli, psychologic patterns, or effects of endogenous and exogenous neurotransmitters. However, most patients recognize only a direct link between a peripheral nociceptive stimulus and its central expression as pain. This layperson's conceptualization brings the patient into rehabilitation with several pre-established attitudes. First, the patient is rarely able to consider causes for the perceived pain other than a single pain-producing lesion somewhere in the spinal area. It is often difficult to educate such a patient about medical concepts that are not observable, such as referred pain or nerve root compression or radiculopathy. Second, the patient has usually been conditioned to expect that any lesion can be identified by state-of-the-art diagnostic technology, and then be "fixed" by the skilled surgical professional.

Another common patient misconception concerning pain is that the patient is able to distinguish its location and severity by monitoring its perceived quality (e.g., the pain is "deep in the bone," or is "right in the disc above the tail bone"). Ample evidence of the lack of sensory specificity in the spinal regions exists, attesting to the inaccuracy of the patient's belief. Finally, and most significantly, pain is a profoundly frightening problem, raising the specter of a life-threatening or disabling disease. Once the patient has been reassured that the painful spinal disorder is a benign problem, the disabling impact on the patient's lifestyle may improve. In the presence of self-doubt about whether the problem is "really in my head," the patient usually develops an additional source of anxiety and pain intensification. Although the patient initially compels the clinician to focus on subjective pain complaints, ultimately the loss of function is the greater concern.

Pain Versus Function

The emphasis on resumption of function rather than pain relief is the primary goal that sets the functional restoration approach apart from other spinal rehabilitation programs. The patient's pain is acknowledged as real in any spinal rehabilitation program, often based on an injury perceived by the patient at some point in time and structural damage demonstrated by imaging techniques. It is medically recognized that the specific pain source and relation to an injury can usually neither be demonstrated nor denied. Yet, in the absence of objective evidence to the contrary, the patient's perception concerning injury should be accepted, unless the clinician has reasons to doubt the veracity of the patient. In rare circumstances, evidence may cast doubt on a patient's truthfulness, but this information is almost always provided after the fact. As medical professionals, the physician and rehabilitation team must be patient advocates, accepting the patient's self-report and evaluating its content in the context of a complete evaluation before forming conclusions.

The overriding goal of the staff is to restore functioning, not to produce a totally pain free individual. As in other sports medicine rehabilitation approaches, the patient must push through pain in order to obtain the advertised benefits. Patients must understand that decrease in pain perception is ultimately proportional to increase in physical capacity into the anticipated range for that individual. Waiting for the pain to go away first guarantees failure to progress physically, as well as failure to ensure ultimate pain relief.

Hurt is Not Necessarily Equivalent to Harm

One of the most difficult concepts to impart to patients is that a pain flare does not equal injury once pain has become chronic. Patients often attempt to distinguish between acute pain, which signals new tissue overload, and chronic pain, which does not necessarily provide such information. However, they must understand that increased pain with increased activity is actually a sign of progress rather than regression. Quantification of function becomes extremely important in demonstrating to the patient that, in spite of his subjective feelings, he is in fact progressing physically as evidenced by the quantified measurements.

Addressing Pain Issues with the Patient

In helping the patient negotiate the sometimes challenging rehabilitation process, the treatment team must balance its efforts in trying to keep the patient as comfortable as possible. They must constantly emphasize function rather than pain, and they must attempt to decrease the patient's dependence on health care professionals. It is important that staff members listen to pain complaints in a concerned and open minded fashion. They must reinforce the patients' new pain self-management tools, including the use of stretching, ice, relaxation, and anti-inflammatory drugs. By observing the pace of training and comparing the patient's current pain report with the initial self-reports, one can determine if the problem represents the normal side effects of the physical progression, or in fact represents an overtraining syndrome. Because of the substantial fear of reinjury experienced by many of these patients, it is essential that staff members share their diagnostic and treatment rationale with the patient at these times. Moreover, sharing this information helps the patient learn to distinguish between chronic pain, flare-ups, and acute muscle strains.

Medication Issues

Along with continuous use of bedrest after the acute phase of injury has passed, the lingering use of opiates, semisynthetic analgesics, or tranquilizers may contribute to the patient's increasing disability. Besides their central pain-relieving effects, these medications have substantial hypnotic effects that add to the patient's deactivation. They also reinforce passive reliance on external sources of relief and "cure." Moreover, they have significant addictive potential and capacity for pain sensitization.

The use of opiates, muscle relaxants, tranquilizers, and sedatives is basically incompatible with a rehabilitation program. Patients must be alert and physically responsive in order to derive full benefit. Furthermore, patients must be aware of kinesthetic and proprioceptive feedback that takes place during exercise. Because most patients are already emotionally depressed, eliminating the central nervous system depressant effects of these medications helps them to begin to control their affective disorder. The avoidance of pain killers also reinforces treatment emphasis on functional restoration, rather than pain relief, as the primary goal.

During the initial phase of rehabilitative treatment such medications are gradually tapered. The rationale of tapering is explained carefully to the patient. In place of these medications, other nonhabituating medications may be substituted as discussed elsewhere in this volume. A basic knowledge of antidepressants, anxietolytics, and anti-inflammatory agents is necessary for any physician involved in spine rehabilitation. Specialized knowledge of additional psychoactive drugs may prevent more complex psychiatric problems from interfering with basic program goals. Medication to peripherally block inflammation is important as patients increase physical activity. Patients whose depression produces vegetative signs of sleep disturbance, low energy, irritability, and memory problems will be more difficult to motivate to participate in rehabilitation without the assistance of antidepressant medication. The psychoactive medication should always be coupled with individual counseling to provide increased patient confidence in the benefits of exploring psychosocial issues remaining as barriers to overall recovery.

In contrast to the medication-dependent individual reluctant to give up drugs that have a substantial central effect, one may encounter patients with a generally negative view about medications. These patients may be easier to work with in a completely drug-free state. However, the treatment team must be alert to medication avoidance as a "red flag" of treatment resistance in patients who would clearly benefit from the use of certain medications.

Another "red flag" individual becoming evermore prevalent in our society is the patient whose primary issue is pre-existing substance abuse or alcoholism manifested as progressive irritability and work maladjustment. Overcoming deep-seated substance abuse problems in a spine rehabilitation program may be impossible. However, the resistance cannot be dealt with in a meaningful way if the treatment team fails to recognize the existence of the drug problem as part of the disability process. In certain instances, a contract must be negotiated with the patient, by which periodic random testing takes place to monitor the tapering and elimination of habituating substances. Lest the treatment team become too messianic in the cause of drug suppression, it is important to point out, once again, that all pre-existing psychosocial deficits of disabled patients cannot be addressed in the context of overcoming disability. As such, given adequate progress in functional restoration, combined with patient compliance and motivation to deal with substance abuse problems, referral to appropriate agencies for long-term maintenance of the drug-free state should be considered.

SUMMARY

Rehabilitation cannot be subsumed under the term conservative care. The latter should not be used generically to cover all nonsurgical care, but instead should be seen as a specific term for dealing with the large majority of patients with acute, subacute, and episodic problems relatively free of disability, psychosocial issues, or progressive deconditioning. Rehabilitation deals with the smaller groups of patients who manifest these complications. It must be "end of the line" treatment, which requires clear identification of remaining surgical options prior to the rehabilitation, and identification of maximum medical improvement, impairment or disability, and physical or work capacity at the conclusion of the treatment process. Pain clinic programs and functional restoration programs are two available options; a multitude of conservative care options and combinations have been described in earlier sections.

Patients entering rehabilitation must face a variety of issues. These are summarized as *physical progression issues, barriers to recovery, pain issues,* and *medication issues.* Each of these problems is discussed in greater detail elsewhere in this section of the text. Rehabilitation treatment generally involves a comprehensive program provided by an interdisciplinary team of physical therapists, occupational therapists, psychologists, nurses, and rehabilitation specialists. The supervising position of the physician is a key factor in achieving the specific goals of this form of treatment.

REFERENCES

1. Fordyce, W., Roberts, A., Sternbach, R.: The behavioral management of chronic pain: a response to critics. Pain 22:112–125, 1985.
2. Turk, D., Meichenbaum, D., Genest, M.: Pain and Behavior Medicine: A Cognitive-Behavior Perspective. New York, Gilford Press, 1983.
3. Fordyce, W., Fowler, R., Lehmann, J., DeLateur, B.: Some implications of learning in problems of chronic pain. J Chronic Dis 21:179–190, 1968.
4. Sternbach, R., Tursky, B.: Ethnic differences among housewives in psychophysical and skin potential response to electric shock. Psychophysiol 1:241–246, 1965.
5. Sternbach, R.: Pain Patients: Traits and Treatment. New York, Academic Press, 1974.
6. Gatchel, R., Baum, A.: Introduction to Health Psychology. New York, Random House, 1983.
7. Mayer, T., Gatchel, R.: Functional Restoration for Spinal Disorders: The Sports Medicine Approach. Philadelphia, Lea & Febiger, 1988.
8. Mayer, T., et al.: A prospective two-year study of functional restoration in industrial low back injury: an objective assessment procedure. JAMA 258: 1763–1767, 1987.
9. Mayer T, et al.: Objective assessment of spine function following industrial accident: a prospective study with comparison group and one-year follow-up. Spine 10:482–493, 1985.
10. Hadler, N.: Legal ramifications of the medical definition of back disease. Ann Intern Med 84:922–999, 1978.
11. Rockey, P., Fantel, J., Omenn, G.: Discriminatory aspects of pre-employment screening: low back x-ray examinations in the railroad industry. Am J Law Med 5:197–214, 1979.
12. Beals, R.: Compensation and recovery from injury. West J Med 140:233–237, 1984.
13. DeLorme, T., Watkins, A.: Progressive Resistance Exercise: Technic Medical Application. New York, Appleton Century Crofts, 1951.

Robert J. Gatchel

36

Psychosocial Assessment and Disability Management in the Rehabilitation of Painful Spinal Disorders

Low back pain is one of the most important public health problems affecting industrialized societies. Next to the common cold, low back pain is the greatest cause of lost work time and the most costly benign disease in the United States. Fortunately, though, almost 90% of low back pain patients regain normal function within 2 months of onset of pain. Yet, of those whose symptoms persist for more than a few months, about 50 to 60% continue to be disabled at the end of the year, and the majority of the group continue to be disabled even after 2 years. These individuals often go on to extensive medical treatment, compensation costs, and settlement awards that make their contribution to the problem disproportionate to that of the entire group suffering from acute low back pain. In fact, 10% of the cases cost about 80% of the money in a variety of industries.[1] It is this chronic group which is the focus of this chapter.

The development of sophisticated techniques of diagnosis, such as roentgenography, myelography, computer tomography, and technetium bone scanning has improved our ability to define anatomic sites of injury. However, these findings often do not correlate with the patient's pain symptoms. Moreover, surgical release of the anatomic lesion does not always eliminate the symptomatic complaints. Thus, it is often difficult to isolate specific structural entities that cause low back pain. Therefore, clinicians are often faced with frustration when treating patients with low back pain. This is not a common phenomenon we experience when treating patients with musculoskeletal problems in the extremities.

With the introduction of the gate control theory of pain in 1965 by Melzack and Wall, the scientific community came to accept the importance of central, psychologic factors in the pain perception process. In the chronic pain patient, these psychologic factors are often difficult for clinicians to evaluate and can seriously limit the success of treatment programs. It should be emphasized that chronic pain is a complex and interactive psychophysiologic behavior pattern that cannot be broken down into distinct, independent psychologic and physical components. Psychologic assessment should *not* be used to try to differentiate "organic" from "functional" causes.[1] Rather, the assessment should be directed at evaluating the important psychological characteristics of each individual patient in order to help guide the treatment and rehabilitation process, as well as to help predict therapeutic outcome. This psychologic assessment evaluates not only the patient's self-reported pain, but also evaluates overall psychologic functioning in order to help treatment personnel effectively integrate each patient into a comprehensive therapeutic regimen. Quantified changes in many of these measures can then be used to document therapeutic improvement.

The first part of the chapter is devoted to an overview of the various psychologic assessment devices that can prove sensitive in evaluating chronic low back pain patients. The latter part of the chapter discusses how this psychosocial evaluation can then be

441

used to guide the patient effectively through a comprehensive disability management program, as well as to evaluate the patient's cognitive and psychologic resources that may affect response to treatment.

PSYCHOSOCIAL ASSESSMENT

At the outset, it should be clearly noted that no one psychologic device can reliably be used in the assessment process. Indeed, one of the major misapplications of psychologic measures in the field of medicine has been the assumption that one psychologic instrument can be used as a sole conclusive predictive or descriptive variable. As I have noted in discussing the field of personality psychology, such data should be viewed as just one source of information to be used with other types of information in helping to make a probability statement concerning the prediction of some behavior.[2] It is extremely rare to be able to make a totally accurate prediction of some behavior based upon a single psychologic instrument. Following is a brief overview of available assessment devices that can provide valuable information when dealing with chronic low back pain patients. Table 36–1 lists the important issues and information that can be obtained on the basis of a competent psychosocial assessment of a low back pain patient.

Table 36–1
Important Issues and Information Obtained on the Basis of a Thorough Psychosocial Assessment

Quality of current psychologic functioning

Personal and family history of psychologic functioning or disturbance

Formal diagnosis of psychopathology

Personality characteristics that may affect the treatment process

Severity of psychosocial stressors

Subjective distress to physical symptoms

Cognitive factors (e.g., intelligence level and cognitive distortion) that may affect the treatment process

Work-related variables (e.g., job satisfaction) that may affect return-to-work

Social reinforcers for illness behavior (e.g., financial disincentives)

Lifestyle characteristics that may affect the treatment process

Substance abuse issues

Psychological Tests

Minnesota Multiphasic Personality Inventory

This inventory is one of the oldest and most frequently used tests of psychological functioning. Often in the past, however, it was used simply because "everyone else uses it." By itself, it does not offer much help in choosing among treatment options. However, in a comprehensive evaluation using several types of assessment tools, the MMPI can add valuable information regarding psychologic functioning.

Of the 10 major clinical scales by which the MMPI responses are classified, the Hysteria (Hy), Depression (D), and Hypochondriasis (Hs) scales are the most important when evaluating a chronic pain patient. Elevation of the Hysteria and Hypochondriasis scales with a normal Depression scale produces the so-called *Conversion V*. This test profile was thought to be associated with pain that has a large psychologic component. It generally flags patients who are neurotic and anxious, and who magnify their symptoms while remaining somewhat indifferent to the limitations of their behavior produced by these symptoms. They often have little insight into their own problems and often use denial as a defense against facing such problems. On the other hand, patients who have a *neurotic triad* (Hysteria, Depression, and Hypochondriasis scales all elevated) are more aware that their symptoms have a psychologic component and are better able to express their anxiety and stress.

Barnes, et al.,[3] evaluated changes in MMPI profile scores before and after successful functional restoration treatment. Figure 36–1 presents these two profiles. It shows a substantial decrease in the elevation of scales after treatment. Note that these figures represent *averaged* profile scores across many patients (104 at pretreatment and 69 at followup). Wide individual differences exist whenever viewing any one particular patient profile. Similar MMPI changes have been reported by Naliboff, et al.,[4] following behavioral treatment. As I noted in Chapter 26 of this text, these results suggest that the elevations of MMPI scores are most likely caused by the trauma and stress associated with the chronic pain condition and not to some stable pre-existing "pain-personality" trait. When successfully treated, these elevations disappear.

Over the years, numerous other scales have been developed for the MMPI. The McAndrew scale, initially standardized on an outpatient population of alcoholics, helps one to recognize the patient with an alcoholic or drug-dependent personality type. Therefore, it can determine those patients who are

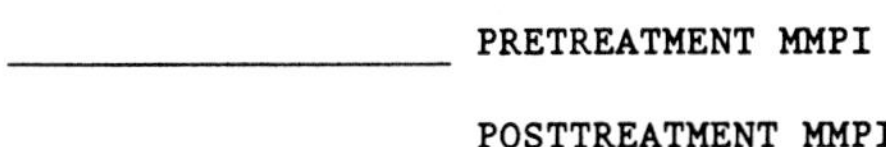

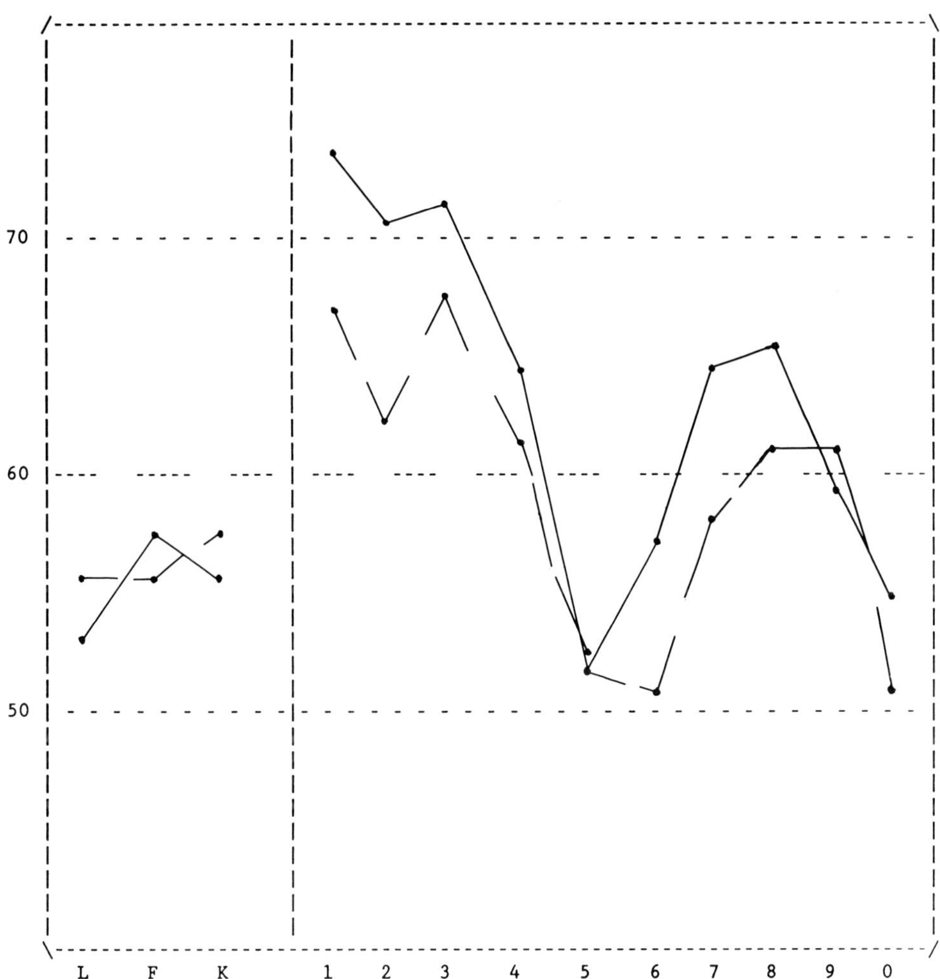

Figure 36–1. MMPI profiles scores of patients before and after successful functional restoration treatment. (From Mayer, T.G., Gatchel, R.J.: Functional Restoration for Spinal Disorders: The Sports Medicine Approach. Philadelphia, Lea & Febiger, 1988.)

at high risk for drug abuse, before habituation occurs. Patients not actively taking drugs may have a positive score on the McAndrew scale, and reformed substance abusers often score high. This scale is useful in evaluating acute low back pain patients to select out those who may be particularly susceptible to long periods of hospitalization for bed rest and excessive intramuscular analgesic use.

Patients scoring high on this test scale also tend to be prolonged users of oral opiate analgesics and tranquilizing muscle relaxants as their pain becomes more chronic. Because the personality profile of the dependent drug abuser bears some resemblance to that of many chronic pain patients, abnormalities on this scale can raise a "red flag" for clinicians to beware of early adverse behavioral changes.

The ego strength scale is another special scale that can help identify patients who have limited emotional resources. Patients who exhibit particularly low ego strength, along with other psychologic problems, are less likely to benefit from treatment regimens that demand motivation and personal responsibility than are patients who score higher on the ego strength scale.

In terms of the MMPI as a whole, there are certain practical drawbacks to the test. It is lengthy and somewhat disturbing for patients to take, sometimes producing a conviction that their physicians think "it's all in my head." Efforts must be made to convince patients that the reason they are being asked to take the test is to provide an overall picture of general psychologic functioning, and not to categorize them into any psychiatric pigeonholes. In addition, the test was standardized on a psychiatrically disturbed population of English speaking subjects, predominantly of Scandinavian heritage. Therefore, the test has substantial built-in biases based on race, national origin, language, and psychiatric disease.

In spite of these above biases, however, the MMPI is extremely useful because it provides a meaningful psychologic profile of a patient that can be invaluable in helping to deal with many of the psychologic and behavioral issues that accompany chronic low back pain (to be discussed later in this chapter). Also, a great wealth of clinical research data can be drawn from the scientific literature when dealing with issues of utility, reliability, and validity of various scales or combination of scales that one might be interested in when attempting to make a diagnostic decision or prediction.

It should be noted that, as an alternative to the MMPI, the Symptom Check List 90-Revised (SCL-90-R) can be administered. This test was developed to measure psychopathology in both psychiatric and medical outpatients,[5] and has been demonstrated to have a high degree of convergence with the MMPI. Although it is not as discriminating as the MMPI,[6] it can provide a good overall index of psychological functioning. It takes only 20 minutes to complete, and provides an alternative to the more time consuming MMPI. At the Productive Rehabilitation Institute of Dallas for Ergonomics (PRIDE), however, we still prefer using the MMPI.

Millon Behavioral Health Inventory (MBHI)

Millon, Green, and Meagher[7] devised a 150 question true or false test based on 20 clinical scales that reflect medically related concerns, such as compliance with treatment regimens and reaction to treatment personnel. This test was intended as an alternative to the MMPI. Unlike the MMPI, however, which was originally designed for a psychiatric population, the MBHI was developed and standardized on an actual medical population. One advantage the MBHI has over the MMPI is that it requires only about 20 minutes to complete. Moreover, most patients find it to be less threatening than the MMPI because it includes questions related to medical care.

The MBHI is still too new to have substantial evidence to document its reliability. We do not yet know as much about this instrument as we do about others. One of the reasons why the test has not been used as widely as it could be is that scoring keys for the test are not available, and scoring must be contracted through National Computer Services, Inc. The cost of this has resulted in limited use of the MBHI and has impeded the development of a larger data base. In addition, a critical review of its test construction procedures[8] may have also stimulated some caution regarding its use.

Nevertheless, this inventory has been found useful as part of an overall assessment of patients with low back pain.[1] A number of scales have been found to be clinically meaningful. For example, we have generally found that subjects who score low on the cooperative style scale and high on the sensitive style scale demonstrate poor outcome. These individuals tend not to follow advice and can be unpredictable and moody. Obviously, such characteristics can be detrimental to the treatment process. In contrast, patients scoring high on the cooperative and sociable scales demonstrate excellent outcome. We have also found that patients scoring high on the emotional vulnerability scale usually require additional psychologic help in dealing with their disabilities. Finally, some of our preliminary research has suggested that individuals scoring high on the premorbid pessimism and forceful style scales often seek out surgical treatment as an alternative.

Beck Depression Inventory (BDI)

The BDI consists of 21 items with a cumulative scoring system focusing on manifestations such as sleep disturbance, sexual dysfunction, weight change, and anhedonia. It was originally developed by Beck[9] as a means of assessing the cognitive components of depression.

The simplicity of the BDI also makes it attractive. Patients can complete the form in less than 5 minutes; scoring takes less than 1 minute. The BDI can also be repeated at subsequent visits to chart progression of the patient's depressive symptoms and the effects of treatment programs.

Depression, like anxiety, is a frequent concomitant of long-term back dysfunction. Although it is unclear whether depression precedes or follows the onset of low back symptoms in the majority of cases, knowledge of its presence can be helpful. Offering depressed patients pharmacologic treatment may encourage greater patient motivation and compliance with therapy. Indeed, the adjunctive use of antidepressant medication has become increasingly popular in the treatment of chronic pain. The recognition that the antidepressants have an effect not only on the clinical depression frequently associated with chronic pain, but also on the pain itself,[10] should not leave the unsuspecting clinician to conclude that there may still be a "magic pill" to cure chronic pain. Antidepressants should be used only on a short-term basis with only carefully selected patients.

When the BDI is used in conjunction with a psychosocial interview, grossly exaggerated or underplayed scores may give significant insight into a patient's defense mechanisms and approach to pain, and may suggest the need for psychiatric or psychologic referral. For instance, patients who deny the existence of depressive symptoms (those with low BDI scores) but have considerable pain and functional impairment are often defensive about accepting any psychologic aspect of their illness. On the other hand, patients who have excessively high scores often are fragile psychologically. Those with a high BDI score, but low functional impairment, generally are dependent and feel overwhelmed by all stressors.

It should be noted that the BDI primarily measures cognitive factors in depression. For careful evaluation of vegetative signs of depression, such as loss of appetite, or sleep, the Hamilton Rating Scale for Depression can be used.[11] The major drawback of this scale is that an interviewer has to be trained to administer it verbally.

Other Self-Report Measures

Quantified Pain Drawing

Mooney, Cairns, and Robertson[12] developed the pain drawing as a nonverbal assessment of pain location, severity, and subjective characteristics. The pain drawing allows the patient to express freely all of his symptoms on a plain front and back drawing of a person (Fig. 36–2). In a later modification, a 10-cm line for indicating intensity of pain was also added to the drawing. A carefully constructed overlay has been designed at the University of Texas Southwestern Medical Center at Dallas to quantitate the pain display. Boxes that are bilaterally symmetric and of approximately equal area cover the pain drawing, but also quantitate pain extending "outside the body." Two scores, one for the "trunk" and the other for "extremities," allow differentiation of localized mechanical and referred or radicular pain patterns. Maximum trunk and extremity scores are 72 boxes each.

Many factors involved in pain perception are assessed by the pain drawing. Anxiety, a major factor in chronic low back dysfunction, often leads to a more dramatic display and higher pain drawing scores. Pain that extends outside the body usually identifies a person as a pain magnifier. Rarely, "outside the body" pain is seen in a patient who is experiencing somatic delusions.

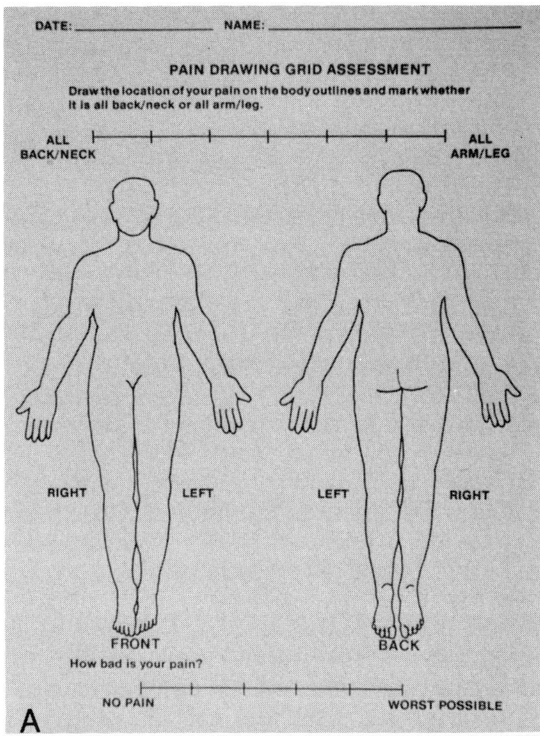

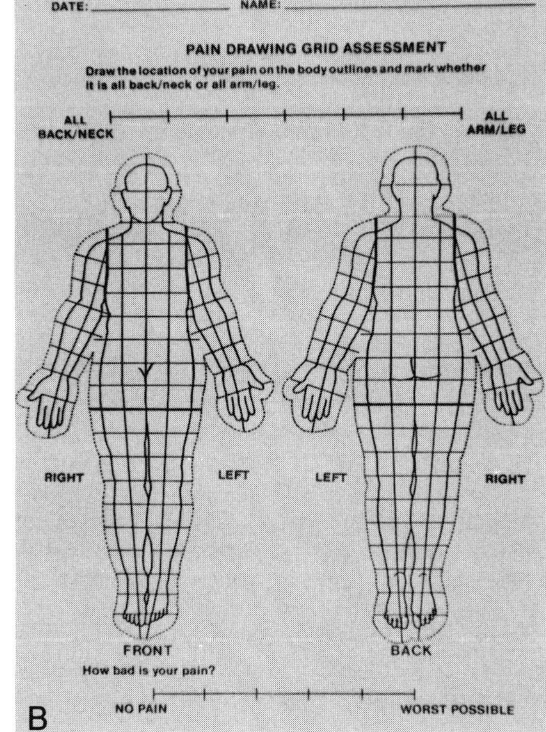

Figure 36–2. A. The quantitated pain drawing. **B.** Drawing with the transparent grid overlay. (From Mayer, T.G., Gatchel, R.J.: Functional Restoration for Spinal Disorders: The Sports Medicine Approach. Philadelphia, Lea & Febiger, 1988.)

Changes in a patient's pain score can document the patient's changing pain perception and shifting pain pattern. However, comparisons of drawings for different patients are of little value, except in alerting the clinician that a patient may be exaggerating.

Million Visual Analog Scale

Million, et al.,[13] published a validated visual analog scale, consisting of 15 questions, that span the gamut of responses, e.g., "Do you have a pain in the back? How severe is it?" A score for each of the 15 questions can be quickly derived using a ruler or grid superimposed on the paper (Fig. 36–3). Visual analog scales are desirable because of their high degree of reproducibility and opportunity for nonverbal expression. Good correlation is found between the subjective analog scores and the objective findings of the clinician. Because the test focuses primarily on pain and the functional limitations pain imposes, it can be used on multiple occasions to assess the patient's symptomatic improvement. In addition, exaggerated responses that do not correlate with the physician's assessment of the patient may lead to further psychologic evaluation.

Oswestry Low Back Pain Disability Questionnaire

This self-rating scale was originally developed by Fairbank, Davies, Couper, and O'Brien.[14] It can be administered and scored in less than 5 minutes, and illustrates the degree of functional impairment the patient is experiencing. This scale, however, has not yet been adequately correlated with objective findings or used in an analysis of therapeutic modalities. Therefore, if it is to be used, it should be as a global clinical index, integrated with other assessment measures.

The primary advantage of the Oswestry Scale is that it has only 10 questions, with responses for each scored from zero to five, providing a simple percentage score that can be compared with the scores of tests given on other occasions. Its grading scale categorizes the degree of functional loss. It also indicates a score above which symptom magnification has likely occurred.

A comparison of results on the Oswestry Scale and the BDI can sometimes offer an index of the patient's level of denial and indicates those patients who are symptom magnifiers. Patients with high scores on the Oswestry (high functional loss) and low scores on the BDI (low depression) often want to receive a medical cure and reject the possibility of an emotional component to their pain.

The Sickness Impact Profile (SIP)

The Sickness Impact Profile was developed by Bergner, Bobbitt, Carter, and Gibson,[15] and was designed to document the disability and behavioral impact across a wide range of groups and illnesses of varying types and severities. It consists of 136 items contained within 12 scales ranging from physical, psychosocial, and independent (i.e., home management) categories. Some impressive reliability and validity data for several patient populations have been reported.[15,16]

Although this instrument is still too new to determine its effectiveness, some research has already been conducted demonstrating its usefulness for assessing disability in chronic low back pain patients.[17] It therefore appears to be a promising assessment tool for measuring disability in these patients. Further validation of its sensitivity to changes in health status and treatment effects is needed.

Other Specific Psychologic Tests and Self-Report Measures

There are many other tests and self-report measures that have been developed and used with chronic low back pain patients. Table 36–2 provides

Table 36–2
Other Psychologic Tests and Self-Report Measures Useful in the Psychosocial Assessment of Chronic Low Back Pain Patients

Back Pain Classification Scale (Leavitt, 1983)[19]

Chronic Illness Problem Inventory (Kames, et al., 1984)[20]

Cognitive Errors Questionnaire (Smith, et al., 1986)[21]

Disability Questionnaire (Roland and Morris, 1983)[22]

Functional Rating Scale (Evans and Kagan, 1986)[23]

Hendler Screening Test (Hendler, et al., 1979)[24]

Health Assessment Questionnaire (Fries, 1983)[25]

Illness Behavior Questionnaire (Pilowsky and Spence, 1975)[26]

McGill-Melzack Pain Questionnaire (Melzack, 1975)[27]

McGill Comprehensive Pain Questionnaire (Monks and Taenzer, 1983)[28]

Pain Disability Index (Tait, Pollard, Margolis, Duckro, and Krause, 1987)[29]

Vanderbilt Pain Management Inventory (Brown and Nicassio, 1987)[30]

West Haven-Yale Multidimensional Pain Inventory (Kerns, et al., 1985)[31]

DATE____________________   NAME____

PLEASE MAKE AN "X" ALONG THE LINE TO SHOW HOW FAR FROM NORMAL TOWARD THE WORST POSSIBLE SITUATION YOUR PAIN PROBLEM HAS TAKEN YOU

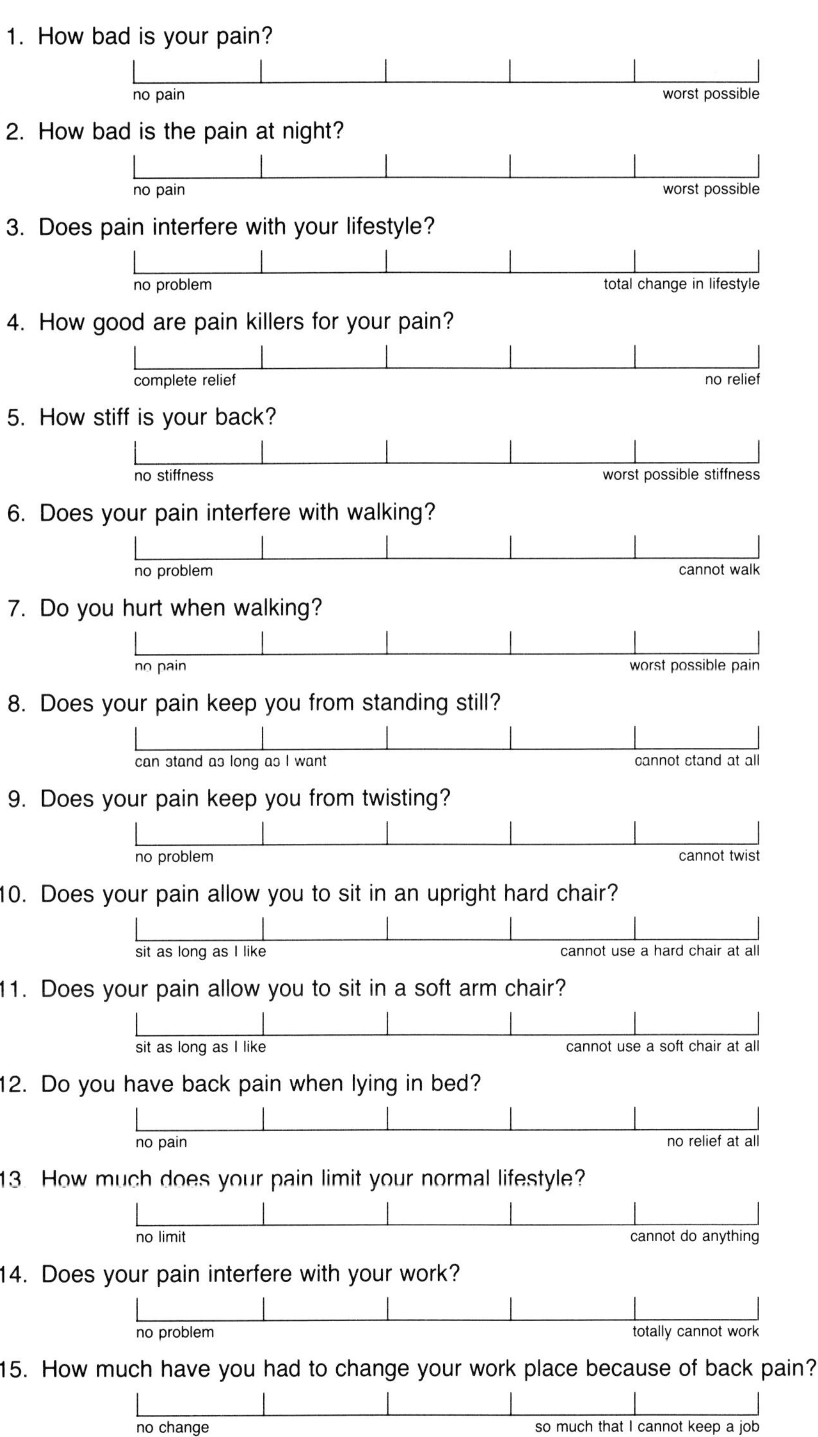

Figure 36–3. The Million visual analog scale. The scores for each line are added together. The highest possible score is 150; the lowest possible score is 0. (From Mayer, T.G., Gatchel, R.J.: Functional Restoration for Spinal Disorders: The Sports Medicine Approach. Philadelphia, Lea & Febiger, 1988.)

447

a brief summary of these tests. Williams[18] has recently provided a useful review of many of these tests and measures. There are advantages and disadvantages to these various tests and measures, and the ones selected depend upon the patient population and environment one is working in.

The Clinical Interview

The most powerful clinical assessment tool is the psychosocial interview. In evaluating chronic low back pain patients, this also holds true. In addition to the traditional areas assessed in clinical history-taking, a number of other areas are explored. These are listed in Table 36–3.

An important covert part of the interview is to determine the patient's motivation for change. Patients with chronic back pain have often restricted their lives by avoiding any risk of pain, through immobilization and use of analgesics. Those patients who are not candidates for surgical intervention (for any reason), and who refuse to work toward active rehabilitation, clearly have suspect motivation that must be carefully evaluated. Obviously, this motivation factor is important for potential success in the functional restoration program.

The clinical interview also allows one to contrast the patient's current psychosocial functioning with past functioning, and to compare the psychologic testing data with the interview data. As I discussed

Table 36–3
Areas Explored in a Clinical Interview

Potential signs of depression

Signs of anxiety and stress

Patient and family mental health history

Patient and family history of substance abuse

History of head injury, convulsions, and impairment of function

Stressful changes in lifestyle or mental status before or since injury

Availability of social and family support systems

Optimism or pessimism about improvement

Faith vs. distrust in the medical system

Financial history, comparing current income to current cost of living

Work history, including explanation of job losses, job changes, and work-integration issues

Any litigation pending related to the patient's current medical problems

in Chapter 26 of this text, there is often a wide array of behavioral and psychologic reactions and problems, such as learned helplessness depression, anger, distrust, and somatization, which are the result of suffering with the chronic pain. The form these problems take primarily depends on the premorbid or pre-existing personality and psychologic characteristics of the individual, as well as current socioeconomic and environmental conditions. This is *not* to say that there is a consistent pre-existing "pain personality." Indeed, a great deal of research has not found any such consistent personality syndrome.[1] Rather, patients bring with them certain predisposing personality and psychologic characteristics that are exacerbated by the stress of attempting to cope with the chronic pain. The clinical interview can provide the first pieces of data to help determine the degree of psychologic disturbance present, which can significantly affect the treatment process. It is the norm, rather than the exception, that a layer of psychological and behavioral problems requires as much attention as the physical issues for the treatment program to be effective (see Chapter 26 of this text). Without a clear delineation of the psychologic issues, the physical component of the treatment process usually will be stalled.

The DSM-III-R Multiaxial Classification and the Structured Clinical Interview for the DSM-III-R

Of course, the degree to which a clinical interview is structured or standardized can vary greatly. An unstructured format can present a problem if one is interested in comparing the content and material gathered from certain patients by different interviewers. The different experiences and clinical skills of the interviewer will make comparisons of interview data difficult, if not impossible. Moreover, comparison will not lead to any standard diagnostic statement. In view of this, Reich, Rosenblatt, and Tupin[32] have cogently argued that a uniform diagnostic nomenclature must be used in order to develop a more accurate means for classifying patients with chronic pain. They suggest that the DSM-III (now the DSM-III-R, American Psychiatric Association)[33] would be a useful way to categorize chronic pain patients. They point out that using the DSM-III-R multiaxial classification criteria allows clinicians and researchers to consider both the physiologic and psychologic components of chronic pain in a systematized manner. The test can be performed with a greater degree of reproducibility than the currently available descriptive method. However, despite the above suggestions on the potential usefulness of the DSM-III-R nomenclature, to date it has not been frequently used in the chronic pain area.

The DSM-III-R sorts the physical, psychologic,

and historical components of a problem behavior into five categories or axes (Table 36–4). The first axis (Axis I) consists of clinical syndromes, and is used to designate major thought disorders and psychiatric problems such as schizophrenia, affective disorders, and substance abuse disorders. Axis II designates personality disorders (adults) and specific developmental disorders (children and adolescents). Some examples of Axis II diagnoses would be obsessive-compulsive and antisocial personalities. Axis III denotes the patient's medical diagnosis. The DSM-III-R considers knowledge of the general physical health of the person to be a major part of the total diagnostic picture. A patient with a herniated nucleus pulposus would have that diagnosis listed under Axis III. However, if a specific organic or pathophysiologic diagnosis cannot be made, the pain problem would be noted under Axis III, but this time by the patient's symptoms. Axis IV, Severity of Psychosocial Stressors, enables the clinician to rate specific psychosocial events that are judged to be significant contributors to the development or exacerbation of the present disorder. For example, death of a spouse, financial condition, and occupational status may have etiologic significance and, therefore, be considered psychosocial stressors. Finally, Axis V, Global Assessment of Functioning, allows the clinician to rate the patient's overall psychological, social, and occupational functioning on the Global Assessment of Functioning Scale, which assesses mental health or illness. Ratings on this scale are made for two time periods: current (level of functioning at the time of evaluation) and past year (the highest level of functioning for at least a few months during the past year).

Thus, a primary strength of the DSM-III-R is to allow multiaxial diagnoses. By ensuring that a diagnosis is based on all five axes, the DSM-III-R reduces the probability that a single diagnostic category will be used to represent a unique individual. The fact that patients with a similar psychiatric diagnosis differ significantly on a host of dimensions was often lost in traditional diagnostic systems. Moreover, unlike prior systems, the internal structure of the DSM-III-R is well delineated, with individual diagnoses defined in a relatively precise manner. It also, for the first time, provides a method by which to integrate concurrent psychiatric and physiologic diagnoses. As Reich, et al.,[32] note, this more precise classification of psychologic and medical diagnoses of patients with chronic pain syndromes will significantly aid in expanding our knowledge of these syndromes, as well as increasing our therapeutic skills in treating them.

One of the traditional problems encountered in studies attempting to diagnose psychiatric disorders, even those using the new DSM-III-R nomenclature, resides in the use of semistructured clinical interviews. Because the manner in which such clinical interviews are conducted can vary from clinician to clinician, it is difficult to make comparisons on the reliability and validity of the diagnoses of these studies. As a means of overcoming this major problem, the use of structured clinical interviews has been advocated. One such type is the Structured Clinical Interview for DSM-III-R (SCID).[34] The SCID requires that the interviewer ask the same set of questions to all patients, to either rule in or rule out various DSM-III-R diagnoses. In research studies, the SCID has the advantage over semistructured interviews because it insures that all patients are asked the same questions to make a diagnosis. Moreover, the SCID has a further advantage in that research has shown it to have good reliability (New York State Psychiatric Institute)[35] and promising validity.[36] In future studies, if investigators use the same diagnostic interview, it will be easier to compare results across different clinical settings and populations. Indeed, this was a major intent of the developers of the SCID.

The advantage of using the SCID for DSM-III-R diagnoses is that it allows a structured means of making more precise statements concerning the presence of any major psychiatric or personality disorders that can affect the course of treatment. At PRIDE and The University of Texas Southwestern Medical Center at Dallas, we are beginning to incorporate this into our clinical practice. This will not only provide useful clinical information, but will generate important data concerning the prevalence rates of various psychiatric and personality disorders in a chronic low back pain population. To date, there are not a great deal of data on this important issue.

Table 36–4
DSM-II-R Multiaxial Classification System

AXIS I:	Clinical syndromes
AXIS II:	Developmental disorders Personality disorders
AXIS III:	Physical disorders and conditions
AXIS IV:	Severity of psychosocial stressors
AXIS V:	Global assessment of functioning

BARRIERS TO RECOVERY

Pilowsky[37] originally formulated the concept of *Abnormal Illness Behavior* as a useful method for understanding and treating patients with physical symptoms or complaints for which there were no clearly diagnosed organic underpinnings. This formulation stemmed from earlier "sick role"[38] and "illness behavior"[39] models that focused on aspects of behavior associated with being sick—what people do when they are sick. The sick role has both advantages and disadvantages. On the one hand, sick people are stigmatized with all the attendant social awkwardness and decreased attractiveness that being sick entails. On the other hand, however, they are excused from their normal responsibilities and obligations. Indeed, some people may be highly motivated to seek the protection that being sick entails, as a way of evading responsibilities and being exempted from social obligations. This may become a potent reinforcer for not becoming "healthy."

According to Pilowsky,[37] a patient has a legitimate illness when he or she fulfills the requirements of an appropriate social group for admission to the sick role (usually the medical network or physician). However, a physician may begin to evaluate illness behavior as abnormal when a discrepancy exists between a patient's complaints or symptoms and observed disease or the patient's reaction to it. Because the determination of *abnormal* illness behavior is based on the judgment made by the physician, considerable authority is obviously placed in the physician's hand. Unfortunately, because a lack of definitive information often exists about the range of normal illness behaviors and what is really "normal," this judgment can be subjective. The physician then has the difficult task of unraveling "barriers to recovery" or disincentives for becoming "healthy" again.

With the help of the earlier reviewed assessment materials, a clinician will be in a better position to determine such barriers to recovery, which include psychologic, physical, financial, legal, social, and work-related issues, that can significantly interfere with a patient discarding the sick role and reassuming full functioning and a productive lifestyle. Psychologically, barriers include traditional concepts such as secondary gain (e.g., the chronic disability may be allowing the individual to avoid an unpleasant job situation); symptom magnification (an increased sensitivity and concern about physical symptoms as a means of justifying continued disability); and resistance to change. At other times, real interfering circumstances may be used as smoke screens or excuses for suboptimal performance and failure to adhere to the treatment regimen.

Treatment staff members must also be alert to potential secondary gains of continued disability, whether legal, financial, familial, or job-related. It is important that members of the treatment team are knowledgeable of all psychosocial issues while the patient is in rehabilitation. This knowledge allows staff members not only to better understand and

serve the patient, but also to be more effective in problem solving when the patient is not physically progressing as expected. Indeed, failure to progress physically generally represents psychosocial barriers to recovery, because the muscles and joints will not fail to respond if they are being exercised and trained appropriately as planned (unless rare denervation or ankylosis has occurred).

These barriers to recovery issues must be effectively assessed and brought to the attention of the entire treatment team. Steps can then be taken to understand their origins and avoid their interference with treatment goals. Table 36–5 lists these issues. They are individually discussed below.

General Psychologic Issues

Chronic pain and back dysfunction are more than just physical phenomena. One can safely assume that the majority of patients who are in a chronic pain population (and who are not working or receiving compensation) are depressed and demoralized by their present physical, psychologic, and socioeconomic status. Only a small percentage of patients are consciously malingering or "faking" for personal gains. Indeed, most researchers agree that true malingering as a voluntary attempt to falsify symptoms and as a means of achieving some specific goal such as a case settlement is a relatively rare phenomenon.[12,40]

By the time most patients reach a comprehensive rehabilitation program, their lack of progress has left them frustrated, discouraged, with low self-esteem, and almost always with significant and severe financial hardship. Most patients have been to several physicians, often receiving conflicting information in the process, resulting in frustration and distrust of medical systems. In addition, adversarial interactions in the work place or with insurance companies may have left many patients feeling betrayed and cheated. Furthermore, long-standing work, family, and self-esteem issues come into play when the pa-

Table 36–5
Barriers to Recovery: Important Issues to Consider in the Treatment of Chronic Low Back Pain

General psychological issues

Compliance or resistance issues

Financial disincentives

Somatization or symptom magnification

General emotional reactions: depression anxiety and fear anger entitlement

tient is injured and not fulfilling his usual social roles. All of these experiences can lead to psychologic barriers to recovery. Once assessed, these barriers must be directly dealt with through a variety of interventions.

Compliance and Resistance Issues

Unlike athletes, who usually have to be held back from doing too much too quickly, chronic back-disabled patients tend to be reluctant to "work through" their pain. Often this is related to fears of reinjury, depression, or other psychosocial barriers to recovery. In the early stages of treatment, when fear and trust are usually major issues for the patients, noncompliance or failure to progress is dealt with in a supportive and educational manner. A great deal of time and effort is put into explaining the treatment rationale to the patients and working with them in a collaborative manner. At the same time, however, staff members establish their roles as trained and experienced professionals who are experts so that they can push patients to greater physical activity.

Financial Disincentives

A major set of barriers to recovery revolves around financial disincentives. Indeed, there can be no doubt that financial compensation is a critical factor in the persistence of disability.[41] Such disincentives serve as secondary gains for not getting better. Many patients entering a treatment program or evaluation procedure are receiving some type of financial supplement, which will cease once the patient is no longer medically restricted from working. When the amount of the supplement approaches the patient's usual earnings, or is sufficient to support the patient's lifestyle, the economic incentive for returning to work is often removed. Patients may be involved in some type of injury-related litigation, which may or may not be affected by appearing "disabled" and in pain. An anticipated monetary settlement may alter the patient's customary behavior patterns, slowing recovery and increasing pain complaints. In many cases such behaviors, if not arrested early, may lead to "illness behaviors" that are difficult to reverse.

Other financial disincentives or secondary gains for not getting better include hoping for early retirement, having loans paid by disability insurance, and hoping for a new or better job based on the patient's being too "disabled" to perform the old job. The specifics of these financial issues vary, depending on state laws and whether the patient is involved in

state, federal, Social Security, long-term disability, or FELA compensation systems. The Treatment staff must be aware of financial disincentives for each patient because these issues have a major influence on motivation, pain reports, and adherence to treatment.

Somatization and Symptom Magnification vs. Malingering

As a result of multiple barriers to recovery, progressing the patient toward full physical functioning may at times be difficult. Moreover, psychosocial influences may lead the patient to be irritable, dependent, passive, or noncompliant, all of which may significantly tax the patience of health care professionals. There is a temptation at these times to view these patients as malingerers and fakes. In order to maintain a sense of respect for the patient that is vital in this type of intensive treatment, it is important to understand that these individuals use their physical symptoms as a way of dealing with, and communicating about, their emotional lives (*somatization*). That is to say, in this type of symptom magnification, physical symptoms may be easier to accept as causing current unhappiness and discontent than admitting that some psychologic reason is contributing to it. Only rarely is a patient consciously "faking" disability, although many times symptoms may be exaggerated consciously or unconsciously. Symptoms may also be magnified as a way of "saving face" and justifying continued disability after such a long period of dysfunction. This may therefore reflect conscious or unconscious illness affirming aspects of the abnormal illness behavior syndrome discussed earlier. These processes are most apparent in the realm of self-report pain measures. It is essential for treatment personnel (e.g., the psychologist) to carefully delineate such issues and develop an appropriate strategy to effectively deal with them. It should also be noted that this issue of symptom magnification, because it is so important in the area of chronic pain and disability, is generating a great deal of research interest.[40]

General Emotional Reactions

Certain emotional reactions can be expected in most chronic low back pain patients. The intensity of these reactions must be adequately assessed for all patients because it can greatly affect the treatment process. That is why the assessment devices reviewed earlier in this chapter are essential for developing a comprehensive clinical picture of a patient. Indeed, adequately assessing and dealing with the emotional fallout of the patient's upheaval in lifestyle is important in every treatment approach, including functional restoration. These important emotional reactions are described below.

Depression

Almost all chronic back patients will be depressed to some degree (whether they can acknowledge these feelings or not) because of the multiple losses they have sustained. Besides material and financial losses, these patients have lost jobs, family roles, important sources of their self-image and self-esteem, and, in some cases, their belief in "the system" (medical and otherwise). A severe, debilitating level of depression may have to be temporarily dealt with through antidepressant medication. This will have to be carefully evaluated and monitored by the medical and psychological staff.

Anxiety and Fear

Along with depression, almost all patients experience some degree of anxiety and fear. Often, a great fear of reinjury may significantly affect effort in the physical reconditioning component of the program. Also, in terms of general anxiety, this emotional state is hardly surprising given the level of disruption that patients experience in their lives. Furthermore, lack of closure regarding the long-term effects of their injury on finances, careers, relationships, and physical capacity adds to their concerns.

Anger

Reactions involving anger are perhaps the most obvious among this population. There is usually a great deal of anger at the workplace, which may be long-standing, or may result from real or perceived mistreatment since the injury. By the time most of these patients reach a comprehensive rehabilitation program, they have also developed an adversarial relationship with their insurance company, leading to an intensification and generalization of anger. Frustration with the lack of physical progress and lack of consistency in medical treatment can produce dissatisfaction with medical systems in general. This same lack of progress leads to anger at family and friends, who may imply that they are faking the injury because of the invisible nature of the physical handicap. It is important for staff to be sensitive to this anger and to defuse it whenever possible.

Entitlement

Along with a sense of anger, patients often have a sense of entitlement. This comes not only from long-standing psychologic issues mentioned earlier, but from a sense of feeling misunderstood, cheated, and betrayed. The financial and material losses they have sustained add to the belief that someone (or everyone) involved in the compensation process "owes me." Again, this emotional reaction must be adequately assessed because it can seriously jeopardize progression through a rehabilitation program.

DISABILITY MANAGEMENT

The above barriers to recovery and emotional reactions obviously need to be dealt with in order for rehabilitation to progress smoothly. Often, when a suboptimal effort is being shown in physical rehabilitation or when compliance is a problem, the barrier to recovery and emotional issues need to be addressed. There have been various psychologic treatment techniques developed and proven to be successful in dealing with these issues.

I have described a Multimodal Disability Management Program (MDMP) elsewhere.[1] It is based on a cognitive-behavioral approach to crisis intervention, and focuses on overcoming physical and psychosocial difficulties that interfere with returning to a productive, functional lifestyle. Treatment issues deal with events in the present or the recent past, and patients are helped in understanding how thoughts contribute to feelings and behaviors. Within this framework, therapists also maintain an awareness of early learning experiences and long-standing psychologic issues that can affect reactions to recent life experiences. For example, many patients come from family backgrounds where there was some significant emotional deprivation. As a result, many experience chronic feelings of anger, depression, and low self-esteem. Relatedly, they also have a sense of entitlement stemming from a frustrated search for an idealized caretaker. These issues, along with the cognitions and emotions accompanying them, are rekindled quickly when the patients find themselves involved in a medical/compensation/disability system that fosters dependency.

It should be noted that this MDMP approach differs from many typical "pain clinics," now estimated at 2000 in the United States, with a variety of treatment approaches. The early proliferation of pain clinics was stimulated primarily by a philosophy of focusing on "quality of life outcome criteria," rather than those outcomes having socioeconomic impact.[42] However, not only did such clinics proliferate in a nonstandardized manner, but when the rare scrutiny of treatment effectiveness was undertaken, results were sometimes no better than those for a placebo.[42] Indeed, as Fordyce and colleagues[42] indicate, the tendency of pain clinics to merely treat the experience of pain, and not the disability associated with pain behavior, has often led to unsuccessful treatment. Such overly narrow approaches were also frequently accompanied by the lack of recognition of physical capacity deficits such as the deconditioning syndrome,[1] as well as the lack of technology to measure it. This lack of effectiveness has led to a general perception, particularly among third party carriers, that rehabilitation for chronic back pain may be ineffective and, in fact, may be no better than placebo in attaining specific societal goals, such as return to work.[43]

The MDMP approach is an alternative to many of these unsuccessful pain clinics, with the major focus on the disability associated with the pain behavior, and not merely the experience of pain. In past publications, we discussed aspects of MDMP in some detail.[1,43,44] Basically, there are four major areas: (1) Individual and group counseling emphasizing a crisis intervention model (e.g., coping with family problems and unemployment). (2) Family counseling, during which family members are encouraged to take an active part in the rehabilitation process and are provided with information about the philosophy and specific details of MDMP. (3) Behavioral stress management training that involves initial training in muscle relaxation, followed by exercises in guided imagery in which patients practice relaxing while imagining themselves in various stressful situations. Patients also receive EMG/temperature biofeedback sessions during which they refine their relaxation skills, with the understanding that these skills will help them cope more effectively with residual pain and discomfort. (4) Cognitive-behavioral skills training that includes instruction in assertiveness, rational versus irrational thinking, and stress and time management.

Besides involvement in the four treatment components of MDMP, the maintenance by the psychologic staff of a positive therapeutic environment is important. Part of the therapeutic environment maintenance is accomplished with each patient individually evaluated and then managed through counseling and educational interventions. Moreover, frequent and clear communication between the psychologic staff and all members of the treatment team working with a particular patient is essential. This active disability management approach emphasizes the return of the patient to his previous productive lifestyle as quickly as possible through aggressive functional restoration.

These above cognitive-behavioral treatment methods have been found to be effective when used in the overall context of a functional restoration treatment approach.[1] In administering such treatment, however, it should be clearly kept in mind that each patient is unique and must be individually evaluated

so that the treatment program can be carefully tailored. Blindly administering the same disability management program to all patients regardless of unique individual needs will guarantee failure. Careful psychosocial assessment, as discussed earlier in this chapter, must be conducted first. Individually tailored treatment can then be effectively administered.

REFERENCES

1. Mayer, T.G., Gatchel, R.J.: Functional Restoration for Spinal Disorders: The Sports Medicine Approach. Philadelphia. Lea & Febiger, 1988.
2. Gatchel, R.J., Mears, F.G.: Personality: Theory, Assessment, and Research. New York, St. Martin's Press, 1982.
3. Barnes, D., Gatchel, R.J., Mayer, T.G., Barnett, J.: Changes in MMPI profile levels of chronic low back pain patients following successful treatment. J Spine Dis. In press.
4. Naliboff, B.D., McCreary, C.P., McArthur, D.L., Cohen, M.J., Gottlieb, H.J.: MMPI changes following behavioral treatment of chronic low back pain. Pain 35: 271–277, 1988.
5. Derogatis, L.R., Lipman, R.S., Covi, L.: The SCL-90: an outpatient psychiatric rating scale. Psychopharm Bull 9:13–28, 1973.
6. Kinney, R., Gatchel, R.J., Mayer, T.G.: The SCL-90R: an alternative to the MMPI for psychological screening of chronic low back pain patients. Presented at the annual meeting of the International Society for the Study of the Lumbar Spine, Kyoto, Japan, May, 1989.
7. Millon, T., Green, C.J., Meagher, R.B.: Millon Behavioral Health Inventory. 3rd Ed. Minneapolis, Interpretive Scoring System, 1982.
8. Mitchell, J. (ed.): The Ninth Mental Measurements Yearbook. Lincoln, University of Nebraska Press, 1985.
9. Beck, A.: Depression: Clinical, Experimental and Theoretical Aspects. New York, Harper & Row, 1967.
10. Ward, N.: Tricyclic antidepressant for chronic low back pain: mechanism of action and predictors of response. Spine 11:661–665, 1986.
11. Hamilton, M.: A rating scale for depression. J Neurol Neurosurg Psychiat 23:56–62, 1960.
12. Mooney, V., Cairns, D., Robertson, J.: A system for evaluating and treating chronic back disability. West J Med 124:370–376, 1976.
13. Million, R., et al.: Evaluation of low back pain and assessment of lumbar corsets with and without back supports. Ann Rheumat Dis 40:449–454, 1981.
14. Fairbank, J.C., Davies, J.D., Couper, J., O'Brien, J.P.: The Oswestry low back pain disability questionnaire. Physiotherapy 66:271–273, 1980.
15. Bergner, M., Bobbit, R.A., Carter, W.B., Gibson, B.S.: The sickness impact profile: development and final version of a health status measure. Med. Care 19:787–805, 1981.
16. Bergner, M.: The sickness impact profile. In Assessment of Quality of Life in Clinical Trials of Cardiovascular Therapies (Edited by N.K. Wenger, M.E. Mattson, and C.D. Furberg). New York, LeJacq Publishing, pp. 152–159, 1984.
17. Follick, M., Smith, T., Ahern, D.: The sickness impact profile: a global measure of disability in chronic low back pain. Pain 21:67–76, 1985.
18. Williams, R.C.: Toward a set of reliable and valid measures for chronic pain assessment and outcome research. Pain 35: 239–251, 1988.
19. Leavitt, F.: Detecting psychological disturbance using verbal pain measurement: the back pain classification scale. In Pain

Measurement and Assessment (Edited by R. Melzack). New York, Raven Press, 1983.

20. Kames, L.O., Naliboff, B.D., Heinrich, R.L., Schag, C.C.: The chronic illness problem inventory: problem-oriented psychological assessment of patients with chronic illness. Int J Psychiat Med 14:65–75, 1984.

21. Smith, T.W., Aberger, E.W., Follick, M.J., Ahern, D.K.: Cognitive distortion and psychological distress in chronic low back pain. J Consult Clin Psychol 54:573–575, 1986.

22. Roland, M., Morris, R.: A study of the natural history of back pain. I: development of a reliable and sensitive measure of disability in low back pain. Spine 8:141–144, 1983.

23. Evans, J., Kagan, A.: The development of a functional rating scale to measure the treatment outcome of chronic spinal patients. Spine 11:277–281, 1986.

24. Hendler, N., Vierstein, M., Gucer, P., Long, D.: A preoperative screening test for chronic back pain patients. Psychosomatics 20:801–808, 1979.

25. Fries, J.F.: Toward an understanding of patient outcome measure. Arthr Rheumatol 26:687, 1983.

26. Pilowsky, I., Spence, N.D.: Patterns of illness behavior in patients with intractable pain. J Psychosom Res 19:279–287, 1975.

27. Melzack, R.: The McGill Pain Questionnaire: major properties and scoring methods. Pain 1:277–299, 1975.

28. Monks, R., Taenzer, P.: A comprehensive pain questionnaire. In Pain Measurement and Assessment (Edited by R. Melzack). New York, Raven Press, pp. 233–237.

29. Tait, R.C., Pollard, A., Margolis, R.B., Duckro, P.N., Krause, J.J.: The pain disability index: Psychometric and validity data. Arch Phys Med Rehabil 68:438–441, 1987.

30. Brown, G., Nicassio, P.: (1987). Development of a questionnaire for the assessment of active and passive coping strategies in chronic pain patients. Pain 31:53–64, 1987.

31. Kerns, R.D., Turk, D.C., Rudy, T.F. The West Haven-Yale Multidimensional Pain Inventory (WHYMPI). Pain 23:345–356, 1985.

32. Reich, J., Rosenblatt, R.M., Tupin, J.: The DSM-III: A new nomenclature for classifying patients with chronic pain. Pain 16:201–206, 1983.

33. American Psychiatric Association: Diagnostic and Statistical Manual of Mental Disorders, 3rd Ed. Washington, DC, APA, 1987.

34. Spitzer, R.L., Williams, J.B.W., Gibbon, M., First, M.B.: Structured Clinical Interview for DSM-III-R. New York, New York State Psychiatric Institute, 1988.

35. New York State Psychiatric Institute: Scoop on SCID reliability. SCID Newsletter, July 1, p. 2, 1988.

36. Skodol, A.E., Rosnick, L., Kellman, D., Oldham, J.M., Hyler, J.E.: Validating structured DSM-III-R personality disorder assessment using longitudinal data. Am J Psychiatry, In press.

37. Pilowsky, I.: Psychodynamic aspects of the pain experience. In The Psychology of Pain (Edited by R.A. Steinbach). New York, Raven Press, 1978.

38. Parsons, T.: Social Structure and Personality. London, Collier-MacMillan, 1964.

39. Pilowsky, I.: A general classification of abnormal illness behavior. Br J Med Psychiatry 51:131–137, 1978.

40. Mechanic, D.: The concept of illness behavior. J Chron Dis 15:189–194, 1962.

41. Matheson, L.N.: Symptom magnification syndrome. In Work injury: Management and prevention (Edited by S.J. Isernhagen). New York, Aspen Publishers, 1988.

42. Beals, R.: Compensation and recovery from injury. West J Med 140:233–237, 1984.

43. Fordyce, W., Roberts, A., Sternbach, R.: The behavioral management of chronic pain: a response to critics. Pain 22:112–125, 1985.

44. Mayer, T., et al.: Objective assessment of spine function following industrial injury: a prospective study with comparison group and one-year follow-up; Volvo Award in Clinical Sciences. Spine 10:482–493, 1985.

45. Mayer, T., et al.: A prospective randomized two year study of functional restoration in industrial low back injury utilizing objective assessment. JAMA, 258:1763–1769, 1987.

Patrick R. Johnson
Wilbert E. Fordyce

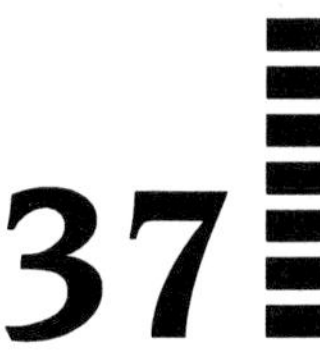

History of Pain Management Treatment

The aim of this chapter is to recount briefly the development of multidisciplinary, behaviorally based treatment for chronic pain related to spinal cord injury (SCI) and present an overview of its component parts. To meet those ends, the problem of chronic pain among SCI patients is described, after which a short history of the development of multidisciplinary pain treatment is presented. Effort will be made to describe the behavioral aspect of pain clinic treatment in some detail; more traditional medical approaches are discussed elsewhere in the text, and it is, after all, the emphasis on behavioral issues that distinguishes the multidisciplinary pain clinic from other treatment settings. The discussion then focuses on the ways in which pain problems are now assessed and diagnosed in the pain clinic, how treatment plans are typically developed and carried out, and what difference a multidisciplinary approach has made in terms of overall ability to manage chronic pain related to SCI.

Description of Chronic Pain Among SCI Patients

Estimates of the prevalence of disabling or incapacitating SCI chronic pain have varied from less than 20% to as much as 50% of all patients with SCI. Incidence of some level of chronic pain, not necessarily disabling, has been reported in excess of 90%. Disabling pain seems relatively rare, and severity of pain is not always associated with the degree of spinal damage the individual has suffered. Also, the presence of severe pain does not appear to be consistently related to a history of surgical rather than conservative treatment.

Although disabling pain may be rare among SCI patients in a relative sense, the absolute number of spinal-injured individuals who also have chronic pain is likely on the order of tens of thousands. For such individuals, limitations imposed by their spinal injuries are augmented by limitations caused by pain. As a result, their ability to participate in normal daily activities—working, family outings, sports and leisure activities, sex, relaxation—is severely curtailed. The successful rehabilitation of these patients is expensive, so that fiscally and in terms of loss of quality of life, disabling pain among SCI patients is a costly problem.

The Need for a Multidisciplinary Approach

Historically, chronic pain among SCI patients has been as poorly understood, and therefore as poorly managed, as any other chronic pain problem. Although clinicians have recognized for decades that unresolved pain is a common complaint of individuals who suffer spinal injuries, such pain problems have often gone undertreated and, in some cases, untreated entirely.

Prior to the development of what might be called "the pain clinic approach," traditional treatments for pain related to spinal injury may have included any combination of the following: neurosurgery (laminectomy, neurolysis, lumbar sympathectomy, cordotomy, anterior rhizotomy); physical therapy modalities (e.g., Hubbard tank, microwave, infrared, ultrasound, massage, heat and cold); medications for pain (morphine, meperidine hydrochloride, ASA, codeine, acetophenetidin); and, as a last resort, psychotherapy. Medications for muscle spasm have also been commonly used (e.g., nicotinic acid, tranquilizers, diphenhydramine hydrochloride) either because of the relationship of pain to spasticity, or because of the patient's perception that such medications directly lead to pain relief.

Historically, each of these treatments, either used alone or in combination with others, has only limited usefulness in the management of chronic SCI pain. As far back as 1948, Munro[1] observed that pain related to SCI was typically associated with unknown causes and unsuccessful operations. Similarly, in 1962, at about the time that Dr. John Bonica was establishing the first chronic pain treatment program at the University of Washington in Seattle (described below), Kaplan, Grynbaum, Lloyd, and Rusk[2] wrote that, "the satisfactory nonsurgical treatment of pain and spasticity has proved to be elusive." The complexity of the problems was well appreciated.

Although it had been observed that complicated psychosocial or behavioral issues, such as psychopathology and inappropriate narcotic and alcohol use, were often concomitants of pain, there was little consensus among early scientists and clinicians regarding the reason for treatment failures. They often were attributed to technically inadequate neurosurgical procedures rather than an emotional imbalance or the development of a "pain pattern" by the patient. On the other hand, some physicians only reluctantly considered radical therapy (i.e., surgery) for pain because of the relative minority of patients who had pain and a strong bias that patients may use pain in a functional conversion sense. This conclusion was based in part on the observation that pain often developed in new anatomical areas following surgical ablation of afferent structures in the initially painful site, at a time when there was no physiologic model for understanding how this could happen.

Various schemes have been developed for classifying SCI chronic pain according to its possible locus. These have been summarized in Table 37–1. It is important, and unfortunate, to observe that the same fundamental error regarding the putative reason patients have pain is present in the SCI literature that is seen in other writings about chronic pain: a dualistic insistence that pain is either caused by "objective" physical causes or is somehow psychogenic, the product of the patient's unconscious needs, emotionality, or psychopathology.

The error inherent in this point of view is partly in the dichotomy it poses (i.e., that pain is either physical or mental), and partly relates to a misunderstanding about the ways that cognition and behavior contribute to pain problems. Burke[3] was one of the first authors to recognize and describe significant psychological components of pain related to spinal injury in a way that is consistent with current thinking. He reported, for example, that the incidence of premorbid drug use and narcotic use was high among patients who later complained of unresolved pain. He found females and older patients to be over-represented, consistent with some current reports, and suggested that pain may be strongly related to histories of multiple operations, commonly

Table 37–1
Summary of Possible Sources or Causes of Chronic Pain Related to Spinal Cord Injury

1. Musculoskeletal: Often related to spasticity
2. Visceral
3. Root
4. Sympathetic: Sometimes relievable by sympathectomy
5. Diffuse pain with sensory loss: Includes causalgia and phantom pain
6. Psychic: Perhaps as an overlay to other types of pain; difficult to treat

seen in American but not Australian patients. Burke also identified other factors that exacerbate pain, including depression and inactivity among patients who lay in bed for weeks and months (often as a means of treating bed sores), delays in rehabilitation following injury that result in significant periods of deactivation, and overuse of narcotic analgesics. He further observed that patients successful in dealing with pain seemed more motivated and determined to fight back than did unsuccessful patients. Thus, he concluded that pain with organic correlates may well be exaggerated by psychologic factors.

In general, Burke's[3] findings have paralleled the reports of others that higher levels of pain and increasing interference with daily activities are associated with greater age, anxiety, depression, and distress, and with worse psychosocial environment. Therefore, there has been a clear need for a more sophisticated, nondualistic model of pain that accounts for complex emotional, behavioral, and psychosocial issues that no doubt influence resistance to traditional treatment.

The Development of the "Pain Clinic" Approach

In order to appreciate the complexity of appropriate treatment for chronic pain, it is useful to understand what a pain clinic is, what it is not, and what multidisciplinary treatment encompasses.

Systematic examination of pain in its own right and not just as a symptom of some other problem began with the pioneering work of John J. Bonica at the University of Washington. In 1961, Bonica and a neurosurgeon, Lowell White, began weekly clinics focusing on analysis of chronic pain problems. Several medical disciplines became involved (e.g., orthopaedic surgery, oral surgery, and psychiatry). These early efforts were largely diagnostic in nature, and patients were often then shunted into various treatment tracks offered by the professionals involved.

A few years later (1967), coincidentally also at the University of Washington but in the Department of Rehabilitation Medicine, Fordyce, Fowler, Lehmann, and DeLateur began almost serendipitously to experiment with modifying the nature of the health care professional's attention to a complaining pain patient. This constituted altering the social consequences of pain behaviors or complaints. Instead of attending closely and sympathetically, they simply responded to statements about pain by, literally, looking out the window. The effects were startling. The patient ended several days of refusing to participate in physical therapy because of intense pain by rising, dressing, and resuming treatment. Although far from sure that modified attention responses accounted for the patient's sudden change in behavior, they devised a set of approaches based on altering consequences or contingencies to various forms of pain behaviors. These approaches involved shifting analgesic consumption from prn, or pain behavior contingent, to a time contingent regimen and shifting the exercise-rest relationship from the more traditional mode of working to tolerance to one of working to quota. That is, rest became contingent upon completing a certain amount of effort rather than being controlled by how the patient felt.

These approaches were then tried with a chronic back pain patient. Again, the results were startling. Prescribed narcotic addiction was eliminated, as was consumption of analgesics. Instead of significant deactivation, activity level rapidly climbed to normal levels. The patient returned to operating his somewhat physically arduous business.

The plan was then applied to yet another patient: a woman in her early 40s who had undergone four back operations for low back pain, was addicted to prescribed analgesics, and was deactivated to the point of spending approximately 23 hours per day reclining. Within a few weeks under the behavioral regimen, she ceased taking analgesics, reduced reclining to approximately 8 hours per day, and returned to her homemaking activities, all the while walking with great speed and vigor. This was the beginning of the so-called operant conditioning approach to chronic pain.

Two years previously, this patient had been evaluated by the Bonica/White Pain Clinic but without their finding a successful treatment program. The two programs discussed these results and decided to join forces. For several years, the two programs, the Pain Clinic and the Operant Program in Rehabilitation Medicine, functioned separately but interactively. Subsequently, in 1983, the two were merged into what is now termed the Multidisciplinary Pain Center.

The central point of this history is that it reflects a symbiotic and synergistic merger of medical science and behavioral science to address one of the most costly and vexatious problems in health care: chronic pain.

The Pain Clinic Approach Compared to Traditional Medicine

As a first approximation, the "pain clinic approach" could be defined as a truly multidisciplinary effort that incorporates the expertise of physicians, behavioral scientists, nurses, physical, occupational, and recreational therapists, and vocational counselors as their expertise is required for the effective management of the complex of problems related to chronic pain. Not all patients require help from each of these disciplines, although, in our experience, at a minimum, a physician and psychologist need to be involved.

Philosophically and in practice, what distinguishes a pain clinic from a more traditional approach is its rejection of the traditional disease model of treatment in favor of a more comprehensive behavioral model that stresses the individual's personal responsibility for getting well. The basis for this model is a central feature of chronic pain: the observation that there is not a one-to-one correspondence between the relative degree of significant illness or injury that is perceived by the clinician, and the amount of pain the patient complains of or the degree of impairment he or she may demonstrate. Stated differently, patients receiving treatment for chronic pain are likely to hurt out of proportion to the objective physical findings related to their pain problem. (In fact, physical findings that could conceivably account for the individual's pain are often absent.)

A corollary of this behavioral model is that pain and suffering are best construed as a focus of treatment, rather than as symptoms or indices of underlying disease. To understand why this is so, it may be useful to consider some basic definitions, now widely accepted, of the components of the experience of pain.

Definitions

First, chronic pain is a distinctly different experience and distinctly different clinical problem from acute pain. Although chronic pain is often defined in terms of months of duration, a more useful definition is that chronic pain is simply pain that persists after healing is known to have taken place. Loeser[4] has described four aspects of the experience of pain, acute or chronic, that are interrelated but distinct (Fig. 37-1).

Nociception is the neural impulse that conveys information to the brain regarding potential or actual tissue damage. It is nothing more nor less than a bioelectric response of nerves of a certain type.

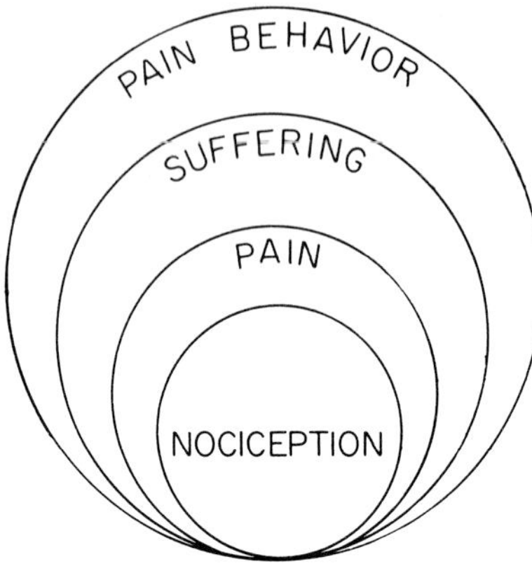

Figure 37–1. Loeser's schematic for describing the components of chronic pain.[1] (From Loeser, J.D.: Concepts in pain. In Chronic Low Back Pain. Edited by M. Stanton-Hicks and R.A. Boas. New York, Raven Press, 1982.)

When the nociceptive input reaches the brain, it is typically, but not always, experienced as pain. Thus, *pain* is defined as a perceptual response, an activity of the cortex. Pain may or may not have nociception as an immediate antecedent, however. When people hurt, they say and do things that communicate to others that they are hurting. These actions are called *pain behaviors*, and represent a very powerful class of social communication. Finally, *suffering* is the emotional response of the individual to the perception of pain and is often also communicated via pain behaviors.

As a means of describing how these four aspects of pain interact, an alternative to Loeser's model is presented in Figure 37–2. It merits some explanation. First, there is not complete overlap among nociception, pain, and pain behaviors, indicating that it is possible for a patient to experience or manifest any one or two of these without input from the others. Thus, although nociception is likely to produce pain, it does not in every case. Under some extraordinary circumstances, for example when an individual has undergone a nerve block or is completely distracted by an engrossing task, tissue damage may have taken place with nociceptive input from the site of the damage that is never perceived as pain. Further examples of this kind of phenomenon can be found in Melzack and Wall.[5]

It is also possible to experience pain in the absence of nociception. As a rule, nociception is not considered to be a common contributing factor to problems of chronic pain because nociception relates to tissue injury that, by definition, is typically no longer present among chronic pain sufferers except as may derive from disuse. Although SCI patients with chronic pain may complain of burning pains, phantom pains, or disesthesias that no doubt are residual

to their spinal injuries, these problems are understood not to be the product of nociceptive input because the injury sites are long healed.

Whether or not nociception is a significant factor, it is critically important to appreciate that the pain behaviors the individual engages in, including complaining of pain as if it were caused by tissue damage, are typically the same. Patients do not make a distinction based on the presence or absence of nociception. Unfortunately, clinicians sometimes attempt to make such a distinction according to the erroneous belief described above that "real pain" is related to "objective findings" and pain in the absence of a lesion of some sort is "not real." It is a de facto assumption of the pain clinic approach that pain behaviors always serve to communicate suffering related to pain, whatever the source of the patient's pain perceptions.

It is the core of the pain clinic approach to focus on behaviors that communicate pain related to suffering as the target of treatment. Partly this is by default. The only possible way of making inferences about the suffering of others is by observing their overt behaviors. It has been rightly observed that the perception of pain is a private experience, and can only be appreciated by others according to what one says and does to communicate his or her pain perceptions. More to the point, however, pain be-

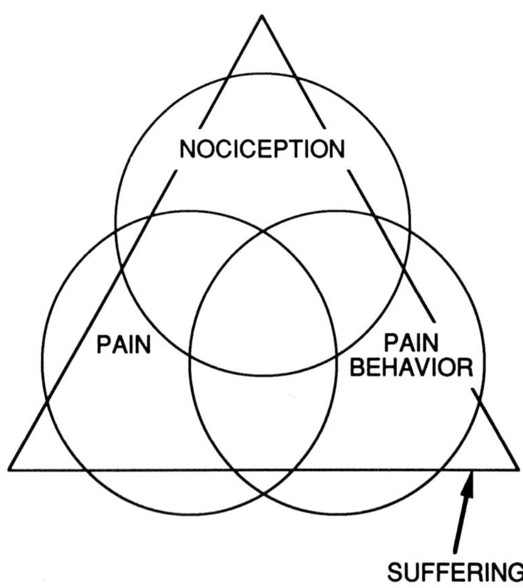

Figure 37–2. An elaboration on Loeser's model. Interactions among nociception, pain, and pain behavior are complex. Suffering, represented as a triangle, will vary in intensity at any given time, and sometimes not be a part of the patient's experience at all. For example, muscle pain following physical therapy that is related to nociception and is evidenced by rubbing the muscle (a pain behavior) may not be related to significant suffering.

haviors, like any other behavior, are under the control of the rules of operant learning to a significant degree. This is as true of pain related to SCI as to any other injury or problem, and some basic terminology about operant learning should be reviewed in order to proceed.

An analysis of pain behaviors related to chronic pain begins with a search for contingencies in the patient's environment that may influence the strength and frequency of specific behaviors. The question in the mind of the clinician might be, "What are the learning-based factors driving this person's pain behaviors other than nociception?" *Reinforcement* of pain behaviors occurs whenever the outcome following the performance of that behavior is positive in some way for the individual. It has the effect of increasing the likelihood that the behavior will be performed again under similar circumstances in the future. Increased attention and nurturance from others, significant amounts of rest and time out from aversive activities, and the pleasant effects of medications can all be powerful reinforcers of pain behavior when they are made available based on the strength or frequency of the performance of the behavior. *Punishment*, on the other hand, occurs whenever the outcome following a behavior is negative or unpleasant in some way and results in a decreased likelihood that the behavior will be performed. It is an axiom of the operant approach that behaviors that persist over time are assuredly being reinforced, either by being followed directly by reinforcing consequences or because they result in successful avoidance of anticipated aversive consequences. Those behaviors that the patient drops out are those that do not encounter reinforcing consequences, a process known as extinction.

Several learned patterns of pain behaviors based on particular kinds of reinforcement have been identified. Pain behaviors are sometimes said to be under social control, a generic term referring to reinforcements deriving from events outside the skin, e.g., in interactions with others. For example, responding to the pain complaints of another by being extraordinarily affectionate and not demonstrating a similar amount of affection when the individual does not complain will almost certainly put that person at risk for engaging in more or stronger pain complaints. As a result, he or she will suffer more.

Pain behaviors may also escalate under certain stimulus conditions. It is not unusual, for example, for an individual originally injured in a motor vehicle accident to complain of worse pain while riding in or driving a car. In such a case, pain behaviors are referred to as being under *stimulus control* and might be thought of as a type of learned fear or phobic response. Not uncommonly, such learned fear often interferes with rehabilitation efforts, in this case

perhaps learning to drive with manual controls.

Pain behaviors may also be shaped and maintained by a process of *avoidance learning.* In the narrowest sense, pain behaviors that result in limiting one's activities are inherently reinforced by the fact that rest and relaxation are, to a point, pleasant. Moreover, movement is often inherently punishing because most chronic pain sufferers are significantly deactivated and virtually any attempts at mobilization and strengthening result in increased pain. In a wider sense, however, avoidance learning may contribute to the constriction of other kinds of behaviors as well. As an example, a physician's order of bed rest is, among other things, a signal to those around the patient to significantly lower their expectations about the patient's abilities to fulfill his or her responsibilities. To the extent that any part of meeting one's responsibilities is aversive, and being granted time out from them is pleasurable, the pain behaviors that initially obtained the sanction for time out will likely be reinforced. Or, to put it simply, if a patient no longer does housework because of pain in his extremities, and housework is aversive for him, he might, over time, display increasingly flagrant pain behaviors and actually hurt more in situations that in the past have been associated with doing housework.

It may be tempting to conclude from this last comment that pain behaviors persist because of some malingering or deceitful manipulation on the part of the patient. Such a conclusion would, however, be patently false. Patterns of operant behavior develop automatically, without regard either to the individual's level of intelligence, or even what behaviors are in his or her best interest. Behaviors, even very maladaptive ones, persist because they have a history of being reinforced.

In the context of the development and maintenance of pain behaviors though, no contingency or outcome is absolutely reinforcing. To begin with, pain behaviors are unpleasant for everyone, including the patient, and it would be difficult to argue that there is much about their performance that is inherently reinforcing. Though bed rest and increased affection from others may have been initially pleasant or rewarding, patients seen for treatment typically complain of being miserable with their lifestyles. Despite their complaints, however, some aspects of the lifestyle are sufficiently reinforcing to overcome the effects of negative outcomes, otherwise the disabled behaviors would not persist.

To understand how an acute pain problem may become chronic, consider the role of *anticipatory learning.* In the acute phase, pain as a signal of damage usually results in guarding behaviors that protect the individual from further injury. It seems likely that a predisposition for learning to protect ourselves is present from birth such that the reinforcement value associated with guarding behaviors is high. Patterns of overguarding tend to carry over into chronicity. Movement should be prescribed as a treatment rather than being avoided, but often it is not. Because movement hurts, increased pain becomes associated with reactivation and becomes a powerful barrier to rehabilitation. Witness the difficulty physical therapists often have trying to help SCI patients with chronic pain to improve their performance in exercise programs. Fearful of reinjury and worse tissue damage, and naturally reluctant to undergo the suffering inherent in movement, such patients learn to anticipate that exercise of any kind may harm them or lead to increased suffering, be it a gentle stretch or a part of a program aimed at getting them back to work. Again, such learning is automatic and insidious, and has no relationship to what the patient might say or intend for himself as a long range treatment goal.

Other ways of learning to hurt, often associated with cognitive processes, are likely at work in the maintenance of pain behaviors as well. For example, the entrenched belief that movement is dangerous is often associated with a strong somatic focus and a powerful disease or *illness conviction,* defined as the equally entrenched belief that chronic pain is caused by some occult cause that the clinicians have overlooked and could be easily treated with a procedure or medication if only the cause could be tracked down. In our experience, such a belief system can only be altered through structured reactivation, such as the physical therapy quota system outlined above. Simple instruction, rational argument, or admonitions are usually futile: Information is a low-power way to change behavior.

Such illness conviction is often seen among chronic pain patients and exemplifies the critical role of labelling in determining one's response to pain. The strong belief that pain is an indication of ongoing physical harm, even pain of years' duration, will always be associated with worse suffering. Conversely, patients who learn to view their pain as benign suffer less, even though their pain may at times be severe. Hence, it might be said that decreasing ambiguity about the meaning of pain is likely to reduce the patient's suffering. This is certainly consistent with the clinical experience of many of the health care professionals who work in pain clinic settings.

Notice in this discussion that reference is often made to suffering, described above as the emotional reaction to pain. Strictly speaking, it is suffering that pain behaviors communicate, of which pain is only one component. In fact, it is the confounding of pain and suffering in the life of the pain patient that complicates the clinical picture and necessitates a sophisticated approach to treatment. As evidence for this assertion, consider the problem of depression, widely acknowledged to be persistent among pain sufferers.

When patients are described as "depressed," a statement is being made about how they behave. Their sleep cycles and eating habits are often disrupted, they sometimes have difficulty concentrating or remembering, they may move and speak slowly, and often pursue pleasurable activities less. Using the shorthand of the clinic, we say they have "vegetative symptoms." In addition, such patients often describe themselves as feeling sad or down, and reliably report that when they are feeling worst emotionally their pain is also at its worst. By observation, they also display a more flagrant and varied panoply of pain behaviors. In the language of operant contingencies, depression describes a pattern of behaviors associated with a certain affect (i.e., sadness, irritability) that stems from the loss of reinforcements and imposition of punishments related to pain and disability.

As should be evident, the suffering and depression almost inevitably associated with assimilation of severe physical disability, as in SCI, is at great risk to be confounded with pain. The SCI patient is suffering, and probably experiencing degrees of nociception, as well. That patient will be hard put to differentiate pain from suffering and often cannot. Pain or suffering behaviors are emitted. Those around the patient, including health care professionals, are equally at risk to be unable to differentiate reliably pain from the suffering associated with assimilation of disability. Like the patient, they may, and indeed, often do, take actions designed to minimize pain, e.g., prescribing or sanctioning rest and guarding of movement. In doing so, they inadvertently contribute directly to the evolution of chronic pain problems in their SCI patients. This issue of confounding pain with suffering is probably the major reason behavioral concepts are so central to pain in SCI. Moreover, difficulties that patients encounter during their rehabilitation efforts, for example, meeting goals of occupational therapy or resuming regular patterns of social interaction, often serve as palpable reminders of limitations imposed by their disability. Such reminders are negative outcomes that may diminish the patient's continued effort in a rehabilitation program through avoidance learning. Thus, the patient says he or she cannot finish physical therapy because it hurts too much.

DIAGNOSIS

Introduction and Case History

In this section, more specific information is presented regarding the application of the principles described above to the analysis of complex pain problems related to SCI. To do this, reference is made to the case history of a patient treated using a multidisciplinary approach. LB was a 46-year-old, Caucasian male who has been paraplegic since December 1980 when he was shot in the back by his wife following an argument. This detail is mentioned because it bears on some of the psychosocial issues related to his history. His spinal cord injury was at the level of T-4, and it left him with spasticity in his abdomen, buttocks, and lower extremities, in addition to chronic pain. His pain was mainly in his buttocks and thighs. He described it as an ache most of the time, although it tended to take on an intense burning quality whenever it became severe.

LB was initially referred to the pain clinic from the department of neurosurgery, where his physicians had been unsuccessful in managing his pain. For about 18 months, he had been treated by traditional approaches. A variety of treatments were tried, including antispasmodics (e.g., Baclofen) and an epidural electrical stimulator, which failed. He appeared to get the greatest relief from Percodan, although tolerance and resulting overuse tended to be problems.

As is often the case with pain related to spinal injury, LB's symptoms were initially treated as if they were primarily the result of some physiological or mechanical abnormality. Specifically, he was diagnosed as having a "central pain state," understood to be a pattern of afferent input that is mediated by the central nervous system and is not caused by nociceptive input from the site of the injury. Because a medical model was initially invoked to account for his symptoms, however, progress in the treatment of his pain and suffering was at first limited. When other factors contributing to his suffering were later identified, progress with treatment improved. For example, LB had a history of depression stemming from his injury that had been well described by the pain clinic. At the time that he was referred to one of the psychologists in the clinic for evaluation, his symptoms of depression, including sleep disturbance, social withdrawal, loss of pleasure in activities, and dysphoria, had worsened. He even had suicidal ideation and some thought of a suicidal plan as recently as 4 or 5 weeks prior to the evaluation. Although he had been tried on an antidepressant medication in the past (Amitriptyline 100 mg HS), with some improvement in his symptoms, it had been discontinued because of problems with weight gain. He was, however, still taking Percodan, at a higher than prescribed rate, as well as Lioresal 20 mg, 5 per day for spasticity.

From a behavioral point of view, there were several factors apparently contributing to LB's complaints of pain and suffering, in addition to the contribution of his alleged central pain syndrome. Concurrent with a significant flare-up in pain, he had been having some significant, intense, and abrasive conflicts with his wife. Although they had remained married following the shooting incident, they were now separated and she had temporary custody of their two teenage children. This was not an entirely amiable split, and the patient had been left feeling used and abandoned, and, as a result, angry and resentful. At this same time, his aging father was seriously ill, and LB was taking primary responsibility for his care with little help from other family members.

In terms of daily activities, LB had become something of a shut-in. In sharp contrast to his description of himself before his injury as a "workaholic" (he had been a construction superintendent working 60 to 70 hours a week on average), an athlete, and an involved parent, he now tended to keep to himself and avoid social activities, ostensibly in an effort to avoid inconveniencing others with his disability. From a cognitive behavioral perspective, it might be said that he was closing himself off from the opportunity for reinforcements derived from pleasurable activities that he had pursued in the past. He elected not to date, return to work, socialize with friends, or participate in athletics, all of which were in fact possible for him, despite his disability.

LB had also developed two methods for attempting to deal with pain flare-ups that, in fact, probably worsened the problem rather than helping. The first had to do with pacing his level of activity throughout the day. Consistent with other aspects of his reclusive lifestyle, he tended to spend much of his free time working on home improvement projects, alone. He often tended to work long hours at a fairly rapid pace, until his pain level increased to the point that he was compelled to stop. Thus, level of activity became an infallible predictor of worsening pain. In other instances, he reported stepping up his work pace deliberately, in an effort to "take [his] mind off the pain." Although using distraction is often an effective means of coping with pain, using it this way further solidified the learned connection between activity and pain while also minimizing neurophysiologic based discomfort.

The second behavioral problem LB had developed related to a habit of locking the front door, drawing the curtains, unplugging the telephone, and sitting for hours alone in a darkened room, attempting to gain control over escalating pain and spasm. Predictably, these episodes occurred most frequently when family conflicts were more intensely felt, and this means of closing himself off from external inputs only produced more suffering. It was not difficult to understand that he had begun relying more and more on narcotic analgesics in an effort to manage these complicated problems.

Based on this evaluation, it was apparent that a multimodal approach to his care was needed. From this point on, treatment decisions were made jointly by the neurosurgeon and the psychologist, integrating cognitive behavioral with medical concepts.

Overview of Diagnostic Issues

The pre-eminent issue related to the diagnosis and treatment of any pain problem, including SCI pain, is the determination of the factors that elicit the pain behaviors observed. The first step in making that determination involves resolving the question of medical stability. A medical problem is said to be stable when it is judged that healing has taken place, no other invasive procedures are likely to produce significant improvement, and not treating the problem will not result in further deterioration. Note that medical stability says nothing about pain or disability.

Most patients with chronic pain are medically stable. This generally includes patients with SCI pain, although their conditions are not always static. Although LB was medically stable, for example, he described changes in sensation in his lower extremities, including changes in pain, apparently related to regeneration of damaged neural tissue, even more than 8 years after his injury. Although such changes in perception somewhat complicated the course of his treatment, they tended to have little impact on diagnostic decisions.

Because most SCI patients with chronic pain are medically stable, nociception from the site of the initial injury is not a contributor to the problem. Diagnostic options, in terms of a medical model, are therefore limited to pain caused by central mediation (which may reflect learning-based changes in the central nervous system), or pain caused by the degeneration of tissue above the site of the spinal lesion. Although the latter diagnosis is more straight forward and suggests specific treatments, it is unfortunately rare among SCI patients.

An analysis of behavioral factors thus takes on central importance. These include environmental contingencies that reinforce pain and disability behaviors as described above. Referring back to the case of LB, to the extent that he was uncomfortable in social interactions because of diminished self-esteem or concerns about being perceived as an inconvenience to others, he ran the risk of having pain behaviors (e.g., social withdrawal and complaining about his pain) reinforced because they sanctioned

time out from aversive activity. As a result, he likely suffered more.

Other behavioral factors have commonly been observed to contribute to chronic SCI pain. Many of these were relevant to LB, including psychosocial stress, difficulty pacing activities, and depression. He did not have particularly strong illness conviction and generally appreciated that the pain and suffering were interlinked with behavioral patterns. He also had not suffered any cognitive impairment, often seen among SCI patients, and a very difficult problem to manage. In addition to suffering the effects of limitations imposed by brain injury, cognitively impaired patients are at risk for confounding that suffering with pain. As yet another example of the avoidance learning described above, it is more acceptable to forego playing bridge with one's friends because of pain than because of difficulty following the course of the game.

TREATMENT

Multidisciplinary treatment programs reflect the input of all members of the treatment team. For example, the long range care of LB has included both medical and psychological components. Regarding medical treatment, relevant options have been few. No further invasive procedures (e.g., operations or nerve blocks) appear likely to help. He has, however, received some benefit from several specific medications. He has been restarted on Amitriptyline 25 mg HS, to be increased as needed, primarily for sleep disruption related to depression. In addition, because it appeared that he had become somewhat tolerant to Percodan, that medication has been replaced with a pain cocktail containing methadone. The long range plan is to continue that prescription indefinitely, as long as it is supplying good relief.

Based on the behavioral analysis of his pain problem, a treatment plan was outlined that focused on: (1) using a daily schedule to pace activities such that the association between pain level and activity, and spasticity and activity, would be broken up, and (2) developing a plan for managing stresses related to family and relationship issues. Although deactivation had not become a problem, the plan also included exploring ways to become more socially active on a scheduled basis.

Over the course of several weeks of treatment, LB experienced significant reduction in suffering related to pain and improved quality of life. He developed a plan for dealing more effectively with family stressors, that was furthered along by improvement in his father's health. He also learned how to pace his activities more effectively throughout the day, and has achieved some success in monitoring and behaviorally counteracting symptoms of depression. In general, both his mood and his vegetative symptoms have improved considerably.

Progress leading to lasting change is likely to be slow. It has been difficult for LB to identify ways of comfortably learning to be more socially outgoing, and that will continue to be a focus of discussion and planning in long-term treatment. In addition, his progress regarding pacing of activities and managing stressors will be monitored once or twice a month, and modifications to the behavioral plan will be made as needed.

Overview of Treatment Issues

Reflecting on the case of LB as a model, it can be said that the primary goals of multidisciplinary treatment for patients with SCI pain are management of pain, differentiating pain from suffering, restoration of function, enhanced adaptation to one's environment, and prevention of complications that may arise within the first few months of onset if complex behavioral, emotional, and psychosocial factors are ignored. Total eradication of pain is probably not an appropriate goal, for several reasons. First, there are no known procedures or agents, medical or behavioral, that reliably eliminate pain. More important, however, it should be clear from the discussion

above that suffering confounded with pain, not pain per se, is usually what brings patients to the pain clinic, SCI patients and otherwise.

As in other treatment settings, multidisciplinary treatment is based on the assessment information originally used to make a diagnosis. Typically, all conceivable medical treatment options will be tried, usually in the early phases of treatment, either prior to or concurrent with the use of cognitive behavioral strategies. Both kinds of modalities have been summarized in Table 37–2.

Although anecdotal reports and clinical experience suggest that the multidisciplinary pain clinic approach to treatment of these problems is unparalleled in its comprehensiveness and efficacy, empirical data to confirm or refute this claim are lacking. This is unfortunate. Because the multidisciplinary approach relies on input from health care professionals from such varied backgrounds as medicine, clinical psychology, physical therapy, and vocational training, it tends to be very costly. Moreover, there may be something better that can only be identified by careful outcome research. Clearly, much work is needed to fine tune and improve upon the treatment that is now available for these unfortunate patients.

SUMMARY

The appropriate diagnosis and treatment of chronic pain related to spinal cord injury should be multidisciplinary in nature, similar to the treatment approach now commonly used in the management of other chronic pain problems. Although the need for a sophisticated approach to managing such pain problems has been evident for many years, the multidisciplinary pain clinic has only come into existence within the past decade.

The pain clinic approach to managing chronic SCI pain differs from traditional approaches primarily in its scope. Expanding upon the traditional medical model, this approach emphasizes the assessment of the patient's behavioral patterns and cognitive or evaluative processes—as well as the differentiation of pain (nociception) from suffering—all of which combine to influence the level of suffering and disability associated with pain complaints. Such psychological factors need to be addressed concurrent with physiological factors that may contribute to pain, in order for a program of treatment to be effective. As a rule, clinicians treating SCI patients with chronic pain should probably assume that operant factors are contributing significantly to the individual's pain complaints, until the clinical evidence suggests otherwise.

Table 37–2
*Summary of Medical and Behavioral Treatment Modalities
for Chronic Pain Related to Spinal Cord Injury*

Medical
1. Medications (Includes Amitriptyline, sometimes used in combination with Prolixin or Tegretol; antispasmodics and analgesics, including the "pain cocktail," discussed in the text.)
2. Nerve blocks and other invasive anesthetic procedures
3. Neurosurgery (Includes both peripheral and central neuroablative procedures, as well as electrical stimulators.)

Behavioral
1. Management of behavioral contingencies (Includes attention to social and stimulus control issues, as well as specific patterns of behavior such as avoidance and anticipatory learning, discussed in the text.)
2. Attention to pacing of activities
3. Stress management (Includes the use of a variety of relaxation training techniques as well as cognitive restructuring.)
4. Depression management
5. Attention to the labels and meanings attached to the pain problem, as they may exacerbate suffering
6. Assessment and remediation of cognitive deficits, if present
7. Physical reactivation in collaboration with physical therapy
8. Vocational retraining

REFERENCES

1. Munro, D.: Rehabilitation of veterans paralyzed as the result of injury to the spinal cord and cauda equina. Am J Surg *IXXV*:3, 1948.
2. Burke, D.C.: Pain in paraplegia. Paraplegia *10*:207, 1973.
3. Loeser, J.D.: Concepts of pain. *In* Chronic Low Back Pain (Edited by M. Stanton-Hicks and R.A. Boas). New York, Raven Press, 1982.
4. Melzack, R., Wall, P.D.: The Challenge of Pain: Exciting Discoveries in the New Science of Pain Control. New York, Basic Books, 1983.
5. Kaplan, L.I., Grynbaum, B.B., Lloyd, K.E., Rusk, H.A.: Pain and spasticity in patients with spinal cord dysfunction: results of a follow-up study. JAMA *182*:120, 1962.

Peter B. Polatin

38

Psychoactive Medications as Adjuncts in Functional Restoration

The patient who presents for functional restoration treatment is frequently someone who has a significant amount of emotional distress. The pain and disability processes may have taken their toll with an increased presence of anxiety, pain sensitivity, avoidance behavior, and emotional pessimism. As mentioned in Chapter 14, it is well acknowledged clinically and in the literature that a high incidence of depression occurs in this patient population. Whether this represents a specific depressive syndrome, or a constellation of symptoms of somatization, anxiety, and discouragement must be clarified in each individual case. Additionally, poor premorbid coping skills, maladaptive behavior, and inherent distrust may contribute to complications in medical management. It is, therefore, a therapeutic challenge to assess these patients behaviorally and psychologically, and to use psychotropic medication to facilitate the goals of rehabilitation. In so doing, it is critically important to monitor the therapeutic benefits while minimizing side effects which will subvert rehabilitation goals, particularly those which may result in oversedation, cognitive disturbance, or excessive anticholinergic or extrapyramidal symptoms.

Specifically then, it is important for the clinician to be able to assess anxiety, depression, substance and alcohol abuse, and other maladaptive behavior, and to use psychotropic medication as a resource to control these problems. This represents the first criterion for the use of psychoactive medications in functional restoration and is similar to their use in a general psychiatric practice, in which psychiatric assessment then dictates the choice of appropriate medication. However, the second criterion by which some of these medications may be used in these patients is more specifically in the context of pain management. The heterocyclic antidepressants have been well documented to have a positive effect on chronic pain, frequently at doses lower than the standard antidepressant dosage, and with a more rapid onset of action.[1-11] The anxiolytics, by modifying anxiety, distress, and associated muscle tension and spasm, will mitigate pain.[12] The antipsychotics, though with no inherent effect on pain, may nevertheless alter pain perception by altering distressing delusional, hallucinatory, or other cognitively distorted symptoms.[12]

MAJOR CATEGORIES OF PSYCHOTROPIC MEDICATIONS

Psychotropic medications may be divided into specific categories, based on primary therapeutic effect. This is summarized in Table 38–1. In considering the use of these medications there may be some confounding issues which make the choice less clear cut. For example: Is a patient not sleeping because of a primary sleep disturbance or because of an underlying depressive disorder? Is an individual who is complaining of stress and presenting with significant anxiety in need of an anxiolytic agent or an antidepressant? Is an agitated patient with multiple psychologic symptoms also presenting with a subtle, and as yet undetected, psychotic disorder that might benefit from a low dose neuroleptic? Is treatment resistance reflective of an underlying personality disorder that may benefit from some short term medication controls aimed at decreasing target symptoms such as anxiety and depression, but which in the long term will remain essentially unchanged and re-

Table 38–1
Categories of Psychotropic Medications

Sedatives

Anti-anxiety agents

Antidepressants

Antipsychotic agents

Mood stabilizing agents

quire more ongoing counseling and behavioral management?

A decision tree for the use of psychotropic medications is summarized in Figure 38–1. The first issue to assess from a pharmacologic perspective is whether the patient is abusing drugs or alcohol. This is a critical piece of information for treatment for several reasons. In the first place, any rehabilitation effort has a poorer prognosis if chemical abuse continues. In addition, compliance with psychotropic medication will be questionable and potential pharmacologic benefit may be neutralized even if the medicine is taken as directed. This is most dramatically illustrated in the case of alcoholism with antidepressants. High doses of alcohol decrease therapeutic levels of heterocyclic antidepressants and also increase the incidence of anticholinergic effects and arrhythmias. Opiates with antidepressants synergistically contribute to an increased incidence of anticholinergic effects as well as central nervous system (CNS) depression. The sedatives and anti-anxiety agents may have additional CNS depression effects with the underlying substance abused and create additional risk of morbidity for the patient.

Once the issue of substance abuse has been addressed and the clinician is dealing with a relatively compliant individual who has tapered his analgesics and muscle relaxants, or has reduced his drinking to an acceptable level, if not total abstinence, then the issue of psychotropic medication can be seriously entertained.

Antidepressants

Table 38–2 summarizes the various categories of antidepressant medications. It is largely the heterocyclics that have direct application to the functional restoration process. These agents have the most clearly documented effect on chronic back pain in a number of clinical studies.[1,3,4,10,11,13] The heterocyclics are thought to exert a therapeutic effect by blocking the re-uptake of biogenic amines at the neurosynaptic junction in various areas of the brain. These transmitters include norepinephrine, serotonin, and dopamine, though it is believed that the former two are the agents most specifically effected in depression. Individual drugs vary in their specificity for norepinephrine versus serotonin (Table 38–3). Although some agents have equal effects on both, others are thought to act more exclusively on norepinephrine (nortriptyline maprotiline) or serotonin (trazodone, fluoxetine). Currently, it is also felt that the pain relieving effect these agents may exert is related to their serotonin effects in specific areas of the spinal cord and the brainstem, though the mechanism of action may be different than the antidepressant action.

The MAO inhibitors exert their antidepressant effect by a different mechanism. Specifically, they inhibit monoamine oxidase activity in the central nervous system, thereby blocking oxidative deamination of naturally occurring monoamines. However, in the treatment of depression, they are considered to be a

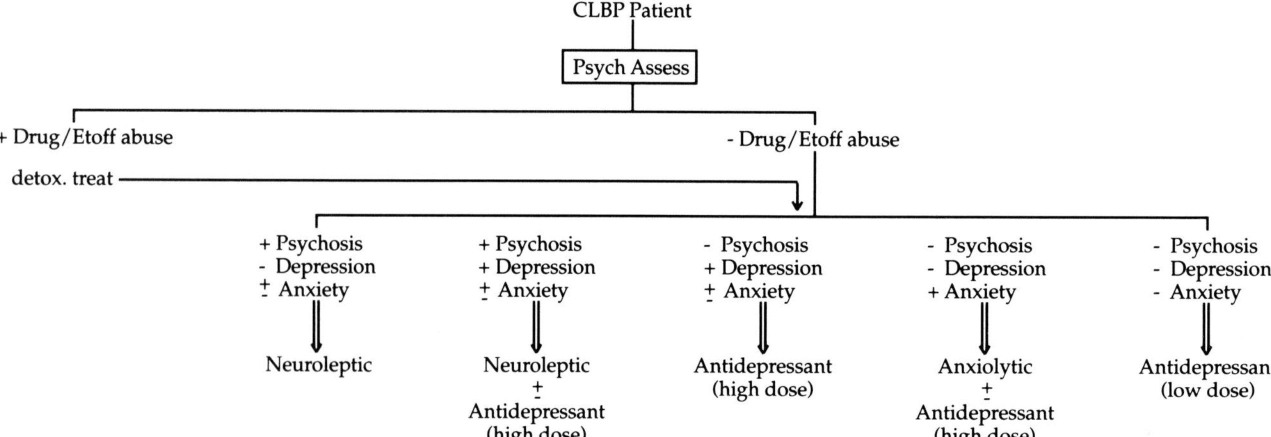

Figure 38–1. A decision tree for the use of psychotropic medications.

Table 38–2
Categories of Antidepressants

Heterocyclics
  imipramine (Tofranil)
  amitriptyline (Elavil)
  doxepin (Sinequan)
  nortriptyline (Pamelor)
  desipramine (Norpramine)
  clomipramine (Anafranil)
  trazodone (Desyrel)
  fluoxetine (Prozac)
  maprotiline (Ludiomil)

MAO Inhibitors
  phenelzine (Nardil)
  tranylcypromine (Parnate)
  isocarboxide (Marplan)

---

second line drug because of the increased incidence of side effects; to prevent these side effects patients must be placed on a tyramine-free diet. In the patient population requiring functional restoration, the necessity of closely monitoring a special diet makes this category of anti-depressant a less desirable option. However, there is no question that these agents have significant and potent antidepressant effects and have been found, in the research literature, additionally to have some beneficial effect on chronic pain.

Use and Choice of Antidepressants

The decision to use an antidepressant (i.e., a heterocyclic) in a candidate for functional restoration rehabilitation depends on the presence of significant chronic pain, which may be somewhat reduced by the use of one of these agents or the presence of clinical depression. One or both of these features should be present. Depression can clearly be established by a careful history as well as by the use of various self-report and clinician administered tests that are helpful for both initially establishing the diagnosis and then monitoring response to antidepressant medication. These assessment techniques have been described in Chapter 36, and consist of such instruments as the Beck Depressive Inventory (BDI), the Hamilton Rating Scale, the Zung Rating Scale and Scale 2 on the MMPI. From a practical perspective, we have found the BDI and the Hamilton Rating Scale to be the most useful in monitoring progress.

The choice of an individual heterocyclic agent is frequently not unequivocal. Individual clinicians are best advised to familiarize themselves with two or three different heterocyclic antidepressants. The choice might be determined by the following factors: (1) All heterocyclics have demonstrated antidepressant activity, but some more than others have been well studied in regard to their effects on chronic pain. Those that have demonstrated a pain relieving effect in a number of clinical trials include amitriptyline, desipramine, doxepin, and clomipramine (recently available in the USA).[1–4,6–8,10,11] (2) On the basis of current theory on the mechanism of action of heterocyclic antidepressants on chronic pain, it would be assumed that those agents with more pure serotoninergic action would be more useful in treating chronic pain.[14] These include trazodone (Desyrel) and fluoxetine (Prozac). There are several other serotoninergic agents being used experimentally, but not yet available in the United States. (3) Some heterocyclic antidepressants have primarily a sedative effect, whereas others have a more alerting or energizing effect. Therefore, patients who present in a more agitated, anxious, sleep disturbed state, might be more likely to benefit from a sedative heterocyclic, whereas a patient presenting as significantly slowed down with low energy and general psychomotor retardation might benefit from a more energizing heterocyclic. The sedative versus the energizing heterocyclics are delineated in Table 38–4.

Within these considerations, it is best to be familiar with a primarily serotoninergic agent and a primarily noradrenergic agent, as well as a more sedative agent versus a more activating agent.

Potential Side Effects

It is also important to be aware of the potential side effects of these medications (Table 38–5). The primarily noradrenergic agents tend to have a higher

---

Table 38–3
Specificity of Serotonin vs. Norepinephrine Re-uptake Blockade of Different Heterocyclics

Pure Serotonin		Serotonin + Norepinephrine Equally	Pure Norepinephrine
trazodone	clomipramine	doxepin	maprotiline
fluoxetine	amitriptyline	imipramine	desipramine
			nortriptyline

Table 38–4
Sedative Spectrum of Heterocyclics

Low Sedation		High Sedation
desipramine	imipramine	amitriptyline
fluoxetine	maprotiline	doxepin
	nortriptyline	trazodone

Table 38–5
Side Effects of Heterocyclics

Autonomic:	*dry mouth *blurred vision retarded ejaculation *decreased intestinal mobility & constipation *urinary retention pathologic sweating anorexia insomnia psychomotor stimulation
Central Nervous System	*sedation psychomotor slowing muscle weakness nervousness *headaches *agitation vertigo tremor ataxia dysarthria nystagmus lowered seizure threshold toxic delerium (central anticholinergic syndrome) *withdrawal syndrome
Cardiac:	*postural hypotension tachycardia arrhythmia EKG changes (flattened T waves, prolonged QT intervals, depressed ST segments)
Ocular:	worsening of narrow angle glaucoma
Gastric:	heartburn *nausea
Hematologic:	leukocytic effects, purpura agranulocytosis
Skin:	rash petechiae photosensitivity urticaria
Miscellaneous:	priapism (trazodone) tinnitus increased appetite edema alopecia

*Commonly seen

incidence of autonomic effects, whereas the serotoninergic agents are more frequently associated with headaches, gastric symptoms, and agitation. Side effects must be monitored closely, not only because of the clinical discomfort and distress they may cause, but additionally because at a mild, tolerable level they may be indicative of the adequacy of the dosage, particularly to attain an antidepressant effect.

As mentioned previously, the antidepressant dosage is significantly higher than the pain dosage of the same agent. The onset of action for pain is much shorter, generally within a week or two, frequently associated with improved sleep pattern. The antidepressant effect, on the other hand, may not be evident for 3 or 4 weeks at adequate dosage, which will be considerably higher. Table 38–6 illustrates demonstrative doses for different heterocyclic agents, comparing their pain-relieving to their antidepressant dosages.

Side effect profile additionally may guide the clinician to a choice of one agent in a particular patient with, for example, cardiac disease. Because cardiac arrhythmia is a potential risk in all of these agents, the least cardiotoxic drug would be chosen in a cardiac patient: this would be either doxepin, trazodone, or fluoxetine. Similarly, when confronted with a patient with significant narrow angle glaucoma, the choice of heterocyclic agent would be restricted to a serotoninergic agent with no significant anticholinergic effects, either trazodone or fluoxetine.

It should be emphasized that these drugs are effective and can be safely administered. However, it is essential that the physician is thoroughly familiar with the side effect profile of any of these agents. For example, trazodone, which is an effective antidepressant, as well as having primarily serotonin reuptake activity, does have the idiosyncratic side effect of priapism in a small number of males, which has not been described with any of the other heterocyclics. Because in the Physicians Desk Reference for Desyrel, this particular side effect is emphasized in capital letters, it is advisable that the physician at

Table 38–6
Heterocyclic Antidepressant Dosages

	Pain	Depression
Desipramine	75 mg	75–200 mg
Nortriptyline	50–100 mg	75–150 mg
Maprotiline	?	75–300 mg
Doxepin	50–100 mg	150–300 mg
Imipramine	50–75 mg	150–300 mg
Amitriptyline	75–150 mg	150–300 mg
Trazodone	?	150–400 mg
Fluoxetine	?	20–80 mg

least mention it when prescribing the medication initially to a male patient.

Clinically, the best way of monitoring a patient's response to a heterocyclic agent is by carefully inquiring about anticipated side effects on regular medical follow up and by serially assessing self-report measures of chronic pain or depression, depending upon the target symptoms being treated. It is also possible to draw blood levels which, with some of these agents (nortriptyline, desipramine, amitriptyline, doxepin), have been found to correlate with antidepressant effect within a dose-response curve. In the case of nortriptyline, a "therapeutic window," below or above which an antidepressant effect may not be seen, has been demonstrated. However, while blood levels confirm that a patient is taking medication as prescribed, the dose-response curve has not been confirmed with all heterocyclics. Regular monitoring of blood levels in all patients may not be useful, but certainly is helpful in problematic cases in which an ambiguous response has been seen, or where compliance is in question.

Similarly, the dexamethasone suppression test (DST), believed to be a "biological marker" of depression, is not valuable in this patient population. Many individuals will be on a variety of medications, which may interfere with the validity of the test. The decision to use an antidepressant will not be exclusively based on strict psychiatric criteria for diagnosis of depression or even for an antidepressant effect. Good and careful clinical assessment has been found to be more relevant. The DST is specific, but not clinically sensitive enough.

Anti-Anxiety Agents

As shown in Table 38–7, a variety of anxiolytic medications exist that are effective in controlling the core symptoms of anxiety. The benzodiazepines (Table 38–8) are the most commonly used and are well tolerated by most patients. The minimal side effects

Table 38–7
Anti-Anxiety Agents

benzodiazepines
buspirone (Buspar)
propranolol (Inderal)
barbiturates
meprobamate (Equanil, Miltown)
antihistamines (Hydroxyzine, Atarax)

Table 38–8
Benzodiazepines (Anxiolytics)

	Dosage Equiv. (mg)	Absorption Rate	Half-life
lorazepam (Ativan)	1	intermediate	short
oxazepam (Serax)	15	slow	short
alprazolam (Xanax)	0.5	intermediate	short
chlordiazepoxide (Librium)	10	intermediate	intermediate
clorazepate (Tranxene)	7.5	fast	longest
diazepam (Valium)	5	fastest	long
prazepam (Centrax)	10	slowest	longest

consist of drowsiness and ataxia. Less frequently reported are psychomotor impairment, sedation, short-term memory loss, and behavioral disinhibition with hostile acting out. All of these are reversible by either lowering the dosage or discontinuing the drug. There is the risk of tolerance and dependency, particularly in individuals with a previous history of chemical abuse.

Clinicians should be aware of the potential for a withdrawal syndrome when a benzodiazepine is discontinued, requiring gradual tapering. Current recommendations are to reduce the dosage by 5 to 10% each day. Recurrence of pretreatment anxiety several weeks after the drug has been discontinued is noted in some cases, requiring a more protracted tapering period, particularly with alprazolam.

The mechanism of action of the benzodiazepine is not fully understood, but they are believed to interact with brain "benzodiazepine" receptors in the limbic system and thalamus, facilitating increased activity of the inhibitory neurotransmitter gamma-aminobutyric acid (GABA).

For the short term treatment of anxiety in the functional restoration setting these agents are the treatment of choice. Buspirone (Buspar), an anxiolytic of a different drug class, has a different mechanism of action, with a slower onset of effect. Because it does have a moderate affinity for brain dopamine receptors, among its other actions, it has the potential for extrapyramidal side effects, including tardive dyskinesia, requiring more careful monitoring, and may not be as satisfactory in the rehabilitation treatment setting. The beta blockers, particularly Inderal, are effective in controlling the peripheral symptoms of anxiety on an ongoing, long term basis, but again, are not the agents of choice in a rehabilitation setting, particularly given their effect on heart rate. Barbiturates, meprobamate, and Atarax, although useful for the treatment of anxiety, are simply not as effective as the benzodiazepines. Additionally, some of the antidepressants have an anxiolytic effect, particularly in the more florid panic disorders. This has been described particularly for imipramine and for Nardil, but is probably true of most of these agents, both heterocyclic and mono-amine oxidate (MAO) inhibitors. However, for ease of administration and rapid onset of therapeutic benefit with safety, the benzodiazepines are preferable.

Again, the clinician is advised to become very familiar with one or two of the benzodiazepines. Agents with a relatively longer half life may have more clinical usefulness with less of a risk of severe or late-emerging withdrawal syndrome. Examples of these are chlordiazepoxide, chlorazepate and diazepam.

These drugs are usually administered on a BID to QID dosage. Preferably, they should not be used in an open-ended manner, but over a period of a few weeks or months to control disturbing symptoms and then tapered slowly when other effective measures have been brought into the treatment program. Examples of effective nonpharmacologic interventions for symptoms of anxiety are biofeedback, self-hypnosis, relaxation training, behavioral therapy, and some cognitive therapy approaches. These may be used within the context of functional restoration rehabilitation.

The addictive potential of the benzodiazepines, particularly diazepam, should never be overlooked, particularly when treating sociopathic or previously chemically dependent patients.

The benzodiazepines themselves are not believed to have the direct effect on chronic pain that has been documented for the antidepressants. However, by reducing stress and muscle tension they indirectly modify pain, and may mitigate somatic focus and symptom magnification in the chronic pain patient.[12]

Antipsychotic Agents

Table 38–9 lists the major tranquilizers, or neuroleptics, by pharmacologic category and dosage range. These medications have a potent effect on psychotic behavior and agitation, primarily by their action of blockading dopamine receptors in various pathways within the brain. Although the clinician supervising functional restoration infrequently requires the use of these agents, it is best to be familiar with one or two that may be used on an occasional basis. There is one spectrum of antipsychotic potency on which to conceptualize these medications. Using chlorpromazine, the prototype drug, as a standard of comparison, lower potency, higher dos-

Table 38–9
Antipsychotic Agents

Phenothiazines	Equivalent dosage (mg)*
chlorpromazine (Thorazine)	100
thioridazine (Mellaril)	100
trifluoperazine (Stelazine)	5
fluphenazine (Prolixin)	2–5
perphenazine (Trilafon)	10
Thioxanthenes	
thiothixene (Navane)	5
Butyrophenones	
haloperidol (Haldol)	2–5
Dibenzoxazepines	
loxepine (Loxitane)	15
Dihydroindolones	
molindone (Moban)	10

*Usual antipsychotic dosage range for an acutely ill schiozophrenic is 300–1200 mg qd of chlorpromazine or equivalent.

age agents, generally tend to be more sedative and additionally have a lower incidence of extrapyramidal side effects. Examples of these would be chlorpromazine and thioridazine. The higher potency, lower dose agents, such as haloperidol and fluphenazine, although used in a much lower dosage range than the sedative group, also tend to have a higher incidence of extrapyramidal effects (Table 38–10).

It should be emphasized that the neuroleptics (or antipsychotics) have a firm place in psychiatry in the control of psychotic behavior and delusional and

Table 38–10
Spectrum of Side Effects Neuroleptics

High Potency (Ex-fluphenazine)	Low Potency (Ex-chlorpromazine)
Extrapyramidal reactions	
Neuroleptic malignant syndrome	
	Sedation
	Postural hypotension
	Decreased seizure threshold
	EKG changes
	Skin pigmentation
	Photosensitivity
	Agranulocytosis
	Anticholinergic Effects
	Cholestatic jaundice

hallucinatory thinking, as well as the associated psychomotor agitation. Although these agents have also been studied with regard to their efficacy in controlling chronic pain, they have not been found to be that useful, though they have augmented opiate analgesia in some studies.

Side Effects

The extrapyramidal effects must be monitored carefully. Acute dystonia, akathisia, and parkinsonism are relatively early side effects in this category. Tardive dyskinesia, which is of later onset and associated with chronic dosage, is particularly troublesome in that it is sometimes irreversible. Therefore, within the functional restoration context, these agents should be used carefully, for short periods of time, in problematic cases which may require psychiatric consultation.

Additionally, the lowest effective dose should be used, such that rehabilitation can continue to be performed. In this clinician's experience, the most useful of these agents tend to be the nonsedating ones: i.e., haloperidol, thiothixene, trifluoperazine, and perphenazine.

If an individual patient on one of these medications develops an extrapyramidal syndrome, this may be well controlled with antiparkinsonian agents, which should then be used along with the neuroleptic (See Table 38–11). A detailed discussion of the administration of the neuroleptics is beyond the scope of this chapter, but references for further information are included in the bibliography.[12,15–18]

Mood Stabilizing Agents

Mood stabilizing agents will be infrequently administered in the rehabilitation context. The most representative and best known of these medications are lithium carbonate and lithium citrate, the first

Table 38–11
*Antiparkinsonian Agents that may be Used with a Neuroleptic
to Prevent Extrapyramidal Side Effects*

	Daily Dosage (in mg)
amantidine (Symmetrel)	100–300
benztropine (Cogentin)	1–6
biperiden (Akineton)	2–6
diphenylhydramine (Benadryl)	25–200
procyclidine (Kemadrin)	6–20
trihexyphenidyl (Artane)	1–10

treatment of choice for bipolar affective disorder (manic depressive illness), particularly in the manic phase. The only use for one of these medications in the functional restoration context is for the emergence of manic behavior, when the diagnosis of bipolar affective illness has been made. Treatment should probably be best initiated by a psychiatrist, but can be monitored by a rehabilitation physician familiar with the side effects of lithium.

Carbamazepine (Tegretol) is also found to have mood stabilizing effects, but is used as a second line drug in the control of manic depressive illness, because it also has a high incidence of significant side effects which require careful monitoring by a clinician, and probably is not recommended for use within the functional restoration context.

These agents themselves do not have inherent pain relieving effect, although lithium carbonate has been found to be effective in cluster headaches, but certainly not in back pain. Therefore, the only justification for use in the rehabilitation arena is for the control of the emerging psychiatric symptoms reflective of mania.

Sedatives

The range of medications used for nocturnal sedation and the treatment of insomnia, are listed in Table 38–12. A number of different drug categories are used, ranging from Trofan (serotonin precursor) and Benadryl (an antihistamine) to the benzodiazepines and barbiturates. In choosing a sedative one must first rule out the etiologic effect of underlying depression on sleep. An individual who presents with a sleep disturbance and clinical depression is best treated with an antidepressant, because therapeutic response will manifest itself with improvement in sleep pattern. Conversely, a highly anxious, extremely stressed individual may benefit from an anxiolytic and manifest sleep improvement as his anxiety is brought under control. However, for the nondepressed, nonanxious patient with chronic pain, the least addictive medication should be tried first. Frequently, excellent sedative response is obtained with Benadryl at a range of 50 to 150 mg hs. Unfortunately, Trofan recently has been found to cause eosinophilic myalgia syndrome, and is therefore no longer recommended, although it is an excellent sedative.

Benzodiazepines are believed to be the most effective of the sedatives because of the least disruption of REM sleep, and the widest margin of safety in their use. Therefore, if insomnia persists in spite of a first line sedative choice, consideration might be given to flurazepam, temazepam, or triazolam. There have been some reports in the literature about

Table 38–12
Sedatives

Benzodiazepines
    fluorazepam (Dalmane)
    temazepam (Restoril)
    triazolam (Halcion)

Barbiturates
    amobarbital (Amytal)
    pentobarbital (Nembutal)
    secobarbital (Seconal)

Chloral derivatives
    chloral hydrate (Noctec)

Antihistamines
    diphenyl hydramine (Benadryl)

Not recommended
    glutethimide (Doriden)
    methyprylon (Noludar)
    methaqualone (Qualude)
    ethchlorvyne (Placidyl)
    ethinamate (Valmid)
    tryptophan (Trofan)

temporary and reversible cognitive deficits with benzodiazepines, as well as disinhibition resulting in violent behavior associated with triazolam use. An individual with poor impulse control should be monitored carefully if placed on a benzodiazepine, whether it be for anxiety or insomnia.

SUMMARY

Psychotropic agents are useful adjuncts to facilitate functional restoration in particularly symptomatic individuals. Although the response to a judiciously used antidepressant or anxiolytic may be dramatic, it is not in itself curative, but merely facilitates the necessary rehabilitation that must occur to ensure that treatment goals are attained. The physician's role here is as the psychopharmacologist, aided by the behavioral observations of the other team members, particularly the managing psychologist. However, although the physician requires the feedback of other members of the team, he must be hypervigilent about issues involving side effects, toxicity, lack of therapeutic response or worsening clinical picture. A detailed "hands on" manual of how to use psychotropic medication is beyond the scope of this chapter. However, the clinician should consult the references in the bibliography for more detailed knowledge of each of these agents.[16–18]

REFERENCES

1. Alcoff, J. et al.: Controlled trial of imipramine for chronic low back pain. J Fam Pract 14(5):841–846, 1982.
2. France, R., Houpt, J., Ellinwood, E.: Therapeutic effects of antidepressants in chronic pain. Gen Hosp Psychiatry 6:55–63, 1984.
3. Hameroff, S., et al.: Doxepin effects on chronic pain, depression, and serum opioids. Anesth Analg 61,2:187, 1982.
4. Hameroff, S., et al.: Doxepin's effects on chronic pain and depression: a controlled study. J Clin Psychiatry 45:47–52, 1984.
5. Lee, R., Spencer, P.: Antidepressants and pain: a review of the pharmacological data supporting the use of certain tricyclics in chronic pain. J Int Med Res 5(Suppl):146–156, 1977.
6. Pilowsky, I., et al.: Controlled study of amitriptyline in the treatment of chronic pain. Pain 14:169–179, 1982.
7. Stauffer, J.: Antidepressants and chronic pain. J Fam Pract 25(2):167–170, 1987.
8. Tollison, C., Kriegel, M.: Selected tricyclic antidepressants in the management of chronic benign pain. South Med J 81(5):562–564, 1984.
9. Walsh, T.: Antidepressants in chronic pain. Clin Neuropharmacol 6(4):271–295, 1983.
10. Ward, N., Blume, V., Friedel, R.: The effectiveness of tricyclic antidepressants in the treatment of co-existing pain and depression. Pain 7:331–341, 1979.
11. Ward, N., et al.: Antidepressants in concomitant chronic back pain and depression: doxepin and desipramine compared. J Clin Psychiatry 45:54–57, 1984.
12. France, R., Krishnan, K.: Psychotropic drugs in chronic pain. In Chronic Pain (Edited by R. France and K. Krishnan). Washington, D.C., American Psychiatric Press, 1988.
13. Goodkin, C., Gullion, C.: A critical review of clinical trials using heterocyclic antidepressants for the relief of chronic pain syndromes with a focus on chronic low back pain. Ann Behav Med, in press.
14. Silvestrini, B.: Trazedone and the mental pain hypothesis of depression. Neuropsychobiology 15(Suppl) 1:2–9, 1986.
15. Atkinson, J.: Psychopharmacological agents in the treatment of pain syndromes. In The Handbook of Chronic Pain Management (Edited by C. Tollison). Baltimore, Williams & Wilkins, 1989.
16. Baldessatini, R.: Chemotherapy in Psychiatry. Cambridge, Harvard University Press, 1977.
17. Bassuk, E., Schoonover, S., Gelenberg (eds): The Practitioner's Guide to Psychoactive Drugs, 2nd Ed. New York, Plenum, 1984.
18. Klein, Gittelman, R., Quitkin, F., Rifkin, A.: Diagnosis and Drug Treatment of Psychiatric Disorders: Adults and Children. Baltimore, Williams & Wilkins, 1980.

William Kermond
Robert J. Gatchel
Tom G. Mayer

39

Functional Restoration Treatment for Chronic Spinal Disorder or Failed Back Surgery

As noted in various other chapters in this text, chronic low back pain is the most expensive benign condition in industrialized countries. It is also the number one cause of disability in persons under age 45. Over this age, it is the third leading cause of disability, becoming progressively less important during the later years when function and productivity become less important than survival. This phenomenon of chronic low back pain has also been recalcitrant to traditional treatment techniques. The often discouraging summaries of surgical procedures have tended to dissuade many surgeons from devoting much time to the practice of spine surgery with these patients.[1]

Through analysis of the effects on the central nervous system of psychosocial, economic, and stress factors, a series of behavioral treatments, based on the perspective that chronic low back pain has cognitive and physical, components, have been developed.[2-4] The behavioral conceptual framework has led, over the past 25 years, to a proliferation of pain clinics devoted to management, among other things, of chronic low back pain using a form of multidisciplinary assessment and treatment. They have succeeded in focusing attention on many important psychosocial issues, especially those related to pain medication abuse and, more recently, to treatment of depression. However, as these clinics began to proliferate over the years, there was a tendency to lump all "hidden disabilities," such as low back and neck pain, headaches and phantom limb pain, into a vast dissimilar array, all supposedly yielding to the same behavioral or psychologic approach. It is not surprising, then, that many pain clinics failed to alter the critical societal outcomes dealing with the financial and human cost of low back pain. In fact, the vast pain clinic literature that subsequently developed rarely demonstrated an interest in exploring its accountability regarding disability, litigation, and cost, preferring instead to focus on "quality of life" issues generally based on subjective patient self-report. Because such patient report is generally viewed as notoriously unreliable, and subject to change from one moment to the next, reports of outcome have been viewed with a great deal of skepticism among the legal, insurance, and medical communities not directly involved in pain management.

FUNCTIONAL RESTORATION: AN OVERVIEW

An approach termed functional restoration has been developed that has been demonstrated to have unique efficacy in spinal rehabilitation. Chapter 40 reviews the positive outcome studies conducted to date evaluating this approach. It should be noted that the term "functional restoration" refers not merely to a treatment methodology for chronic low back pain, but to a wider conceptualization of the entire problem, its diagnosis, and management. Rather than accepting current methods of history-taking based on patients self-report of pain and diagnosis through skeletal imaging technology, the functional restoration methodology involves reliance on more objective information. Structured inter-

473

views, quantified self-report measures, and batteries of psychosocial tests provide problem-oriented information for patient management. Moreover, objective assessment of physical capacity and effort, with comparison to a normative database, adds a new dimension to diagnosis. This permits the development of treatment programs of varied intensity and duration aimed primarily at restoring physical functional capacity and social performance. The previous goals of merely attempting to alter pain complaints, decreasing medications, and "improving the quality of life" are greatly enlarged by a focus on the vast societal problems associated with low back pain. This attention to realistic goals has already helped to alter the focus of treatment programs, as well as the evaluation process for its effectiveness.

The functional restoration treatment process involves a team approach modeled after that usually applied when dealing with more catastrophic musculoskeletal rehabilitation. However, because of the lack of physical visual feedback and the desperate psychologic, social, and economic factors peculiar to the low back "hidden disability," even closer staff intercommunication is essential. The critical elements of such a program are physical therapy, occupational therapy, psychology, nursing, and physician direction. In the program originally developed at the Productive Rehabilitation Institute of Dallas for Ergonomics (PRIDE), certain specific roles have evolved for staff over the years. The unique effectiveness of this program attests to the appropriateness of such roles, though clearly there is room for development of other role-types. The much abused term "interdisciplinary" may also be applicable, although it often implies a hodge-podge of inputs to a program with no coherent guiding principles (i.e., multiple physician specialties providing consultation in areas such as psychiatry and neurology are often termed interdisciplinary). Staffing of patients, guided by a physician-arbiter, is essential. The leadership ability of the physician in cutting to the heart of the critical "barriers to functional recovery" present in some patients, and focusing the team's attention on objective assessment rather than pain complaints, can make the treatment process an exciting and rewarding one for all the participants. The higher the quality of individual staff members, and the more incisive they are in "getting to the issues," the more successful the treatment is likely to be.

Pain Versus Function

Because the functional restoration approach stresses treating disability as opposed to merely attempting to lower the patient's level of self-reported pain, a sharp distinction is drawn between pain and function. Thus, success is defined in terms of the extent to which function is restored and begins to approach levels sufficient to allow resumption of normal activities, a goal that typically involves the patient re-entering the work force at the completion of treatment. In this sense, functional restoration can be viewed as a "sports medicine" approach to rehabilitation of the spine. Accordingly, little stress is placed upon altering the patient's self-reported pain which, in contrast to functional capacity, is not subject to objective assessment and is often influenced by a host of psychological, legal, and financial factors. In fact, a temporary increase in pain often occurs when one is regaining function, a common finding in anyone undergoing a new physical conditioning program (i.e., no pain, no gain). However, significant decreases in self-reported pain are found as the patient progresses through the program.

Functional Restoration and the Quantification of Function

Functional restoration has as its primary goals the elimination of disability and the restoration of functioning. Traditionally, the absence of visual feedback to the low back area has been the major factor forcing us to accept the evidence of radiographic screening in spite of its inconsistencies. Patient pain complaints in the spine are unverifiable and fail to lead to a pain source that can be noted on a physical examination, unlike other musculoskeletal conditions. In a knee, for instance, the location of pain and tenderness may correlate with findings such as instability or a meniscal click. In the spine, however, we are confounded by peculiar deep seated anatomy with its small, complex hidden joints and muscles, and an absence of a contralateral side for comparison. In fact, our only standardized physiologic test available for the back is range-of-motion, which has become the standard for determining disability under both American Medical Association and American Academy of Orthopedic Surgeons guidelines. Other important factors that have been found to have substantive impact on function of extremity joints, such as periarticular strength, stability, endurance, cardiovascular fitness and coordination have been virtually ignored. It is one of the central contentions of the functional restoration approach that new technology may provide an insight to the physiology of the lumbar musculoskeletal system. Furthermore, it appears clear that deficits of physical functional capacity may play a substantial role in explaining a major part of the dysfunction and persistent pain in chronic back pain cases, and that correction of such deficits may lead to major alterations in outcome.

There are now methods available to objectively

quantify the degree of deconditioning. However, one must carefully select the appropriate type of test for such quantification. For example, isometric lifting tests have been used to "measure back strength."[5,6] In fact, though engineering principles require that the force of an isometric test be transmitted through the body from hands to foot or floor contact, the spine can often be placed into such a position that virtually no spinal musculature strength is required to support the load.[7] This exemplifies the first criteria for any functional evaluation: the test must be *relevant* to the physical capacity being measured. If you wish to assess isolated spinal muscle strength, then measures of trunk torques in flexion and extension and rotation or lateral bend must be sought, not whole body tasks such as lifting.

A second critical principle of measurement is the need to know the *validity* and *reproducibility* of the measurement. Validity is related to the accuracy of the test device itself, whereas reproducibility refers to the ability of the test (device plus subject) to give a repeatable and precise measure of a clinical variable. *A valid test is not necessarily reproducible and vice versa.* An invalid test is simply useless, but an irreproducible test may reflect actual clinical reality (such as comparing inter-subject body weight or changes in spinal mobility before and after exercise in the same individual). As in the examples, reproducibility problems can often be corrected by restructuring the test protocol.

Once a functional test has been found to be valid, reproducible, and relevant, an *effort factor* must be defined. Without the ability to identify suboptimal effort, invalid low readings may be accepted as true physical deficits. Although suboptimal effort may reflect a clinical abnormality (such as low motivation or personality disorder leading to conscious malingering), the clinician must be able to assess whether he is dealing with a true physical deficit or not.

Finally, once the appropriate device and test protocol have been chosen, a *normative database* must be compiled on a large population sample to permit comparisons to be drawn to a patient grouping. Degree of deviation from "normal" may significantly affect treatment protocols. Although more should be said about measurement criteria, it is most important to select the optimal measurement device in the first place, to avoid the tedious task of collecting additional normative data.

THE FUNCTIONAL RESTORATION PROGRAM

The Interdisciplinary Treatment Team Approach

With the above issues clearly in mind, we can now discuss the treatment team approach to func-

tional restoration. (Mayer and Gatchel have provided a detailed review of this approach[1]). It should be apparent from the discussion so far that the functional restoration approach encompasses all aspects of the complex physical and psychosocial interaction impinging on the back-disabled patient. The success of this approach lies in the coordinated efforts of the interdisciplinary treatment team. The use of the team allows the staff to thoroughly address the numerous issues facing each patient. Furthermore, patients are treated in a consistent manner by staff members who share a unified philosophy and reinforce the importance of each of the other departments. The functional restoration system involves physical therapy, occupational therapy, psychology, medical and nursing professionals. Table 39–1 lists the major components and characteristics of a functional restoration program.

Department Responsibilities

Physical Therapy

The physical therapy department is responsible for the instruction and supervision of patients in individualized physical therapy programs. The physical therapists focus on retraining the specific injured area of the body and treating the spine as a functional unit. Indeed, the functional restoration approach has as its cornerstone the systematic quantification of function, which "drives" the treatment process. In all, five aspects of function are quantified and used as barometers of a patient's progress toward increasing physical capacity.[1] True spinal range of motion (both flexion and extension) is quantified using a computerized inclinometer. Trunk strength is quantified using a device that assesses isometric and isotonic trunk strength by isolating the torque produced by the lower back. Cardiovascular endurance is assessed and quantified through the use of bicycle exercise and upper body ergometry. This type of exercise is suited to the low level of cardiovascular fitness typically encountered in patients who have been inactive for long periods

Table 39–1
Characteristics of a Functional Restoration Program

1. Quantification of physical capacity.
2. Quantification of psychosocial function.
3. Reactivation for restoration of fitness.
4. Reconditioning of the injured functional unit.
5. Retraining in multi-unit task performance.
6. Work simulation.
7. Multimodal disability management approach.
8. Vocational and societal reintegration.
9. Formalized outcome tracking.

of time. In order to assess how the body as a whole performs during a functional lifting task, a device that measures the overall force exerted when lifting from the floor to a height of 7 feet is used. The device stabilizes speed, which enables one to overcome inertia, thereby permitting a better measurement of the individual's true strength capacity. In contrast to the measurement of trunk strength, which involves isolation of one part of the lifting chain—indeed, often the weakest part—the measurement of overall functional lifting capacity allows patients to use their extremities to produce their maximum output of force. This often results in discrepancies between trunk strength and lifting capability. Well motivated patients may demonstrate lifting capacities proportionally greater than their trunk strength, whereas poorly motivated or cautious patients may evidence lifting capacities well below the level predicted by their trunk strength. Finally, an isoinertial or psychophysical lifting protocol is used that allows the assessment of a patient's frequent lifting capacity, another valuable measure of functional task performance. During this timed task, the patient progressively lifts greater amounts of weight. This allows the calculation of peak weight lifted, force to body weight, endurance time, and final heart rate.

All of the tests used to quantify function have two important features: a normative database with which to compare test results and an effort factor used to determine whether a patient has manifested optimal effort during the testing. By comparing a patient's test results with a normative database, one can determine the extent to which the demonstrated level of function falls below normal. Test values are typically expressed in terms of "percent normal," thereby facilitating a quick assessment of the patient's deficits. Though patients often begin with levels of functional capacity well below normal, it is not unusual for them to demonstrate normal or even supernormal levels of function by the time they finish the treatment program. By taking into account the effort factors for each test, which constitute a type of "validity scale," one can assess the extent to which a patient's demonstrated level of function approaches his or her true functional capacity. So-called "malingering" is only one reason why a test

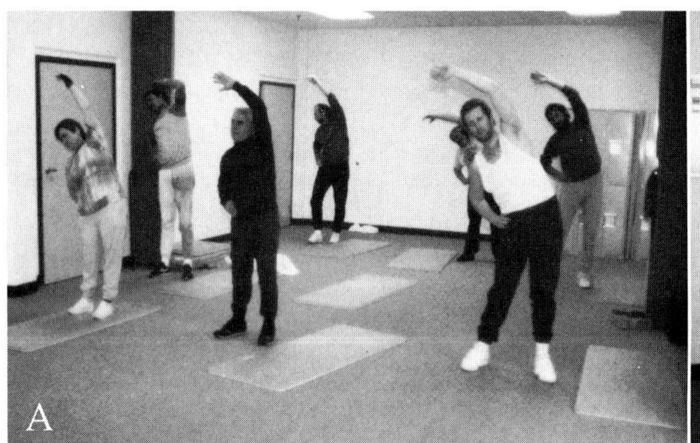
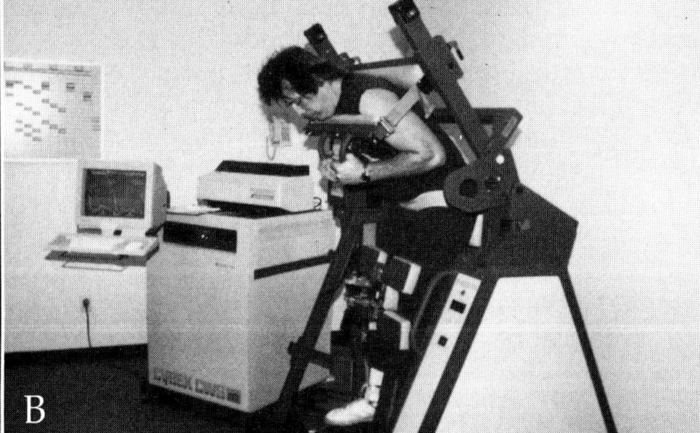
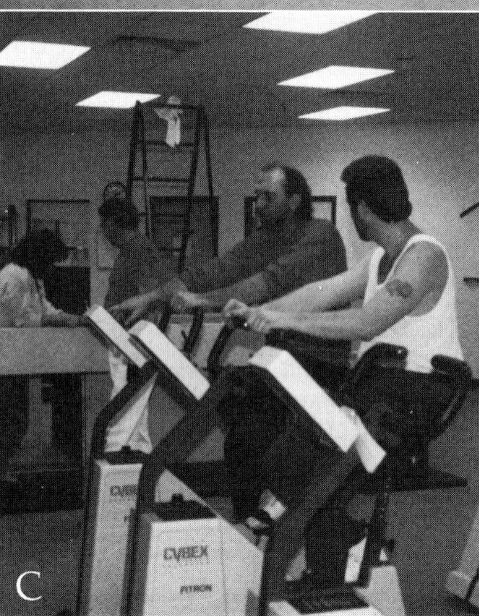

Figure 39–1. Physical reconditioning is initially directed at increasing range-of-motion **(A)**, strength **(B)**, and endurance **(C)**.

result might appear invalid. Often, suboptimal effort is not a result of conscious dissimulation, but rather reflects factors such as anxiety, depression, or fear of reinjury. In general, lower global effort ratings make the test results less credible, and may necessitate retesting after a staff psychologist has had an opportunity to address the psychosocial issues causing the patient to manifest suboptimal effort.

Occupational Therapy

Occupational therapy also supervises physical reconditioning, but focuses on functional tasks through work hardening and work simulation (Fig 39-2). Additionally, the occupational therapists are involved in addressing the financial, legal, and work-related barriers to recovery that might interfere with the ultimate return to work goal for each patient.

As is true in other parts of the program, pain may interrupt the patient's ability to perform these tasks, though the therapist needs to be persistent in educating the patient that training develops capacity to perform these physical tasks, just as it does the more general physiological aspects of mobility and strength. For a variety of reasons related to structural damage, personality, emotional and socioeconomic factors, patients may feel a need to continue to enunciate pain complaints through the process. Most will acknowledge, however, after a period of training, that gradual improvement seems to be occurring, although there are still frequent "bad days." In evaluating the frequency and severity of pain complaints, the therapist must constantly be on the watch for barriers to functional recovery.

It is vital that the occupational therapy staff members understand enough about the treatment technique and rationale of other departments to reinforce their approaches with the patients. Although occupational therapists are not expected to perform as psychologists, physical therapists, or nurses, they should be alert to the behavior and issues that affect the patient's performance in these departments. When the therapist becomes aware of problems relevant to other departments, this must be relayed to them. The customary way in which this is done is at the biweekly staffing conference, the major source for internal communication and discussion. However, on an "emergency" basis, the communication should take place directly between the involved parties, or perhaps even in a small conference with the patient.

Conversely, the occupational therapist receives a great deal of input from other departments. In some ways, occupational therapy sits at the fulcrum of the patient's physical and psychosocial functioning, binding physical reconditioning and disability management, as well as their own unique contributions in these areas. Because of this position, the occupational therapist must rely on team work in order to avoid becoming overwhelmed with the multiple issues involving each patient. This situation becomes progressively more intense as patients approach program completion, and a variety of employment and compensation issues must be dealt with.

Work issues frequently motivate a variety of hidden agendas and other barriers to recovery to which the therapist must be alert. Because patients tend to focus on the recent conflicts they have been experi-

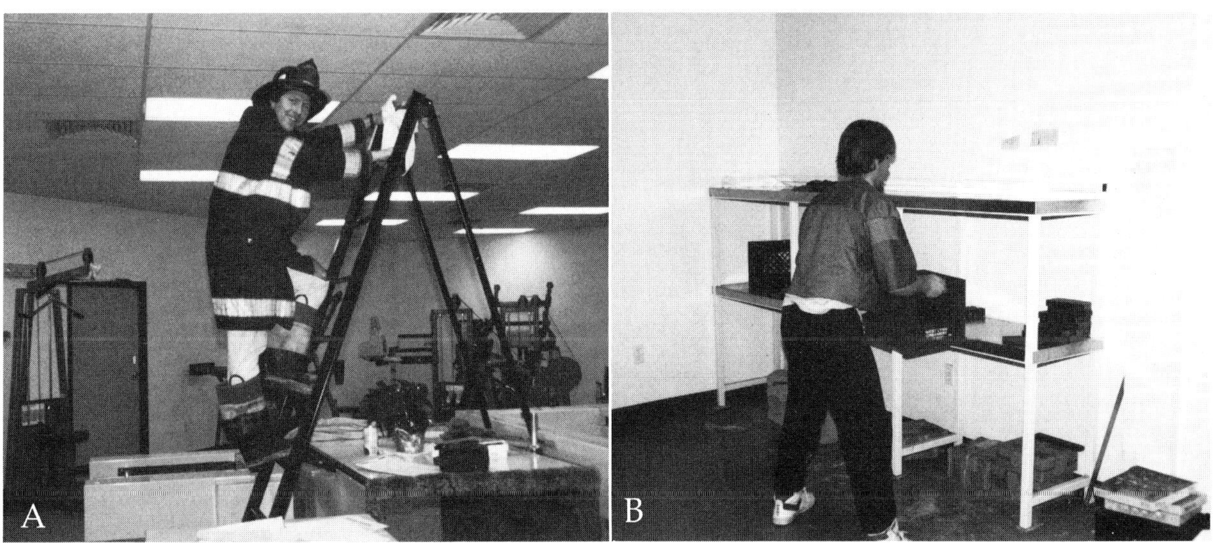

Figure 39–2. Functional tasks such as climbing **(A)** and lifting **(B)** are used for work hardening and work simulation.

encing relative to the work place, it is often fruitful to focus on the wider role of work. Work fills many needs and represents many things besides earning a living. For most people, work carries a certain amount of status, is a place to belong, a place to feel productive, and an important social network outside of the family. It is a place to experience feelings of self-esteem over a job well done, and a place to establish a self-image as a worker and producer. Most people lose sight of these important aspects of the workplace because of the recent conflicts they have been experiencing, but usually recognize some sense of loss regarding this part of their lives as the length of disability increases. Exceptions to this might occur in individuals who have never really established a firm work relationship, and this should be sought in the patient's history. The "habitual housewife," who had only a few short-term or part-time jobs, or the individual probably involved in elicit industries who hides true sources of income, are examples of this group. It is generally useless to attempt to reform these individuals, who will be "failures" of treatment in one sense. However, disability management calls for an end to compensation issues and a return to some level of productivity within a societal framework, and this partial success can generally be achieved.

Psychology

Psychologic services address psychosocial and behavioral issues that affect patients during this time of upheaval in their lives. These issues are dealt with through a MultiModal Disability Management Program (MDMP) approach. Again, Mayer and Gatchel have discussed aspects of this approach in detail elsewhere.[1] Basically, this approach has four major sections:

1. Individual and group counseling emphasizing a crisis-intervention model (e.g., coping with family problems or unemployment). Group counseling is conducted on a daily basis; the amount of individual counseling depends on the particular needs of the patient.
2. Family counseling, which is conducted on a weekly basis. During these sessions, family members are encouraged to take an active part in the rehabilitation process and are provided with information about the philosophy and specific details of MDMP.
3. Behavioral stress management training that involves initial training in muscle relaxation, followed by exercises in guided imagery in which patients practice relaxing while imagining themselves in various stressful situations. They also receive daily electromyography and temperature biofeedback sessions during which they refine their relaxation skills, with the understanding that these skills will help them cope more effectively with residual pain and discomfort.
4. Cognitive-behavioral skills training that includes instruction in assertiveness, rational versus irrational thinking, and the management of stress and time.

Besides involvement in the four treatment components of MDMP, the psychologic staff works to maintain a positive therapeutic environment. Part of this therapeutic environment maintenance is accomplished with each patient individually through counseling and educational interventions. Moreover, frequent and clear communication between the psychologic staff and all members of the treatment team working with a particular patient is essential.

Nursing

The nursing department functions as an extension of the program physician, assessing and dealing with the patient's physical and medical needs. It acts as a triage without direct physician involvement as much as possible to avoid "overpathologizing" the patients. The nurse serves as an extension of the physician, with responsibilities such as checking and ordering medications, injections, and initial evaluation of medical problems affecting a patient's ability to engage in the physical reconditioning program. The nursing department also serves as an important conductor of information between the physicians and other members of the treatment team.

Treatment Program Time Format

The program typically consists of four phases, as presented in Table 39–2. As noted in the table, each program is divided into a variety of comparable phases. The comprehensive program focuses on the most important and expensive chronically disabled cases, i.e., those generally unable to work. Under certain circumstances working patients may be admitted into the comprehensive program, as discussed below.

In the preprogram phase (Phase I), issues of pain and barriers to functional recovery, specifically those related to compliance and willingness to get well, are the focus. Phase II is the major portion of the program. It consists of 3 weeks of daily 10-hour sessions involving patient participation. The followup phase varies in length, based primarily on such factors as patient proximity to home, degree of deconditioning, and ergonomic demands of the patient's anticipated work. Finally, there is an outcome track-

Table 39–2
Phases of Treatment Programs

Phases	Comprehensive Program	Outpatient Programs
I. Preprogram	4–8 sessions (may begin with QFE)	1–2 sessions
II. Core (intensive) program	3 weeks (full day)	6–24 sessions, over 3–6 weeks
III. Followup	0–20 sessions, over 0–6 weeks	1–2 sessions Home program instruction
IV. Outcome tracking	Physician re-referral	
	Periodic repeat QFEs	
	Structured telephone interview annually	

ing phase involving periodic Quantified Functional Evaluations (QFEs) to assess maintenance of physical capacity. Patients are referred back to their original physicians, generally return to a productive lifestyle, but are also followed at length to be sure that treatment goals are maintained in various outcome areas. This program may involve using structured telephone interviews at specified intervals.

ASSISTANCE AND SUPPORT AFTER THE COMPREHENSIVE PROGRAM

Continued contact and support are needed to ensure the maintenance of treatment gains and long-term compliance with the program's philosophy and prescribed lifestyle adjustments after discharge. Before discussing in detail the methods employed to maintain physical capacity gains, a review of some additional overall strategies of assistance and support in helping patients re-establish themselves as productive members of their environment will be provided.

One useful support mechanism is the telephone hotline service that allows patients to get in contact with program personnel when a significant problem arises. Issues and concerns can be discussed over the phone, and, if necessary, an appointment can be made to have the patient come into the clinic. Also, if a referral is needed, this can be accomplished over the telephone. The knowledge that this mechanism is available can be reassuring to patients who need to "touch base" with a member of the treatment team after being back on their own.

Another important assistance mechanism is serving as a referral source for patients. After leaving the program, a patient may encounter a major emotional crisis with which he or she needs help. Referral to an appropriate counseling or therapy facility can be provided. For example, there are many self-help groups in the community, such as Alcoholics Anonymous and Weight Watchers, to which individuals can be referred. Likewise, referral to an appropriate health care professional for related physical problems and concerns can also be made. A significant aspect of post-treatment assistance is that patients come to see the treatment program facility as an important resource if they encounter a significant problem in their lives.

Another area of assistance can be in the realm of vocational rehabilitation. Many times, the employment plans of a patient may suddenly be subject to change. Although vocational retraining or education is a less desirable goal than returning the patient to work because it may leave the patient in a dependent student role, such may be the only alternative available. Part-time employment may be necessary in conjunction with training or school. Additional assistance is usually required in these cases to maintain living standards during the retraining, and the program staff can provide assistance in helping patients get in contact with the appropriate facilities such as the local State Rehabilitation Counseling Agency. Occupational therapy can play an important role in this process.

It should also be noted that in some cases, a patient may be too old, unskilled, or severely damaged by multiple operations or cognitive deficits to resume competitive employment. Given sufficient motivation, a wide variety of home industries are available that can supply limited incomes, decreasing the burden to insurers or government for subsidizing this individual. We have constantly been amazed at the ingenuity of patients in finding self-employment opportunities once conventional employment is recognized to be too difficult to attain or sustain. Support during this transition can be helpful.

Maintaining Physical Capacity

Obviously, the maintenance of physical capacity gains is an important goal of functional restoration. This section discusses how this can be accomplished.

Periodic Testing

A Quantitative Functional Evaluation (QFE) is performed on multiple occasions as part of the PRIDE post-program to continue feedback to the patient concerning maintenance of physical capacity. Periodic testing of strength, flexibility, endurance, and task performance capability shows whether the recovering patient or athlete continues to maintain physical performance at a desired level. In Phase IV of the program, increase in patient pain complaints is frequently accompanied by gradual decrease in QFE scores. It is up to the program physician to evaluate whether a setback has been caused by the patient's specific musculoskeletal problem, inattention to exercise protocols, or psychosocial crises. If home exercise protocols are at fault, the feedback afforded by the QFE permits the physical or occupational therapist to provide advice to the patients for working harder on the specific areas of deficit. If, on the other hand, a major psychosocial stressor has produced the decrement in measured physical capacity or effort, appropriate counseling intervention can be arranged to assist with the relevant present crisis. Most organic musculoskeletal problems can be identified specifically, resulting in conventional orthopedic management, e.g., injections or non habituating medications. However, the patient with unusual pain responses who maintains high levels of physical capacity should be thoroughly investigated with appropriate diagnostic tests for previously unsuspected pathologic conditions.

First Aid for Recurrent Pain Episodes

Recurrent back pain episodes are endemic among the entire population, and those who have been chronically disabled are no exception. From a pathologic point of view, the scarring or derangement from injury or surgery that originally produced the biomechanical dysfunction that led to the chronic low back pain, is still latent and may produce additional episodes. However, it is an important function of the back school process for the subacute individual, or the full-blown educational process in the comprehensive treatment program, to instruct the patient in dealing with a new acute episode to prevent it from becoming more long term. If one assumes that the process that led to chronic disability in the first place is a concurrence of maladaptive physical and psychosocial processes for which the patient was not provided with adequate intervention and education, then future episodes likely can be prevented as part of the rehabilitation training.

A secondary benefit of the pain increase initially experienced as part of overcoming the deconditioning syndrome is the need to be educated to "work through pain" in overcoming the disability. As such, the groundwork is set for maintaining the highest possible levels of activity with recurrent episodes. Patient self-help measures are taught first, including appropriate stretching exercises, use of anti-inflammatory and over-the-counter analgesics, limited bedrest and judicious use of heat and cold. By overcoming the episode through self-analysis, calmness, and patience, rather than immediate reliance on health professionals, passive care, or habituating medications, self-pride is instilled during the followup phase of the program. Demonstrated confidence in the patient's ability to handle a new acute episode is one way in which the treatment staff can evaluate the patient's level of understanding of functional restoration.

Home Fitness Programs and Devices

Numerous programs and products are available to help the patient maintain fitness at home. Unfortunately, patients are also bombarded with conflicting advice from the mass media, friends, and a variety of medical and paramedical professionals. At this point, it should be clear to the reader that jogging or riding an exercise bicycle is *not* sufficient to maintain back health if the primary deficit is in true spine mobility or sagittal or rotational strength. Even when all physical capacity deficits noted on initial evaluation have been corrected, those areas of greatest deficiency tend to be those that recur without attention to home maintenance. It is true that people usually do the things that come easiest to them. The same is true for the injured back patient who will find most distasteful those exercises that are most necessary. For example, many individuals vigorously pursue aerobic activities in spite of excellent aerobic capacity, but avoid the specific stretching or strengthening exercise most necessary for their functional restoration maintenance.

Most home programs are nonspecific generic fitness programs. It is up to the therapists delivering the instructions at the conclusion of followup to provide the patients with specific information regarding special areas to emphasize in his own program. The information provided is generally reassessed at the time of each subsequent postprogram QFE, with additional recommendations being made if the patient has been unsuccessful in improving the deficient physical characteristic, or if backsliding has occurred in a given area. Generally, patients ultimately reach a plateau at which they neither increase nor decrease their physical capacity substantially. At this stage, they have reached a balance between their daily activities, exercise, and natural abilities that is usually sufficient to keep their symptoms under control most of the time. Only those individuals motivated to extremely high work or athletic performance will push physical capabilities beyond this point.

A plethora of home exercise devices is available with new ones constantly appearing. Exercise bicycles, free weight equipment, Roman chairs, dynamic back flexion and extension devices, and a variety of spring or elastic controlled tension devices may be obtained to maintain program goals. Such devices in the home have a definite advantage because their presence tends to act as a constant reminder and motivator about exercise. If equipment is available to deal with the specifically deficient dimension and element of performance, it can be useful, indeed. Cost, availability, and utility are factors in determining purchase of such equipment.

On the other hand, certain individuals may benefit greatly from participation in a health club or fitness center. Such facilities frequently have extensive variable resistance strength training equipment very similar to that on which the patient has trained in functional restoration. Utilization of such equipment on a regular basis may continue to build, and then maintain, the patient's high level of function. Such devices are usually more efficient than those purchased for home use, and in the environment of a health club the patient is more likely to exert maximally in exercise maintenance than he would at home. Subtle decreases in capability can be recognized by the patient as a decrease in force or torque generation on a given machine, something that is not usually recognized in a completely unquantified home exercise program. The disadvantage of such equipment involves persistence with the program. The dropout rate of health clubs and fitness centers is high because of the inconvenience inherent in the need to drive to the center, change clothes, and shower after exercise. The postprogram individual must commit significant time to such adventures, and if it is not part of his or her daily routine, adherence to the maintenance program will gradually diminish. Furthermore, as the patient returns to a more normal lifestyle with work, home, and social responsibilities, it becomes more and more difficult to squeeze in the substantial time commitment required for participating in a health club. On the other hand, certain patients will find fitness center participation improves their social lives and will make the necessary commitment. Therefore, a sufficient trial period to evaluate the patient's adherence to such a program should be instituted before recommending a high-cost, long-term membership.

"Reasonable" Ergonomics

One of the disadvantages of current ergonomic training is the teaching of conflicting principles, as

discussed previously in this text. In attempting to teach safe lifting methods, the public has taken advice concerning the lifting of very heavy loads, and translated it as appropriate behavior for all situations. For example, we have previously extensively discussed rationale for the bent back "hanging on its ligaments" as a more efficient way of lifting medium loads than the "straight back, bent knee" position involving substitution of the lower extremity functional unit for the lumbopelvic functional unit.[1] The patient who has paid attention to training principles learned in functional restoration will self-select the style of lifting to provide safety at the highest loads, but also provide efficiency and sufficient training to maintain physical capacity under appropriate circumstances. Most machines cannot be left idle for extended periods of time, nor can they be run at their highest performance levels indefinitely. However, regular running of a new machine under a variety of speeds and loads is generally felt to provide the highest level of preventive maintenance. In fact, we generally "run in" a new engine by alternating speeds and loads in a prescribed manner for a specified period of time. It is likely that the human machine is no different, and that each patient who has completed functional restoration needs to continue a prescribed "run-in period" for a similar period of time. Athletes talk of getting their bodies "in the groove" for specific activities. Restoring function of the human spine in coordination with other parts of the body and in relation to its multiple physiological determinants would appear to be equally important parts of the maintenance process.

REFERENCES

1. Mayer, T., Gatchel, R.: Functional Restoration for Spinal Disorders: The Sports Medicine Approach. Philadelphia, Lea & Febiger, 1988.
2. Fordyce, W., Roberts, A., Sternbach, R.: The behavioral management of chronic pain: a response to critics. Pain 22:112–125, 1985.
3. Sternbach, R.: Pain Patients: Traits and Treatments. Academic Press, New York, 1983.
4. Turk, D., Meichenbaum, D., Genest, M.: Pain and Behavioral Medicine: A Cognitive-Behavioral Perspective. Gilford Press, New York, 1983.
5. Chaffin, D.: Pre-employment strength testing: an updated position. J Occup Med 10:105–110, 1978.
6. Kishino N., et al.: Quantification of lumbar function part 4: isometric and isokinetic lifting simulation in normal subjects and low back dysfunction patients. Spine 10:921–927, 1985.
7. Gracovetsky, S., Farfan, H.: The optimum spine. Spine 11:543–573, 1986.

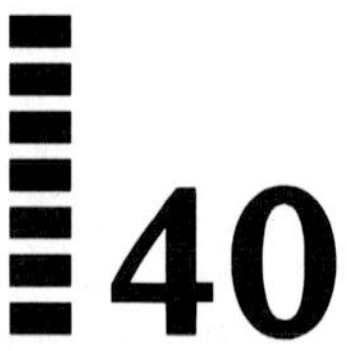

40

Rowland G. Hazard

Functional Restoration Treatment Outcomes

HISTORICAL AND CONCEPTUAL BACKGROUND

Despite our best efforts, the prevalence of chronic disabling back pain is increasing in the United States. According to data from the National Center for Health Statistics, between 1971 and 1981 the number of people with disabling back pain increased by 168% while the population increased by only 12.5%. Although the vast majority of people with acute back pain recover uneventfully, the bulk of costs associated with back pain compensation, lost productivity, and health care is devoted to the relatively small number of patients with chronic disability. Most patients with chronic back pain do not have a specific pathophysiologic diagnosis that can be predictably treated. Others may have had an initial anatomic lesion that has not responded to decompression or fusion surgery.

Unfortunately, of the myriad nonsurgical therapies available, few have been proven effective in valid clinical trials.[1] Low back schools have become a popular method of dealing with the increasing number of patients with back pain, though the effectiveness of this intervention is unclear. Although the patient's levels of knowledge may improve with education, clear evidence of reduced health care visits, work absence, and pain complaints are as yet forthcoming.[2]

Similarly, multidisciplinary pain units have been established worldwide since Bonica's early work in this area. Although a wide variety of treatments including manual therapy, passive physical modalities, acupuncture, spinal injection, and counseling techniques have been used in these centers, they are generally characterized by primary goals of pain reduction and improved coping skills. Because a multitude of difficulties exist in measuring outcomes from pain centers, their effectiveness is inconclusive.[3]

Fordyce and Roberts have given a positive review of behavioral modification programs considering outcomes such as medication usage, activity level, and performance of daily living tasks. However, they did not find conclusive evidence of pain reduction.[4]

Problems in Measuring Treatment Outcomes: Back Pain as a Biopsychosocial Phenomenon

The problems in measuring the outcome of various treatments for chronic low back pain begin with the lack of specific anatomic and pathophysiologic diagnoses in the majority of cases. Because we are unable to control for specific underlying conditions, studies of treatment efficacy frequently include patients with segmental instability, facet joint syndrome, and idiopathic pain without investigating the impact these different underlying conditions may have on outcome. As Waddell has reported, chronic low back pain is more complex than a simple pain-stimulating anatomic derangement.[4] Once the patient has been disabled by his pain for more than a few months, a plethora of physical and psychosocial problems may beset him. These include physical deconditioning, loss of employment and usual wage, disordered family dynamics, depression, somatic anxieties, and legal and economic issues relating to worker compensation or personal injury rewards. While there may well have been an initial nociceptive event, in the chronic phase of disability, psychologic distress and related illness behaviors take on increasingly important roles and clearly influence the patient's response to treatments ranging from physical rehabilitation to surgical fusion. How much of a given patient's problem is "in his mind" is not only a key, if unanswerable, clinical question, it also determines the kinds of measurements of outcome that make sense for a given patient or in the context of a major clinical trial.[5] Fordyce has reported poor correlations between self-assessed pain severity and measured physical activity levels in patients with chronic low back pain.[6] This discrepancy between symptoms and functional capacities is common among chronic pain sufferers, and confounds treatment outcome measurement.[4,7,8] For instance, if a given treatment improves self-assessments of pain but decreases physical capacity, what is the most appropriate tool for outcome measurement? In this sense, the results sections of clinical trials in low back pain therapy are frequently incomparable because they differ in focus between physical and psychologic criteria.

The appropriateness of various outcome measures depends largely on the observer's perspective. Patients who view pain as the most obvious issue in their overall suffering may view self-assessments of pain as the best outcome measure. A vocational or rehabilitation specialist, whose goals for the patient include the establishment of an occupational plan, may be more interested in work capacity. Under the rubric of work capacity, it may be unclear whether one should measure the patient's physical impairment against some statistical norm for legal and administrative purposes, or to compare this combined physical and psychosocial capacity to the estimated demands of specific occupations. The difference in these approaches becomes almost comic when a patient asks for the maximum impairment rating for worker compensation case settlement, but not such a high assessment that by implication he is disqualified from the specific job he is pursuing. The patient's attorney may be interested in physical capacity limitations in order to calculate impairment in a worker compensation case, but may be more interested in self-assessed pain and suffering and prognosis for future work loss if his client's pain began with a personal injury. A prospective employer may be less interested in self-assessments of pain and even measured physical capacity than in the patient's risk for future injury as he sees his company's worker compensation insurance premiums skyrocket. The patient's insurance carrier may be interested in the effect of a given treatment on health care use in addition to improvements in pain and physical activity levels.

Studies of actual medical expenditures before and after treatment are rare.[9] The majority of costs associated with occupational low back pain are nonmedical, so a claims manager may be more interested in the rate of case settlement in assessing treatment outcome. The documentation of cost-effectiveness in treating low back pain is extremely difficult because the total cost in a given case may include health expenses from multiple sources, wage loss compensation, wage level demotion on return to work, family

dynamic impact, and retraining of the patient or training of his replacement.

Return to work may be the single best measurement of treatment outcome for patients with chronic low back disability. Return to work implies that the patient and his physician mutually consent that the patient has sufficient pain relief or control and adequate physical capacity to resume work with an acceptable risk of future injury. Return to work is often the cornerstone of legal and administrative settlements as well. Therefore, return to work rate generally accounts for biologic, psychologic, social, and economic features of low back disability and serves as a practical index of recovery.

Unfortunately, there are several drawbacks to using return to work as a yardstick for comparing different treatments. Local employment conditions may vary both in job availability as measured by unemployment rate and in the kinds of jobs available. Outcomes for the same treatment might vary considerably between a geographic area with high unemployment and a high percentage of heavy labor and an area where light duty jobs are plentiful. As patients approach retirement age, return to work probably loses much of its significance as an outcome measure. Because previous work experience, level of training, education, and job satisfaction have profound impact on employability, treatment outcomes may be affected by variations in these attributes in otherwise comparable patient populations. Return to work rates may vary between studies that account differently for the following questions: How many hours per week must the patient work to be declared re-employed? Does it count if a prior $17/hour mason is forced to work as a fast food handler at minimum wage? Is on-the-job training with supplemental wage compensation or a full-time academic curriculum considered employment? What if the patient recovers sufficiently to be fit for work, but can't find a suitable job? Finally, return to work data do not necessarily correlate with improvements in social and recreational activity levels outside the workplace. Nevertheless, inasmuch as return to work combines biologic, psychologic, social, and economic features of chronic low back pain and disability, it is a useful measure of outcome.

Measurement Tools and Techniques

The fundamental enigma in outcome measurement resides in our inability to measure the chief complaint: pain. Laboratory measurements of serum endorphins, pain peptides, neurotransmitters, and neuroelectric function are clinically impractical. Radiographic evaluation frequently does not correlate with symptoms and disability level, and suffers from a considerable degree of inter-observer variation. In the past several years, quantification of functional capacity has drawn increasing research and clinical attention. Given the difficulties in measuring the subjective, existential experience of pain, and the poor correlation between pain and function, functional measurements have become essential in guiding and assessing treatment. The predominant physical deficits in patients with chronic low back disability include trunk stiffness, trunk and extremity muscular weakness, and cardiovascular deconditioning. Probably the most accurate measurement of trunk flexibility involves the use of goniometers as described by Mayer, et al.[10] The popularity of isokinetic trunk flexion and extension strength measurement appears to be increasing following early reports of the technique's repeatability, reliability, and safety.[11] Lifting capacity may also be measured isokinetically.[12] Repetitive isoinertial lifting capacity is less expensive and probably more directly applicable to real-world physical demands.[13] Cardiovascular endurance may be measured using upper and lower extremity cycle ergometers while monitoring heart rate response. Psychologic measures include the Minnesota Multiphasic Personality Inventory (MMPI), depression scales, somatic perception questionnaires, locus of control and self-efficacy questionnaires, and job and life satisfaction scales. More specific to the point of measuring the patient's chief complaint, visual analog scales and multiple choice questionnaires are most commonly used to quantify self-assessments of pain and disability. The editors of the journal *Spine* recommend the Million Behavioral Health Index, MMPI, Waddell, Oswestry, and visual analog techniques.[14] Socioeconomic parameters include insurance carriers' tabulations of medical expenses, physician's office visits, tests, procedures, days in hospital, and compensation costs.[9] One of the key issues in assessing the outcome of treatment for any medical condition is "generalizability."[15] The population considered in a given study must be defined thoroughly enough so the reader can compare the subjects in the study to his own patients. Again, in an editorial that appeared in the journal *Spine,* Drs. Nachemson and LaRocca request that future studies include a clear explanation of treatment, outcome assessment by an unbiased observer, sufficient duration of followup, and qualification of any results consisting of less than 90% of the initial treatment population.[14]

RESULTS OF FUNCTIONAL RESTORATION PROGRAMS

In 1983, Tom G. Mayer, M.D., assembled a group of psychologists and physical and occupational therapists in Dallas, TX. They developed a program of multidisciplinary therapy, The Productive Rehabilitation Institute of Dallas for Ergonomics (PRIDE), for patients with chronic low back pain and disability. Their program was distinquished by reliance on state-of-the-art measurements of physical capacity. Quantification of lumbar flexibility, lifting capacity, trunk strength, and general cardiovascular conditioning provided objective feedback to patients and therapists to guide the restoration of the patient's capacities for the functional tasks required by their anticipated return to work. In 1986, a similar program was established in Burlington, VT. The remainder of this chapter summarizes the results of these two programs and briefly outlines issues for future consideration.

Functional Restoration: The PRIDE Experience

In their original study,[16] Dr. Mayer and his group studied 111 patients with chronic back pain whose disability had lasted at least 4 months and who had no clear evidence of a surgically correctable lesion. Of these patients, 73 entered the treatment program, with 7 subsequently dropping out before completion of treatment. Thirty-eight of the original patients were denied financial authorization for treatment by their insurance companies, and became a "no treatment" comparison group. The treatment program graduates, drop-outs, and denials were roughly comparable in age, sex, number of operations, duration of symptoms, duration of work absence, worker compensation status, and medications. All patients entering the treatment program underwent measurement of spinal range of motion, isometric and isokinetic trunk strength, cardiovascular fitness, obstacle course performance, static lifting, dynamic lifting, and global effort. All patients were administered the Beck Depression Inventory, Million Visual Analog Scale, and Quantitative Pain Drawing. The treatment program consisted of behavioral pain management training, cognitive-behavioral skills training, and individual, group and family counseling, along with physical exercise and work hardening. The program began with an intensive 3-week, 57-hours per week session, and was followed by an average of 5 weeks of followup treatment, consisting of 2 hours per day from 0 to 4 days per week. Program graduates were encouraged to return 3 months after discharge for quantification of self-assessed pain, disability, and depression, and for functional capacity measurements. At the end of one year, work status was ascertained by a structured telephone interview for all three groups. At least some data were available for 100% of the treatment group,

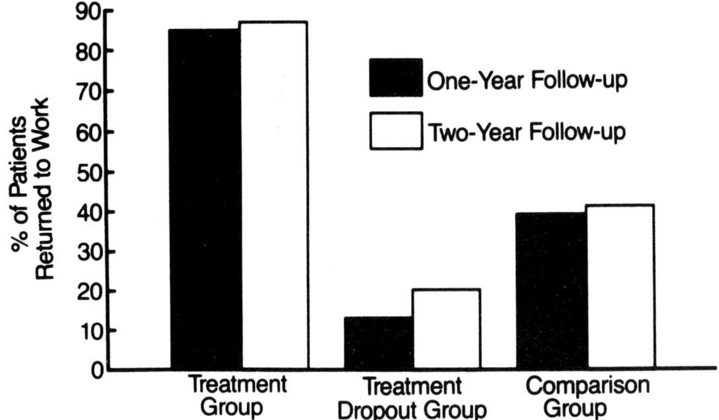

Figure **40–1.** Percentage of patients who returned to work in each of three groups at one- and two-year followups. (From Mayer, T.G., et al.: A prospective two-year study of functional restoration in industrial low back injury. An objective assessment procedure. JAMA 258:1765, 1987. Copyright, 1987, American Medical Association.)

98% of the comparison group, and 86% of the treatment drop-out group.

At the end of one year, 86% of the program graduates were either working or in a training program supported by the Texas Rehabilitation Commission. Forty-five percent of the untreated comparison group and 20% of the drop-out group were employed. Thirty-three percent of the treatment dropout group underwent additional surgery, whereas only 7% of the program graduates and 6% of the comparison patients underwent operations. Of the patients in the study with worker compensation cases, all but 14% of the treatment group had settled their litigation, whereas 32% of the comparison patients and 33% of the program drop-outs had litigation pending. Significant improvements resulted in isokinetic trunk strength, frequent dynamic lifting, and lumbar flexibility. Furthermore, significant improvements were seen in self-reported pain, according to the Million Analog Scale, along with improvements in depression self-reports. Unfortunately, correlations between year-end return-to-work status and followup isokinetic trunk strength and flexibility could not be made with statistical significance be-

cause of an attrition in the number of patients available for followup testing.

In 1987, the PRIDE group expanded their study to include 116 consecutive patients and 72 nontreatment comparison patients.[17] The study design was similar to that described above, except that the followup period was extended to 2 years. Over 85% of the program graduates and comparison patients were evaluated. Eighty-seven percent of the treatment group were working compared to 41% of the nontreatment group at the end of the two years (Fig. 40–1). Although 20% of the comparison group underwent additional surgery, only 9% of the treatment group did so during this two-year period (Fig. 40–2). Health care visits were more than twice as frequent among the comparison patients, when followup visits with the original referring physician or PRIDE physician were excluded (Fig. 40–3). Only 6% of the treatment group patients suffered reinjury, whereas 12% of the comparison patients developed new or recurrent back injuries. Although improvements in isokinetic trunk strength, trunk flexibility, and self-assessments of pain, disability, and depression were reported, statistical correlation

Figure **40–2.** Percentage of additional surgeries for three groups at two-year followup. (From Mayer, T.G., et al.: A prospective two-year study of functional restoration in industrial low back injury. An objective assessment procedure. JAMA 258:1765, 1987. Copyright, 1987, American Medical Association.)

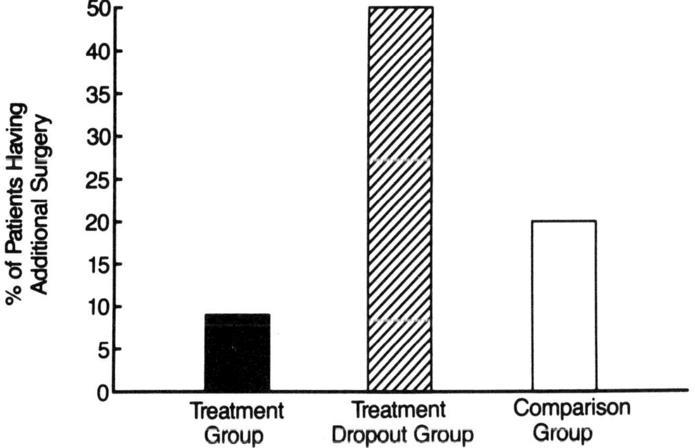

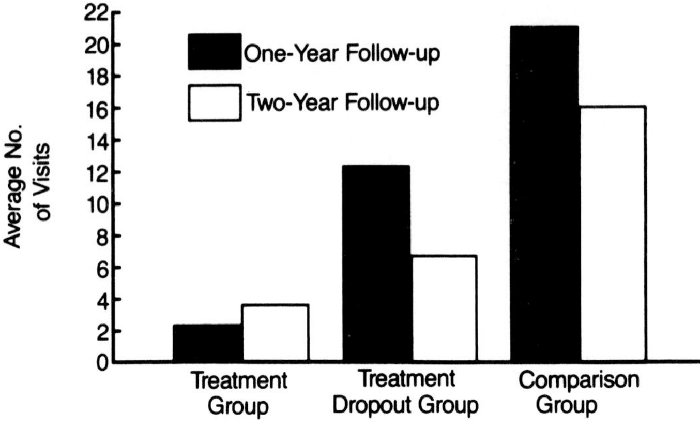

Figure 40–3. Percentage of patients visiting health care professionals for three groups at one- and two-year followups. (From Mayer, T.G., et al.: A prospective two-year study of functional restoration in industrial low back injury. An objective assessment procedure. JAMA 258:1766, 1987. Copyright, 1987, American Medical Association.)

of these parameters with eventual return-to-work status was not possible. The authors concluded that the "systematic application of the entire comprehensive program" produced these outstanding results, rather than single, isolated elements of the physical, psychologic, and occupational treatments.

The New England Back Center Experience

In 1989, the New England Back Center group reported a similar prospective investigation designed to assess return-to-work status of functional restoration program graduates and a comparison group in a different socioeconomic and geographic setting.[18] In addition, this study included functional capacity and self-assessment data at the end of one year following treatment. With these data, the authors were able to assess the persistence of immediate treatment benefits and to compare long-term physical and self-assessment outcomes with return to work status. Because Fordyce had reported poor correlation between self-assessments of pain and physical capacities during exercise therapy, it stood to reason that similar discrepancies might persist following functional restoration.

Ninety patients with at least 4 months of continuous disability because of back pain and absence of a surgically correctable lesion and psychiatric disorder precluding participation in group treatment were studied. As in the studies described above, these patients were divided into program graduates (59), program drop-outs (5) and comparison patients (17). In addition, 6 cross-over patients were denied program authorization for at least 6 months, then treated and followed for at least 6 months. Three patients declined participation in the treatment program. No significant initial differences existed among the participant groups in terms of age, sex, spinal operations, medications, smoking history, education, self-assessments of pain, disability, and de-

pression, trunk flexibility, frequent lifting, isokinetic trunk strength, and cycling endurance. Worker compensation was somewhat more frequent in the treatment group.

At the end of one year following treatment, 81% of the program graduates, 40% of the program dropouts, and 29% of the comparison group had returned to work. All 6 cross-over patients were working 6 months after treatment. Continued disabling pain, pregnancy, retirement, schooling, cardiac disability, and inability to find work characterized the program graduates who remained unemployed.

Self-assessments of pain, disability, and depression improved dramatically in the course of treatment as did measured physical capacities. At year-end, the significant improvements in self-assessments among program graduates immediately following treatment persisted through the year. Program graduates had major improvements in trunk flexibility, frequent lifting, cycling endurance, and isokinetic trunk strength, and these improvements persisted through the year with the exception of partial attrition in frequent lifting, cycling endurance, and isokinetic trunk extension strength. The program graduates' year-end, self-assessments did not correlate well with work status, except that those who were working had significantly better Oswestry Pain Questionnaire Scores than those who were unemployed. The only physical capacity measurements that correlated with work status at any testing interval were year-end trunk flexibility and cycling endurance at all testing intervals, both of which were higher in the employed program graduates.

Overall, the PRIDE and New England Back Center studies demonstrated significant improvements in return-to-work status for patients undergoing intensive functional restoration with behavioral support compared to nonrandom, but clinically similar, patients with chronic disabling low back pain. Both research groups concluded that a comprehensive approach to the multifaceted physical and psychosocial problems of these patients was required for successful treatment. Given the lack of demonstrated correlation between most of the physical and self-assessment outcomes and return-to-work status in the New England Back Center study, it may well be that efforts to match patients' re-employment plans with measured physical capacities, work aptitudes and desires provide the cornerstone for successful reemployment.

FURTHER RESEARCH

If individual portions of the treatment programs are more significant for certain kinds of patients, how can these patients be identified so that more efficient and economical focusing of treatment becomes feasible? How can we identify patients earlier in the course of their disabilities, apply perhaps limited amounts of functional restoration or behavioral support in order to avoid long-term pain behaviors and work loss? How important are the expensive and highly technical measurements of physical capacity, particularly, isokinetic strength measurements, in quantifying function and directing rehabilitation? What are the optimal physical training techniques for patients with disabling back pain? How rapidly and intensively can such patients be trained without undue risk of soft tissue injuries common to injured athletes during retraining? How can we more accurately assess the economic impact of this intensive treatment approach? Which underlying pathophysiologic conditions respond best to functional restoration? Which psychologic features characterize successful outcomes? These and many other questions demand further research in this most promising field of functional restoration with behavioral support.

REFERENCES

1. Deyo, R.A.: Conservative therapy for low back pain: Distinguishing useful from useless therapy. JAMA *250* (8):1057, 1983.
2. Linton, S.J., Kamwendo, K.: Low back schools: a critical review. Phys Ther *67*(9):1375, 1987.
3. Aronoff, G.M., Evans, W.O., Enders, P.L.: A review of follow-up studies of multidisciplinary pain units. *In* Evaluation and Treatment of Chronic Pain (Edited by G.M. Aronoff). Baltimore, Urban and Schwarzenberg, 1985.
4. Fordyce, W.E., Roberts, A.H., Sternbach, R.A.: The behavioral management of chronic pain: a response to critics. Pain *22*:113, 1985.
5. Waddell, G.: A new clinical model for the treatment of low-back pain. Spine *12*(7):632, 1987.
6. Waddell, G., et al.: Chronic low-back pain, psychologic distress, and illness behaviour. Spine *9*(2):209, 1984.
7. Fordyce, W., et al.: Pain complaint—exercise performance relationship in chronic pain. Pain *10*:311, 1981.
8. Deyo, R.A.: Measuring the functional status of patients with low back pain. Arch Phys Med Rehabil *69*:1044, 1988.
9. Waddell, G., Main, C.J.: Assessment of severity in low-back disorders. Spine *9*(2):204, 1984.
10. Simmons, J.W., Arant, W.S., Demski, J., Parisher, D.: Determining successful pain clinic treatment through validation of cost effectiveness. Spine *13*(3):342, 1988.
11. Mayer, T.G., Tencer, A.F., Kristoferson, S., Mooney, V.: Use of noninvasive techniques for quantification of spinal range-of-motion in normal subjects and chronic low-back dysfunction patients. Spine *9*(6):588, 1984.
12. Smith, S., Mayer, T.G., Gatchel, R.J., Becker, T.J.: Quantification of lumbar function. Part 1: Isometric and multispeed isokinetic trunk strength measures in sagittal and axial planes in normal subjects. Spine *10*(8):757, 1985.
13. Mayer, T.G., et al.: Progressive isoinertial lifting evaluation: I. A standardized protocol and normalized data base. Spine *13*(9):993, 1989.
14. Nachemson, A.L., LaRocca, H.: Editorial: spine, 1987. Spine *12*(5):427, 1987.
15. Bloch, R.: Methodology in clinical back pain trials. Spine *12*(5):430, 1987.
16. Mayer, T.G., et al.: Objective assessment of spine function following industrial injury: a prospective study with comparison group and one-year followup. Spine *10*(6):482, 1985.
17. Mayer, T.G., et al.: A prospective two-year study of functional restoration in industrial low back injury. JAMA *258*(13):1763, 1987.
18. Hazard, R.G., et al.: Functional restoration with behavioral support: a one-year prospective study of patients with chronic low-back pain. Spine *14*(2):157, 1989.

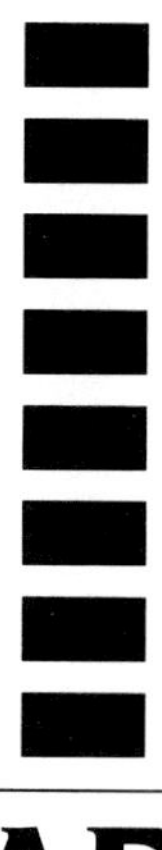

PART VIII

Special Issues in Spinal Care

Patty Newton
Steven Carter

41

Vocational Rehabilitation

The average wage earner sets aside at least one third of his day to pursue his chosen vocational path.[1] In terms of time expenditure alone, work is a major part of life. But, more than that, work establishes the sense of self-esteem and, perhaps more than any other factor, the societal prestige and worth of the individual. The onset of disability is a blow not only to the body of the worker, but to his self-perception and to the value placed on him by society.[2]

The Vocational Rehabilitation (VR) movement is a mirror of society's perception of the injured worker. VR has ranged from a minor social movement, reflecting a type of benevolent stinginess,[3] to a major bureaucratic enterprise. Funding and emphasis of vocational rehabilitation has changed to reflect the political nuances of government, although the needs of the injured client have not changed from the usual desire to rejoin society as a productive worker. The goal of VR is to facilitate the injured worker's re-entry into the world of work.

HISTORICAL PERSPECTIVE

Most people in colonial America were of European descent, usually from England. This meant that the early Americans were also replete with European perspectives of superstition, sorcery, alchemy, and witchcraft. Physical and mental aberrations were viewed with suspicion.[4] The physically disabled were thought to be the victims of demonic possession or the targets of divine wrath. Obviously, the prospects for rehabilitation did not bode well for the disabled persons of the era. Medical technology of the day also did not promote chances of successful recovery even from relatively minor injuries.

Rehabilitation progressed slowly during the eighteenth and early nineteenth centuries until the work of several pioneers brought the needs of specific disability groups to the forefront. The work of Thomas Gallaudet with the deaf, Samuel Howe with the blind and mentally retarded, and Dorothea Dix with the mentally ill, began to bring the plight of the disabled to the attention of the nation.

The beginnings of the workers' compensation programs and the rehabilitation of the physically disabled can be traced to the disabled veterans of the Civil War, Spanish-American War, and World Wars I and II. Gradually, medical technology evolved to the point that more veterans survived their war wounds, only to find their attempts to return to a productive role in society frustrated. Responding to the needs of these veterans, Congress, on June 27, 1918, passed Public Law 178. Often referred to as the Smith-Sears Act, the legislation provided for the vocational training and placement of individuals disabled as a result of service in the armed forces. Although Smith-Sears did not apply to civilians, it set a precedent and provided the service provision pattern, which was later followed by the Smith-Fess Act of 1920.

Smith-Fess launched the civilian vocational rehabilitation program, but the program remained small and ineffective until World War II produced large numbers of disabled service men.[3] Medical advances had allowed war casualties to live longer. Individuals with spinal cord injuries, burns, and multiple amputations no longer died quickly from complications.[5]

When Smith-Fess was passed in 1920 it was written as a temporary program, which was extended by Congress in 1924. Rehabilitation continued to be funded as a temporary program until 1935 when the Social Security Act made rehabilitation a permanent program. Under the Social Security Act, federal funding for rehabilitation was $2 million annually.[6]

Workers' Compensation legislation frequently paralleled rehabilitation legislation but was largely separate. The Federal Employee's Compensation Act (FECA) was passed by Congress in 1908. The act was designed to provide assistance to civil employees of the federal government. In 1916, FECA was amended to institute a consistent program for all civil employees of the United States.[7] Early workers' compensation laws made no allowance for vocational rehabilitation, but the laws had an indirect effect on the funding for vocational rehabilitation programs. Oberman[8] stated that workers' compensation was more dangerous than life in the army during a war. Legislators began to see the importance of vocational rehabilitation programs to deal with the injuries resulting from the industrial revolution.

The first compulsory state workers' compensation law in the US was passed by the New York State Legislature in 1910. When Mississippi passed a workers' compensation program in 1948, all of the states had some type of workers' compensation program.

In the 1980s, rehabilitation found itself being the victim of closer legislative scrutiny, and has fallen victim to the fiscal ax of the executive branch many times. This resulted in the need for closer monitoring of rehabilitation costs and increased the emphasis on program evaluation. Rehabilitation programs have found the need to demonstrate their value by followup and other program evaluation techniques.[9]

THE ROLE AND FUNCTION OF THE REHABILITATION COUNSELOR

If the role and function of the rehabilitation counselor is to be addressed, first an understanding of how the rehabilitation counselor differs from other counselors must be developed. Thomason and Barrett[11] describe the rehabilitation counselor as the individual who works in a face-to-face relationship with a disabled person in order to help him develop a better understanding of his problems and potentials. Williamson[10] maintains that the rehabilitation counselor differs from generic counseling because the rehabilitation counselor is required to blend three streams of thought in understanding and assisting the disabled person. First, the medical model, which explains the disabling condition and the restorative services that are necessary. Second, the vocational guidance model that is used to provide direction for vocational decision making. Finally, the mental health model, which addresses personal and social adjustment needs.

Rubin and Roessler[3] point out the vast discrepancy between the role of the rehabilitation counselor as it should be versus the way it really is. The center of the controversy is the notion of whether the counselor should act as a counselor, a coordinator, or both.[12] Patterson advocated the use of rehabilitation counselors as therapeutic counselors, whereas other counselors are specifically assigned the duties of coordination of basic case management issues. Phillips, et al., identifies some movement toward spe-

cialization of the roles of different rehabilitation workers, but for the most part rehabilitation counselors are expected to be jacks-of-all-trades in order to be effective.[13] Richardson, et al.,[14] conducted a survey that showed the basic subroles of rehabilitation counselors.

In this survey, Richardson found that counselors' routines are dominated by administrative duties such as information acquisition and provision. The increasing size of the public rehabilitation counselor's caseload and, on average, the decreasing size of his budget per client, has precipitated major changes in the way rehabilitation counselors conduct business. Today, the client can principally view the rehabilitation counselor as a coordinator of services, rather than a classical counselor.[3] Recognizing the trend, the National Council on Rehabilitation Education (CORE), in its recent position statement on undergraduate rehabilitation, emphasized the importance of basic skills other than traditional counseling. These skills usually include interpretation of information provided by other professionals such as the physician, psychologist, and vocational evaluator, and purchasing necessary services, such as aides, adaptive devices, and training.

DIAGNOSIS AND INTERVENTION IN VOCATIONAL REHABILITATION

Early intervention for physical needs is vital to the recovery and rehabilitation of any person, as is early intervention in addressing the individual's vocational needs. Often, within the disability service and delivery system, the injured worker becomes caught up in a power struggle among many players. Some of the players in the struggle are insurance representatives, attorneys and other legal professionals, physicians, and the rehabilitation counselor. For the client to receive the services he needs, it is often necessary to allow him to work through the power system. The counselor can often be an ally by providing information to the client about alternatives. The rehabilitation counselor can act as a coordinator, gathering information from the available resources and keeping lines of communication open.

If the role of information gatherer is considered one of the principal roles of the rehabilitation counselor,[14] then the interpretation of information is a necessary skill for the rehabilitation counselor. This information can come from a variety of sources, as noted in Table 41–1.

Efficient and effective use of information depends largely on the approach the counselor uses for such information. If the counselor approaches the information with the desire to identify all possible limitations and thereby eliminate inappropriate job

Table 41–1
Sources of Information Used by the Rehabilitation Counselor

Medical and psychological data.

Complete work history.

Education history.

An analysis of hobby interests.

Transferable skills analysis.

Job analysis.

Work hardening reports.

Vocational evaluation.

Job development and job placement information.

Retraining or on-the-job training.

choices, the counselor may find the process overwhelming and frustrating. Working with clients in the negative perspective of limitations never helps to identify job choices, rather it acts only to rule out choices. The effective rehabilitation counselor approaches each bit of information searching for assets. Each bit of information builds on others, eventually forming a pattern that may suggest specific alternatives. Then client needs can be approached in the manner in which they can be accommodated, rather than how they limit the client.

The medical report may be somewhat difficult for the novice counselor to approach in terms of this positive approach because much of the information is presented as limits; however, limits also suggest abilities. A medical limitation suggesting an individual should not lift more than 50 pounds suggests the functional capacity to lift forty pounds. Similarly, other medical information should be used as means of selection rather than means of exclusion.

The psychological report can be used to provide data about the client's ability to process varying kinds of information. If the Wechsler Adult Intelligence Scale-Revised is administered, differences in verbal and performance scores can be illustrative of the client's optimum learning mode. Performance scores suggest visual and tactile learning, whereas verbal scores reflect auditory processing. These differences can be used to aid decision making between didactic programs and applied training programs.[15,16] Personality measures and behavior observations can aid in selecting work environments; withdrawn individuals obviously make poor sales representatives.

One of the most valuable tools of the rehabilitation counselor, and one of the most underused, is the personal interview. Interviews can be effective tools, particularly if planned ahead of time. Rubin

and Farley[17] described the effective interview as involving an efficient plan of action. According to Rubin and Farley this planning involves determining objectives and developing strategies to achieve those objectives. The result of the planning process is the development of one or more of the following types of objectives:

1. General objectives. Objectives that are to be accomplished with every client.
2. Specific objectives. Objectives that are developed for a specific client. These are highly individualized and differ from client to client.
3. Moment-to-moment objectives. These are objectives that arise as the result of interaction during the interview.

The end result of the evaluation should be a basic understanding of the client's educational and vocational histories. The educational history should tell the counselor what educational or training programs were completed and also about class performance, grade averages, favorite courses, problem courses, and educational goals and aspirations (short- and long-term). Similarly, the vocational history should provide more than job titles. The routine duties of the individual are more important than the title. Often, company titles are not consistent with the duties performed. The individual's feeling about different jobs, the durations of jobs (longevity), and the relationships with supervisors and co-workers should be explored. Work-related goals held by the individual prior to disability onset also are important. These goals are often more indicative of real interests than the post-disability goals, which are likely to be influenced by what others think the individual can do now.

VOCATIONAL EVALUATION

One tool of the rehabilitation counselor is the vocational evaluation. A thorough vocational evaluation can give the counselor an indication of work habits, abilities, stamina, interests, and personality factors that influence the individual's ability to work and his work readiness. The Tenth Institute on Rehabilitation Services (1972) Study Group III defined vocational evaluation as a comprehensive process that uses work, real or simulated, as the focal point for assessment and that uses vocational counseling to assist individuals in vocational development. Vocational evaluation, according to the study group, incorporates medical, psychological, social, vocational, educational, cultural, and economic data to assist in attaining the goals of the evaluation process.

Among the results gained from the vocational evaluation is a general assessment of the client's work readiness. Work readiness, according to Power[18] refers to the individual's personal attributes to the world of work. Job readiness, in contrast, refers to the extent to which an individual's qualifications fit the requirements of a specific job. Methods for determining work readiness and job readiness vary. Table 41–2 presents the approaches often used:

In the typical vocational evaluation, a combination of the methods shown in Table 41–2 is used in order to arrive at a judgment of the individual's work readiness. Commonly, this is done through a battery or series of exercises, tests, work samples, job tryouts, and interviews. McCarron and Dial[16] identified five predictor factors to be measured in the vocational evaluation process: verbal, spatial, and cognitive abilities; sensory abilities; motor abilities; emotional and behavioral variables; and integration and coping abilities. Verbal, spatial, and cognitive abilities are defined as the individual's ability to use language, to process verbal and spatial information and to learn. The sensory factor, according to McCarron and Dial, pertains to the basic mechanisms of receiving and perceiving information from the environment and responding in a purposeful, adaptive manner. The motor factor consists of four basic facets: speed, coordination, strength, and balance. Emotional variables affect work performance substantially because they represent the ability to interpret social cues and to appropriately respond to those cues. Integration-coping is defined as the individual's knowledge and skills related to activities of daily living, personal and social life, and work adjustment. These abilities are often referred to as adaptive behaviors. Most evaluations include some measures of these variables, as well as other information derived from work samples and interest tests.

Work samples are of two primary types: worker trait samples and job samples. Worker trait samples are those which measure characteristics common to many jobs, such as eye-hand-foot coordination or range-of-motion. Job samples measure traits more specifically associated with a particular job, such as a drafting or electronic assembly work sample.

The most common source of information about worker traits is the Dictionary of Occupational Titles (DOT) and the Selected Characteristics of Occupations Defined in the Dictionary of Occupational Titles (SCO). Most work sample systems use the references as the basis for skills measured within the system. The DOT contains important defining information about approximately 20,000 occupations. The SCO provides information on each job, including its physical demands, environmental conditions, mathematical and language development, specific vocational preparation, and occupational aptitude patterns (OAPs). Physical demands include specific demand areas and classifications, as listed in Table 41–3.

Working conditions used to classify occupations in the SCO are listed in Table 41–4; Specific Vocational Preparation (SVP) times are shown in Table 41–5.

Aptitude factor scores are used to cluster occupations into patterns of related occupations; these patterns are referred to as Occupational Aptitude Patterns. The scores used for clustering occupations were derived from the nine aptitudes on the General Aptitude Test Battery (GATB). These aptitudes include: general learning, verbal ability, numerical aptitude, spatial aptitude, form perception, clerical perception, motor coordination, finger dexterity, and manual dexterity. Other commonly used multiple aptitude tests include: the Non-Reading Apti-

Table 41–2
Approaches for Determining Work Readiness and Job Readiness

Analysis of work, education, and social histories.

Interviews with the client and family.

Medical and psychiatric consultation.

Psychological testing.

Work evaluation.

Situational assessment.

On-the-job tryout.

Table 41–3
Specific Physical Demand Areas and Classifications

1—Strength (Lift, carry, push, pull):

		Maximum Lift	Frequent Lift/Carry
S	Sedentary	10 lbs.	
L	Light	20 lbs.	Up to 10 lbs.
M	Medium	50 lbs.	Up to 25 lbs.
H	Heavy	100 lbs.	Up to 50 lbs.
V	Very Heavy	Over 100 lbs.	Over 50 lbs.

2—Climb and balance

3—Stoop, kneel, crouch, and crawl

4—Reach, handle, finger, and feel

5—Talk, hear

6—See (Acuity, depth perception, field of vision, accommodation)

Table 41–4
Working Conditions Used to Classify Occupations in the SCO

I—Inside (75% or more)

O—Outside (75% or more)

B—Both

Extremes of cold plus temperature changes

Extremes of heat plus temperature changes

Wet and humid

Noise and vibration

Hazards

Fumes, odors, toxic conditions, dust, poor ventilation

tude Test Battery (and adaptation for nonreaders), the Differential Aptitude Test, and the Career Ability Placement Survey.

Often, work sample systems use more involved mechanisms to measure worker traits and aptitudes. Many times these mechanisms are designed to more accurately reflect actual work-related tasks or activities than are represented on the paper and pencil tests described above. Power[18] described many of the more commonly used work evaluation systems. Examples and descriptions of these systems are as follows:

SYSTEM	DESCRIPTION
JEVS Work Samples	28 work samples for special needs populations; administered over 5 to 7 days.
VIEWS	16 work samples designed for the mentally retarded.
VALPAR	19 work samples for normal and special populations.

Table 41–5
Specific Vocational Preparation (SVP) Times and Codes

9	Over 10 years
8	4 to 10 years
7	2 to 4 years
6	1 to 2 years
5	6 months to 1 year
4	3 to 6 months
3	30 days to 3 months
2	Short demonstration (30 days)
1	Short demonstration only

Vocational interest measures are also critically important in determining the vocational path to pursue. Interest exploration can stimulate counseling by suggesting occupations that had not previously been considered by the rehabilitation client or the counselor.[18] Super[19] described three different kinds of interest:

1. Expressed interest. A verbal indication of liking a given stimulus.
2. Manifest interest. The evidence of participation in an activity or task that others can witness.
3. Tested interest. Interests measured through objective approaches.

Interest inventories frequently have one of two common formats. The first format is based on a Likert-type rating scale and requires the examinee to rate the item, occupation, or task in a degree of likability. The second format requires a forced choice between occupations or activities, "Which task would you prefer, if you had to choose?"

An obvious concern for the rehabilitation counselor is how to deal with discrepancies between interests and abilities. Homework can often be used to deal with this issue. If the client investigates, on his own, the requirements of a job, he may find the occupation does not suit him. Assignments to library materials or to speak with employers in the field may help in this respect. A second approach is to discuss related occupations with fewer restrictive requirements in order to identify one that meets the interest related needs of the client and is consistent with his capabilities. These jobs are likely to be received better if there is a clear career path. An office clerk position, for example, might be an entry position for eventual office management.

TREATMENT PLANS: VOCATIONAL AND OCCUPATIONAL EXPLORATION

Once arriving at a job choice for a client, the rehabilitation counselor must begin to formulate a treatment plan. In the public sector, this usually is referred to as an Individualized Written Rehabilitation Program (IWRP). This program details the steps to be taken to prepare the client for work or to increase his work readiness. The IWRP goals are agreed upon jointly by the rehabilitation counselor and client. The agreement identifies the vocational objective and key subobjectives, including physical restoration, counseling, educational preparation, work adjustment, and vocational training. Private sector or medical facilities may refer to this planning simply as a job plan or a return-to-work plan.

When a client is disabled and unemployed for a

long period, his stamina and work tolerances are likely to suffer. In fact, as Kiluk and Farrell[20] point out, the earlier the intervention, the more likely its success. Edelman,[21] for example, points out that there is a significant learning component to the development of chronic pain. Frequently, then, it is necessary to unlearn the chronic pain behaviors. The use of classical and operant conditioning models has improved the individual's ability to deal with the experience of chronic pain. Involvement of the family has also been reported to be crucial in the process of unlearning the pain response.[22] The rehabilitation counselor must be prepared to deal appropriately with pain responses through close interaction with the client's physician and other professionals. Work hardening is the term commonly applied to programs that use conditioning tasks that are graded to progressively improve the biomechanical, neuromuscular, cardiovascular, metabolic, and psychosocial functions of the individual in conjunction with real and or simulated work activities (Commission on Accreditation of Rehabilitation Facilities, 1989). Perhaps a better term for the process is functional restoration.[23] This differs somewhat because the important element is the restoration of function rather than the elimination of pain. As Mayer and Gatchel describe the process, it is an aggressive individualized physical reconditioning program patterned after sports medicine. The functional restoration differs from pain management principally in that it is an approach with positive goals—regaining function—rather than the negative goals of elimination of pain. It avoids some of the loaded qualities of "How are you feeling?" for the more objective "What can you do?" This approach more closely follows the overall rehabilitation goal of focusing on residual abilities rather than on limitations.

VOCATIONAL COUNSELING AND CHRONIC SPINAL DISORDERS

The Social Security Administration has predicted that by the year 2000 the population of the US will have reached a population of over 300 million, with approximately 4% of that population experiencing chronic spinal injuries. With 80% of dollars expended for treatment of the injuries, it is becoming more important for vocational rehabilitation to be an integral part of the treatment outcome. Physical rehabilitation will deteriorate if the person reverts back to inactivity following treatment. Therefore, productivity becomes the continuation of physical reconditioning. Productivity includes work.

In treatment of the chronic spinal disorder patient, traditional vocational counseling returns. Even though the vocational counselor continues to use those basic skills of case management, the interpretation and use of information provided by other professionals (physicians, physical therapists, occupational therapists, nurses, psychologists, and vocational evaluations) can only be successful through counseling. The vocational counselor must be proficient in counseling in order to build a trust and rapport with the patient. It is in this way that information regarding strengths and weaknesses is given. The successful identification of these strengths and weaknesses in regard to a return to productivity requires the vocational counselor to obtain:

1. A complete medical history (from the physician, physical therapist, occupational therapist, and nurses).
2. A complete work history with job duties (responsibilities, length of time of each job and wages, and vocational education).
3. Job analysis of job at the time of disability (vocational evaluation).
4. Behavior and socioeconomic barriers to recovery (psychological).

Through effective counseling, the vocational counselor can assist the person to objectively assess and plan re-entry to a productive lifestyle.

Goals for Re-Entry

Work hardening functional simulation is proving to be a means of returning the back-injured patient to work. The Commission on Accreditation of Rehabilitation Facilities (CARF) definition of work hardening is:

> Work hardening programs are interdisciplinary in nature, use conditioning tasks that are graded to progressively improve the biomechanical, neuromuscular, cardiovascular/metabolic, and psychosocial functions of the individual in conjunction with real or simulated work activities. Work hardening provides the transition between acute care and return to work while addressing the issues of productivity, safety, physical tolerances, and work behaviors. Work hardening is a highly structured, goal oriented, individualized treatment program designed to maximize the individual's ability to return to work.

Functional simulation includes most of these same components but is expanded to include quantitative evaluation and functional restoration. It is suggested that the back-injured person experiences more difficulty in returning to preinjury jobs. Through the functional simulation approach, the patient is more successful in return to work efforts.

The work hardening included in a functional restoration program results in the back-injured patient working up to the physical demands of the pre-injury job. It becomes a "team effort" of vocational rehabilitation. The team includes the above-mentioned professional team members, the back-injured person, the pre-injury employer, the worker compensation carrier, the legal system, and the vocational counselor. In this team, the vocational counselor remains the case manager, with the task of collecting and disseminating information to each of the team members, while leading the communication between all team members.

It is important to complete a job analysis with both the employer and the worker. Physical demands are listed in Table 41–6. Work hardening functional simulation addresses these physical demands. Including the injured worker when designing the activities, makes him more confident of his ability to return to work in the pre-injury job.

Functional simulation leads the back-injured patient to functional readiness. Through the counseling process, the vocational counselor, works with the back-injured patient toward job readiness. The vocational evaluation has provided the vocational counselor and the patient information regarding the skills this person must possess to return to gainful productivity (work). The grid for work status is presented in Table 41–7.

Note that retraining and on-the-job training are not the first choices of this grid. The vocational counselor uses this grid to document the patient's return-to-work status. Should the person be unable physically to return to work at the preinjury job, the vocational counselor explores the transferrable skills defined through the vocational assessment of skills and counsels the patient in this regard. The vocational counselor also determines job availability with the preinjury employer for a less physically demanding job or for a graduated return to work for the back-injured worker, thus allowing the worker to continue the work hardening, but in a real work environment.

Enhancing the worker's ability to seek jobs is important. Many persons who work in physically demanding jobs previously located work in nontraditional ways, or have had the same job for a number of years and feel insecure in their ability to locate appropriate employment. Vocational counseling also opens the way for injured workers to express concerns of peer relationships in regard to the injury and the employer's doubts of the injured worker's physical ability to do the job. The vocational counselor can facilitate communication to the employer, including the levels of physical abilities. The vocational counselor also counsels the injured worker by providing information to the employer to allow that employer to become comfortable with the worker, both in physical abilities, as well as skills for the job.

Formal retraining of a back-injured person usually is less effective than return to work. Few worker compensation laws include this benefit for injured workers. Without regular income, the injured worker is unable to provide for self and family and does not have money for tuition and books. On-the-job training (OJT) becomes a more acceptable means of learning a new trade. In an OJT placement, the worker is paid a wage to learn the new skills required for the occupational change.

The vocational counselor must be knowledgeable of the labor market and employer attitudes toward hiring the back-injured worker. He or she must be ready to counsel both the employer and employee in ways of cooperative work plans. Headley[24] reports a common thought expressed by the disability system is that a "green back poultice" is an instant cure for the chronic back injured patient, but there appears to be evidence that this is not the case. In reviewing outcome studies from various treatment programs, state worker compensation reports, and other reports, it appears that returning the spinal-injured individual to employment is the more cost effective and overall positive means of finalizing the case. Roberts[25] responds to rehabilitation outcomes in the 1987–1988 annual report from the Victorian Accident Rehabilitation Council in Melbourne (Australia): ". . . due to rehabilitation intervention . . . conservative estimates of $7 saved for each $1 invested for cases closed with a worker returning to work . . . The Council is of the firm view that rehabilitation must be a participatory process. Injured workers, employers, and rehabilitation providers must be motivated to actively engage in the rehabilitation." The Northwestern National Life Insurance Company reports, ". . . rehabilitating workers disabled on or off the job can save companies $30 for every $1 spent on rehabilitation services that return a worker to work." The United States Social Security Administration research indicates ". . . rehabilitation of a disability beneficiary produces a return of $10 for every $1 spent in returning a beneficiary to work."

Table 41–6
Work Status

Current Employment Status?

0. Never returned to work.

Working Codes   1. Same employer/same job.
                            2. Same employer/different job.
                            3. Different employer/same job.
                            4. Different employer/different job.
                            5. Vocational training or school/retraining.
                            6. Self-employed.

Table 41–7
JOB ANALYSIS

PATIENT ____

EMPLOYER/COMPANY ____________________________ Date _________

CONTACT PERSON/SUPERVISOR _______________________________

PHONE NUMBER _____________________________

PATIENT'S JOB TITLE ______________________ AVERAGE NUMBER OF HOURS WORKED DAILY ______

Please check the appropriate job-related task and the frequency which applies to the above mentioned patient and job:

	N/A	OCCASIONAL (0–33% of workday)	FREQUENT (34-66% of workday)	CONSTANT (67–100% of workday)
Sitting	—	___________	___________	___________
Standing	—	___________	___________	___________
Walking	—	___________	___________	___________
Climbing	—	___________	___________	___________
Kneel/Squat Stoop	—	___________	___________	___________
Bending	—	___________	___________	___________
Twisting	—	___________	___________	___________
Push/Pull	—	___________	___________	___________
Reaching	—	___________	___________	___________
Lifting (floor to waist)	—	___________ (indicate lbs.)	___________ (indicate lbs.)	___________ (indicate lbs.)
Lifting (waist to shoulder)	—	___________ (indicate lbs.)	___________ (indicate lbs.)	___________ (indicate lbs.)

Is there any body part which is used repeatedly? ___ Yes ___ No

If so, what body part is used? _______________

COMMENTS:

____
Case Manager

By encouraging the spinal-injured person to understand himself, his injury, and his functional capacities, the vocational counselor becomes an integral component of this cost-effectiveness. As previously mentioned, it is important for the full team (medical professionals, injured individuals, employer, insurance carrier, and justice system) to work together for a positive outcome.

SUMMARY

In summary, the rehabilitation programs of the 1990s must move forward in the direction of focusing on abilities rather than disabilities. This focus should lead to more ease in developing work goals and in improving client satisfaction with the rehabilitation process. Certainly, it is more satisfying for an individual to be aware of what he can do rather than what he is unable to do. Also, job development and placement become easier if potential employers are apprised of a person's abilities rather than his disabilities. The spine-injured person requires complete and objective diagnosis with appropriate intervention. This intervention should always include a structured assessment of the person's physical abilities and skills for returning to gainful productivity.

REFERENCES

1. Black, B.J.: Principles of Industrial Therapy for the Mentally Ill. New York, Grune & Stratton, 1968.
2. Steers, R.M.: Introduction to Organizational Behavior. Glenview, IL, Scott, Foresman, & Co., 1981.
3. Rubin, S.E., Roessler, R.T.: Foundations of the Vocational Rehabilitation Process. Austin, TX, Pro-Ed, 1987.
4. Wright, G.N.: Total Rehabilitation. Boston, Little, Brown, & Co., 1980.
5. Allan, W.S.: Rehabilitation: A Community Challenge. New York, John Wiley, 1958.
6. MacDonald, M.E.: Federal Grants for Vocational Rehabilitation. Chicago, University of Chicago Press, 1944.
7. Matkin, R.E.: Insurance Rehabilitation. Austin, TX, Pro-Ed, 1985.
8. Oberman, C.E.: A History of Vocational Rehabilitation in America, Minneapolis, MN, Dennison, 1965.
9. Carter, S., Chan, F., Lam, C.S., Parker, H.J.: Program evaluation in an intensive work adjustment program. Vocational Eval Work Adjustment Bull, 20:3–6, 1987.
10. Williamson, E.: Vocational Counseling. McGraw Hill, NY, 1965.
11. Thomason, B., Barrett, A.M.: Casework performance in vocational rehabilitation. GTP Bull 1—Rehabilitation Services Series 505. Washington, DC, US Department of Health, Education, and Welfare, Office of Vocational Rehabilitation, 1959.
12. Patterson, C.H.: Power, prestige, and the rehabilitation counselor. Rehabil Res Pract Rev 1(3), 1–7, 1970.
13. Field, T., Emerer, W.G.: Rehabilitation counseling in the 80's: the coming of camelot. J Appl Rehabil Counsel 12(2):44–46, 1982.
14. Richardson, B.K., Rubin, S.E., Bolton, B.: Counseling interview behavior of empirically derived subgroups of rehabilitation counselors. Arkansas Studies in Vocational Rehabilitation, Series 1, Monograph 7. Fayetteville, AR, University of Arkansas, Rehabilitation Research and Training Center, 1973.
15. Aiken, L.R.: Psychological Testing and Assessment. Boston. Allyn and Bacon, 1985.
16. McCarron, L., Dial, J.G.: McCarron-Dial Evaluation System Manual. Dallas, TX, McCarron-Dial Systems, 1986.
17. Rubin, S.E., Farley, R.C.: Intake Interview Skills for Rehabilitation Counselors. Fayetteville, AR, University of Arkansas, Rehabilitation Research and Training Center, 1980.
18. Power, P.W.: A Guide to Vocational Assessment. Baltimore, University Park Press, 1984.
19. Super, D.: Vocational Interests of Men and Women. Stanford, Stanford University Press, 1959.
20. Kiluk, D.J., Farrell, A.D.: The efficacy of early treatment of the chronic low back patient in an outpatient multiple disciplinary pain clinic. Pain 2:260, 1984.
21. Edelman, R.I.: The Chronic Pain: A Guide to Rehabilitation. New York, Matthew Bender, 1985.
22. Dew, D.W., Phillips, B., Reiss, D.: Assessment and early planning with the family in vocational rehabilitation. J Rehabil 55:1, 1989.
23. Mayer, T.G., Gatchel, R.J.: Functional Restoration for Spinal Disorders: The Sports Medicine Approach. Philadelphia, Lea & Febiger, 1988.
24. Headley, B.J.: Delayed recovery: taking another look. Rehabil 55:61–67, 1989.
25. Roberts, B.: Vocational rehabilitation of the industrially injured worker—A New Approach. NARPPS News 10:6, 1989.

42

Gary D. Herrin

Ergonomic Considerations in Workplace Design and Worker Selection

There are fundamentally only two approaches to matching employees to manual materials handling tasks in industry. Either the person can be evaluated in terms of his or her work capacities and then selectively conditioned or trained to fit the job; or the workplace must be modified to fit the prospective worker. The later strategy is of an engineering type, dealing with methods to assure that the workplace and work tasks are specified in ways that minimize injurious stresses, and is the only long-term solution to control musculoskeletal injuries in the workplace. Both strategies rely on knowledge of the physical requirements of the job. These requirements must be carefully evaluated by knowledgeable observers using prescribed measurements and analysis procedures. The relevant techniques for analyzing prospective workplaces and workforces is the topic of this chapter. Some simple suggestions for workplace design or redesign are also presented.

ERGONOMICS

The term ergonomics is based on two Greek words *ergon* meaning work and *nomus* meaning law. It is commonly associated with the study of humans at work. Ergonomics focuses on understanding the complex relationships among people, machines, job demands, and work methods. All work places both physical and mental stresses on the worker. As long as these stresses are maintained within reasonable limits, work performance is satisfactory and the worker's health and well being are maintained. On the other hand, if stresses exceed capacities, undesirable outcomes may occur in the form of work avoidance, increased errors, accidents, injuries, or some decrement in health or well being.

Ergonomists are primarily concerned with evaluating the stresses that occur in the work environment and the ability of people to cope with these stresses. The goal of ergonomics is to design facilities, equipment, tools, and jobs compatible with human dimensions, capabilities, limitations, and expectations.

Over the years, ergonomics has emerged from five major disciplines: psychology, anthropometry, physiology, mechanics, and epidemiology.

Engineering Psychology

Human factors engineering, also called engineering psychology, is a discipline of ergonomics concerned with the informational requirements of work. Since the industrial revolution, this discipline has developed to understand increasingly sophisticated equipment and systems in the work environment. Successful operation of these advanced systems often places high information processing loads and decision making demands on the worker. If these stresses are excessive, human error may occur, resulting in an accident. Actions based on confusing arrays of alarms, lights, and gauges actually contribute to the adverse outcomes of an accident. It is assumed that all accidents can be prevented if better human factors engineering is practiced in the design and operation of facilities.

Anthropometry

Anthropometry is fundamental to ergonomics practice. Measures of human body dimensions are central to designing facilities, equipment, furniture, tools, and personal protective devices, to accommodate the variability in human size.

The design of work can be approached either mechanically or empirically. In the mechanical approach, the body is treated as a system of links connected at joints (kinematics). By summing the links, it is possible to determine where objects should be located to be within reach. In the empirical approach, the dimensions of the body do not correspond to individual link lengths, but are combinations of links functionally related to a given task. Examples include the reach envelop of a seated operator and the spatial requirements of holding a screwdriver.

Physiology

Work physiology is the subdiscipline of physiology concerned with stresses resulting in fatigue. From an ergonomic perspective, fatigue is a temporary decrease in the desire or capability to work. Fatigue may be limited to a small number of muscles that have been overly stressed (i.e., localized fatigue) or may affect the entire body (i.e., cardiovascular fatigue).

Local Muscle Fatigue

The short-term effects of static work are fatigue and pain. Tremor, for example, may interfere with a person's ability to perform precise manipulation tasks. Static muscular work performed only on an occasional basis, is unlikely to precipitate permanent disorders. However, if job demands repeatedly place excessive static stresses on the same muscles on a daily basis over a long period of time, deterioration can take place in the joints, tendons, and ligaments adjacent to the muscle. Because the postures needed to perform some jobs require prolonged static work on a daily basis (e.g., a grocery checker continuously leaning forward to retrieve and scan items), occupational postural stresses can potentially contribute to the development of permanent musculoskeletal disorders.

Whole Body Fatigue

Aerobic capacity (also called maximum oxygen uptake) is the maximum rate at which an individual can use oxygen to fuel muscle metabolism. Many personal factors are related to aerobic capacity: age, sex, body weight, heredity, and physical fitness. Variability between people is an important consideration in evaluating fatigue potential. For a job that is performed over an 8-hour shift, the average energy expenditure rate should not exceed 33% of a person's aerobic capacity. Assuming an "average" 60-year-old female, for example, has an aerobic capacity of about 9 kcal/min, for an 8-hour workshift, the rate of energy expenditure by this worker should not exceed 3 kcal/min.

Jorgenson[1] reviewed the literature on permissible loads based on energy expenditure criteria. Asfour, et al.,[2] examined the association between endurance and strength training programs on lifting capabilities. Khalil, et al.,[3] Mital and Ayoub,[4] and Asfour, et al.,[5,6] examined metabolic and cardiovascular responses to a variety of manual materials tasks. Their results estimate the oxygen consumption and heart rate increases associated with the increase of load, frequency, height range, box length, and box width. A comprehensive database of metabolic and cardiac costs is developing to provide easy and useful data for guidance in the design of work tasks.

Mechanics

Occupational biomechanics is a subdiscipline of ergonomics that focuses on understanding mechanical properties of human tissue and the resistance of tissues to mechanical stresses. Mechanical stresses in the environment can cause acute injuries (e.g., a concussion when a worker is struck in the head by a dropped object) or cumulative trauma injuries. Acute hazards are often recognized and controlled through safety engineering techniques such as machine guarding and personal protective equipment. Cumulative trauma stresses in the environment on the other hand, are more subtle and often overlooked.

Chaffin[7] summarizes the development of occupational biomechanical models for studying and reducing the consequences of injuries to the low back. Current biomechanical spinal stress models of dynamic load lifting activities are mostly restricted to sagittal plane motions, as described by Freivalds et al.,[8] McGill and Norman,[9] and Ekholm, et al.[10] Three-dimensional static models of the lumbar motion segments have been developed, as typified by the models of Schultz and Andersson[11] and Bean, et al.[12] These three-dimensional spinal motion segment models, however, are restricted to static analysis over a limited range of motion, and do not include passive tissue stiffness responses that have been shown recently to be important when modeling the motion segments throughout their ranges of motion.[13]

These models assume rather simplified muscle actions to stabilize and move the spinal column. Chaffin and Andersson,[14] Andersson,[15] and Garg, et al.[16] discuss low back stress during static loading and slow speed dynamic sagittal plane lifting. The ability to accurately predict muscle and spinal column forces during normal speed dynamic and asymmetric lifting has not been demonstrated.[9,12,17–19]

Epidemiology

Epidemiology has been important to the development of ergonomics because it helps us to understand the personal and occupational risk factors associated with low back pain. Major epidemiologic studies of the past decade included studies by Andersson,[20] Frymoyer, et al.,[21] and Bigos, et al.[22–24] These studies link a variety of individual and work factors to occupational low back pain.

The National Institute of Occupational Safety and Health guidelines[25] cite studies revealing that musculoskeletal injury rates (i.e., number of injuries per man-hours on the job) and severity rates (i.e., number of hours lost because of injury per man-hours on job) increases significantly when: (1) Heavy objects are lifted. (2) The object is bulky. (3) The object is lifted from the floor. (4) Objects are frequently lifted.

Niskanen[26] reported on a study to clarify the differences between concrete reinforcement workers and painters in the frequency, causes, and types of accidents and minor accidents affecting the musculoskeletal system. David's[27] study of drilling accidents found elevated heart rates and intratruncal pressure associated with high incidence rate jobs.

Bergquist-Ullman and Larson [28] found a strong relationship between low back pain caused by lifting and the duration of sickness absence. Chaffin and Park[29] found that over a one year period low back pain was eight times greater in workers who performed heavy lifting work. Snook, Campanelli, and Hart[30] concluded that the proper design of lifting tasks could reduce up to one-third the incidence of LBP; however, simply training workers in good lifting technique was ineffective.

Long-term physiologic changes accompany heavy lifting. Hult[31] showed that long-term heavy lifting was related to osteophyte formation in the spine. One proposed mechanism for osteophytic formation relates to the annular bulging of the spinal discs that occurs in lifting or bending. Fibers of the annulus of the disc attach at the disc margins and are placed under tension when lifting, twisting, or bending, stimulating new bone formation at the site.

Numerous investigations have indicated an increase in absence caused by sickness with low back pain and an increase in low back symptoms in jobs generally considered as physically heavy work.[32–34]

Snook[35] found that a worker was three times more susceptible to compensable low-back injury if exposed to excessive manual handling tasks. Unskilled laborers had the highest prevalence rate for disc prolapse and lumbago in the Dutch study by Valkenburg and Haanen.[36] Svensson and Andersson[37] found heavy physical work to be strongly associated with the occurrence of low back pain, and the highest prevalence of low back pain in their cross-sectional study was in men with professions involving physically heavy work.

WORK EVALUATION SYSTEMS

In order to effectively apply the aforementioned ergonomics knowledge to the workplace, it is essential that work requirements are evaluated. Unfortunately, there is a paucity of such systems in the available literature. As one might suspect, there is general disagreement on what, precisely, should be measured. One survey of the available research literature disclosed that each of the following physical workplace factors have been identified as important.[38]

1. Loads—measures of the vector forces and moments (e.g., lifting, pushing, or pulling) acting on the body during materials handling.
2. Dimensions—measures of size, shape, and form of the objects handled.
3. Distribution of loads—measures of the location of the object's center of gravity with respect to the worker.
4. Couplings—measures of the interfacing between the worker and the load (e.g., handle design parameters such as size, shape, location, coating, and texture).
5. Stability of load—measures of the consistency of the load's center of mass (as in handling liquids and bulky materials).
6. Workplace geometry—measures of the spatial properties of the task such as movement distances; directions and extent of motion paths; obstacles; nature of the destination (each affect worker posture).
7. Temporal factors—measures of the frequency, duration, and pace of work activities over the short- and long-term.
8. Complexity—measures of manipulation requirements; objective of activity, tolerances for motion error.
9. Environment—measures such as temperature, humidity, lighting, noise, vibration, foot traction, and toxic agents.
10. Organization—measures of administrative factors such as the use of teamwork, machine pacing, work incentives, extended work shifts, job rotations, and personal protective devices.

Although this list is far from complete, it does suggest that work evaluation can require detailed

Table 42–1
Work Evaluation Systems Relevant to Low Back Pain Causes

Synthetic Time Prediction Systems

Physical Stress Checklists and Surveys

NIOSH Lifting Guidelines

Static Strength Analysis

Biomechanical Job Analysis

Psychophysical Strength Analysis

Job Posture Analysis

and complex data collection. Further, the evaluation must consider the interaction of many simultaneous work factors. A practical difficulty with evaluation of workplaces for potential risks of low back pain is that the available literature is unclear about whether the problems are, indeed, attributable to acute or cumulative trauma.

If the cause is normally a long-term, degenerative, "wear and tear" process, then presumably the workplace evaluation should include the temporal aspects of work, such as frequencies and durations of exertions, fatigue, work and rest regimes, and so forth. If, on the other hand, the cause is predominantly acute trauma, as in slipping and falling or being struck, then infrequent, unpredictable, atypical aspects of work, such as emergency procedures, maintenance and machine setup, and perhaps leisure time activities, should receive primary analysis and documentation attention. It is apparent that the risks of both acute and cumulative trauma are major concerns in industry; hence, it is necessary to apply multiple evaluation procedures.

Herrin, et al.,[39] summarizes a variety of contemporary work evaluations applicable to design of manual materials handling jobs. Some of the more popular analysis systems which are important because they quantify work stressors related to low back pain are shown in Table 42–1. A brief discussion of each of these approaches follows.

Synthetic Time Prediction Systems

Synthetic, predetermined motion-time systems first emerged in the 1930s. Today they are ostensibly only used for planning staffing requirements for new workplaces before they become operational. Once a workplace is operational, direct observation techniques (such as time study) can be used to refine the actual work methods and procedures.

A survey of the use of such techniques reported by Karger and Bayha[40] disclosed that about two-thirds of firms sampled use some form of work measurement system, and that about 56% of these used a predetermined motion-time measurement system (MTM). One of the original and most popular systems, used by thousands of practitioners throughout the world, is referred to as MTM-1. To use this particular motion classification system with accuracy and consistency requires training in a special course comprised of 24 to 80 classroom hours (offered and certified by the MTM Association). For a detailed discussion of the use of such systems, the reader should consult the referenced textbooks.[40–44]

Conventional work measurement approaches rarely record the variability of work in such terms as loads handled and distances moved; hence, extreme deviations about the atypical average are often ignored. The fact that the total time required to complete a particular task is relatively insensitive (or robust) to this variability does not lessen the importance of this aspect in the cause of low back pain. Further, these systems virtually ignore posture except for the grossest classifications (such as standing versus seated work). The most important shortcoming relative to low back pain is the concentration on time accounting. No attention is given to infrequent or nonroutine work. Typically, tasks that require less than 5% of the total workday such as occasional machine setups, maintenance or cleanup, or emergency procedures, are neither rigorously documented nor analyzed. Many accident and injury reports suggest that these unusual, undocumented, infrequent job tasks account for a large number of overexertion injuries.

Physical Stress Checklists

Physical task checklists sometimes can be used to document the job's general physical requirements. In such a procedure a job analyst observes the worker and "checks" those activities performed from a list of common manual tasks (e.g., bend trunk, pull with arm(s), lift with back).[45] Such lists have been used to improve job placement procedures for individuals with physical impairments.[46]

It should be clear that such physical stress survey data are important when identifying jobs that could be potentially hazardous to a worker's musculoskeletal system. They are also applicable to jobs that are not highly repetitive, wherein traditional methods are weak. In this sense, the surveys indicate when special in-depth studies may be warranted. Such surveys are especially useful when combined with injury data analysis to motivate more intensive evaluations.

NIOSH *Lifting Guidelines*

A federal guide entitled, *Work Practices Guideline for Manual Lifting*[25] offers specific recommendations for evaluating human lifting limitations in particular. The Guide is intentionally simplistic in approach and application because it was intended for general industry use. Due to its widespread interest and application, it will be discussed in some detail here. The guideline is based on four criteria:

1. Epidemiology—the occurrence of low-back pain in the workplace.
2. Biomechanics—the mechanical stresses acting upon the low back created by muscle exertions and external loads.

3. Psychophysics—the muscular strength-producing capabilities of the workforce.
4. Physiology—whole body fatigue potential.

The guideline allows the evaluation of manual lifting tasks by defining the following task measurements (Fig. 42–1):

1. Object weight (L)—measured in pounds. If this varies from lift to lift, the average and maximum are necessary.
2. Horizontal location of the hands (H)—measured in inches forward of the midpoint between the ankles at the origin of the lift (i.e., where the hands grip the object or the location of the object's center of gravity).

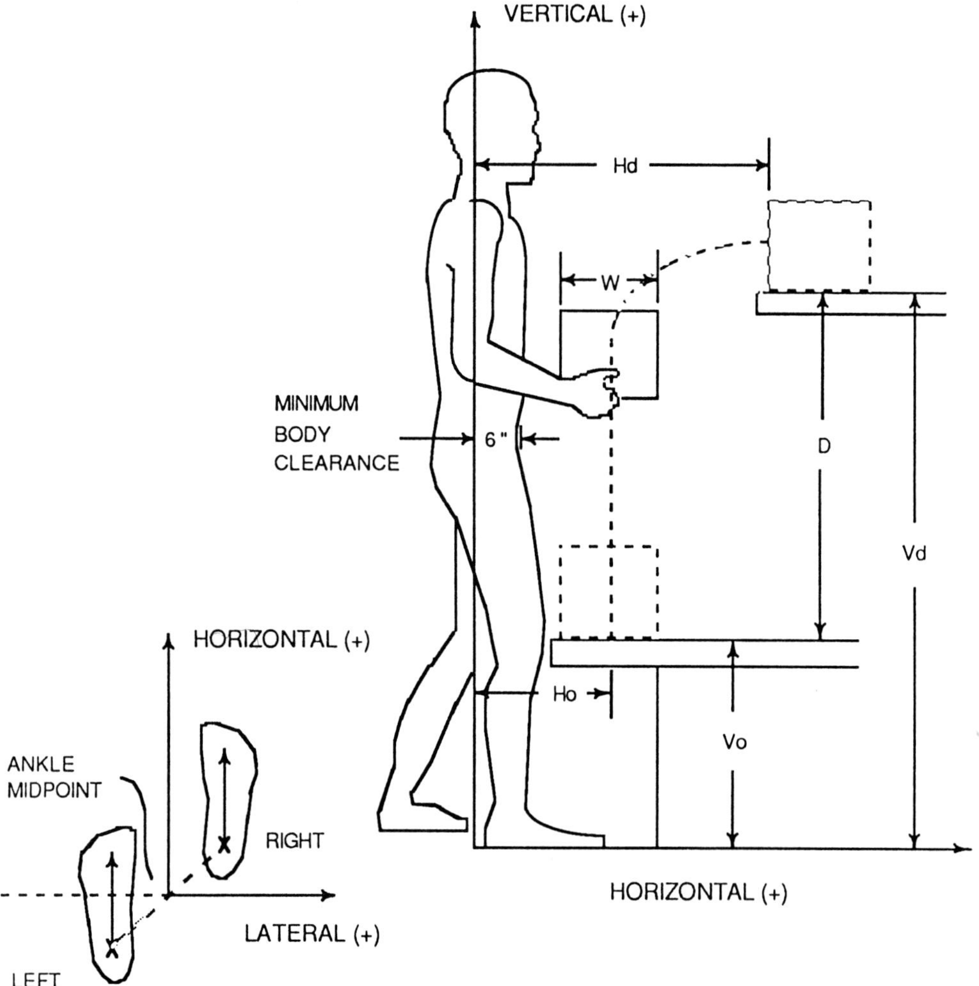

Figure 42–1. Illustration of lifting task variables. (Adapted from NIOSH, 1981.)

3. Vertical location of the hands (V)—measured in inches from the floor to the origin of the lift.
4. Vertical travel distance (D)—measured in inches from the origin to the destination of the lift.
5. Frequency of lifting (F)—measured in lifts per minute assuming continuous lifting.
6. Duration or period of lifting (P)—assumed to be either occasional (less than one hour during the day) or continuous (for the entire 8 hours).

The guideline establishes two lifting limits based on the epidemiologic, biomechanic, physiologic, and psychophysical criteria. The limits and their criteria are:

1. Maximum permissible limit (MPL), in pounds—this limit reflects a lift that produces 1430 pounds of compression on the L5–S1 disc, or creates a metabolic load of 5.0 kcal per minute, or is within the strength capabilities of only 25% of men and virtually no women.
2. Action limit (AL), in pounds—this limit is algebraically equal to one-third of the MPL. It creates 770 pounds of compression on the L5–S1 disc, and requires less than 3.5 kcal per minute, and is within the strength capabilities of at least 75% of women and virtually all men.

These two limits define three lifting task hazard zones.

1. Above the MPL—those tasks that most people cannot perform without hazard, requiring engineering controls.
2. Below the AL—tasks that are presumably of acceptable stress and risk to most people.
3. Between the AL and MPL—tasks that some people cannot perform without specific risk, and that require either engineering controls or administrative controls.

The guideline oversimplifies the true stresses involved in lifting by making the following assumptions:

1. Smooth lifting. The guide assumes minimal accelerations of the load and human body. High accelerations or "jerk" lifts increase the stress to the low back.
2. Two-handed, symmetric lifting in the sagittal plane. The guide assumes that lifting is two dimensional with both hands directly in front of the body and no twisting throughout the lift.
3. Moderate width object. The hands are assumed to be separated no more than shoulder width. The handling of extremely wide objects (such as a standard sheet of plywood, for example) would be outside the scope of the guide.

4. Unrestricted, standing posture. The guide assumes that no obstructions interfere with the movement of the object and no props or aids are used to assist the individual. Lifting style is not considered beyond simple stoop versus squat techniques.
5. Good couplings or handles on the object. The guide assumes that good gripping surfaces or handles are used and that the worker is standing on a slip-resistant surface.
6. Favorable environmental conditions. The guide assumes that heat and cold stress are not contributing to the burden on the individual.
7. No other major physical work activities. The guide assumes that the worker is essentially at rest when not lifting (i.e., doing no significant carrying, pushing, pulling, or holding).

Figure 42–2 illustrates the three manual lifting regions formed by the Action Limit (AL) and the Maximum Permissible Limit (MPL) boundaries. In this figure, the task requires infrequent lifting (F < .2 lifts per min or 1 lift every 5 min) of an object from the floor to approximately knuckle height (V = 6 in. and D = 24 in.). The figure displays the inverse relationship of horizontal hand location and weight lifted with the AL and MPL.

The AL and MPL can be calculated as follows, using the algebraic form of the two limits:

$$\text{AL (lbs.)} = 90 \times (6/H) \times (1.0 - .01|V - 30|) \times (.7 + 3/D) \times (1 - F/F_{max})$$
$$\text{MPL (lbs.)} = 3 \times (\text{AL})$$

These task variables or measurements have the following limits:

1. H must be between 6 and 32 in. Objects cannot be held closer than 6 in. without interference with the body. For most people, 32 in. is the maximum reachable horizontal distance.
2. V must be between 0 and 70 in. This represents the range of vertical reach for most people.
3. D must be between 10 and (80 − V) in. For travel distances less than 10 in., set D at 10 in.
4. F must be between .2 (one lift every 5 min) and F_{max} (Table 42–2). For lifting frequencies below .2, set F at 0.
5. F_{max} can be determined using Table 42–2. Its value depends on the average vertical location of the load (V) and the duration of activity or period (P).

The most effective method for reducing low back injuries is to implement engineering controls such as reducing the size and weight of the object being

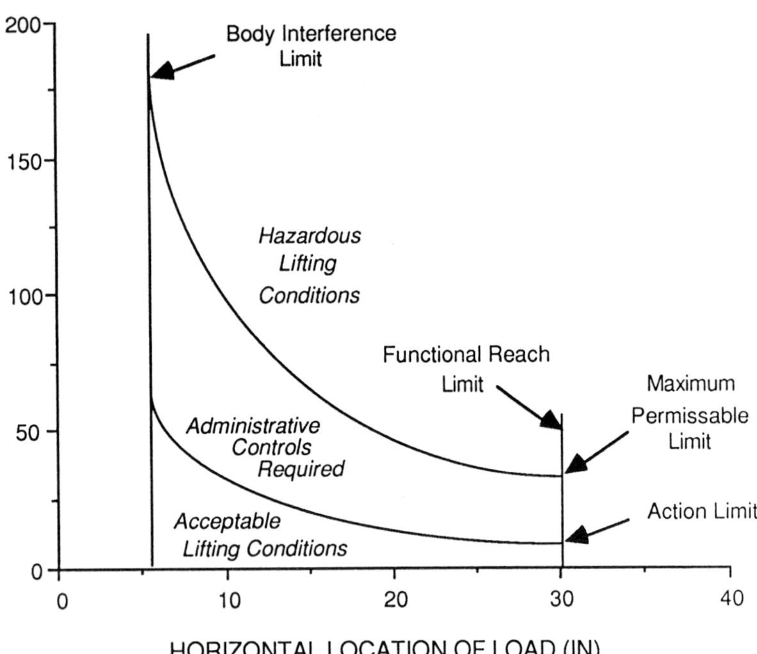

Figure 42–2. Weight lifted versus horizontal location for infrequent lifting from floor to knuckle height. (Adapted from NIOSH, 1981.)

lifted, redesigning the work station to reduce horizontal and vertical distances, or reducing the task frequency. If these are impractical, the installation of automated material handling equipment (e.g., hoists, conveyors, and lift tables) can be used to reduce the biomechanical stresses on the worker. If engineering changes do not bring the job within the acceptable zone defined by NIOSH, administrative controls should be implemented. Administrative controls include training, use of two people for heavy lifting, or selection and placement testing. Several studies have shown that functional tests that accurately simulate a job can be used to effectively match the job to the employee and to reduce musculoskeletal injuries.

Table 42–3 shows the emphasis of each criteria (biomechanical, physiological, and psychophysical) for each lifting task variable. Figure 42–3 is a simple nomogram for identifying discounting factors associated with each lifting task variable. To use this nomogram, identify the task variable (e.g., H = 12 in.) on the horizontal axis, then look up discount on the vertical axis (e.g., horizontal factor = .5). In this ex-

ample, the horizontal location would lead to a discount of 50% from maximum capacities.

Example. Lifting a stock reel onto a punch press. Figure 42–4 shows a worker lifting a reel of stock onto a punch press. The worker performs this task by lifting the reel, taking one step forward and placing the reel on the press. This task is repeated every 5 minutes for a half hour once during the 8-hour work shift.

Table 42–2
F_{max} *Table* (NIOSH, 1981)

	Average Vertical Location (in.)	
Period	*V > 30 in.* *Standing*	*V < = 30 in.* *Stooped*
1 Hour	18	15
8 Hours	15	12

Table 42–3
The Emphasis of Task Variables on Various Types of Physical Stress Associated with Manual Lifting

Lifting Task Variable	Low Back Stress (Biomechanics)	Whole Body Fatigue (Work Physiology)	Localized Muscle Fatigue (Psychophysics)
Object Weight (L)	x	x	x
Horizontal Location (H)	x	x	x
Vertical Location (V)	x	x	x
Travel Distance (D)		x	x
Frequency of Lift (F)		x	x
Duration or Period (P)		x	

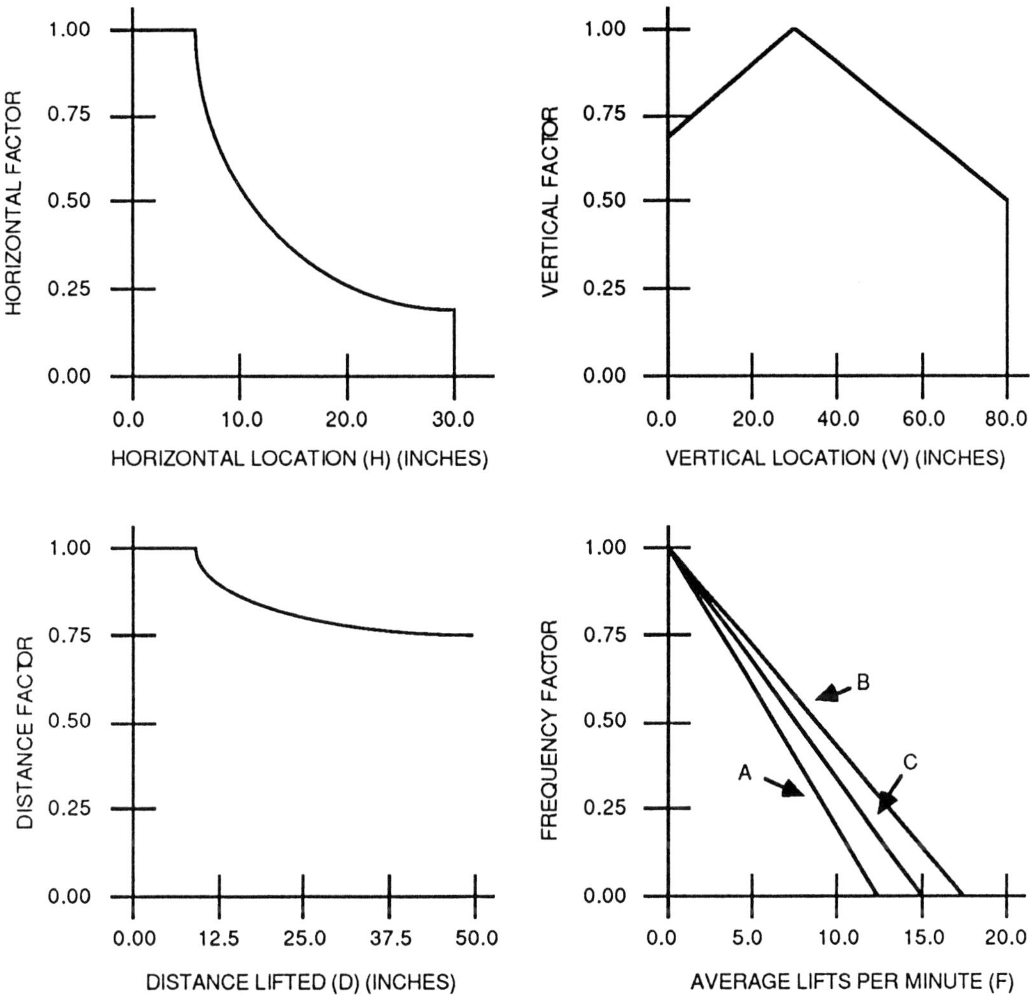

Figure 42–3. Nomogram for determining lifting discounting factors.

The task variables are:

Object weight (L) = 44 lbs.
Horizontal hand location (H_{origin}) at the origin of the lift = 20 in.
Vertical hand location (V_{origin}) at the origin = 15 in.
Horizontal hand location ($H_{destination}$) at the destination of the lift = 30 in.
Vertical hand location ($V_{destination}$) at the destination of the lift = 63 in.
Frequency of lifting (F) = .2 lifts per min (1 lift every 5 min)
Duration or period of lifting task (P) = less than 1 hour

The AL and MPL are calculated as:

$$AL = 90 \; (HF) \; (VF) \; (DF) \; (FF)$$
$$= 90 \; (.30) \; (.85) \; (.76) \; (.99) = 17.3 \text{ lbs}$$
$$MPL = 3 \; (AL) = 3 \; (17.3) = 51.9 \text{ lbs}$$

Because the weight of the stock reel is close to the task's MPL, engineering controls also are recommended to reduce the risk of injury associated with the task.

Often jobs involve a variety of lifting tasks. In this case two separate analyses are required; one to consider the "worst case" exertion and a second "composite evaluation." This later case is especially important in assessing fatigue potential.

Guideline Applications

Muthuswamy, et al.,[47] considered the design of work and rest schedules as an administrative and engineering control for jobs between the AL and MPL. Nicholson[48] examined the degree of coherence between the four main lifting criteria: psychophysical, biomechanical, intra-abdominal pressure, and metabolic. His results showed some agreement on

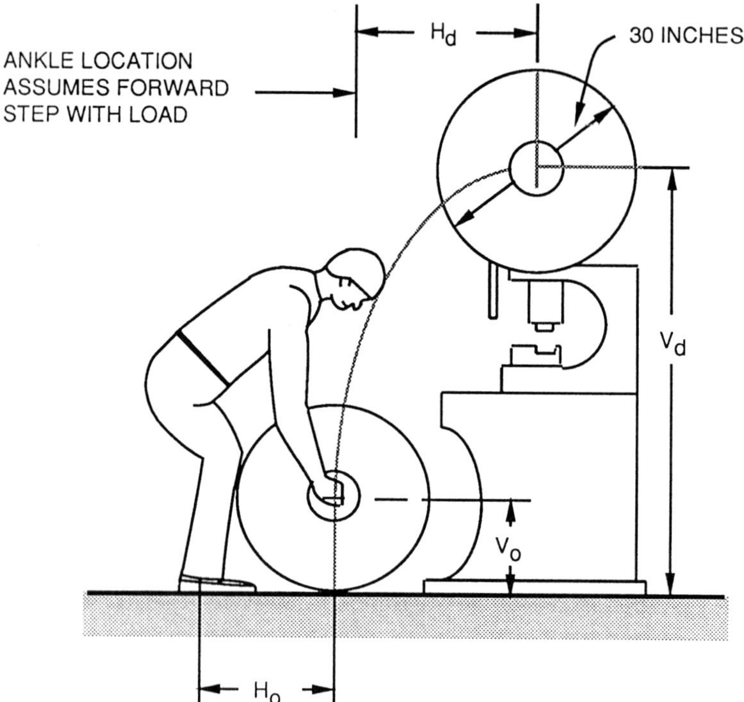

Figure 42–4. A worker lifting a reel of stock onto a punch press. (Adapted from Niosh, 1981.)

recommended load limits according to the different criteria, but considerable disagreement for many manual handling tasks, as expected. Subsequently, Nicholson and Clark[49] applied the NIOSH guidelines to analyze baggage handling facilities at Heathrow Airport, London. Their results showed an unacceptable handling burden on ground service crews, primarily caused by extended horizontal reach requirements.

Static Strength Analysis

Because the NIOSH guidelines only apply to symmetric lifting in the sagittal plane, a more generalized analysis scheme is often necessary to describe and evaluate manual work. One such scheme concentrates on static strength predictions.

A model developed at the University of Michigan[7,50] compares the load moments produced at various body joints during any task to population capabilities. The job analysis requirements are comparable to the NIOSH procedures but can be extended to pushing and pulling in other than orthogonal directions. A complete description of this job analysis can be found in Chaffin & Andersson.[14]

A detailed discussion of the strength prediction and L5–S1 compression force model and computer algorithm is available in Garg and Chaffin[50] and

Chaffin and Andersson.[14] The methods for assessing isometric strength in industry and predicting population norms are discussed in Stobbe[51] and Herrin.[52]

Biomechanical Job Analysis

Over the last 10 years, several static biomechanical models have been developed to predict the strength capability of a population and to quantitatively identify physical acts required in highly stressful jobs. In applying static biomechanical models to a dynamic act, such as lifting, it is assumed that the effects of acceleration and momentum are negligible. In a detailed dynamic biomechanical simulation of lifting psychophysically determined maximum loads, Garg, Chaffin, and Freivalds[16] showed that the compressive force at the low back and peak task moments at various body joints were approximately two to three times greater than those based on a static biomechanical simulation. The resulting trade-offs between the static and dynamic biomechanical simulations of lifting are discussed. Also, maximum voluntary isometric lifting strengths are compared with the maximum weights acceptable to the subjects.

A laboratory study was conducted by Garg, et al.,[53] to assess the effects of lift angle on biomechanical stresses to the musculoskeletal system, and in particular, on the lower back. There were large differences between the maximum acceptable weights and the "maximum permissible limits" recommended by NIOSH. The estimated compressive force on the lumbar spine was, on the average, 11% lower for lifting at an angle as compared with a straight vertical lift.

Biomechanical models are often used to quantify spinal stress. Static models reveal the postural effects caused by gravity, whereas dynamic models also take into account inertial factors. Leskinen[54] used both dynamic and static models to evaluate the lumbosacral compression.

In lieu of intradisc pressure measurements, intra-abdominal pressure measurements have received attention as criteria for work design, especially in the United Kingdom. Davis[55] outlined a study of the correlation between intra-abdominal pressure measurements and intradiscal pressures and myoelectric activity of the trunk muscles and as determinants of spinal stress. Measurements made in industrial situations used a radio pill to observe stresses imposed by different tasks. Earlier, Davis and Stubbs[56] proposed safe levels of manual forces for young males based on intra-abdominal pressure measurements. Nordin, et al.,[57] measured intra-abdominal pressures with a wireless radio pill. Measurements were made during common postures, simple activities, and static and dynamic lifting.

Psychophysical Strength Analysis

The psychophysical approach to assessment of strength does not assume an underlying mechanical model of a body nor does it relate to spinal loading per se. Rather, it focuses directly on the individual's perception of manual capability when doing a task.

Psychophysical scales have been developed in many practical problem areas. For example, the scales of effective temperature, loudness, and brightness were all developed with a psychophysical methodology.[58-60] Psychophysics has also been used by Borg[61,62] in developing rating scales of "perceived exertion" (PRE); by the Air Force in studies of lifting;[63,64] by the Army in studies of treadmill walking;[65,66] and in developing effort scales.[67,68]

A series of seven studies conducted at Liberty Mutual Research Center and summarized by Snook,[69] stand out for their comprehensiveness in the area of manual materials handling capacities, as does the study of Ayoub, et al.[70] The latter study was restricted to lifting tasks only. Snook and his associates also provided the first analysis to relate psychophysical strength predictions to the increased risk of low back injury.

In order to evaluate the effectiveness of job design

in the reduction of injuries (as well as the effectiveness of selection techniques and training procedures), 191 cases of low back injury from 32 states were investigated by Snook, Campanelli, and Hart.[30] Questionnaire results revealed that about 25% of policy holder jobs involve manual materials handling tasks that (on a psychophysical rating scale) are acceptable to less than 75% of the workers. However, half of the low back injuries were associated with these jobs, indicating that a worker is three times more susceptible to low back injury if performing a manual handling task that is acceptable to less than 75% of the working population. This suggests that, at best, two out of every three low back injuries associated with heavy manual handling tasks can be prevented if the tasks are designed to fit at least 75% of the population. The third injury will apparently occur anyway, regardless of the job. The other low back injuries not associated with heavy manual handling tasks will also occur. It can be concluded that up to a third of industrial back injuries can be obviated by the careful and proper design of manual handling tasks.

A similar study by Ayoub, et al.,[70] provided prediction models for maximum psychophysical lifting capacity as a function of worker and task variables. Six regression equations were generated for each lifting region: floor to knuckle, floor to shoulder, floor to reach, knuckle to shoulder, knuckle to reach, and shoulder to reach. Experiments were conducted at frequencies of 2, 4, 6, and 8 lifts per min and box sizes of 12, 18, and 24 in. (30.5, 45.7 and 61.0 cm, respectively) in the sagittal plane. A series of job stress indices (variations of the ratio of weight lifted to individual lifting capacities aggregated across tasks) were developed in an effort to predict lost time resulting from injury. None of these indices was strongly correlated with the injury experience, in part because of the small sample size.

Mital[71-73] provided a series of reports on the development of maximum acceptable weight of lift databases for male and female industrial workers for a variety of work situations (e.g., 8- vs. 12-hour work periods, restricted space, differing material densities, center of gravity location, hand preference, and frequency). Garg and Ayoub[74] performed a literature survey on recommendations for the maximum weight of the work load. Their comparison revealed:

1. Recommendations based on a given criterion are not in agreement.
2. The maximum permissible weights of the loads, based on psychophysical studies, are lower than those based on biomechanical criteria.
3. The psychophysical fatigue criteria, as compared to physiologic fatigue criteria, result in greater work loads at higher frequencies of lifting.

Load and pace trade-off and effects of lifting technique and location of load on acceptable work loads are also examined.

Job Posture Analysis

Awkward trunk posture during work can be caused by a number of controllable factors, including poor work station layout, inappropriate design of tools and equipment, and incorrect work methods. If not eliminated, these postures can cause fatigue and contribute to the development of pain and disorders in the lower back. Keyserling, et al.,[75] presents results of a study of trunk postures at work and the incidence of back pain.

A computer-aided system was developed to evaluate trunk posture during work by measuring the time spent in neutral and non-neutral postures. This system was used to assess postural risk factors in a case study of back disorders in an automobile assembly plant. The use of non-neutral trunk postures, such as forward flexion, lateral bending, and axial twisting, was associated with reports of back pain.

The results of this study suggest that job redesign or other methods for controlling non-neutral posture be implemented to reduce the risk of back pain on industrial jobs. A general approach to work station design, based on a mechanical model of the human skeletal system, is described. This model is used to develop specific job design guidelines to prevent awkward trunk posture.

Keyserling[76] developed a method to evaluate postural stress of the shoulders and trunk for various work activities. When completed, the system can generate a posture profile and posture-task graph. The posture profile helps determine if a job requires the shoulders or trunk to assume non-neutral postures for excessive periods of time.

The posture-task graph simultaneously displays the task analysis and the trunk and shoulder postures. The graph can help identify specific work elements associated with non-neutral postures. Once identified, the tasks can be redesigned to minimize muscle fatigue, discomfort, and musculoskeletal disorders.

An approach to recording potentially stressful postures was developed by Corlett, et al.,[77] and is referred to as posture targeting. This procedure requires the job analyst to observe a worker at random times during the workday and record the angular configuration of various body segments with the aid of the "body diagram."

Corlett and Manenica[78] have also demonstrated that this procedure is useful in evaluating workplace layouts when combined with worker reports of lo-

calized musculoskeletal pain obtained at several intervals during a workday.

Priel[79] proposed a system to allow postures to be numerically defined and recorded on a "posturegram." Another system developed in Finland, the Ovaco Working Posture Analysis System (OWPAS), is a practical method for identification and evaluation of unsuitable working posture.[80,81]

A method similar to OWPAS is a technique developed by Berns and Milner[82] for analyzing moving work postures (TRAM). Both OWPAS and TRAM record the postures at regular intervals on a recording sheet. By using various combinations of the basic posture, a wide range of postures can be described.

A new Swedish system called ARBAN was developed by Holzmann.[83] ARBAN is a method for ergonomic analysis of work, including work situations involving greatly differing body postures and loads.

These observation techniques can be used together with discomfort and comfort scales[84] and different biomechanical analysis techniques. Finally, Grieve[85] has suggested a method to determine potential mechanical constraints during static exertions based on equilibrium (body balance) considerations reflected in a postural stability diagram.

WORKPLACE DESIGN

The preceding literature on biomechanics, physiology, psychophysics, and epidemiology provides a wealth of data upon which to base work designs. The basic principles from the models lead to some simple guidelines for work. Chaffin[86] and Keyserling, et al.,[75] provide detailed discussions of ergonomics as design approaches.

Devices to Assist Materials Handling

When an object is large and heavy it is often desirable to use a hoist or crane to assist in its movement. If an overhead mounted hoist is used that is manually pulled from one location to another, sufficient time must be provided to the operator to avoid sudden jerking motions that will result in an uncontrolled swinging of the object being moved. It is not uncommon for hoist operators to suffer back injuries by attempting to stop an uncontrolled swing motion of an object supported by the hoist. It also is possible for an object to slip from the hoist or overload the hoist when swinging.

Carts and manually powered trucks also are used to move heavy objects in the workplace. The risk of low back pain being induced while using such devices arises from two hazards. First is the overexertion hazard associated with pushing or pulling on a load that is too heavy. To avoid this situation, it is important to assure that the pushing or pulling hand force requirements are below 50 lbs. and that the hands are at about hip to waist level when making a maximum exertion (thus minimizing the spinal load moments).

These requirements can be satisfied best in the design of a workplace by specifying a cart that: (1) has vertical handles that can be grasped at varying heights, (2) uses large rubber tires with good bearings that will not "hang up" on irregular surfaces, (3) has wheels that easily pivot, and (4) is designed to handle the intended load. Furthermore, it is just as important to assure that the floor surface is smooth, clean, and has little or no grade inclination.

The second hazard to the back when pushing or pulling carts comes from the increased risk of slipping during such activities. It is not uncommon for the required coefficient of friction (ratio of foot shear force divided by normal force) to exceed 1.0 during pushing and pulling activities. Hence, floor surfaces should be kept clean and dry and workers should be instructed to use, or be provided with, high traction shoes.

Winkel[87] studied the manual handling of wide-body carts used in civil aircraft. The findings in his experiments caused the Swedish National Board of Occupational Safety and Health to reduce its recommended limit for repetitive push and pull in this task from 200 N to 100 N. As a result, the handling of wide-body carts in the DC-9 would be delayed until at least 14 to 15 minutes after take off to fulfill the new recommendations. On short flights, for which the DC-9 is used, however, this was not possible without reducing the level of service. Hence, a followup project on the development of an improved cart was required, incorporating ergonomics into the design.

Container Design

The weight and dimensions of a load to be lifted are primary risk factors. Containers should be compact so a worker can minimize the spinal load moment by keeping the object's center of mass close to the body. The dimensions of a container also are important if a person must ascend or descend stairs while carrying the object. If the container is too large, it will impair vision, resulting in an increased risk of a trip or fall.

If the container must be lifted from the floor, and it is too large to pass between the knees, the person must lift the object in front of the knees. This causes a larger spinal load moment than would be the case if the object could be lifted between the knees. Any object larger than about 12 inches cannot be lifted easily between the knees.

Container design must also include a means by which to firmly grasp it. This is important not only to lift the container properly but also to avoid sudden spinal inertial loads that occur when one attempts to regain control of an object slipping from the hands. In general, a forceful grasp of an object is provided by either a "hook grip," whereby the fingers wrap around the object but without thumb opposition, or a "power grip," whereby the thumb assists in retention of the object by overlapping the fingers. The power grip requires less upper muscle action to maintain the coupling because the handle is fully secured between the fingers and the thumb. To provide such a handle requires consideration of hand anthropometry.

Bag handling was studied by Smith, et al.,[88] who used physiologic and psychophysical research approaches to determine the effects of two levels of fullness (70% and 95%) and the use of handles on bag lifting tasks. The maximum acceptable weight lifted was significantly higher when performing a bag lifting task either with handles or when the bag was 95% full. The maximum acceptable weight of lift for bag lifting tasks was higher (2.21 kg) than for box lifting tasks under the conditions studied.

Garg and Saxena[89] performed a laboratory study to evaluate the effects of handles, shape of the container, and dimensions of the container on maximum acceptable weight of lift using a psychophysical methodology. It is concluded that the recommendations for maximum acceptable weight of the load based on boxes with handles must be adjusted when applied to boxes without handles or to some other types of containers.

Legg[90] studied the heart rate and intra-abdominal pressure (IAP) while handling cylinders for 15 min in an enclosed compartment. These results support the hypothesis that physical training may help to offset the additional physiological strain of wearing protective clothing during materials handling tasks, and suggest that the development of higher peak IAPs during lifting following physical training may be part of a spinal protective mechanism.

Drury, et al.,[91] surveyed more than 2000 different box handling tasks, performed by workers in nine factories, and offered many insightful recommendations.

Hand Tools

The recent literature has indicated that the use of large hand tools may contribute to the incidence of low back disorders among workers. A study by Marras[92] used electromyography to evaluate the effects of spine loading caused by tool characteristics and method of tool use. Spine loading indices were defined, which provide relative measures of compression, shear, and torsion for 40 male subjects. The method of tool use was found to influence the components of spine loading.

Workspace Design

One of the primary concerns when designing a workspace to prevent low back disorders is to allow the person to stand or sit erect. This requirement means that workers should not have to reach beyond comfortable arm reach in front and to the side of the body, especially if the manual activity required is lifting of heavy materials. This means that obstructions over which a worker must lean to reach an object or place an object must be eliminated. If a heavy object is to be lifted, it should be located so that the worker can lift it without bending down or leaning forward. In practice, this may require the following:[75,86]

1. Roller conveyors that allow objects to be pulled toward the body before lifting or powered conveyors to bring containers to the worker.
2. Gravity-fed slides (or shelves), such as used in airline baggage claim areas, which present items to the worker.
3. Machine designs that have the workpiece or part being manufactured located close to the operator.
4. Tilting of large stock bins to present parts closer to the operator.
5. Enough room for a worker to walk around large bins or pallets of parts to avoid having to reach and lean forward to remove parts from the opposite side.

In order to minimize awkward trunk posture, the workplace design recommendations are similar:

1. Use work benches and parts bins that are adjustable in height, or use anthropometric data to determine the optimal height for specific tasks, tools, and equipment. Consider using tiltable benches or bins to reposition work closer to operators' reach limits.
2. Never store manually handled objects on the floor. Use devices such as benches, conveyors, lift tables, and hoists to deliver objects to the worker at a comfortable height.
3. If possible, position objects and other devices that must be grasped (e.g., hand rails, handles, and control knobs) at least 29 in. above the floor. This allows even tall workers (up to 95th percentile males) to grasp the object without stooping.
4. Minimize required horizontal reach distances.

Provide foot space under benches to allow workers to get closer to objects that must be grasped. Eliminate any barriers that unnecessarily restrict horizontal reaches.
5. Discourage axial twisting of the spine through improved work station layout. Eliminate situations that require workers to turn the body 180° to perform sequential operations. If the work station layout cannot be improved, train workers to turn their bodies by moving their feet instead of twisting the spine.

WORKER EVALUATION

The assessment of an individual who performs manual materials handling must include specific tests of physical capability. The medical justification for such tests is recognized by all concerned with controlling the potential for overexertion strain and sprain injuries and illnesses.

Criteria for Testing

Strength and work capacity assessments have been implemented as part of medical examinations in a number of industries as experimental medical procedures with varying success. In evaluating any medical assessment the following criteria are of paramount importance:

1. Is the test safe to administer?
2. Is it reliable and reproducible?
3. Is it practical to administer?
4. Is it predictive of capability and risk?
5. Is it specific to the requirements of the job?
6. Is it ethically and legally defensible?

Taking of medical history is generally regarded as safe; x rays and strength testing programs, on the other hand, have inherent risks. The test and retest measurement errors and inter-rater reliability can have large effects on accuracy and precision of assessments and subsequent decisions. Some test procedures are relatively inexpensive in time and effort; others are quite expensive. At present, cost-benefit analyses of alternative test protocols do not exist.

Four measures of test quality (accuracy, specificity, sensitivity, and prevalence) must be jointly considered before a test can be deemed valid. Two kinds of errors can occur: rejection of qualified applicants (e.g., a concern of EEOC), and hiring unqualified people (e.g., a concern of management, reflected by health and safety concerns). In terms of functional capacity testing, both are consequences of professional malpractice. There is a fundamental difference between impairment and disability evaluation.

Each of these criteria must be kept in mind when evaluating any proposed examinations and in future studies designed to refine and validate the approach. The interested reader should consult Rothstein,[93] Miner and Miner,[94] and Pope, et al.[95]

Strength Assessment

Human muscle strength assessments have long been recognized as valuable clinical assessment tools, and testing has been conducted on populations from adolescence[96–100] to old age.[101–106]

Sports medicine has concentrated on training conditioning and rehabilitation. Table 42–4 identifies a

Table 42–4
*Strength Assessments in Sports Medicine**

Exercise Conditioning Programs
Hickson, Rosenkoetter, and Brown (107)
Sullivan and Portney (108)
Wood, et al. (109)
Grossi (110)
Hamberg, et al. (111)
Kanehisa and Miyashita (112)
Vegso, Genuario, and Torg (113)
Roxin, Venge, and Friman (114)
Wirth and Lohman (115)
Knutsson and Martensson (116)
Clarkson, et al. (117)
Maughan, Watson, and Weir (118)
Steroids
Bergman and Leach (119)
Cycling
Westerling (120)
Rowing
Bompa (121)
Soccer
Ekstrand and Gillquist (122)
Oberg, et al. (123)
Tennis
Strizak, et al. (124)

**Numbers in parentheses indicate references.*

Table 42–5
*Evaluation of Musculoskeletal Disorders**

ALS	Harrington, Hallett, and Tyler (125)
Diabetic Neuropathy	Jaspan, et al. (126)
Down's Syndrome	Morris, Vaughan, and Vaccaro (127)
Duchenne's Dystrophy	Allsop and Ziter (128)
	Cohen, et al. (129)
	Lane, et al. (130)
Ehlers-Danlos Syndrome	Bilkey, et al. (131)
Low Limb Disability	Kofsky, et al. (132)
Multiple Sclerosis	Armstrong, et al. (133)
Nerve Compression Syndromes	Gelberman, et al. (134)
Neuromuscular Disease	Griffin, McClure, and Bertorini (135)
	Wiles and Karni (136)
Orthopedic Disorders	Odensten, et al. (137)
Paraplegia	Sanderson and Sommer (138)
Parkinson's Disease	Koller and Kase (139)
Polymyositis	Braun, Arora, and Rochester (140)
	Davies, Jones, and Shearer (141)

**Numbers in parentheses indicate references.*

few representative articles. Further, orthopaedic rehabilitation medicine has actively used muscle strength to evaluate a wide variety of musculoskeletal disorders, as summarized in Table 42–5. The allied health professions have also found strength relevant to a number of issues as reflected in Table 42–6. These three tables are not intended to reflect comprehensive compilations, but rather to act as starting points for exploring the research literature.

Selection and Placement Testing

In applying strength testing technology to the workplace, the literature is more limited. This section reviews some of those efforts.

Chaffin, et al.,[152,153] proposed that assessment of a worker who performs manual labor must include specific tests of physical capability. These studies reported on the results of an industrial study of the viability of static strength tests as pre-employment criteria and subsequent prevalence of occupational low back pain. Chaffin, et al.,[154] discuss the use of isometric strength as an indicator of a person's capacity

Table 42–6
*Strength Research in Allied Health Care**

Biofeedback	Shiavi, et al. (142)
Hemodialysis	Saiki, et al. (143)
Hypobaric Hypoxia	Young, et al. (144)
Occupational Environment	Redmond and Breslin (145)
Pain	Mills and Edwards (146)
	Sedlak (147)
Postoperative Deterioration	Edwards, Rose, and King (148)
Smoking	Orlander, Kiessling, and Larsson (149)
Stroke	Hamrin, et al. (150)
Wheelchair Use	Davis, et al. (151)

*Numbers in parentheses indicate references.

to safely perform tasks requiring high physical effort. In a followup study, Keyserling, et al.,[155] performed an investigation of the use of isometric strength tests to select workers for strenuous jobs. It was concluded that isometric strength tests can be used to reduce occupational injuries and should be considered for implementation in industries with strenuous jobs.

In a three part paper, Ayoub[156] discussed the control of manual lifting hazards via pre-employment screening. With a screening procedure, lifting stresses can be controlled by effecting a match between job demands and human work capacity. This is predicated on the principle that jobs cannot be redesigned or changed to lower their demands. Accordingly, the hazard control strategy becomes one of selecting only those individuals with the capacity to perform the given job without excessive risk. An integrative screening program suited for physically demanding jobs is presented. Prerequisites for implementation of the program include: (1) step testing at submaximal levels, (2) strength testing using three standard postures (arms, back, and legs), and (3) determination of job demands expressed in terms of work output and strength requirements. The criteria for screening are based on the level of utilization of each of the principal determinants of human work capacity (energy expenditure, heart rate, and strength capability).

Static ergonomic strength testing (SEST) was employed by Harber and SooHoo[157] as part of a multidisciplinary evaluation program for occupational back pain, providing a quantitative description of lift ability in several positions. Comparison of intrasubject with intersubject variation confirmed that SEST truly measured a personal characteristic. The expected degree of intrasubject variability is independent of the degree of impairment and provides a guide for detecting inadequate subject efforts. The technique allows worker-specific work restriction limitations to be recommended.

Two additional studies of the importance of physical fitness by Cady, et al.,[158,159] concluded that physical fitness and conditioning of firefighters were preventive of back injuries. Kamon and Goldfuss[160] performed an in-plant evaluation of the muscle strength of workers. Later, Kamon, et al.,[161] compared dynamic and static strength measurements to maximal actual lifting and to static lifting strength of steelmill workers.

Celentano, et al.,[162] developed an intensive task analysis approach for three physically demanding military occupations (trades). The methodology used was: (1) survey trade experts (incumbents) to obtain information on the physically demanding aspects of the trade; (2) quantify representative trade tasks; (3) relate operator performance on these representative trade tasks with performance on a selected battery of physical tests from the literature; and (4) determine valid job selection standards from predictive tests. The results of the study demonstrated that static strength and anthropometric measurements were successful in predicting work performance in the trade tasks.

Schultz,[163] in an assessment of the ability of workers with upper extremity injuries to return to work, noted that occupational therapists specializing in the rehabilitation of persons with upper extremity injuries have established an evaluation procedure to determine if and when an injured worker has the physical capacity to go to work. The return to work evaluation has three components: (1) a physical evaluation; (2) a biomechanical analysis of the job; and (3) a work simulation. The therapist documents the patient's response to the work simulation and formulates recommendations to the physician regarding the patient's ability to safely return to work.

Hultman, et al.,[164] examined the influence of a preventive educational program on trunk flexion in janitors. The study emphasizes that it is possible to alter movement patterns of the spine, and thereby decrease the load during janitorial work, by a suitably designed educational program. McGarvey, et al.,[165] examined the reliability of isometric strength testing based on temporal factors and strength variation. Pytel and Kamon[166] outlined a study to develop a practical and reliable test to predict the maximum lifting capacity of an individual.

Kroemer[167] developed an isoinertial technique to assess individual lifting capability. Based on this evaluation, a new dynamic testing technique has been developed and used in experiments with 39 subjects. The new isoinertial test has proven to be easily applied and reliable in its results.

Markhede and Grimby[168] developed a standard procedure for measurement of hip muscle strength with an isokinetic dynamometer. The coefficient of variation when measuring one test subject at ten different occasions was smaller with isokinetic than with isometric measurements. Maxwell, et al.,[169] developed a portable chair for testing isometric muscle strength.

Hansson, et al.,[170] studied safety of isometric strength testing by following reports of back discomfort and back injuries during testing. A biomechanical analysis was compared to EMG force predictions and intravital disc pressure measurements were used for the calculations of the loads in four persons. The calculations indicated compressive loads on L3 ranging from 5000 to 11,000 N during squat and torso lifting. Such loads in vitro have been found to cause structural failures of the vertebral endplates. Similar loads also may result in damage to the spine in vivo.

Strength Prediction

Considerable attention has focused on prediction of muscle strength. These models are important if test results are to be extrapolated and interpolated from clinic to industrial setting. The multifactorial nature of strength capacity, in particular, makes valid predictions challenging.

An early study by Poulsen[171] developed predictive formulas, based on measurements of the back muscle strength, for prediction of maximum loads to be lifted. From tests with 50 male and female subjects, the simplest prediction formulas for maximum loads were as follows: for men, maximum load = 1.10 × isometric back muscle strength; for women, maximum load = 0.95 × isometric back muscle strength minus 8 kg.

Ayoub, et al.,[172] Mital,[173] Mital and Ayoub,[174] and Mital, et al.,[175] examined a variety of regression modeling approaches to predicting psychophysical lifting capacity. Taboun and Dutta[176] developed a polynomial regression model to predict the maximum acceptable handling weights for both individual and combined MMH activities. This model provides a relationship of the total weight (body + handling weight) with subject anthropometric characteristics, task variables, and isometric static strength capabilities.

Yates, et al.,[177] examined static lifting strength and maximal isometric voluntary contractions of back, arm, and shoulder muscles. Regression analysis, using maximal isometric tray lifting strength as the dependent variable and the five muscle group strengths and anthropometric data as independent variables, revealed the insufficiency of a single multivariate predictor. Arm and shoulder strengths were suggested as limiting factors in lifting because they appeared in 19 of the 24 regression equations (12 each for men and women). Isometric back extension strength appeared in 10 of the equations. Height seemed to be an important factor for men in lifts above waist level (134 cm or above).

Karwowski and Mital[178] present a concept of a safety index (SI) for assigning a worker to a particular manual lifting task and developed a simple formula for its calculation. Karwowski, et al.,[179] present simple prediction models for psychophysically selected loads lifted by males while sitting at a workbench.

Detecting Deceitful Tests

A problem within the industrial setting for many years has been determining whether certain injured workers were truly incapable of performing physically exertive tasks or whether they were exhibiting less than genuine exertions. Experiments were performed by Marras[180] to provide testing criteria for this distinction. Significant correlations were found between strength onset and slope-strength. However, the findings with respect to strength variability were less conclusive. Subsequently, Kroemer and Marras[181] described experiments performed with 30 subjects that indicated that the rate of strength build-up in repeated exertions may provide objective criteria to judge whether or not a subject exerts full muscular strength in a routine test.

Waikar, et al.,[182] evaluated strength tests for evaluating low back injuries. This research investigated differences in the strength exertions of healthy and injured populations. They observed that the coefficient of variation could discriminate healthy from injured workers.

Isometric, Isokinetic, and Isoinertial Testing

The choice of appropriate strength measurements have received considerable attention in the literature. The following studies attempted to correlate alternative measures and develop relational models.

Knapik and Ramos[183] studied the relationship between isokinetic and isometric torque, and maximum voluntary contractions. Their data suggest that the torque elicited at low velocity isokinetic contractions can be predictive of the torque elicited during isometric contractions. Faster velocities were less related to isometric strength. Garg, et al.,[184] also reported on a laboratory study to determine if job-specific static strength could be used to predict dynamic lifting capability (maximum acceptable weight of lift) based on psychophysical methodology. The findings of a later study, based on 9 college students, were inconclusive.

Smith, et al.,[185] reported on a multipart study designed to: (1) evaluate the repeatability of a method of measuring trunk strength; (2) measure isometric and isokinetic strength of trunk flexors, extensors, and rotators; (3) explore relationships among these muscle groups; and (4) compare a torque to body weight adjustment measure to lean body weight.

Zeh, et al.,[186] observed strength measurements from more than 1000 volunteers in an industrial back pain study. It was concluded that one exertion in each test position for each subject provided a reasonably good indication of the subject's strength in that position, but strength in one position was not predictable from strength in a different position.

Legal Obstacles

There are several legal obstacles to employee selection and placement based on physical work capacity, including OSHA Act (1970), Rehabilitation Act (1973), state handicapped laws, Civil Rights Act (1964), Title VII, EEOC, Worker's Compensation and Common Law Personal Injury Actions, and Federal Workers Compensation Laws (FECA and FELA)

Under OSHA (1970), employees may not assume risk nor consent to work in conditions that are unsafe. Section 11(c) of the act provides that "No person shall discharge or in any manner discriminate against any employee . . . because of the exercise by such employee on behalf of himself or others any right afforded by this Act."

The employer has five main duties for protection of employees:

1. To provide a safe place to work.
2. To provide safe appliances, tools, and equipment for work.
3. To give warnings of dangers.
4. To provide a sufficient number of suitable fellow employees.
5. To promulgate and enforce work rules for conduct of employees that make the work safe.

OSHA's only attempt to regulate effects of medical examinations involves medical removal protection (MRP) and rate retention (RR). These two provisions have met mixed court reception relative to overlap with other agencies charged with improved employment terms, such as the National Labor Relations Board (NLRB), and opportunities for high risk employees, such as EEOC and Handicapped/Rehabilitation Laws.

An estimated 40 to 60 million handicapped individuals are covered by the Rehabilitation Act of 1973. Under these regulations (section 504), an employer may not make pre-employment inquiry about whether the applicant is handicapped or about the nature or severity of existent handicap unless a pre-employment medical exam is required of all applicants, and the information obtained from the examination is relevant to the applicant's ability to perform job-related functions. If the employer's job qualification requirements "tend to screen out qualified handicapped individuals, the requirements shall be related to the specific job or jobs for which the individual is being considered and shall be consistent with the business necessity and the safe performance of the job."

There is no requirement under section 504 prohibiting discrimination against qualified handicapped but the medical procedure must have a high predictive value or be within accepted medical practice. However (under section 503 mandating affirmative action of federal contracts), the medical exam must have a scientifically valid basis, have a high predictive value, and be the least onerous and most accurate alternative.

In the case of OFCCP vs. E.E. Black, Ltd. the Labor Department found that pre-employment back x ray procedures tended to disqualify handicapped applicants despite their current ability to perform the job. The term impairment was extended to be "any condition which weakens, restricts, or otherwise damages an individual's health, physical, or mental activity" resulting in a bar to employment that the individual is currently capable of performing. The court concluded that the applicant was subject to protections of the Act because:

1. The back condition was found to be an impairment, or at least was regarded so by the employer.
2. The impairment was found to be substantial because it precluded essentially all apprentice carpenters jobs in the country.
3. The court rejected the employers claim that the Act was not intended to protect applicants denied employment based on risk of future injury.

Equal employment opportunities are assured under Title VII of the Civil Rights Act of 1964. Historic cases such as Griggs vs. Duke Power Co. (where requirement of a high school diploma affected employment of blacks) led to the concept of disparate impact. Employment practices that result in under representation of females, for example, although facially neutral, are forbidden unless they can be justified by business necessity.

Defense must show "the tests in question have a manifest relationship to employment in question." Plaintiff may rebut this evidence by demonstrating that "other tests or selection devices, without similarly undesirable racial effect, would also serve employer's legitimate interest in efficient and trustworthy workmanship."

In the case of Albermarle Paper Co. vs. Moody, the Supreme Court found "discriminatory tests are impermissible unless shown by professionally acceptable methods to be predictive of or significantly correlated with important elements of work behavior which comprise or are relevant to the job or jobs for which candidates are being evaluated."

Job relatedness under this law has a somewhat narrower scope, concerning whether an employer's criteria bear a reasonable relationship to the demands of the job. In order to create a Bonafide Occupational Qualification (BFOQ) for an occupation, the employer must prove reasonable cause to believe that all or substantially all individuals in a protected group (such as females) would be unable to perform safely and efficiently the duties of the job involved.

Worker compensation is a form of "strict liability," whereby the employer is charged with the injuries arising out of its business without regard to fault. Resort to the compensation system is the exclusive remedy of injured workers. As a result, employers are reluctant to hire individuals with pre-existing infirmities or disabilities because of fear of liability for future worker compensation. In five states, the agencies permit employee waivers of their rights, another 15 permit waivers for aggravation of an existing condition. Others expressly disallow any such waivers whatsoever (e.g., Massachusetts). Employee capacity tests that would diagnose pre-existing infirmities or be predictive of future injuries would obviously improve the fairness of administration of these laws.

The Federal Employees Liability Act (FELA) provides the exclusive remedy for injury and death of interstate railroad employees caused by the negligence of the employer. Unlike FECA (Federal Employees Compensation Act), which provides benefits regardless of fault, the FELA provides for the recovery of damages—including pecuniary loss, medical expenses, and pain and suffering. The employer is usually permitted to assert comparative negligence to mitigate the damage award. In this regard, employee capacity testing could be used to mitigate damages. However, virtually no one is developing such selection and placement tests.

CONCLUSIONS

The matching of workers and jobs via applied ergonomics concepts has potential to eliminate many of the overexertion injuries common in industry today. A cursory review of the disciplines of ergonomics reveals a burgeoning technical literature. The engineering emphasis on fitting the job to the person offers hope for a long term solution to overexertion injury control. However, lacking total automation and work mechanization, a substantial number of occupations will continue to require significant manual materials handling requirements for the foreseeable future. Consequently, there will continue to be a requirement to also fit people to jobs.

The assessment of an individual who performs manual materials handling must include specific tests of physical capability. Such tests must meet certain criteria to be accepted as medically, economically, and legally justified. The medical and economic justification for such tests is recognized by all concerned with controlling the excessive costs and human suffering associated with overexertion strain, sprain injuries, and illness. The legal basis for such tests, however, is not well established. Further, it will not exist until a documented history of success or failure is developed for a variety of tests.

REFERENCES

1. Jorgenson, K.: Permissible loads based on energy expenditure measurements. Ergonomics *28*(1), 1985.
2. Asfour, S.S., Ayoub, M.M., Mital, A.: Effects of an endurance and strength training program on lifting capability of males. *Ergonomics 27*(4), 1984.
3. Khalil, T.M., Genaidy, A.M., Asfour, S.S., Vinciguerra, T.: Physiological limits in lifting. *Am Ind Hyg Assoc J 46*(4):220–224, 1985.
4. Mital, A., Ayoub, M.M.: Effect of task variables and their interactions in lifting and lowering loads. *Am Ind Hyg Assoc J 42*, 1981.
5. Asfour, S.S., Ayoub, M.M., Genaidy, A.M., Khalil, T.M.: A database of physiological responses to manual lifting. *Trends Ergonom Hum Factors* 801–809, 1986.
6. Asfour, S.S., Ayoub, M.M., Genaidy, A.M.: A database of physiological responses to manual lowering. *Trends Ergonom Hum Factors* 811–818, 1986.
7. Chaffin, D.B.: Biomechanical modelling of the low back during load lifting. *Ergonomics 31*(5):685–697, 1988.
8. Freivalds, A., Chaffin, D.B., Garg, A., Lee, K.S.: A dynamic biomechanical evaluation of lifting maximum acceptable loads. *J Biomech 17*(4):251–262, 1984.
9. McGill, S.M., Norman, R.W.: Dynamically and statically determined low back moments during lifting. *J Biomech 18*(12):877–885, 1985.
10. Ekholm, J., Arborelius, U.P., Nemeth, G.: The load on the lumbo-sacral joint and trunk muscle activity during lifting. *Ergonomics 25*(2):145–161, 1982.
11. Schultz, A.B., Andersson, G.B.J.: Analysis of loads on the lumbar spine. *Spine 6*(1):76–82, 1981.
12. Bean, J.C., Chaffin, D.B., Schultz, A.B.: Biomechanical model calculation of muscle contraction forces: a double linear programming method. *J Biomech 21*(1):59–66, 1988.
13. Miller, J.A.A., Schultz, A.B., Warwick, D.N., Spencer, D.L.: Mechanical properties of lumbar spine motion segments under large loads. *J Biomech 19*(1):79–84, 1986.

14. Chaffin, D.B., Andersson, G.: Occupational Biomechanics. Wiley, New York, 1984.
15. Andersson, G.B.J.: Correlations for computed muscle forces and EMG during heavy loads. *Trans Orthop Res Soc* 11: 1986.
16. Garg, A., Chaffin, D.B., Freivalds, A.: Biomechanical stresses from manual load lifting: a static and dynamic evaluation. *IEE Trans* 14(4):272–281, 1982.
17. Marras, W.S., Wongsam, P.E., Rangarajulu, S.L.: Trunk motion during lifting: the relative cost. *Int J Ind Ergon* 1:103–113, 1986.
18. Mital, A., Kromodihardjo, S.: Kinetic analysis of manual lifting activities: part 2—Biomechanical analysis of task variables. *Int J Ind Ergon* 1:91–101, 1986.
19. Chaffin, D.B., Andersson, G.B.J., Page, G., Bloswick, D.: Low-back muscle models: a sensitivity analysis. *Proceedings of the American Society for Biomechanics*, Ann Arbor, MI, 1985.
20. Andersson, G.B.J.: Epidemiologic aspects on low-back pain in industry. *Spine* 6(1):53–60, 1981.
21. Frymoyer, J.W., et al.: Epidemiologic studies of low back pain. *Spine* 5(5):419–423, 1980.
22. Bigos, S.J., et al.: Back injuries in industry: a retrospective study I: overview and cost analysis. *Spine* 11(3):241–245, 1986.
23. Bigos, S.J., et al.: Back injuries in industry: a retrospective study II. injury factors. *Spine* 11(3):246–251, 1986.
24. Bigos, S.J., et al.: Back injuries in industry: a retrospective study III. Employee-related factors. *Spine* 11(3):252–256, 1986.
25. National Institute for Occupational Safety and Health. A work practices guide for manual lifting (Report 81–122), US Dept. of Health and Human Services. Cincinnati, Ohio, NIOSH, 1981.
26. Niskanen, T.: Accidents and minor accidents of the musculoskeletal system in heavy (concrete reinforcement work) and light (painting) construction work. *J Occup Med* 7:17–32, 1985.
27. David, G.C.: Ergonomic design could promote safer drilling. *Technology* 103:95–98, 1984.
28. Bergquist-Ullman, M., Larson, U.: Acute low-back pain in industry: a controlled prospective study with special reference to therapy and confounding factors. *Acta Orthop Scand (Suppl)* 170:1–117, 1977.
29. Chaffin, D.B., Park, K.Y.S.: A longitudinal study of low back pain as associated with occupational weight lifting factors. *Am Ind Hyg Assoc J* 34:513–525, 1973.
30. Snook, S.H., Campanelli, R.A., Hart, J.W.: A study of three preventative approaches to low back injury. *J Occup Med* 20(1):478–481, 1978.
31. Hult, L.: Cervical, Dorsal and Lumbar Spinal Syndromes. *Acta Orthop Scand (Suppl)* 17:1–102, 1954.
32. Lawrence, J.S.: Rheumatism in coal miners: occupational factors. *Br J Ind Med* 12:149–161, 1955.
33. Ikai, M., Steihous, A.H.: Some factors modifying the expression of human strength. *J Appl Physiol 16:* 1961.
34. Magora, A.: Investigation of the relation between low back pain and occupation, part 1 and part 2. *Ind Med Surg* 39:21–28, 1970.
35. Snook, S.H.: Low-back pain in industry. *In* Symposium on Idiopathic Low-back Pain (Edited by A.A. White and S.L. Gordon). St. Louis, Mosby, 1982.
36. Valkenberg, H.A., Haanan, H.C.M.: The epidemiology of low-back pain. *In* Symposium on Low-Back Pain (Edited by A.A. White and S.L. Gordon). St. Louis, Mosby, 1982.
37. Svensson, H., Andersson, G.B.J.: Low-back pain in forty to forty-seven year old men: work history and work environment factors. *Spine* 8:272–276, 1983.
38. Herrin, G.D.: A taxonomy of manual materials handling hazards. *In* Safety in Manual Materials Handling. (Edited by C. Drury). National Institute for Occupational Safety and Health, Pub 78–185, 1978.
39. Herrin, G.D., Chaffin, D.B., Anderson, G.B.J., Pope, M.H.: Workplace evaluation. *In* Occupational Low Back Pain (Edited by M.H. Pope, J.W. Frymoyer, and G. Andersson). New York, Praeger 1984.
40. Karger, D.W., Bayha, F.H.: Engineered Work Measurement. New York, Industrial Press, 1986.
41. Barnes, R.M.: Motion and Time Study: Design and Measurement of Work, 6th Ed. New York, Wiley and Sons, 1980.
42. Niebel, B.W.: Motion and Time Study, 5th Ed. Homewood, IL, R.D. Irwin, 1972.
43. Karger, D.W., Hancock, W.M.: Advanced Work Measurement. New York, Industrial Press, 1982.
44. Konz, S.: Work Design. Columbus, Grid Publishing, 1979.
45. Loyl, F.F., Marsters-Hanson, P.: Age, Physical Ability and Work Potential. Washington, DC, US Dept. of Labor, Manpower Administration, 1973.
46. Smith, P., Armstrong, T.J., Lizza, G.D.: IE's can play crucial role in enabling handicapped employees to work safely, productively. *Ind Engineer* 14(4):98–105, 1982.
47. Muthuswamy, S., Asfour, S.S., Vinciguerra, T., Genaidy, A.M.: The design of work/rest schedules as an ergonomic component in manual materials handling. *Trends Ergonom/Hum Factors* 871–878, 1986.
48. Nicholson, A.S.: Manual handling limits: a comparative study modeling. *Trends Ergonom/Hum Factors* 793–800, 1986.
49. Nicholson, A.S., Clark, A.G.: The use of load handling guidelines in assessing baggage handling facilities. *Trends Ergonom/Hum Factors* 855–862, 1986.
50. Garg, A., Chaffin, D.B.: A biomechanical computerized simulation of human strength. *Am Inst Ind Eng Trans* 7:1–15, 1975.
51. Stobbe, T.: The development of a practical strength testing program for industry. Doctoral Thesis, The University of Michigan, 1982.
52. Herrin, G.D.: Standardized strength testing methods for population descriptions. *In* Anthropometry and Biomechanics—Theory and Application. (Edited by R. Easterby, K.H.E. Kroemer, and D.B. Chaffin) NATO Conference Series 16. New York, Plenum Press, 1982.
53. Garg, A., Sharma, D., Chaffin, D.B., Schmidler, J.M.: Biomechanical stresses as related to motion trajectory of lifting. *Hum Factors* 25(5):527–539, 1983.
54. Leskinen, T.P.J.: Comparison of static and dynamic biomechanical models. *Ergonomics* 28(1):285–291, 1985.
55. Davis, P.R.: The use of intra-abdominal pressure in evaluating stresses on the lumbar spine. *Spine* 6(1):90–92, 1981.
56. Davis, P.R., Stubbs, D.A.: Safe levels of manual forces for young males, part I. *Appl Ergonom* 8(3), 1977.
57. Nordin, M., Elfstrom, G., Dahlqvist, P.: Intra-abdominal pressure measurements using a wireless radio pressure pill and two wire connected pressure tranducers: a comparison. *In* Methods for Studying Workload (Edited by M. Nordin). Goteborg, 63–72, 1982.
58. Houghton, F.C., Yagloglou, C.P.: Determination of the comfort zone. *Am Soc Heating Ventil Eng* 29:515–536, 1923.
59. Stevens, S.S.: The direct estimation of sensory magnitudes loudness. *Am J Psychol* 69(1):1–25, 1956.
60. Stevens, S.S.: The psychophysics of sensory functions. *Am Scientist* 48:226–253, 1960.
61. Borg, G.A.V.: Physical Performance and Perceived Exertion. Copenhagen, Ejnar M. Munksgoard, 1962.
62. Borg, G.A.V.: Perceived exertion: a note on "history" and methods. *Med Sci Sports* 5:90–93, 1973.
63. Emanuel, J., Chafee, J., Wing, J.: A study of human weight lifting capabilities for loading ammunition into the F-86 H aircraft. US Air Force (WADC-TR 056–367). Wright Patterson Air Force Base, OH, 1959.
64. Switzer, S.A.: Weight lifting capabilities of a selected sample of human males. Aerospace Medical Research Laboratory

Report AD 284054. Wright Patterson Air Force Base, OH, 1962.

65. Evans, W.O.: A titration schedule on a treadmill. US Army Medical Research Laboratory Report 525. Fort Knox, KY, 1961.

66. Evans, W.O.: The effect of treadmill grade on performance decrement using a titration schedule. US Army Medical Research Laboratory, Report 535. Ft. Knox, KY, 1962.

67. Caldwell, L.S., Smith, R.P.: Subjective estimation of effort, reserve, and ischemic pain. US Army Medical Research Laboratory Report 730. Ft. Knox, KY, 1967.

68. Caldwell, L.S., Grossman, E.E.: Effort scaling of isometric muscle contractions. *J Motor Behav, 5*(1):9–16, 1973.

69. Snook, S.H.: The design of manual handling tasks. *Ergonomics 21*(12):963–985, 1978.

70. Ayoub MM, et al.: Determination and Modeling of Lifting Capacity. Washington, DC, Dept. of Health and Human Services, NIOSH, 1978.

71. Mital, A.: Maximum weights of lift acceptable to male and female industrial workers for extended work shifts. *Ergonomics 27*(11):1115–1126, 1984.

72. Mital, A.: Models for predicting maximum acceptable weight of lift and heart rate and oxygen uptake at that weight. *J Occup Med* 1984.

73. Mital, A., Vinayagomoorthy, R.: Three-dimensional dynamic strength measuring device: a prototype. *Am Ind Hygiene Assoc J 45*:9–10, 1984.

74. Garg, A., Ayoub, M.M.: What criteria exist for determining how much load can be lifted safely? *Hum Factors 22*(49):475–86, 1980.

75. Keyserling, W.M., Punnett, L., Fine, L.J.: Trunk posture and back pain: identification and control of occupational risk factors. *Appl Ind Hyg 3*:87–92, 1988.

76. Keyserling, W.M.: Postural analysis of the trunk and shoulders in simulated real time. *Ergonomics 4*:569, 1986.

77. Corlett, E.N., Madeley, S.J., Manenica, L.: Postural targeting: a technique for recording working postures. *Ergonomics 22*(3):357–366, 1979.

78. Corlett, E.N., Manenica, L.: The effects and measurement of working postures. *Appl Ergonom 11*(1):7–16, 1980.

79. Priel, V.Z.: A numerical definition of posture. *Hum Factors 16*(6):576–584, 1974.

80. Karhu, O., Kansi, P., Kuorinka, L.: Correcting working postures in industry: a practical method for analysis. *Appl Ergonom 18*:199, 1977.

81. Karhu, O., Harkonen, R., Sorvali, P., Vepsalainen, P.: Observing working postures in industry, *Appl Ergonom 12*(1):13–17, 1981.

82. Berns, T.A.R., Milner, N.P.: TRAM—A technique for the recording and analysis of moving work posture. *In* Methods to Study Work Posture (Edited by N.P. Milner). Stockholm, Sweden, Ergolabs Report *80*:22–26, 1980.

83. Holzmann, P.: ARBAN—A new method for analysis of ergonomic effort. *Appl Ergonom 13*(2):82–86, 1982.

84. Corlett, E.N., Bishop, R.P.: A technique for assessing postural discomfort. *Ergonomics 19*(2):175–182, 1976.

85. Grieve, D.W.: The postural stability diagram (PSD): personal constraints on the static exertion of force. *Ergonomics 22*(10):1155–1164, 1979.

86. Chaffin, D.B.: Manual materials handling and the biomechanical basis for prevention of low-back pain in industry—an overview. *Am Ind Hyg Assoc J 12*:989–996, 1987.

87. Winkel, J.: On the manual handling of wide-body carts used by cabin attendants in civil aircraft. *Appl Ergonom 14*(3):162–168, 1983.

88. Smith, J.L., Jiang, B.C.: A manual materials handling study of bag lifting. *Am Ind Hyg Assoc J 45*(8):505–508, 1984.

89. Garg, A., Saxena, U.: Container characteristics and maximum acceptable weight of lift. *Hum Factors 22*(4):487–495, 1980.

90. Legg, S.J.: Cardiovascular and spinal strain of a complex materials handling task in a confined space: influences of protective clothing and physical training. *Trends Ergonom Hum Factors* 819–825, 1986.

91. Drury, C.G., Law, C.H., Pawenski, C.S.: A survey of industrial box handling. *Hum Factors 24*(5):553–565, 1982.

92. Marras, W.S., Rockwell, T.H.: An experimental evaluation of method and tool effects in spike maul use. *Hum Factors* 1986.

93. Rothstein, M.A.: Medical screening of workers. Washington DC, Bureau of National Affairs, 1984.

94. Miner, M.G., Miner, J.B.: Employee selection within the law. Washington DC, Bureau of National Affairs, 1978.

95. Pope, M.H., Frymoyer, J.W., Andersson, G.B.J.: Occupational Low Back Pain. New York, Praeger 274–291, 1984.

96. Davis, P.R., Stubbs, D.A.: Safe levels of manual forces for young males. *Appl Ergonom 8*(3), 1977.

97. Davies, C.T., White, M.J., Young, K.: Muscle function in children. *Eur J Appl Physiol 52*(1):111–114, 1983.

98. Baldauf, K.L., Swenson, D.K., Medeiros, J.M., Radtka, S.A.: Clinical assessment of trunk flexor muscle strength in healthy girls 3 to 7 years of age. *Phys Ther 64*:1203–1208, 1984.

99. Lefkof, M.B.: Trunk flexion in healthy children aged 3 to 7 years. *Phys Ther 66*(11):39–44, 1986.

100. Parizkova, J., Adamec, A.: Longitudinal study of anthropometric, skinfold, work, and motor characteristics of boys and girls, three to six years of age. *Am J Phys Anthropol 52*(3):387–396, 1980.

101. Landin, R.J., Linnemeier, T.J., Rothbaum, D.A., Chappelear, J., Noble, R.J.: Exercise testing and training of the elderly patient. *Cardiovasc Clin 15*(2):201–218, 1985.

102. Danneskiold-Samsoe, B., et al.: Muscle strength and functional capacity in 78–81-year-old men and women. *Eur J Appl Physiol 52*:310–314, 1984.

103. Murray, M.P., Duthie, E.H. Jr., Gambert, S.R., Sepic, S.B., Mollinger, L.A.: Age-related differences in knee muscle strength in normal women. *J Gerontol 40*, 1985.

104. Aniansson, A., Sperling, L., Rundgren, A., Lehnberg, E.: Muscle function in 75-year-old men and women. A longitudinal study. *Scand J Rehabil Med* (Suppl) *9*:92–102, 1983.

105. Aniansson, A., Rundgren, A., Sperling, L.: Evaluation of functional capacity in activities of daily living in 70-year-old men and women. *Scand J Rehabil Med 12*(4):145–154, 1980.

106. Nishimura, J.: The relationship between perceived exertion of daily activities and aging of physical function (author's translation). *Shinrigaku Kenkyu 52*(4):219–225, 1981.

107. Hickson, R.C., Rosenkoetter, M.A., Brown, M.M.: Strength training effects on aerobic power and short-term endurance. *Med Sci Sports Exerc 12*(5):336–339, 1980.

108. Sullivan, P.E., Portney, L.G.: Electromyographic activity of shoulder muscles during unilateral upper extremity proprioceptive neuromuscular facilitation patterns. *Phys Ther 60*:283–288, 1980.

109. Wood, G.A., Lockwood, R.J., Cresswell, A.G., Henstridge, J.: Motor unit activity and muscle strength development. *Aust Phys Eng 6*:71–75, 1983.

110. Grossi, J.A.: Effects of an applied kinesiology technique on quadriceps femoris muscle isometric strength. *Phys Ther 61*:1011–1016, 1981.

111. Hamberg, P., Gillquist, J., Lysholm, J., Oberg B.: The effect of diagnostic and operative arthroscopy and open meniscectomy on muscle strength in the thigh. *Am J Sports Med 11*:289–292, 1983.

112. Kanehisa, H., Miyashita, M.: Effect of isometric and isokinetic muscle training on static strength and dynamic power. *Eur J Appl Physiol 50*:365–371, 1983.

113. Vegso, J.J., Genuario, S.E., Torg, J.S.: Maintenance of ham-

string strength following knee surgery. *Med Sci Sports Exerc* 17:376–379, 1985.

114. Roxin, L.E., Venge, P., Friman, G.: Variations in serum myoglobin after a 2-min isokinetic exercise test and the effects of training. *Eur J Appl Physiol* 53:43–47, 1984.

115. Wirth, J.C., Lohman, T.G.: Vitamin B6 status and static muscle function: 2 case reports. *Ann Nutr Metab* 28:240–244, 1984.

116. Knutsson, E., Martensson, A.: Isokinetic measurements of muscle strength in hysterical paresis. *Electroencephalogr Clin Neurophysiol* 61:370–374, 1985.

117. Clarkson, P.M., Zigon, S.T., Kamen, G.: Post vibratory effects on fractionated reaction time and maximum isometric strength. *Am J Phys Med* 59:271–279, 1980.

118. Maughan, R.J., Watson, J.S., Weir, J.: Strength and cross-sectional area of human skeletal muscle. *J Physiol* 338:37–49, 1983.

119. Bergman, R., Leach, R.E.: The use and abuse of anabolic steroids in olympic-caliber athletes. *Clin Orthop* 198:169–172, 1985.

120. Westerling, D.: A study of physical demands in riding. *Eur J Appl Physiol* 50:373–382, 1983.

121. Bompa, T.O.: Technique and muscle force. *Can J Appl Sport Sci;* 5:245–249, 1980.

122. Ekstrand, J., Gillquist, J.: The avoidability of soccer injuries. *Int J Sports Med* 4:124–128, 1983.

123. Oberg, B., Ekstrand, J., Moller, M., Gillquist, J.: Muscle strength and flexibility in different positions of soccer players. *Int J Sports Med* 5:213–216, 1984.

124. Strizak M., Gleim, G.W., Sapega, A., Nicholas, J.A.: Hand and forearm strength and its relation to tennis. *Am J Sports Med* 11: 1983.

125. Harrington, H., Hallett, M., Tyler, H.R.: Ganglioside therapy for amyotrophic lateral sclerosis: a double-blind controlled trial. *Neurology* 34:1083–1085, 1984.

126. Jaspan, J., Maselli, R., Herold, K., Bartkus, C.: Treatment of severely painful diabetic neuropathy with an aldose reductase inhibitor: relief of pain and improved somatic and autonomic nerve function. *Lancet* 2:758–762, 1983.

127. Morris, A.F., Vaughan, S.E., Vaccaro, P.: Measurements of neuromuscular tone and strength in down's syndrome children. *J Ment Defic Res* 26:41–46, 1982.

128. Allsop, K.G., Ziter, F.A.: Loss of strength and functional decline in duchenne's dystrophy. *Arch Neurol* 38:406–411, 1981.

129. Cohen, L., et al.: A statistical analysis of the loss of muscle strength in duchenne's muscular dystrophy. *Res Commun Chem Pathol Pharmacol* 37:123–138, 1982.

130. Lane, R.J., et al.: An evaluation of some carrier detection techniques in duchenne muscular dystrophy. *J Neurol Sci* 43:377–394, 1979.

131. Bilkey, W.J., Baxter, T.L., Kottke, F.J., Mundale, M.O.: Muscle formation in ehlers-danlos syndrome. *Arch Phys Med Rehabil* 62:444–448, 1981.

132. Kofsky, P.R., Davis, G.M., Shephard, R.J., Jackson, R.W., Keene, G.C.: Field testing: assessment of physical fitness of disabled adults. *Eur J Appl Physiol* 51:109–120, 1983.

133. Armstrong, L.E., et al.: Using isokinetic dynamometry to test ambulatory patients with multiple sclerosis. *Phys Ther* 63:1274–1279, 1983.

134. Gelberman, R.H., Szabo, R.M., Williamson, R.V., Dimick, M.P.: Sensibility testing in peripheral-nerve compression syndromes: an experimental study in humans. *J Bone Joint Surg* 65:632–638, 1983.

135. Griffin, J.W., McClure, M.H., Bertorini, T.E.: Sequential isokinetic and manual muscle testing in patients with neuromuscular disease: a pilot study. *Phys Ther* 66:32, 1986.

136. Wiles, C.M., Karni, Y.: The measurement of muscle strength in patients with peripheral neuromuscular disorders. *J Neurol Neurosurg Psychiatry* 46:1006–1013, 1983.

137. Odensten, M., Tegner, Y., Lysholm, J., Gillquist, J.: Knee function and muscle strength following distal ileotibial band transfer for antero-lateral rotatory instability. *Acta Orthop Scand* 54:924–928, 1983.

138. Sanderson, D.J., Sommer, H.J.: Kinematic features of wheelchair propulsion. *J Biomech* 18:423–429, 1985.

139. Koller, W., Kase, S.: Muscle strength testing in parkinson's disease. *Eur Neurol* 25:130–133, 1986.

140. Braun, N.M., Arora, N.S., Rochester, D.F.: Respiratory muscle and pulmonary function in polymyositis and other proximal myopathies. *Thorax* 38:616–623, 1983.

141. Davies, C.W., Jones, D.M., Shearer, J.R.: Hand grip—a simple test for morbidity after fracture of the neck of femur. *J Royal Soc Med* 77:833–836, 1984.

142. Shiavi, R.G., Champion, S.A., Freeman, F.R., Bugel, H.J.: Efficacy of myofeedback therapy in regaining control of lower extremity musculature following stroke. *Am J Phys Med* 58: 185–194, 1979.

143. Saiki, J.K., Vaziri, N.D., Naeim, F., Meshkinpour, H.: Dialysis-induced changes in muscle strength. *J Dial* 4:191–201, 1980.

144. Young, A., Wright, J., Knapik, J., Cymerman, A.: Skeletal muscle strength during exposure to hypobaric hypoxia. *Med Sci Sports Exerc* 12:330–335, 1980.

145. Redmond, C.K., Breslin, P.P.: Comparison of methods for assessing occupational hazards. *J Occup Med* 17:313–317, 1975.

146. Mills, K.R., Edwards, R.H.: Investigative strategies for muscle pain. *J Neurol Sci* 58:73–78, 1983.

147. Sedlak, K.: Low-back pain: perception and tolerance. *Spine* 10:440–444, 1985.

148. Edwards H., Rose, E.A., King, T.C.: Postoperative deterioration in muscular function. *Arch Surg* 117:899–901, 1982.

149. Orlander, J., Kiessling, K.H., Larsson, L.: Skeletal muscle metabolism, morphology and function in sedentary smokers and nonsmokers. *Acta Physiol Scand* 107:39–46, 1979.

150. Hamrin, E., et al.: Muscle strength and balance in post-stroke patients. *Ups J Med Sci* 87(1), 1982.

151. Davis, G.M., Kofsky, P.R., Kelsey, J.C., Shephard, R.J.: Cardiorespiratory fitness and muscular strength of wheelchair users. *Can Med Assoc J* 125: 1981.

152. Chaffin, D.B., Herrin, G.D., Keyserling, W.M.: Pre-employment strength testing: an updated position. *J Occup Med 20:* 1978.

153. Chaffin, D.B., Freivalds, A.: On the validity of an isometric biomechanical strength model. *Proc AIIE Annu Conf* 1981.

154. Chaffin, D.B., Lee, M., Freivalds, A.: Muscle strength assessment from EMG analysis. *Med Sci Sports Exercise 12:* 1980.

155. Keyserling, W.M., Herrin, G.D., Chaffin, D.B.: Isometric strength testing as a means of controlling medical incidents on strenuous jobs. *J Occup Med 22:* 1980.

156. Ayoub, M.A.: Control of manual lifting hazards: III. Preemployment screening. *J Occup Med* 24:751–761, 1982.

157. Harber, P., SooHoo, K.: Static ergonomic strength testing in evaluating occupational back pain. *J Occup Med 26:* 1984.

158. Cady, L.D., Bischoff, D.P., O'Connell, E.R., Thomas, P.C., Allan, J.H.: Strength and fitness and subsequent back injuries in firefighters. *J Occup Med 21(4):* 1979.

159. Cady, L.D., Thomas, P.C., Karwasky, R.J.: Program for increasing health and physical fitness of fire fighters. *J Occup Med* 27:110–114, 1985.

160. Kamon, E., Goldfuss, A.J.: In-plant evaluation of the muscle strength of workers. *Am Ind Hyg Assoc J* 39:801–807, 1978.

161. Kamon, E., Kiser, D., Pytel, J.L.: Dynamic and static lifting capacity and muscular strength of steelmill workers. *Am Ind Hyg Assoc J* 43:853–857, 1982.

162. Celentano, E.J., Nottrodt, J.W., Saunders, P.L.: Relationship

between size, strength and task demands. *Ergonomics* 27:481–488, 1984.

163. Schultz, K.S.: Assessing the upper extremity injured workers' ability to safely return to the workplace. *Trends Ergonom/Hum Factors, Part B*, 1986. 641–649.

164. Hultman, G.A., Nordin, M., Ortengren, R.: The influence of a preventive educational program on trunk flexion in janitors. *In* Methods for Studying Workload (Edited by M. Nordin). Goteborg; 35–47, 1982.

165. McGarvey, S.R., Morrey, B.F., Askew, L.J., An, K.N.: Reliability of isometric strength testing. Temporal factors and strength variation. *Clin Orthop 185*:301–305, 1984.

166. Pytel, J.L., Kamon, E.: Dynamic strength test as a predictor for maximal and acceptable lifting. *Ergonomics 24*(9):663–672, 1981.

167. Kroemer, K.H.E.: An isoinertial technique to assess individual lifting capability. *Hum Factors 25*:493–506, 1983.

168. Markhede, G., Grimby, G.: Measurement of strength of hip joint muscles. *Scand J Rehabil Med 12*:169–174, 1980.

169. Maxwell, J.D., Hodt, P., Taylor, W.H.: Portable chair for testing isometric muscle strength. *Lancet 1*:18–19, 1984.

170. Hansson, T.H., Bigos, S.J., Wortley, M.K., Spengler, D.M.: The load on the lumbar spine during isometric strength testing. *Spine 9*:720–724, 1984.

171. Poulsen, E.: Back muscle strength and weight limits in lifting burdens. *Spine 6:* 1981.

172. Ayoub, M.M., Dryden, R., McDaniel, J., Knipfer, R., Dixon, D.: Predicting lifting capacity. *Am Ind Hyg Assoc J 40*:1075–1084, 1979.

173. Mital, A.: Generalized model structure for evaluating/designing manual materials handling jobs. *Int J Prod Res 21*:401–412, 1983.

174. Mital, A., Ayoub, M.M.: Equation for predicting lifting capabilities of people. *Trends Ergonom/Hum Factors, Part B*, 767–774, 1986.

175. Mital, A., Karwowski, W., Mazouz, A.B., Orsarh, E.: Prediction of maximum acceptable weight of lift in the horizontal and vertical planes using simulated job dynamic strengths. *Am Ind Hyg Assoc J 47*:288–292, 1986.

176. Tabourn, S.M., Dutta, S.P.: Modeling psychophysical capacities for combined manual materials handling activities. *Trends Ergonom/Hum Factors, Part B*, 785–791, 1986.

177. Yates, J.W., Kamon, E., Rodgers, S.H., Champney, P.C.: Static lifting strength and maximal isometric voluntary contractions of back, arm, and shoulder muscles. *Ergonomics 23:* 1980.

178. Karwowski, W., Mital, A.: Validation of a fuzzy model for the assessment of human operator responses to manual lifting tasks. *Proc 28th Annu Conf Hum Factors Soc* 408–412, San Antonio, 1984.

179. Karwowski, W., Yates, J.W., Pongpatanasuegsa, N.: Prediction models for maximum acceptable loads while sitting at a workbench. *Trends Ergonom/Hum Factors, Part B*, 775–783, 1986.

180. Marras, W.S.: Tests to distinguish between "true" and "faked" maximum muscle strength exertions. *Proc 22nd Annu Meet Hum Factors Soc*, Detroit, MI, Oct. 16–19, 1978. Santa Monica, CA, Human Factors Society 461–468, 1978.

181. Kroemer, K.H.E., Marras, W.S.: Evaluation of maximal and submaximal static muscle exertions. *Hum Factors 23:* 1981.

182. Waikar, A.M., Schlegel, R.E., Lee, K.S.: Strength tests for evaluating low back injuries. *Trends Ergonom/Hum Factors Part B*, 667–674, 1986.

183. Knapik, J.J., Ramos, M.U.: Isokinetic and isometric torque relationships in the human body. *Arch Phys Med Rehabil 61*:64–67, 1980.

184. Garg, A., Mital, A., Asfour, S.S.: Comparison of isometric strength and dynamic lifting capability. *Ergonomics 23*:13–27, 1980.

185. Smith, S.S., Mayer, T.G., Gatchel, R.J., Becker, T.J.: Quantification of lumbar function part 1: isometric and multispeed isokinetic trunk strength measures in sagittal and axial planes in normal subjects. *Spine 10*(8):1985.

186. Zeh, J., Hansson, T., Bigos, S., Spengler, D., Battie, M., Wortley, M.: Isometric strength testing: recommendations based on a statistical analysis of the procedure. *Spine 11:* 1986.

43

Michele C. Battié
Stanley J. Bigos

The Role of Pre-Employment Screening in Prevention

Industry has been attempting to prevent back injuries in the workplace for more than 60 years.[1,2] Medical expenses, work absence, and the hidden costs of lost productivity all contribute to the financial implications of back problems.[3] Steadily rising health care costs and insurance premiums in the United States also have contributed to industry's interest in prevention.[4]

Now, more than ever, industry recognizes medicine's inability to solve the complex problem of industrial back injury claims and related disability.[4] Despite increasing medical costs and a multitude of treatment approaches, recovery from back pain in the working population appears to be more a product of the expected natural history than specific medical treatment.[5]

Industries have typically approached the dilemma of back injuries through:

1. Safety and health programs designed to reduce the risk of back problems in employees.
2. Preplacement screening programs to identify individuals thought to be at higher risk.
3. Risk management through insurance companies directed at controlling the costs of back problems once reported.

Unfortunately, the growth of the problem over the past few decades attests to the inadequacies of these attempts.[6,7]

Industry has relied on safety and insurance records for most information about back problems. The inherent biases in these types of records may have added to the confusion surrounding the causes and prevention of back problems within industry.[8,9] Attempts to prevent back "injuries" also have failed to face some basic flaws of logic. First, population studies indicate that physical limitations caused by back symptoms affect nearly all workers at some time before retirement.[10–13] Second, the onset of back pain generally is not triggered by uncommon activities or specific precipitating events.[12,14,15] Third, little prospective scientific information has been available about risk factors to help guide health promotion programs or preplacement exams.[16]

The limitations in current knowledge of the pathological condition responsible for most back symptoms, as well as related risk factors, constrains prevention efforts. The difficulties in identifying factors clearly associated with increased risk for back problems may be partially attributed to the tendancy to group all categories of back problems together when considering risk factors. Although the cause of back problems is seldom known, it may be helpful to differentiate study findings based on predicting general complaints of back problems, hospitalizations because of herniated discs, back injury reports within the workplace, and long-term disability from back problems.

PREDICTING FUTURE BACK PROBLEMS

The great majority of studies investigating back problems, and factors affecting them, have been retrospective in nature, examining various factors after back problems have been reported. Although such studies have introduced a variety of variables as potential risk factors, they do not allow the determination of cause and effect, and the potential for bias is great. Considering the limitations of retrospective studies, it is not surprising that results have been so varied and conflicting. Such studies are most useful for developing hypotheses to be tested in subsequent prospective efforts.

Repeated calls have been made for the need to identify and further the understanding of risk factors for back problems and back injury reporting

522

through prospective longitudinal studies. Yet, only a small number of such prospective studies have been cited in the scientific literature. The findings from these studies can be categorized as applying to: (1) general complaints of low back pain or trouble, (2) hospitalization for the diagnosis of herniated disc, and (3) back "injury" reports at the workplace.

These categories appear to represent different entities in terms of incidence. Experiencing low back pain or trouble is common, as is demonstrated by the one-year incidence of subsequent problems reported in the studies below (26 to 47%),[17–19] whereas filing a back pain report at the workplace is much less common (2 to 5% per year).[20] Even more rare is the diagnosis of herniated disc leading to hospitalization. As the incidence of these entities varies, risk factors also must be expected to vary.

Risk Factors for General Back Problems

Gyntelberg, in 1974, reported the first prospective, longitudinal study of risk factors for back problems.[18] The study involved 5249 Danish men, age 40 to 59, who underwent questioning and an examination that included measurements of height, weight, blood pressure, and predicted maximal oxygen uptake. One year later they were questioned about low back problems occurring since they had been examined. At this point, one year after the examination, 4753 men (91%) provided followup information and 26% reported experiencing back problems during that time. The men reporting back problems were more likely to be slightly taller (>181 cm), but did not tend to be particularly obese or thin, as compared to men who did not report back problems. There was no association between fitness level, as judged through predicted maximal oxygen uptake, and back problems. However, an association was present between back pain complaints and reports of other symptomatic health problems.[18]

Biering-Sorensen published one of the more extensive studies in 1984.[17] Over 900 individuals were questioned about prior back troubles and underwent a physical examination, which included anthropometric measurements, such as height, weight, and possible leg length discrepancies, as well as flexibility and trunk muscle strength and endurance. One year after the examination, the subjects were questioned about low back trouble experienced during the year since the examination. The strongest indicators of low back trouble during this time were previous reports of similar problems. The individual physical factors that were significantly associated with first-time low back troubles among men were less back muscle endurance and greater lumbosacral

flexion. Similar trends were not found among women.

In 1987, Troup and co-workers reported on a prospective study of the predictive value of a number of pre-employment screening tests.[19] Nearly 3000 British men and women were questioned about their perception of physical exertion at work and about prior experiences of low back pain. They also underwent a battery of tests that included anthropometric measurements, back flexibility, maximal lifting strength, respiratory function, and psychophysical tests. The authors stated that "none of the tests were of any value in predicting new cases of low back pain." However, when prior history of back problems was known, which was the strongest predictor of subsequent back problems, the test results enhanced prediction. Interestingly, psychophysical tests were reportedly as accurate in predicting low back pain as were direct measurements of strength or mobility.

From the prospective studies discussed above, individual physical factors alone would appear to have little influence on future risk of experiencing low back pain. Anthropometric factors, isometric strength, psychophysical tests, sagittal flexibility, and estimated maximal aerobic capacity, among others, were deemed to be of little or no predictive value.[17–19] However, there was a suggestion of higher risk for first-time occurrences in men who had greater flexibility in flexion and less back muscle endurance.[17] It also appears that there may be an association between complaints of back pain and reports of other symptoms.[18]

Risk Factors for Disc Herniation

Two prospective studies of hospitalizations resulting from herniated lumbar discs have included anthropometric measurements as risk factors. The first study examined anthropometric measurements obtained at the time of induction of 1095 United States military recruits who later were hospitalized with the diagnosis of herniated disc.[21] When compared to controls matched by age and period of military service, the hospital cases tended to be taller and heavier. Military rank and occupational specialty also appeared to influence risk.

A more recent prospective study considering height, weight, and relative weight (weight/height^2) as risk factors for 332 cases of herniated discs, found taller men and women more likely to be hospitalized with the diagnosis of disc herniation than matched controls during an 11-year followup period. An association between relative weight (weight/height^2) and hospitalizations for disc problems was less clear.[22]

Both studies of risk factors for disc herniations

found an association between hospitalizations for herniated discs and slightly greater than average height.[21,22] Greater weight also was a risk factor among men in Hrubec's study, and Heliovaara identified a similar trend among men, but not women.[22]

Risk Factors for Industrial Back Pain Reports

Because of the effect of back problems on the ability to work, back pain reports have received considerable attention within industry. Yet, only a small number of prospective, longitudinal studies have attempted to identify risk factors for back injury claims occurring in the workplace.

In 1973, Chaffin reported on a longitudinal study of low back pain in association with isometric lifting strength and occupational lifting requirements.[23] Isometric lifting strength in relation to job demands was evaluated among 411 people employed in 103 different jobs. During the 1-year followup period, 25 low back incidents among the study group were reported to the company medical department. The incidence rate was approximately three times greater among individuals who were unable to demonstrate strength equal to or greater than that required by the job, as compared to individuals demonstrating greater relative strength. However, this difference was not reported as statistically significant, perhaps because of the small number of subjects and back incident reports involved. Age and weight were not associated with back pain reporting.

In 1980, Keyserling, et al., reported on two longitudinal studies of isometric lifting strength with respect to job requirements and injury reports. The first study compared medical reports among two groups of employees of a tire and rubber plant. One group was selected for job positions based on strength levels that matched job requirements. The other group did not undergo strength testing prior to employment. Subjects who were not matched to the job on the basis of strength tended to have more medical complaints during the followup year (p = 0.10). Too few musculoskeletal and back problems were reported at the workplace to allow analysis of these subsets.[24]

Another study involving aluminum reduction workers found that those who were required to lift more than 75% of their maximum capacity, as tested in some job simulations, tended to have an increased risk for medical complaints and musculoskeletal injury reports. However, the relationship between inadequate strength to meet job demands and increased medical reports did not hold true for all strength testing positions. Employees with strength that matched job requirements in the arm lift position actually had the highest incidence rate.[25]

This finding emphasizes the importance of pilot testing a program before its widespread use in decision making, and indicates that such an approach may not lead to the desired outcome in at least some cases.

Neither of these studies examined back problems separately from other musculoskeletal problems. Another consideration that came to light in a later prospective study of isometric strength testing was the potential for injury complaints as a result of testing.[26,27]

In 1979, Cady, et al., presented their findings from a prospective study of physical fitness in relation to subsequent back pain reports among 1652 firefighters.[28] An overall fitness score was derived from several isometric strength, flexibility, and cardiovascular endurance measures. They found an association between back pain reporting and fitness level, and concluded that "physical fitness and conditioning are preventive of back injuries." Unfortunately, other factors that varied significantly between fitness groups, such as age, were not controlled during the analyses, making interpretation less clear.

Several years later, MacDonald, et al., reported on a prospective study of industrial back pain reports and spinal canal diameter among miners.[29] Canal measurements were obtained by ultrasonography for 204 of 373 miners solicited, with a subsequent followup at 3 years. The medical and work attendance records for the 3 years prior to the ultrasound examinations also were reviewed. Miners who left the industry with records indicating prior back problems or related time loss had significantly narrower canals as compared to other subjects. Unfortunately, a reduction in the labor force led to well over half of the subjects leaving the industry within the followup period, which limited the analyses and conclusions.

A more comprehensive prospective, longitudinal study of back injury reports within the Boeing Company recently has been reported.[30-36] The purpose of the study was to examine a wide variety of workplace, individual physical, demographic, and psychosocial variables as potential predictors of back pain reports in 3020 Boeing aircraft manufacturing employees.

At the time of induction into the study, employees underwent a physical examination entailing measures of anthropometric variables, flexibility, isometric lifting strength, and estimated aerobic capacity. A back examination also was conducted, including lower extremity girths, straight leg raise testing, and reflex testing, among other measures. At the time of the physical examination, medical history, demographic, and psychosocial information also was requested. The study participants then were tracked for future industrial back pain reports.

Questioning upon entrance into the study revealed that treatment for back problems had been sought by 39% of the aircraft manufacturing workers, and 2% had prior back surgery. Twelve percent reported current back problems at the time of testing or back-related work loss during the prior 6 months.[34] Subsequently, during the average followup period of 3 years, 279 employees participating in the study reported back problems.

The incidence of future back pain reporting was similar among men and women. Age was related to incidence, with younger employees significantly more likely to report a back problem at the workplace than older employees.

A history of back problems has been recognized for some time as an important risk factor for future problems. The Boeing study findings support this association: Of all the factors studied, the report of current or recent back problems was the variable most significantly related to future back injury reports.[34] This finding is consistent with previous reports that individuals experiencing back problems are at highest risk for recurrences during the 2 to 3 years following an episode.[19,37] Additionally, a history of treatment for back problems, chiropractic visits, doctor visits, and medical prescriptions for pain problems of any kind were associated with increased risk of industrial back injury reports.[36]

It was notable how few of the many individual physical variables examined were significantly associated with increased risk of future back pain reports. None of the strength, flexibility, and aerobic capacity measures obtained were significantly associated with an increased or decreased incidence of back pain reports, whether examined independently or in multivariate models. Furthermore, among employees without a reported history of back problems, no individual physical factors were associated with increased risk. Among subjects reporting a history of back problems, the only premorbid physical examination variable to be highly associated with future back pain reporting was back pain elicited on straight leg raising. This relationship is not surprising, because it would appear to indicate the presence of some degree of back irritation or complaints at the time of testing, from which followup began. Once the presence or absence of back pain elicited on SLR was known, no other physical measures had any significant additional predictive value, with the exception of increased weight in women, which slightly increased the risk for future back pain reporting.[33]

Similar to a number of other studies,[22,38–40] smoking was found to be a risk indicator.[32] The relative risk for a smoker was 1.4 times that of a nonsmoker for reporting an industrial back injury report in the followup period. A number of possible explanations have been introduced for this association. Among

them are possible microfractures caused by decreased bone mineral content and osteoporosis, increased coughing and intradiscal pressure, changes in vertebral body blood flow affecting discal metabolism, and certain demographic and psychosocial characteristics that may be associated with both smoking and greater risk of back injury complaints.[32,39,40]

One of the most interesting findings of the Boeing Study was the influence of work perceptions and psychosocial factors on back pain complaints.[35] With the exception of reporting current back pain or recent back disability, the strongest predictors of subsequent reports were perceptions of the workplace, such as low job enjoyment, and certain psychosocial responses identified on the Minnesota Multiphasic Personality Inventory (MMPI). Reports of hardly ever enjoying job tasks and relatively high scale 3 scores on the MMPI, indicating tendencies toward somatic complaints or denial of emotional distress, were associated with subsequent back injury reports. These findings emphasize the importance of adopting a broader approach to understanding and dealing with the multifaceted problem of back pain complaints that interfere with work, and offer an explanation of why past efforts focusing on purely physical or injury factors have met with little success.

Most of the prospective studies of work-related back pain reports have been limited in scope, focusing on individual physical capacities among workers in occupations with high physical demands. One study suggests an association between industrial back pain reports and insufficient isometric strength relative to job demands.[23] Another indicates that spinal canal diameter may play a role in the risk of back pain reporting and related absenteeism in miners.[29] A negative correlation between work-related back incident reports and overall fitness, in terms of strength, flexibility, and cardiovascular fitness factors, appears to exist in firefighters.[28] However, similar associations between physical factors and back pain reporting were not corroborated within aircraft manufacturing workers with generally less extreme physical job demands. When perceptions of work and other psychosocial factors also were considered, they were found to play a greater role in back pain reporting than the wide array of physical measures studied.[35]

Risk Factors for Long-Term Disability

Prevention of chronic back pain disability could dramatically reduce the costs and the amount of suffering and loss of livelihood experienced by individuals and their families. Of those who file claims, 90% follow the expected course of natural recovery, return to work rapidly, and account for only 20% of back injury claims costs.[3,41] Conversely, 80% of the disability costs are accounted for by the 10% of claims involving individuals who experience continued problems and disability for 3 months or longer.[3] Chronic back pain disability is thus the most expensive and devastating component of the industrial back problem.[3,16,41]

Retrospective studies have revealed psychosocial and environmental difficulties associated with prolonged disability.[8,42,43] Yet, no prospective, longitudinal studies of chronic disability have been reported to date. Such studies would be most enlightening in identifying risk factors that could guide intervention strategies to effect this most significant aspect of back problems within industry.

A REVIEW OF PREVIOUS ATTEMPTS AT SCREENING

A logical basis for designing risk screening programs is a knowledge of factors that increase an individual's chances of experiencing the disease or problem of interest. Unfortunately, as discussed previously, few risk factors have been clearly and consistently identified for various categories of back complaints. Yet, despite scientific evidence, or the lack thereof, various screening procedures have been introduced and used over the years.

In 1929, pre-employment x ray screening was introduced as a potential tool to identify anatomical variations that might compromise the back's resistance to injury.[1,2] Studies involving more than 27,000 sets of lumbosacral spine films indicate that findings from standard radiographs are not predictive of future back problems.[15,44–51] Although radiographs are still used in some industries, their popularity has waned, as reflected by Rowe's position paper that concluded, "routine spinal roentgenograms of industrial workers are not cost- or risk benefit-effective."[52] A recent review by Gibson adds further support to this conclusion.[53]

Some regard a pre-employment medical history and physical examination as an important step in selecting employees for physical labor.[23,54–56] The primary objective is to identify individuals with previous back problems, because a high incidence of recurrent episodes is expected.[12,19,23,57–61] However, the chances are small that individuals with prior back problems will be identified through physical examination unless a surgical scar is present.[62] Furthermore, the reliability of information gathered through a pre-employment history is questionable.[55,63,64]

More recently, back pain prevention has focused on individual physical capacities, such as strength, cardiovascular fitness, and flexibility. Using a variety of research designs, Chaffin, Cady, Keyserling, Biering-Sorensen, Nicoliasen, and others have measured and studied strength as a potential risk factor for back problems.[17,23,25,28,31,65–68] Despite these studies, the relationship between a person's strength and the occurrence of back pain is not well understood. Cardiovascular fitness also has been evaluated with respect to back problems[18,28,32,69,70] and controversies remain regarding its role in prevention as well.

Similar controversies surround spinal flexibility. A common perception is that greater spinal flexibility is associated with improved back health and lower risk of injury. This perception is evidenced by the stretching programs that are being promoted for back pain prevention in the general public and within many workplaces.[71] Additionally, increasing spinal range of motion is a specific goal of many treatment and rehabilitation programs, although the efficacy of this approach remains uncertain.[72–77] The role of flexibility in uncovering past back problems or predicting future problems is dubious.[17,19,30]

Spinal canal diameter, as measured through ultrasonography, also has been introduced as a possible risk factor for back problems, particularly those associated with root entrapment symptoms. Its proposed use in screening is based on the assumption that individuals with relatively narrow canals, who are thought to be at greatest risk, have significantly fewer back problems if they avoid jobs with high physical demands.[29,78,79] However, questions remain about the ability to predict subsequent back problems based on canal diameter as measured by ultrasound. Moreover, controversy surrounds the reproducibility of measurements to detect the relatively small variations in diameter that would be necessary for screening determinations.[80,81]

PRACTICAL CONSIDERATIONS IN PLANNING PREVENTION STRATEGIES

Prevention through pre-employment screening faces many practical challenges. Limited knowledge of clear risk factors is an obvious constraint. In addition, many of the clinical tests used in the past lack acceptable reliability, and they are poor indicators of notable prior back problems. The sensitivity and specificity of the tests are poor for predicting those individuals who will subsequently report back problems during followup. Also, predictors of back pain incidents may not be the same or carry the same weight as predictors of resultant long-term disability. If the overall problem of work-related back pain is to be significantly improved, we must effectively curb long-term disability.

Of the few known risk indicators, most can be

identified only by questioning the individual, as opposed to taking simple measurements of physical attributes. These indicators for future back pain reports include a sometimes self-incriminating history of back and other health problems, responses to straight leg raising, psychosocial questionnaires, and inquiries about the workplace. We must keep in mind that these associations were identified in environments where confidentiality of responses was assured, such that employment would not be jeopardized. Thus, it may not be realistic to expect the same degree of candor in a pre-employment screening setting where responses may be perceived as affecting employment opportunities.

Conversely, few directly measurable physical attributes have been identified as important indicators of risk. Of the few that have, such as height, weight, and age, the findings have not been consistent between studies. Such inconsistencies also apply to measures of strength, flexibility, and aerobic capacity.

We are limited in our ability to predict individuals who will report back problems, even when using multivariate techniques that consider a number of potential risk factors simultaneously. These techniques also are subject to the difficulties posed by requiring verbal responses. For example, in the Boeing Study, history of back problems and other painful health conditions, work perceptions, and psychosocial responses contributed most to multivariate modeling.[35,36] Troup, et al., also found that a history of back symptoms, as well as perceptions of work capacity, enhanced prediction.[19] All of these factors depend on candid responses by the individuals.

Another practical issue in pre-employment screening relates to the accuracy with which the tests can identify individuals who will report back problems during the employment period in question. How poorly even those factors that are strongly associated with back injury predict such complaints is exemplified in the Boeing Study. Back pain elicited on straight leg raising was strongly associated with back pain reports during the 4-year followup period (p < 0.0001). However, nearly four-fifths of persons citing back symptoms on SLR at the time of the initial volunteer screening did not report subsequent work-related back problems.[33] Furthermore, given that positive findings on straight leg raising are fairly rare (2.9% of workers), back pain reports from that group composed only 6.5% of all subsequent back injury reports.

Another important consideration with respect to screening procedures is that approximately 80% of the costs from industrial back problems arise from 10% of the back injury claimants.[3] At this time, we do not know whether risk factors identified as important for reporting an incident of back pain also

will be important in identifying those who go on to long-term disability. Thus, activities to reduce risk of incidence may or may not have a considerable impact on the most devastating aspect of the problem—long-term disability.

RECOMMENDATIONS FOR A MORE PRODUCTIVE COURSE OF ACTION

Past limitations of pre-employment screening are evident from the growth in back pain disability over past decades, during which such screening has been a major component of prevention efforts.[7,82] Considering the dearth of scientific evidence identifying clear indicators of future risk, the overall failure of pre-employment screening is not surprising.

One exception is that screening may offer some benefit in jobs of uncommonly high physical demands by ensuring that an individual's physical capacities meet the rigorous job requirements.[23–25,28] However, as service occupations and automation in manufacturing continue to expand in the developed countries of the world, jobs of extreme physical demands become less common. For those few remaining jobs that are extremely physically demanding, it may be prudent to consider some type of matching of physical abilities to job demands. However, despite a variety of expensive capacity testing equipment on the market, the benefits of using such equipment over more simple job simulation methods is not always clear.[83]

Pre-employment screening may have a place in encouraging improved health, particularly in the area of cardiovascular fitness, but there is little basis supporting its value for most workforces in preventing the occurrence of back problems. Although we should continue the quest for risk factors and causes of different types of back problems, achieving primary prevention through pre-employment screening based on present knowledge does not appear to be realistic. However, using current information, we can advocate several steps that may offer more immediate benefits in minimizing the impact of back problems within industry:

1. Encourage early, positive communication between the workplace and the employee once an injury has been reported. The goal of this communication should be to express support and concern for the employee's well being, and to send the message that the employee is valued and needed at the workplace.[84–86]
2. Recognize the value of maintaining as normal a lifestyle as possible throughout the recovery period and encourage gradual resumption of normal activities. Promote the use of temporary light

duty or modified job tasks, if necessary, to allow an employee experiencing back problems to continue working during recovery.[84,85,87,88]

3. Use knowledge of ergonomics to decrease the level of stress on the spine so that a job can be performed with minimal exacerbation of back symptoms, and thus promote continued work or rapid return to work for those having back discomfort. Such adaptations also would have the added benefit of opening jobs up to workers with a greater range of physical abilities.

4. Evaluate ways of bolstering employees' perceptions of the workplace and of their personal resources to discourage maladaptive ways of handling problems.[35] Recognize psychosocial problems at home or at the worksite that may contribute to delayed return to work.

5. Use current information on the effectiveness of various treatment approaches to caution individuals about the potential debilitation of excessive bed rest, the dangers of dependence on strong pain medications, and the inadvisability of surgery without strong preoperative indications.[88–90] Provide positive expectations based on knowledge of the natural history and encourage progressive activity, recognizing the benefit of return to work to the overall restoration process.[37,91]

Considering the limited resources that industry has available to spend on back problems, efforts could be directed in a more beneficial vein than pre-employment screening. Directing limited resources toward assisting all employees who are experiencing problems conveys a more caring stance, as opposed to spending resources on ineffectively picking out the "bad apples." At present, we must focus on preventing long-term disability by encouraging approaches that have reportedly yielded positive results in a variety of industries, rather than continuing our ineffective focus on prevention of back pain.[84–86,88]

REFERENCES

1. Bohart, W.H.: Anatomic variations and anomalies of the spine: relation to prognosis and length of disability. JAMA 92:698–701, 1929.
2. Cushway, B.C., Mayer, R.J.: Routine examination of the spine for industrial employees. JAMA 93:701–704, 1929.
3. Spengler, D.M., et al.: Back injuries in industry: a retrospective study. I. Overview cost analysis. Spine 11(3):241–256, 1986.
4. Stamper, M.: Good health is not for sale. Ergonomics 30(2):199–206, 1987.
5. Deyo, R.A.: Conservative therapy for low back pain: distinguishing useful from useless therapy. JAMA 250(8):1057–1062, 1983.
6. Grazier, K.L., Holbrook, T.L., Kelsey, J.L., Stauffer, R.N.: The frequency of occurrence, impact, and cost of musculoskeletal conditions in the United States. Chicago; American Academy of Orthopaedic Surgeons, 1984.
7. US Social Security Administration, Social Security Suppl HE3.3/3:979. Washington DC, Government Printing Office, 1977–1979.
8. Anderson, B.J.: Epidemiological aspects of low-back pain in industry. Spine 6:53, 1981.
9. Bigos, S.J., Battié, M.C.: Surveillance of back problems in industry. In Clinical Concepts in Regional Musculoskeletal Illness (Edited by N.M. Hadler). New York, Grune & Stratton, 1987.
10. Mortality and Morbidity Weekly Report 34:521, 1985.
11. Nachemson, A.L., Bigos, S.J.: The low back. In Adult Orthopaedics (Edited by R.L. Cruess and W.R. Rennie). New York, Churchill Livingstone, pp. 843–937, 1985.
12. Vallfors, B.: Acute, subacute and chronic low back pain: clinical symptoms, absenteeism and working environment. Scand J Rehab Med Suppl 11:1–98, 1985.
13. Vincente, P.J.: The Nuprin report: a summary, part I. Skokie, IL, American Pain Society Newsletter, 1988.
14. Green, M., Battié, M.C., Bigos, S.J.: The role of acute injury in the onset of lower back problems. Submitted, J Spinal Disorders.
15. Rowe, M.L.: Low back pain in industry: a position paper. J Occup Med 11:161–169, 1969.
16. Snook, S.H.: Low back pain in industry. In Symposium on Idiopathic Low Back Pain (Edited by A.A. White and S.L. Gordon). St. Louis, C.V. Mosby, 1982.
17. Biering-Sørenson, F.: Physical measurements as risk indicators for low-back trouble over a one-year period. Spine 9(2):106–119, 1984.
18. Gyntelberg, F.: One year incidence of low back pain among male residents of Copenhagen age 40–59. Danish Med Bull 21:30–36, 1974.
19. Troup, J.D.G., Foreman, T.K., Baxter, C.E., Brown, D.: The perception of back pain and the role of psychophysical tests of lifting capacity. Spine 12(7):645–657, 1987.
20. Waddell, G.: Clinical model for the treatment of low-back pain. Spine 12(7):632–644, 1987.
21. Hrubec, A., Nashbold, B.S. Jr: Epidemiology of lumbar disc lesions in the military in World War II. Am J Epidemiol 102:366–376, 1975.
22. Heliövaara, M.: Body height, obesity, and risk of herniated lumbar intervertebral disc. Spine 12(5):469–472, 1987.
23. Chaffin, D.B., Park, K.S.: A longitudinal study of low-back pain associated with occupational weight lifting factors. Amer Ind Hyg Assoc J 34:513–525, 1973.
24. Keyserling, W.M., Herrin, D.G., Chaffin, D.B.: Isometric strength testing as a means of controlling medical incidents on strenuous jobs. J Occup Med 22:332–336, 1980.
25. Keyserling, W.M., Herrin, D.G., Chaffin, D.B., Armstrong, T.J., Foss, M.L.: Establishing an industrial strength testing program. Am Ind Hyg Assoc J 41:730–736, 1980.
26. Hansson, T.H., Bigos, S.J., Wortley, M.D., Spengler, D.: The load on the lumbar spine during isometric strength testing. Spine 9(7):720–723, 1984.
27. Zeh, J., et al.: Isometric strength testing, recommendations based on a statistical analysis of the procedure. Spine 11(1):43–46, 1986.
28. Cady, L.D., Bischoff, D.P., O'Connell, E.R., Thomas, P.C., Allan, J.H.: Strength and fitness and subsequent back injuries in firefighters. J Occup Med 21:269–272, 1979.
29. MacDonald, E.B., Porter, R., Hibbert, C., Hart, J.: The relationship between spinal canal diameter and back pain in coal miners: ultrasonic measurement as a screening test? J Occup Med 26:23–28, 1984.
30. Battié, M.C., et al.: The role of spinal flexibility in back pain complaints within industry: a prospective study. Spine 15(8):768–773, 1990.

31. Battié, M.C., et al.: Isometric lifting strength as a predictor of industrial back pain. Spine *14*:141–147, 1989.
32. Battié, M.C.: A prospective study of the role of cardiovascular risk factors and fitness in industrial back pain complaints. Spine *14*(2):141–147, 1989.
33. Battié, MC, et al.: Anthropometric and clinical measurements as predictors of industrial back pain complaints: a prospective study. J Spinal Dis *3*:195–204, 1990.
34. Battié, M.C.: The reliability of physical factors as predictors of the occurrence of back pain reports: a prospective study within industry. Doctoral Thesis, Gothenburg University, Gothenburg, Sweden, 1989.
35. Bigos, S.J., et al.: A longitudinal, prospective study of acute industrial back problems: the influence of work perceptions and psychosocial factors. Submitted, J Occup Med.
36. Bigos, S.J., et al.: A prospective evaluation of commonly used pre-employment screening tools for acute industrial back pain. Submitted, N Eng J Med.
37. Nachemson, A.L.: The natural course of low back pain: American Academy of Orthopaedic Surgeons symposium of idiopathic low back pain. St. Louis, CV Mosby, pp. 46—49, 1982.
38. Frymoyer, J.W., et al.: Epidemiologic studies of low-back pain. Spine *5*:419–423, 1980.
39. Frymoyer, J.W., et al.: Risk factors in low-back pain. J Bone Joint Surg *65*:213–218, 1983.
40. Svensson, H., Vedin, A., Wilhelmsson, C., Andersson, G.B.J.: Low-back pain in relation to other diseases and cardiovascular risk factors. Spine *8*:277–285, 1983.
41. Leavitt, S.S., Johnson, T.L., Beyer, R.D.: The process of recovery: patterns in industrial back injury, part 1: Costs and other quantitative measures of effort. Ind Med Surg *40*:7, 1971.
42. Beals, R.K., Hickman, N.W.: Industrial injuries of the back and extremities. J Bone Joint Surg *54A*: 1593, 1972.
43. Flynn, J.C., Hoque, M.P.A.: Anterior fusion of the lumbar spine. End result study with long-term follow-up. J Bone Joint Surg *61-A*:1143–1161, 1979.
44. Diveley, R., Oglevie, R.R.: Pre-employment examination of the low back. JAMA *160*:856–858, 1956.
45. Fullenlove, T.M., Williams, A.J.: Comparative roentgen findings in symptomatic and asymptomatic backs. Radiology *68*:572–574, 1957.
46. LaRocca, H., MacNab, I.: Value of pre-employment radiographic assessment of the lumbar spine. Can Med Assoc J *101*:49–54, 1969.
47. Magora, A., Schwartz, A.: Relation between low back pain syndrome and x-ray findings, 2. transitional vertebra (mainly sacralization). Scand J Rehab Med *10*:135–145, 1978.
48. Redfield, J.T.: The low back x-ray as a pre-employment screening tool in the forest products industry. Occup Med *13*:219, 1971.
49. Runge, C.F.: Pre-existing structural defects and the severity of compensation back injuries. Ind Med Surg *27*:249–252, 1958.
50. Splitoff, C.A.: Lumbosacral junction: roentgenographic comparison of patients with and without backaches. JAMA *152*:1610–1613, 1953.
51. Valkenburg, H.A., Haanen, H.C.N.: The epidemiology of back pain. *In* Symposium on Idiopathic Low Back Pain, (Edited by A.A., White, and S.L. Gordon). St. Louis, CV Mosby, pp. 9–22, 1982.
52. Rowe, M.L.: Are routing spine films on workers in industry cost- or risk-benefit effective? J Occup Med *24*:41–43, 1982.
53. Gibson, E.S.: The value of preplacement screening radiography of the low back. Occup Med (State of the Art Reviews) *3*(1):91–107, 1988.
54. Alexander, D.C., Pulat, B.M.: Industrial ergonomics: a practitioner's guide. Norcross, GA, Industrial Engineering and Management Press, 1985.
55. Rowe, M.L.: Low back pain disability in industry: updated position. J Occup Med *13*:476, 1971.
56. Schussler, T., Kaminer, A.J., Power, V.L., Pomper, I.H.: The preplacement examination. J Occup Med *17*:254, 1975.
57. Bergquist-Ullman, M., Larsson, U.: Acute low back pain in industry. Acta Orthop Scand Suppl *170*:1–117, 1977.
58. Biering-Sørenson, F., Thomsen, C.: Medical, social and occupational history as risk indicators for low-back trouble in a general population. Spine *11*(7):720–725, 1986.
59. Dillane, J.B., Fry, J., Dalton, G.: Acute back syndrome—a study for general practice. Br Med J *2*:82, 1966.
60. Svensson, H.O.: Low-back pain in 40–47 year old men: some socioeconomic factors and previous sickness absence. Scand J Rehabil Med *14*:54–59, 1982.
61. Troup, J.D.G., Martin, J.W., Lloyd, D.C.E.F.: Back pain in industry: a prospective study. Spine *6*:61–69, 1981.
62. Glover, J.R.: Prevention of back pain. *In* The Lumbar Spine and Back Pain (Edited by M. Jayson). New York, Grune and Stratton, pp. 47–54, 1976.
63. Biering-Sørenson, F., Hilden, J.: Reproducibility of the history of low-back trouble. Spine *9*(3):280–286, 1984.
64. Riihimäki, H., Videman, T., Tola, S.: Reliability of retrospective questionnaire data on the history of low back trouble. Presented at the International Society for the Study of the Lumbar Spine meeting, Kyoto, Japan, May 15–19, 1989.
65. Chaffin, D.B., Herrin, G.D., Keyserling, W.M.: Preemployment strength testing—an updated position. J Occup Med *20*:403–408, 1978.
66. Doolitle, T.L., Kaiyala, K.: Strength and musculo-skeletal injuries of firefighters. Proc nineteenth Annu Conf Hum Factors Assoc Can, Vancouver, BC, 1986.
67. Nachemson, A.L., Lindh, M.: Measurement of abdominal and back muscle strength with and without low back pain. Scand Rehabil Med *1*:60–65, 1969.
68. Nicoliasen, N., Jørgenson, K.: Trunk strength, back muscle endurance and low-back trouble. Scand J Rehab Med *17*:121–127, 1985.
69. Brennan, G.P., et al.: Physical characteristics of patients with herniated intervertebral lumbar discs. Spine *12*:699–702, 1987.
70. Cady, L.D., Thomas, P.C., Karwasky, R.J.: Program for increasing health and physical fitness of firefighters. J Occup Med *2*:111–114, 1985.
71. Locke, J.C.: Stretching away from back pain, injury. Occup Health Saf *52*:8–13, 1983.
72. Davies, J.E., Gibson, R., Tester, L.: The value of exercises in the treatment of low back pain. Rheumatol Rehabil *18*:243, 1979.
73. Kendell, P.H., Jenkins, J.S.: Exercise for backache: a double-blind controlled trial. Physiotherapy *54*:154, 1968.
74. Kraus, H., Nagler, W., Melleby, A.: Evaluation of an exercise program for back pain. Am Fam Physician *28*(3):153–158, 1983.
75. Lindstrom, A., Zachrisson, M.: Physical therapy on low back pain and sciatica: an attempt at evaluation. Scand J Rehab Med *2*:37–42, 1970.
76. Mayer, T.G.: Rehabilitation of the patient with spinal pain. Orthop Clin North Am *14*(3):623–637, 1983.
77. Tollison, C.D., Kriegel, M.L.: Physical exercise in the treatment of low back pain. Part II: A practical regimen of stretching exercise. Orthop Rev *17*(9):913–923, 1988.
78. Porter, R.W., Hibbert, C.S., Wicks, M.: The spinal canal in symptomatic lumbar disc lesions. J Bone Joint Surg *60-B*(4):485–487, 1978.
79. Porter, R., Hibbert, C., Wellman, P.: Backache and the lumbar spinal canal. Spine *5*:99–105, 1980.
80. Battié, M.C., et al.: The reliability of measurements of the lumbar spine using Ultrasound B-scan. Spine *11*(2):144–148, 1986.
81. Howie, D.W., Chatterton, B.E., Hone, M.R.: Failure of ultrasound in the investigation of sciatica. J Bone Joint Surg *65B*:144–147, 1983.

82. Snook, S.H., Campanelli, R.A., Hart, J.W.: A study of three preventive approaches to low back injury. J Occup Med *20*:478–481, 1978.

83. Hazard, R.G., et al.: Functional restoration with behavioral support: a one-year prospective study of patients with chronic low-back pain. Spine *14*(2):157–161, 1989.

84. Fitzler, S.L., Berger, R.A.: Attitudinal change: the Chelsea back program. Occup Saf Health *51*:24–26, 1982.

85. Fitzler, S.L., Berger, R.A.: Chelsea back program: one year later. Occup Saf Health *52*:52–54, 1983.

86. Wood, J.W.: Design and evaluation of a back injury prevention program within a geriatric hospital. Spine *12*(2):77–82, 1987.

87. Nachemson, A.L.: Work for all: for those with low back pain as well. Clin Orthop Res *179*:77–85, 1983.

88. Weisel, S.W., Feffer, H.L., Rothman, R.H.: Industrial low back—a prospective evaluation of a standardized diagnostic and treatment protocal. Spine *9*:199–203, 1984.

89. Deyo, R.A., Diehl, A.K., Rosenthal, M.: How many days of bed rest for acute low back pain? A randomized clinical trial. NEJM *315*(17):1064–1070, 1986.

90. Spengler, D.M., et al.: Low-back pain following lumbar spine procedures: failure of initial selection? Spine *5*:356–360, 1980.

91. Fordyce, W.E., Brockway, J.A., Bergman, J.A., Spengler, D.M.: Acute back pain: a control group comparison of behavioral versus traditional management methods. J Behav Med *9*(2):127–140, 1986.

Gunnar B.J. Andersson

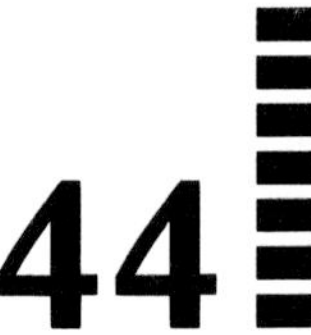

44

Impairment Evaluation Issues and the Disability System

INTRODUCTION AND HISTORICAL PERSPECTIVE

Several chapters in this book are related to impairment and disability. Although these issues may not be of significant interest to the physician in general, they are an important part of the social, legal, and political system in which we exist. By definition, therefore, they vary between countries, and even within the same country when, as is the case in the US, local legislation and social and political concerns vary.

Regardless of background and type of practice, physicians with interest in low back disorders will all be exposed to some aspects of disability evaluation. To many, this is an unpleasant and unaccustomed obligation for which he is unprepared, and which requires not only considerations of medical facts, but also of occupational, social, and economic factors. Disability evaluation is needed, not for medical reasons, but because society has created compensation programs to support those with reduced capacity for everyday activities and gainful employment. Large segments of the population are compensated for disability. For example, more than four million Americans receive support from the Social Security Disability Insurance (SSDI) and Supplemental Security Income (SSI) programs, and each year there are more than 2 million worker's compensation disability claims. In addition, disability evaluations are required by personal disability insurances and personal injury litigation.

Compensation is one of the social and legal characteristics of civilization.[1] Medical negligence appears to be the earliest example. Thus, the Code of Hammurabi (about 1752 B.C.) stated that if a slave

died as a result of treatment, the surgeon had to replace him, and if a free man died the surgeon lost his right hand. Worker's compensation laws date back to Roman times, and by Roman law, a worker could claim compensation for accidental injury both against an employer and a fellow employee. Even slave owners had to care for injuries to slaves. Successful litigation required identifying a responsible party, and monetary rewards were accepted between equals.

Although some compensation laws existed during the middle ages, it was not until the industrial revolution that compensation for negligent accidental injury became a significant issue. Thus, the first successful personal injury case in the English High Court dates back to 1836.[1] Proof of negligence was necessary, and litigation was invalid if there was contributory negligence, or if the accident was caused by "ordinary risk." Already the following year, however, the "fellow-servant" doctrine was accepted by English Courts, stating that an employer was not responsible for negligence on the part of another employee or "fellow-servant." Another step toward modern compensation laws was the English "Fatal Accident Act," which required compensation to the family of a person killed by accident. About the same time German law made railway companies responsible for any accidents on the Berlin-Potsdam Railroad.

Parallel development in Germany and England during the 1880s resulted in more comprehensive insurance laws. Bismarck introduced a comprehensive social insurance system in Germany, which included worker's compensation, and compulsory insurance was introduced in England through the Employer's Liability Act (1880). Up until this time, fault had to be proven by the injured worker. This was abolished in England by the Workman's Compensation Act (1887), which, by 1911, covered all workers and not only those injured in accidents but also those with industrial diseases and sickness as well.

In Europe, the industrial liability was part of a social security and welfare system, whereas acceptance of employer responsibility in the US developed as a separate, no fault system. In 1908, the Federal Employees Compensation Act passed, and in 1914 the California Industrial Accident Act. Employers were sold on insurance coverage by the promise of immunity from liability suits on behalf of an employee. By 1949, worker's compensation systems existed in all states, and, in 1954, the Social Security Disability Act was passed, creating a second major disability compensation system.

Legal aspects of disability are discussed elsewhere in this text. The purpose of this chapter is to discuss alternative systems of disability and impairment evaluation, with particular reference to the US situation.

DEFINITIONS

All systems of work incapacity distinguish between *disability* and *impairment*. The term *impairment* denotes a physical or mental limitation of function resulting from disease or injury. Impairment is a quantifiable anatomic or functional loss, which can be permanent or temporary. Impairment is determined by a physician. *Disability*, on the other hand, is reduced capacity to meet certain demands of everyday work activities. It is the loss of capacity to be gainfully employed as a result of an impairment. Disability, therefore, is a broad term and includes not only the physical or mental impairment but also motivation, education level, work experience, psychologic factors, age, socioeconomic factors, and financial status. Disability reflects the interaction between impairment and economic and social aspects. It is ultimately an administrative decision, often made by an agency and based on information other than the physician's measure of impairment.

Handicap is the disadvantage resulting from impairments and disabilities, i.e., a description of the interaction between the impaired and the environment, relative to peers and social norms. It focuses on social roles, including physical independence, mobility, occupation, social integration and economic independence.

A peculiarity of some impairment evaluation systems is the "whole man" concept. First introduced in Russia in 1907,[2] the "whole man" concept immediately became the basis for the US worker's compensation system. By this principle, a certain percentage is assigned to different impairments of parts of the body. In the American Medical Association's *Guides to the Evaluation of Permanent Impairment*,[3] for example, amputation of a finger at the proximal interphalangeal joint represents an 80% impairment of the finger, 4% of the hand, and 2% of the whole person. A person assessed to have complete loss of spine function, i.e., a 100% spinal impairment, has only partial impairment of the "whole man."

LOW BACK IMPAIRMENT EVALUATION SYSTEMS

Three different impairment evaluation systems have evolved: the anatomic, based on physical examination; the diagnostic, based on diagnosis; and the functional, based on measures of function and work capacity. All have advantages and disadvantages. Ideally, a disability evaluation should validly measure disability (content validity); should result in the same measure if used by several people (reproducibility); should remove subjective influence as much as possible (objective); should be simple enough to be used in a physician's office; should not require expensive equipment; should allow for recognition of differences between levels of disability (discriminating); should allow for changes as technology advances (flexibility); should be acceptable to different disability evaluation requiring bodies; should result in numerical values that can be handled by computer; should be universal in scope, and should be related to work.

Anatomic systems were the earliest forms of disability evaluation in use.[2,4] They were at first based on amputation and ankylosis, and as such, were simple, accurate, objective, and reproducible. They were also limited because they covered only a small part of impairment disorders. Predictably, the simple, early systems were expanded to include loss of motion, weakness, and loss of sensation. At the same time, some of the accuracy, objectivity, and reproducibility were sacrificed.

An example of a modified anatomic system is the American Medical Association (AMA) *Guides to the Evaluation of Permanent Impairment*,[3] which was first published in 1958, and is now in its third revision. It is not purely anatomic, but includes some diagnostic features as well. Thus, the spine section includes a "short" list of diagnoses that are combined with range of motion measurements.

Another predominantly anatomic system was published by the American Academy of Orthopaedic Surgeons (AAOS) in 1962,[5] and is a modification of the AMA System. It included additional orthopaedic disorders and a scale for pain in patients with documented organic disorders, but still focused on range of motion. This *Manual for Orthopaedic Surgeons in Evaluating Permanent Physical Impairment* is currently being revised.

The advantages of a diagnostic system are objectivity, simplicity, and reproducibility. If diagnostic criteria can be agreed upon and are strictly enforced, reproducibility should be excellent. This is not as simple for spinal conditions as for many other musculoskeletal conditions because of disagreements on classification. Even so, the degree of impairment and disability for a given diagnosis can be highly variable.[6] A diagnosis-based system is currently used by the Social Security Administration,[7,8] and in Minnesota, for Worker's Compensation Disability evaluation (MMA).[9] Diagnoses are also partially used by the AMA and AAOS Systems. The SSA requires diagnoses, history, physical examination, and laboratory evaluation (when applicable). It is oriented toward disease more than injury. The MMA System also requires history, physical examination, and x ray evaluation, and grossly evaluates subjective complaints.

Although a functional system would be the most desirable in terms of actually measuring disability, no such system is currently in use. California has an industrial accident system that is partly functional because it requires recommendations of work restrictions. Subjective and objective findings are submitted to an agency along with recommended work restrictions, and then a disability percentage is awarded by a disability evaluation specialist. Anatomic, pathologic, functional, age, and pain factors all enter into the decision. The physician may be required to provide estimates of postural ability, lifting capacity, and similar functions. These functions are not measured, however, but merely estimated, which results in large variations in evaluation of the same disease or accident. Table 44–1 summarizes some of the systems currently in use in the United States.

The Physician's Responsibility

A physician has at least four responsibilities in the disability evaluation process.[10] The first is to establish a causal relationship between the injury event and the resulting impairment. This process is important in worker's compensation and personal injury cases, although it is not central to social security. A causal relationship can be direct, or can be an aggravation of an existing condition. The physician's responsibility at this stage is to record the events as described, and to assess whether a reasonable causal relationship exists. The minimum necessary information includes a description of the alleged accident, including information about where and when it occurred. The problem of establishing causality for spinal disorders is well established.[11–14]

The second responsibility is to determine the end of the healing period, defined as the time beyond which no reasonable progress toward resolution will be made. It is important that both physician and patient understand this definition, which does not imply that normal function has been restored. Unfortunately, with many back conditions the healing period is poorly defined. This is particularly true for the so-called "soft tissue injuries" often referred to as sprains and strains. Unfortunately, the physician tends to prolong the healing period "to be on the safe side," which, as discussed in previous chapters, can lead to deconditioning and chronic pain.

The third responsibility is to determine if at the time of maximum medical improvement any impairment exists, and if so to rate this impairment. Irrespective of the system that is used, the contribution of a pre-existing condition (apportionment) must be assessed at this time. The AMA Guide[3] identifies five types of aggravation.

1. An occupational disorder aggravated by a supervening nonoccupational disorder.
2. An occupational disorder aggravated by another

Table 44–1
Comparison of Impairment (Disability)

System	Symptoms	ROM*	Diagnosis	Other Physiologic	Functional Evaluation
Social Security[8]	X	X		X	
California[18]	X	X	X	X	X
Minnesota[9]	X		X		
American Medical Association[3]		X	X		
American Academy Orthopaedic Surgeons[5]	X	X	X		

*ROM = Range of motion

supervening industrial condition arising out of and in the course of employment by a different employer.

3. An occupational disorder aggravated by another supervening occupational condition arising out of and in the course of employment by the same employer.

4. An occupational disorder aggravated by a pre-existing nonoccupational condition.

5. An occupational disorder aggravating a pre-existing nonoccupational condition.

An impairment rating can be legally challenged by the injured worker, employer or insurance carrier who can request an independent medical examination (IME). The physician providing the IME examines the patient (claimant) to provide a second opinion on causation, treatment plan, ability to work, permanence of disability and, rate of impairment.

The fourth responsibility relates to work capacity. Often, the physician is asked to estimate work capacity and outline restrictions, temporarily or permanently. The quality of this information varies greatly, because the physician's ability to determine work capacity is limited. The precision by which work capacity is outlined varies, from a simple statement of "light work" to specific limitations. The technology to assess work capacity is discussed elsewhere in this book, and will not be described further here. Clearly, further validation is required before this technology can be put to general use. Nonetheless, in some areas it provides a clear improvement over current estimates based more on "an educated guess,"[15,16] than on objective evaluation.

Variability in Impairment Rating

Ideally, an individual's impairment should be rated equal by different physicians. In the spinal area this is not the case. Brand and Lehmann[16] found wide variation among orthopaedists in Iowa when the same spine condition was rated, and Greenwood[17] found a similar variation between physicians in West Virginia. Ratings were influenced by factors such as the patient's personality, the level of education, and the social environment.[16,17] Brand and Lehmann[16] concluded that "any method of rating impairment is arbitrary at best and incorrect and unfair at worst." In spite of the variation (which in West Virginia was from 5 to 35%) the mean was similar in both states: 13% in Iowa and 12% in West Virginia. Clark, et al.,[18] provided California IME physicians, who by definition are trained and experienced in evaluations, with hypothetical patient records, and asked them to rate impairment. Large differences occurred. For example, in one patient the rat-

Table 44–2
Disability Rating of the Same Hypothetical Patient by 65 Independent Medical Examiners in a Specialty Dealing with Back Pain

Assuming a 55-year-old person with uncomplicated laminotomy for disc at L4–5 and a successful L4–S1 fusion, x rays show mild generalized osteoarthritis at L5–S1 disc space narrowing; operative result considered good: one year postoperatively, what do you think the disability rating should be according to California Disability Evaluation Schedule?

Number of IMEs selecting	Disability Rating
2	0%
1	10%
4	15%
5	20%
20	25%
13	30%
16	50%
3	60%
1	70%
Total 65	

ing ranged from 0 to 70%. Clark's group then developed a list of rating factors and asked the IME physicians to assign weights based on importance. Agreement was considerable, and a weighting scale was developed (Table 44–2), along with a standardized scoring system. Although the difference between examiners was still as high as 10 to 15 points, much better agreement was found when this new system was again tested on IME physicians.

These studies indicate the difficulty inherent in an impairment rating based on patient history and physical examination. Value judgements result in variation and contribute to measurement errors. This was the reason that a diagnostic system was adopted in Minnesota instead.[9] As discussed previously, however, this system, although it has the potential to reduce rating differences resulting from examination interpretation, still will result in differences unless criteria for diagnostic entities are extremely tight, which is difficult because the cause of spinal disease is often uncertain.

SUMMARY

The ideal disability evaluation system does not exist at the present time. A functionally based system would be desirable, but technology is not sufficiently advanced and validated at the present time. Lacking hard objective criteria, physicians tend to combine clinical examination data and perceptions of motivation, pain, education, and social environment to arrive at their evaluation. Interesting new systems such as the diagnosis based system in Minnesota and the more functionally directed system in

California, along with modified systems from the AMA and AAOS, will need constant revisions to mature. Whichever system is used, delay in assigning disability should be avoided. Unfortunately, the delay in assigning low back disability and impairment has negative consequences for rehabilitation.

REFERENCES

1. Allan, D.B., Waddell, G.: An historical perspective on low back pain and disability. Acta Orthop Scand Suppl *234*:1–23, 1989.
2. Luck, J.V.: History and Comparative Analysis of Disability Evaluation Systems Manuscript. Orthopaedic Hospital, Los Angeles, 1987.
3. Guides to the Evaluation of Permanent Impairment, 3rd Ed. (Edited by A. Edelson). Chicago, American Medical Association, 1988.
4. Kessler, H.H.: Disability Determination and Evaluation. Philadelphia, Lea & Febiger, 1970.
5. Manual for orthopaedic surgeons in evaluating permanent impairment. Chicago, American Academy of Orthopaedic Surgeons, 1966.
6. McBride, E.: Disability Evaluation. Philadelphia, J.B. Lippincott, 1963.
7. US Bureau of Disability Insurance: disability evaluation under social security. A handbook for physicians. Washington, DC, US Government Printing Office, 1970.
8. Social Security Administration: Disability Evaluation under Social Security. Washington, DC, US Government Printing Office, pp. 1–22, 1979.
9. Minnesota Medical Association: Worker's Compensation Permanent Partial Disability Schedule. Minneapolis, Minnesota Medical Association, 1984.
10. Frymoyer, J.W., Haldeman, S., Andersson, G.B.J: Impairment rating—The US perspective. *In* Occupational Low Back Pain. (Edited by M.H., Pope, J.W., Frymoyer, G.B.J., Andersson, and D.B. Chaffin). Chicago, Mosby, 1990.
11. Hadler, N.M.: Occupational illness: the issue of causality. J Occup Med *26*:587–593, 1984.
12. Carey, T.S.: Disability determination: the challenge. *In* Clinical Concepts in Regional Musculoskeletal Illness. (Edited by N. Hadler). Orlando, Grune & Stratton, Inc., pp. 247–261 1987.
13. Haddad, G.H.: Analysis of 2932 workers' compensation back injury cases: the impact on the cost to the system. Spine *12*:765, 1987.
14. Lehmann, T.R., Brand, R.A.: Disability in the patient with low back pain. Orthop Clin North Am *13*:559, 1982.
15. Burd, J.G.: The educated guess: doctors and permanent partial disability percentage. J Tenn Med Assoc *73*:441, 1980.
16. Brand, R.A., Lehmann, T.R.: Low back impairment rating practices of orthpaedic surgeons. Spine *8*:75, 1983.
17. Greenwood, J.G.: Low-back impairment-rating practices of orthopaedic surgeons and neurosurgeons in West Virginia. Spine *10*:773, 1985.
18. Clark, W.L., et al.: Back impairment and disability determination: another attempt at objective, reliable rating. Spine *13*:332, 1988.

45

George Preston

Legal Issues and Concepts
of Disability

Disability as a discrete topic has been given little room in legal literature. The two major encyclopedias in the legal world, *American Jurisprudence, 2nd Ed.* and *Corpus Juris Secundum*, amply illustrate this. *American Jurisprudence 2D* has no chapter on disability or impairment. *Corpus Juris Secundum* devotes just over four pages to disability and three short paragraphs to impairment. To the extent that disability receives attention in the legal forum it does so under the umbrella topic of damages. By way of contrast, both of these legal encyclopedias devote a full volume to damages.[1]

Disability is a fluid term in law because its contours are determined by the circumstances causing it. An automobile accident that occurs while on vacation, and which causes a disability, will have a different framework than the same injury caused while operating a vehicle during the course and scope of one's employment.

LEGAL CAUSATION—PROXIMATE CAUSE AS THE BASIS FOR LIABILITY

Outline of the Personal Injury System

A person who is injured by another party is entitled to damages if: (1) the other party violated a legal right (e.g., ran a red light), which (2) constituted negligence, which in turn (3) was the proximate cause of damages. The damages may include past lost wages, future loss of earnings capacity, past physical pain and mental anguish, future physical pain and mental anguish, reasonable and necessary past medical expenses, reasonable and necessary future medical expenses, miscellaneous expenses such as loss of consortium, loss of household services, and disfigurement.

For legal liability to exist there must be tortious conduct on behalf of the person or entity sued. A tort is a violation of a legal right not arising out of contract. The tortious act or omission must be the legal cause (cause in fact) of the injury. This legal cause is known as the "proximate cause." It is variously defined as a cause that, in a natural and continuous sequence, produces an event, and without which cause such event would not have occurred. The act or omission complained of must be such that a person using ordinary care would have foreseen that the event, or some similar event, might reasonably result. There can be more than one proximate cause of the event. Negligence is "conduct which falls below the standard established by law for the protection of others against unreasonable risk of harm."[2]

But none of this explains why disability is a function of damages in the legal field. Consider an individual who, through the fault of a third party, suffers a herniated disc that leaves him so disabled that he cannot return to his previous employment in a warehouse. His disability is his lack of physical ability to return to his past relevant work. Because neither the legislature nor the courts can give the man a new back, he is entitled to such damages as were "proximately" caused by the negligence of the person or entity that caused his injury. This is the most the law can do, the only way he can be made whole.

DISABILITY VS. IMPAIRMENT

The concept of disability is treated so little in the legal community that the terms "disability" and "impairment" are used often as though they were interchangeable. Doctors' reports as well frequently use the terms as if they were synonymous.

The functional definition of impairment is a deviation from the norm, a loss, or an abnormality of a person's mental process, or of the anatomic structure or function of the body. An impairment is deviation from the norm in that individual's case. Disability is a restriction or a lack of ability to perform an activity in a manner considered normal for humans, or for that particular individual because of a physiologic or anatomic impairment. For example, if a right-handed history professor loses his left ring finger, he may have a 1% physical impairment to the body as a whole from this loss. But his disability from the loss may be nil unless he was in the habit of composing lectures on his word processor, in which case he would then suffer some disability.

A more hackneyed example is that of Van Cliburn losing his left small finger. The disability from this minor impairment to most of the populous would be minute. It would obviously end the career of any concert pianist, resulting in 100% disability for that particular individual as far as pursuing past relevant work. The damages would be very high.

A handicap may result from an impairment or a disability. Handicap is "a disadvantage for a given individual, resulting from an impairment or a disability that limits or prevents fulfillment of a role that is normal (depending upon age, sex, and social and cultural factors) for that individual."[3] The handicaps that may result from an impairment or disability may be one of orientation, physical independence, mobility, occupation, social integration, economic self-sufficiency, or other handicaps.

DISABILITY IN A TYPICAL NEGLIGENCE CASE

The most common negligence situation results when an individual has been injured in an automobile collision because of the failure of another party to exercise reasonable care, which proximately causes physical injuries that result in physical impairment. The physical impairment in turn causes a disability that has an adverse economic impact on the automobile injury victim.

For illustrative purposes we shall assume that at the time of injury this citizen was a 45-year-old warehouse employee, and that the accident caused a herniated disc at the L5-S1 level. Assume further that he worked 40 hours per week at $13.00 per hour, which gave a gross salary of $520.00 per week. Assume that he also received pension and health insurance contributions from his employer totaling $110.00 per week. His true income is $630.00 per week when his benefit package is factored in. Because of resulting spinal instability, this particular individual underwent a fusion at L4-L5 and L5-S1,

but afterward was left with low back pain and some radiculopathy caused by postsurgical scarring. As a result, he was unable to return to his job of lifting, bending, carrying, pushing, and pulling in the warehouse. He was off work for 1 year prior to obtaining a new job at $8.00 per hour as a helper in a camera shop. The camera shop provided neither health insurance nor pension contributions.

The time off from work left the man in deep financial straits, and the pain caused by the herniated disc, surgery, and postsurgical scarring left him with some depression. Moreover, prior to the injury he belonged to a company bowling league. He bowled in the league 7 months of the year, and bowled with his family the other 5 months of the year. This was his only "sport" outside of work. He can sit for only 45 minutes at a time before he becomes uncomfortable, and he now takes two days on the weekends to do his yardwork, whereas before he could mow, edge, and trim his yard in a morning. He has grandchildren whom he now cannot play with in the same fashion that he could prior to his injury, and he misses lifting them up, rolling around with them on the living room floor, and sometimes running with them. Although the back injury did not create any sexual dysfunction, the man now finds that sex is always accompanied by pain. In the automobile accident he was thrown forward into the windshield and received a cut on his forehead that left a permanent scar. Because of loss of income the man and his wife had to sell a piece of property in the country to which they were going to retire and build a home.

The automobile accident occurred when the man was going through a green light on the way home from work. His car was suddenly and without warning broadsided by another individual. He now has fears of proceeding through intersections, driving his car home from work, and has never gone through the same intersection since the accident. His family doctor believes he has a form of posttraumatic stress disorder.

Legal Consequences

Variously, this individual is entitled to monetary damages for:

1. Past and future physical pain and mental anguish.
2. Loss of past and future earnings capacity.
3. Reasonable and necessary medical expenses incurred in the past and to a reasonable probability will incur in the future.
4. Past and future physical impairment and loss of enjoyment of life.
5. Damages for physical disfigurement.

Past and Future Physical Pain and Mental Anguish

Physical pain and mental anguish consist of anxiety, humiliation, shock, and pain while the individual is conscious, depression, post-traumatic stress disorder, grief resulting from lost income, lost job, loss of companionship that he had at his job, and loss of his dream retirement home in the country. How are such damages proved and how much can be awarded? Generally, these damages are supported by the injured party's testimony before the jury regarding how he feels about this new station in life caused by his physical impairment. His wife, neighbors, parents, and friends may also testify about the postinjury changes they have observed.

The final monetary award by the jury is entirely within its discretion as long as the award is reasonably related to the evidence before the jury. There is no formula or exact measure by which a jury can equate a certain amount of pain, grief, and mental anguish with any sum of money.

In this hypothetical situation, testimony from a physician concerning the mechanical causes of pain and their *likely effects on performance* would be invaluable, and provide a solid factual basis for a jury's monetary award.

The standard of evaluation by which an award for pain and suffering is measured is such an amount that a reasonable person would estimate to be fair compensation when that amount appears to be in harmony with the evidence when considered without passion or prejudice.[4] One of the factors a jury will probably be invited to look at in cases such as this hypothetical one, are the life expectancy tables published by the federal government.[5] In this instance the man's life expectancy is 29.4 years, and the jury can legitimately be asked to consider this many years of physical pain and mental anguish in computing its award.

Past and Future Loss of Earnings Capacity

The general rule in cases involving an impairment of earnings capacity is that the measure of damages will be the difference between the amount that the plaintiff was capable of earning before his injury and that which he is capable of earning thereafter. Damages should be estimated based on the person's ability to earn money, rather than what he actually earned before his injury. The difference between the actual earnings of the plaintiff before and after the injury does not constitute the measure,[6] although the jury does not have to ignore it.

The plaintiff in the hypothetical case had a high school education, no vocational training, but over the years had obtained on his own some knowledge of photography, which qualified him for the job he currently holds in the camera store.

The $13.00 per hour and the $110.00 a week in benefits was probably the highest preinjury figure that this man could have earned in an open and competitive job market. Thus, the one year of missed work would entitle this man to compensation for the full value of what he lost, or $32,760.00 ($630.00 × 52 weeks).

Assuming that the plaintiff was 45 years old at the time of injury and has a work life expectancy of 23 years (until age 68), the loss of future earnings capacity must be proved to the jury to the extent that it is reasonably being capable of being proved. The jury can deduce this from the testimony of the plaintiff alone, or from the plaintiff's testimony in conjunction with that of a vocational expert or economist. Assuming that a vocational expert would state that the highest earnings capacity that the plaintiff has after the injury and resulting impairment is $8.00 per hour (his current earnings), then his future loss of earnings capacity is $310.00 per week ($630.00 per week preinjury earnings minus $320.00 [40 hours × $8.00 per hour]).

At this point, the plaintiff can either present these figures to the jury or use yet another expert, this time an economist, to project his future damages under the loss of earnings capacity category. The economist would be given the date of birth of the injured party, his past training, his past earning history, any special training or education, paid vacation time, employer contributions to health insurance, employer pension contributions, any other benefits of his past work, and his current income and benefits. He would then be told how long the man planned to work, e.g., to age 60, 62, or 68.

If an economist or other expert found that the man planned to work for 23 more years and that his increases in his current job would be offset by inflation, then there would be no need to reduce the future award to its present value, which is done by taking the gross amount and applying a discount factor to that figure. In this particular instance, 23 years times an annualized loss of $16,200.00 ($310.00 per week times 52 weeks) equals $370,760.00.

Looking at another example, suppose an injured party had a past relevant work experience as an executive secretary, including use of a word processor and computer, such that these skills could be brought back to a competitive level in a short period of time. Assume that this party suffered an injury that left her with a residual functional capacity of performing less skilled jobs. If this person had not worked for the past five years, it is still determinable from the job market what her earnings capacity was for that period of time. Assume that she was married to someone with a good income and was not working at the time of her injury. Some would ask what her real damages are because she does not need to work and probably was not planning to work any time in the future. But suppose a year after the accident her husband died with no insurance, leaving her with two minor children. If she were able to earn \$29,000.00 before the injury and \$16,000.00 after the injury, her loss becomes real, and demonstrates why loss of earnings capacity is compensable under the law.

Past and Future Physical Impairment

Some of the consequences of the physical injuries that the hypothetical automobile injury victim suffered are not addressed under the heading of physical pain and mental anguish. These include the ability to continue to bowl, hunt, play with grandchildren, cut, edge, and trim the lawn, have sex on a regular and enjoyable basis, and other daily and regular activities. These changes in his life fall under the heading of physical impairment or loss of enjoyment of life.

At least 13 states hold that loss of enjoyment of life or physical impairment is a separate element of damages.[7] Depending on the jurisdiction, one practical consequence may be that the jury will make a separate award for this element of damages. In other words, in the written instructions given to the jury there will be a separate line on which to write in a dollar figure for physical impairment, and another line for physical pain and mental anguish.

Other states and some of the federal courts of appeals hold that this is not a separate element of damages and is to be compensated within the confines of the physical pain and mental anguish area of damages. Some of these jurisdictions allow an instruction to the jury for "pain and suffering and inconvenience including the effect of the injuries upon 'the normal pursuits and pleasures of life.' "[8]

Past and Future Medical Expenses

Assume that the hypothetical auto crash victim was treated conservatively for six months, had a myelogram, CT scan, x rays, EMG, two days of hospitalization, 11 office visits to his orthopaedist, and prescriptions for anti-inflammatory drugs and analgesics. Assume that the total amount of pre-surgical medical bills was \$4000.00, that the surgery and hospitalization cost \$15,000.00, and that up until the time of trial physical therapy and followup doctor visits and medications totalled \$4000.00. Pretrial medical expenses thus total \$23,000.00.

The plaintiff can get these figures before the jury by several methods, but will be required to prove that the medical expenses were causally related to the injuries he received in the accident. Equally important, he must prove that the expenses were reasonable and that the goods and services provided were medically necessary for his care.

If the medical expenses are proved through the testimony of the treating physician, in most jurisdictions the treating physician will be asked several critical and necessary questions to connect the injury and consequential damages. First, he would be asked if the history of the injury as told to him by the patient was consistent with the injuries he has treated. He could also be given a hypothetical situation that sets forth the facts of the accident and subsequent physical complaints and asked if these facts were consistent with the injuries he has treated.

Second, the physician should be asked if he was familiar with the charges in his locale for the treatment that he rendered, if his charges were reasonable in relation to them, and if the treatment he rendered was necessary to the plaintiff's medical well being. He could be asked to detail future medical care and its anticipated cost. This would provide a basis for the jury to find future medical damages. Some states allow the jury to infer from the nature of the injury and the plaintiff's past medical treatment history that he will continue to need medical treatment in the future. Life expectancy tables are used to project the number of years of treatment that would be necessary. Because future medical costs are impossible to prove with exact certainty, the plaintiff need only prove them to the extent that circumstances will allow. The requirements of proof run from proving that there is a reasonable probability that medical expenses will be necessary in the future,[9] to proving a reasonable medical certainty that future medical services will be necessary.[10]

Damages for Disability When the Plaintiff has a Pre-existing Impairment that was Aggravated by the Conduct of the Defendant

The law says that a defendant takes a plaintiff as he finds him. Restated, this means that if an injured individual has a low tolerance for pain, then the responsible party may have to pay more for past and future physical pain than to someone who has a high pain tolerance.

Assume that the warehouse employee of the hypothetical situation in the previous section had a laminectomy and partial discectomy 5 years prior to the automobile injury, and that the automobile injury added instability to his back by injuring the facet joints at the L4-L5 and L5-S1 levels, and that there was a reherniation at the L5-S1 level. Assume that for the previous 5 years the plaintiff, although he had returned to his work as a warehouse worker, did not perform heavy duty work or repetitive physical labor because he had been elected dock steward and thus only drove a forklift. This presents an interesting situation for both plaintiff and defendant. The plaintiff is, of course, going to argue that his future earning capacity has dropped from $13.00 an hour and $110.00 in benefits to roughly $320.00 a week, the amount he would make if he had been forced to enter the competitive job market.

The defendant is in the position to argue that when the plaintiff suffered his original back injury he no longer had the physical capacity to go back to his old job performing full duties in the warehouse because of his impairment, and thus 5 years ago his earnings capacity was lower than he is currently willing to admit. The plaintiff wants the full year's worth of salary he lost, and the defendant wants to pay as little money as possible. The defendant can argue that the real capacity for earnings dropped five years before the defendant injured him. The point is that earnings capacity is not necessarily legally determined by actual earnings.

Assume that the plaintiff, instead of having an injured back from the automobile accident, had a bad knee that had undergone arthroscopic surgery, which left him with some minor limitations of lifting and bending. In most jurisdictions, the jury would be instructed upon request of defense counsel that the defendant was liable for only that part of the increased ill effects caused by the defendant.[11]

Postaccident Aggravation of Injury

In most jurisdictions, the defendant is liable for any subsequent aggravation of an injury when the aggravation is a "proximate result" of the original injury.[12] An example is an injured party who, because of an injury to his foot, subsequently twisted his leg and injured his knee. If the plaintiff was not negligent in his actions, then the defendant would be liable for this injury because it is reasonably foreseeable that this was a natural consequence of the original foot injury.

Subsequent Injury or Aggravation by a Treating Physician

The general rule in tort cases in United States jurisprudence is that a person injured by the tort of another is not entitled to recover damages for any harm that he could have avoided by the use of a reasonable effort or expenditure after the commission of the tort.[13] Restated, the law imposes a duty on the injured party to mitigate damages.

When a reasonable and prudent person would have sought medical treatment but did not do so, the defendant will not be held liable for additional damages the plaintiff visited upon himself. In our hypothetical situation, one could posit the situation in which the plaintiff, even though he had medical insurance, failed to seek treatment for 10 months. At the end of this time he had permanent and irreversible nerve damage to his leg, which could have been avoided by earlier surgery. The defendant, in the written instructions to the jury, would be entitled upon request to an instruction to the jury to not include any amount of money for any condition resulting from the failure of the plaintiff to have acted as a person of ordinary prudence would have under the same or similar circumstances in caring for and treating the injuries that resulted from the occurrence made the basis of the lawsuit.[14]

If, however, the plaintiff instead sought immediate medical treatment and the physician is the one who made his condition worse by giving him a myelogram which caused complications, then the defendant will be held liable for this. This assumes that the physician who administered the myelogram acted as a reasonable and prudent physician would have under the same or similar circumstances. Assuming *arguendo* that no medical malpractice was involved, the untoward consequences of the myelogram were a natural and probable consequence of the original tort-feasor's negligence, and the defendant would be held liable for this additional injury in most jurisdictions. The one qualification to this rule is that the doctor must be selected by the injured party in good faith and with ordinary care. In other words, if the plaintiff picked a doctor with a notorious reputation for slipshod and dangerous work, the defendant would not be held legally responsible for the exacerbation of the plaintiff's condition stemming from this doctor's work.

Assume that the doctor who administered the myelogram had been guilty of negligence. In this case, the defendant would have a defense to the new injury to the plaintiff under the theory that the medical malpractice was an independent and superseding cause, which was not reasonably foreseeable, and for which he should not be held liable. In the majority of American jurisdictions, the defendant could obtain an instruction to the jury on this defensive issue. More simply stated, the defendant probably will not get out from under liability unless the medical provider does something foolish that constitutes serious medical malpractice.

The Plaintiff's Loss of Earnings Capacity After Returning to the Same Job for the Same Pay

When an injured individual returns to the same job with the same pay, his projected loss of earnings capacity remains theoretical until he is placed in the open job market where he has to actively compete for gainful work. The question, which is purely theoretical in this situation, is the amount of earnings *capacity* that has been lost.

In the hypothetical situation we have used throughout this section it is undeniable that the 45-year-old high school graduate with no specialized training and a spinal fusion has few opportunities to match his past earnings given his age, education, residual impairments, past relevant work experience, and lack of transferability of skills, with a job that pays a similar salary, were he to enter the job market anew. In the case of a man who returns to the same job, questions regarding what he could earn in the open market place must be answered by expert testimony, either from a vocational expert, from members of the state employment commission, or from other people whose specialty is employment requirements and opportunities. This is a situation that arises with some regularity in the setting of workers' compensation cases.

The Plaintiff's Duty to Mitigate Damages

It is a universal rule in American jurisprudence that an injured person has a duty to mitigate damages. The injured party will be held to the standard of what a reasonable and prudent person would have done under the same or similar circumstances. The obligation to mitigate damages is not unique to the field of tort law. Those who sue for breach of contract are required to mitigate damages as well. In the field of tort law this means that the injured party must take reasonably good care of his person and continue to earn as much money as he is reasonably capable of.

FEDERAL STATUTORY CAUSES OF ACTION

The FELA and Jones Act cases differ from common law negligence cases significantly in that:

1. For the employer to be liable, it has to play only a slight role in causing injury as opposed to proximately causing injury, which must be proved in common law negligence cases.
2. The Federal Tort Claims Act allows for suit against the government under limited circumstances and does not include intentional torts such as assault, nor discretionary functions of the government.

Federal Employers' Liability Act

The Federal Employers' Liability Act (FELA) was enacted in 1908.[15] FELA covers employees of common carriers engaged in interstate commerce (e.g., railroads), and provides recovery for injury or death caused in whole or in part by the negligence of any of the officers, agents, or employees of common carriers, or for violations of the Safety Appliance Act[16] or the Boiler Inspection Act.[17] When the Safety Appliance Act or the Boiler Inspection Act have been violated contributory negligence by the employee does not diminish his recovery. This is because the duty imposed by the statute is absolute. In other words, there are no excuses for any violation no matter how careful the railroad was.

In common law negligence cases the defendant must proximately cause the injuries to the defendant before being held legally responsible. But in FELA cases, the Supreme Court has ruled that when the employer's negligence played even the slightest role in the causation of the injury to the employee, the defendant is liable.[18] The damages that are recoverable are for mental anguish and physical pain, past and future, loss of past earnings, the reasonable present cash value of future lost earnings capacity, past and future medical expenses, and disfigurement.

The Jones Act

Seamen who are injured or killed in the course of employment are covered by the Jones Act,[19] which incorporates many of the provisions of the FELA. Thus, such defenses as assumption of the risk and injury by a fellow servant do not bar recovery by a seaman or his heirs. When the seaman is contributorily negligent, he is still not barred from receiving damages, but damages are proportionately reduced according to the amount of his contributory negligence.

To be entitled to recover damages under the Jones Act one must be a seaman who is a member of a crew, and thus must be originally on board ship in aid of navigation and have a reasonably permanent connection with the vessel.[20] Longshoremen are generally not individuals who are covered by the Jones Act except when they are performing the traditional activities of a seaman. The ship owner has an absolute and nondelegable duty to provide a seaworthy vessel. This duty extends to equipment on the vessel and its crew. These duties exist independent of all precautions and care taken by the ship owner. The damages under the Jones Act are largely the same as those under FELA cases.

The Federal Tort Claims Act

The Federal Tort Claims Act[21] permits a recovery of monetary damages from the federal government for injury or loss of property, personal injury or death, caused by the negligent or wrongful act or omission of any employee of the government while acting within the scope of his office or employment to the same extent that the United States, if it were a private person, would be liable to the claimant in accordance with the law of the place where the act or omission occurred.[22] These suits may be filed only in federal court.[23]

The interesting aspect of the Federal Tort Claims Act is that the liability of the United States depends upon the substantive law of the state where the wrongful act or omission of the government occurred.[24] An injured person may not sue the government for a variety of intentional torts including assault, battery, false imprisonment, false arrest, malicious prosecution, abuse of process, libel, slander, misrepresentation, or interference with contract rights.[25] However, if an employee is empowered by law to execute searches, to seize evidence, or to make arrests for violation of federal law, the injured party is permitted to file suit for intentional torts sustained during the operation of those persons in the course and scope of their job. Exceptions to liability under the Act include failing to deliver letters and injuries caused by the imposition or establishment of a quarantine by the United States.

DISABILITY IN SOCIAL SECURITY CASES

The Sequential Evaluation of a Social Security Disability Claim

Claimants are entitled to disability benefits under the Social Security Act only under limited circumstances. The claimant must have a severe impairment that meets or equals an impairment listed in the Code of Federal Regulations. This impairment must prevent the claimant from performing past relevant work, or from performing other work, considering the claimant's residual functional capacity.

The Administrative Law Judges (ALJs) who hear Social Security cases after the initial denial by the Social Security Administration do not have the leeway that juries have with personal injury cases in deciding a person's level of disability. The ALJ proceeds through a five-step sequence in order to determine whether or not claimants qualify for Social Security disability benefits. The sequential process is set forth in abbreviated form in Table 45–1.

Table 45–1
The Sequential Process of Determining Disability

1. Is the claimant engaging in substantial gainful activity (i.e., work involving significant physical or mental activities for profit or pay)? If no, then proceed to Step 2.
2. Does the claimant have a severe impairment or combination of impairments? If yes, then proceed to Step 3.
3. Does the severe impairment meet or equal those impairments listed in the Listing of Impairments? (If so, disability is presumed and benefits awarded.)
4. Does the impairment prevent the performance of the claimant's past relevant work activity? If it does, then the government must present evidence to rebut this, or the claimant wins.
5. Is there work in the national economy that the claimant can perform and that exists in significant numbers?

The Social Security rules, as codified in the Code of Federal Regulations (CFR), state two apparently conflicting rules: first, that residual functional capacity is a medical assessment,[26] and second, that the ALJ is responsible for deciding the claimant's amount of residual functional capacity.[27] The residual functional capacity determination is one that is made primarily from the medical symptoms, signs and laboratory results. The medical records in a social security disability case are therefore critical. However, the medical records rarely supply all the information the ALJ needs to make a favorable decision. A narrative from the doctor is necessary to supply all the elements for a favorable finding. In the case of an orthopaedic injury, the narrative should state all of the tests that the doctor saw, such as x rays, CT scans, or discograms, which demonstrate an anatomic impairment and a basis for pain, limitation of movement, and weight lifting limitations. It must further set a limit on the number of pounds the claimant can lift, and the number of hours the claimant can sit and stand on a regular, sustained basis.

Medical-Vocation Guidelines (The Grids)

The Medical-Vocational Guidelines, which are called Appendix 2, Subpart P, (20 C.F.R. §404) are popularly known as the "Grids" (Table 45–2). The Grids have three tables. The first one deals with situations in which the administrative law judge finds that the maximum sustained work ability of the claimant is limited to sedentary work; the second table applies when the residual functional capacity of the claimant is limited to light work; and the third table is related to claimants with a residual functional capacity for medium work.

Sedentary, light, and medium work have specific meanings.[28] Sedentary work involves lifting no more

Table 45–2
Medical-Vocational Guidelines (Grids)

The Medical-Vocational Guidelines (Grids) call for a finding of disabled, and therefore entitle the claimant to disability benefits under the following situations: Individuals Limited to Sedentary Work as a Result of Severe Medically Determinable Impairment(s)

Age	*Evaluation*	*Previous Work Experience*	*Decision*
Advanced age (55 or older)	Limited or less	Unskilled	Disabled
Advanced age	High School graduate or more, but does not provide for direct entry into skilled work	Unskilled or none	Disabled
Advanced age	High School graduate or more, but does not provide for direct entry into skilled work	Skilled or semiskilled, but skills not transferable	Disabled
Closely approaching advanced age (49–54)	Limited or less	Unskilled or none	Disabled
Closely approaching advanced age (49–54)	High School graduate or more, but does not provide for direct entry into skilled work	Unskilled or none	Disabled
Closely approaching advanced age (49–54)	High School graduate or more, but does not provide for direct entry into skilled work	Skilled or semiskilled, but skills not transferable	Disabled
Younger individual	Illiterate or unable to communicate in English	Unskilled or none	Disabled
Individuals Limited to Light Work as a Result of Severe Medically Determinable Impairment(s)			
Advanced age	Limited or less	Unskilled or none	Disabled
Advanced age	Limited or less	Skilled or semiskilled, but skills not transferable	Disabled
Advanced age	High School graduate or more, but does not provide for direct entry into skilled work	Unskilled or none	Disabled
Closely approaching advanced age (49–54)	Illiterate or unable to communicate in English	Unskilled or none	Disabled

than 10 pounds at a time, and occasionally lifting or carrying articles such as docket files, ledgers, and small tools. Jobs are sedentary if walking and standing are required occasionally and other criteria are met. Work must be performed primarily in a seated position and entail no significant stooping. The general rule is that most unskilled sedentary jobs require use of the hands and fingers for repetitive hand-finger action. Standing is required "occasionally," and the periods of standing or walking should generally total no more than two hours of an eight-hour work day.

Light work is defined as lifting no more than 20 pounds at a time with frequent lifting or carrying objects weighing up to 10 pounds. If prolonged walking or standing is required the job becomes light work as opposed to the "occasional" ambulatory requirement of sedentary work. If some pushing and pulling of arm/hand or leg/foot controls is called for that requires greater exertion than in sedentary work, such as mattress sewing or machine or motor-grader operating, then the job qualifies as light work. Few unskilled light jobs are performed in a seated position. "Frequent" means occurring from one-third to two-thirds of the time. Thus, to be eligible to perform light work, the claimant must be able to stand or walk, off and on, for a total of approximately six hours of an eight-hour work day. The lifting requirements for the majority of light jobs can be accomplished with occasional, rather than frequent stooping. Because many light jobs are performed in one location, the ability to stand may be more critical than the ability to walk. These jobs require the use of arms and hands to grasp, hold, and turn objects, and generally do not require the use of fingers to perform fine motor skill activities.

Medium work is defined as a job requiring the lifting of no more than 50 pounds at a time with frequent lifting and carrying of objects weighing up to 25 pounds. The full range of medium work requires standing or walking, off and on, for a total of approximately six hours in an eight-hour work day, as well as the aforementioned lifting requirements. Sitting may occur intermittently during the remaining time. The use of arms and hands is necessary to grasp, hold, and turn objects, as opposed to the finer activities of much kinds of sedentary work, which require the precise use of the fingers as well as the use of the hands and arms. Frequent bending and stooping is required to perform the full range of medium work. The ability to frequently lift or carry objects weighing up to 25 pounds is often more critical than the ability to lift up to 50 pounds at a time.[29]

Each Grid has four components. They are the maximum exertion level, age, education, both remote and recent, and previous work experience. The Grids act like a flow chart and direct the administrative law judge where to proceed upon making or failing to make a finding for each category. For example, if the claimant has a residual functional capacity for light work, this means that the second table is applicable. If the claimant is 54 years old, which is defined as "closely approaching advanced age," has less than a high school education, and a past relevant work experience of unskilled medium work, then although it is conclusive that he can no longer perform his former work, he would be denied benefits because of a presumed ability to perform some type of sedentary work. However, if the same person were illiterate in English, then the flow chart would direct a finding of disabled. Similarly, if the individual were 55 years old, which qualifies as advanced age, he would receive benefits under the Grids.

For Social Security purposes the fact that an individual cannot perform his past relevant work does not mean that he is unemployable. The question for the Social Security ALJ is whether the work skills acquired from past relevant work are transferrable to a significant number of other jobs. The applicable Social Security regulations[30] provide that transferability is most probable in jobs that require the same or a lesser degree of skill, use the same or similar tools and machines, and involve the same or similar raw materials, products, processes, or services.

The most important Social Security ruling[31] on transferability states that all functional limitations included in the residual functional capacity, both exertional and nonexertional, must be considered in determining transferability of previously acquired work skills. An exertional limitation, for example, may prevent the claimant from operating machinery or using tools associated with primary work activities of his or her past relevant work. Similarly, environmental, manipulative, postural, or mental limitations may prevent a claimant from performing semiskilled or skilled work activities necessary for a job. The examples given by the Social Security Administration are a watchmaker who has hand tremors, a house painter who has a severe allergic reaction to paint fumes, a craftsman who has lost proper hand-eye coordination, a construction equipment operator whose back impairments will not permit the return to work in equipment with no suspension, or a business executive who suffers brain damage that notably lowers his IQ. For individuals who are 55 or older, who are limited to sedentary work exertion, and who possess skills that are transferable to other occupations, the rule is that little, if any, vocational adjustment must be required in terms of tools, work processes, work settings, or industry. The same is true for individuals who are age 60 or older and are limited to light work exertion.

DISABILITY AND WORKERS' COMPENSATION

When a worker is injured in the course and scope of his employment and suffers damage or harm to the physical structure of his body, this triggers a workers' compensation claim. The insurance company that provides workers' compensation coverage (termed "the carrier") is obligated after an initial waiting period of typically 1 to 2 weeks to provide both reasonable and necessary medical benefits to the injured worker, and a certain percentage of the average weekly wage of the employee in weekly benefits, with a certain maximum dollar figure set by the legislature.

In an era of tort reform, a lot of theories are tossed around concerning the origin and purpose of workers' compensation. Workers' compensation began in Prussia in 1884, and was quickly instituted in other industrialized countries such as England (1897), France (1898), Italy (1898), and Belgium (1903). In the United States, the first major workers' compensation act was passed in New York, modeled largely after the 1897 British legislation. By the end of 1911, 10 more states had passed workers' compensation legislation, including New Jersey, Ohio, California, and Massachusetts. Other states followed suit quickly thereafter, such as Texas in 1913. Although some today think that the system promotes time away from work and inflicts a massive and unfair burden for the employer, a review of the history of workers' compensation and of its present day consequences may relieve some prejudices.

When workers' compensations statutes were originally enacted any contributory negligence by the employee was a complete defense to the employer for any injuries received. For example, no matter how lax or dangerous the premises or working conditions of the employer were, if the employee was even 1% negligent, the employer had a complete defense. When the workers' compensation statutes were enacted manufacturing jobs took a heavy toll on the human body. It was a period when there was little or no job protection, except for the occasional union contract, no federal or state statutes regarding handicapped hiring, and no safety regulations, such as those propounded by OSHA. Although today many people still have no job protection, most workers' compensation acts provide protection for the worker who files a workers' compensation claim. The acts provide that filing a claim cannot be used as a pretextual reason for firing the employee.

The employer gets certain benefits from the purchase of a worker's compensation policy. Specifically, the employer has purchased insurance that is obligated to pay the entire amount of medical bills that the employer might otherwise have been obligated to pay if it were negligent. Moreover, and more important, the employer escapes common law liability for its negligence, such as providing unsafe tools or dangerous working conditions.

Are there drawbacks for the worker? Many times there are. Assume, for example, that the worker had a $15.00 per hour job as a machine press operator, but had to work with a machine press that had no mechanism or guards to protect his hands from the crushing force of the press. Assume that one day the worker, in order to meet the productivity levels required by the employer, lost both hands in the press, and that he was the fifth worker to do so that year. Unless the worker could sue the manufacturer of the machine in a products liability case, the only remedy provided by law for the worker is to collect his workers' compensation benefits. The employer is immune from suit because it purchased insurance. In all probability this worker will be unemployable and the money he receives for workers' compensation will be only a small fraction of what he could have received had he been able to sue his employer in common law negligence for providing unsafe machinery. Clearly, in this instance, it is cheaper to purchase workers' compensation insurance than to be sued by an employee and be exposed to a work life's worth of lost wages, medical care, and the physical pain and mental anguish associated with this traumatic loss.

In the states where workers' compensation coverage is not mandatory upon employers and the employee is injured, the law provides that the employer loses virtually all common law defenses should it be sued, the most important being any contributory negligence of the employee (Table 45–3).

MEDICAL IMPAIRMENT VS. ECONOMIC WAGE LOSS: COMPETING THEORIES OF COMPENSATION

Within the field of workers' compensation there exists a real tension both in theory and in practice regarding individuals who have similar injuries with different results in their work life. For example, the warehouse employee discussed in the previous section who returned to his company earning the same

Table 45–3
The Common Law Contrasted with Workers' Compensation

	Common Law	Workers' Compensation System
Employee negligence	If the employee is negligent, no recovery. Modified by introduction of comparative negligence.	As long as the employee doesn't intentionally injure himself, insurance pays benefits.
Employer negligence	Employee can sue.	Employer immune from suit.
Damages	Lost wages, loss of earnings capacity, pain and suffering, medical expenses, physical impairment, disfigurement are all items of damages.	Employee entitled only to weekly benefits, medical treatment, and such disability benefits that are set by statute.
Adversarial vs. administrative	Common law tort cases are purely adversarial.	In most states administrative guidelines are administered by a state agency. The appeals are limited in scope. The process is less adversarial, although the claimant is dealing with an insurance company desiring to make a profit underwriting workers' compensation.

wages provides a good example. If the theory behind compensation is actual wage loss, then he would be entitled to no money even though he underwent a back operation solely because of a job injury. But if loss of earnings capacity is the test, what should the man get? He is earning the same wages because of the job protection he had under a union contract coupled with his good fortune in getting elected dock steward and driving a forklift as opposed to moving freight by hand all day. His doctor says that his postoperative condition is such that repetitive physical activities involving lifting, twisting and bending are not possible. Because of this man's age, education, residual functional capacity, and lack of transferability of skills to a more sedentary and skilled job, his current value on the open job market is a fraction of what it was prior to the injury.

Another variation is the individual who, through courage and determination, returns to a job that is more physically demanding than is reasonable for him to be expected to perform. Yet, he does the job to feed his family and to maintain his dignity. It would assuredly be unfair to penalize this person because he has returned to his old job and is making the same wages as he did preinjury.

By way of contrast, one must include in these examples the worker who has a back injury and who misses work for such an extended period of time that his position is filled with a younger worker. Assuming that this worker is over 45 years old and has a past relevant work experience of unskilled to semi-skilled jobs that called upon the use of his physical strength, this man will have a difficult time obtaining a job. The reasons are several. First, he is over 40 applying for work involving demanding and repetitive physical labor and he has to compete with younger uninjured workers. Second, many job applications inquire about both previous work-related and nonwork-related injuries. A truthful applicant in this situation will be relegated to progressively lower paying and less skilled jobs with few or no benefits, such as health insurance and pension contributions. In other words, one finds side by side people who have serious impairments but little or no loss of actual wages, and those with vague diagnoses (e.g., lumbar syndrome) and nonsurgical problems, but who suffer large economic consequences in the labor market.

The general rule throughout America is that the award to the claimant is based upon a comparison between actual earnings preinjury, and the earnings capacity postinjury. Therefore, actual wages after the injury are not determinative of the amount of earnings capacity. The example of the dock worker turned forklift driver shows why. Because of this rule, the fact finder, be it a jury, judge, or adminis-

trative body, can legitimately make a finding that the claimant has suffered a large loss of earnings capacity even though he may be making more money after the injury.

If the system was based on actual wages it would be arguable that the claimant who made more money after an injury because he switched jobs, for example, would owe money to the insurance carrier because the injury ultimately put him in a better financial posture. However, there is a growing trend away from the correlation between awards based on loss of earnings capacity. A move is underway toward recoveries based on percentages of bodily impairment. This system more or less conclusively presumes that a certain percentage of impairment, irrespective of past relevant work, age, and education, translates into an equitable award to replace what the wage earner has lost. The premise is questionable at best, but presumably makes for an easier administrative process because all one need do to calculate the compensation amount is plug the impairment rating from the physician into a formula.

Typical of this scheme are Florida and California. In California, for injuries that occur before 1992, if a person has a permanent disability incurred of, for example, 30 to 49.75%, he will receive 6 weeks of workers' compensation benefits (two-thirds of the average weekly wage) for each percentage of disability.[32] The Florida statute uses the word impairment rather than disability, and specifically refers to the *Guides to the Evaluation of Permanent Impairment* as the final say of the impairment ratings, pending adoption of a permanent schedule.[33]

One should remember that in receiving workers' compensation coverage the worker has given up any right to sue his employer, no matter how negligent the employer may have been. When the claimant returns to the same or better job and manages his life well the tradeoff is beneficial. When he is permanently relegated to a lower paying job with fewer benefits, he has given up much more than he has gained.

Injuries to Specific Bodily Members

An interesting aspect of workers' compensation is that most states provide for specific payments for injuries to, or losses of, various bodily members, e.g., fingers, arms, legs. These payments occur regardless of the claimant's work status, wage losses, or loss of earnings capacity, past or future. The theory is that certain losses have an absolute fixed value, such as the loss of an arm is worth so many weeks of compensation. This is generally true in most states whether or not they have an impairment-based award system or loss of earnings capacity system. The underlying presumption necessarily is that all body parts are worth the same to all people. The driving force behind the law is administrative convenience and economic efficiency.

A farm worker who loses his left little finger might lose a week or so of work and get a windfall from this loss. If a symphony pianist had the same loss because of a tuba falling on and severing his little finger, the result would be devastating. Still, with few exceptions, this is the law.

Originally, most state statutes provided for payment only for total loss of a bodily member. The injustices occasioned by this rigidity gave way to payments for a percentage of loss of use of that member. This has naturally led to a war of numbers and contest of experts.

When the effects of the injury to a specific member extend to and affect other parts of the body the schedule award is no longer applicable. An example would be a hand injury that caused a reflex sympathetic dystrophy. Here the strict schedule would not apply because the injury had extended to the torso.

Proving Loss of Earnings Capacity

One of the two most contested areas in workers' compensation is how much earnings capacity has, in fact, been lost. The other area is the extent and duration of a claimant's impairment. The hypothetical examples given previously provide some insight into the types of issues and situations that arise.

The framework used by the Social Security Administration in deciding the factors that are important in evaluating disability are not only useful, but are also the theoretical underpinnings of most employment experts' opinions. Age, residual functional capacity, transferability of skills, education level, and past relevant work experience are the factors that provide a basis for demonstrating a person's ability to obtain and maintain employment in the job market.

The Practical Effects of Surgery

It is both fortunate and unfortunate that orthopaedic surgery improves a claimant's opportunity for a larger recovery. It is fortunate because the claimant has had his body cut and his chances of getting another job that requires any physical exertion may well be diminished. It is unfortunate because the weakest parts of the system (doctors and lawyers who put their bank accounts ahead of the welfare of the patient or client) take advantage of this fact.

Adjusters, who hold the purse strings of the insurance companies, almost universally view a claimant who has undergone surgery as someone who has a case with more merit than someone who did not have surgery but is otherwise similarly situated. The reasons for this strong bias in the system are several. The first is that everyone is looking in the rearview mirror to times when operations cured one problem but left another just as great, when physical rehabilitation was up to the patient, and when less may have been expected of someone who had a serious operation. Time and medical advances have not made this bias obsolete or unreasonable, but it does cause discrimination against those who, wisely or not, elect not to have surgery. The second reason is that deep in the psyche we associate the violation of a person's body with the surgeon's tools as something called for in grave situations. The case will always stay in the shadow of the operation.

In personal injury cases, surgery enhances the case value because the doctors' and hospital bills amount to so much money. Adjusters tend to think of settling cases in terms of multiples of the monies actually expended or lost (e.g., lost wages). Such evidence as the claimant can marshall in each area is helpful to prove his case.

END NOTES

1. See, for example, 22 Am.Jur. 2d Damages (1988); 25, 25A C.J.S. Damages (1966).
2. Restatement (Second) of Torts §282 (1965).
3. P.H.N. Wood, E.M. Bradley, *People With Disabilities-Toward Acquiring Information Which Reflects More Sensitively Their Problems and Needs,* Word Rehabilitation Fund (New York, 1980).
4. *Fudge v. City of Kansas City,* 720 P.2d 1093 (Kan.1986).
5. *Vital Statistics of the United States,* 1980, Life Tables, Volume II, Section 6 (1984) (Department of Health and Human Services Publication Number PHS 84-1104).
6. *Robinson v. Greely and Hansen,* 114 Ill. App. 3d 720, 449 N.E.2d 250 (1983).
7. The states are Colorado, Florida, Georgia, Indiana, Maryland, Michigan, Minnesota, Nebraska, New Jersey, New York, Tennessee, Texas and Washington.
8. See, for example, *Grunenthal v. Long Island R. Co.,* 388 F.2d 480, reversed on other grounds, 393 U.S. 156 (2d Cir. 1968).
9. *Keller Industries, Inc. v. Reeves,* 656 S.W.2d 221 (Tex. App.-Austin 1983, writ ref'd n.r.e.).
10. *Calavera v. Vix,* 356 N.W. 2d 901 (N.D.1984).
11. See, for example, *Sterrett v. East Texas Motor Frt. Lines,* 236 S.W.2d 776 (Tex.1951).
12. *City of Port Arthur v. Wallace,* 171 S.W. 2d 480 (Tex. 1943).
13. Restatement (2nd) of Torts §918(1) (1979).
14. 1 State Bar of Texas, Texas Pattern Jury Charges §7.09 (1988).
15. 45 U.S.C. §§51-60 (1982).
16. 45 U.S.C. §116 (1982).
17. 45 U.S.C. §§22-34 (1982).
18. *Gallick v. Baltimore & Ohio R.R. Co.,* 372 U.S. 108 (1963).

19. 46 U.S.C. §688 (Supp. 1989).
20. *Senko v. LaCrosse Dredging Company*, 352 U.S. 370 (1957).
21. 28 U.S.C. §§2671-2680 (1976).
22. 28 U.S.C. §1346(b) (1976).
23. *Richards v. U.S.*, 369 U.S. 1 (1962).
24. 28 U.S.C. §2680(a) (1965).
25. 28 U.S.C. §2680(h) (Supp.1987).
26. 20 C.F.R. §404.1545(a).
27. 20 C.F.R. §404.1546.
28. 20 C.F.R. §404.1567(a) (b) (c).
29. Vocational Experts—Testifying at Disability Hearings: A Self Study Guide (SSA Pub. No. 70-009, 1987). PP. 67–70. SSR 83–10.
30. 20 C.F.R. §404.1568.
31. SSR 82-41.
32. CAL. LAB. CODE §4658 (West, Supp.1990).
33. FLA. STAT. ANN. §440.15 (3)(a)3. (West, Supp.1989).

James R. Fricton
Andrew Nelson
Matthew Monsein
David Florence

46

Assessment of Pain in Disability Determination

Pain, by definition, is an unpleasant subjective experience of hurt that is perceived or felt only by the individual. Because of this subjectivity and the lack of reliable physiologic techniques for measurement, pain is difficult to prove, disprove, or quantify. As a result, many physicians find pain difficult to assess when determining the severity of a condition in disability determination and, therefore, primarily consider objective medical findings, such as radiographic changes or neurologic abnormalities, in determination of impairment for disability compensation. In many chronic pain states, particularly soft tissue pain, complaints of pain are often not fully corroborated by objective medical findings and are complicated by significant behavioral and psychosocial problems. Although the functioning of these individuals can be severely affected by the pain, the inability to objectively validate the severity of their disorder prevents an accurate appraisal of their functional status. Consequently, some patients with complaints of chronic pain are unfairly labeled as malingerers or as having a psychiatric disorder, and denied disability benefits; others who purposefully complain excessively and exhibit exaggerated pain behavior receive compensation. This situation has created unfairness, complaints, and increased litigation in both the Social Security Administration and the workers' compensation disability programs.

The purpose of this chapter is to discuss pain and its implications for the disability determination process of the Social Security Administration (SSA) and workers' compensation and to propose new methods for collecting data to clarify the patient's allegations of pain and its effect on work capacity in an effort to be more fair and efficient.

CHRONIC PAIN AND DISABILITY

In both the workers' compensation and SSA programs, the problem of chronic pain has caused many problems and significant costs. In the workers' compensation system, the majority of benefits are paid to a minority of injured workers with permanent disability. For example, in Minnesota, 80% of loss dollars are paid to less than 6% of claimants, most of whom have chronic back pain.[1] The vast majority of the permanency claims involve injured workers who fall under the category of delayed recovery syndrome. In this situation, the worker, often with a work-related back injury, does not improve with standard treatment. The primary care doctor and other specialists find no objective evidence of a continuing physical problem. Yet, the worker continues to complain of severe pain and insists that he could not work with this pain. If the worker is eventually denied benefits, and still cannot work, he or she can apply for Social Security disability. In 1984, 1.5 million claimants applied for Social Security Disability. Of these, 82 thousand claimants suffered from what was defined as a "chronic pain syndrome."[2] In other words, these individuals claimed that they were unable to work, or perform normal physical, social, or emotional functions because of pain. In these cases, no medically determinable condition could be found sufficient for the complaints of pain. Many of these claimants contend that the pain is real and causes disability. This has resulted in many appeals, litigation, and inefficiencies in the SSA disability determination system. To better understand the underlying factors responsible for claimants with a delayed recovery syndrome, a discussion of the characteristics of chronic pain syndrome is necessary.

Acute pain is self-limiting and temporary, has a specific observable cause and purpose, and generally has no persisting psychologic reactions. Chronic pain, on the other hand, is not self-limiting, appears to be permanent, serves no discernable biologic purpose, and can involve multiple psychosocial problems that confound the patient and clinician and perpetuate the problem.[3-6] A patient may feel helpless, hopeless, and desperate in his inability to obtain relief. Such patients may become hypochondriacally obsessed and worried about any symptom or sensation they perceive in their bodies. Vegetative symptoms and overt depression may set in, with sleep and appetite disturbances. Irritability, confusion, and mood fluctuations are common. Loss of self-esteem, libido, and interest in life's activities add to the patient's misery. All this may erode personal relationships with family, friends, and health professionals. Patients may focus much of their energy on analyzing and alleviating the pain problem and believe that it is the cause of all their problems. They shop from doctor to doctor, desperately searching for an organic or external cure. They can become belligerent, hostile, and manipulative in seeking care, particularly to obtain analgesics for their sole periods of relief. Many clinicians make gallant attempts with multiple drug regimens, extensive physical therapy, or multiple surgical procedures, but failure frustrates the clinician and adds to the patient's ongoing depression while adding dependencies or the potential for complications.

Near the end of this progression, many patients with chronic pain, in addition to their pain problem, can experience multiple drug dependencies, high stress levels, loss of relationships, loss of vocation, impaired ability to perform social or recreational functions, involvement in litigation, and permanent disability, much of which is iatrogenically produced. In addition to these unfortunate personal consequences, chronic pain is a significant societal problem because of the high costs of health care and disability benefits associated with it. Bonica has estimated that chronic pain costs our society over 60 billion in lost wages, health care, and medication.[7]

Because pain is assumed to be a symptom of an underlying disease, determining the source of the pain using objective medical tests has been the subject of much debate. Most authors contend that the majority of chronic pain is musculoskeletal in nature.[8,9] In studies of back pain, imaging studies have been found to be an unreliable marker of chronic musculoskeletal pain. For example, both MRI and CT studies of individuals with no back symptoms often demonstrate signs of disc degeneration and herniation. In a British study, over one-third of 100 asymptomatic women seen in a gynecology clinic were found to have degenerative discs.[10] In another study, three neuroradiologists reviewed CAT scans of the lumbar spine in 52 asymptomatic people with no history of back trouble and found that overall 35.4% of these asymptomatic individuals were noted to have a herniated disc, spinal stenosis, or facet degeneration.[11] The patients over 40 years of age (N = 26) showed a 50% abnormal rate. In this study, the range of abnormal findings varied from 30% from the first radiologist to over 80% from the second radiologist, further indicating the problems of unreliability in interpreting these findings. Likewise, other studies question the reliability of physical examination findings.[12,13] This is particularly true for nonneurologic findings such as tenderness and the presence or absence of "spasm."

Thus, patients with abnormal findings can and do function well, whereas others with little in the way of physical or x ray findings claim to be seriously disabled. This well known and currently unquantifiable situation is the crux of the controversy with chronic pain and is the source of much of the confusion in disability determination and the assessment of patients with chronic pain. At present, disability systems in the United States have dealt with this dilemma by relying almost totally on clinical rather than functional data, the assumption being that the former is more objective.

This confusion is particularly evident in patients with soft tissue pain such as myofascial pain (MFP) and fibromyalgia. These muscular pain disorders have been cited as the most common diagnoses associated with chronic pain. For example, Fishbain, et al.,[14] found MPS to be the primary diagnosis in 85% of 283 consecutive patients presenting to a chronic pain clinic. In a study of 296 consecutive chronic head and neck pain patients, 55.4% had a primary diagnosis of MFP whereas only 21% had a joint disorder.[15] Yet, in contrast to joint disorders, MFP has no truly objective clinical findings to confirm its presence.[16] A diagnosis of MFP is established based on three criteria: (1) The presence of pain. (2) Tender spots (termed trigger points) in taut bands of skeletal muscles that correspond to the area of pain. (3) Reproducible alteration of the pain referral with specific palpation of the trigger point. This third criteria is present only in muscles that are accessible to palpation.[15]

Currently, only a few tests can be used to measure the objective characteristics of MFP. Pressure algometry can be used to reliably determine the pain threshold of trigger points and holds promise to lend objectivity to the diagnosis of MFP (Fig. 46–1). A number of studies have supported the reliability and validity of pressure algometry for use with MFP assessment but further research is necessary to determine its sensitivity and specificity in diagnosis without relying on patient report.[14,15] Thermography also has been proposed to confirm alterations in skin temperature associated with trigger points or referral zones but its reliability and validity as a diagnostic test for MFP has not yet been established.[19–21] However, there is much evidence that MFP begins with trauma or muscle strain, often becomes chronic, and can be quite severe and disabling.[7,22–24] It is this group of patients who fall into the category of a delayed recovery syndrome.[25,26]

Workers with delayed recovery syndrome caused

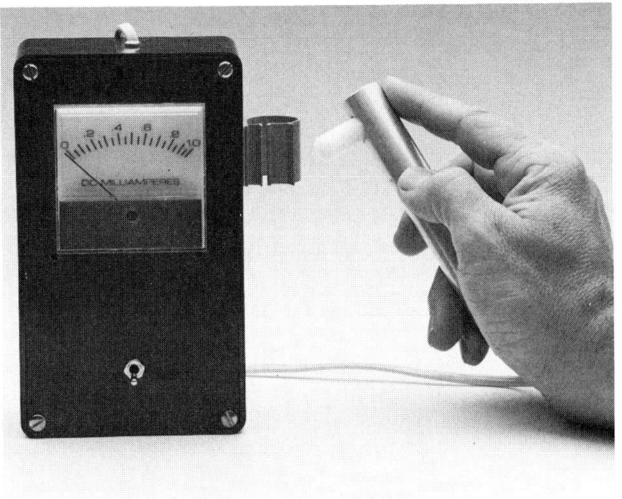

Figure 46–1. Presure algometry can be used to determine the pain threshold of trigger points. It holds promise to lend objectivity to the diagnosis of MPS.

by MFP or other pain disorders with no established objective findings are a heavy burden to both the workers' compensation and the SSA disability programs. Many of these injured workers receive extensive benefits from workers' compensation because of pain, yet have no structural impairment that prevents them from working. Much criticism has been directed at state workers' compensation review boards to revise laws to encourage a more detailed and fair assessment of whether these people can work or not and, if they can work, to help them get back to work.

In the SSA, these people are typically denied disability but have created considerable controversy and expense resulting from litigation and political pressure in an effort to receive benefits. In response to these efforts, the United States Congress passed an amendment to mandate assessment of pain and its effects on the SSA disability determination process. Despite these criticisms and changes, neither system (SSA or workers' compensation) has a mechanism to efficiently and routinely complete comprehensive reliable assessments of clients to describe their characteristics, risk factors, and functional and health status.

To help improve this situation, the disability determination process of the Social Security Administration and many workers' compensation programs is being amended to consider alternative approaches and data collection methods for providing more fair and objective data for assessing pain and functional status in these patients. Assessment instruments are being completed to identify risk factors in the work place that can cause injury or lead to the development of a delayed recovery syndrome if injured.

With this information, comprehensive worker safety programs can target specific risk factors and rehabilitation programs can be designed to be more effective in returning a patient to work. In addition, comprehensive assessment instruments have recently been developed to standardize detailed illness and medical histories and reliably measure claimant characteristics, functional status, and well being. Physicians, claim examiners, adjudicators, employers, insurance companies, and government officials can monitor individual cases more accurately and consistently and improve the fairness and cost effectiveness of the decisions made. These new developments are discussed for the SSA and workers' compensation systems.

SOCIAL SECURITY ADMINISTRATION POLICY

The difficulty of providing a standardized disability determination process with consideration of pain is evidenced in the Social Security Administration (SSA) disability programs, Social Security Disability Insurance (SSDI), and the Supplemental Security Income (SSI), provided for under Title II and Title XVI, respectively, of the Social Security Act. The Social Security Disability Insurance is an earned benefit available to the worker and his dependents. This is paid from the Social Security Disability Trust Fund and the payment is computed based on past earnings. The average monthly SSDI benefit in 1987 was $492 for individuals and $922 for workers with spouse and children. In the Supplemental Security Income (SSI) program, monthly payments are provided based on needs and not as an earned right. There are no work requirements and the payment is set by law. In 1987, the average SSI payment was $251 per month for an individual. However, individuals receiving SSI must meet the disability definitions. SSI is designed to provide minimum income for the needy, aged, blind, and disabled.[27]

Both Social Security disability programs define disability as "the inability to engage in *any* substantial gainful activity, by reason of a *medically determinable* physical or mental *impairment*, which can be expected to result in death, or has lasted, or can be expected to last, for a continuous period of not less than 12 months."

Furthermore, a "physical or mental impairment" is further defined as that which would result from anatomic, physiologic, or psychologic abnormalities that can be shown by *medically acceptable* clinical and laboratory techniques and which, by regulation, must be established by *medical evidence* consisting of symptoms, signs, and laboratory findings.

The regulations define *symptoms* as the claimant's own perception of his or her physical or mental impairments. *Signs* are anatomic, physiologic, or psychologic abnormalities that can be observed through the use of *medically acceptable* clinical techniques. In psychiatric impairments, signs are medically demonstrable abnormalities of behavior, affect, attitude, memory, orientation, and awareness of reality. *Laboratory findings* are manifestations of anatomic, physiologic, or psychologic phenomena demonstrable by replacing or extending the perceptiveness of the observers senses. These include chemical, electrophysiological, imaging, or psychometric tests.

Regulations require that an orderly adjudication process be followed in determining whether an individual meets the definition of disability. This process is called a sequential evaluation process (SEP) and is applicable to the initial entitlement decision. This process has five steps and is completed by the Disability Determination Services (DDS) examiner and medical consultant team including a claim examiner who compiles evidence and a consulting physician who reviews it. A determination of "not disabled" can be made purely on the basis that the individual does not meet one of the factors in the basic definition of disability. The five steps they use to determine disability are.

Step 1

Is the individual currently engaging in substantial gainful activity? This refers to work for pay or profit and is generally evaluated using earning guidelines set forth by regulations. If the individual is not engaging in substantial gainful activity, the examiner must proceed to Step 2.

Step 2

Does the individual have a severe impairment? An individual's impairment and its effect on the ability to perform basic work activities are reviewed at this step. Basic work activities involve the capacity for sitting, standing, walking, lifting, pushing, pulling, handling, seeing, hearing, communicating, understanding, and following simple instructions. If an impairment is found to be not severe, the claim is denied on medical grounds alone without consideration of any additional information such as vocational factors. If the impairment is found to be severe, the examining team must proceed to Step 3.

Step 3

Does the individual have an impairment that meets or equals the listing? The listing of impairments is a compilation of disabling impairments categorized by the major body system. The level of severity is specified in terms of medical signs, symptoms, and findings for each impairment listed.

An individual is said to "meet the listing" when the medical evidence in the file substantiates *all* of the signs, symptoms, and findings called for in a listing. When a finding is made that an individual "meets" a listing, it means that in the absence of substantial gainful work activity, a finding of disability can be made on the basis of medical evidence alone. Conversely, if all criteria are not present, then the individual cannot "meet" the listing. An individual may be found to be disabled on the basis of medical factors alone if the level of severity and duration of the individual's impairments as shown by the signs, symptoms, and findings equal the level of severity and duration of a listed impairment. The DDS medical consultant must make the decision regarding whether the impairment is equal in severity to a listed impairment even if the individual's impairment does not meet or equal criteria of a listed impairment. If impairment is found to meet or equal a listing, the claim is paid on a medical basis alone. If not, the process proceeds to Step 4.

Step 4

Does the individual have residual functional capacity to perform past relevant work? In this step, vocational factors are considered. The residual functional capacity assessment is made to determine the individual's capacity to perform the physical or mental functions of work, despite any limitations caused by medically determinable impairment. Strength, ability to walk, sit, stand, and lift are included in the assessment of the individual's maximum residual functional capacity for sustained activity on a regular basis. Other significant physical functions and sensory characteristics such as seeing, hearing, speaking, exertional functions, and nonexertional limitations (e.g., understand, carry out, remember instructions, and work with coworkers) are also assessed. The capacity to perform past relevant work is usually a sufficient basis for finding that the individual is not disabled. However, if the individual is determined to be unable to perform his past relevant work the examining team must proceed to Step 5.

Step 5

Does the individual have residual functional capacity to perform other work? The inability to perform past relevant work is not in itself a basis for finding a disability. A person who is functionally and vocationally qualified to engage in substantial gainful activity in other work may not be found disabled if the range of work for which he or she is functionally and vocationally suited is sufficiently broad and such jobs exist in significant numbers in the patient's geographic region. To determine the

                                                                                        553

exertional requirements of work, jobs are defined as sedentary, light, medium, heavy, and very heavy. These definitions for classifying the exertional levels are found in the *Dictionary of Occupational Titles*, published by the Department of Labor. Occupations are classified as unskilled, semiskilled, and skilled. In Step 5, along with the residual functional capacity, the individual's age, education, and work experience are taken into consideration. Previous educational level, work experience, age, and the inability to adapt to other work situations also are considered at this level.

Claimants may request reconsideration of a claim denial. This reconsideration is processed through the sequential evaluation process by a different DDS examiner or medical consultant team. A second reconsideration is heard by an administrative law judge. The third level of a claims appeal is heard by the Appeals Council. Denials by the US District Court (fourth level), US Circuit Court (fifth level), and a final appeal are passed on to the Supreme Court.

Current law and SSA policy consider pain important in the disability determination process only if: (1) the claimant has a medically determinable physical or mental impairment that is established by medically acceptable clinical or laboratory diagnostic techniques such as sensory changes, reflex changes, electromyography, and radiographs, and (2) the medically determinable impairment could reasonably be expected to produce the alleged pain.[28] This situation essentially eliminates most patients with myofascial pain syndrome regardless of functional status, unless a concomitant joint or other structural disorder is present.

However, when medical findings do not substantiate physical impairment capable of producing the alleged pain, the possibility of a mental impairment as the basis for the pain can also be investigated. However, few patients with chronic pain have a clinically apparent psychiatric disorder. Only when a medically determinable physical or mental impairment is documented, can the effects of the pain be considered in each step of the sequential evaluation process as described by the SSA and outlined here.[29]

Is the Condition Severe?

To be found disabled, an individual must have a medically determinable severe impairment. To be considered severe, the impairment, or combination of impairments, must have more than a minimal effect on the individual's ability to do basic work activities. In determining whether an impairment is severe, consideration is given to all material evidence, including signs, symptoms (such as pain), and laboratory findings. When the degree of pain reported is consistent with a level that can reasonably be associated with the objective findings presented, the conclusion that the impairment is severe is based on a determination that the evidence, including the alleged pain, establishes that the individual's ability to do basic work activities is significantly limited. However, when the degree of pain is significantly greater than that which can be reasonably anticipated based on the objective findings, such as the case with severe myofascial pain with mild joint disorder, the pain must be shown to produce additional limitations on the individual's functional ability beyond those limitations indicated by the objective findings before any conclusions about severity can be reached.

Are the Findings about the Individual's Impairment Identical to and, thus, Meet Those in the Listing?

Disability may be established on a medical basis alone if the characteristics of an impairment meet the criteria cited in the Listing of Impairments. Some listed impairments include symptoms among the requisite criteria. For example, listing 1.04 requires a history of joint pain and stiffness.[29] When a symptom, such as pain, appears as a criterion, it is necessary that the symptom be present only in combination with the remaining criteria. Unless specifically indicated (as in Listing 1.04, which requires that abduction of both arms at the shoulders, including scapular motion, be restricted to less than 90°), quantification or evaluation of the intensity, or the functionally limiting effects, of that symptom is not required to determine whether the documented findings meet the requisite criteria.

Do the Findings about the Individual's Impairment Equal Those for the Impairment in the Listing?

In considering whether documented findings and symptoms are equivalently severe to the requisite findings and symptoms of a listed impairment, the set of symptoms, signs, and findings must be equal to, or more significant than, those in the listed criteria. However, an alleged or reported increase in the intensity of a symptom cannot be substituted for a missing or deficient sign or finding to elevate impairment severity to equal a listed impairment. For example, a history of severe, persistent joint pain cannot be substituted for the required x ray evidence of either joint space narrowing with osteophytosis or bony destruction (with erosions or cysts) in Listing 1.04 to draw a conclusion of "equal."

In the circumstance of a severe impairment that does not meet or equal a listing, pain can be considered to add to the claimant's limitations and reduce the residual functional capacity. A claimant may become eligible only if there is consistency in the medical evidence regarding the intensity and duration of pain and its effects on residual functional capacity. If no underlying physical or mental impairment is found to affect an individual's ability to do basic work activities, then disability resulting from pain during exertional and nonexertional activities as determined by residual functional capacity assessment cannot be established.

However, if an impairment is found, residual functional capacity assessment can be affected by pain. If the listing is not met or equaled, a residual functional capacity assessment is necessary to determine the effects of the impairment, including any additional limitations imposed by pain, on the claimant's capacity to perform former work or other work. Medical history and objective findings, such as evidence of muscle atrophy, reduced joint motion, muscle spasm, and sensory and motor disruption, are usually used to draw conclusions about the intensity and persistence of pain and the effect such pain may have on the individual's work capacity. Whenever available, this type of objective medical evidence must be obtained and, as expressed in Public Law 98-460, "must be considered in reaching a conclusion as to whether the individual is under a disability." If a particular physician does not recognize or assess severity of pain, then these claimants cannot have the residual functional capacity modified.

However, there are situations in which an individual's alleged symptoms, such as pain caused by myofascial pain suggest the possibility of a greater restriction of the individual's ability to function than can be demonstrated by objective medical findings alone.[29] In such cases, reasonable conclusions about limitations on the individual's ability to do basic work activities can be derived from the consideration of other information in conjunction with medical findings.

In developing evidence of pain or other symptoms, all avenues presented that relate to subjective complaints, including the claimant's prior work record, and information and observations by treating physicians and third parties, must be assessed for the following:

1. The nature, location, onset, duration, frequency, radiation, and intensity of pain.
2. Precipitating and aggravating factors (e.g., movement, activity, environmental conditions).
3. Type, dosage, effectiveness, and adverse side effects of any pain medications.
4. Treatment, other than medication, for relief of pain.
5. Functional restrictions.
6. The claimant's daily activities.

In the residual functional capacity assessment, the medical consultant should describe the relationship between the medically determinable impairment and his conclusions of residual functional capacity that have been derived from the evidence, including a discussion of why reported daily activity restrictions are not reasonably consistent with the medical evidence.

In cases of alleged pain, the determination is based on a thorough discussion and analysis of the objective medical and nonmedical evidence, including the individual's personal reports and the personal observations of those responsible for the development of the claimant's file. The rationale then is to provide a resolution of any inconsistencies in the evidence as a whole and establish a logical determination of the individual's capacity to work.

Many authorities claim that chronic pain alone without an objectively determined physical or mental impairment can cause significant functional difficulties and, thus, should be considered important in the disability determination process. This is the case of patients with myofascial pain and several other diagnoses. As a result, recent court cases have challenged the existing SSA policy on pain in disability determination under SSDI and SSI programs. For example, in the case of Polaski vs. Heckler, the Federal Court of Appeals held that:

> "An adjudicator may not disregard the claimant's subjective complaints solely because objective medical evidence does not fully support them . . . the adjudicator must give full consideration to all of the evidence presented relating to subjective complaints, including the claimant's prior work record and observations by third parties and treating and examining physicians relating to such matters as: (1) the claimant's daily activity, (2) the duration, frequency, and intensity of pain, (3) precipitating and aggravating factors, (4) dosage, effectiveness, and side effects of medication, and (5) functional restrictions."[30]

In response to this situation, Congress passed an amendment to the Social Security Disability Benefits Reform Act (P.L. 98-460) to establish a commission to study the issue of pain in the SSA disability determination process. The secretary of the health and human services appointed a commission on the evaluation of pain in consultation with the Institute of Medicine from the National Academy of Sciences to make recommendations to the SSA regarding evaluation of pain in disability determinations. The statutory language (HR 2660) establishing the existing policy on the evaluation of pain has a "sunset" date of December 31, 1990, to allow time to complete specific recommendations by the commission on the evaluation of pain.[31]

In its report, the pain commission proposed criteria to help establish disability for individuals impaired primarily because of pain. The proposed criteria includes both individuals with a measurable impairment of function with physical tissue damage in body parts specifically related to pain *and* individuals with pain complaints disproportionate or inappropriate in location, intensity, or duration to the physical damage and its normal expected healing time. In the latter case, the individual's pain must be substantiated by the presence of three out of five behavioral manifestations of pain (preoccupation with pain, overuse of health care, persistent excessive medication use, consistent pain displays, and other pain behaviors). In both cases, frequent or persistent alteration in four areas of life functioning (including activities of daily living, social functioning, task completion, and functional capacity) must also be substantiated to be considered for eligibility.

However, implementation of pain commission criteria is premature without establishing reliable and valid instruments and methods to measure these criteria and determine the fiscal impact that their use will have on the SSDI and SSI programs. The SSA is currently involved in a study to design and test appropriate instruments and methods to measure these criteria routinely in the disability determination process. Once research is completed, these methods will be implemented throughout the system to establish a more fair and consistent method of pain assessment in claimants with alleged pain.

WORKERS' COMPENSATION

The issues of pain in assessment of disability within the workers' compensation system differs from the SSA system because it provides benefits for disabled workers who are recently injured at work regardless of the presence of a medically determinable impairment. It provides an earlier source of income and medical benefits than the SSA's SSI and SSDI programs. In both cases, the problematic claimant is one who claims to have severe disabling pain but medical evidence fails to verify it. The SSA problem involves claimants who are not receiving benefits and claim they should be. The workers' compensation problems involve workers who receive short-term benefits, fail to recover, and claim to need long-term benefits. Workers who fail to return to work and fail at rehabilitation are considered

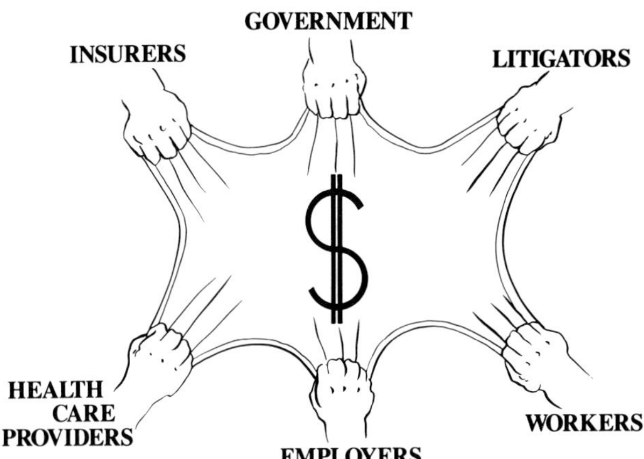

Figure 46–2. The different "players" involved in the cost of pain disability.

to have a delayed recovery syndrome, and most will qualify for permanent lifetime benefits. The remaining workers who do not qualify may apply for benefits through the SSA disability program.

The issues with workers' compensation are fairness and cost. Do workers who have delayed recovery syndrome, with no objective impairment, and who fail to return to work, receive a fair assessment of their ability to work? Is there a method to return these workers to gainful employment and reduce the cost of workers' compensation? The players holding power and interest in the resolution of these issues are the federal and state governments, health care providers, employers, workers, insurers, and litigators (Fig. 46–2). A discussion of the workers' compensation system is needed to examine these issues.

Workers' Compensation Benefits

Workers' compensation provides injured workers with four kinds of benefits:

1. Wage replacement—for the period during which the employee is unable to return to work.
2. Loss of bodily function—payment for the loss of, or permanent damage to, body parts (such as a hand, finger, or leg).
3. Medical costs—all reasonable current and future costs arising from, or connected to, the evaluation and treatment of a work-related injury.
4. Rehabilitation costs—including, but not limited to, counseling, job placement, evaluations and testing, on-the-job training, vocational or formal education, or other activities necessary to prepare the employee to return to his old job or to a new job.

There is increasing recognition that these programs are expensive and cost industry a considerable percentage of pretax profits. Minnesota recently studied the cost of worker's compensation and found that between 1983 and 1986, workers' compensation insurance premiums doubled in Minnesota while countrywide, they increased 54%.[1] About 26% of the premium growth was a result of payroll growth; the remainder was caused by increases in benefits. The total premium for insured and self-insured employers in Minnesota in 1986 was $834 million and is expected to increase annually by 20%.

An analysis of these costs can be made based on the type of injury. In most states, workers' compensation losses are classified as one of five types (listed below). The first three types are frequently grouped together and termed permanent injuries.

  I. Death: An employee is fatally injured.
 II. Permanent total: An employee is permanently injured and can never return to the work force. He receives benefits for the rest of his life.
III. Permanent partial: An employee is injured and has a permanent impairment. The employee may or may not return to work, but in either case the benefits terminate unless the employee is considered permanently unable to perform work. In Minnesota, permanency is rated as a percentage of the whole body and may be as small as 1%.
 IV. Temporary total: An employee loses some time from work but there is no permanency and return to work is relatively quick.
  V. Medical only: The injured employee requires medical treatment but is off work for less than three days.

Other states use two categories: disabled (permanent or temporary) and not disabled. Figures 46–3 and 46–4 show the distribution among these types

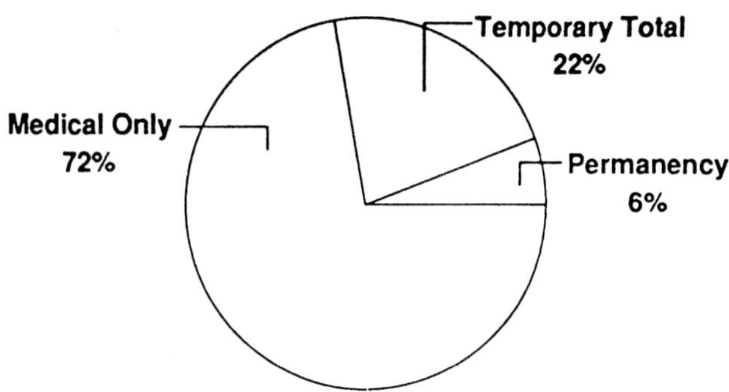

Figure 46–3. Percentage distribution of injuries in Minnesota.

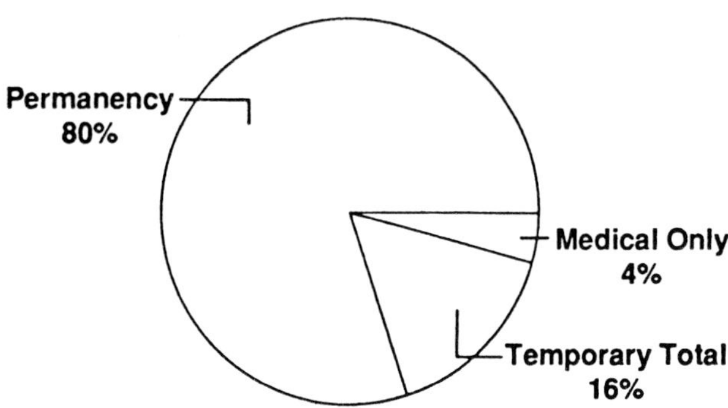

Figure 46–4. Percentage distribution of the cost of injuries in Minnesota.

of injuries in terms of the number of injured employees and the cost of their injuries in Minnesota.[1] Of the 113,000 injuries a year reported by private insurers, 82,000 are medical only, 25,000 are temporary total only, and 6,000 are permanency claims. These figures do not include injuries of employees working for self-insured employers or employers who are exempt from purchasing workers' compensation insurance. The permanent category contains less than 6% of the claimants (Fig. 46–3), but 80% of the loss dollars (Fig. 46–4). The cost of permanent cases may be understated because this distribution does not include supplementary benefits, almost all of which are paid to workers with permanent injuries.

The high cost of the Minnesota system is directly related to the high cost of permanent cases and is consistent with other states. Of the 350 Workers' Compensation Reinsurers Association (WCRA) lifetime pensions each year, about 30 are medically serious cases such as burns and brain and spinal cord injuries or fatalities. Most of the others are back problems associated with delayed recovery syndrome resulting from chronic pain.[1] In these cases, physicians are responsible for establishing the presence of a permanent impairment and its effects on work capacity. Permanent impairment is defined as an anatomic or functional abnormality or loss after maximum medical rehabilitation has been achieved, which abnormality or loss the physician considers stable or nonprogressive at the time of evaluation. This maximum improvement, particularly in the cases of chronic pain, varies considerably because of the presence of specific risk factors.

The reasons for the development of a delayed recovery syndrome vary with the type of occupation, injury, treatment, and personal characteristics. Recently, researchers have studied the risk factors for an injury at work and subsequent failure to return to work. For example, Hall, et al.,[32] studied 179 workers in a garment industry that had an epidemic of absenteeism caused by fainting, nausea, and weakness. Rather than finding a toxic substance responsible for the illnesses, they found high work intensity, mental strain, and work or home problems as the most significant risk factors involved. Hirschfeld and Behan found that certain internal conflicts can lead an individual to cause or be prone to an accident in some cases and perpetuate the injuries because the accident is seen as a solution to current life problems.[33] Derebery and Tulus identified a number of risk factors for delayed recovery syndrome, including continued compensation, patient as the cause of injury, frequent medical appointment cancellations and conflicts, chemical dependency, doctor shopping, and high work absenteeism. Other factors cited as significant risk factors include behavioral and psychosocial factors, such as poor job satisfaction, employer conflicts, and life dissatisfaction.[34–50] Socioeconomic conditions suggestive of economic insecurity such as high unemployment rate, receiving food stamps, and low per capita income, also play a role in encouraging back pain to become disabling.[51]

In reviewing the literature, it becomes apparent that there are many factors involved in the risk of injury and failure to return to work. Physicians, in assessing and treating injured workers, must be aware of these factors early in the rehabilitation process to maximize the potential to heal and return to work. However, in any given patient, the number and complexity of these factors make routine assessment by physicians, occupational therapists, or other clinicians difficult. Failure to identify and change these factors increases the likelihood of developing a delayed recovery syndrome and receiving permanent entitlements. Traditionally, routine assessment of the characteristics and risk factors of injured workers has been difficult and costly because it entails patient interviews. Recently, self-assessment through questionnaires that have gone through psychometric testing have supplemented and improved efficiency of data collection.[2] Physicians also are responsible for assessing patient characteristics and functional status as imposed by the impairment. This entails determining if the impairment prevents an individual from performing certain physical and mental functions. There have been many methods proposed for determining a complete disability evaluation. Gordon provides some guidelines to help standardize an independent medical examination for disability determination. The physician should include a detailed history, including symptoms, emphasizing the details of the injury, how it happened, where it happened, and when. Reading through the history, one should be able to conceptualize the actual mechanism of injury so that a relationship between the episode and injury or illness (causation) can be determined. The physician should also describe in de-

tail symptoms of pain and the affect of pain on physical, psychosocial, and vocational functioning. A physician's disability evaluation report would include the following:

1. History of injuries and treatments
2. Past history, family history, educational and work history, social history
3. Physical examination
4. Medical diagnosis and impressions
5. Summary of objective findings supporting diagnosis
6. Description of impairments
7. Description of functional limitations
8. Relationship of functional limitations to work and job possibilities
9. Relationship of functional limitations to activities of daily living, hobbies, and social roles
10. Causal relationship of injury to impairments
11. Recommended treatment including equipment, environmental modifications, and future medical needs
12. Expected future course of the condition with prognosis
13. Percentage of impairment

Although most physicians include each of these components in an evaluation, the poor reliability of information and decisions from one physician to another has been a source of much criticism and confusion in disability determination. Some physicians are considered patient advocates and others are considered insurance company advocates depending on their particular bias in patient assessment. This fuels controversy regarding individual disability decisions and often results in litigation. To improve this, comprehensive patient assessment instruments have been proposed to improve standardization of data collection and reliability of measurements of functional status.

DEFINING DISABILITY THROUGH SELF-ASSESSMENT

Understanding the person with chronic pain is a complex task that requires gathering data from multiple sources. However, because pain and disability are such personal experiences, it is the person suffering who can yield the most comprehensive and revealing information. The reliability of self-assessment is inherently questionable, particularly if it is used to make decisions regarding benefits to the person involved. For this reason, self-assessment must be corroborated by objective medical evidence and opinions of colleagues, supervisors, or a significant other. In addition, self-assessment must be structured in an interview or questionnaire that demonstrates adequate validity and reliability.

This type of assessment instrument can fulfill many needs. It can provide physicians, other health care providers, litigators, and disability adjudicators with a consistent and in-depth understanding of the patient. Data include demographic characteristics, functional capacity, illness history, behavioral and psychosocial problems, and risk factors for failure to return to work. With this information, all parties have the same information, allowing fairer decision-making and less potential for litigation. Data on patients can be studied in aggregate to increase understanding of the system and allow administrative decisions that are based on detailed, reliable information. It also can be used to enhance rehabilitation outcome and prevent the possibility of reinjury. These advantages have the SSA and many states studying the need for a comprehensive assessment instrument.

A recent report on chronic pain and disability by the Institute of Medicine for the Social Security Administration[2] states that "progress in this field depends on developing and refining uniform definitions and approaches to measuring numerous independent and dependent variables including patient classification, psychosocial variables, the delineation of interventions, and outcomes . . . the committee recommends the use of a standardized pain questionnaire or visual analog scales to systematize information (collection)." The committee further states that this questionnaire should be comprehensive in nature, a minimal burden on the patients, understandable by the patients, yield a wide range of scores with sensitivity to changes resulting from time or interventions, and demonstrate appropriate reliability and validity. In response, the SSA is developing such an instrument.

With costs and litigation escalating in many states, there has also been a call for major changes in workers' compensation laws. The use of a comprehensive assessment system for disability determination is one suggested change. These suggestions focus on measurement of disability in chronic pain patients and identification of risk factors for delayed recovery syndrome. Because a single technique or diagnostic test is too limited, disability determination for injured workers with chronic pain must rely on multidimensional assessments. Disability is a function of many variables. These include not only the degree of tissue damage, but more important, how these nociceptive signals emanating from injured or irritated tissue are modulated by the synaptic pathways in the spinal cord and in the brain and ultimately how these signals interface with the patient's consciousness. Thus, the expression of this process includes not only the sensation of pain but a whole spectrum of behaviors, emotions, and cognitive beliefs

that reflect the patient's limitations. In order to quantify this situation, a biomechanical or disease model that looks at only physical parameters is inadequate.

Rather, a multiaxial or biopsychosocial model is needed to integrate the numerous emotional, psychosocial and environmental variables with the physical findings. As pointed out previously, most disability systems minimize these factors. Rather, the emphasis has been placed on rating disability on the basis of "objective" physical findings and laboratory tests, which presumably prevents the patient from misrepresenting himself. Thus, the belief is that the physical examination and laboratory findings are more accurate representations of function than what the patient reports. However, there is clearly an error in this reasoning. X rays and laboratory findings are measurements of anatomy or physiology, not functioning. As discussed, two individuals with the same level of measurable impairment can experience different levels of pain and can be affected differently both functionally and psychologically because of that experience.

Traditionally, the clinician has relied on the self-report of the patient to assess his condition in terms of severity of symptoms and the impact the condition has on his ability to function. However, rarely is there an attempt to quantify these variables in the same way that laboratory and x rays attempt to quantify impairment.

The development and integration of scientifically valid and reliable self-report instrumentation and functional assessment testing would provide consistency and objectivity in the analysis of the subjective manifestations of pain. Using this information, the physician and the disability administrator would obtain a far more thorough and comprehensive picture of the patients' level of functioning.

A number of valid instruments currently exist to measure various aspects of disability, e.g., activities of daily living scales, health status measures, risk factors, physical symptoms, cognitive belief scales, and instruments that assess emotional, social, cognitive, and behavioral characteristics. In fact, so many instruments are available to measure the parameters of disability outcome that the US Department of Health has established a separate clearing house for health indices. At the present time, however, no specific instrument exists that has been established as the gold standard in the assessment of disability and pain. If an ideal instrument did exist, in theory it should meet the following criteria as proposed by Deyo.[52]

Practicality

It should be administered and scored in a reasonable time frame. Self administration requires the least amount of staff time, but contingencies must be built in for those individuals with poor or no reading skill, and for those who do not understand the language.

Comprehensiveness

The instrument should provide information in the various dimensions associated with the disability determination process, i.e., social, cognitive, emotional, and behavioral characteristics, as well as functional abilities and activities of daily living.

Reliability

The instrument should provide consistency over time, assuming stability in the patient's condition. Reliability refers to the reproducibility of results and does not refer to the accuracy of the instrument in measuring the assumed variables.

Validity

The instrument should quantify in a statistically significant manner and in a consistently predictable

Table 46–1
Items Included in a Comprehensive Assessment of Disability

1. Pain complaints	9. Failure to complete tasks in timely fashion
Location	Concentration/attention
Intensity	Late because of slow pace or persistence
Duration	Independent functioning
Frequency	Understand and remember instructions
Disproportionate to physical findings or expected healing time	Make errors
Does pain come from physical impairment	Taking orders from others
Precipitating and aggravating factors	Coworker interaction
2. Preoccupation with pain	Speaking clearly
Persistent repeated verbal complaints	Leave job undone
Willingness to undergo repeated painful procedures	10. Functional abilities estimation to perform work
3. Utilization of health care	Walking
4. Persistent excessive use of analgesic or sedative drugs (type, dosage, effectiveness, side effects)	Standing
5. Consistent audible and body language displays	Sitting
Verbal complaints	Lifting
Guarded movements	Lifting and carrying
Facial grimace	Simple grasping
Moaning	Firm grasping
Shifting positions	Use of feet and legs
Bracing (abnormal posturing)	Push/pull cart
Use of brace or cane	Push/pull heavy object
6. Other pain related behaviors	Squat down or kneel
Sleep	Crawl
Eating	Climbing stairs or ladder
Sexual dysfunction	Reach above shoulder height
Inactivity	Height restriction
Task avoidance	Moving machinery restriction
7. Significant restrictions in activities of daily living caused by pain	Temperature change restriction
Light household tasks (dusting, dishes)	Driving restriction
Heavy household tasks (yardwork, washing)	Dust, fumes, gas restriction
Light leisure activity (reading, watching TV)	11. Emotional and mental consequences
Moderate leisure activity (bowling, walks)	Anxiety and nervousness
Heavy leisure activity (running, aerobics)	Depression and sadness
Transportation about town	Anger
Personal hygiene	Irritable or crabby
Sleep	Tearful or crying
Ambulation around the house	Low health esteem
Manual dexterity (writing letters, paying bills)	Low self esteem
Shopping	Hopelessness
Dressing self	Suicidal ideation
Being active most of the day	Consistency of emotional factors with degree of pain
8. Significant difficulties in maintaining social functioning	Treated patient for emotional difficulty and outcome
Significant other	Referral to mental health specialist
Friends	Has patient followed through on referral
Family members	Did it help
Work associates	12. Rehabilitation potential
Community (store clerks, etc.)	Candidate for rehabilitation
Social involvement such as church	Motivation
Authority figures (police, boss)	Compliance with treatment
Neighbors	Comfort with situation
	No hope to work

direction, those variables that the instrument has been designed to measure. Validation of an instrument becomes increasingly complex in a manner directly proportional to the number of variables in question. The use of the computer in the development of sophisticated multivariant statistical analysis, however, allows for accurate discernment of the construct validity of the variables in question. A more challenging issue in terms of assessing validity is the lack of a standard or clearly defined objective parameters defining the dimensions that should be used to measure disability. Williams suggests a set of physical, functional, behavioral, emotional, economic, and sociocultural parameters for the evaluation of outcome in patients undergoing treatment in a comprehensive pain clinic.[53] Many of these variables are applicable in the assessment of pain and its relationship to disability (Table 46–1). Although this model is indeed comprehensive, it has not gained wide acceptance, and, moreover, although instruments do exist to measure individual parameters described, use of these multiple instruments would be time-consuming, expensive, and impractical, except perhaps in the setting of a comprehensive pain management clinic or for research.

Sensitivity and Responsiveness

An instrument should be capable of measuring subtle but important clinical changes over time. This is critical if one is to measure the responsiveness to respective therapeutic interventions or the impact the underlying condition has on the patient over time. In addition, the instrument would require sufficient sensitivity to discriminate subtle differences between patients presenting with similar complaints.

With the advent of computers and optical scanner technology, the potential for accomplishing these goals is significantly improved. This will aid in the development of population norms and will allow individual responses to be analyzed and reported with comparative relevance. In addition, the establishment of the resulting database will create an information source for physicians and resource decision-makers.

IMPATH is a comprehensive assessment system for pain and disability assessment.[4,54] It is designed to use both the full capabilities of new assessment technologies and the advantages of a psychometrically sound instrument for the routine assessment of patients in most health care settings. It provides the following:

1. An evaluation of the patient's perception of the pain and its location, intensity, quality, temporal characteristics, and chronology of the pain experience and treatment.

2. A multidimensional evaluation of the contributing factors that may complicate management as classified as biological, behavioral, cognitive, emotional, social, and environmental.

3. An evaluation of the impact of the pain on different aspects of the patient's life, such as in the use of health care, vocation, relationships, and attitudes.

In addition, it is designed to provide statistical analysis and reporting of the results.

The instrument is only one part of a comprehensive assessment regimen for individual patients in order to improve the consistency of the evaluative and decision-making capabilities of clinicians, disability adjudicators, and resource decision-makers. It also provides a clinical research instrument that can be used to determine individual and aggregate treatment effectiveness and predictors of failure.

Although IMPATH is one example of an instrument that can serve the needs of all parties involved in disability determination, it is the concept of collecting comprehensive and reliable data about people applying for disability that is important. With a data collection system in place, informed decisions about people's lives and the entire disability program can be made more fairly and consistently. Costs for disability programs can be better studied and justified. Without proper information, decisions can only be based on opinions and politics by default.

REFERENCES

1. Minnesota Department of Labor and Industry: Report to the Legislature on Workers' Compensation in Minnesota, Jan, 1988.
2. Osterweis, M., Kleinman, A., Mechanic, D.: Institute of Medicine's Committee on Pain, Disability, and Chronic Illness Behavior, Pain and Disability: Clinical, Behavioral, and Public Policy Perspectives. Washington DC, National Academy Press, 1987.
3. Sternbach, R.A.: Pain Patients: Traits and Treatments. New York, Academic Press, 1974.
4. Fricton, J.R., Nelson, A.F., Monsein, M.R.: IMPATH: microcomputer assessment of behavioral and psychosocial factors in craniomandibular disorders. J Craniomandibul Prac 5(4):372–381, 1987.
5. Flor, H., Turk, D.C., Scholz O.B.: Impact of chronic pain on the spouse: marital, emotional, and physical consequences. J Psychosom Res 31(1):63–71, 1987.
6. Brena, S.F., Chapman, S.L., Stegall, P.G., Chyatte, S.B.: Chronic pain states: their relationship to impairment and disability. Arch Phys Med Rehabil 60:387–389, 1979.
7. Bonica, J.J.: Preface: New approaches to treatment of chronic pain: a review of multidimensional pain clinics and pain centers. NIDA Research 36 Monograph Series. Washington DC, US Government Printing Office, pp. 7–10, 1984.
8. Travell, J.G., Simons, D.G.: Myofascial Pain and Dysfunction—The Trigger Point Manual. Baltimore, Williams & Wilkins, 1983.
9. Cunningham, L.S., Kelsey, J.: Epidemiology of musculoskele-

tal impairments and associated disability. Am J Pub Health 74:574–579, 1984.

10. Powell, M.C., Wilson, M., Szypryt, P., Symonds, E.M., Worthington, B.S.: Prevalence of lumbar disc degeneration observed by magnetic resonance in symptomless women. Lancet 2:1366–1367, 1986.

11. Wiesel, S.W., Tsourmas, M., Feffer, H.L., Citrin, C.M., Patronas, N.: A study of computer-assisted tomography: 1. The incidence of positive CAT scans in an asymptomatic group of patients. Spine 9:549–551, 1984.

12. Nelson, M.A., Allen, P., Clampe, S.E., de Dombal, F.T.: Reliability and reproducibility of clinical findings in low-back pain. Spine 4(2):97–101, 1979.

13. Waddell, G., et al.: Normality and reliability in the clinical assessment of backache. Brit Med J 284:1519–1523, 1982.

14. Fishbain, A.A., Goldberg, M., Meagher, B.R., Steele, R., Rosomoff, H.: Male and female chronic patients categorized by DSM-II psychiatric diagnostic criteria. Pain 26:181–197, 1986.

15. Fricton, J.R., et al.: Myofascial pain syndrome of the head and neck: a review of clinical characteristics of 164 patients. Oral Surg 60:615–623, 1985.

16. Fricton, J.R., Awad, E.: Myofascial Pain and Fibromyalgia. New York, Raven Press, 1990.

17. Schiffmann, E., Fricton, J.R., Haley, D., Tylka, D.: A pressure algometer for myofascial pain syndrome: reliability and validity. In Proceedings of the 5th World Congress on Pain, 1988 (Edited by R. Dubner, G.F. Gebhart, and M.R. Bond). Elsevier Science Publishers, New York, pp. 407–413, 1988.

18. Reeves, J., Jaeger, B., Graff-Radford, S.B.: Reliability of pressure algometer as a measure of myofascial trigger point sensitivity. Pain 24:313–321, 1986.

19. Wexler, C.E.: Cervical, thoracic, and lumbar thermography: a clinical evaluation. J Neurol Orthop Surg 2:183–185, 1981.

20. Haberman, J.D., Ehrlich, G.E., Levenson, C.: Thermography in rheumatic diseases. Arch Phys Med Rehabil 49:187–192, 1968.

21. Fischer, A.A.: Documentation of myofascial trigger points. Arch Phys Med Rehabil 69:286–291, 1988.

22. Cailliet, R.: Soft Tissue Pain and Disability. Philadelphia, F.A. Davis, 1977.

23. Simons, D.G., Travell, J.G.: Myofascial origins of low back pain. Parts 1, 2, 3. Postgrad Med 73:66–108, 1983.

24. Travell, J.G., Rinzler, S.H.: The myofascial genesis of pain. Postgrad Med 11:425–434, 1952.

25. Derebury, V.J., Tulus, W.H.: Delayed recovery in patient with work compensable injury. J Occup Med 25(11):829–835, 1983.

26. Enelow, A.J.: Malingering and delayed recovery from injury. In Compensation in Psychiatric Disability and Rehabilitation (Edited by J.J. Leedy). Springfield, Charles C Thomas, pp. 42–46, 1971.

27. Social Security Bulletin, Annual Statistical Supplement, 1988.

28. SSA Policy 20 CFR 404.1529/416.929.

29. SSA Document DI 24515.060D.

30. Polaski vs. Heckler, 751 F2d 943, 8th Circuit, 1984.

31. United States Department of Health and Human Services. Report of the Commission on the Evaluation of Pain (SSA Pub. No. 64-031). Washington, DC, US Government Printing Office, 1987.

32. Hall, E., Johnson, J.: A case study of stress and mass psychogenic illness in industrial workers. J Occup Med 31(3):243–250, 1989.

33. Hirschfeld, A.H., Behan, R.C.: The accident process: I. Etiological considerations of industrial injuries. JAMA 186:193–199, 1963.

34. Frymoyer, J.W., Rosen, J.C., Clements, J., Pope, M.H.: Psychologic factors in low-back pain disability. Clin Orthop 195:178–184, 1984.

35. Holmes, T.H., Wolf, H.G.: Life situation, emotions and backache. Psychosom Med 14:18, 1952.

36. Pope, M.H., Rosen, J.C., Wilder, D.G., Frymoyer, J.W.: The relation between biomechanical and psychological factors in patients with low-back pain. Spine 5:173–178, 1980.

37. Andersson, G.B.: Symposium: low back pain in industry. Spine 6:52–60, 1981.

38. Frymoyer, J.W., Kats, B.W.: Predictors of low back pain disability. Clin Orthop 221:89–98, 1987.

39. Behan, R.C., Hirschfeld, A.H.: The accident process: II. Toward more rational treatment of industrial injuries. JAMA 186:300–306, 1963.

40. Gentry, W.D., Shows, W.D., Thomas, M.: Chronic low back pain: a psychological profile. Psychosom 15(4):174–187, 1974.

41. Braceland, F.J.: Stress and crisis in work and leisure. Psych Ann 12:109–110, 1982.

42. Cady, L.D., et al.: Strength and fitness and subsequent back injuries in firefighters. J Occup Med 21:269–272, 1979.

43. Enelow, A.J.: Industrial injuries: prediction and prevention of psychological complications. J Occup Med 10:683–687, 1968.

44. Kelman, H.: Character and the traumatic syndrome. J Nerv Ment Dis 192:121–152, 1945.

45. Krusen, E.M., Ford, D.E.: Compensation factor in low back injury. JAMA 166:1128–1133, 1958.

46. Martin, R.D.: Secondary gain, everybody's rationalization. J Occup Med 16:800–801, 1974.

47. Meyers, T.J.: Industrial backache. Dis Nerv Sys 28:155–159, 1967.

48. Millen, F.J.: Post-traumatic neurosis in industry. Ind Med Surg 35:929–935, 1966.

49. Nagi, S.Z., Riley, L., Newby, L.: A social epidemiology of back pain in a general population. J Chron Dis 26:769–779, 1973.

50. Rossignol, M., Suissa, S., Abenhaim, L.: Working disability to occupational back pain: 3 year follow-up of 2,300 compensated workers in Quebec. J Occup Med 30(6):502–505, 1988.

51. Volinn, E., Lai, D., McKinney, S., Loeser, J.D.: When back pain becomes disabling: a regional analysis. Pain 33:33–39, 1988.

52. Deyo, R.A.: Measuring the functional status of patients with low back pain. Arch Phys Med Rehabil 69:1044–1053, 1988.

53. Williams, R.C.: Toward a set of reliable and valid measures for chronic pain assessment and outcome research. Pain 35:239–251, 1988.

54. Social Security Administration, Pain Study Design, 1988.

47

Alan L. Engelberg

American Medical Association's Guides to the Evaluation of Permanent Impairment: A Standardized Approach

HISTORICAL PERSPECTIVE

As important as it has always been, the evaluation of impairment and disability as a focus of specialized knowledge within the profession of medicine, remained a subject of research and publication for only a few individuals, such as McBride.[1] In 1956, the board of trustees of the American Medical Association recognized the emerging growth of this area of medicine by creating an ad hoc committee on the medical rating of physical impairment (later renamed the Committee on Rating of Physical and Mental Impairment). It was charged with creating a series of guidelines for the rating of impairment of the various organ systems of the body. This Committee, assisted by many consultants, produced 13 Guides to the evaluation of permanent impairment, which were published in the Journal of the American Medical Association between 1958 and 1970.[2,3] The timeliness of this activity was underscored by the Journal's fulfilling requests for over 225,000 reprints of the individual Guides.

In 1971, the Committee reviewed the 13 articles and compiled them into one publication, the first edition of the Guides to the Evaluation of Permanent Impairment.[4] In so doing, the Committee updated the clinical information that had appeared initially in the separate Journal articles. However, this new publication also gave the Committee the appropriate platform from which to espouse a more unified concept of impairment evaluation. Definitions clearly delineating the differences between impairment and disability, and evaluation of each, were introduced.[4] Furthermore, the "whole man" (later changed to "whole person") approach to impairment rating was introduced, which was a unifying mathematical concept that allowed for the combining of all ratings of impairment, such that all impairments could add up to, at most, 100% of the whole person. In order for such combining to be done, it was necessary to quantify the relationship of an impairment of a body part to the person as a whole. In so doing, the Committee decided that the spine, which in the 1958 Journal article was a separate body part along with the extremities, would be integrated directly into the whole person for the sake of determination of impairment ratings.

PUBLICATION OF THE SECOND EDITION

Although in 1977 the *Guides* was republished, no changes were made. In 1981, the AMA, realizing that during the decade since the publication of the first edition (which itself had clinical information based on the state-of-the-art of the late 1950s and 1960s) great strides had been made in the understanding of impairment of some of the organ systems, conducted a thorough review of the book, and created a second edition for publication in 1984.[5] In this edition, the AMA expanded the preface and created a glossary in order to espouse more completely the basic philosophies of its view of impairment and disability evaluations. For instance, the definitions of impairment and disability were made more clear (Table 47–1). In addition, this edition of the book spelled out for the first time a fundamental concept upon which all guidelines for impairment evaluation and ratings were based since the publication of the initial Journal article, but which had never been put to print: that the evaluation and rating of impairment was based upon how an impairing condition affected a person's ability to carry out his or her "Activities of Daily Living," which are shown in Table 47–2. Thus, although a major use of an impairment evaluation is in workers' compensation systems, in which it is important to understand how impairing conditions affect an individual's ability to perform job-specific tasks (i.e., the individual's abilities and *disabilities* within the job market), the evaluation of impairment is really a measure of a person's total health status at a given point in time, and how that health status affects his or her ability to carry on the routine activities of life that we all learn in childhood and early adulthood. The "Activities of Daily Living" as the underpinning of impairment evaluation, therefore, substantiates the basic philosophies of the *Guides:* (1) that impairment is assessed by physi-

Table 47–2
Activities of Daily Living

Self care and personal hygiene: Urinating, defecating, brushing teeth, combing hair, bathing, dressing oneself, eating.
Communications: Writing, typing, seeing, hearing, speaking.
Normal living postures: Sitting, lying down, standing.
Ambulation: Walking, climbing stairs.
Travel: Driving, riding, flying.
Nonspecialized hand activities: Grasping, lifting, tactile discrimination.
Sexual function: Having normal sexual function and participating in usual sexual activity.
Sleep: Restful nocturnal sleep pattern.
Social and recreational activities: Ability to participate in group activities.

(From American Medical Association Guides to the Evaluation of Permanent Impairment. 3rd Ed. Chicago, American Medical Association, p. 235, 1988.)

cians, whose knowledge of clinical matters includes how impairing conditions affect daily activities and, (2) that impairment evaluation is applicable to many forms of disability evaluation, and not just to an evaluation of ability to carry out job tasks.

IMPAIRMENT EVALUATION REPORTS

There are essentially two individuals who affect the outcome of an impairment evaluation: (1) the evaluator, usually a physician, who is responsible for carrying out an evaluation and reporting its results, and (2) the user, usually a nonphysician, who is responsible for understanding the report and for making a nonmedical, administrative decision based upon the report and other forms of information he or she may gather. Often, the user is faced with two or more reports of evaluations, and must decide how to make use of the information in both. To assist in these matters, another fundamental concept of the AMA *Guides* is the standardization of both the evaluating and reporting processes. (The concept of standardization of evaluation and reporting was first published in the second edition, but was enhanced in the publication of the third edition in 1988.[6]) It is obvious that if two or more physicians use the same evaluation techniques, differences in their measurements can be seen as differences in what they observed at the time they examined the patient, rather than as differences in preferred clinical techniques or of opinions. It should be just as obvious that the thoroughness and coherence of reports of their ob-

Table 47–1
Definitions of Impairment and Disability

Impairment: The loss of, the loss of use of, or derangement of any body part, system, or function.

Permanent impairment: Impairment that has become static or well stabilized with or without medical treatment, or that is not likely to remit despite medical treatment of the impairing condition.

Evaluation or rating of impairment: An assessment of data collected during a clinical evaluation and the comparison of those data to the criteria contained in the *Guides.*

Disability: The limiting loss or the absence of the capacity of an individual to meet personal, social, or occupational demands, or to meet statutory or regulatory requirements. Disability may be caused by medical impairment or by nonmedical factors.

Permanent disability: Occurs when the degree of capacity becomes static or well stabilized and is not likely to increase in spite of continuing medical or rehabilitative measures.

Evaluation or rating of disability: A nonmedical assessment of the degree to which an individual does or does not have the capacity to meet personal, social, or occupational demands, or to meet statutory or regulatory requirements.

(From American Medical Association Guides to the Evaluation of Permanent Impairment, 3rd Ed. Chicago, American Medical Association, p 236, 1988.)

servations would also help establish the reasons for differences in observations and conclusions. For this reason, especially in its third edition, the *Guides* dwells heavily on correct reporting. Table 47–3 shows the four steps of thorough reporting and the contents of each step. The reporting recommendations may seem daunting, but they are essential to follow. Nonmedical persons, in whose hands lies the responsibility to determine the potential outlay of thousands of dollars to individuals, and in the aggregate, millions of dollars to society, must have this type and amount of information to do their jobs with the greatest degree of accuracy.

To assist the evaluator in preparing a comprehensive report and to assist the user of the report who would like to know its contents, the third edition of the Guides provides a report form (Fig. 47–1) summarizing the contents and sources of reporting information. This form brings to light one other axiom of impairment evaluation: that an evaluation is not conducted in a vacuum, but rather is part of the impaired individual's total medical history. Thus, the form allows for (and therefore encourages) the evaluator to obtain and make use of past medical office and hospital records pertaining to the impairing condition. The inclusion of this information is vital, be-

cause if it does not corroborate either the patient's own narrative history, or the observations of the examiner on the day of the evaluation, then the examiner must offer explanations for discrepancies between the history and the presenting symptoms and signs. If the information does corroborate both the narrative history and the observations of that day, the findings and reporting of the findings are all the more substantiated.

EVOLUTION OF SPECIFIC METHODOLOGIES OF EVALUATION OF IMPAIRMENT OF THE MUSCULOSKELETAL SYSTEM

In all editions of the AMA *Guides*, the musculoskeletal system has been divided into four units: the upper extremity, the lower extremity, the spine, and the pelvis. The evaluation of impairment of the pelvis, which is based upon the effects of fractures, has not changed since the first Journal publication of 1958, and is not discussed here. The guidelines for evaluation of the other three units have changed to varying degrees over time. Since 1958, amputation, range of motion and ankylosis, and objectively documented peripheral neuropathy have been the

Table 47–3
Steps and Contents of Report Writing

1. Medical evaluation in accordance with the protocols of the *Guides*, which includes:
    a. A narrative history of the medical condition(s) with specific reference to onset and course of the condition, findings on previous examinations, treatments and responses to treatment.
    b. Results of the most recent clinical evaluation, including (if obtained): physical examination findings, laboratory test results, electrocardiogram, radiographic studies, rehabilitation evaluation, mental status and psychological tests, other specific tests or diagnostic procedures.
    c. Assessment of current clinical status, and statement of plans for future treatment, rehabilitation and reevaluation.
    d. Diagnosis and clinical impressions.
    e. Estimate of the expected date of full or partial recovery.
2. Analysis of findings, which includes:
    a. Explanation of the impact of the medical condition(s) on life's activities.
    b. Narrative explanation of the medical basis for any conclusion that the medical condition has, or has not, become static or well stabilized.
    c. Explanation of the medical basis for a conclusion that the individual is, or is not, likely to suffer sudden or subtle incapacitation as a result of the medical condition.
    d. Explanation of the medical basis for any conclusion that the individual is, or is not, likely to suffer injury or harm or further medical impairment by engaging in activities of daily living or any other activity necessary to meet personal, social, and occupational demands.
    e. Explanation of any conclusion that restrictions or accommodations are, or are not, warranted with respect to daily activities or any other activities that are required to meet personal, social, and occupational demands. If restrictions or accommodations are necessary, there should be an explanation of their therapeutic or risk-avoiding value.
3. Comparison of the results of the analysis with the impairment criteria in the *Guides*, which includes:
    a. A description of specific clinical findings related to each impairment, with reference to how the findings relate to the criteria described in the chapter. Reference to the absence of, or to examiner's inability to obtain, pertinent data is essential.
    b. Comparison of specific clinical findings to the specific criteria that pertain to the particular body system, as they are listed in the *Guides*.
    c. Explanation of each percent of impairment rating, with reference to the applicable criteria.
    d. Summary list of all impairment ratings.
4. Rating of impairment of the whole person (NOTE: this step may or may not be required, depending on the nature of the impairment(s) and the requirements of the disability system in which the evaluation is to be used.)

(From American Medical Association Guides to the Evaluation of Permanent Impairment. 3rd Ed. Chicago, American Medical Association, pp. 9–10, 1988.)

Report of Medical Evaluation (Permanent Medical Impairment)

To: Re:

                                                       Case Number:

                                                       Date of Injury:

1. Past Medical History

		Yes	No
a. Medical Office Records	Reviewed		
	Enclosed		
b. Hospital Records	Reviewed		
	Enclosed		
c. From Patient			
d. From Other Source (describe)			

2. Clinical Evaluation

		Yes	No
a. Physical Examination	Report Enclosed		
b. Laboratory Tests	Reports Attached		
c. Special Tests and Diagnostic Procedures	Reports Attached		
d. Specialty Evaluations	Reports Attached		

3. Diagnoses

a.

b.

c.

4. Stability of the Medical Condition

_____ The clinical condition is not likely to improve with further active medical treatment or surgical intervention—medical maintenance care only is warranted

_____ Employability is not likely to improve with further active medical treatment or surgical intervention

_____ The degree of impairment is not likely to change by more than 3% within the next year

5. Impairment Evaluation—AMA Guides

(Attach a complete report of findings and narrative comments for each body part or system)

Body Part/System	Protocol (Section) No.	Table No.

_____ This patient has been under my care from _____________ to _____________.

_____ I have not provided care for this patient. I have seen this patient _______ time(s) for the purpose of evaluating medical impairment.

_______________________________________, M.D.
(Signature)

Figure 47–1. Report of medical evaluation (permanent medical impairment). (From: Guides to the Evaluation of Permanent Impairment. 3rd Ed. Chicago, American Medical Association, 1988.)

mainstays of evaluation of the extremities and the spine. The two-armed goniometer has been the instrument of choice in assessing range of motion, first because it was thought to be the most objective and accurate method of measurement, and second because it is a simple, inexpensive piece of technology that could be used in any medical care setting. For the extremities, the accuracy and the simplicity of the goniometer still remains, but for the spine, its value has been questioned, as we shall see later. Peripheral nerve deficits, either sensory or motor, which can be shown clinically to relate to specific nerve roots or named peripheral nerves by the distribution of the nerve deficits, have always been important in the evaluation of impairment. However, this was not always evident to the users of the *Guides* because of the placement of the nervous system criteria in a separate section of the book.

The Upper Extremity

While amputation, range of motion, and nervous system deficits continue to be the attributes by which impairment of the upper extremity is evaluated, in the third edition of the *Guides* these attributes were brought together in a system of evaluation that was developed over the past quarter century by Swanson and colleagues.[7] It was adopted for international use by the International Federation of Societies for Surgery of the Hand (IFSSH). In this system, commonly called the "A = E + F" method, A (ankylosis, or total loss of motion) equals E (loss of extension) plus F (loss of flexion), where the measured flexion angle, V_{flex}, equals the measured extension angle, V_{ext}. Similarly, I_A (impairment caused by ankylosis) is equal to I_E (impairment caused by loss of extension) plus I_F (impairment caused by loss of flexion), and I_A varies according to the angle at which V_{flex} equals V_{ext}. This formula allows for a precise mathematical relationship among the impairment ratings for extension, flexion, and ankylosis for each plane of motion of each joint in the upper extremity. An example for one joint is shown in Figure 47–2.

The IFSSH method also allows for mathematically precise ratings of impairment caused by transverse or longitudinal sensory losses, and for disorders of the joints of the upper extremity that do not necessarily result in loss of range of motion. All these disorders can be summarized in a report form provided in the third edition of the *Guides* (Fig. 47–3).

The Lower Extremity

Unlike impairment of the upper extremity, impairment of the lower extremity has not gone through a

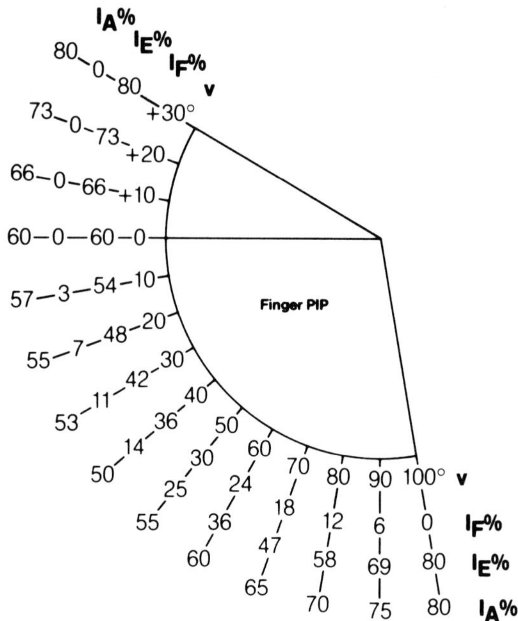

$I_A\%$ = impairment due to ankylosis
$I_E\%$ = impairment due to loss of extension
$I_F\%$ = impairment due to loss of flexion
V   = degrees of motion or ankylosis

Figure 47–2. Chart of finger PIP impairments. (From: Guides to the Evaluation of Permanent Impairment. 3rd Ed. Chicago, American Medical Association, 1988.)

thorough review since the late 1950s. As a result, the guidelines for evaluating impairment of the lower extremity have changed little in 30 years. The 1984 edition of the *Guides* introduced guidelines for disorders of the knee that did not necessarily cause impairment resulting from loss of range of motion, and these guidelines were refined somewhat in the 1988 edition. Beyond that, however, not much has changed, which leaves users of the *Guides* in an unfortunate clinical "time warp," in which evaluation of the upper extremity and the spine has vaulted ahead of evaluation of the lower extremity by 30 years.

The Spine

From 1958 through the publication of the second edition of the *Guides* in 1984, range of motion was the primary method for evaluating and rating impairment of the spine, and the two-armed goniometer was the instrument of choice to measure the range of motion. The earliest Journal article, and subsequently the first edition of the book, allowed for rating of impairment for only one set of diagnosis-based disorders, namely, vertebral fractures. The

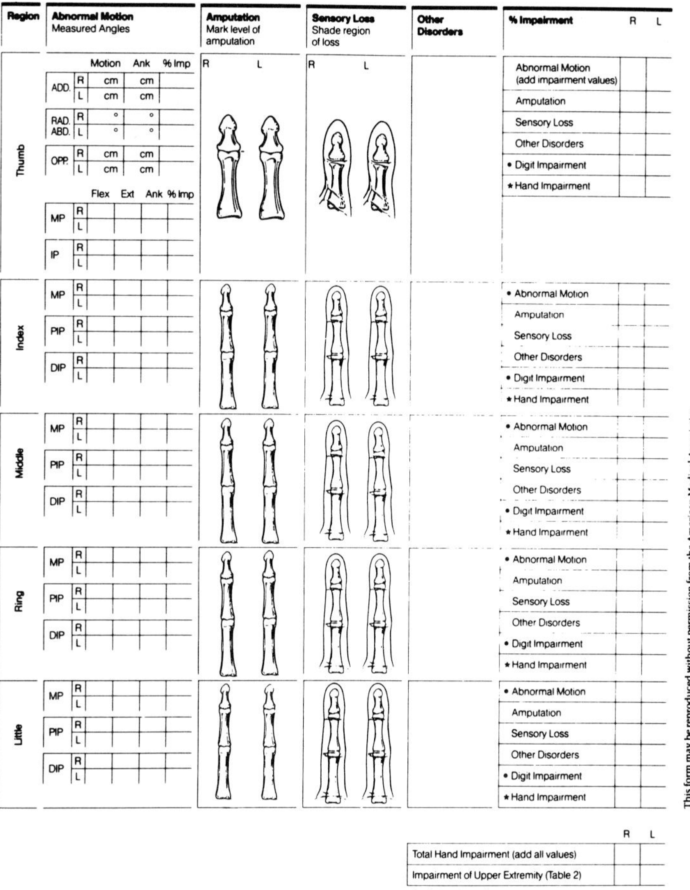

Figure 47–3. Upper extremity impairment evaluation record. (From. Guides to the Evaluation of Permanent Impairment. 3rd Ed. Chicago, American Medical Association, 1988.)

expert panel convened by the AMA to prepare the second edition corrected this by creating a small table of ratings for other diagnosis-based impairments—spondylolysis, spondylolisthesis, and intervertebral disc lesions.[5] The approach was laudable, although the table as it was constructed created difficulties for users of the book.

The third edition changed considerably the method by which spine impairment is evaluated. Mayer and colleagues[8,9] showed that movement of

Table 47–4
Impairments Due to Specific Disorders of the Spine

Disorder	% Impairment of Whole Person		
	Cerv	*Thor*	*Lumb*
I. Fractures			
A. Compression of one vertebral body			
0%-25%	4	2	5
26%-50%	6	3	7
>50%	10	5	12
B. Fracture of posterior elements (pedicles, laminae, articular processes, or transverse processes)	4	2	5
Note: Impairments due to compression of the vertebral body and to fractures of the posterior elements are combined using the Combined Values Chart.			
Note: When two or more vertebrae are compressed or fractured, combine all impairment values.			
C. Reduced dislocation of one vertebra	5	3	6
Note: If two or more vertebrae are dislocated and reduced, combine the impairment values using the Combined Values Chart.			
Note: An unreduced dislocation causes temporary impairment until it is reduced; then the physician should evaluate permanent impairment on the basis of the subject's condition with the reduced dislocation. If no reduction is possible, then the physician should evaluate impairment on the basis of restricted motion and concomitant neurological findings in the spinal region involved.			
II. Intervertebral disc or other soft tissue lesions			
A. Unoperated, with no residuals	0	0	0
B. Unoperated with medically documented injury and a minimum of six months of medically documented pain, recurrent muscle spasm or rigidity associated with none-to-minimal degenerative changes on structural tests	4	2	5
C. Unoperated, with medically documented injury and a minimum of six months of medically documented pain, recurrent muscle spasm, or rigidity associated with moderate to severe degenerative changes on structural tests, including unoperated herniated nucleus pulposus, with or without radiculopathy	6	3	7
D. Surgically treated disc lesion, with no residuals	7	4	8
E. Surgically treated disc lesion, with residual symptoms	9	5	10
F. Multiple operative levels, with or without residual symptoms	Add 1%/level		
G. Multiple operations ("failed back surgery") with or without residual symptoms:			
1. Second operation	Add 2%		
2. Third or subsequent surgery	Add 1%/operation		
III. Spondylolysis and spondylolisthesis, unoperated			
A. Spondylolysis or Grade I (1%-25% slippage) or Grade II (26%-50% slippage) spondylolisthesis, accompanied by medically documented injury and a minimum of six months of medically documented pain, recurrent muscle spasm, or rigidity	7	4	8
B. Grade III (51%-75% slippage) or Grade IV (76%-100% slippage) spondylolisthesis, accompanied by medically documented injury and a minimum of six months of medically documented pain, recurrent muscle spasm, or rigidity	9	5	10
IV. Spinal stenosis, segmental instability, or spondylolisthesis, operated			
A. Single level operation, with no residuals	8	4	9
B. Single level operation, with residual symptoms	10	5	12
C. Multiple levels operated, with residual symptoms	Add 1%/level		
D. Multiple operations ("failed back surgery") with residual symptoms:			
1. Second operation	Add 2%		
2. Third or subsequent operation	Add 1%/operation		

Note: List impairments separately for cervical, thoracic, and lumbar regions.
Note: All impairment ratings above should be combined with the appropriate values of residuals, such as:
1. Ankylosis (fusion) in the spinal area or extremities
2. Abnormal motion in the spinal area (i.e., objectively measured rigidity) or extremities
3. Spinal cord and spinal nerve root injuries, with neurologic impairment
4. Any combination of the above using the Combined Values Chart.

the small, inaccessible spinal joints was not readily observed and measured by the goniometer, and that gross spine movement is a compound movement confounded by motions above and below the point of goniometric measurement. Instead, their studies demonstrated that inclinometers placed above and below the area of measure could provide more accurate and reproducible ranges of motion, and take into account movements of other joints, such as the shoulders or hips, which complement spine motion (Figure 47-4). Thus, the inclinometer was incorporated as the instrument of choice in assessing range of motion of the spine.

The result in the third edition is an amalgam of diagnosis-based impairments and range of motion impairments. Users of the book are first introduced to an expanded table of diagnosis-based impairments[6] (Table 47–4), including vertebral fractures, intervertebral disc lesions and other soft tissue lesions, spondylolisthesis and spondylolysis, and spinal stenosis and segmental instability. The diagnosis-based

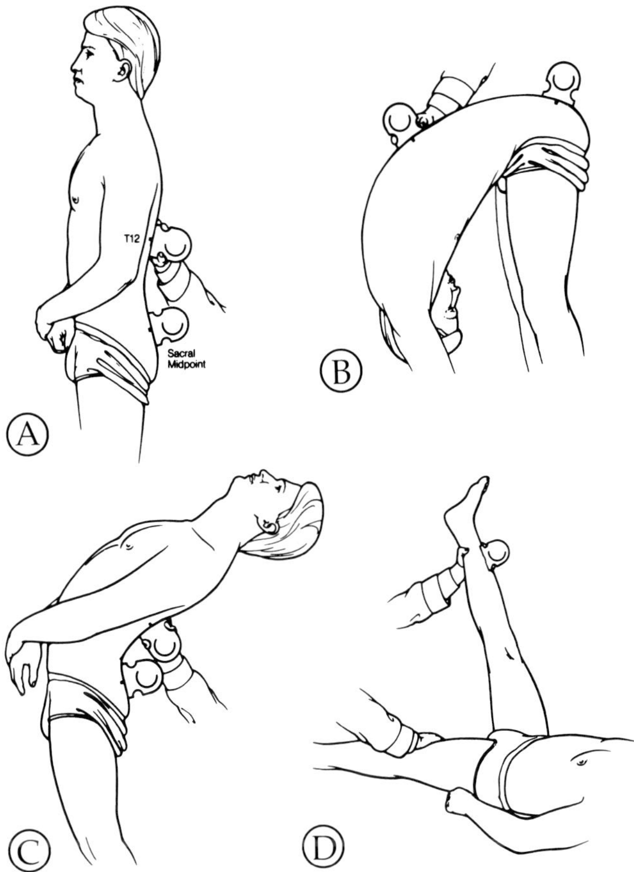

Figure **47–5.** Two inclinometer measurement techniques for lumbosacral flexion/extension. **(A)** Neutral position and **(B)** flexion shown with the inclinometers at T12 and over the sacrum; **(C)** True lumbar extension = T12 inclination—sacral inclination (hip motion); **(D)** Straight leg raise on the tightest side should be within 10° of the total hip motion (hip flexion + hip extension). (From: Guides to the Evaluation of Permanent Impairment. 3rd Ed. Chicago, American Medical Association, 1988.)

impairment evaluation is designed to adhere to two basic premises of the *Guides:* first, that the impairment evaluation must take into account a medical history that documents pain, muscle spasm, and rigidity (i.e., the evaluation is not done "in a vacuum"); and second, that the evaluation should consider impairment resulting from neurologic signs, if present, and combine the ratings for these impairments into the final evaluation (i.e., if clinically appropriate, sections of the book other than the spine section should be used).

It is after the diagnosis-based portion of the spine section that the user finds the more familiar range of motion evaluation guidelines. The inclusion of the inclinometer as the preferred instrument of measurement introduces the possibility of enhancing the reliability of the range of motion tests. First, it more

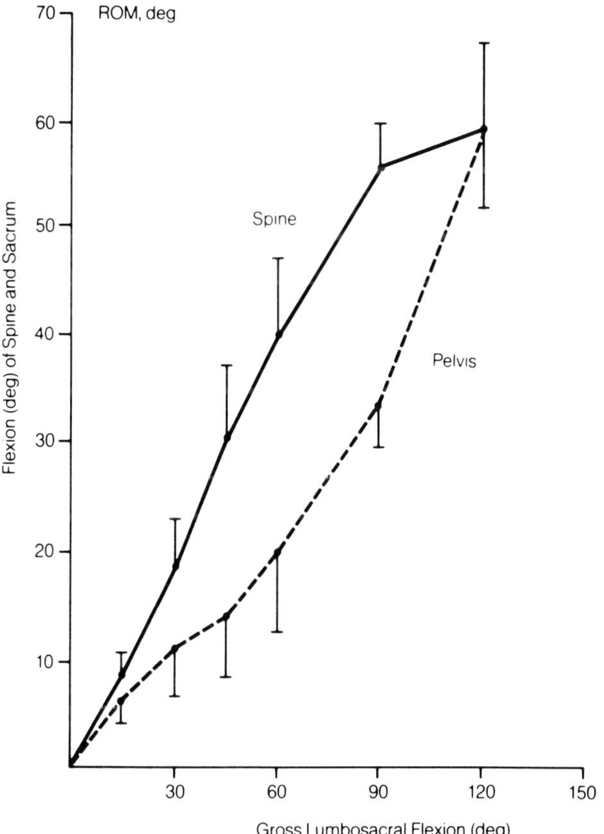

Figure **47–4.** Relationship of spine flexion to sacral (hip) flexion during gross lumbosacral flexion. (Adapted from Mayer, T.G., Tencer, A.F., Kristoferson, S., Mooney, V.: Use of noninvasive techniques for quantification of spinal range of motion in normal subjects and chronic low back dysfunction patients. Spine, 1984.)

accurately measures the movement of the spine and subtracts the complementary movements of neighboring, extra-spinal joints, as noted above. Second, it allows for novel and more appropriate approaches to spine range of motion, such as the "angle of minimum kyphosis" for the thoracic spine, and straight leg raising (a measure of motion of the pelvis) as a test of validity for range of motion of the lumbosacral spine, as shown in Figures 47–5 and 47–6. The accuracy of the inclinometer also allows the evaluator to take multiple measurements of a plane of motion to assess the precision of the measurements as well. This precision can be tested against a recommended guideline of plus or minus 10° or 5% and reported upon in the evaluator's report (Fig. 47–7). In an area of contention, such as spine impairment,

Movement	Description	Range						
Lumbar Flexion	T12 ROM							
	Sacral ROM							
	True lumbar flexion angle							
	±10% or 5°?	Yes	No					
	Maximum true lumbar flexion angle							
	% Impairment							
Lumbar Extension	T12 ROM							
	Sacral ROM							
	True lumbar extension angle							
	±10% or 5°?	Yes	No					
	Maximum true lumbar extension angle			(add Sacral flexion and extension ROM and compare to tightest Straight Leg Raising Angle)				
	% Impairment							
Straight Leg Raising, Right	Right SLR							
	±10% or 5°?	Yes	No	(if tightest SLR ROM exceeds sum of Sacral flexion and extension by more than 10%, Lumbar ROM test is invalid)				
	Maximum SLR Right							
Straight Leg Raising, Left	Left SLR							
	±10% or 5°?	Yes	No	(if tightest SLR ROM exceeds sum of Sacral flexion and extension by more than 10%, Lumbar ROM test is invalid)				
	Maximum SLR Left							
Lumbar Right Lateral Flexion	T12 ROM							
	Sacral ROM							
	Lumbar right lat flexion angle							
	±10% or 5°?	Yes	No					
	Maximum lumbar right lat flexion angle							
	% Impairment							
Lumbar Left Lateral Flexion	T12 ROM							
	Sacral ROM							
	Lumbar left lat flexion angle							
	±10% or 5°?	Yes	No					
	Maximum lumbar left lat flexion angle							
	% Impairment							
Lumbar Ankylosis in Lateral Flexion	Position			(Excludes any impairment for abnormal flexion/extension motion)				
	% Impairment							

Total Lumbar Range of Motion Impairment
(*add* all ROM impairments if no ankylosis;
use ankylosis impairment value if ankylosis is present)

Figure 47–6. Lumbar range of motion. (From: Guides to the Evaluation of Permanent Impairment. 3rd Ed. Chicago, American Medical Association, 1988.)

Disorder	% Impairment of Whole Person		
	Cerv	Thor	Lumb
I. Fractures			
A. Compression of one vertebral body			
0%-25%	4	2	5
26%-50%	6	3	7
>50%	10	5	12
B. Fracture of posterior elements (pedicles, laminae, articular processes, or transverse processes)	4	2	5
Note: Impairments due to compression of the vertebral body and to fractures of the posterior elements are combined using the Combined Values Chart.			
Note: When two or more vertebrae are compressed or fractured, combine all impairment values.			
C. Reduced dislocation of one vertebra	5	3	6
Note: If two or more vertebrae are dislocated and reduced, combine the impairment values using the Combined Values Chart.			
Note: An unreduced dislocation causes temporary impairment until it is reduced; then the physician should evaluate permanent impairment on the basis of the subject's condition with the reduced dislocation. If no reduction is possible, then the physician should evaluate impairment on the basis of restricted motion and concomitant neurological findings in the spinal region involved, according to the criteria in this Chapter and in Chapter 4.			
II. Intervertebral disc or other soft tissue lesions			
A. Unoperated, with no residuals	0	0	0
B. Unoperated with medically documented injury and a minimum of six months of medically documented pain, recurrent muscle spasm or rigidity associated with none-to-minimal degenerative changes on structural tests	4	2	5
C. Unoperated, with medically documented injury and a minimum of six months of medically documented pain, recurrent muscle spasm, or rigidity associated with moderate to severe degenerative changes on structural tests, including unoperated herniated nucleus pulposus, with or without radiculopathy	6	3	7
D. Surgically treated disc lesion, with no residuals	7	4	8
E. Surgically treated disc lesion, with residual symptoms	9	5	10
F. Multiple operative levels, with or without residual symptomatology	Add 1%/level		
G. Multiple operations ("failed back surgery") with or without residual symptoms:			
1. Second operation	Add 2%		
2. Third or subsequent surgery	Add 1%/operation		
III. Spondylolysis and spondylolisthesis, unoperated			
A. Spondylolysis or Grade I (1%-25% slippage) or Grade II (26%-50% slippage) spondylolisthesis, accompanied by medically documented injury and a minimum of six months of medically documented pain, recurrent muscle spasm, or rigidity	7	4	8
B. Grade III (51%-75% slippage) or Grade IV (76%-100% slippage) spondylolisthesis, accompanied by medically documented injury and a minimum of six months of medically documented pain, recurrent muscle spasm, or rigidity	9	5	10
IV. Spinal stenosis, segmental instability, or spondylolisthesis, operated			
A. Single level operation, with no residuals	8	4	9
B. Single level operation, with residual symptoms	10	5	12
C. Multiple levels operated, with residual symptoms	Add 1%/level		
D. Multiple operations ("failed back surgery") with residual symptoms:			
1. Second operation	Add 2%		
2. Third or subsequent surgery	Add 1%/operation		

Note: List impairments separately for cervical, thoracic, and lumbar regions (Figures 83a-c).

Note: All impairment ratings above should be combined with the appropriate values of residuals, such as:

1. Ankylosis (fusion) in the spinal area or extremities

2. Abnormal motion in the spinal area (i.e., objectively measured rigidity) or extremities

3. Spinal cord and spinal nerve root injuries, with neurologic impairment (see Upper Extremity and Lower Extremity sections of Chapter 3 and Peripheral Nervous System section of Chapter 4)

4. Any combination of the above using the Combined Values Chart.

Figure 47–7. Evaluator's report. (From Guides to the Evaluation of Permanent Impairment. 3rd Ed. Chicago, American Medical Association, 1988.)

both the accuracy and the precision of the testing, and the reporting thereof, can enhance the value of an evaluation to the reader of a report, such as a workers' compensation adjudicator.

A NEED FOR THE FUTURE: STANDARDIZATION

A major deficiency with the musculoskeletal portion of the AMA *Guides,* as well as with any other system of evaluation of musculoskeletal impairment currently in use, is the scientific substantiation of the rating values that are given to the clinical parameters that are measured, such as range of motion. The ratings are not grounded in sound epidemiologic studies of large population groups, which would provide normative data to support those ratings. The musculoskeletal system is not the only organ system of the body that suffers from this deficiency. All do, except, perhaps, the pulmonary system.

The lung has only a few ways in which it responds to an insult: (1) an inflammatory process, which may cause airways to the lung to clog up and contract, and the alveolar air sacs perhaps to fill up with fluid and inflammatory cells; (2) an immune response process, which also may cause the airways to contract and fill with fluid, and in the case of hypersensitivity pneumonitis, cause the alveoli to fill with fluid; (3) a degenerative process, in which the walls of both the alveoli and air passages become flabby or nonexistent; (4) a fibrotic process, in which inhaled particles fail to be cleared, embed in the alveolar walls and set up a fibrotic reaction; and, (5) a neoplastic process, in which a tumor is produced. Furthermore, the lung, with its respiratory function of gas exchange, the fluid dynamics of which can be studied, is amenable to a quantifiable physiologic understanding. For the pulmonary system, the five basic processes of response to insult in one way or another affect highly quantifiable parameters, namely, pulmonary function, as measured most simply by spirometers, and gas exchange, as measured not so simply by the diffusing capacity of carbon monoxide.

Added to this quantitative understanding of pulmonary function is the development of techniques that easily measure these functions. Since the late nineteenth century spirometers have been refined to the point that they are compact, transportable, easy to use by both patient and technician, and give accurate and precise readouts of pulmonary function immediately.[10] Even machines that measure the diffusing capacity of carbon monoxide, the D_{CO}, have been refined so that this test can be performed at sites distant from major medical centers, and can yield results that are both accurate and precise.[11]

Thus, for the last 30 years at least, there was never a question that researchers could test for simple pulmonary function in populations large enough to develop statistically-based "normal measurements" according to age, sex, and height.[12]

Added to these is another excellent study instrument that tests the subjective side of respiratory disease, namely, the questionnaire on respiratory symptoms that was developed initially by the British Medical Research Council in the 1950s to study the prevalence and causes of chronic bronchitis in Great Britain.[13] The questionnaire has been validated and modified for use in many nations, including the United States. It provides a standardized manner in which the symptoms of pulmonary diseases, such as cough, wheezing and dyspnea, can be assessed and correlated with pulmonary function testing.

Clearly, the evaluation of the musculoskeletal system does not enjoy this scope of scientific research. For whatever reasons, our society has decided to fund the development of standardized techniques to assess the effects of smoking, occupational dust exposure and environmental air pollution on the lungs in a systematic fashion, but not to fund in a similar fashion techniques to assess the effects of automobile crashes, occupational injuries and recreational injuries on the musculoskeletal system. To develop and carry out large population based studies on this organ system would be an enormous undertaking. Each movable joint would have to be assessed across all age groups, and both sexes, and perhaps across different racial and ethnic groups, with sufficient numbers of people in each category to provide adequate statistical power. Yet, such studies cry out to be done. Each year millions, if not billions, of dollars are spent on disability claims, the clinical substantiation for many of which lie on very shaky ground.

An independent study group commissioned by the US Department of Health and Human Services, the US Preventive Services Task Force, issued a report on the scientific evidence to support or not support preventive services of a clinical nature, such as various immunizations, pap smears, mammography and antismoking interventions.[14] The task force used strict criteria to assess the quality of the scientific evidence upon which it formulated recommendations, shown in Table 47–5. The lower the Roman numeral, the stronger the evidence. Surprisingly, such time honored practices as screening for fecal occult blood were substantiated by studies to only Roman numeral three quality. Clearly, if one were to apply these strict scientific criteria to the evaluation of impairment of most organ systems, the quality of the evidence for the ratings would also be low. One consequence of this was that in its review that led to the third edition of the *Guides,* the expert panel on impairments caused by mental and behavioral disor-

Table 47–5
Quality of Evidence Used By the US Preventive Services Task Force

I:	Evidence obtained from at least one properly randomized controlled trial.
II:	Evidence obtained from well designed controlled trials without randomization.
II-2:	Evidence obtained from well designed cohort or case control studies, preferably from more than one center or research group.
II-3:	Evidence obtained from multiple time series with or without intervention.
III:	Opinions of respected authorities, based on clinical experience, descriptive studies, or reports of expert committees.

(From US Preventive Services Task Force: Guide to Clinical Preventive Services: An Assessment of the Effectiveness of 169 Interventions. Baltimore, Williams & Wilkins, 1989.)

ders concluded that it could not justify any past or present rating schemes for these impairments, and declined to offer one. They stated instead, "Eventually research may support the direct link between medical findings and percentage of mental impairment."[6] This author believes that, although the experts on mental impairment were alone in taking this approach, they were not alone in this predicament. The *direct* link has not been established yet even in the musculoskeletal system. Much work still needs to be done.

REFERENCES

1. McBride, E.D.: Disability Evaluation: Principles of Treatment of Compensable Injuries, 4th Ed. Philadelphia, JB Lippincott, 1948.
2. Guide to the evaluation of impairment of the extremities and back. JAMA, *167*:(special issue), 1958.
3. Guide to the evaluation of impairment of the hematopoietic system. JAMA, *213*:1314, 1970.
4. American Medical Association Committee on the Rating of Physical and Mental Impairment: Guides to the Evaluation of Permanent Impairment, 1st Ed. Chicago, American Medical Association, 1971.
5. American Medical Association Council on Scientific Affairs: Guides to the Evaluation of Permanent Impairment, 2nd Ed. Chicago, American Medical Association, 1984.
6. Guides to the Evaluation of Permanent Impairment, 3rd Ed. (Edited by A.L. Engelberg). Chicago, American Medical Association, 1988.
7. Swanson, A.B., Goran-Hagert, C., de Groot Swanson, G.: Evaluation of impairment in the upper extremity. J Hand Surg 12A:896, 1987.
8. Mayer, T.G., Tencer, A.F., Kristoferson, S., Mooney, V.: Use of noninvasive techniques for quantification of spinal range-of-motion in normal subjects and chronic low-back dysfunction patients. Spine 9:588, 1984.
9. Keeley, J., et al.: Quantification of lumbar function. Part 5: Reliability of range-of-motion measures in the sagittal plane and an in vivo torso rotation measurement technique. Spine *11*:31, 1986.
10. American thoracic society committee on proficiency standards for pulmonary function laboratories: standardization of spirometry-1987 update. Am Rev Respir Dis *136*:1285, 1987.
11. American thoracic society D_{CO} standardization conference: single breath carbon monoxide diffusing capacity (transfer factor): recommendations for a standard technique. Am Rev Respir Dis *136*:1299, 1987.
12. Crapo, R.O., Morris, A.H., Gardner, R.M.: Reference spirometric values using techniques and equipment that meet ATS recommendations. Am Rev Respir Dis *123*:659, 1981.
13. Samet, J.A.: A historical and epidemiologic perspective on respiratory symptoms questionnaires. Am J Epidemiol *108*:435, 1978.
14. US Preventive Services Task Force: Guide to Clinical Preventive Services: An Assessment of the Effectiveness of 169 Interventions. Baltimore, Williams & Wilkins, 1989.